Dietary Reference Intakes (DRIs): Recommended Intakes for Individuals, Elements
Food and Nutrition Board, Institute of Medicine, National Academies

Life Stage Group	Calcium (mg/d)	Chromium (µg/d)	Copper (µg/d)	Fluoride (mg/d)	Iodine (µg/d)	Iron (mg/d)	Magnesium (mg/d)	Manganese (mg/d)	Molybdenum (µg/d)	Phosphorus (mg/d)	Selenium (µg/d)	Zinc (mg/d)
Infants												
0–6 mo	210*	0.2*	200*	0.01*	110*	0.27*	30*	0.003*	2*	100*	15*	2*
7–12 mo	270*	5.5*	220*	0.5*	130*	11	75*	0.6*	3*	275*	20*	3
Children												
1–3 y	500*	11*	340	0.7*	90	7	80	1.2*	17	460	20	3
4–8 y	800*	15*	440	1*	90	10	130	1.5*	22	500	30	5
Males												
9–13 y	1,300*	25*	700	2*	120	8	240	1.9*	34	1,250	40	8
14–18 y	1,300*	35*	890	3*	150	11	410	2.2*	43	1,250	55	11
19–30 y	1,000*	35*	900	4*	150	8	400	2.3*	45	700	55	11
31–50 y	1,000*	35*	900	4*	150	8	420	2.3*	45	700	55	11
51–70 y	1,200*	30*	900	4*	150	8	420	2.3*	45	700	55	11
>70 y	1,200*	30*	900	4*	150	8	420	2.3*	45	700	55	11
Females												
9–13 y	1,300*	21*	700	2*	120	8	240	1.6*	34	1,250	40	8
14–18 y	1,300*	24*	890	3*	150	15	360	1.6*	43	1,250	55	9
19–30 y	1,000*	25*	900	3*	150	18	310	1.8*	45	700	55	8
31–50 y	1,000*	25*	900	3*	150	18	320	1.8*	45	700	55	8
51–70 y	1,200*	20*	900	3*	150	8	320	1.8*	45	700	55	8
>70 y	1,200*	20*	900	3*	150	8	320	1.8*	45	700	55	8
Pregnancy												
≤18 y	1,300*	29*	1,000	3*	220	27	400	2.0*	50	1,250	60	12
19–30 y	1,000*	30*	1,000	3*	220	27	350	2.0*	50	700	60	11
31–50 y	1,000*	30*	1,000	3*	220	27	360	2.0*	50	700	60	11
Lactation												
≤18 y	1,300*	44*	1,300	3*	290	10	360	2.6*	50	1,250	70	13
19–30 y	1,000*	45*	1,300	3*	290	9	310	2.6*	50	700	70	12
31–50 y	1,000*	45*	1,300	3*	290	9	320	2.6*	50	700	70	12

NOTE: This table presents Recommended Dietary Allowances (RDAs) in **bold type** and Adequate Intakes (AIs) in ordinary type followed by an asterisk (*). RDAs and AIs may both be used as goals for individual intake. RDAs are set to meet the needs of almost all (97 to 98 percent) individuals in a group. For healthy breastfed infants, the AI is the mean intake. The AI for other life stage and gender groups is believed to cover individuals in the group, but lack of data or uncertainty in the data prevent being able to specify with confidence the percentage of individuals covered by this intake.

SOURCES: Dietary Reference Intakes for Calcium, Phosphorus, Magnesium, Vitamin D, and Fluoride (1997); Dietary Reference Intakes for Thiamin, Riboflavin, Niacin, Vitamin B-6, Folate, Vitamin B-12, Pantothenic, Biotin, and Choline (1998); Dietary Reference Intakes for Vitamin C, Vitamin E, Selenium, and Carotenoids (2000); and Dietary Reference Intakes for Vitamin A, Vitamin K, Arsenic, Boron, Chromium, Copper, Iodine, Iron, Manganese, Molybdenum, Nickel, Silicon, Vanadium, and Zinc (2001). These reports may be accessed via www.nap.edu.

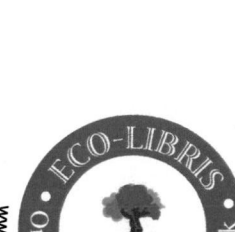
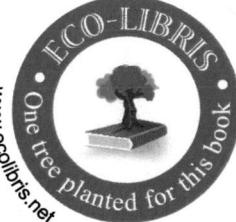

ECO-LIBRIS · One tree planted for this book · www.ecolibris.net

D0071135

Dietary Reference Intakes (DRIs): Recommended Intakes for Individuals, Macronutrients
Food and Nutrition Board, Institute of Medicine, National Academies

Life Stage Group	Carbohydrate (g/d)	Total Fiber (g/d)	Fat (g/d)	Linoleic Acid (g/d)	α-Linolenic Acid (g/d)	Protein[a] (g/d)
Infants						
0–6 mo	60*	ND	31*	4.4*	0.5*	9.1*
7–12 mo	95*	ND	30*	4.6*	0.5*	**13.5**
Children						
1–3 y	130	19*	ND[b]	7*	0.7*	13
4–8 y	130	25*	ND	10*	0.9*	19
Males						
9–13 y	130	31*	ND	12*	1.2*	34
14–18 y	130	38*	ND	16*	1.6*	52
19–30 y	130	38*	ND	17*	1.6*	56
31–50 y	130	38*	ND	17*	1.6*	56
51–70 y	130	30*	ND	14*	1.6*	56
>70 y	130	30*	ND	14*	1.6*	56
Females						
9–13 y	130	26*	ND	10*	1.0*	34
14–18 y	130	26*	ND	11*	1.1*	46
19–30 y	130	25*	ND	12*	1.1*	46
31–50 y	130	25*	ND	12*	1.1*	46
51–70 y	130	21*	ND	11*	1.1*	46
>70 y	130	21*	ND	11*	1.1*	46
Pregnancy						
14–18 y	175	28*	ND	13*	1.4*	71
19–30 y	175	28*	ND	13*	1.4*	71
31–50 y	175	28*	ND	13*	1.4*	71
Lactation						
14–18 y	210	29*	ND	13*	1.3*	71
19–30 y	210	29*	ND	13*	1.3*	71
31–50 y	210	29*	ND	13*	1.3*	71

NOTE: This table presents Recommended Dietary Allowances (RDAs) in **bold type** and Adequate Intakes (AIs) in ordinary type followed by an asterisk (*). RDAs and AIs may both be used as goals for individual intake. RDAs are set to meet the needs of almost all (97 to 98 percent) individuals in a group. For healthy breastfed infants, the AI is the mean intake. The AI for other life stage and gender groups is believed to cover needs of all individuals in the group, but lack of data or uncertainty in the data prevent being able to specify with confidence the percentage of individuals covered by this intake.

[a]Based on 0.8g protein/kg body weight for reference body weight.

[b]ND = not determinable at this time

SOURCES: Dietary Reference Intakes for Energy, Carbohydrate, Fiber, Fat, Fatty Acids, Cholesterol, Protein, and Amino Acids (2002). This report may be accessed via www.nap.edu.

Contemporary Nutrition

Sixth Edition Update

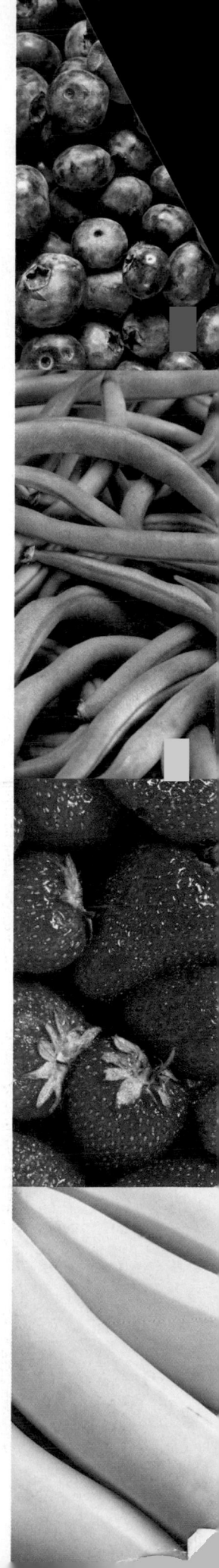

Gordon M. Wardlaw

PH.D., R.D.

Formerly of
Department of Human Nutrition,
College of Human Ecology
The Ohio State University

Anne M. Smith

PH.D., R.D., L.D.

Department of Human Nutrition,
College of Human Ecology
The Ohio State University

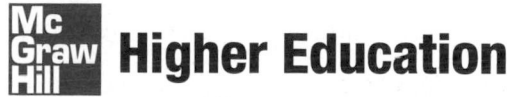

McGraw Hill **Higher Education**

Boston   Burr Ridge, IL   Dubuque, IA   Madison, WI   New York   San Francisco   St. Louis
Bangkok   Bogotá   Caracas   Kuala Lumpur   Lisbon   London   Madrid   Mexico City
Milan   Montreal   New Delhi   Santiago   Seoul   Singapore   Sydney   Taipei   Toronto

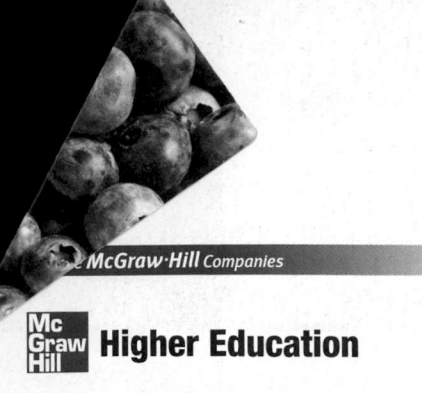

McGraw-Hill Companies

Mc Graw Hill | Higher Education

CONTEMPORARY NUTRITION UPDATE, SIXTH EDITION

Published by McGraw-Hill, a business unit of The McGraw-Hill Companies, Inc., 1221 Avenue of the Americas, New York, NY 10020. Copyright © 2007 by The McGraw-Hill Companies, Inc. All rights reserved. No part of this publication may be reproduced or distributed in any form or by any means, or stored in a database or retrieval system, without the prior written consent of The McGraw-Hill Companies, Inc., including, but not limited to, in any network or other electronic storage or transmission, or broadcast for distance learning.

Some ancillaries, including electronic and print components, may not be available to customers outside the United States.

This book is printed on recycled, acid-free paper containing 10% postconsumer waste.

3 4 5 6 7 8 9 0 WCK/WCK 0 9 8 7

ISBN–13 978–0–07–322580–7
ISBN–10 0–07–322580–0

Publisher: *Colin H. Wheatley*
Senior Developmental Editor: *Lynne M. Meyers*
Marketing Manager: *Tami Petsche*
Project Manager: *Jodi Rhomberg*
Senior Production Supervisor: *Kara Kudronowicz*
Lead Media Project Manager: *Stacy A. Patch*
Media Producer: *Daniel M. Wallace*
Designer: *Rick D. Noel*
Cover/Interior Designer: *Ellen Pettengell*
(USE) Cover Images: Center photo *Anne Dowie*, small detail photos *PhotoDisc*
Senior Photo Research Coordinator: *John C. Leland*
Supplement Producer: *Tracy L. Konrardy*
Compositor: *Carlisle Publishing Services*
Typeface: *10/12 Giovanni Book*
Printer: *Quebecor World Versailles, KY*

The credits section for this book begins on page C-1 and is considered an extension of the copyright page.

Library of Congress Cataloging-in-Publication Data

Wardlaw, Gordon M.
  Contemporary nutrition update / Gordon M. Wardlaw and Anne M. Smith. — 6th ed. [rev.]
    p.;   cm.
  Rev. ed. of: Contemporary nutrition / Gordon M. Wardlaw, Anne M. Smith. 6th ed. © 2006.
  Includes bibliographical references and index.
  ISBN 978–0–07–322580–7 — ISBN 0–07–322580–0 (hard copy : alk. paper)
  1. Nutrition. I. Smith, Anne M., Ph.D. II. Wardlaw, Gordon M. Contemporary nutrition. III. Title.
  [DNLM: 1. Nutrition. QU 145 W266 © 2007]

QP141.W378   2007
612.3—dc22   2005033162
                                              CIP

www.mhhe.com

Brief Contents

Contents

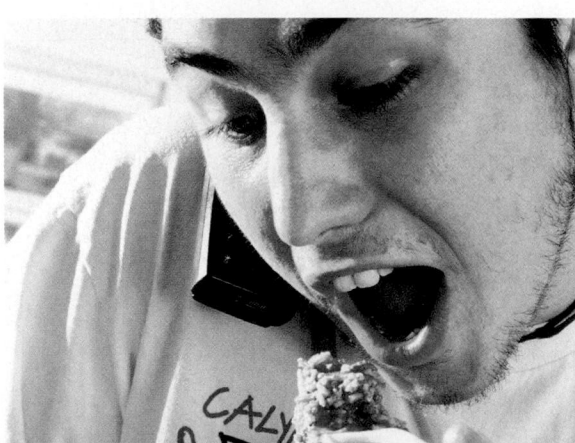

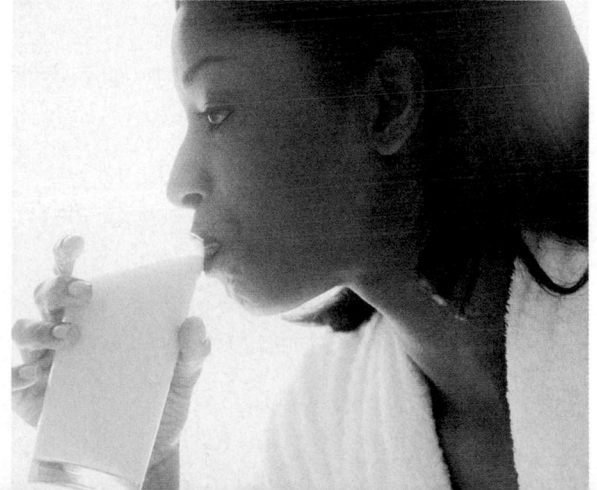

Part Three   Vitamins and Minerals 237

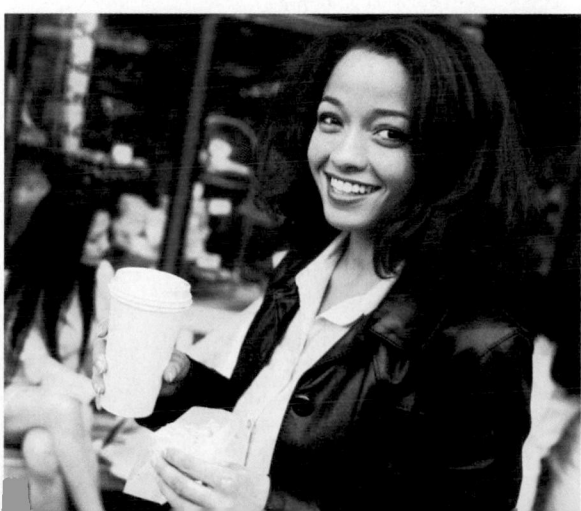

Part Four   Energy: Balance & Imbalance 333

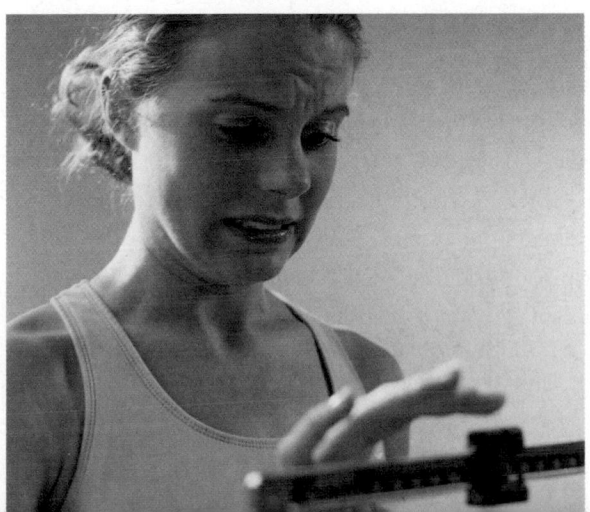

Part Five   Nutrition: A Focus on Life Stages 435

13 Pregnancy and Breastfeeding 435

14 Nutrition from Infancy through Adolescence 467

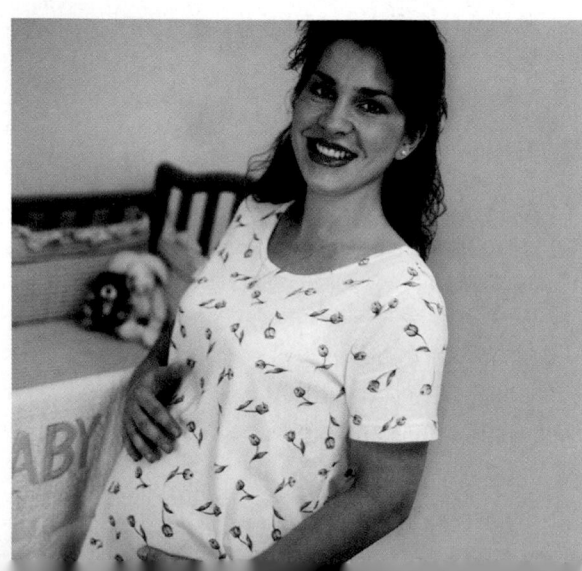

Part Six   Nutrition: Beyond the Nutrients 527

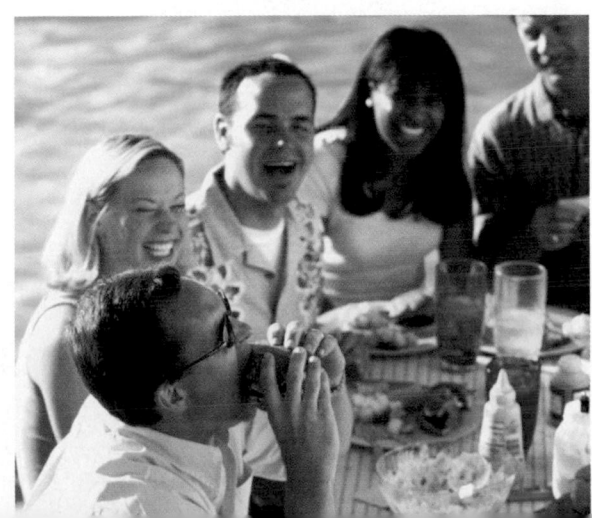

Introducing the *Updated* Sixth Edition

In our efforts to bring up-to-date and reliable nutrition information to you and your introductory students, we would like to present the updated sixth edition of *Contemporary Nutrition*. Because the 2005 Dietary Guidelines for Americans and MyPyramid represent substantial new tools for implementing healthy food choices, we have integrated this content into the updated sixth edition. The following paragraphs showcase the features and strengths of the sixth edition and also describe the new content enhancements related to the Dietary Guidelines and MyPyramid, as well as other recent advances in nutritional science.

Our Approach to Teaching Nutrition

If you teach nutrition, you undoubtedly already find it a fascinating subject. Nutrition, however, can also be a frustrating subject to teach, for a variety of reasons. New research studies seem to emerge at an almost dizzying pace. Claims and counterclaims abound regarding the need for certain constituents in our diets. How does an instructor adequately convey changing and seemingly conflicting messages to introductory students? Our students also commonly bring to class many misconceptions about nutrition, and many have not had a college-level biology or chemistry course. How do we convey complex scientific concepts at a level appropriate for undergraduate students? And finally, how do we help our students meaningfully apply the material we cover in class to their own lives?

■ Keeping Current

The vast amount of research underway is constantly reshaping our knowledge of nutritional science. As authors and teachers, we constantly scour the literature to ensure that students' first exposure to the study of nutrition is reliable, accurate, and as up-to-date as this rapidly changing field allows. Key enhancements featured in this updated version of the sixth edition include integrated coverage of the 2005 Dietary Guidelines for

Americans and the new USDA MyPyramid, as well as other recent data and research findings. We are also aware of conflicting opinions in our field and thus draw on as many reputable sources as possible to create a balanced resource for nutrition information. We strive to present an objective approach to newly emerging or controversial topics so that students learn to carefully scrutinize the nutritional information they read and hear about.

■ Understanding Our Audience

We have written *Contemporary Nutrition* assuming that our students have a limited background in college-level biology, chemistry, or physiology. We have been careful to include the essential science foundation needed to adequately comprehend certain topics in nutrition, such as the basic discussion of protein synthesis in Chapter 6. Scientific discussions have been written in a simple, straightforward manner.

We also take into consideration the fact that students enrolled in introductory nutrition often come from a broad range of majors and interests. We address this by incorporating a thorough system of pedagogical tools, such as critical thinking questions and concept checks, to help them master the material. A variety of applications and real-life examples are interspersed throughout to appeal to students whose majors range from business to education.

■ Personalizing Nutrition

A prominent theme in nutrition today is *individuality*. Not all of us, for example, find that saturated fat in our diets raises our blood cholesterol values above recommended standards. Each person responds differently to nutrients, and we try to reinforce this point throughout the book.

Moreover even at this basic level, the text's discussions do not assume that all nutrition students are alike. Chapter content and features, such as Rate Your Plate, repeatedly ask students to learn more about themselves and their health status and to use their new knowledge to improve their health. After reading this textbook, students will be better equipped to understand how the nutrition information coming from all directions—whether on the evening news, on ready-to-eat cereal boxes, in popular magazines, or from government agencies—applies to them. Our goal is for students to understand that their knowledge of nutrition will allow them to evaluate and personalize nutrition information, rather than to follow every guideline issued for an entire population. After all, a population consists of individuals with varying genetic and cultural backgrounds, and these individuals will have varying responses to diet.

As a final note on bringing nutrition down to a personal level, the book covers important questions students often bring to class, concerning topics such as eating disorders, dietary supplements, vegetarianism, popular weight-loss diets, and diets for athletes. Regardless of topic, the overall emphasis remains the same—the importance of understanding one's food choices and modifying one's diet to best meet personal needs.

Organization

This book remains organized into six parts that reflect the major topics typically covered in an introductory nutrition course:

Part One   Nutrition: A Key to Health
Part Two   The Energy-Yielding Nutrients and Alcohol
Part Three   Vitamins and Minerals
Part Four   Energy: Balance and Imbalance
Part Five   Nutrition: A Focus on Life Stages
Part Six   Nutrition: Beyond the Nutrients

The Table of Contents also reflects the inclusion of two chapters not typically found in introductory textbooks: Chapter 7, Alcohol and Chapter 12, Eating Disorders. The expanded discussion of these topics is the result of feedback from instructors who feel it is important to provide their students with a thorough, balanced discussion of these relevant topics.

Although most frequently used in semester-long courses, the text's organization allows instructors to omit Parts or Chapters to fit the needs of quarter-length courses. We have also tried as much as possible to make each chapter function independently so that instructors can cover the material in the order that best fits their particular course needs.

A Closer Look at the Sixth Edition Update

▮ Streamlined Chapter Features

Despite thoroughly updating the content to reflect latest guidelines and research findings in this update, we have retained changes to the composition of the chapter features. With the help of colleagues, reviewers, symposium participants, and our own students, we determined that, compared to the Fifth edition, the number and length of boxed readings should be reduced. We also learned that most people prefer that the end-of-chapter boxed readings should instead fall within the main body of the chapter (before the sum-

mary, study questions, and the readings). We therefore condensed some of the material previously covered in the boxed readings to focus on essential content. Other boxed reading content was moved into the main body of the text, such as the discussion of dietary fiber in Chapter 4 on carbohydrates. The chapters now typically contain only one or two boxed readings, entitled "Looking Further." We hope that you agree that this arrangement suits the needs of introductory students.

▮ Art and Design Features

Two important enhancements have been made to the visual appeal and pedagogical function of the sixth edition in general. First, the design layout has been streamlined and the colors are more vivid to better capture students' attention; and, more importantly, the sixth edition featured dramatically improved illustrations. Per feedback and suggestions from professors, we made the figures more colorful and simplified the labeling within the figures. One by one, each diagram and photo was scrutinized with an eye toward improving its visual appeal and ability to convey nutrition concepts.

▮ Chapter-by-Chapter Revisions

In response to feedback from instructors using this text, we reduced the complexity and refined the content to better meet the needs of today's students. The following list highlights just some of the changes and in the sixth edition of *Contemporary Nutrition*, as well as those added as part of the update.

Chapter 1: What You Eat and Why

- The Another Bite section briefly introduces *trans* fatty acids, since they are now be listed on the Nutrition Facts panel. All the Nutrition Facts panels in the book have been revised to reflect the addition of *trans* fatty acids.
- Household units are part of the Looking Further box, "Math Tools for Nutrition."
- Figure 1-4 shows the location of the hypothalamus as part of the discussion of satiety.

Chapter 2: Tools for Designing a Healthy Diet

- The entire discussion of diet planning has been rewritten to reflect advice of MyPyramid.
- The 2005 Dietary Guidelines are reviewed in detail.
- Looking Further box, "The Alphabet Soup of Nutrient Needs" contains a figure comparing nutrient standards, such as RDA

and UL, as well as a discussion of the Estimated Energy Requirements recently set by the Food and Nutrition Board.
- Figure 2-5 shows an updated and simplified example of the Nutrition Facts panel on a macaroni & cheese box.
- Another Bite discusses the new types of preliminary health claims allowed by the FDA.

Chapter 3: The Human Body: A Nutrition Perspective

- Figure 3-5, illustrating blood circulation, is enlarged and the corresponding labels simplified.
- Figure 3-6 shows a more detailed depiction of capillary flow.
- There is brief mention of the Heimlich maneuver and a website address for further details.
- Elements in Figure 3-13, and the legend are color-coded to make it easier to identify the specific method for nutrient absorption.
- A figure on enterohepatic circulation is included.
- A brief discussion of gall bladder disease was added to the second Looking Further box.

Chapter 4: Carbohydrates

- Chapter 4 was updated throughout to reflect the latest guidance for carbohydrate intake provided by the Food and Nutrition Board.
- The Carbohydrate MyPyramid figure is new, and is accompanied by a table of 15 common food sources of carbohydrate and the amount provided in a typical serving.
- Fiber is discussed in the body of the text (rather than in a box) and includes the differentiation of *dietary fiber* and *functional fiber*.
- The Looking Further box on diabetes and hypoglycemia includes a table that compares and contrasts type 1 and type 2 diabetes.
- Figure 4-7 is simplified to illustrate the key hormones that regulate blood glucose.
- Table 4-5 provides diet plans containing 25 grams and 38 grams of fiber per the latest recommendations of the Food and Nutrition Board.
- Discussion of glycemic index also includes a discussion of glycemic load.
- The alternative sweetener tagatose was added to the first Looking Further box.

Chapter 5: Lipids

- The Lipid MyPyramid figure is new, and is accompanied by a table of 15 common food sources of lipids and the amount provided in a typical serving.

- The discussion of atherosclerosis is placed in the Looking Further box on cardiovascular disease to simplify the main content of Chapter 5.
- The text has been updated to reflect the inclusion of *trans* fatty acids on Nutrition Facts panels, which are now required on the labels of all U.S. foods.
- Figure 5-3 compares the common food sources for saturated, monounsaturated, and polyunsaturated fats, and *trans* fatty acids.
- Figure 5-9 depicts lipoprotein interactions in the body.

Chapter 6: Proteins

- The Protein MyPyramid figure is new, and is accompanied by a table of 15 common food sources of proteins and the amount provided in a typical serving.
- New Figure 6-1 presents a visually appealing and realistic view of a cell to help students better understand the process of protein synthesis.
- The discussion of soy protein has been updated in the Looking Further box reviewing plant proteins in general.
- Other key illustrations include the following: Figure 6-8 contains a realistic presentation of organs involved in amino acid metabolism; Figure 6-10 conveys the concept of protein balance; Figure 6-11 uses photos to illustrate protein balance in practical terms; and Figure 6-13 includes photos of children afflicted with kwashiorkor and marasmus.
- In Looking Further, "Vegetarian Diets," the discussion of vegan diets was expanded to include infants and children.

Chapter 7: Alcohol

- The illustration on the effects of alcohol abuse (Fig. 7-2) contains a more realistic-looking person, and the content of the labeling is simplified.
- Table 7-4 summarizes the negative effects of binge drinking on society.

Chapter 8: Vitamins

- Coverage throughout Chapter 8 has been thoroughly updated to reflect latest vitamin intake recommendations.
- All previous vitamin pyramids have been redrawn to reflect the MyPyramid format.
- New Figure 8-14 applies a MyPyramid approach to evaluating nutrient supplement use.
- The Looking Further box examines the debate on need for daily multivitamin and mineral supplements by including the latest advice from the U.S. Preventive Services Task Force, as well as opposing advice provided by recent articles in the *Journal of the American Medical Association*.

Chapter 9: Water and Minerals

- The latest nutrient standards for sodium, potassium, chloride, and water have been incorporated.
- All mineral pyramids have been redrawn to reflect MyPyramid format.
- Discussion of the possible health benefits of calcium has been updated to reflect latest findings.
- The Looking Further box on osteoporosis has been thoroughly updated and revised.
- New figures include improved presentation of fluid compartments in the body (Fig. 9-1), a summary of how minerals contribute to body functions (Fig. 9-11), and a chart relating peak bone mass and risk of osteoporosis (Fig. 9-15).

Chapter 10: Energy Balance and Weight Control

- The latest statistics on weight status of North Americans are provided.
- A brief discussion of resting metabolic rate (this term is used in available diet analysis software programs) is included.
- Formulas provided by the Food and Nutrition Board for estimating the energy needs of adults are included.
- Figures of a BodPod and dual energy X-ray absorbtiometry are added to the discussion of diagnosing obesity and determining body composition.
- Figure 10-15 illustrates a typical surgical procedure to treat severe cases of obesity.

Chapter 11: Nutrition: Fitness and Sports

- Figure 11-1 summarizes the health benefits of physical activity.
- Figure 11-2 provides easy-to-follow diagram tracing the flow of energy-yielding nutrients into metabolism.
- The discussion of carbohydrate needs of athletes based on the latest guidance from the American Dietetic Association and the American College of Sports Medicine has been updated.
- Current recommendations for protein intake for athletes have also been updated.
- Table 11-6 summarizes the nutrient content of popular energy bars.

Chapter 12: Eating Disorders: Anorexia Nervosa, Bulimia Nervosa, and Other Conditions

- A second Looking Further box, "Thoughts of an Anorexic Woman," contributes a counterpoint to Looking Further, "Thoughts of a Bulimic Woman."

- Chapter 12 is organized so that binge-eating disorder is introduced before the female athlete triad.

Chapter 13: Pregnancy and Breastfeeding

- There is greater emphasis on the discussion of the importance of adequate folic acid intake prior to pregnancy to reduce the risk of neural tube defects.
- Chapter 13 includes the updated increase in calorie, carbohydrate, and protein needs of pregnant and lactating women recently issued by the Food and Nutrition Board.
- The food plan for pregnant women and lactating women has been updated to reflect the latest guidance provided by MyPyramid.
- Figure 13-5 better illustrates the processes of the let-down reflex.
- The latest American Academy of Pediatrics recommendation that breastfeeding infants be given 200 IU per day of vitamin D is included.

Chapter 14: Nutrition from Infancy through Adolescence

- The latest estimates for calorie, carbohydrate, fat, and protein needs for the appropriate infant age groups recommended by the Food and Nutrition Board and MyPyramid are included.
- Discussion of the causes and treatment of childhood obesity has been updated.
- The latest MyPyramid designed for children is included.

Chapter 15: Nutrition during Adulthood

- The discussion on nutrition and cancer in the Looking Further box is simplified. (This content was previously in Chapter 8.)
- The discussion of alternative medicines and herbal supplements is incorporated within the main body of the text. Table 15-4 lists the benefits and risks of some popular herbal remedies.

Chapter 16: Food Safety

- Table 16-2, which lists the U.S. agencies responsible for monitoring the food supply, is part of an earlier section of Chapter 16 for greater emphasis.
- Table 16-3 focuses on the most important microorganisms involved in foodborne illnesses.

- Figure 16-1 shows the minimum internal temperatures for cooking or reheating foods.
- Table 16-4 lists the caffeine content of common beverages.

Chapter 17: Undernutrition throughout the World

- The discussion of hunger in the United States emphasizes the concept of food insecurity.
- Statistics related to North American and world hunger and health issues have been updated to reflect latest data.
- Figure 17-4 promotes some possible approaches to solving the problem of undernutrition, in part to give a more hopeful tone to Chapter 17.

Special Acknowledgments

We would like to especially thank Angela Collene, M.S., R.D., for all her help with the sixth edition, including proofreading. Many of the text's improvements are the result of her suggestions. Michelle Asp, M.S., R.D., also helped proofread and edit the original manuscript. Our editor, Lynne Meyers, supported and assisted us through every step of the revision and facilitated the many decisions required to accomplish the enhancements of this edition, including the update. Jodi Rhomberg and the rest of the McGraw-Hill production staff carefully oversaw the myriad of tasks needed to create a beautiful and precise sixth edition, as well as this updated textbook.

Thank You to Reviewers and Contributors

As with earlier editions, our goal remains to provide students with the most accurate, up-to-date, and useful textbook possible. These ambitious goals would not be possible without the meticulous, professional assistance of colleagues who have aided us in so many ways. Their advice and suggestions helped us formulate the vision that made the sixth edition a more effective and efficient learning tool. Whether it was reviewing the fifth edition or evaluating materials for the sixth edition, participating in an instructional symposium, or responding to a survey, we owe our sincere thanks to each of these individuals. Along with our editors, we would like to acknowledge these dedicated educators whose contributions did so much to guide the direction of the sixth edition of *Contemporary Nutrition*.

A Request to Professors Who Use Contemporary Nutrition: Issues and Insights

The first edition of this text began with a dream. Each new edition, and this update in particular, is fostered by the excitement that improvements bring, and ends with the satisfaction of knowing that we have produced a dependable tool that will guide students as they begin their study of nutrition. As you might imagine, it is difficult to thoroughly address the vast range of nutrition science, keeping pace with countless new developments and controversies. We try our best but realize that sometimes we miss a side of an argument that deserves attention. As you read this book, if you find content that you question or believe warrants further attention, feel free to contact either of us:

Gordon M. Wardlaw, Ph.D., R.D.
P.O. Box 290
Mendocino, California 95460
Phone: (707) 937-2160
Email: gordonmark.wardlaw@gmail.com

Anne M. Smith, Ph.D., R.D., L.D.
Department of Nutrition
The Ohio State University
325 Campbell Hall
1783 Neil Avenue, Columbus, OH 43210
Phone: (614) 292-0715   Fax: (614) 292-8880
Email: smith.23@osu.edu
Website: www.hec.ohio-state.edu/hn/faculty/smith.html

Reviewers

Liz Applegate
University of California, Davis

Mokhtar Atallah
University of Massachusetts at Amherst

Georgina M. Awipi
The University of Tennessee at Martin

James W. Bailey
University of Tennessee

Beverly A. Benes
University of Nebraska—Lincoln

Ethan A. Bergman
Central Washington University—Ellensburg

Darlene E. Berryman
Ohio University

Debra Boardley
University of Toledo

Brenda Breeding
Oklahoma City Community College

Nancy Brenowitz
University of Maryland

Anne Bridges
University of Alaska, Anchorage

Amy Brown
University of Hawaii at Manoa

Lora Beth Brown
Brigham Young University

Martha S. Brown
Eastern Illinois University

Pat Brown
Cuesta College

Melanie Tracy Burns
Eastern Illinois University

Kathleen Cahill
San Jose State University

Patricia Chisamore
SUNY Orange Community College

Anne C. Cioffi
Hudson Valley Community College

Paula K. Cochrane
Albuquerque TVI

Janet Colson
Middle Tennessee State University

Margaret C. Craig-Schmidt
Auburn University

Robert T. Davidson
Brigham Young University

Earlene Davis
Bakersfield College

Judy A. Driskell
University of Nebraska

Vicki Erdmann
Normandale Community College

Michelle C. Fisher
Camden County College

Pam Fletcher
Albuquerque TVI—Community College

Bernard Frye
University of Texas at Arlington

Juliet M. Getty
University of North Texas

Art Gilbert
University of California, Santa Barbara

Janet W. Gloeckner
James Madison University

Joanne Gould
Kean University

Vivian Haley-Zitlin
Clemson University

Peter Horvath
SUNY University at Buffalo

Beckee Hobson
College of the Sequoias

Thunder Jalili
University of Utah

Molly A. Hoffman Jalufka
The Victoria College School of Vocational Nursing

Judy Kaufman
Monroe Community College

Mary L. Kelso
Antelope Valley College

Laura J. Kruskall
University of Nevada, Las Vegas

Heather Lynne
Mission College

Rick D. Mattes
Purdue University

Marilyn Mook
Michigan State University

Donna H. Mueller
Drexel University

Linda Kautz Osterkamp
University of Arizona

Leonard A. Piche'
Brescia University College

Linda L. Pope
Southwest Tennessee Community College

Ruth A. Reilly
University of New Hampshire

Barbara Reynolds
College of Sequoias

Jennifer Ricketts
University of Arizona

Nidia Romer
Miami Dade Community College—South

Janet Rouslin
Johnson and Wales University

Doris Sabin
Raritan Valley Community College

Tammy Sakanashi
Santa Rosa Junior College

Gretchen Scalpi
Orange Community College

Kevin Schalinske
Iowa State University

Annalisa Sherman
Cosumnes River College

Ingrid A. Skoog
University of Oregon

Linda Strause
University of California, San Diego

Sara W. Sutton
Eastern Kentucky University

Sandra L. Thomas
Coconino Community College

Nancy Vandenberg
Everett Community College

Ruth D. Verhegge
East Tennessee State University

Jennifer Weddig
Metropolitan State College of Denver

Fred H. Wolfe
University of Arizona, Tucson

Cynthia B. Wright
Southern Utah University

Daniel L. Wulff
University at Albany, SUNY

Donna L. Zoss
Purdue University

Nutrition science is constantly evolving. The classroom and students of today place new expectations on instructors. To help you meet these challenges, McGraw-Hill has created a suite of supplements tailored to *Contemporary Nutrition* that are intended to help you maximize your time in and out of the classroom.

Overhead Transparencies

More than 225 illustrations and tables from *Contemporary Nutrition*, as well as other McGraw-Hill nutrition texts, are available to support your classroom presentations. Artwork and labels have been enlarged to aid in classroom viewing.

Instructor's Testing and Resource CD-ROM

This cross-platform CD-ROM provides a wealth of resources for the instructor. Supplements featured on this CD-ROM include a computerized test bank utilizing McGraw-Hill's EZ Test testing software to quickly create customized exams. This user-friendly program allows instructors to search for questions by topic, format, or difficulty level; edit existing questions or add new ones; and scramble questions and answer keys for multiple versions of the same test. Word files of the text bank are included for those instructors who prefer to work outside of the test-generator software.

Other assets on the Instructor's Testing and Resource CD-ROM, such as User's Guides for the diet analysis software, are grouped within easy-to-use folders.

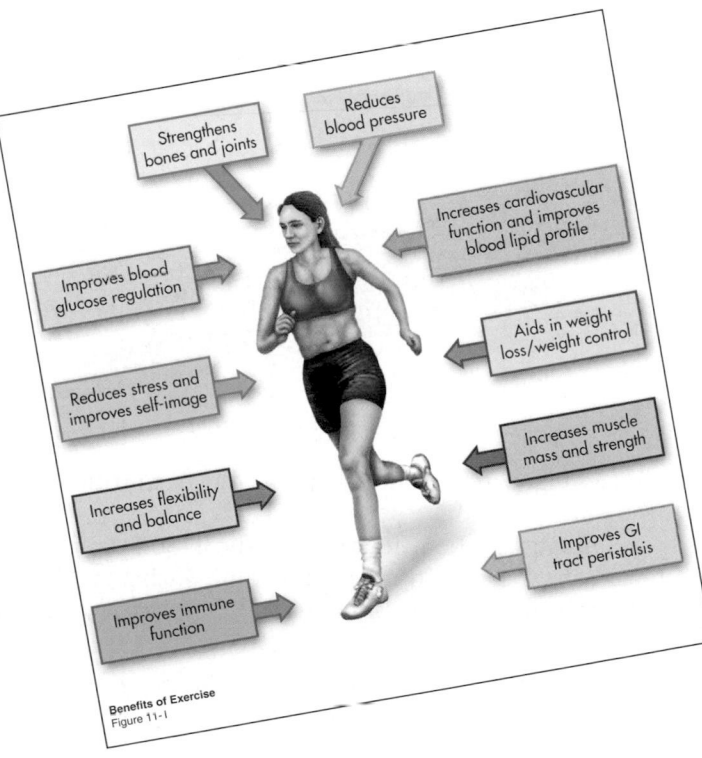

Benefits of Exercise
Figure 11-1

Strengthens bones and joints

Reduces blood pressure

Increases cardiovascular function and improves blood lipid profile

Improves blood glucose regulation

Aids in weight loss/weight control

Reduces stress and improves self-image

Increases muscle mass and strength

Increases flexibility and balance

Improves GI tract peristalsis

Improves immune function

25. All of the following are true about the toxicity of vitamin A
   A) One can experience toxic effects from consuming too m
   B) Fetal malformation can occur.
   C) One is unlikely to get toxic doses from eating food.
   D) Most adverse effects disappear after doses stop.
   Answer: A
   Topic: Vitamin A
   Difficulty: Moderate
   Type: Application
   Page: 245

New Dietary Reference Intakes for Energy, Carbohydrate, Fiber, Fat, Fatty Acid Sodium, Potassium, Chloride, and Water

Source: Dietary Reference Intakes, Institute of Medicine of the National Academies, 2002 and 2004. Press, Washington DC
Available at www.nap.edu

Energy
Boy and Girl Infants and Toddlers
0-3 months   EER (kcal/d) = (89 x Wt [kg] − 100) + 175
4-6 months   EER (kcal/d) = (89 x Wt [kg] − 100) + 56
7-12 months   EER (kcal/d) = (89 x Wt [kg] − 100) + 22
13-35 months EER (kcal/d) = (89 x Wt [kg] − 100) + 20

Boys 3-8 y   EER (kcal/d) = 88.5 − 61.9 x Age [y] + PA x (26.7 x Wt [kg] + 903 x Ht [m]) + 20
Boys 9-18 y   EER (kcal/d) = 88.5 − 61.9 x Age [y] + PA x (26.7 x Wt [kg] + 903 x Ht [m]) + 25

PA = 1.00 Sedentary
1.13 Low active
1.26 Active
1.42 Very Active

Girls 3-8 y   EER (kcal/d) = 135.3 − 30.8 x age [y] + PA x (10 x Wt [kg] + 934 x Ht [m]) + 20
Girls 9-18 y EER (kcal/d) = 135.3 − 30.8 x age [y] + PA x (10 x Wt [kg] + 934 x Ht [m]) + 25

PA = 1.00 Sedentary
1.16 Low active
1.31 Active
1.56 Very active

If you have questions about *Contemporary Nutrition* supplements, please contact your local McGraw-Hill representative. To find your local representative, check out www.mhhe.com.

Online Learning Center (www.mhhe.com/wardlawcont6)

The Online Learning Center for *Contemporary Nutrition* offers instructors an array of useful online teaching aids, such as chapter objectives, best teaching practices, as well as links to important nutrition sites organized by chapter.

Combine these resources with animations and interactivities and you have a powerful suite of tools to assist you in a traditional classroom or an online course.

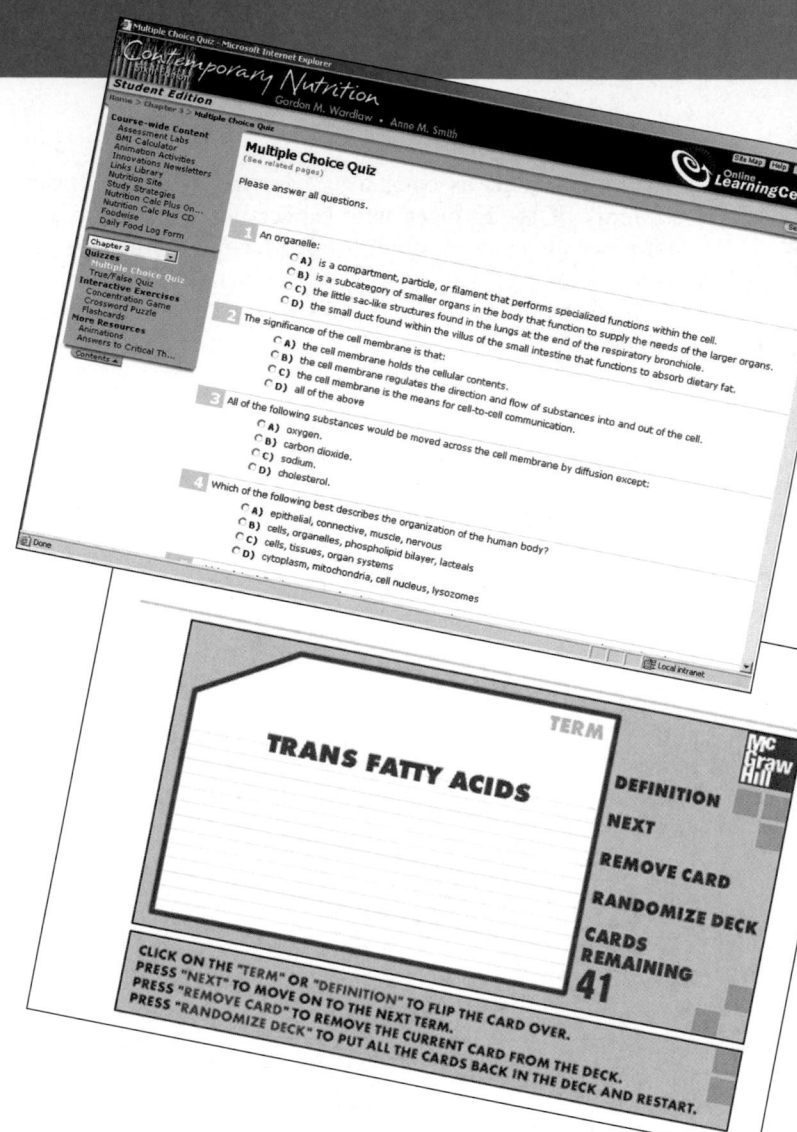

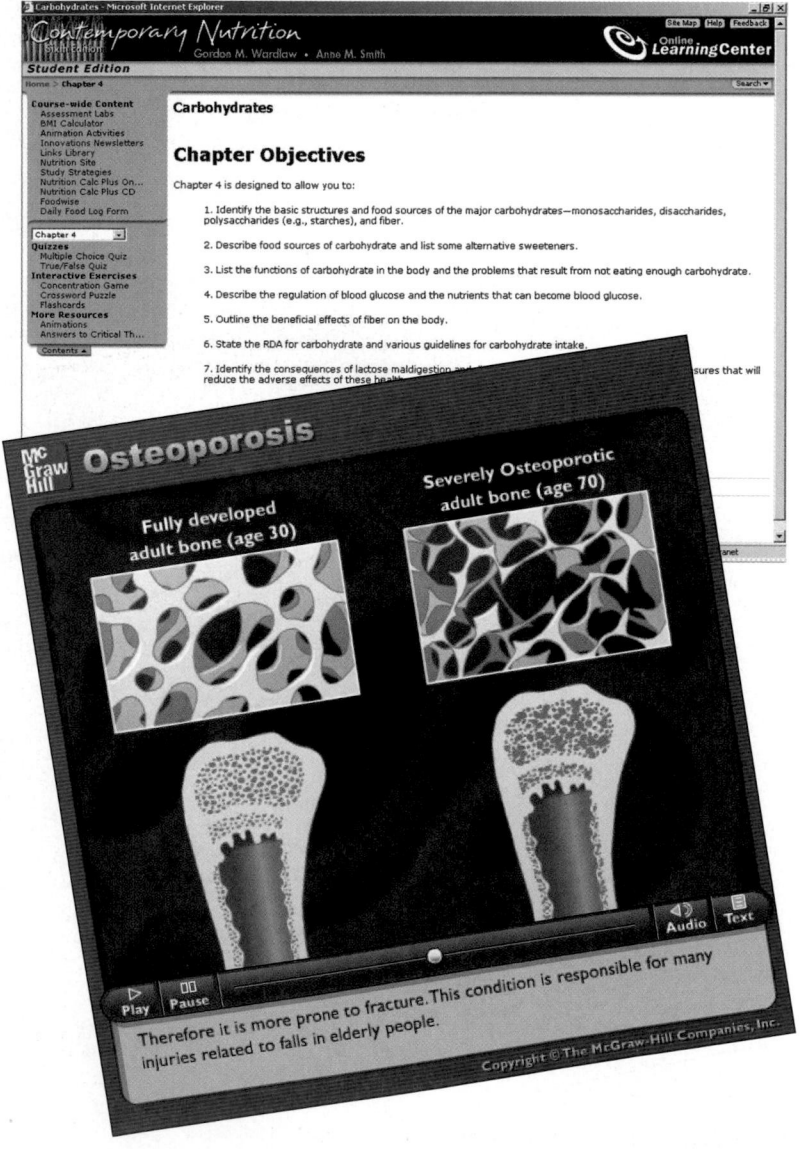

Getting better grades—and healthier nutrition—are what it's all about!

Students also benefit from a variety of tools designed to make the most out of their study time, such as multiple-choice; true/false, and animation quizzes; links to current nutrition articles, and nutrition animations.

Diet Analysis Software

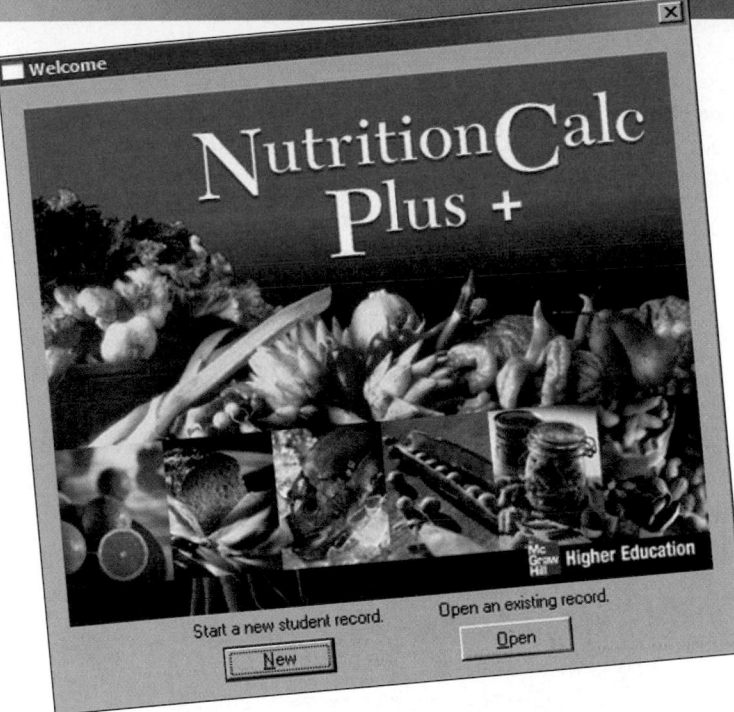

Diet Analysis Software

McGraw-Hill offers you the choice of three software programs. These programs can be packaged with *Contemporary Nutrition* at money-saving discounts.

◀ **NutritionCalc Plus 2.0 CD-ROM (Windows)** is a powerful tool to help students learn to analyze and monitor their diets. It features the reliability of the ESHA food database and a wide variety of reports to match your course assignments.

NutritionCalc Plus 2.0 Online offers all of the above with the addition of a colorful, easy-to-use interface and the ability to email reports to the professor. ▶

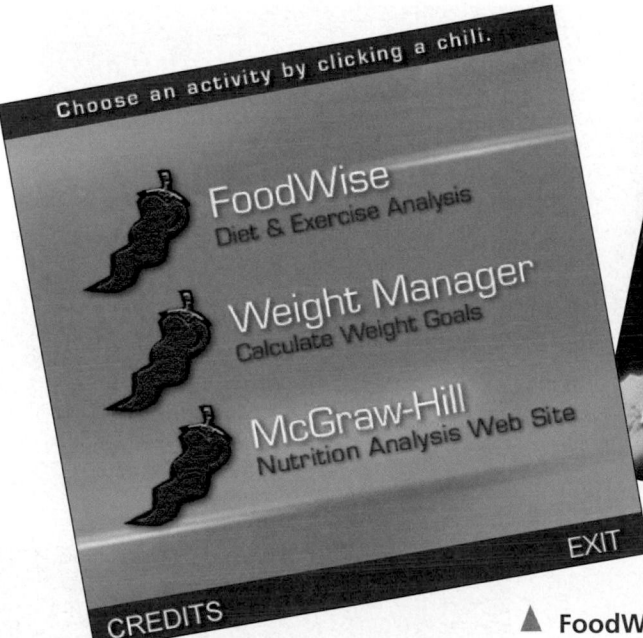

▲ **FoodWise CD-ROM** also allows students to track their food intake, daily exercise, and weight management.

xi

Digital Content Manager CD-ROM

Digital Content Manager CD-ROM

Imagine everything you need to create powerful, compelling lectures in one easy-to-use resource. Imagine animations that capture dynamic scientific processes in action. Imagine having the ability to modify the size, labels, and colors of illustrations with a click of your mouse. The Digital Content Manager for *Contemporary Nutrition* gives you the power of all this and more. This practical tool also includes hundreds of illustrations, photographs, tables, and animations to incorporate into your lecture presentations, handouts, or quizzes. With digital assets from *Contemporary Nutrition* and other McGraw-Hill nutrition texts, you simply click on the chapter folder, select an asset and you're ready to import that asset into the application of your choice. *It's that simple!*

New Animations cover an even broader range of nutrition topics. Approximately 30 dynamic new animations allow you to harness the visual impact of nutrition processes in motion.

▼

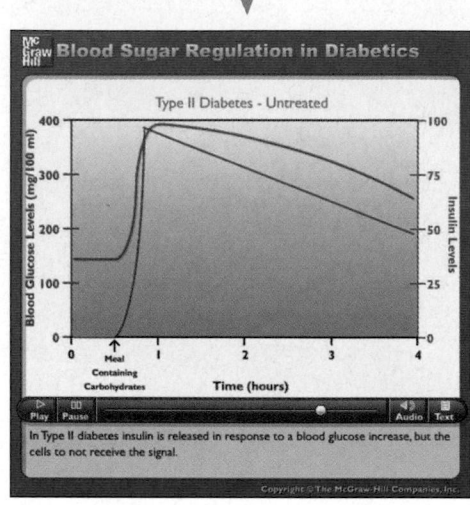

PowerPoint Lecture Outlines have been prepared for each chapter and already contain illustrations and animations to enliven any lecture. Use the outline as is or modify to suit your specific course needs.

▼

Full-color digital files of **Illustrations, Photos,** and **Tables** from *Contemporary Nutrition* allow you to easily customize your classroom materials.

What is a Calorie?

- Measurement of energy
- "the amount of heat it takes to raise the temperature of 1 gram of water by 1 d
- 1,000 Calori

Sample Calculation of a Nutrition Label

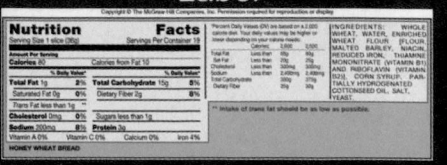

- Per serving
  - Carbohydrate: 15g x 4 kcal/g = 60 kcal
  - PRO: 3g x 4 kcal/g = 12 kcal
  - FAT: 1g x 9 kcal/g = 9 kcal
  - TOTAL: 81 kcal, rounded down to **80**

1 - 22

Active Art

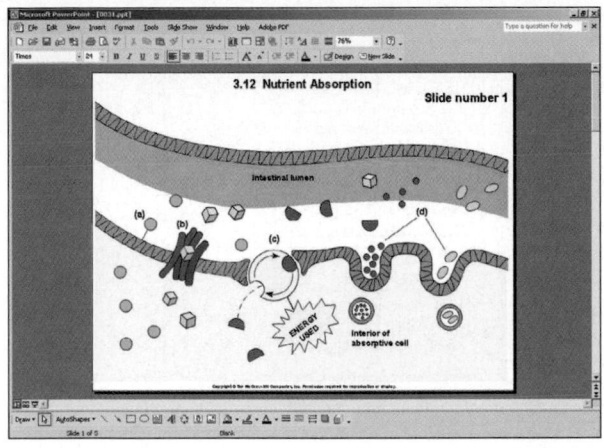

Active Art

Active Art allows you to customize key figures from the text to complement your lecture! Figures have been broken into smaller digestable parts so each piece can be used in whatever order or format chosen. Using Microsoft PowerPoint's ungroupable art feature, instructors can also move, resize, or change the color of any or all objects in a piece of art.

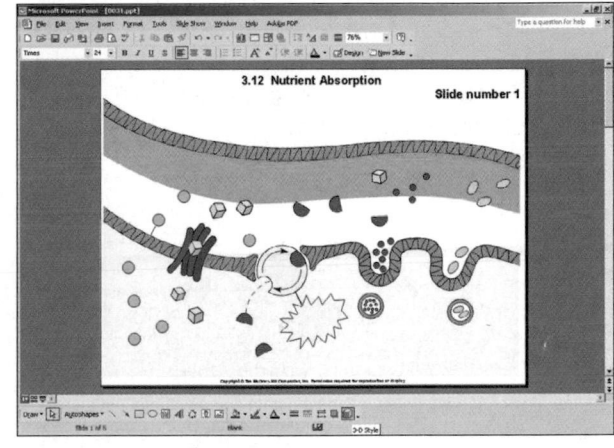

Remove Labels Labels and leader lines can be easily repositioned, edited, or removed. Your customized images can then be used for course assignments or additional quizzing for your students.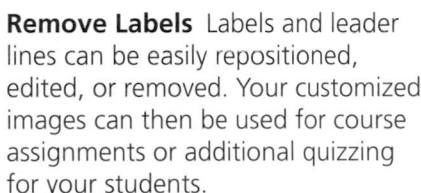

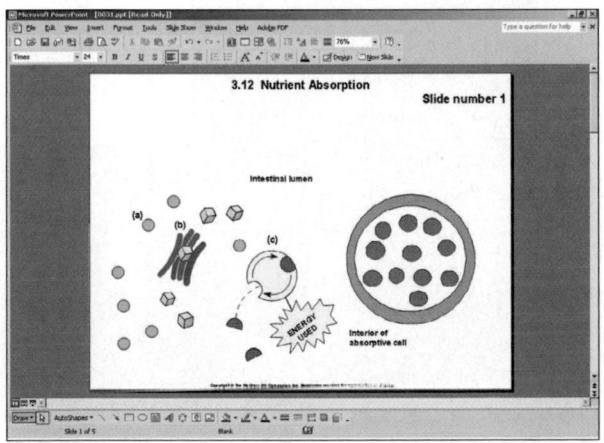

Resize Objects The entire image or parts of the image can be made larger or smaller depending on what you choose to emphasize.

Change Colors Colors can be removed and/or changed from any Active Art slide or object.

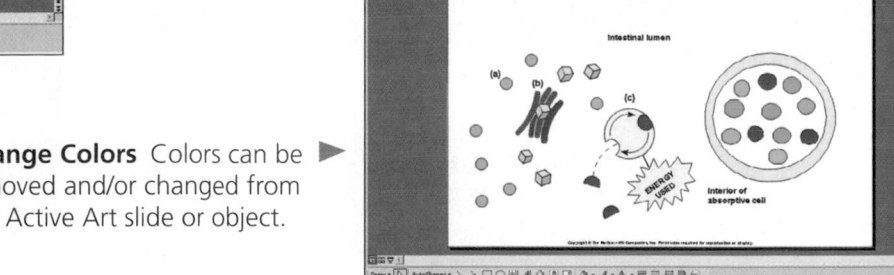

Dynamic New Illustrations

Line Drawings • Graphs •

Enhanced Art Program

Check out the figure comparisons for examples of the dramatic improvements we have made to the sixth edition illustrations.

- More Vibrant Colors
- Streamlined Labeling
- Remarkable Realism
- Striking New Photographs

• Fifth Edition

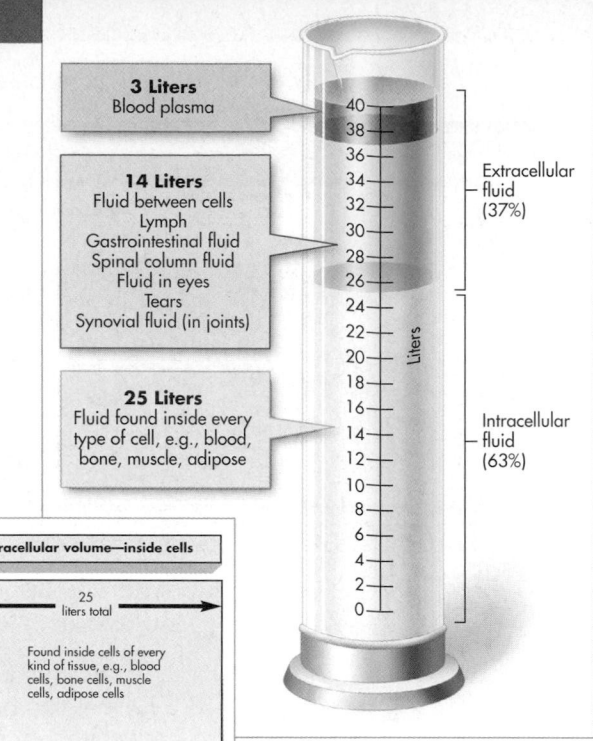

Extracellular volume—outside cells		Intracellular volume—inside cells
17 liters total		25 liters total
3 liters	14 liters	
Blood plasma	Fluid between cells Lymph Gastrointestinal fluids Spinal column fluid Fluid in eyes Tears Synovial fluid (in joints)	Found inside cells of every kind of tissue, e.g., blood cells, bone cells, muscle cells, adipose cells

3 Liters
Blood plasma

14 Liters
Fluid between cells
Lymph
Gastrointestinal fluid
Spinal column fluid
Fluid in eyes
Tears
Synovial fluid (in joints)

25 Liters
Fluid found inside every type of cell, e.g., blood, bone, muscle, adipose

Extracellular fluid (37%)

Intracellular fluid (63%)

Liters

• Sixth Edition

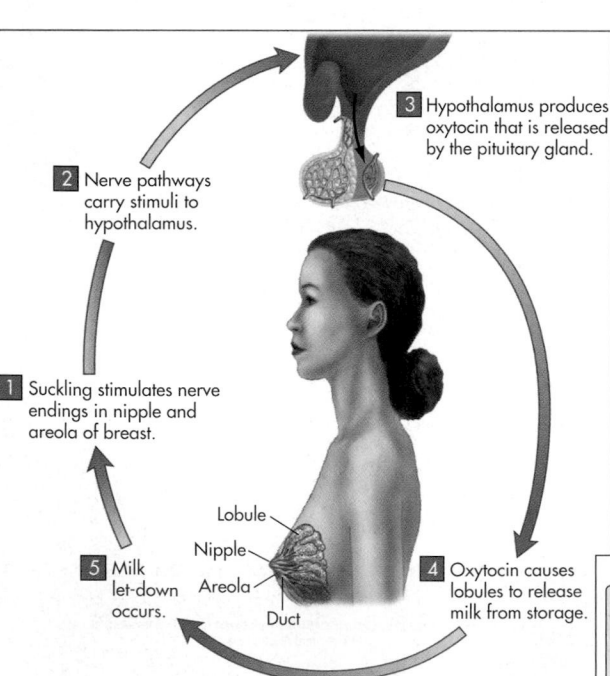

2 Nerve pathways carry stimuli to hypothalamus.

3 Hypothalamus produces oxytocin that is released by the pituitary gland.

1 Suckling stimulates nerve endings in nipple and areola of breast.

5 Milk let-down occurs.

4 Oxytocin causes lobules to release milk from storage.

Lobule
Nipple
Areola
Duct

• Sixth Edition

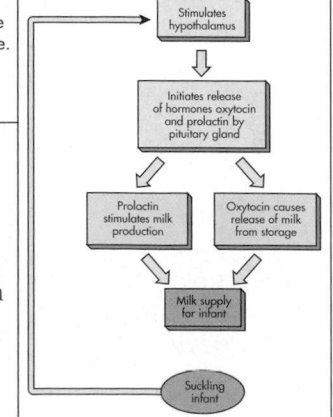

Stimulates hypothalamus

Initiates release of hormones oxytocin and prolactin by pituitary gland

Prolactin stimulates milk production

Oxytocin causes release of milk from storage

Milk supply for infant

Suckling infant

• Fifth Edition

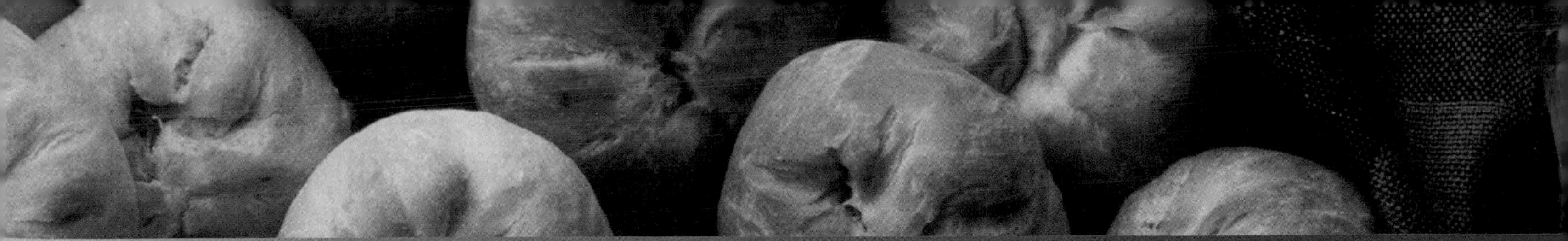

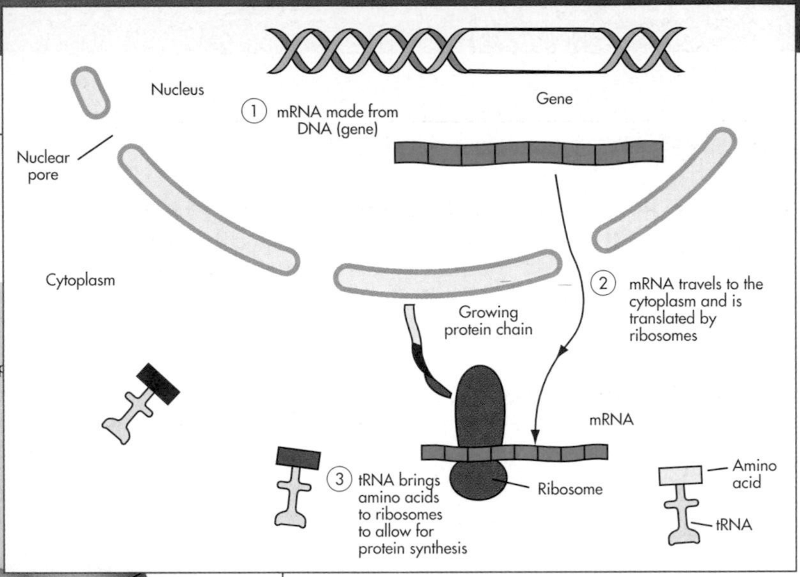

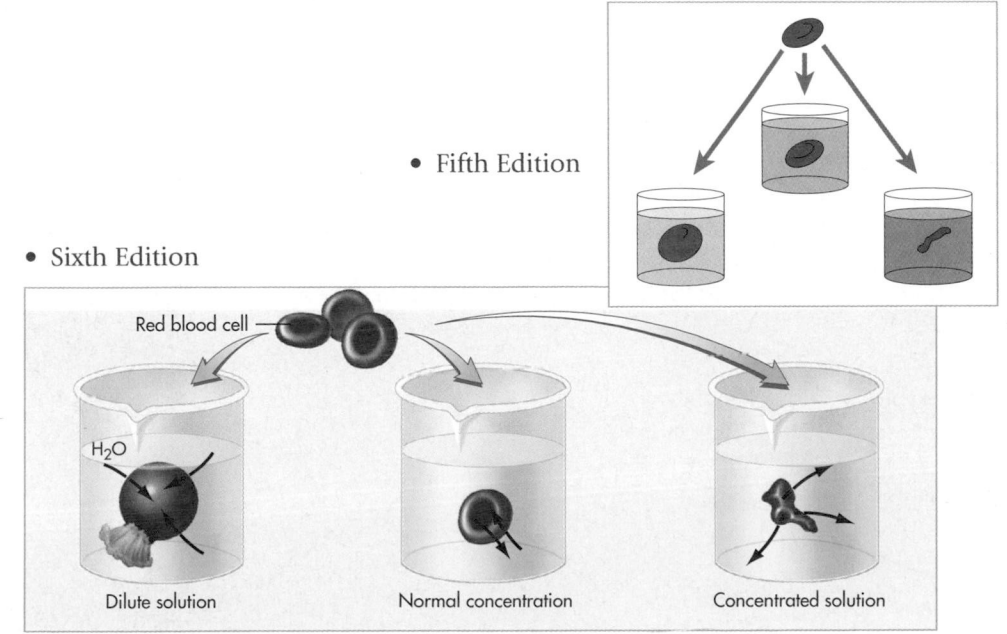

Sixth Edition (protein synthesis diagram):

1 DNA contains the information necessary to produce proteins.

2 Transcription of DNA results in mRNA, which is a copy of the information in DNA needed to make a protein.

3 The mRNA leaves the nucleus and goes to a ribosome.

4 Amino acids, the building blocks of proteins, are carried to the ribosome by tRNAs.

5 In the process of translation, the information contained in mRNA is used to determine the number, kinds, and arrangement of amino acids in the protein.

DNA strand 1

mRNA strand 2 **Transcription**

Nucleus

Cytoplasm

3

Amino acid pool 4

tRNA

Ribosome

Translation 5

Protein chain

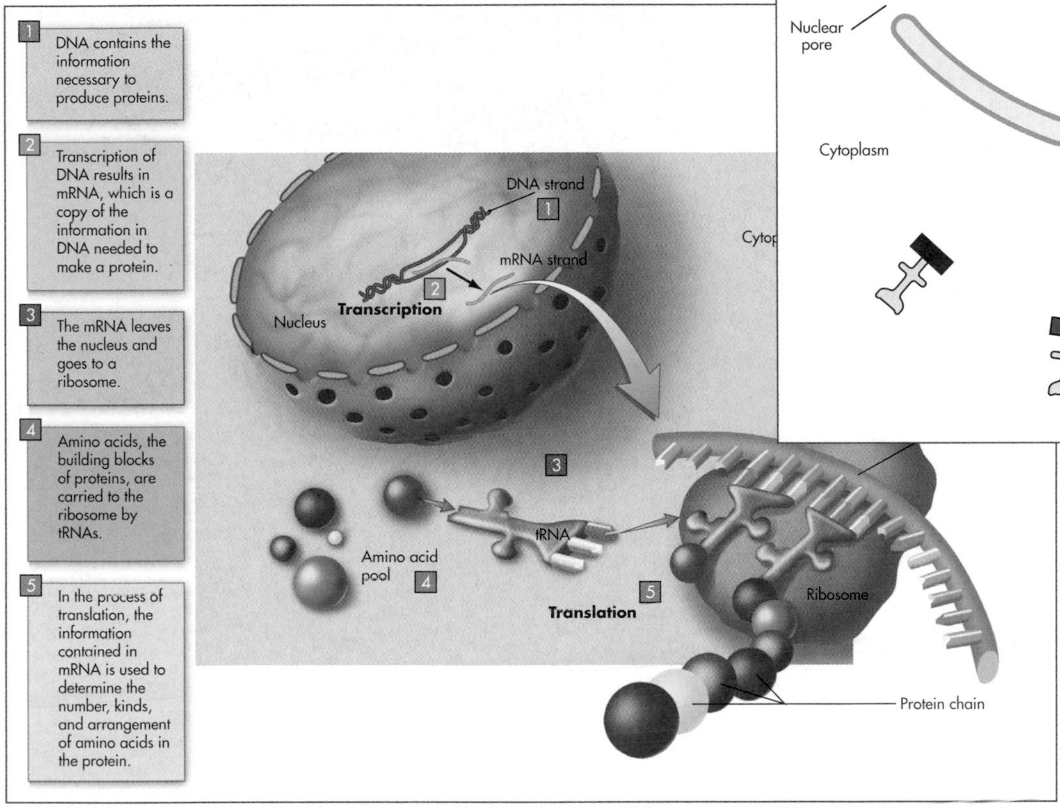

• Sixth Edition

Fifth Edition (protein synthesis diagram):

Nucleus

Nuclear pore

Cytoplasm

Gene

1 mRNA made from DNA (gene)

2 mRNA travels to the cytoplasm and is translated by ribosomes

Growing protein chain

mRNA

3 tRNA brings amino acids to ribosomes to allow for protein synthesis

Ribosome

Amino acid

tRNA

• Fifth Edition

Fifth Edition (osmosis diagram)

• Fifth Edition

Sixth Edition (osmosis diagram)

• Sixth Edition

Red blood cell

H_2O

Dilute solution

Normal concentration

Concentrated solution

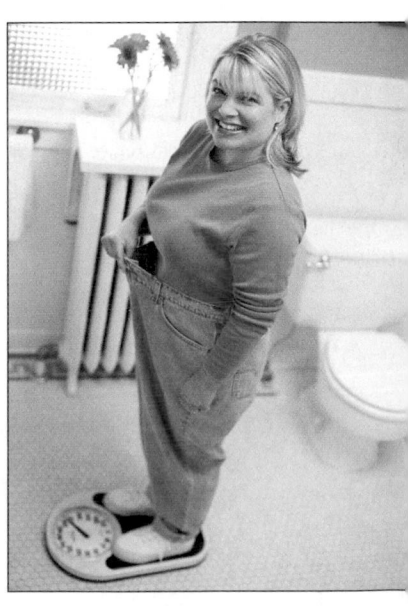

Personalized Guide to Nutrition

Rate Your Plate • Real Life Scenarios • Personal Assessments

Nutrition for the Individual

The authors provide ample opportunities for students to apply concepts and guidelines to their own lives. Real-life examples and activities help make the material relevant and provide the tools needed for students to carefully assess nutrition information on their own.

Real Life Scenarios introduce nutrition topics to be covered in context of a real person. The questions raised in the Real Life Scenario are discussed later in the chapter once the student has achieved an understanding of the concepts involved.

Rate Your Plate sections are activities that students can work through as a group or individually. All are designed to encourage students to actively analyze their own eating habits.

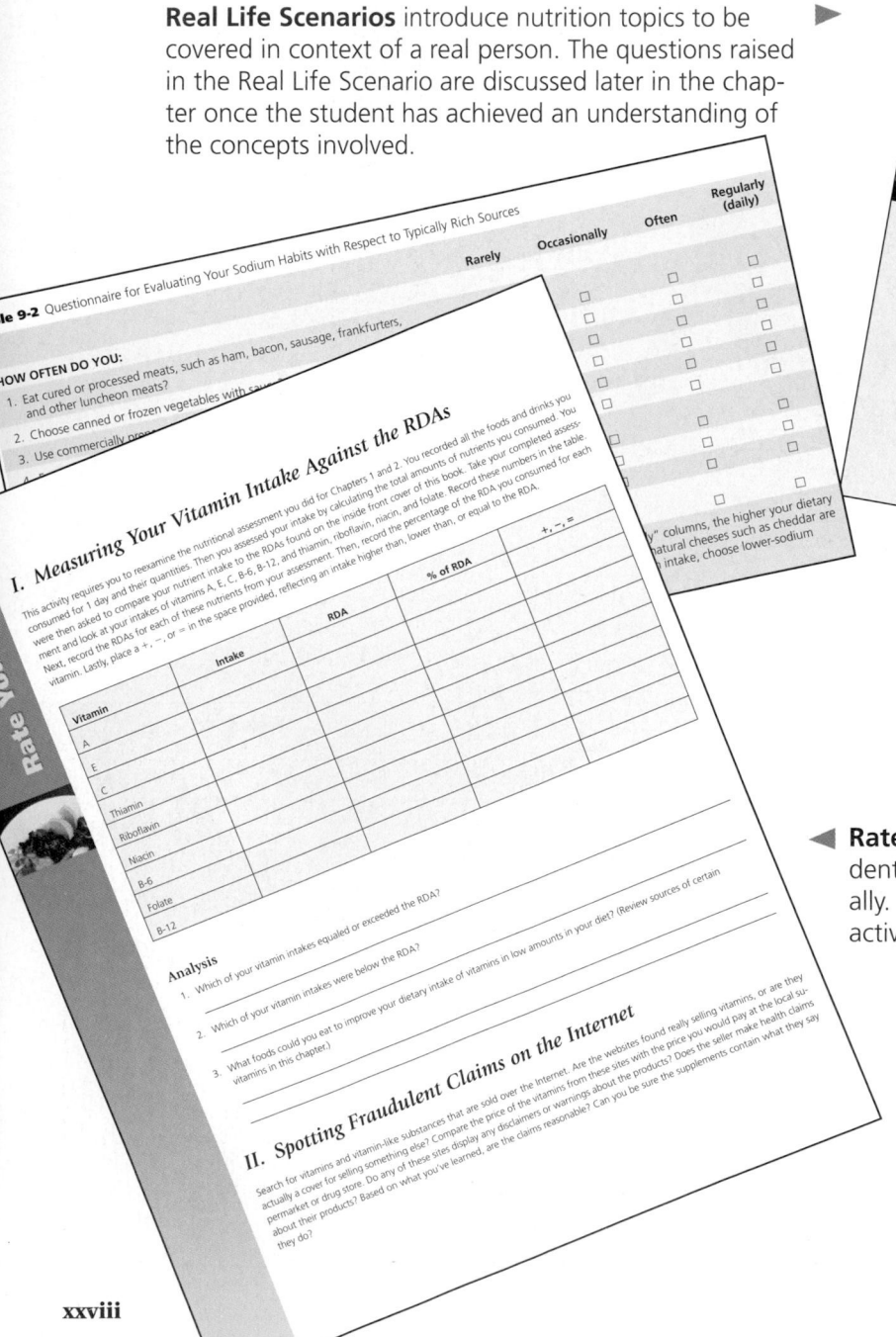

Part 3 Vitamins and Minerals

Vitamins

8

Real Life Scenario

Kristen works nights at a local package distribution center to pay her way through college. The combination of college and work is a source of stress for her. It also make it important that she not become ill. On a recent visit, a co-worker suggested she take supplements to avoid colds and other illnesses. She recommends that Nutramega is ideal for health maintenance. Kristen looks at the Supplement Facts panel and finds that each tablet contains (as percent of the Daily Value) 700% vitamin C, 100% vitamin A (three-quarters of which is preformed vitamin A), 700% vitamin C, 100% selenium, and 100% zinc. A month's supply also costs about $15. Should Kristen use this product? Are there health risks with this product, especially considering the dosage recommended on the label?

Check out the **Contemporary Nutrition Online Learning Center** at www.mhhe.com/wardlawcont6 for quizzes, flash cards, other activities to further help you learn about vitamins.

Real Life Scenario *Follow-*

Use of *Nutramega* poses some health risks for Kristen. Taking two tablets every 3 hours would mean taking at least 16 tablets per day. This alone would provide an intake of vitamin A, vitamin C, and zinc well in excess of the Upper Levels for these nutrients. Intake of preformed vitamin A would be 1.3 times the Upper Level, intake of vitamin C would be 3.4 times the Upper Level, and intake of zinc would be 3 times the Upper Level. Intake of selenium, however, falls well below the Upper Level set for that nutrient. This is how the math works out.

Vitamin A
33% (0.33) times the Daily Value of 1000 micrograms RAE equals 330 micrograms RAE per tablet. Sixteen tablets would yield 5280 micrograms RAE. The Upper Level is 3000 micrograms RAE for preformed vitamin A. Since 75% of the vitamin A is preformed vitamin A, this yields 3960 micrograms RAE of preformed vitamin A (5280 × 0.75 = 3960), or 1.3 times the Upper Level (3960/3000 = 1.3).

Vitamin C
700% (7) times the Daily Value of 60 milligrams equals 420 milligrams per tablet. 16 tablets would yield 6720 milligrams. The Upper Level is 2000 milligrams. This would then yield 3.4 times the Upper Level (6720/2000 = 3.4).

235

Table 9-2 Questionnaire for Evaluating Your Sodium Habits with Respect to Typically Rich Sources

HOW OFTEN DO YOU:	Rarely	Occasionally	Often	Regularly (daily)
1. Eat cured or processed meats, such as ham, bacon, sausage, frankfurters, and other luncheon meats?			☐	☐
2. Choose canned or frozen vegetables with sauce?		☐	☐	☐
3. Use commercially prepared...	☐	☐	☐	☐
	☐	☐	☐	☐
		☐	☐	☐
	☐	☐	☐	☐
	☐		☐	☐
	☐	☐		☐
		☐		☐

" columns, the higher your dietary ...natural cheeses such as cheddar are ...intake, choose lower-sodium

I. Measuring Your Vitamin Intake Against the RDAs

This activity requires you to reexamine the nutritional assessment you did for Chapters 1 and 2. You recorded all the foods and drinks you consumed for 1 day and their quantities. Then you assessed your intake by calculating the total amounts of nutrients you consumed. You were then asked to compare your nutrient intake to the RDAs found on the inside front cover of this book. Take your completed assessment and look at your intakes of vitamins A, E, C, B-6, B-12, and thiamin, riboflavin, niacin, and folate. Record these numbers in the table. Next, record the RDAs for each of these nutrients from your assessment. Then, record the percentage of the RDA you consumed for each vitamin. Lastly, place a +, −, or = in the space provided, reflecting an intake higher than, lower than, or equal to the RDA.

Vitamin	Intake	RDA	% of RDA	+, −, =
A				
E				
C				
Thiamin				
Riboflavin				
Niacin				
B-6				
Folate				
B-12				

Analysis

1. Which of your vitamin intakes equaled or exceeded the RDA?

2. Which of your vitamin intakes were below the RDA?

3. What foods could you eat to improve your dietary intake of vitamins in low amounts in your diet? (Review sources of certain vitamins in this chapter.)

II. Spotting Fraudulent Claims on the Internet

Search for vitamins and vitamin-like substances that are sold over the Internet. Are the websites found really selling vitamins, or are they actually a cover for selling something else? Compare the price of the vitamins from these sites with the price you would pay at the local supermarket or drug store. Do any of these sites display any disclaimers or warnings about the products? Does the seller make health claims about their products? Based on what you've learned, are the claims reasonable? Can you be sure the supplements contain what they say they do?

280

Latest Available Information

Current DRIs • Up-To-Date Science • Topics of Interest

Keeping Pace with Today's Nutrition

Becoming knowledgeable consumers of nutrition information means that students need to be aware of the rapidly changing nature of nutritional science and how they can responsibly evaluate and apply such information to their lives.

Throughout the text the latest Dietary Reference Intakes and guidelines have been updated to expose students to the most up-to-date information available. ▶

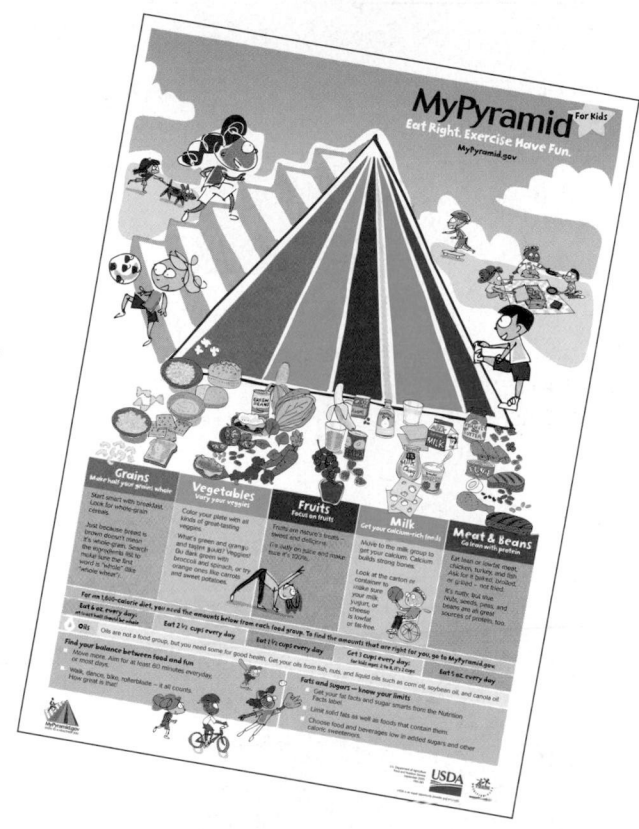

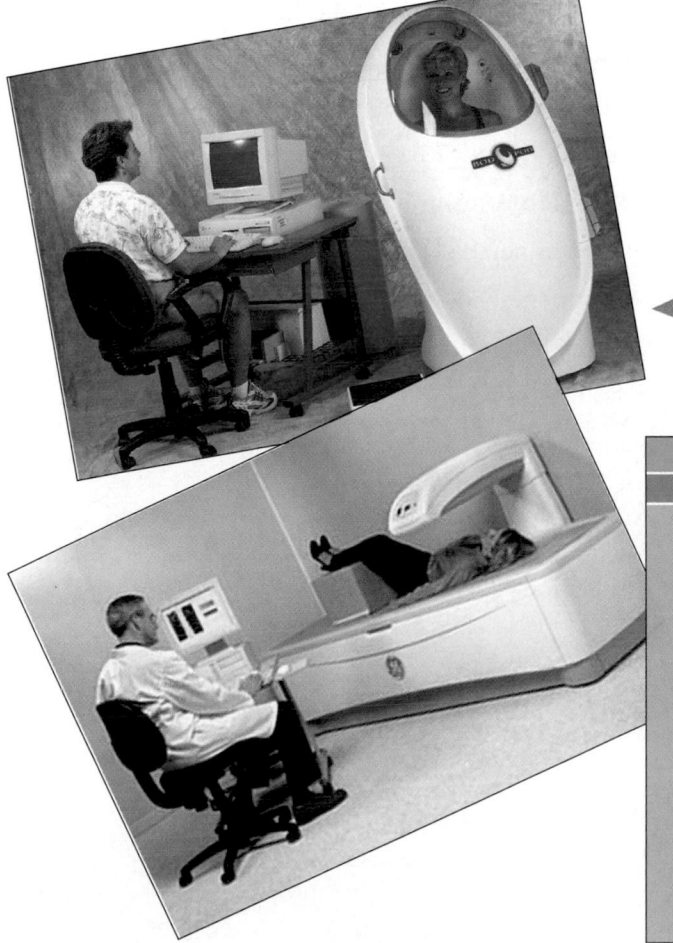

The latest nutrition issues and data reported in the media are explained in clear and accurate scientific terms. Students are given the knowledge needed to look beyond the headlines to make sound nutrition judgments. ▼

Estimated % of Cancer Deaths for 2004		
Male		**Female**
<1%	Brain	2%
4%	Esophagus and stomach	<1%
32%	Lung	25%
	Breast	15%
3%	Liver	<1%
5%	Pancreas	6%
9%	Leukemia and lymphomas	9%
10%	Colon and rectum	10%
6%	Urinary	
	Ovary	6%
10%	Prostate	
	Uterus and cervix	3%
25%	All others (e.g., oral and skin) (e.g., oral, skin, and bladder)	24%

About the Authors

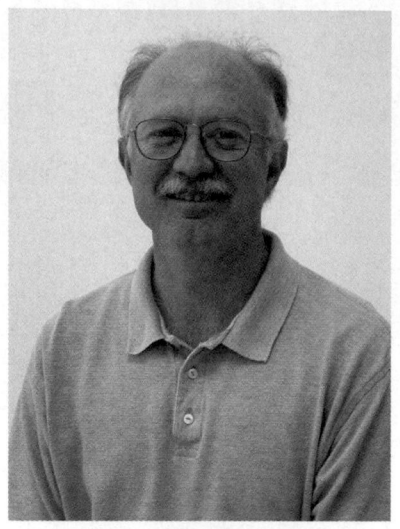

GORDON M. WARDLAW, Ph.D., R.D. has taught introductory nutrition courses to students in the Department of Human Nutrition at The Ohio State University, and as well at other colleges and universities. Dr. Wardlaw is the author of many articles that have appeared in prominent nutrition, biology, physiology, and biochemistry journals and was the 1985 recipient of the American Dietetic Association's Mary P. Huddleson Award. Dr. Wardlaw is a member of the American Society for Nutritional Sciences and is certified as a Specialist in Human Nutrition by the American Board of Nutrition.

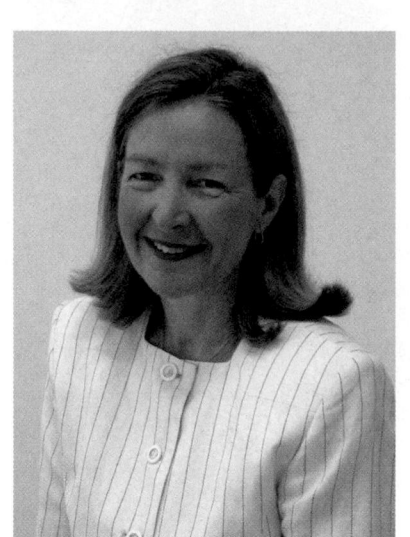

Anne M. Smith, Ph.D., R.D., L.D. currently teaches nutrition to nutrition majors and non-majors at The Ohio State University and was the recipient of the 1995 Outstanding Teacher Award from the College of Human Ecology. Dr. Smith is the Director of the Didactic Program in Dietetics in the Department of Human Nutrition, College of Human Ecology, of The Ohio State University and received the 1998 Emerging Dietetic Leader Award from The American Dietetic Association. Dr. Smith conducts research in the area of vitamin and mineral metabolism and was awarded the 1996 Departmental Research Award from the Ohio Agricultural Research & Development Center. Dr. Smith's research articles have appeared in prominent nutrition journals. She is a member of the American Society for Nutritional Sciences, the American Society for Clinical Nutrition, and the American Dietetic Association.

What You Eat and Why

1

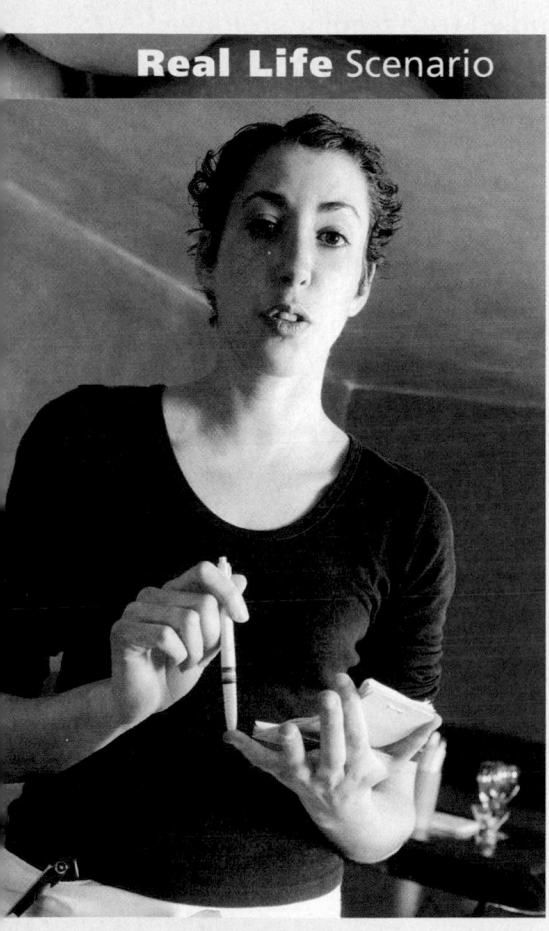

While Brenda was driving to campus last week, she heard an advertisement for a supplement containing a plant substance recently imported from China. It supposedly gives people more energy and helps one cope with the stress of daily life. This advertisement caught Brenda's attention because she has been feeling run down lately. She is taking a full-course load and has been working 30 hours a week at a local restaurant to try to make ends meet. Brenda doesn't have a lot of extra money. Still, she likes to try new things and this recent breakthrough from China sounded almost too good to be true. After searching for more information about this supplement on the Internet, she discovered that the recommended dose would cost $60 per month. Because Brenda is looking for some help with her low energy level, she decides to order a 1-month supply. Does this extra expense make sense to you?

Chapter 1 Objectives

Chapter 1 is designed to allow you to:

1. Define the terms *nutrition, carbohydrate, protein, lipid (fat), alcohol, vitamin, mineral, water, kilocalorie (kcal),* and *fiber.*

2. Use the caloric values of energy-yielding nutrients to determine the total calories (kcal) of a food or diet.

3. Outline the basic units of the metric system used in nutrition and calculate a percentage value, such as percent of calories from fat in a diet.

4. List the major characteristics of the North American diet and the food habits that often need improvement.

5. Describe how our food habits are affected by body physiological processes, meal size and composition, early experiences, ethnic customs, health concerns, advertising, social class, and economics.

6. Identify diet and lifestyle factors that contribute to the 10 leading causes of death in North America.

7. Understand the basis of the scientific method as it is used in developing hypotheses and theories in the field of nutrition.

8. Identify reliable sources of nutrition information.

Check out the **Contemporary Nutrition Online Learning Center**
www.mhhe.com/wardlawcont6 *for quizzes, flash cards, other activities, and web links designed to further help you learn about what you eat and why.*

Chapter 1 Outline

Do you need to take a balanced multivitamin and mineral supplement? Are you eating too much saturated fat, *trans* fat, and cholesterol? Are carbohydrates in our diets the cause of most of our health problems? Is much of what you eat unsafe? Are some foods actually *junk foods*? Should you become a vegetarian? If you have asked yourself any of these questions and are confused about what you should eat, you are not alone. Chapter 1 will help you sort out some of these issues as you are introduced to the science of nutrition.

And, as you begin this study of nutrition, keep this in mind. Research over the last 40 years has shown that a healthy diet—especially one rich in fruits, vegetables, and whole grains—coupled with regular prolonged, vigorous exercise and some strength-building exercise—can both prevent and treat many age-related diseases. Overall, it is clear that the nutritional lifestyles of some (but not all) North Americans are out of balance with their physiology. And, since we live longer than our ancestors did, preventing the age-related diseases that develop later in life is a more important focus today than in the past.

By optimizing dietary choices, we can strive to bring the goal of a long, healthy life within reach. This is the primary theme not just of Chapter 1 but throughout the entire book.

Refresh Your Memory

As you begin your study of what you eat and why in Chapter 1, you may want to review:

- The metric system in Appendix I.

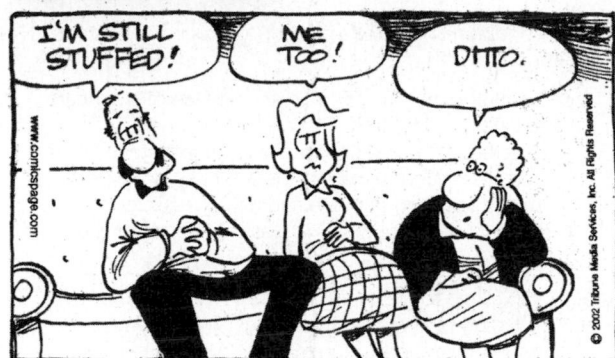 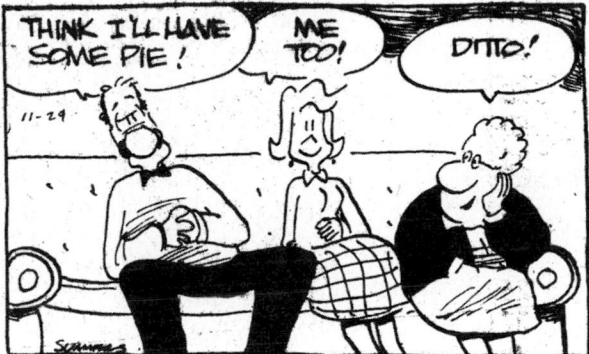

What influences daily food choices? How important is taste? Appearance? Nutrition? Convenience? Cost (Value)? Do these daily food choices go on to influence long-term health? If so, to what extent? Chapter 1 provides some answers.

Nutrition and Your Health

In your lifetime, you will eat about 70,000 meals and 60 tons of food. Chapter 1 will take a close look at the general classes of nutrients supplied by this food, the role research plays in sorting out which food components are essential for the maintenance of health, and the powerful effect of dietary habits in determining overall health.

What Actually Is Nutrition?

The Council on Food and Nutrition of the American Medical Association defines *nutrition* as "The science of food, the nutrients and the substances therein, their action, interaction, and balance in relation to health and disease, and the process by which the [human] organism ingests, digests, absorbs, transports, utilizes, and excretes food substances."

Nutrients Come from Food

What is the difference between food and **nutrients?** Food provides both the energy and the materials needed to build and maintain all body cells. Nutrients are the nourishing substances we, for the most part, must obtain from food. These substances are vital for growth and maintenance of a healthy body throughout life. For a substance to be considered an **essential nutrient,** three characteristics are needed:

- First, its omission from the diet must lead to a decline in certain biological functions, such as production of blood components.
- Second, if the omitted nutrient is restored to the diet before permanent damage occurs, those biological functions hampered by its absence should regain normal function.
- Third, the specific biological function(s) of the nutrient in the body must be identified.

Why Study Nutrition?

Nutrition is one key to developing and maintaining a state of health that is optimal for you. A poor diet and a sedentary lifestyle are known to be **risk factors** for life-threatening

nutrients Chemical substances in food that contribute to health, many of which are essential parts of a diet. Nutrients nourish us by providing calories to fulfill energy needs, materials for building body parts, and factors to regulate necessary chemical processes in the body.

Some nutrients that perform life-sustaining functions can be produced by the body if they are missing from the diet. The essential nature of such nutrients sometimes is not clear-cut. For example, humans require vitamin D, but the body is capable of synthesizing its own vitamin D upon exposure of the skin to sunlight. This reduces the need for vitamin D from dietary sources among people who experience regular sun exposure (see Chapter 8).

Table 1-1 Glossary Terms to Aid Your Introduction to Nutrition*

Term	Definition
Cancer	A condition characterized by uncontrolled growth of abnormal cells.
Cardiovascular (heart) disease	A general term that refers to any disease of the heart and circulatory system. This disease is generally characterized by the deposition of fatty material in the blood vessels (hardening of the arteries), which in turn can lead to organ damage and death. Also termed coronary heart disease (CHD), as the vessels of the heart are the primary sites of the disease.
Cholesterol	A waxy lipid found in all body cells; it has a structure containing multiple chemical rings. Cholesterol is found only in foods of animal origin.
Chronic	Long-standing, developing over time. When referring to disease, this term indicates that the disease process, once developed, is slow and lasting. A good example is cardiovascular disease.
Diabetes	A group of diseases characterized by high blood **glucose.** Type 1 diabetes involves insufficient or no release of the hormone insulin by the pancreas; requires daily insulin therapy. Type 2 diabetes results from either insufficient release of insulin or general inability of insulin to act on certain body cells, such as muscle cells. Persons with type 2 diabetes may or may not require insulin therapy.
Hypertension	A condition in which blood pressure remains persistently elevated. Obesity, inactivity, alcohol intake, excess salt intake, and genetics may each contribute to the problem.
Kilocalorie (kcal)	Unit that describes the energy content of food. Specifically, a kilocalorie (kcal) is the heat energy needed to raise the temperature of 1000 grams (1 liter) of water 1° Celsius. A single calorie would do the same for 1 gram of water. Kcal is also written as Calorie, with a capital C, signifying a 1000 calorie unit of measurement.
Obesity	A condition characterized by excess body fat.
Osteoporosis	Decreased bone mass related to the effects of aging, genetic background and poor diet in both genders, and hormonal changes of menopause in women.
Risk factor	A term used frequently when discussing the factors contributing to the development of a disease. A risk factor is an aspect of our lives—such as heredity, lifestyle choices (e.g., smoking), or nutritional habits.

*All bold terms in the book are defined in the glossary for this book. Many bold terms are also defined in the page margins within each chapter.

The energy content of a food is commonly referred to as calories. Because it is a familiar term, we will use it as such in this book.

glucose A six-carbon monosaccharide that exits in a ring form; found as such in blood, and in table sugar bound to fructose; also known as *dextrose*, it is one of the simple sugars.

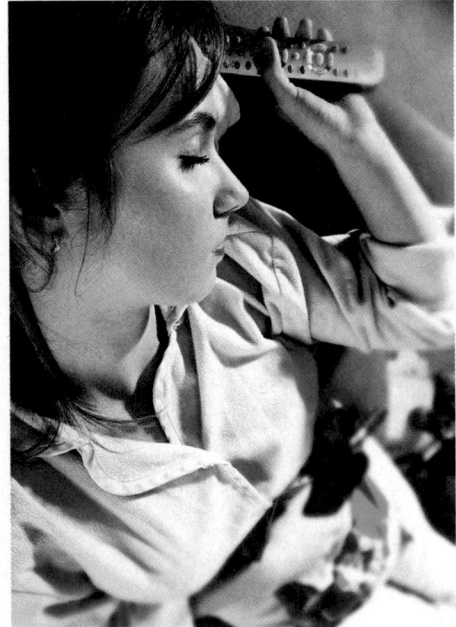

The major health problems in North America are largely caused by a poor diet, excessive calorie intake, and not enough physical activity.

chronic diseases such as **cardiovascular (heart) disease, hypertension, diabetes,** and some forms of **cancer** (Table 1-1). Together, these and related disorders account for two-thirds of all deaths in North America (Table 1-2). Not meeting nutrient needs in younger years also makes us more likely to suffer health consequences, such as bone fractures from the disease **osteoporosis,** in later years. At the same time, taking too much of a nutrient supplement—such as vitamin A—can be harmful. Another dietary problem, drinking too much alcohol, is associated with many health problems.

All of these consequences of modern living are partly an "affliction of affluence." Note, however, that these diseases are often preventable. Age fast or age slowly: It is partly your choice. U.S. government scientists have calculated that a poor diet combined with a lack of sufficient physical activity contributes up to 365,000 fatal cases

Table 1-2 Ten Leading Causes of Death in the United States

Rank	Cause of Death	Percent of Total Deaths
	All causes	100
1	Diseases of the heart (primarily coronary heart disease)*†#	29
2	Cancer*‡	22
3	Cerebrovascular diseases **(stroke)***†‡#	7
4	Chronic obstructive pulmonary diseases and allied conditions (lung diseases)‡	5
5	Accidents and adverse effects†	4
	Motor vehicle accidents	(2)
	All other accidents and adverse effects	(2)
6	Diabetes*	3
7	Influenza and pneumonia	3
8	Alzheimer's disease*	2
9	Kidney disease*‡	2
10	Blood-borne infections	1

From Centers for Disease Control and Prevention, *National Vital Statistics Report,* accessed October 9, 2002. Canadian statistics are quite similar.

*Causes of death in which diet plays a part

†Causes of death in which excessive alcohol consumption plays a part

‡Causes of death in which tobacco use plays a part

#Diseases of the heart and cerebrovascular disease are included in the more global term "cardiovascular disease."

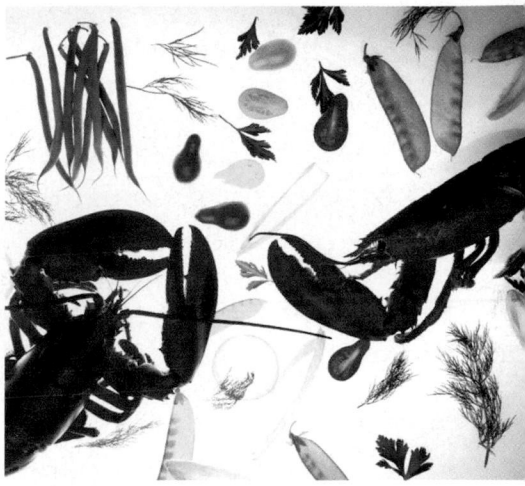

Many foods are rich sources of nutrients.

of cardiovascular disease, cancer, and diabetes each year among adults in the United States. Thus, the combination of poor diet and too little physical activity may be the second leading cause of death in the United States. In addition, **obesity** is considered the second leading cause of preventable death in North America (smoking is the first). Put together, obesity and smoking spell even more trouble healthwise. And as you will learn in Chapter 10, surgery to help treat obesity costs about $20,000 to $40,000. Compare that to the cost of prevention: none.

As you gain understanding about your nutritional habits and increase your knowledge about nutrition, you will have the opportunity to dramatically reduce your risk for many common health problems. For additional help, the U.S. federal government provides two websites that contain links to many sites providing health and nutrition information (www.healthfinder.gov and www.nutrition.gov). Other useful sites are webmd.com, www.navigator.tufts.edu, and www.eatright.org.

Classes and Sources of Nutrients

To begin the study of nutrition, let's start with an overview of the six classes of nutrients. You are probably already familiar with the terms **carbohydrates, lipids** (fats and oils), **proteins, vitamins,** and **minerals.** These, plus **water,** make up the six classes of nutrients found in food (Fig. 1-1).

Nutrients can then be assigned to three functional categories: (1) those that primarily provide us with calories to meet energy needs (expressed in **kilocalories [kcal]**); (2) those that are important for growth, development, and maintenance; and (3) those that act to keep body functions running smoothly. Some overlap exists among these groupings. The energy-yielding nutrients make up a major portion of most foods (Table 1-3).

Let's now look more closely at these six classes of nutrients (Table 1-4).

stroke A decrease or loss in blood flow to the brain that results from a blood clot or other change in arteries in the brain. This in turn causes the death of brain tissue. Also called a *cerebrovascular accident.*

carbohydrate A compound containing carbon, hydrogen, and oxygen atoms. Most are known as *sugars, starches,* and *fibers.*

lipid A compound containing much carbon and hydrogen, little oxygen, and sometimes other atoms. Lipids dissolve in ether or benzene, but not in water, and include fats, oils, and cholesterol.

protein Food and body components made of amino acids; proteins contain carbon, hydrogen, oxygen, nitrogen, and sometimes other atoms, in a specific configuration. Proteins contain the form of nitrogen most easily used by the human body.

vitamin Compound needed in very small amounts in the diet to help regulate and support chemical reactions in the body.

mineral Element used in the body to promote chemical reactions and to form body structures.

water The universal solvent; chemically, H_2O. The body is composed of about 60% water. Water (fluid) needs are about 9 (women) or 13 (men) cups per day; needs are greater if one exercises heavily.

Carbohydrate	Lipid	Protein

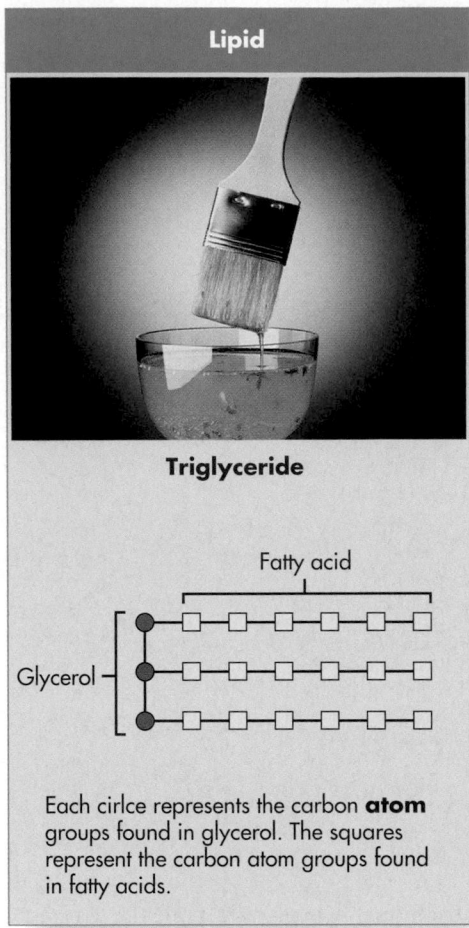

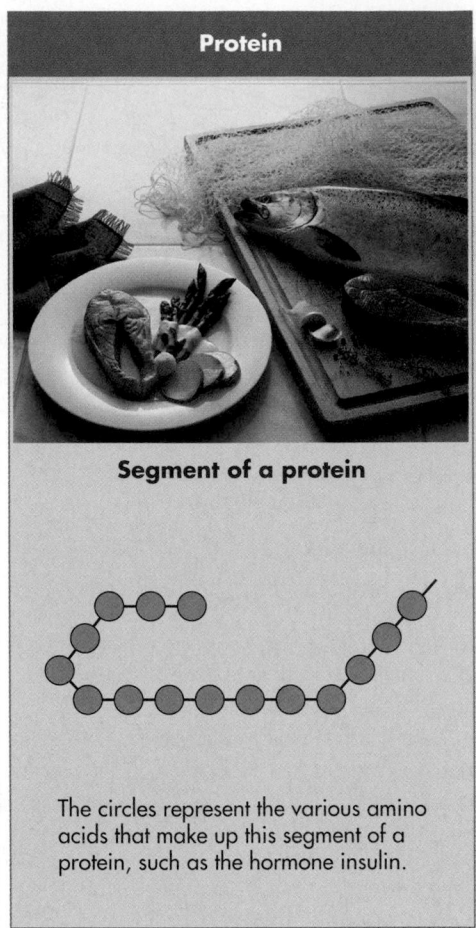

Figure 1-1 Two views of carbohydrates, lipids, and proteins—chemical and dietary perspectives.

Table 1-3 Major Functions of the Various Classes of Nutrients

Nutrient Classes That Provide Energy	Nutrient Classes That Promote Growth, Development, and Maintenance	Nutrient Classes That Regulate Body Processes
Most carbohydrates	Proteins	Proteins
Proteins	Lipids	Some lipids
Most lipids	Some vitamins	Some vitamins
	Some minerals	Some minerals
	Water	Water

Carbohydrates, proteins, lipids, and water are needed in relatively large amounts, so they are called **macronutrients.** Vitamins and minerals are needed in such small amounts in the diet that they are called **micronutrients.**

■ Carbohydrates

Chemically, carbohydrates are composed mainly of the **elements** carbon, hydrogen, and oxygen. Carbohydrates provide a major source of calories for the body, on average 4 kcal per gram. Carbohydrates can exist as simple sugars and complex carbohydrates. **Simple sugars,** sometimes referred to simply as *sugars,* are relatively small molecules. The smallest simple sugars are called monosaccharides. They consist of a single sugar unit. The sugar in your blood, **glucose** (also known as *blood sugar* or *dextrose*), is an example of a monosaccharide. Other simple sugars are made by joining two

atom Smallest combining unit of an element, such as iron or calcium. Atoms consist of protons, neutrons, and electrons.

element A substance that cannot be separated into simpler substances by chemical processes. Common elements in nutrition include carbon, oxygen, hydrogen, nitrogen, calcium, phosphorus, and iron.

macronutrient A nutrient needed in gram quantities in a diet.

micronutrient A nutrient needed in milligram or microgram quantities in a diet.

monosaccharides together to form a **disaccharide.** Table sugar, sucrose, is an example of a disaccharide because it is formed from fructose and glucose (both monosaccharides). Joining many monosaccharides—often found as repeating units—forms **polysaccharides,** also known as **complex carbohydrates.** For example, plants store carbohydrates in the form of **starch,** a polysaccharide made up of hundreds of repeating glucose units (review Fig. 1-1).

Aside from enjoying their taste, we need sugars and other carbohydrates in our diets primarily to help satisfy the calorie needs of our body cells. Glucose, a simple sugar that the body can derive from most carbohydrates, is a major source of calories in most cells. When not enough carbohydrate is consumed to supply sufficient glucose, the body is forced to make glucose from proteins—not a healthy change.

Digestion of complex carbohydrates begins in the mouth. The digestive process continues in the small intestine until starches are broken down into single sugar molecules (such as glucose), which are absorbed via **cells** lining the small intestine into the bloodstream (see Chapter 3 for more on digestion and absorption). However, the **bonds** between the sugar molecules in certain complex carbohydrates cannot be broken down by human digestive processes. These carbohydrates are part of what is called **fiber.** This instead passes through the small intestine undigested to provide bulk for the stool (feces) formed in the large intestine (colon). Chapter 4 focuses on carbohydrates.

▪ Lipids

Lipids (mostly fats and oils) are composed primarily of the elements carbon and hydrogen; they contain fewer oxygen atoms than do carbohydrates. Because of this difference in composition, lipids yield more calories per gram than do carbohydrates—on the average, 9 kcal per gram. Lipids dissolve in certain solvents (e.g., ether and benzene) but not in water.

The basic structure of most lipids is the **triglyceride.** Triglycerides provide a key calorie source for the body (e.g., **fatty acids**) and are the major form of fat in foods. They are also the main form for energy storage in the body. In this book, the more familiar terms *fats* or *fats and oils* will generally be used, rather than lipids or triglycerides. Roughly speaking, fats are lipids that are solid at room temperature and oils are lipids that are liquid at room temperature.

Most lipids can be separated into two basic types—saturated fat and unsaturated fat—based on the chemical structure of their dominant fatty acids. Saturated fats are rich in **saturated fatty acids.** These fatty acids do not contain carbon-carbon double bonds. Unsaturated fats are rich in **unsaturated fatty acids.** These fatty acids contain one or more of carbon-carbon double bonds.

The presence of carbon-carbon double bonds determines whether the lipid is solid or liquid at room temperature. Think of a double bond as a "kink" somewhere along the carbon chain of a fatty acid. Having one or more kinks limits the extent to which fatty acids can pack tightly together, and therefore how solid a mass of fatty acids can be. Plant oils tend to contain many unsaturated fatty acids—this makes them liquid at room temperature. Animal fats are often rich in saturated fatty acids—this makes them solid at room temperature. Almost all foods contain a variety of saturated and unsaturated fatty acids.

Another Bite

Some foods contain *trans* **fatty acids,** also called *trans* fats. These fats are commonly found in processed foods, and especially those that are deep-fried, such as doughnuts and French fries. Large amounts of *trans* fats in the diet pose certain health risks, so intake should be minimized (see Chapter 5 for details). For now, note that if partially hydrogenated fat or partially hydrogenated oil is listed on a food label, the food contains *trans* fat. All food labels in the United States and Canada have to list *trans* fat content.

cell A minute structure; the living basis of plant and animal organization. In animals it is bounded by a cell membrane. Cells contain both genetic material and systems for synthesizing energy-yielding compounds. Cells have the ability to take up compounds from and excrete compounds into their surroundings.

bond A linkage formed by the sharing of electrons, or attractions between two atoms.

fiber Substances in plant foods that are not digested by the processes that take place in the human stomach or small intestine. These add bulk to feces. Fiber naturally found in foods is also called dietary fiber.

triglyceride The major form of lipid in the body and in food. It is composed of three fatty acids bonded to glycerol, an alcohol.

fatty acid Major part of most lipids; primarily composed of a chain of carbons flanked by hydrogen.

saturated fatty acid A fatty acid containing no carbon-carbon double bonds.

unsaturated fatty acid A fatty acid containing one or more carbon-carbon double bonds.

Much attention has been given to saturated fat in the past few years. This is because saturated fat bears a great deal of the responsibility for raising blood **cholesterol.** High blood cholesterol leads to clogged arteries and can eventually lead to cardiovascular disease (see Chapter 5).

trans fatty acids A form of an unsaturated fatty acid, usually a monounsaturated one when found in food, in which the hydrogens on both carbons forming that double bond lie on opposite sides of that bond, rather than on the same side (typical of fatty acids). Stick margarine, shortenings, and deep fat-fried foods in general are rich sources.

Table 1-4 Essential Nutrients in the Human Diet and Their Classes*

Energy-Yielding Nutrients			Water
Carbohydrate	**Lipids†**	**Protein**	
Glucose (or a carbohydrate that yields glucose)‡	Linoleic acid a-Linolenic acid	Amino acids	

Certain unsaturated fatty acids are essential nutrients that must come from our diet. These key fatty acids that the body can't produce, called essential fatty acids, perform several important functions in the body: they help regulate blood pressure and play a role in the synthesis and repair of vital cell parts. However, we need only about four tablespoons of a common vegetable oil (such as the canola or soybean oil found in supermarkets) each day to supply these essential fatty acids. A serving of fatty fish, such as salmon or tuna, at least twice a week is another healthy source of essential fatty acids. The unique fatty acids in these fish complement the healthy aspects of common vegetable oils. This will be explained in greater detail in Chapter 5, which focuses on lipids.

■ Proteins

enzyme A compound that speeds the rate of a chemical process but is not altered by the process. Almost all enzymes are proteins (some are made of genetic material).

Like carbohydrates and fats, proteins are composed of the elements carbon, oxygen, and hydrogen. But, unlike the other energy-yielding nutrients, all proteins also contain nitrogen. Proteins are the main structural material in the body. For example, proteins constitute a major part of bone and muscle; they are also important components in blood, body cells, **enzymes,** and immune factors. Furthermore, proteins can also

Vitamins		Minerals		
Water-soluble	**Fat-soluble**	**Major**	**Trace**	**Questionable minerals**
Thiamin	A	Calcium	Chromium	Arsenic
Riboflavin	D§	Chloride	Copper	Boron
Niacin	E	Magnesium	Fluorideǁ	Nickel
Pantothenic acid	K	Phosphorus	Lodide	Silicon
Biotin		Potassium	Iron	Vanadium
B-6		Sodium	Manganese	
B-12		Sulfur	Molybdenum	
Folate			Selenium	
C			Zinc	

*This table includes nutrients that the current *Dietary Reference Intakes* and related publications list for humans. Some disagreement exists over the essential nature of some minerals, and certain other minerals not listed. Fiber could be added to the list of essential substances, but it is not a nutrient (see Chapter 4). Alcohol is a source of calories but is not a nutrient per se.

†The lipids listed are needed only in small amounts, about 5 to 10% of total calorie needs (see Chapter 5).

‡To prevent ketosis and thus the muscle loss that would occur if protein were used to synthesize carbohydrate (see Chapter 4).

§Sunshine on the skin also allows the body to make vitamin D for itself (see Chapter 8).

ǁPrimarily for dental health (see Chapter 9).

provide calories for the body—on average, 4 kcal per gram. Typically, however, the body uses little protein for the purpose of meeting daily calorie needs. Proteins are formed by bonding together **amino acids.** Twenty or so common amino acids are found in food; nine of these are essential nutrients for adults, and one additional amino acid is essential for infants.

Most North Americans eat about one and a half to two times as much protein as the body needs to maintain health. In a healthy person (i.e., no evidence of cardio-vascular disease, kidney disease, diabetes or family history of colon cancer or kidney stones), this amount of extra protein in the diet is generally not harmful—it simply reflects the standard of living and the dietary habits of most North Americans. The excess is used for calorie needs or ultimately contributes to storage of fat or carbohydrate. Chapter 6 focuses on proteins.

amino acid The building block for proteins containing a central carbon atom with nitrogen and other atoms attached.

chemical reaction An interaction between two chemicals that changes both chemicals.

organic Any substance that contains carbon atoms bonded to hydrogen atoms in the chemical structure.

inorganic Any substance lacking carbon atoms bonded to hydrogen atoms in the chemical structure.

electrolytes Substances that separate into ions in water and, in turn, are able to conduct an electrical current. These include sodium, chloride, and potassium.

solvent A liquid substance in which other substances dissolve.

metabolism Chemical processes in the body by which energy is provided in useful forms and vital activities are sustained.

Critical Thinking

Believing that supplements provide the nutrition her body needs, Janice regularly takes numerous supplements while paying relatively little attention to daily food choices. How would you explain to her that this practice may lead to health problems?

For suggested answers to the Critical Thinking questions in this and every chapter, refer to the Online Learning Center at www.mhhe.com/wardlawcont6.

■ Vitamins

Vitamins exhibit a wide variety of chemical structures and can contain the elements carbon, hydrogen, nitrogen, oxygen, phosphorus, sulfur, and others. The main function of vitamins is to enable many **chemical reactions** to occur in the body. Some of these reactions help release the energy trapped in carbohydrates, lipids, and proteins. Remember, however, that vitamins themselves provide no usable calories for the body.

The 13 vitamins are divided into two groups: four are **fat-soluble** in that they dissolve in fat (vitamins A, D, E, and K); nine are **water-soluble** in that they dissolve in water (vitamin C and the B vitamins). The two groups of vitamins often act quite differently. For example, cooking destroys water-soluble vitamins much more readily than it does fat-soluble vitamins. Water-soluble vitamins are also excreted from the body much more readily than are fat-soluble vitamins. Thus, the fat-soluble vitamins, especially vitamin A, are much more likely to accumulate in excessive amounts in the body, which then can lead to toxicity. Vitamins are the focus of Chapter 8.

■ Minerals

All of the nutrients discussed so far are **organic** compounds, whereas minerals are structurally very simple, **inorganic** substances, which exist as groups of one or more of the same atoms. These terms, *organic* and *inorganic*, have nothing to do with agriculture but are based on simple chemistry concepts (see Chapter 2 for use of the term organic on food labels). Inorganic substances for the most part do not contain carbon atoms.

Minerals typically function independently in the body (Na^+, K^+), or as parts of simple mineral combinations, such as bone mineral [$Ca_{10}(PO_4)_6 OH_2$]. Because of their simple structure, minerals are not destroyed during cooking, but they can still be lost if they leach into the water used for cooking and that water is then discarded. Although minerals themselves yield no calories as such for the body, they are critical players in nervous system functioning, other cellular processes, water balance, and structural (e.g., skeletal) systems.

The amounts of the 16 or more essential minerals that are required in the diet for good health vary enormously. Thus, they are divided into two groups: **major minerals** and **trace minerals,** based on dietary needs. If daily needs are less than 100 milligrams, the mineral is classified as a trace mineral, otherwise, it is a major mineral. The actual dietary requirement for some trace minerals has yet to be determined. Minerals that conduct electricity when dissolved in water are also called **electrolytes;** these include sodium, potassium, and chloride. Minerals are the focus of Chapter 9.

■ Water

Water is the sixth class of nutrients. Although sometimes overlooked as a nutrient, water (chemically, H_2O) has numerous vital functions in the body. It acts as a **solvent** and lubricant, as a vehicle for transporting nutrients and waste, and as a medium for temperature regulation and chemical processes. For these reasons, and because the human body is approximately 60% water, the average man should consume about 3 liters—equivalent to 3000 grams or about 13 cups—of water and/or other fluids containing water every day. Women need closer to 2200 grams or about 9 cups per day.

Water is not only available from the obvious sources, but it is also the major component in some foods, such as many fruits and vegetables (e.g., lettuce, grapes, and melons). The body even makes some water as a by-product of **metabolism.** Water is examined in detail in Chapter 9.

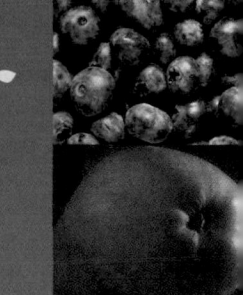
Y ou will use a few mathematical concepts in studying nutrition. Besides performing addition, subtraction, multiplication, and division, you need to know how to calculate percentages and convert English units of measurement to metric units.

Percentages

The term *percent* (%) refers to a part of the total when the total represents 100 parts. For example, if you earn 80% on your first nutrition examination, you will have answered the equivalent of 80 out of 100 questions correctly. This equivalent could be 8 correct answers out of 10; 80% also describes 16 of 20 (16/20 = 0.80 or 80%). The decimal form of percents is based on 100% being equal to 1.00. The best way to master this concept is to calculate some percentages. Some examples follow:

Question	Answer
What is 6% of 45?	6% = 0.06 0.06 × 45 = 2.7
What is 32% of 8?	32% = 0.32 0.32 × 8 = 2.6
What percent of 16 is 6?	$\frac{6}{16}$ = 0.375 or 37.5% (0.375 × 100)
What percent of 99 is 3?	$\frac{3}{99}$ = 0.03 or 3% (0.03 × 100)

Joe ate 15% of the adult Recommended Dietary Allowance (RDA) for iron at lunch. How many milligrams did he eat? (RDA = 8 milligrams)

$$0.15 \times 8 \text{ milligrams} = 1.2 \text{ milligrams}$$

It is difficult to succeed in a nutrition course unless you know what a percentage means and how to calculate one. Percentages are used frequently when referring to menus and nutrient composition.

The Metric System

The basic units of the metric system are the meter, which indicates length; the gram, which indicates weight; and the liter, which indicates volume. Appendix I in this textbook lists conversions from the metric system to the English system (pounds, feet, cups) and vice versa. Here is a brief summary:

One **meter** (m) is 39.4 inches long, or about 3 inches longer than 1 yard (3 feet).
A meter can be divided into 100 units of centimeters, or into 1000 units of millimeters.
A millimeter (mm) is about the thickness of a dime.
There are 2.54 centimeters (cm) in 1 inch and about 30 centimeters in 1 foot.
A person 6 feet tall is equivalent to 183 centimeters tall.

A gram (g) is about 1/30 of an ounce (28 grams to the ounce).
5 grams of sugar or salt is about 1 teaspoon.
A pound (lb) weighs 454 grams.
A kilogram (kg) is 1000 grams, equivalent to 2.2 pounds.
To convert your weight to kilograms, divide it by 2.2.
A 154-pound man weighs 70 kilograms (154/2.2 = 70).
A gram can be divided into 1000 milligrams (mg) or 1,000,000 micrograms (µg or mcg).
10 milligrams of zinc (approximately adult needs) would be a few grains of zinc.

Liters are divided into 1000 units called milliliters (ml).
One teaspoon equals about 5 milliliters (ml), 1 cup is about 240 milliliters, and 1 quart
(4 cups) equals almost 1 liter (L) (0.946 liter to be exact).

If you plan to work in any scientific field, you will need to learn the metric system. **For now, remember that a kilogram equals 2.2 pounds, an ounce weighs 28 grams, 2.54 centimeters equals 1 inch, and a liter is almost the same as a quart.** In addition, know what the prefixes micro (1/1,000,000), milli (1/1000), centi (1/100), and kilo (1000) represent.

▮ Household Units

Common household units are listed below with their metric equivalents. Note that ounces and fluid ounces differ. Ounces are a measure of weight, while fluid ounces are a measure of volume. Fluid ounces are based on the corresponding volume of water as the standard; 1 ounce of water by weight equals one fluid ounce. Any fluid that is more or less dense than water will yield a different number of fluid ounces per ounce of material.

3 teaspoons	= 1 tablespoon	= 15 grams
4 tablespoons	= ¼ cup	= 60 grams
5⅓ tablespoons	= ⅓ cup	= 80 grams
8 tablespoons	= ½ cup	= 120 grams
10⅔ tablespoons	= ⅔ cup	= 160 grams
16 tablespoons	= 1 cup	= 240 grams
1 tablespoon	= ½ fluid ounce	= 15 milliliters
1 cup	= 8 fluid ounces	= 240 milliliters
1 cup	= ½ pint	= 240 grams
2 cups	= 1 pint	= 480 grams
4 cups	= 1 quart	= 960 grams
2 pints	= 1 quart	= 960 grams
4 quarts	= 1 gallon	= 3840 grams

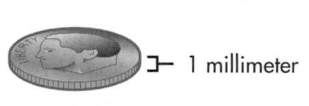
2 centimeters
or about 1 inch

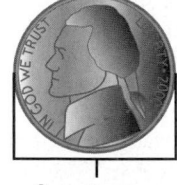
1 millimeter

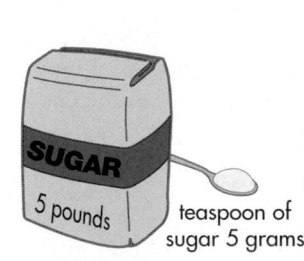
teaspoon of
sugar 5 grams

2 kilograms

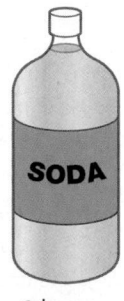
2 liters or
about 8 cups

Nutrient Composition of Diets and the Human Body

The quantities of the various nutrients that people consume vary widely, and the nutrient amounts present in different foods also vary a great deal. The total daily intake of protein, fat, and carbohydrate amounts to about 500 grams (about 1 pound). In contrast, the typical daily mineral intake totals about 20 grams (about 4 teaspoons), and the daily vitamin intake totals less than 300 milligrams (1/15 of a teaspoon). Although each day we require a gram or so of some minerals, such as calcium and phosphorus, we need only a few milligrams or less of other minerals. For example, we need about 10 milligrams of zinc per day, which is just a few specks of the mineral.

Figure 1-2 contrasts the relative proportions of all the major classes of nutrients in a lean man and a lean woman with the proportions of these nutrients in both a cooked steak and french fries. Note how the nutrient composition of the human body differs from the nutritional profiles of the foods we eat. This is because growth, development, and later maintenance of the human body are directed by the genetic material (DNA) inside body cells. This genetic blueprint determines how each cell uses the essential nutrients to perform body functions. These nutrients can come from a variety of sources. Cells are not concerned about whether available amino acids come from animal or plant sources. The carbohydrate glucose can come from sugars or starches. Thus, you really aren't what you eat. Rather, the food that you eat provides cells with basic materials to function according to the directions supplied by the genetic material (**genes**) housed in body cells (see the Looking Further feature in Chapter 3).

genes A specific segment on a chromosome. Genes provide the blueprints for the production of cell proteins.

alcohol Ethyl alcohol or ethanol (CH_3CH_2OH).

compound A group of different types of atoms bonded together in definite proportion.

ion An atom with an unequal number of electrons and protons. Negative ions have more electrons than protons; positive ions have more protons than electrons.

Energy Sources and Uses

Humans obtain the energy we need to perform body functions and do work from various calorie sources: carbohydrates, fats, and proteins. Foods generally provide more than one calorie source. Plant oils are one exception; these are 100% fat.

Alcohol is also a source of calories for some of us, supplying about 7 kcal per gram. It is not considered an essential nutrient, however, because it has no required function. Still, alcoholic beverages, such as beer—generally also rich in carbohydrate—are a contributor of calories to the diet of many adults.

The body transforms the energy trapped in carbohydrate, protein, and fat (and alcohol) into other forms of energy in order to:

- Build new **compounds.**
- Perform muscular movements.
- Promote nerve transmissions.
- Maintain **ion** balance within cells.

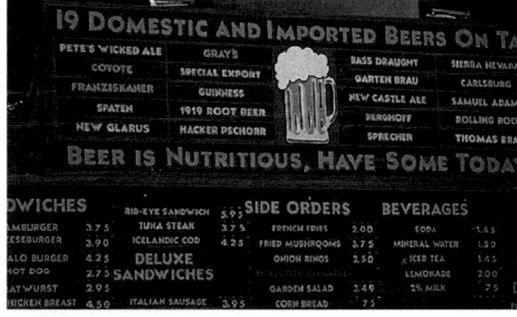

Alcoholic beverages are calorie-rich, but alcohol is not a nutrient per se.

Composition (percent of weight)				
Nutrient	French fries	Steak	Healthy man	Healthy woman
Carbohydrate	37%	0%	<1%	<1%
Protein	4%	27%	16%	13%
Fat	17%	18%	16%	25%
Minerals	1%	1%	6%	5%
Water	41%	54%	62%	57%

Figure 1-2 You aren't what you eat. The proportions of nutrients in the healthy human body compared to those found in typical foods—animal or vegetable. Note that the amount of vitamins found in the body is negligible.

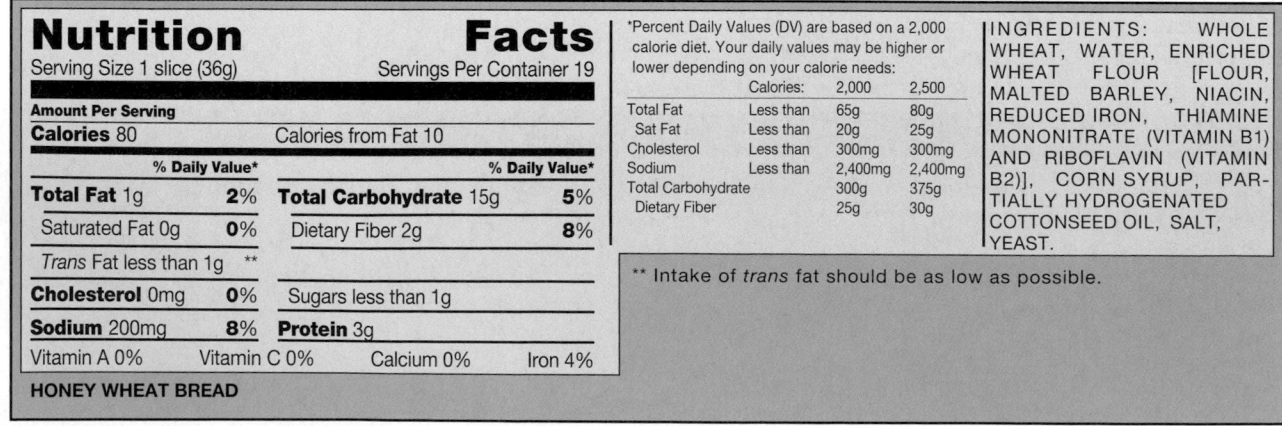

Chapter 11 describes how that energy is released from the chemical bonds in energy-yielding nutrients and then used by body cells to support the processes just described.

You have likely noticed on food labels that the energy in food is often expressed in terms of calories. As defined earlier, a calorie is the amount of heat energy it takes to raise the temperature of 1 gram of water 1 degree **Celsius** (1 °C, centigrade scale). (Chapter 10 has a diagram of the instrument that can be used to measure calories in foods [bomb calorimeter].) Because a calorie is such a tiny measure of heat, food energy is more accurately expressed in terms of the kilocalorie (kcal), which equals 1000 calories. (If the "c" in calories is capitalized, this also signifies kilocalories.) A kcal is the amount of heat energy it takes to raise the temperature of 1000 grams (1 liter) of water 1 °C. The abbreviation *kcal* is used throughout this book. On food labels, the word *calorie* (without a capital "C") is also used loosely to mean *kilocalorie*. Any values given on food labels in calories are actually in kilocalories (Fig. 1-3). A suggested intake of 2000 calories per day on a food label is really 2000 kcal.

Carbohydrate
4 kcal per gram

Protein
4 kcal per gram

Energy sources for body functions

Alcohol
7 kcal per gram

Fat
9 kcal per gram

Another Bite

Use the 4-9-4 estimates for the calorie content of carbohydrate, fat, and protein introduced over the last few pages to determine calorie content of a food. Consider a typical deluxe hamburger sandwich:

Carbohydrate	39 grams × 4 = 156 kcal
Fat	32 grams × 9 = 288 kcal
Protein	30 grams × 4 = 120 kcal
Total	564 kcal

You can also use the 4-9-4 estimates to determine what portion of total calorie intake is contributed by the various calorie-yielding nutrients. Assume that one day you consume 290 grams of carbohydrates, 60 grams of fat, and 70 grams of protein. This consumption yields a total of 1980 kcal ([290 × 4] + [60 × 9] + [70 × 4] 5 = 1980). The percentage of your total calorie intake derived from each nutrient can then be determined:

$$\% \text{ of kcal as carbohydrate} = (290 \times 4) \div 1980 = 0.59 \ (\times 100 = 59\%)$$
$$\% \text{ of kcal as fat} = (60 \times 9) \div 1980 = 0.27 \ (\times 100 = 27\%)$$
$$\% \text{ of kcal as protein} = (70 \times 4) \div 1980 = 0.14 \ (\times 100 = 14\%)$$

Check your calculations by adding the percentages together. Do they total 100?

Nutrition Facts

Serving Size 1 slice (36g)   Servings Per Container 19

Amount Per Serving

Calories 80   Calories from Fat 10

	% Daily Value*			% Daily Value*
Total Fat 1g	**2%**	**Total Carbohydrate** 15g		**5%**
Saturated Fat 0g	**0%**	Dietary Fiber 2g		**8%**
Trans Fat less than 1g	**			
Cholesterol 0mg	**0%**	Sugars less than 1g		
Sodium 200mg	**8%**	**Protein** 3g		
Vitamin A 0%	Vitamin C 0%	Calcium 0%		Iron 4%

HONEY WHEAT BREAD

*Percent Daily Values (DV) are based on a 2,000 calorie diet. Your daily values may be higher or lower depending on your calorie needs:

	Calories:	2,000	2,500
Total Fat	Less than	65g	80g
Sat Fat	Less than	20g	25g
Cholesterol	Less than	300mg	300mg
Sodium	Less than	2,400mg	2,400mg
Total Carbohydrate		300g	375g
Dietary Fiber		25g	30g

INGREDIENTS: WHOLE WHEAT, WATER, ENRICHED WHEAT FLOUR [FLOUR, MALTED BARLEY, NIACIN, REDUCED IRON, THIAMINE MONONITRATE (VITAMIN B1) AND RIBOFLAVIN (VITAMIN B2)], CORN SYRUP, PARTIALLY HYDROGENATED COTTONSEED OIL, SALT, YEAST.

** Intake of *trans* fat should be as low as possible.

Figure 1-3 Use the nutrient values on the Nutrition Facts label to calculate calorie content of a food. Based on carbohydrate, fat, and protein content, a serving of this food (Honey Wheat Bread) contains 81 kcal ([15 × 4] + [1 × 9] + [3 × 4] = 81). The label lists 80, suggesting that the calorie value was rounded down.

Concept Check

Nutrition is the study of food and nutrients—their digestion, absorption, and metabolism, and their effect on health and disease. Food contains the vital nutrients that are essential for good health: carbohydrates, lipids (fats and oils), proteins, vitamins, minerals, and water. Nutrients have three general functions in the body: (1) to provide materials for building and maintaining the body; (2) to act as regulators for key metabolic reactions; and (3) to participate in metabolic reactions that provide the energy necessary to sustain life. A common unit of measurement for this energy is the kilocalorie (kcal). On average, carbohydrates and protein provide 4 kcal per gram of energy to the body, while lipids provide 9 kcal per gram. Although not considered a nutrient, alcohol provides about 7 kcal per gram. The other classes of nutrients do not supply calories but are essential for proper body functioning.

In the fifth century B.C., Hippocrates said "Let food be your medicine and medicine be your food."

Current State of the North American Diet and Overall Health

If we ignore alcohol, North American adults consume about 16% of their calorie intake as proteins, 50% as carbohydrates, and 33% as fats. These percentages are estimates and vary slightly from year to year and from person to person. This pattern falls within the 10% to 35%, 45% to 65%, and 20% to 35% distribution of calories from protein, carbohydrate, and fat, respectively, advocated in the latest advice from the Food and Nutrition Board of the National Academy of Sciences. (Note that these standards apply to both people in the United States and Canada.) Note also that recommendations for different distributions of calorie intake among protein, carbohydrate, and fat come and go in the popular press.

Animal sources supply about two-thirds of protein intake for most North Americans; plant sources supply only about one-third. In many other parts of the world, it is just the opposite: plant proteins—from rice, beans, corn, and other vegetables—dominate protein intake. About half the carbohydrate in North American diets comes from simple sugars; the other half comes from starches (such as in pastas, breads, and potatoes). About 60% of dietary fat comes from animal sources and 40% from plant sources.

The Food and Nutrition Board of the National Academy of Sciences also suggests minimizing saturated fat, *trans* fat, and cholesterol intake when putting their diet guidelines into place (see Chapter 5).

■ Assessing the Current North American Diet

With the aim of finding out what and when North Americans eat, federal agencies collect data about food and nutrient consumption, as well as connections between diet and health, through survey-based programs. In the United States, the U.S. Department of Health and Human Services monitors food consumption with the National Health and Nutrition Examination Survey (NHANES). In Canada, this information is gathered by Health Canada in conjunction with Agriculture and Agrifood Canada.

Results from national nutrition surveys and other studies show that North Americans consume a wide variety of foods, but often do not choose the right balance of foods to meet their nutrient needs. Chapter 2 will look at this situation in more detail. For now, note that more attention should be focused on foods that are rich in iron, calcium, potassium, magnesium, various B vitamins, vitamin C (especially smokers), vitamin D, vitamin E, and fiber. Daily intake of a balanced multivitamin and mineral supplement is one strategy to help meet nutrient needs, but does not make up for a poor diet in all respects. Also keep in mind that taking numerous dietary supplements can lead to health problems (see Chapter 8).

Routinely, experts also recommend that we pay more attention to balancing calorie intake with needs. An excess intake of calories is usually tied to overindulgence in

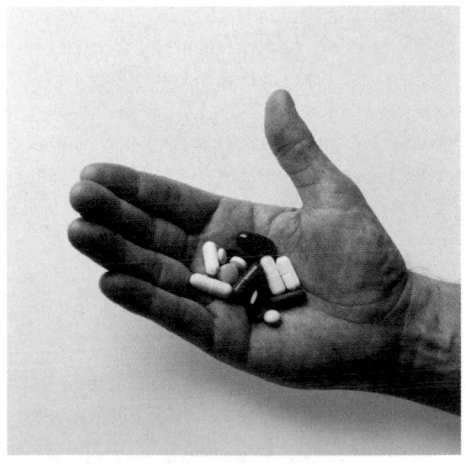

Taking numerous nutrient supplements can lead to health problems.

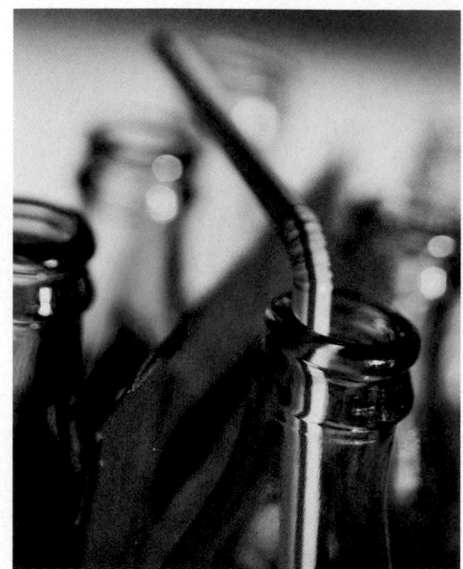

Today, soft drinks are more popular than milk, but not as beneficial to the diet. Soft drinks account for about 10% of the calorie intake of teenagers in North America, and in turn contribute to generally poor calcium intakes seen in this age group.

C urrently, the most agreed-upon measure of a healthy weight is **body mass index (BMI)**. This should range from 18.5 to 24.9, with a waist circumference of no more than 35 inches (88 centimeters) in women and 40 inches (102 centimeters) in men. Body mass index is based on a person's weight (in kilograms) divided by height (in meters) squared. Use Table 10-1 in Chapter 10 to determine your body mass index.

sugar, fat, and alcoholic beverages. African-Americans and Hispanics in particular may need to take notice of the amount of **salt** (sodium chloride) and alcohol in their diets. This is because they have a greater chance of developing hypertension than do other ethnic groups in North America, and these substances are two of the many factors linked to that health problem. Actually, a careful look at salt and alcohol intake— along with saturated fat, *trans* fat, cholesterol, and total calorie intake—is a recommended practice for all adults.

Many North Americans would benefit from a healthier balance of food in their diets. Moderation is the key for some foods, such as sugared soft drinks and fried foods. For other foods, such as fruits and vegetables, increased variety is warranted. Few adults currently meet the "5-a-day" minimum recommendation promoted for total servings of vegetables and fruits.

■ Health Objectives for the United States for the Year 2010 Include Numerous Nutrition Objectives

Health promotion and disease prevention have been public health strategies in North America since the late 1970s. One part of this strategy is *Healthy People 2010*, a report issued in 2000 by the U.S. Department of Health and Human Services' Public Health Service. This report outlines health promotion and disease prevention objectives for the nation for the year 2010 and assigns each of the objectives to appropriate U.S. federal agencies to address. Many nutrition-related objectives are part of the overall plan (Table 1-5). The main objectives of *Healthy People 2010* are to promote healthful lifestyles and to reduce preventable death and disability. The following Internet site provides more details on the *Healthy People* program: www.health.gov/healthypeople.

Another way to promote your health and prevent chronic diseases in the future is to observe the recommendations listed in Table 1-6. In total, these contribute to maximal health and prevention of disease.

Table 1-5 A Sample of Nutrition-Related Objectives from *Healthy People 2010*

	Target	Current Estimate
Increase the proportion of adults who are at a healthy weight.	60%	35%
Reduce the proportion of children and adolescents who are overweight or obese.	5%	10%
Increase the proportion of persons age 2 years and older who consume:		
• At least 2 daily servings of fruit.	75%	28%
• At least 3 daily servings of vegetables, with at least one-third being dark green or deep yellow vegetables.	50%	3%
• At least 6 daily servings of grain products, with at least 3 being whole grains (e.g., whole wheat bread and oatmeal).	50%	7%
• Less than 10% of calories from saturated fat.	75%	36%
• Six grams or less of salt (2400 milligrams or less of sodium) daily.	65%	5%
• Enough calcium (see inside cover of this book).	75%	46%
Reduce iron deficiency among young children and females of childbearing age.	6%	10%

Note: In later chapters, we will explore additional nutrition-related objectives, such as those addressing osteoporosis, various forms of cancer, diabetes prevention and treatment, food allergies, cardiovascular disease, low birth weight, nutrition during pregnancy, breastfeeding, eating disorders, physical activity, and alcohol use.

Table 1-6 Recommendations for Health Promotion and Disease Prevention: What Can Adults Expect from Adequate Nutrition and Good Health Habits?

Diet

Consuming enough essential nutrients, including a variety of fruits and vegetables, while moderating calorie, saturated fat, *trans* fat, cholesterol, and alcohol (if used) intake can result in:

Improvements in:
- Body weight
- Bone density
- Digestion
- Eye health
- Dental health

Reduced Risk of:
- Cardiovascular diseases
- Type 2 diabetes
- Some types of cancer
- Osteoporosis
- Micronutrient deficiencies

Physical Activity

Adequate, regular physical activity (60 minutes or more on most days of the week is optimal, but any amount is beneficial) can result in:

Improvements in:
- Body weight
- Bone density
- Muscle tone
- Flexibility
- Stamina

Reduced Risk of:
- Cardiovascular diseases
- Type 2 diabetes
- Colon and breast cancers
- Osteoporosis
- Premature aging

Lifestyle

Limiting alcohol intake (no more than two drinks per day for men and one drink per day for women and adults of both sexes over the age of 65) can result in:

Improvements in:
- Nutrient intake

Reduced Risk of:
- Accidents
- Liver disease

Never starting/cessation of use of cigarettes, cigars, or other types of tobacco can result in:

Improvements in:
- Oral health
- Sense of taste
- Sense of smell
- Pregnancy outcome

Reduced Risk of:
- Lung cancer/lung diseases
- Kidney disease
- Cardiovascular diseases
- Degenerative eye disease

In addition, minimum use of medication, no illicit drug use, adequate sleep (7 to 8 hours), adequate water and related fluid intake (about 9 (women) or 13 (men) cups per day), and a reduction in stress (practice better time management, meditate, relax, listen to music, have a massage, and stay physically active) provide a more complete approach to good nutrition and health. Add to this maintaining close relationships with others and a positive outlook on life. Finally, consultation with health care professionals on a regular basis is important. This is because early diagnosis is especially useful for controlling the damaging effects of many diseases. Overall, prevention of disease is an important investment of one's time, including during college years.

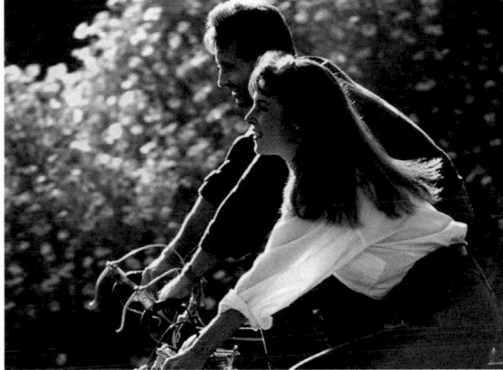

Regular physical activity complements a healthy diet. Whether it's all at once or in segments throughout the day, ideally incorporate 30 to 60 minutes or more of such activity into your daily routine.

Concept Check

Surveys in the United States and Canada show that we generally have a variety of foods available to us. However, some of us could improve our diets by focusing on rich food sources of various vitamins, minerals, and fiber. In addition, many of us should reduce our consumption of calories, sugar, protein, saturated fat, *trans* fat cholesterol, salt, and alcoholic beverages. These recommendations are consistent with an overall goal to attain and maintain good health.

hunger The primarily physiological (internal) drive to find and eat food, mostly regulated by innate cues to eating.

appetite The primarily psychological (external) influences that encourage us to find and eat food, often in the absence of obvious hunger.

satiety State in which there is no longer a desire to eat; a feeling of satisfaction.

Why Am I So Hungry?

Understanding what drives us to eat and what affects food choice will help put your study of nutrition into greater focus. This especially helps you understand the complexity of factors that influence eating, especially the effects of ethnicity and societal change. You can then see why foods may have different meanings to different people. In turn, this allows for greater appreciation of food habits that differ from yours.

Two drives, **hunger** and **appetite,** influence our desire to eat. These differ dramatically. Hunger our primarily physical biological drive to eat, is controlled by internal body mechanisms. For example, as nutrients are processed by the stomach and small intestine, these organs communicate with the liver and brain to reduce further food intake.

Appetite, our primarily psychological drive to eat, is affected by external food choice mechanisms, such as seeing a tempting dessert. Fulfilling either or both drives by eating sufficient food normally brings a state of **satiety,** temporarily halting our desire to continue eating.

∎ The Hypothalamus Contributes to Satiety

The **hypothalamus,** a region of the brain, helps regulate satiety (Fig. 1-4). Imagine a game of tug-of-war in the brain: two sites in the hypothalamus—the *feeding center* and the *satiety center*—work opposite each other to promote adequate availability of nutrients at all times. When stimulated, cells in the feeding center of the hypothalamus signal us to eat. As we eat, cells in the satiety center are stimulated, and we stop eating.

What stimulates these two centers of the hypothalamus? The amounts of macronutrients in the blood probably stimulate both the satiety and feeding centers. For example, when we haven't eaten for a while, stimulation of the feeding center causes us to eat. When the macronutrient content in the blood rises after a meal, we no longer have a strong desire to seek food. (Exactly how the two are interrelated is under study.) Certain chemicals, surgery, and some cancers can destroy either center in the hypothalamus. Without satiety center activity, laboratory animals (and humans) eat their way to obesity. Without feeding center activity, the opposite happens and weight is lost.

Admittedly, this concept of a tug-of-war between the feeding and satiety centers is an oversimplification of a very complex process. Overall, the entire system depends on the hypothalamus to process the signals generated by nerves throughout the body that are influenced in various ways by recent food intake. In reality, the hypothalamus has numerous sites crisscrossed with a network of nerves that are constantly receiving and passing on information about the body's nutritional state.

∎ Meal Size and Composition Affect Satiety

The effects of stomach expansion from food intake combined with the later intestinal absorption of nutrients during a meal likely reduce our desire to eat more food. These actions of the **gastrointestinal (GI) tract** contribute to a feeling of satiety. In fact, a meal is generally terminated before significant amounts of nutrients are made available for metabolism and storage. Putting this information into practice, researchers have recently shown that bulky meals (high in fiber and water) produce much more satiety than do more concentrated meals. As the fiber and water content of the foods increase, humans experience increased satiety and thus do not seek another meal as quickly. Consider how you would feel if you ate five pieces of whole fruit versus a small serving of French fries (each yielding about 380 kcals).

(a) Hypothalamus

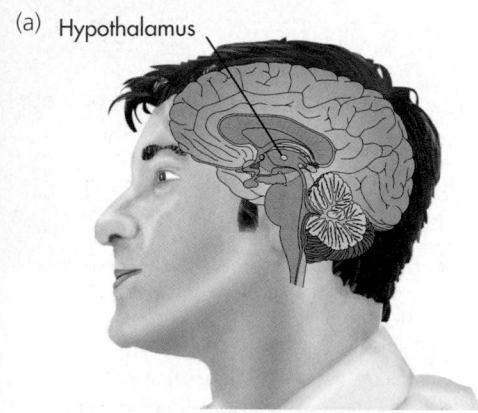

(b)

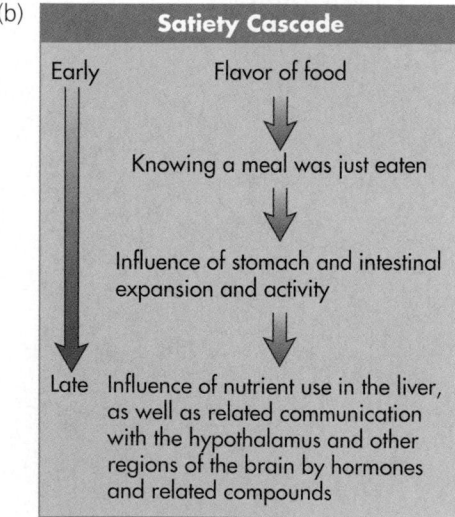

Figure 1-4 The hypothalamus and satiety. (a) The hypothalamus is one important region in the brain that influences whether we eat or not. (b) The process of satiety starts with eating food and concludes with actions in the hypothalamus and other regions in the brain.

■ Hormones Affect Satiety

Hormones and hormone-like compounds in our body influence whether we eat or not. Those that increase hunger include **endorphins, ghrelin,** and **neuropeptide Y.** Those that cause satiety include **leptin** (working in conjunction with the hormone insulin), **serotonin,** and **cholecystokinin (CCK).** Research is underway to produce weight control medications that will increase the action of satiety-inducing hormones or block the action of hunger-related hormones. Initially, researchers were hopeful that the use of leptin would curb hunger and lead to weight loss. However, the excitement about leptin has waned since clinical trials have not supported its general usefulness. This is likely because researchers have found leptin primarily works to prevent weight loss, rather than to prevent weight gain. Low amounts of leptin in the brain signal a low amount of body fat, and hunger is stimulated in response. In contrast, high amounts of leptin do not appear to contribute to a feeling of satiety.

■ Does Appetite Affect What We Eat?

Various feeding and satiety messages from body cells do not single-handedly determine what we eat. Almost everyone has encountered a mouthwatering dessert and devoured it, even on a full stomach. Appetite can be affected by a great variety of external forces, such as environmental and psychological factors as well as social customs (Fig. 1-5).

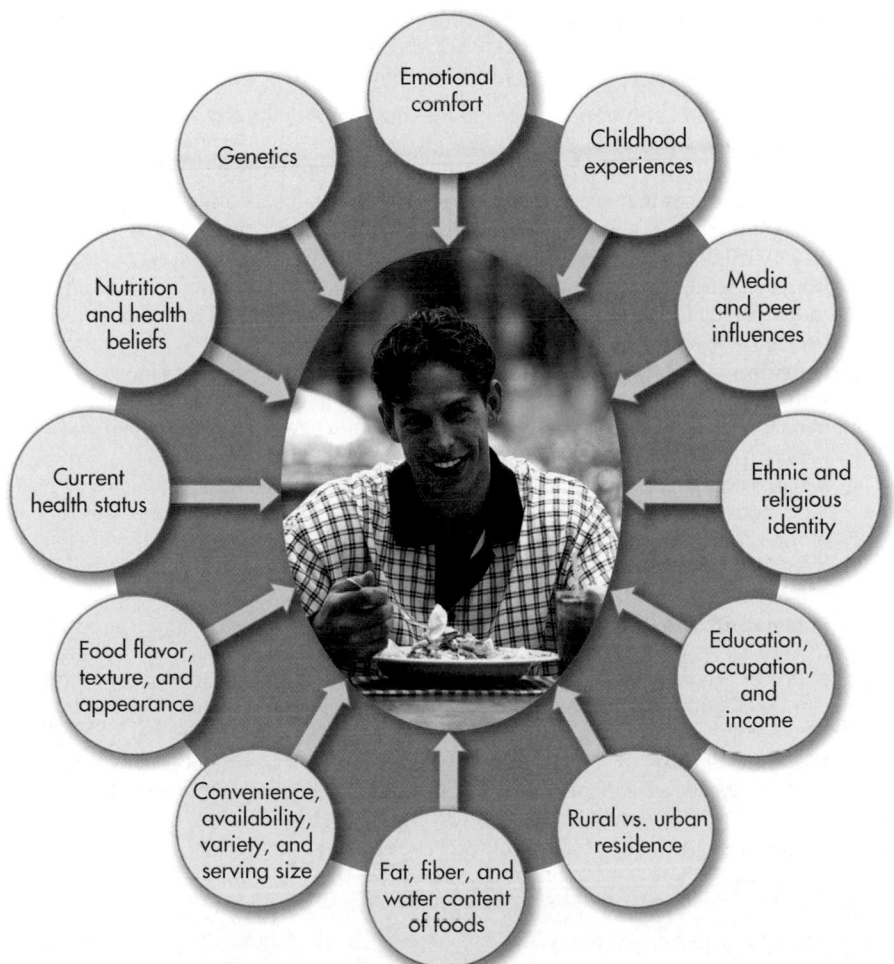

hypothalamus A region at the base of the brain that contains cells that play a role in the regulation of hunger, respiration, body temperature, and other body functions.

gastrointestinal (GI) tract The main sites in the body used for digestion and absorption of nutrients. It consists of the mouth, esophagus, stomach, small intestine, large intestine, rectum, and anus. Also called the digestive tract.

hormone A compound secreted into the bloodstream by one type of cells that acts to control the function of another type of cells. For example, certain cells in the pancreas produce insulin, which in turn acts on muscle and other types of cells to promote uptake of nutrients from the blood.

endorphins Natural body tranquilizers that may be involved in the feeding response.

ghrelin A hormone made by the stomach that increases the desire to eat.

neuropeptide Y A chemical substance made in the hypothalamus that stimulates food intake. The hormone leptin inhibits neuropeptide Y production.

leptin A hormone made by **adipose tissue** in proportion to total fat stores in the body that influences long-term regulation of fat mass. Leptin also influences reproductive functions, as well as other body processes, such as release of the hormone insulin.

adipose tissue A group of fat storing cells.

serotonin A neurotransmitter synthesized from the amino acid tryptophan that affects mood (sense of calmness), behavior, and appetite, and induces sleep.

cholecystokinin (CCK) A hormone that participates in enzyme release from the pancreas, bile release from the gallbladder, and hunger regulation.

Figure 1-5 Food behavior is influenced by many sources. Which are important in your life?

Scientists suspect we are born with a taste for sweets and over time acquire a taste for fat.

We often eat because food confronts us. It smells good, tastes good, and looks good. We might eat because it is the right time of day, we are celebrating, or we are seeking emotional comfort to overcome the blues. After a meal, memories of pleasant tastes and feelings reinforce appetite. If stress or depression sends you to the refrigerator, you are mostly seeking comfort, not food calories. Appetite may not be a biological process, but it does influence food intake. Table 1-7 lists additional social and other related factors that influence food choices.

Another Bite

Satiety associated with consuming a meal may actually reside primarily in our psychological frame of mind. We become accustomed to a certain amount of food at a meal. Providing less than that amount leaves us wanting more. One way to put this observation into practice for weight-control purposes is to train the eye to expect less food by slowly decreasing serving sizes to more appropriate amounts (see Figure 2-5 in Chapter 2 for some examples). Our appetites then readjust as we expect less food.

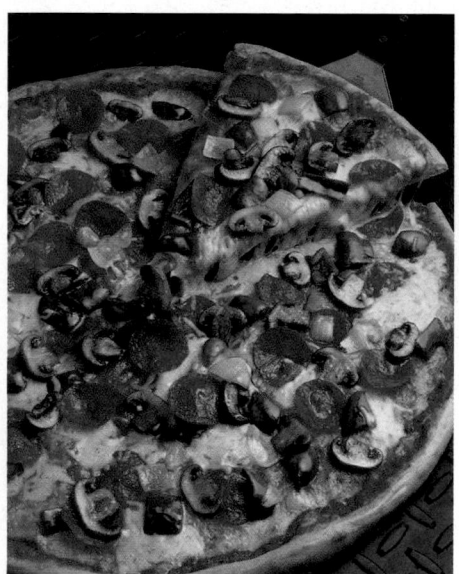

A market research firm surveyed the eating habits of people in 2000 United States households. The top meal choice was pizza, followed by ham sandwich, hot dog, peanut butter and jelly sandwich, steak, macaroni and cheese, turkey sandwich, cheese sandwich, hamburger on a bun, and spaghetti.

Table 1-7 What Else Influences Our Food Choices?

Food means so much more to us than simply nourishment—it reflects much of what we think about ourselves. In the course of our lives, we spend a total of 13 to 15 years eating. Beyond simple hunger and emotions, why do we choose what we eat?

- **Flavor, texture, and appearance** are the most important factors determining our food choices. Creating more flavorful foods that are both healthy and profitable is a major focus of the food industry (referred to as "better for you" products).
- **Early influences** that expose us to various people, places, and events have a continuing impact on our food choices. Many aspects of various ethnic diet patterns begin as we are introduced to foods during childhood.
- **Routines and habits** are tied to some food choices. Most of us eat from a core group of foods: About 100 basic items account for 75% of an individual's total food intake. Food habits, food availability, and convenience strongly influence choices.
- **Nutrition,** or what we think of as "healthy foods," directs our food purchases. North Americans who tend to make health-related food choices are often well-educated, middle-class professionals. These same people are generally health-oriented, have active lifestyles, and focus on weight control.
- **Advertising** is a major media tool for capturing the food interest of the consumer. The food industry in the United States alone spends well over $33 billion on advertising. Some of this advertising is helpful, as it promotes the importance of calcium and fiber in our diets. However, the food industry also advertises highly sweetened cereals, cookies, cakes, and soft drinks because they bring in the greatest profits.
- **Restaurants** have long been a growth industry in North America. Today, about 45% of all food dollars is spent on meals outside the home. This food is often very calorie-dense and of poorer nutritional quality compared to foods made at home. However, in response to consumer demands, restaurants have placed healthier items on their menus over the past ten years.
- **Social changes** are leading to a general time shortage for many of us. This creates the need for convenience. Supermarkets now supply already-prepared meals, microwave entrees, and various quick-prep frozen products.
- **Economics** play a minor role in our food choices. The average North American spends only about 12% of after-tax income on food (will be greater for low-income people). However, as income increases, so do meals eaten away from home.

Overall, daily food intake is a complicated mix of social and biological influences. The first Rate Your Plate activity in Chapter 1 asks you to keep track of what influences your food intake on a daily basis. This assessment is an important part of developing a plan to improve your diet as necessary. How do you compare to the typical North American?

■ Putting Hunger and Appetite into Perspective

The next time you pick up a candy bar or ask for second helpings, remember the physical influences on eating behavior. Body cells (brain, stomach, small intestine, liver, and other organs), macronutrients in the blood, hormones (like leptin and ghrelin), brain chemicals (like serotonin and neuropeptide Y), and social customs all influence food intake. When food is ample, appetite—not hunger—mostly triggers eating. Keep track of what triggers your eating for a few days. Is it primarily hunger or appetite? Note as well that satiety regulation is not perfect; body weight can fluctuate.

Concept Check

Hunger is the primarily physical or internal desire to find and eat food. Appeasing it creates satiety—no further desire to eat exists. Satiety is influenced by hunger-related (internal) forces in the brain, gastrointestinal tract, liver, and other organs, as well as fiber and water content of the foods in the meal. Various hormones and hormone-like compounds participate. Food intake is also affected by appetite-related (external) forces like social customs, time of day, flavor, appearance, texture, and being with others. Recently, factors such as health concerns, economics, convenience, seeking emotional comfort, and social changes are also becoming important dietary determinants. North Americans probably respond more to external, appetite-related forces than to hunger-related ones in choosing when and what to eat.

■ Improving Our Diets

While more efforts by the general public are needed to lower saturated fat, *trans* fat, and cholesterol intake and to improve variety in our diets, our cultural diversity, varied cuisines, and generally high nutritional status should be points of pride for North Americans. Today we can choose from a tremendous variety of food products, the result of continual innovation by food manufacturers.

We are eating more breakfast cereals, pizza, pasta entrees, stir-fried meats and vegetables served on rice, salads, tacos, burritos, and fajitas than ever before. Sales of whole milk are down, while in the same time period sales of fat-free and 1% low-fat milk have increased. Consumption of frozen vegetables, rather than canned vegetables, is also on the rise.

Another Bite

One recent trend by food manufacturers has been to promote meal replacement bars (also called "energy" bars). These bars typically contain about 180 to 250 kcal, with a protein:carbohydrate:fat ratio typical of common diets. However, some bars replace much of the carbohydrate with protein. All of the bars are fortified with vitamins and minerals in amounts ranging from about 25% to 100% of typical human needs. Some people find these bars provide a convenient way to consume a meal (or snack) on the run, while also focusing on certain nutrients they may underconsume, such as the B vitamin folate or the mineral calcium. These bars generally cost $1 to $2. Typical brands are Ensure® bar, Balance® bar, Gatorade® Energy bar, Slim-Fast® bar, Genisoy® bar, Luna™ bar, Cliff™ bar, PowerBar®, and Centrum® bar. Critics suggest these products are essentially just the nutritional equivalent of a low-fat yogurt and piece of fruit.

Critical Thinking

Sarah is majoring in nutrition and is well aware of the importance of a healthy diet. She has recently been analyzing her own diet and is confused. She notices that she eats a great deal of high-fat foods, and few fruits, vegetables, and whole grains. She also has developed quite a "sweet tooth." What three factors may be influencing Sarah's food choices? What advice would you give her on how to have her diet match her needs?

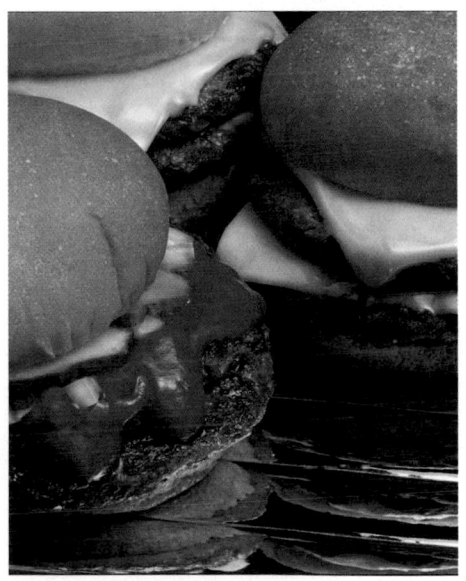

One trend in North America has been large serving sizes for foods, especially in restaurants. Consumers might see these as a bargain, but few need the extra calories supplied by the increased serving sizes. One option is to share the oversized portion with another person.

A dietary objective that deserves more attention is to try to eat with others more often. Mealtime is a key social time of the day. The Japanese are ahead of us in recognizing that food's powers go beyond the realm of nutrition. Their national dietary guidelines, which like ours stress the importance of eating a variety of foods, maintaining healthy weight, and moderating fat in the diet, also advise people to make all activities pertaining to food and eating pleasurable.

Today, North Americans live longer than ever before and enjoy better general health. Many also have more money and more diverse food and lifestyle choices to consider. The nutritional consequences of these trends are not fully known. Deaths from various forms of cardiovascular disease, for example, have dropped dramatically since the late 1960s, partly because of better medical care and diets. Still, if affluence leads to sedentary lifestyles and high intakes of saturated fat, *trans* fat, cholesterol, salt, and alcohol, this lifestyle pattern can lead to problems such as cardiovascular disease, hypertension, and obesity. Because of better technology and greater choices, we can have a much better diet today than ever before—if we know what choices to make.

The goal of this book is to help you find the best path to good nutrition. Nutrition experts generally agree that there are no "good" or "bad" (i.e., "junk") foods, but some foods provide relatively few nutrients in comparison to calorie content and thus contribute to fewer nutritious food behaviors. One's overall diet is the proper focus in a nutritional evaluation. Chapter 2 will emphasize this point and show you how to balance your diet. As you reexamine your nutritional habits, remember your health is largely your responsibility. Your body has a natural ability to heal itself. Offer it what it needs, and it will serve you well. In addition, eating a healthy diet is one way to affirm that you care about your health.

Confusing and conflicting health messages hinder diet change. Nutrition science does not have all the answers, but as you will see, enough is known to help you (1) set a path to good health and (2) put diet-related recommendations you hear in the future into perspective.

Concept Check

Healthy food habits developed and strengthened throughout life can provide many benefits. Many of us should pay more attention to this observation.

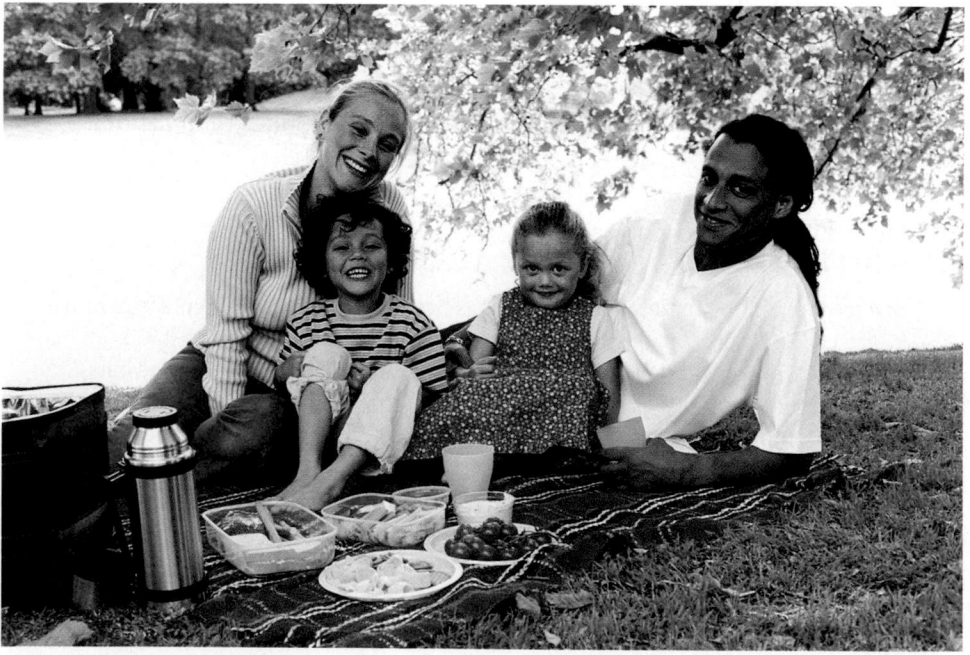

A healthy diet benefits people of all ages.

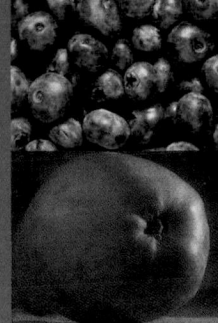
How do we know what we know about nutrition? How has this knowledge been gained? In a word, *research*. Like other sciences, the research that sets the foundation for nutrition knowledge has developed through the use of the *scientific method*, a testing procedure designed to detect and eliminate error. The first step is the observation of a natural phenomenon. Scientists then suggest possible explanations, called **hypotheses,** about its cause. Distinguishing a true cause-and-effect relationship from mere coincidence can be difficult. For instance, early in the past century, many patients in mental hospitals in the southern United States suffered from the disease **pellagra,** which suggested a possible relationship between the climate in that region (and, in particular, the mosquitoes that thrived in the climate) and this disease. In time, it became clear that this supposed connection was simply coincidental; the real culprit was the poor diet common to rural people at that time and a resulting vitamin deficiency.

To test hypotheses and eliminate coincidental explanations, scientists perform controlled scientific **experiments.** The data gathered from these experiments may either support or refute each hypothesis. If the results of many experiments support a hypothesis, the hypothesis becomes generally accepted by scientists and can be called a **theory** (such as the theory of gravity). Very often, the results from one experiment suggest a new set of questions to be answered (Fig. 1-6).

The scientific method requires a skeptical attitude. Scientists must not accept proposed hypotheses and theories until they are supported by considerable evidence, and they must reject those that fail to pass critical analysis. Likewise, students should adopt a healthy skepticism and be critical of many current ideas about nutrition.

A recent example of this need for skepticism involves stomach **ulcers.** Not so many years ago, "everyone knew" that stomach ulcers were caused by a stressful lifestyle and a poor diet. Then, in 1983, an Australian physician, Dr. Barry Marshall, reported in a respected medical journal that ulcers are usually caused by a common **microorganism** called *Helicobacter pylori*. Furthermore, he stated that a cure is possible using antibiotics. At first, other physicians were skeptical about this finding and continued to prescribe medications such as antacids that reduce stomach acid. But, as more studies were published demonstrating that patients using antibiotics were cured of ulcers, the medical profession eventually accepted the findings. Today, ulcers are managed for the most part by medications that destroy the microorganism. Overall, we can expect that sound scientific discoveries will always be subject to challenge and change.

In sum, you will see that sound scientific research requires that:

1. Questions are asked.
2. Hypotheses are generated to explain the phenomena.
3. Research is conducted (experiments).
4. Incorrect explanations are rejected.
5. The most likely explanation for an observation is proposed.
6. The research results are subjected to review by other scientists and published in a scientific journal.
7. The research results are confirmed by more experiments.

hypotheses Tentative explanations by a scientist to explain a phenomenon.

pellagra A deficiency disease characterized by inflammation of the skin, diarrhea, and eventual mental incapacity; results from an insufficient amount of the vitamin niacin in the diet.

experiments Tests made to examine the validity of a hypothesis.

theory An explanation for a phenomenon that has numerous lines of evidence to support it.

ulcer Erosion of the tissue lining, usually in the stomach (gastric ulcer) or the upper small intestine (duodenal ulcer). As a group these are generally referred to as peptic ulcers.

microorganism Bacteria, virus, or other organism that is invisible to the naked eye, some of which cause diseases. Also called *microbes.*

Asking Questions and Generating Hypotheses

Historical events have provided clues to important relationships in nutrition science. In the fifteenth and sixteenth centuries, for example, many European sailors on the long voyages to the Americas developed the disease scurvy. The sailors ate very few fruits and vegetables, and

scurvy The deficiency disease that results after a few weeks to months of consuming a diet that lacks vitamin C; pinpoint sites of bleeding on the skin are an early sign.

epidemiology The study of how disease rates vary among different population groups.

eventually a British naval surgeon, Dr. James Lind, discovered that lime juice prevented or cured **scurvy.** After this, sailors were given a ration of lime juice, earning them the nickname "limeys." This simple practice ensured a healthy workforce for the British navy and helped it dominate the seas worldwide. About 200 years later, scientists identified vitamin C, the nutrient present in the lime juice and other fruits and vegetables that prevents scurvy.

In a related approach to using historical observation, scientists establish nutritional hypotheses by studying the dietary and disease patterns among various populations in today's world. If one group tends to develop a certain disease but another group does not, scientists can speculate about the role diet plays in this difference. The study of diseases in populations is called **epidemiology,** and ultimately forms the basis for many laboratory studies.

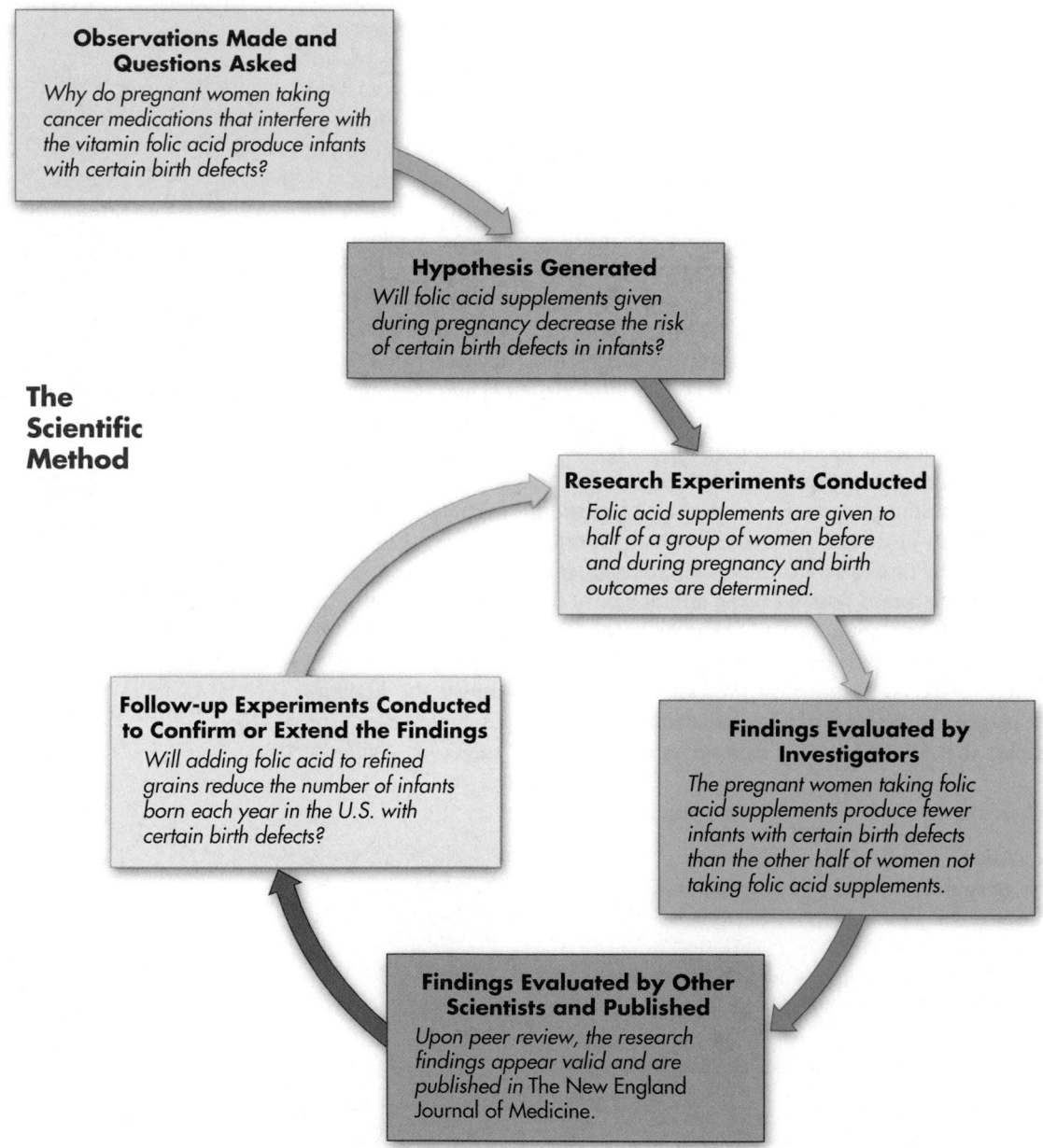

The Scientific Method

Observations Made and Questions Asked
Why do pregnant women taking cancer medications that interfere with the vitamin folic acid produce infants with certain birth defects?

Hypothesis Generated
Will folic acid supplements given during pregnancy decrease the risk of certain birth defects in infants?

Research Experiments Conducted
Folic acid supplements are given to half of a group of women before and during pregnancy and birth outcomes are determined.

Findings Evaluated by Investigators
The pregnant women taking folic acid supplements produce fewer infants with certain birth defects than the other half of women not taking folic acid supplements.

Findings Evaluated by Other Scientists and Published
Upon peer review, the research findings appear valid and are published in The New England Journal of Medicine.

Follow-up Experiments Conducted to Confirm or Extend the Findings
Will adding folic acid to refined grains reduce the number of infants born each year in the U.S. with certain birth defects?

Figure 1-6 Implementing the scientific method using the vitamin folic acid (part of a group of compounds referred to as folate) as an example. Scientists consistently follow these steps in conducting scientific research. It is important not to embrace a nutrition or other scientific concept until it has been thoroughly tested using the scientific method. Incidentally, the answer to the follow-up experiment question regarding folic acid was *yes* (see Chapter 8 for details).

In the 1920s, an observation by an American physician exemplified the epidemiological approach. Dr. Joseph Goldberger noticed that inmates in mental hospitals suffered from the disease pellagra (discussed earlier). However, their caretakers showed no signs of the disease. He reasoned that, if pellagra were an **infectious disease**, both groups would suffer from it. Since this was not the case, he hypothesized that pellagra is probably caused by a dietary deficiency.

Historical and epidemiological findings can suggest hypotheses about the role of diet in various health problems. Proving the role of particular dietary components, however, requires controlled experiments. For instance, once the high **incidence** of pellagra in mental institutions during the 1920s was linked to poor diet, various foods were given to patients who had the disease. These experiments showed that yeast and high-protein foods could cure pellagra in these patients if the disease was not in its final stage, indicating that pellagra results from a deficiency of some nutrient present in these foods. Eventually, this nutrient was found to be the vitamin niacin (formerly called vitamin B_3).

Laboratory Animal Experiments

When scientists cannot test their hypotheses by experiments with humans, they often use animals. Much of what we know about human nutritional needs and functions has been generated from animal experiments. Still, human experiments are the most convincing to scientists. In the 1930s, scientists showed that a pellagra-like disease seen in dogs, called *blacktongue*, is cured by nicotinic acid. Only when nicotinic acid actually cured pellagra in humans were scientists convinced that nicotinic acid, later identified as a vitamin and called niacin, was the critical dietary factor.

The use of animal experiments to study the role of nutrition in certain human diseases depends on the availability of an **animal model**—a disease in laboratory animals that closely mimics a particular human disease. However, most chronic diseases do not occur naturally in laboratory animals. Often, however, if no animal model is available and human experiments are ruled out, scientific knowledge often cannot advance beyond what can be learned from epidemiological studies.

Human Studies

Various experimental approaches are used to test research hypotheses in humans, including case-control and double-blind studies.

■ Case-Control Study

In a **case-control study,** scientists compare individuals who have the condition in question, such as lung cancer, are compared with individuals who do not have the condition. Comparisons are made only between groups that are matched for other major characteristics (e.g., age, race, and gender) not being studied. You can think of such a protocol as a mini-epidemiological study. This type of study may identify factors other than the disease in question, such as fruit and vegetable intake, that differ between the two groups, thus providing researchers with clues about the cause, progression, and prevention of the disease. However, without a controlled experiment, researchers cannot definitively prove cause and effect.

■ Double-Blind Study

An important approach for more definitive testing of hypotheses is the **double-blind study**, in which a group of participants—the experimental group—follows a specific protocol (e.g., consuming a certain food or nutrient), and participants in a corresponding **control group** follow their normal habits. People are randomly assigned to each group, such as by the flip of a coin. Scientists then observe the experimental group over time to see if there is any effect that is not found in the control group. Sometimes individuals are used as their own control: First they are observed for a period of time, and then they are treated and their responses noted.

infectious disease Any disease caused by invasion of the body by microorganisms, such as bacteria, fungi, or viruses.

incidence The number of new cases of a disease in a defined population over a specific period of time, such as 1 year.

animal model Study of disease in animals that duplicates human disease. This can be used to understand more about human disease.

case-control study Individuals who have the condition in question, such as lung cancer, are compared with individuals who do not have the condition.

double-blind study An experimental design in which neither the participants nor the researchers are aware of each participant's assignment (test or placebo) or the outcome of the study until it is completed. An independent third party holds the code and the data until the study has been completed.

control group Participants in an experiment who are not given the treatment being tested.

Two features of a double-blind study help reduce the introduction of bias (prejudice), which can easily affect the outcome of an experiment. First, neither the participants nor the researchers know which individuals are in the experimental group and which are in the control group. Second, the expected effects of the experimental protocol are not disclosed to the participants or researchers until after the entire study is completed. This approach reduces the possibility that researchers may see the change they want to see in the participants to prove a certain "pet" hypothesis, even though such a change did not actually occur. This approach also reduces the chance that the persons participating begin to feel better simply because they are involved in a research study or are receiving a new treatment, a phenomenon called the *placebo effect.*

In a double-blind experiment, the control group often receives a sugar pill (or other placebo treatment) to camouflage who is in which group and thereby eliminate the bias introduced by the placebo effect. During the course of the experiment, neither the researchers nor the participants know who is getting the real treatment and who is getting a placebo.

A recent example illustrates the need to test hypotheses based on epidemiological observations in double-blind studies. Epidemiologists using primarily case-control studies found that smokers who regularly consumed fruits and vegetables had a lower risk for lung cancer than smokers who ate few fruits and vegetables. Some scientists proposed that beta-carotene, a pigment present in many fruits and vegetables, could reduce the damage that tobacco smoke creates in the lungs. This hypothesis helped fuel sales of supplements of beta-carotene.

However, in double-blind studies involving heavy smokers, the risk of lung cancer was found to be higher for those who took beta-carotene supplements than for those who did not (note that this is not true for the small amount of beta-carotene found naturally in foods). Some investigators criticized this research, arguing that the beta-carotene was given too late in the smokers' lives to be of much use, but even these critics did not suspect that the supplements would increase cancer risk. Soon after these results were reported, the U.S. federal agency supporting two other large ongoing studies that employed beta-carotene supplements called a halt to the research, stating that these supplements are ineffective in preventing both lung cancer and cardiovascular disease.

Overall, health and nutrition advice provided by grandparents, parents, friends, and other well-meaning individuals can't be verified unless it is put to the ultimate scientific test—blinded studies. Until that is done, we can't be sure that the substance or procedure in question is truly effective. When people say, "I get fewer colds now that I take vitamin C," they overlook the fact that many cold symptoms disappear quickly with no treatment; the apparent curative effect of vitamin C or any other remedy is often coincidental rather than causal to the natural healing process.

All consumers need to become more sophisticated about science, its accepted standards of evidence, and its current limitations. Failure to do so leads many to a frantic pursuit of fraudulent remedies. To ignore science is to follow an inferior path—the road of hard knocks. Those who follow this road learn about the dangers of various health practices primarily from the experiences of being harmed by them. Medical science does not ignore novel approaches to disease prevention and cure. Anecdotes and personal experiences are important clues leading to fruitful experimentation, but they are not credible evidence.

Peer Review of Experimental Results

Once an experiment is complete, scientists summarize the findings and seek to publish the results in scientific journals. Generally, before articles are published in scientific journals, they are critically reviewed by other scientists familiar with the subject. The objective of this peer review is to ensure that only high-quality research findings are published. This is an important step because most scientific research in this country is funded by the federal government, nonprofit foundations, drug companies, and other private industries. All of these funding sources can have strong expectations about the research outcomes. In theory, the scientists conducting these research studies will be fair in evaluating their results and will not be influenced by their sponsors. Peer review helps ensure that the researchers are as objective as possible. Be assured that the results published in **peer-reviewed journals,** such as the *American Journal of Clinical Nutrition, The*

placebo Generally a fake medicine used to disguise the treatments given to the participants in an experiment.

peer-reviewed journal A journal that publishes research only after two or three scientists who were not part of the study agree it was well conducted and the results are fairly represented. Thus, the research has been approved by peers of the research team.

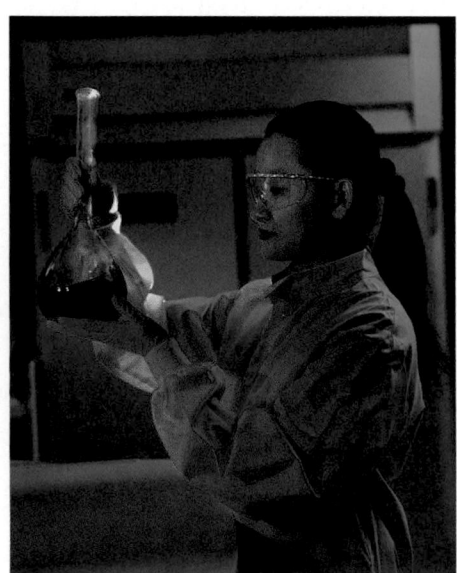

Careful research contributes to nutrition knowledge, more so than personal experience.

New England Journal of Medicine, and the *Journal of the American Dietetic Association,* are much more reliable than those found in popular magazines or promoted on television talk shows.

Follow-Up Studies

Even if an acceptable protocol has been followed and the results of a study have been accepted by the scientific community, one experiment is never enough to prove a particular hypothesis or provide a basis for nutritional recommendations. Rather, the results obtained in one laboratory must be confirmed by experiments conducted in other laboratories, and possibly under varying circumstances. Only then can we really trust and use the results. The more lines of evidence available to support an idea, the more likely it is to be true (Fig. 1-7). It is important to avoid rushing to accept new ideas as fact or incorporating them into your health habits until they are proved by several lines of evidence.

How to Use This Knowledge to Evaluate Nutrition Claims and Advice

Based on what has been covered so far, the following suggestions should help you make healthful and logical nutrition decisions:

1. Apply the basic principles of nutrition as outlined in this chapter (along with the 2005 Dietary Guidelines for Americans and related resources in Chapter 2) to any nutrition claim including those on websites. Do you note any inconsistencies? Do reliable references support the claims? Beware of the following:

   - Testimonials about personal experience
   - Disreputable publication sources
   - Dramatic results (rarely true)
   - Lack of evidence from supporting studies made by other scientists

2. Examine the background and scientific credentials of the individual, organizations, or publication making the nutritional claim. Usually, a reputable author is one whose educational background or present affiliation is with a nationally recognized university or medical center that offers programs or courses in the field of nutrition, medicine, or a closely allied specialty.

3. Be wary if the answer is "Yes" to any of the following questions about a health-related nutrition claim:

   - Are only advantages discussed and possible disadvantages ignored?
   - Are claims made about "curing" disease? Do they sound too good to be true?
   - Is extreme bias against the medical community or traditional medical treatments evident? Physicians as a group strive to cure diseases in their patients, using what proven techniques are available. They do not ignore reliable cures.
   - Is the claim touted as a new or secret scientific breakthrough?

4. Note the size and duration of any study cited in support of a nutrition claim. The larger it is and the longer it went on, the more dependable its findings. Also consider the type of study: epidemiology versus case-control versus double-blind. Check out the group studied; a study of men or women in Sweden may be less relevant than one of men or women of Southern European, African, or Hispanic descent, for example. Keep in mind that "contributes to," "is linked to," or "is associated with" does not mean "causes."

5. Beware of press conferences and other hype regarding the latest findings. Much of this will not survive more detailed scientific evaluation.

6. When you meet with a nutrition professional, you should expect that he or she will do the following:

   - Ask questions about your medical history, lifestyle, and current eating habits.
   - Formulate a diet plan tailored to your needs, as opposed to simply tearing a form from a tablet that could apply to almost anyone.

Recently major nutrition organizations put together 10 red flags that they consider signals for poor nutrition advice:

1. Recommendations that promise a quick fix
2. Dire warnings of dangers from a single product or regimen
3. Claims that sound too good to be true
4. Simplistic conclusions drawn from a complex study
5. Recommendations based on a single study
6. Dramatic statements that are refuted by reputable scientific organizations
7. Lists of "good" and "bad" foods
8. Recommendations made to help sell a product
9. Recommendations based on studies published without peer review
10. Recommendations from studies that ignore differences among individuals or groups

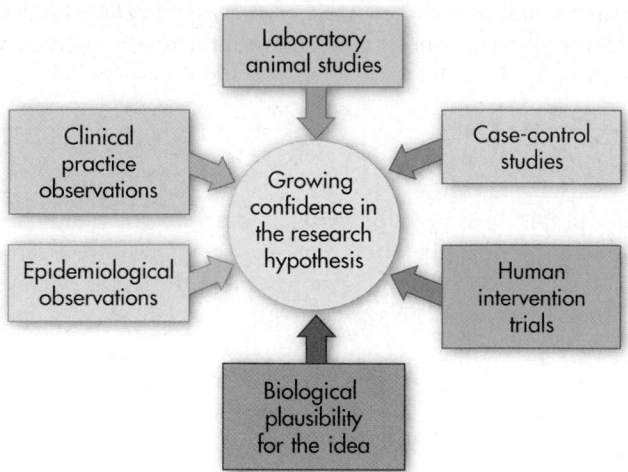

Figure 1-7 Data from a variety of sources can come together to support a research hypothesis. For example, epidemiological studies show that type 2 diabetes is characteristically found in obese populations, compared with leaner populations. Physicians notice in clinical practice that type 2 diabetes is much more likely in their obese patients, compared with their leaner patients. Laboratory animal studies show that overfeeding that eventually leads to obesity often leads to the development of type 2 diabetes. Case-control studies show that obese patients are much more likely to have type 2 diabetes than the learner comparison group that is matched for other characteristics. Finally, human intervention trials show that weight loss can correct type 2 diabetes in many people. Laboratory researchers also show that the enlarged adipose cells associated with excess fat deposition and obesity are much less responsive to the hormonal signals involved in blood glucose regulation. All of these lines of data come together with biological plausibility from various laboratory studies to support the research hypothesis that obesity can lead to type 2 diabetes.

megadose Intake of a nutrient beyond estimates of needs or what would be found in a balanced diet; 2 to 10 times human needs is a starting point.

- Schedule follow-up visits to track your progress, answer any questions, and help keep you motivated.
- Involve family members in the diet plan, when appropriate.
- Consult directly with your physician and readily refer you back to your physician for those health problems a nutrition professional is not trained to treat.

7. Avoid practitioners who prescribe **megadoses** of vitamin and mineral supplements for everyone.
8. Examine product labels carefully. Be skeptical of any product promotion not clearly stated on the label. A product is not likely to do something that is not specifically claimed on its label or package insert (legally part of the label).

This cautious approach to nutrition-related advice and products is even more important today because of sweeping changes in U.S. federal law passed in 1994.

The Dietary Supplement Health and Education Act (DSHEA) of 1994 classified vitamins, minerals, amino acids, and herbal remedies as "foods," effectively restraining the U.S. Food and Drug Administration (FDA) from regulating them as heavily as drugs and food additives. According to this act, rather than the manufacturer having to prove a dietary supplement is safe, FDA must prove it is unsafe before preventing its sale. In contrast, the safety of food additives and drugs must be demonstrated to FDA's satisfaction before they are marketed.

FDA can act, however, if evidence accumulates showing that a product is harmful. This has been true for some herbal remedies marketed as dietary supplements, such as ephedra.

Currently, a dietary supplement (or herbal product) can be marketed in the United States without FDA approval if (1) there is a history of its use or other evidence that it is expected to be reasonably safe when used under the conditions recommended or suggested in its labeling, and (2) the product is labeled as a dietary supplement. It is permissible for the labels on such products to claim a benefit related to a classic nutrient-deficiency disease, describe how a nutrient affects human body structure or function (called structure/function claims), and claim that general well-being results from consumption of the ingredient(s). Examples could be "maintains bone health" or "improves blood circulation." However, the label of products bearing such claims also must prominently display in boldface type the following disclaimer: "This statement has not been evaluated by the Food and Drug Administration. This product is not intended to diagnose, treat, cure, or prevent disease" (Fig. 1-8). Despite this warning, when consumers find these products on the shelves of supermarkets, health-food stores, and pharmacies, they may mistakenly assume FDA has carefully evaluated the products.

The fact remains that many of us are willing to try untested nutrition products and believe in their miraculous actions. Popular products claim to increase muscle growth, enhance sexuality, boost energy, reduce body fat, increase strength, supply missing nutrients, increase longevity, and even improve brain function. Clearly, many nutritional products commonly found in stores are not strictly regulated in terms of effectiveness. The amount and potency are also often in question. (In general, national brands are more reliable.) Few have been thoroughly evaluated by reputable scientists.

If you embark on a self-cure by means of such products, you will probably waste money and possibly risk ill health. A better approach is to consult a physician or **registered dietitian** first. You can find a registered dietitian in North America by consulting the Yellow Pages in the telephone directory, contacting the local dietetic association, calling the dietary department of a local hospital, or visiting www.eatright.org/find.html or www.dietitians.ca. Make sure the person has the credentials "R.D." after his/her name ("R.D.N." is also used in Canada). This indicates the person has completed rigorous classroom and clinical training in nutrition and participates in continuing education. Appendix H also lists many reputable sources of nutrition advice for your use. Finally, the following websites can help you evaluate ongoing nutrition and health claims:

www.eatright.org
www.acsh.org
www.quackwatch.com
www.ncahf.org
dietary-supplements.info.nih.gov
www.fda.gov
navigator.tufts.edu.

Overall, nutrition is a rapidly advancing field and there are always new findings.

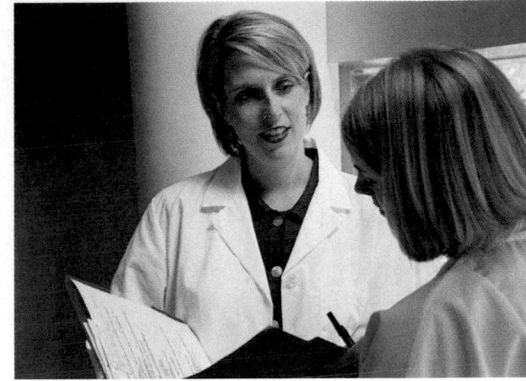

Registered dietitians are a reliable source of nutrition information.

registered dietitian (R.D.) A person who has completed a baccalaureate degree program approved by the American Dietetic Association, performed at least 900 hours of supervised professional practice, and passed a registration examination.

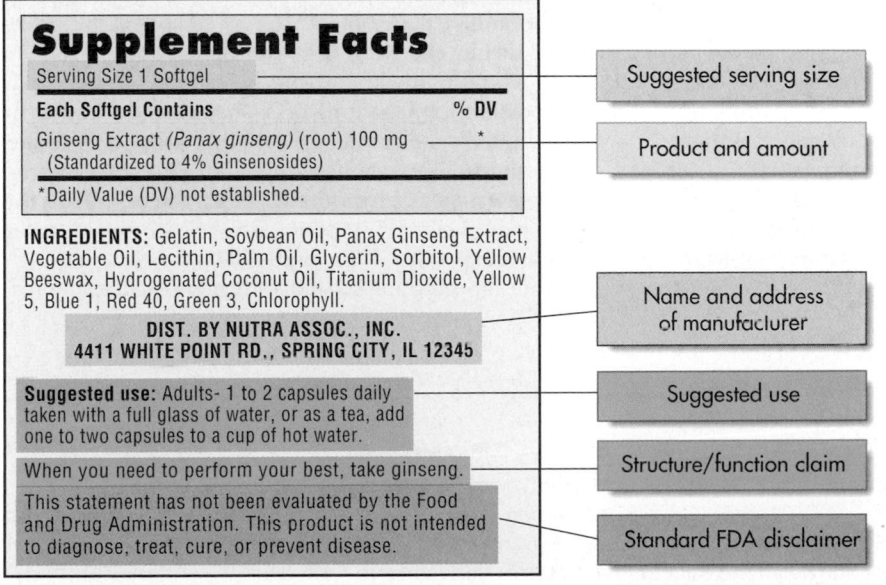

Supplement Facts

Serving Size 1 Softgel — Suggested serving size

Each Softgel Contains	**% DV**
Ginseng Extract *(Panax ginseng)* (root) 100 mg (Standardized to 4% Ginsenosides)	*

Product and amount

*Daily Value (DV) not established.

INGREDIENTS: Gelatin, Soybean Oil, Panax Ginseng Extract, Vegetable Oil, Lecithin, Palm Oil, Glycerin, Sorbitol, Yellow Beeswax, Hydrogenated Coconut Oil, Titanium Dioxide, Yellow 5, Blue 1, Red 40, Green 3, Chlorophyll.

DIST. BY NUTRA ASSOC., INC.
4411 WHITE POINT RD., SPRING CITY, IL 12345

Name and address of manufacturer

Suggested use: Adults- 1 to 2 capsules daily taken with a full glass of water, or as a tea, add one to two capsules to a cup of hot water.

Suggested use

When you need to perform your best, take ginseng.

Structure/function claim

This statement has not been evaluated by the Food and Drug Administration. This product is not intended to diagnose, treat, cure, or prevent disease.

Standard FDA disclaimer

Figure 1-8 Supplement Facts label on an herbal product. Note the structure/function claim and the FDA disclaimer. Any nutrients or other food constituents would also be listed if contained in the product.

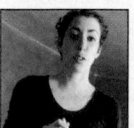

Real Life Scenario Follow-Up

Brenda should be cautious about taking any supplement, especially one advertised as a "recent breakthrough." As you have read, dietary supplements are not closely regulated by FDA; a general statement such as "increases energy" would be considered a structure/function claim and therefore does not require prior approval by FDA with regard to product labeling. Furthermore, FDA will not have evaluated either the safety or effectiveness of such a product, and even harmful dietary supplements are difficult for FDA to recall. There is even a chance that the supplement, if effective, would contain little or none of the purported active ingredient. Unfortunately, Brenda will find out all of this the hard way and will be out $60. Her hard-earned money would be better spent on a medical checkup at the Student Health Center. Currently all consumers need to be cautious about nutrition information, especially regarding dietary supplements marketed as cure-alls and breakthroughs—Let the buyer beware!

Summary

1. Nutrition is the study of the food substances vital for health and the study of how the body uses these substances to promote and support growth, maintenance, and reproduction of cells.

2. Nutrients in foods fall into six classes: (1) carbohydrates, (2) lipids (mostly fats and oils), (3) proteins, (4) vitamins, (5) minerals, and (6) water. The first three, along with alcohol, provide calories for the body to use.

3. The body transforms the energy contained in carbohydrate, protein, and fat into other forms of energy that in turn allow the body to function. Fat provides, on average, 9 kcal per gram, whereas both protein and carbohydrate provide, on average, 4 kcal per gram. Vitamins, minerals, and water do not supply calories to the body but are essential for proper body function.

4. A basic plan for health promotion and disease prevention includes eating a varied diet, performing regular physical activity, not smoking, not abusing nutrient supplements (if used), consuming adequate water and other fluids, getting enough sleep, limiting alcohol intake (if consumed), and limiting or coping with stress.

5. The primary focus of nutrition planning should be on food, not on dietary supplements. The focus on foods to supply nutrient needs avoids the possibility of severe nutrient imbalances.

6. Results from large nutrition surveys in the United States and Canada suggest that some of us need to concentrate on consuming foods that supply more of certain vitamins, minerals, and fiber. Daily use of a balanced multivitamin and mineral supplement is another strategy that helps address some of these shortcomings but does not substitute for a healthy diet.

7. Groups of cells in the hypothalamus and other regions in the brain affect hunger, the primarily internal desire to find and eat food. These cells monitor hormonal and nerve signals from digestive organs as well as amounts of nutrients and other substances in the blood to control satiety.

8. A variety of external (appetite-related) forces affect satiety. Hunger cues combine with appetite cues, such as easy availability of food, to promote food intake.

9. The flavor, appearance, and texture of foods primarily influence our food choices. Several other factors also help determine food habits and choices: our upbringing, various social and cultural factors, the image we want to project to others, economics, convenience, emotional state, and concerns about health.

10. There are no true "good" or "bad" foods, but some food choices are healthier than others. The focus should be on balancing a total diet by choosing many nutritious foods.

11. The scientific method is the procedure for testing the validity of possible explanations of a phenomenon, called hypotheses. Experiments are conducted to either support or refute a specific hypothesis. Once we have much experimental information that supports a specific hypothesis, it then can be called a theory. All of us need to be skeptical of new ideas in the nutrition field, waiting until many lines of experimental evidence support a concept before adopting any suggested dietary practice.

Study Questions

1. Name one chronic disease associated with poor nutrition habits. Now list a few corresponding risk factors.

2. Explain the concept of calories as it relates to foods. What are the values used to calculate kcals from grams of carbohydrate, fat, protein, and alcohol?

3. Identify three ways that water is used in the body.

4. Wendy's Big Bacon Classic contains 44 grams carbohydrate, 36 grams fat, and 37 grams protein. Calculate the percentage of calories derived from fat.

5. Describe two types of fat and explain why the differences are important in terms of overall health.
6. According to national nutrition surveys, which nutrients tend to be underconsumed by many North Americans? Why do you think this is the case?
7. List four health objectives for the United States for the year 2010. How would you rate yourself in each area? Why?
8. Describe the various organs and hormones that control hunger and satiety in the body. List other factors that influence our food patterns.
9. Describe how your own food preferences have been shaped by the following factors:
   a. Exposure to foods at an early age
   b. Advertising (what is the newest food you have tried?)
   c. Eating out
   d. Peer pressure
   e. Economic factors
10. What products in your supermarket reflect the consumer demand for healthier foods? For convenience?

Further Readings

1. ADA Reports: Position of the American Dietetic Association: Total diet approach to communicating food and nutrition information. *Journal of the American Dietetic Association* 102:100, 2002.

   The American Dietetic Association states that there are no good or bad foods, only good or bad diets or eating styles. No single food or type of food insures good health, just as no single food or type of food is necessarily detrimental to health. Adults should emphasize adequacy of the total diet over time, the importance of obtaining nutrients from foods, and portion control, coupled with weight control and regular physical activity.

2. ADA Reports: Position of the American Dietetic Association: Food and nutrition misinformation. *Journal of the American Dietetic Association* 102:260, 2002.

   Much food and nutrition misinformation pervades North American society. Individuals should carefully consider the training of those who give such advice, and be assured that registered dietitians are a reliable source.

3. ADA Reports: Position of the American Dietetic Association and Dietitians of Canada: Nutrition and women's Health. *Journal of the American Dietetic Association* 104:984, 2004.

   Comprehensive look at health issues related to nutrition that women often face. Diets rich in fruits, vegetables, and whole grain breads and cereals, with some low fat dairy and lean meat choices, is widely advocated. Individual nutrients likely to be under consumed include calcium, iron, vitamin D, vitamin E and folate.

4. Cotton PA and others: Dietary sources of nutrients among U.S. adults, 1994 to 1996. *Journal of the American Dietetic Association* 104:921, 2004.

   The five leading calorie sources for American adults are (in order): yeast bread, beef, cakes/cookies/quick breads/doughnuts, soft drinks/soda, and milk. The cake, etc category also has been moving up in the order compared to the 1980's. Clearly many adults need to improve their dietary choices.

5. Cordain L and others: Origins and evolution of the Western diet: health implications for the 21st century. *American Journal of Clinical Nutrition* 81:341, 2005.

   Throughout man's existence the overall diet has included a greater number of foods rich in refined sugars, refined flours, salt, and animal fat. This has resulted in a decline in diet quality for many of us in the modern world.

6. de Graaf C and others: Biomarkers of satiation. *American Journal of Clinical Nutrition* 79:946, 2004.

   The feeling of satiety depends on a constellation of factors, such as stomach distention, the action of various hormones, such as ghrelin, and communication between various organs and the brain. This article reviews the latest findings with regard to these and other factors affecting satiety.

7. Food and Nutrition Board: *Dietary reference intakes for energy, carbohydrate, fiber, fat, fatty acids, cholesterol, protein, and amino acids.* Washington DC: The National Academy Press, 2002.

   This report provides the latest guidance for macronutrient intakes. With regard to the amounts of carbohydrate, fat, and protein in a diet, this should be 45% to 65%, 20% to 35%, and 10% to 35%, respectively.

8. How much exercise is enough? *UC Berkeley Wellness Letter*, p. 5, September 2003.

   A minimum amount of physical activity is considered to be 30 minutes at least five times per week. Increasing the amount to 60 minutes per day is even more health-promoting, especially if weight loss/control is an issue. For both recommendations, bouts of physical activity can be broken up into a few sessions in a day.

9. Junk food or junky choices? *Tufts University Health & Nutrition Letter*, p. 3, September 2003.

   Some sweet or high-fat foods can be safely incorporated into an otherwise healthy diet. This healthy diet should be rich in fruits, vegetables, and whole-grain breads and cereals, and contain some low-fat and fat-free dairy choices and lean protein sources. A person's total dietary intake is what determines the quality of a diet.

10. Lubin F and others: Lifestyle and ethnicity play a role in all-cause mortality. *Journal of Nutrition* 133:1180, 2003.

    Dietary habits that reduce all-cause mortality include focusing on both high-fiber foods and those low in saturated fat and cholesterol. Positive lifestyle habits include regular physical activity and avoiding smoking and obesity.

11. Mokdad AH and others: Actual causes of death in the United States, 2000. *Journal of the American Medical Association* 291:1238, 2004.

    Smoking is the leading cause of preventable death in the United States, with obesity a close second. A combination of a poor diet and inactive lifestyle may account for about 1/3 of all deaths in the United States.

12. Olshansky SJ and others: A potential decline in life expectancy in the United States in the 21st century. *The New England Journal of Medicine* 352:1138, 2005.

    The growing problem of overweight and obesity in our society is likely to lead to more overall premature deaths. An alarming concern is that this widespread increase in body weight could result in a life expectancy of fewer years for today's children compared to their parents. Reversing this trend of greater overweight and obesity thus is crucial.

13. Paeratakul S and others: Fast-food consumption among U.S. adults and children: Dietary and nutrient intake profile. *Journal of the American Dietetic Association* 103:1332, 2003.

    Regular intake of fast-food contributes a lot of fat and calories to a diet. Such foods can also crowd out more healthful foods in a diet. Regular fast-food consumers would be wise to focus on lower-fat items, and greatly limit or avoid sugared soft drinks and French fries.

14. Tholin S and others: Genetic and environmental influence on eating behavior: the Swedish Young Male Twins Study. *American Journal of Clinical Nutrition* 81:564, 2005.

    Genetics plays a distinct role in the development of eating habits, such as emotional eating or restrained eating. This may be linked to the amount of various hormones and other physiological factors that can influence eating habits.

I. *Examine Your Eating Habits More Closely*

Choose one day of the week that is typical of your eating pattern. Using the first table found in Appendix E, list all foods and drinks you consumed for 24 hours. In addition, write down the approximate amounts of food you ate in units, such as cups, ounces, teaspoons, and tablespoons. Check the food composition table in Appendix J for examples of appropriate serving units for different types of foods, such as meat and vegetables. After you record the amount of each food and drink consumed, indicate in the table why you chose to consume the item. Place the corresponding abbreviation in the space provided to indicate why you picked that food or drink.

FLVR	Flavor/texture	ADV	Advertisement	PEER	Peers
CONV	Convenience	WTCL	Weight control	NUTR	Nutritive value
EMO	Emotions	HUNG	Hunger	$	Cost
AVA	Availability	FAM	Family/cultural	HLTH	Health

There can be more than one reason for choosing a particular food or drink.

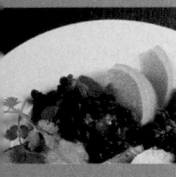

Application

Now ask yourself what your most frequent reason is for eating or drinking. To what degree is health or nutritive value a reason for your food choices? Should you make these higher priorities?

II. *Observe the Supermarket Explosion*

Today's supermarkets carry up to 60,000 items, compared to 20,000 items 10 years ago. Think about your last grocery shopping trip and the items you purchased to eat. Following is a list of 20 newer food products added to supermarket shelves. Check the items that you have tried. Then use the key from Part I of the Rate Your Plate exercise to identify why you might have chosen these products.

_____ Prepackaged salad greens (variety packs other than iceberg lettuce) _____

_____ Gourmet salad oils (e.g., walnut, almond, olive, or sesame oil) _____

_____ Gourmet vinegars (e.g., balsamic or rice) _____

_____ Prepackaged lunch products (e.g., nacho, pizza, taco, and tortilla Lunchables) _____

_____ Precooked frozen turkey patties _____

_____ Bean soup mixes (e.g., lentil, black bean, combination bean soups) _____

_____ Microwaveable sandwiches (e.g., Hotpockets, frozen sandwiches) _____

_____ Refrigerated, precooked pasta (e.g., tortellini, fettucini) and accompanying sauces (e.g., pesto, tomato basil) _____
_____

_____ Imported grain products (e.g., risotto, farfalline, gnocchi, fusilli) _____

_____ Frozen dinners (list your favorite of any of the wide variety) _____

_____ Imported sauces for food preparation (e.g., hoisin or brown bean sauce, mandarin marinade, sesame, curry, or fire oils) _____
_____

_____ Bottled waters (flavored or unflavored) _____

_____ Trendy juices (e.g., draft apple cider, hurricane punch) _____

_____ Roasted and/or flavored coffees (e.g., beans, ground, or instant) _____

_____ Gourmet jelly beans and candies (e.g., gummi coca-colas or imported chocolates) _____

_____ Instant hot cereal in a bowl (add water and go!) _____

_____ "Fast-shake" pancake mix (add water, shake, and ready to cook) _____

_____ Breakfast bars (e.g., granola or fruit-flavored bars) _____

_____ Meal replacement/fitness products (e.g., "energy" bars, high-protein bars, sports drinks) _____

_____ Low-carbohydrate meat and pasta dishes _____

Finally, identify three new food products that are not on this list that you have seen in the past year. Discuss the appeal of these products to the North American consumer.

Tools for Designing a Healthy Diet

2

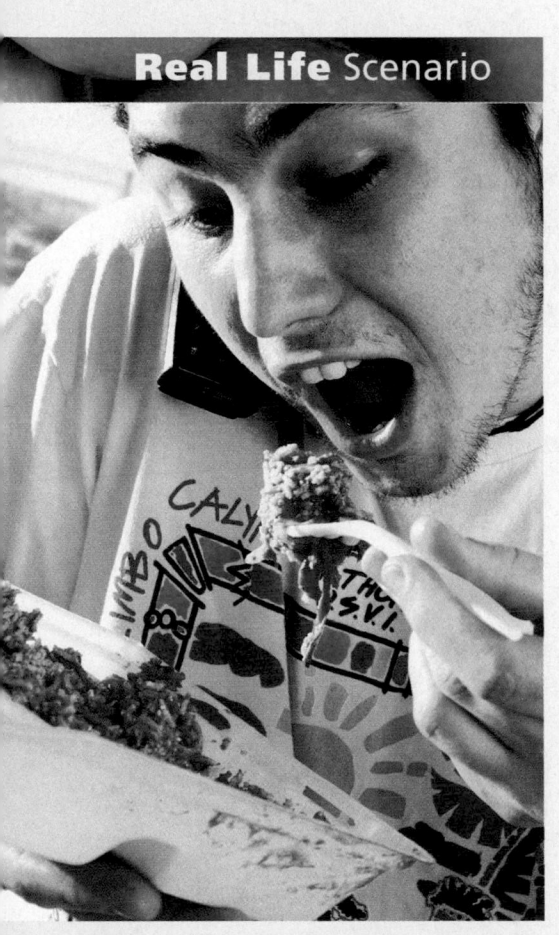

Andy is like many other college students. He grew up on a quick bowl of cereal and milk for breakfast and a hamburger, French fries, and cola for lunch, either in the school cafeteria or at a local fast-food restaurant. At dinner, he generally avoided eating any of his salad or vegetables, and by 9 o'clock he was deep into bags of chips and cookies. Andy has taken most of these habits to college. He prefers coffee for breakfast and possibly a chocolate bar. Lunch is still mainly a hamburger, French fries, and cola, but pizza and tacos now alternate more frequently than when he was in high school. One thing Andy really likes about the restaurants surrounding campus is that, for just about half a dollar more, he can *supersize* his meal. This helps him stretch his food dollar; searching out value meals for lunch and dinner now has become part of a typical day.

Can you provide some dietary advice for Andy? Start with his positive habits and then provide some constructive criticism, based on what you now know.

Chapter 2 Objectives

Chapter 2 is designed to allow you to:

1. Develop a healthy eating plan.
2. Outline the ABCDEs of nutrition assessment: *a*nthropometric, *b*iochemical, *c*linical, *d*ietary, and *e*conomic.
3. Describe what the Recommended Dietary Allowances (RDAs) and other dietary standards represent.
4. Learn the food groupings used in MyPyramid.
5. List the Dietary Guidelines and the diseases these guidelines are designed to prevent or minimize.
6. Describe what a nutrition label currently consists of and the various health claims and label descriptors that are allowed.

Check out the **Contemporary Nutrition Online Learning Center**

www.mhhe.com/wardlawcont6 *for quizzes, flash cards, other activities, and web links designed to further help you learn about various tools for diet planning.*

How many times have you heard wild claims about how healthful certain foods are for you? As consumers focus more and more on diet and disease, food manufacturers are asserting that their products have all sorts of health benefits. Supermarket shelves have begun to look like an 1800s medicine show. "Take fish oil capsules to avoid a heart attack." "Eat more olive oil and oat bran to lower blood cholesterol." Hearing these claims, you would think that food manufacturers have solutions to all of our health problems.

Advertising aside, nutrient intakes that are out of balance with our needs—such as excess calories, saturated fat, cholesterol, *trans* fat, salt, alcohol, and sugar intakes—are linked to many leading causes of death in North America, including obesity, hypertension, cardiovascular disease, cancer, liver disease, and type 2 diabetes. Physical inactivity is also too common. In Chapter 2, you will explore the components of a healthy diet and lifestyle—an approach that will minimize your risks of developing nutrition-related diseases. The goal is to provide you with a firm understanding of these concepts before you study the nutrients in detail.

Refresh Your Memory

As you begin your study of diet planning in Chapter 2, you may want to review:

- The terms in the margin in Chapter 1 and Table 1-1.
- The impact of the Dietary Supplement Health and Education Act (DSHEA) on certain label claims in Chapter 1.

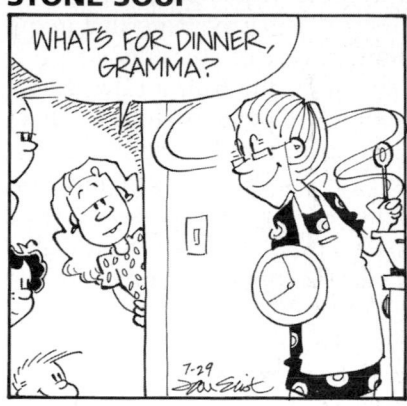 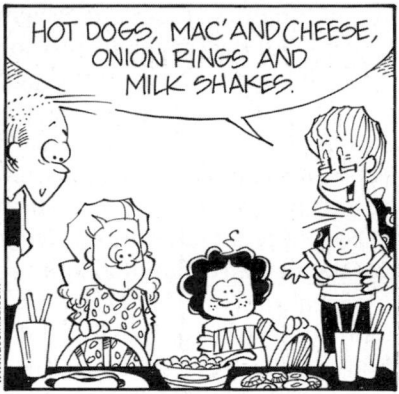 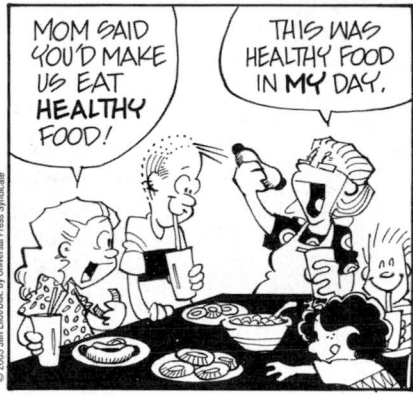

On what do nutrition experts generally agree regarding a healthy food or diet? Why is a diet rich in fiber that includes some fish and is low in fried foods and animal fat emphasized, along with at least 30 minutes or more of physical activity on most or all days of the week? Are North Americans generally following this plan? What are the potential consequences for those who do not? Chapter 2 provides some answers.

A Food Philosophy That Works

You may be surprised to learn that what you should eat to minimize the risk of developing the common nutrition-related diseases seen in North America is exactly what you've heard many times before: *Consume a variety of foods balanced by a moderate intake of each food.* A variety of foods is best because no one food meets all your nutrient needs. Meat provides protein and iron but little calcium and no vitamin C. Eggs also provide protein but little calcium because the calcium is mostly in the shell. Cow's milk contains calcium, but very little iron. And none of these foods contains fiber. Thus you need a variety of foods in your diet because the required nutrients are scattered among many foods.

Health professionals have recommended the same basic diet and health plan for the past 40 years: Control how much you eat, focus on the major food groups, and stay physically active. Whole-grain breads and cereals, fruits, and vegetables have always been among the foods emphasized for our diet for these past 40 years.

It is disappointing, however, that according to a recent survey conducted by the American Dietetic Association, two of five people in the United States believe that following a healthful diet means completely giving up foods they enjoy. To the contrary, a healthful diet requires only some simple planning and doesn't have to mean deprivation and misery. Besides, eliminating favorite foods typically doesn't work for "dieters" in the long run. The best plan consists of learning the basics of a healthful diet—a variety and balance of foods from all food groups and moderate consumption of all foods. Let's now fine-tune this advice by focusing on variety, balance, moderation, nutrient density, and energy density.

Variety Means Eating Many Different Foods

Variety in your diet means choosing a number of different foods within any given food group rather than eating the "same old thing" day after day. Variety makes meals more interesting and helps ensure that a diet contains sufficient nutrients. For example, carrots—a rich source of a pigment that forms vitamin A—may be your favorite vegetable; however, if you choose carrots every day as your only vegetable source, you may miss out on the vitamin folate. Other vegetables, such as broccoli and asparagus,

Some people would like to live mostly on French fries. What is the nutrient content of French fries? Check the food composition table in Appendix J for the vitamin C content of French fries. How many servings would you need to eat to meet vitamin C needs (75 to 95 milligrams)?
(Answer: 4 to 5 servings)

Monitoring total calorie intake is also important for many of us, especially if unwanted weight gain is taking place.

35

phytochemical A chemical found in plants. Some phytochemicals may contribute to a reduced risk of cancer or cardiovascular disease in people who consume them regularly.

Some research suggests that increasing variety in a diet can lead to overeating. Thus, as one incorporates a wide variety of foods in a diet, attention to total calorie intake is also important to consider.

Foods rich in phytochemicals are now part of a family of foods referred to as **functional foods.** A functional food is a food that provides health benefits beyond those supplied by the traditional nutrients it contains. Since a tomato contains the phytochemical lycopene, it can be called a functional food. You may hear this term more from the food industry in the future.

are rich sources of this nutrient. This concept is true of all classes of foods: fruits, vegetables, grains, and so on. Different foods within each class vary somewhat in the nutrients they contain, but they generally provide similar types of nutrients.

An added bonus of variety in the diet, especially within the fruit and vegetable groups, is the inclusion of a rich supply of what scientists call **phytochemicals.** These plant components are not considered essential nutrients in the diet. Still, many of these substances provide significant health benefits. Considerable research attention is focused on various phytochemicals in reducing the risk for certain diseases (e.g., cancer). You can't just buy a bottle of phytochemicals—they are generally available only within whole foods. Current multivitamin and mineral supplements contain few or none of these beneficial plant chemicals.

Numerous population studies show reduced cancer risk among people who regularly consume fruits and vegetables. This is true for cancer of the gastrointestinal (GI) tract, breast, lung, and bladder. Researchers surmise that some phytochemicals present in the fruits and vegetables block the cancer process. The cancer process and the specific roles of some phytochemicals in this regard are described in the Looking Further section in Chapter 15. For now, realize that cancer develops over many years via a multistep process. If an agent such as a phytochemical can block any one of the steps in this process, the chances that cancer will ultimately appear in the body are reduced. Some phytochemicals also have been linked to a reduced risk of cardiovascular disease. Could it be that, because humans evolved on a wide variety of plant-based foods, the body developed with a need for these phytochemicals, along with the various nutrients present, to maintain optimal health?

It will likely take many years for scientists to unravel the important effects of the myriad of phytochemicals in foods, and it is unlikely that all will ever be available or effective in supplement form. For this reason, leading nutrition and medical experts suggest that a diet rich in fruits, vegetables, and whole-grain breads and cereals is the most reliable way to obtain the potential benefits of phytochemicals. Table 2-1 lists

Table 2-1 Some Phytochemical Compounds Under Study

Phytochemical	Food Sources
Allyl sulfides/organosulfurs	Garlic, onions, leeks
Saponins	Garlic, onions, licorice, legumes
Carotenoids (e.g. lycopene)	Orange, red, yellow fruits and vegetables (egg yolks are a source as well)
Monoterpenes	Oranges, lemons, grapefruit
Capsaicin	Chili peppers
Lignans	Flaxseed, berries, whole grains
Indoles	Cruciferous vegetables (broccoli, cabbage, kale)
Isothiocyanates	Cruciferous vegetables, especially broccoli
Phytosterols	Soybeans, other legumes, cucumbers, other fruits and vegetables
Flavonoids	Citrus fruit, onions, apples, grapes, red wine, tea, chocolate, tomatoes
Isoflavones	Soybeans, other legumes
Catechins	Tea
Ellagic acid	Strawberries, raspberries, grapes, apples, bananas, nuts
Anthocyanosides	Red, blue, and purple plants (eggplant, blueberries)
Fructooligosaccharides	Onions, bananas, oranges (small amounts)
Resveratrol	Grapes, peanuts, red wine

Some related compounds under study are found in animal products, such as sphingolipids (meat and dairy products) and conjugated linoleic acid (meat and cheese). These are not phytochemicals per se because they are not from plant sources, but they have been shown to have health benefits.

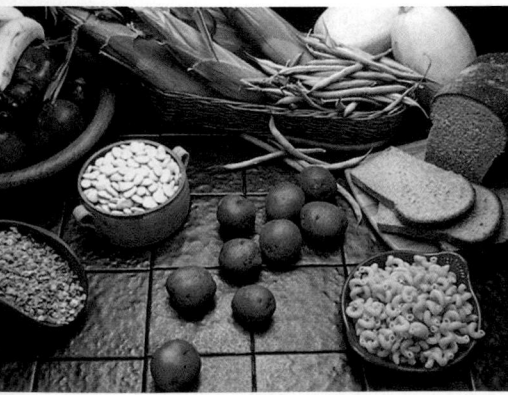

Fruits, vegetables, beans, and whole-grain breads and cereals are typically rich in phytochemicals.

some phytochemicals under study, with their common food sources. Table 2-2 provides a number of suggestions for including more phytochemicals in your diet, as does the website www.5aday.com and 5aday.nci.nih.gov.

■ Balance Means Not Overconsuming Any Single Type of Food

One way to balance your diet as you consume a variety of foods is to select foods from the six major food groups every day:

- Grains
- Vegetables
- Fruits
- Milk
- Meat & Beans
- Oils

A dinner consisting of a bean burrito, lettuce and tomato salad with oil and vinegar dressing, a glass of milk, and an apple covers all groups.

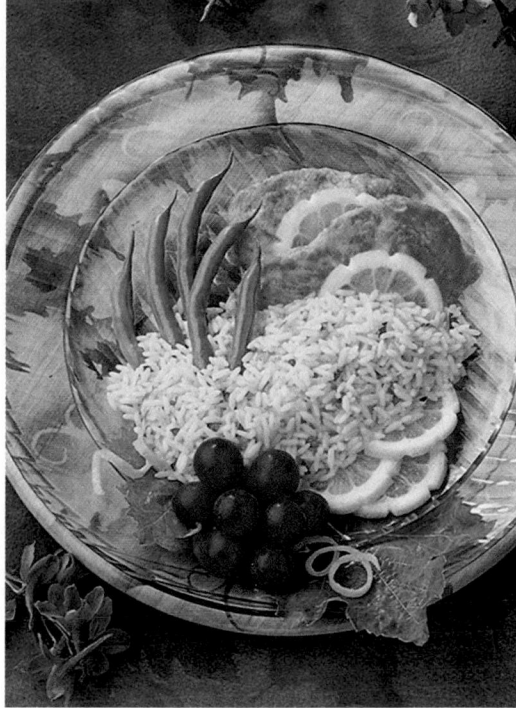

Focus on nutrient-rich foods as you strive to meet your nutrient needs. The more colorful your plate, the greater the content of nutrients and phytochemicals.

Table 2-2 Tips for Boosting the Phytochemical Content of a Diet

- Include vegetables in main and side dishes. Add these to rice, omelets, potato salad, and pastas. Try broccoli or cauliflower florets, mushrooms, peas, carrots, corn, or peppers.

- Look for quick-fixing grain side dishes in the supermarket. Pilafs, couscous, rice mixes, and tabbouleh are just a few that you'll find.

- Choose fruit-filled cookies, such as fig bars, instead of sugar-rich cookies. Use fresh or canned fruit as a topping for puddings, hot or cold cereal, pancakes, and frozen desserts.

- Put raisins, grapes, apple chunks, pineapples, grated carrots, zucchini, or cucumber into coleslaw, chicken salad, or tuna salad.

- Be creative at the salad bar: Try fresh spinach, leaf lettuce, red cabbage, zucchini, yellow squash, cauliflower, peas, mushrooms, or red or yellow peppers.

- Pack fresh or dried fruit for snacks away from home instead of grabbing a candy bar or going hungry.

- Add slices of cucumber, zucchini, spinach, or carrot slivers to the lettuce and tomato on your sandwiches.

- Try one or two vegetarian meals per week, such as beans and rice or pasta; Chinese vegetable stir fry; or spaghetti and tomato sauce.

- When daily protein intake more than meets recommended amounts, reduce the meat, fish, or poultry in casseroles, stews, and soups by one-third to one-half and add more vegetables and legumes.

- Keep a bowl of fresh vegetables in the refrigerator for snacks.

- Choose fruit or vegetable juices instead of soft drinks, and preferably 100% juice varieties.

- Substitute tea for coffee or soft drinks on a regular basis.

- Have a bowl of fruit on hand.

- Switch from crisphead lettuce to leaf lettuce, such as romaine.

- Use salsa as a dip for chips in place of creamy dips.

- Choose whole-grain breakfast cereals, breads, and crackers.

- Add flavor to your plate with ginger, rosemary, basil, thyme, garlic, onions, parsley, and chives in place of salt.

- Incorporate soy products, such as tofu, soy milk, soy protein isolate, and roasted soybeans into your meals (see Chapter 6).

Critical Thinking

Andy, described in the Real Life Scenario, would benefit from more variety in his diet. What are some practical tips he can use to increase his fruit and vegetable intake?

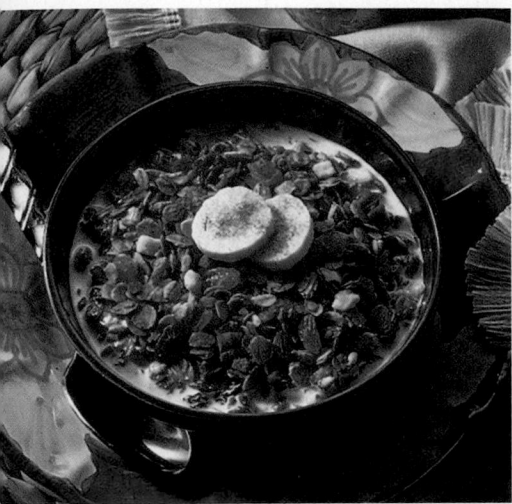

Choosing whole-grain cereals is an excellent way to increase the nutrient content of a diet. Ideally, the cereal should have at least 3 grams of fiber per serving.

nutrient density The ratio derived by dividing a food's contribution to nutrient needs by its contribution to calorie needs. When its contribution to nutrient needs exceeds its calorie contribution, the food is considered to have a favorable nutrient density.

energy density A comparison of the calorie (kcal) content of a food with the weight of the food. An energy-dense food is high in calories but weighs very little (e.g., many fried foods), whereas a food low in energy density has few calories but weighs a lot, such as an orange.

■ Moderation Refers Mostly to Portion Size

Although moderating portion size is a good practice, eating moderately also requires planning your entire day's diet so that you don't overconsume nutrient sources. For example, if you eat something relatively high in fat, salt, and calories, such as a bacon cheeseburger, you should eat other foods that are less concentrated sources of the same nutrients by incorporating foods such as fruits and salad greens at other meals that same day. This helps balance one's diet. If you prefer whole milk to low-fat or fat-free milk, reduce the fat elsewhere in your meals. Try low-fat salad dressings, or use jam rather than butter or margarine on toast. Overall, strive to simply moderate—rather than eliminate—serving sizes of some foods.

As noted in Chapter 1, many nutrition experts agree that there are no exclusively "good" or "bad" foods. Even so, many North Americans have diets that lack the foundations of a healthy food plan—variety, balance, and moderation. Consuming diets that are overloaded with foods high in fatty meats, fried foods, sugared soft drinks, and refined starches can result in substantial risk for nutrition-related chronic diseases.

■ Nutrient Density Focuses on Nutrient Content

Nutrient density has gained acceptance in recent years for assessing the nutritional quality of an individual food. To determine the nutrient density of a food, simply compare its vitamin or mineral content with the amount of calories it provides. A food is said to be nutrient dense if it provides a large amount of a nutrient for a relatively small amount of calories (compared with other food sources). The higher a food's nutrient density, the better it is as a nutrient source. Comparing the nutrient density of different foods is an easy way to estimate their relative nutritional quality. Generally, nutrient density is determined with respect to individual nutrients. For example, many fruits and vegetables have a high content of vitamin C compared with their modest calorie content: That is, they are nutrient-dense foods for vitamin C. Moreover, as Figure 2-1 shows, fat-free milk is much more nutrient dense than sugared soft drinks for many nutrients.

As noted previously, menu planning focuses mainly on the total diet—not on the selection of one critical food as key to an adequate diet. Nonetheless, nutrient-dense foods—such as fat-free and low-fat milk, lean meats, legumes (beans), oranges, carrots, broccoli, whole-wheat bread, and whole-grain breakfast cereals—do help balance less nutrient-dense foods—such as cookies and potato chips—which many people like to eat. The latter are often called empty-calorie foods because they tend to be high in sugar and/or fat but few other nutrients.

Eating nutrient-dense foods is especially important for people who tend to consume few calories. This includes some older people and those following weight-loss diets.

■ Energy (kcal) Density Especially Influences Calorie Intake

Energy density is a concept that has captured the attention of nutrition scientists in recent years. Energy density of a food is determined by comparing the calorie (kcal) content with the weight of food. A food that is rich in calories but weighs relatively little is considered energy dense. Examples include nuts, cookies, fried foods in general, and fat-free snacks, such as fat-free pretzels. Foods with low energy density include fruits, vegetables, and any food that incorporates lots of water during cooking, such as oatmeal (Table 2-3).

Researchers have shown that eating a meal with many foods of low energy density promotes satiety without contributing many calories. This is probably because we consume a constant weight of food at a meal, rather than a constant number of calories. How this constant weight of food is regulated is not known, but careful

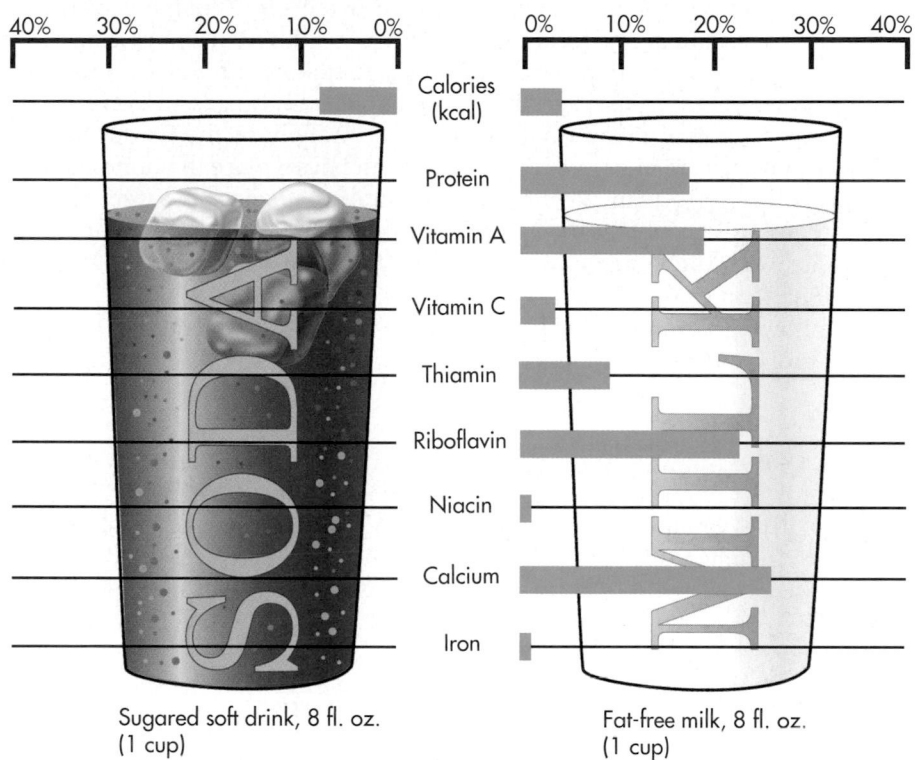

Percent Contribution to Adolescent Female RDAs

Calories (kcal)
Protein
Vitamin A
Vitamin C
Thiamin
Riboflavin
Niacin
Calcium
Iron

Sugared soft drink, 8 fl. oz. (1 cup)

Fat-free milk, 8 fl. oz. (1 cup)

Figure 2-1 Comparison of the nutrient density of a sugared soft drink with that of fat-free (i.e., nonfat or skim) milk. Choosing a glass of fat-free milk makes a significantly greater contribution to nutrient intake than does a sugared soft drink. An easy way to determine nutrient density from this chart is to compare the lengths of the bars indicating vitamin or mineral contribution with the bar that represents calorie contribution. For the soft drink, no nutrient surpasses calorie content. Fat-free milk, in contrast, has longer nutrient bars for protein, vitamin A, the vitamins thiamin and riboflavin, and the mineral calcium. Including many nutrient-dense foods in your diet is a good way to meet nutrient needs.

Table 2-3 Energy Density of Common Foods (Listed in Relative Order)

Very Low Energy Density (less than 0.6 kcal per gram)	Low Energy Density (0.6 to 1.5 kcal per gram)	Medium Energy Density (1.5 to 4 kcal per gram)	High Energy Density (greater than 4 kcal per gram)
Lettuce	Whole milk	Eggs	Graham crackers
Tomatoes	Oatmeal	Ham	Fat-free sandwich cookies
Strawberries	Cottage cheese	Pumpkin pie	Chocolate
Broccoli	Beans	Whole-wheat bread	Chocolate chip cookies
Salsa	Bananas	Bagels	Tortilla chips
Grapefruit	Broiled fish	White bread	Bacon
Fat-free milk	Fat-free yogurt	Raisins	Potato chips
Carrots	Ready-to-eat breakfast cereals with 1% low-fat milk	Cream cheese	Peanuts
Vegetable soup		Cake with frosting	Peanut butter
		Pretzels	Mayonnaise
	Plain baked potato	Rice cakes	Butter or margarine
	Cooked rice		Vegetable oils
	Spaghetti noodles		

Data adapted from Rolls B, Barnett RA: *Volumetrics*. New York: HarperCollins, 2000.

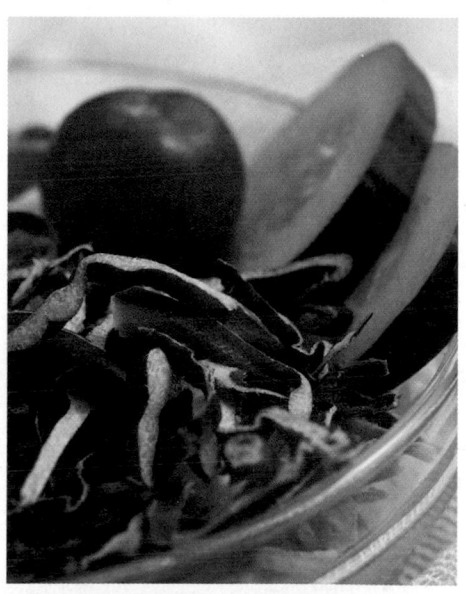

Salads are low in energy density if we limit additional calories from salad dressing, and especially minimize bacon bits, cheese crumbles or cubes, and croutons.

One more dietary strategy to consider is increased meal frequency. Eating smaller, more frequent meals and snacks provides benefits to the body—such as lower blood glucose, cholesterol, and triglycerides—since body metabolism is not as overwhelmed as is seen with large meals. In addition, fasting for much of a day may lead to overeating once eating resumes. As long as overall calorie intake remains appropriate, spreading food throughout the day is a healthy practice. One idea is to pack a lunch and consume it throughout the day, rather than all at once at noontime.

laboratory studies show that people consume fewer calories in a meal if most of the food choices are low in energy density, compared with foods high in energy density. Following a diet low in energy density can aid in losing (or maintaining) weight.

Overall, foods with lots of water and fiber provide a low-energy-density contribution to a meal and help one feel full, whereas foods with high energy density must be eaten in greater amounts in order to contribute to fullness. This is one more reason to support a diet rich in fruits, vegetables, and whole-grain breads and cereals, a pattern that also is typical of many rural ethnic diets throughout the world. Still, favorite foods, even if they are high in energy density, can have a place in your dietary pattern, but you will have to plan for them. For example, chocolate is a very energy-dense food, but a small portion at the end of a meal can supply a satisfying finale. In addition, foods with high energy density can help people with poor appetites, such as some older people, to maintain or gain weight.

The following sections of Chapter 2 describe various states of nutritional health and provide tools and nutrient guidelines for planning healthy diets to support overall health.

Concept Check

Basic diet-planning concepts include consuming a variety of foods, balancing a diet by consuming foods from each of the five food groups, and moderating portion size with each food choice, so that the diet is not excessive in calories. Choosing nutrient-dense foods, such as fat-free milk, fruits, vegetables, and whole-grain breads and cereals, helps supply a diet with many nutrients but not excessive calories. Many of these foods are also rich sources of phytochemicals, supplying an even greater health benefit to the diet. Consuming foods of low energy density, such as fruits and vegetables, may also help in weight control, in that these provide satiety after a meal because of their large weight but relatively few calories.

States of Nutritional Health

The body's nutritional health is determined by the sum of its **nutritional state** with respect to each needed nutrient. Three general categories are recognized: desirable nutrition, undernutrition, and overnutrition. Maintaining a state of desirable nutrition is the basis for establishing human nutrient needs and the diet plans to meet those needs that are discussed later in Chapter 2. The common term **malnutrition** can refer to either **overnutrition** or **undernutrition.** Neither state is conducive to good health.

■ Desirable Nutrition

The nutritional state for a particular nutrient is desirable when body tissues have enough of the nutrient to support normal metabolic functions as well as surplus stores that can be used in times of increased need. A desirable nutritional state can be achieved by obtaining essential nutrients from a variety of foods.

■ Undernutrition

Undernutrition occurs when nutrient intake does not meet nutrient needs. Any surpluses are then put to use and health begins to decline. Many nutrients are in high demand due to the constant cycles of cell loss and later regeneration in the body, such as in the gastrointestinal tract. For this reason, certain nutrient stores are exhausted rapidly, including many of the B vitamins. In turn, a regular intake is needed. In addition, some women in North America do not consume sufficient iron to meet monthly losses and eventually deplete their iron stores (Fig. 2-2).

nutritional state The nutritional health of a person as determined by anthropometric measurements (height, weight, circumferences, and so on), biochemical measurements of nutrients or their by-products in blood and urine, a clinical (physical) examination, a dietary analysis, and economic evaluation; also called nutritional status.

malnutrition Failing health that results from long-standing dietary practices that do not coincide with nutritional needs.

overnutrition A state in which nutritional intake greatly exceeds the body's needs.

undernutrition Failing health that results from a long-standing dietary intake that is not enough to meet nutritional needs.

Undernutrition   **Desirable Nutrition**   **Overnutrition**

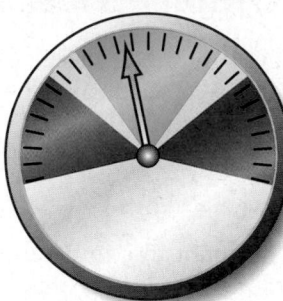

Decline in body functions associated with a decline in nutrient status. With iron deficiency, iron-containing proteins and in turn oxygen supply to body tissues is reduced. This then leads to clinical symptoms, such as fatigue upon exertion.

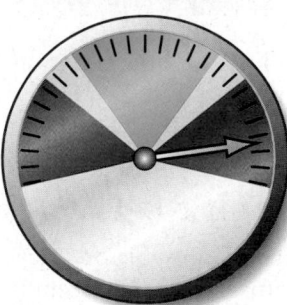

Adequate stores of nutrients, such as iron, and adequate blood values, such as for iron-related compounds.

Toxic damage to the body. In iron toxicity, liver cells in particular are affected.

Figure 2-2 The general scheme of nutritional status. Green reflects good status, yellow marginal status, and red poor status undernutrition or overnutrition. This general concept can be applied to all nutrients. Iron was chosen as an example because you are likely familiar with this nutrient and iron deficiency is the most common nutrient deficiency worldwide.

Once availability of a nutrient falls sufficiently low, biochemical evidence indicates that the body's metabolic processes have slowed or stopped. At this state of deficiency there are no outward symptoms, thus it is termed a **subclinical** deficiency. A subclinical deficiency can go on for some time before clinicians are able to detect its effects.

Eventually clinical **symptoms** will develop, sometimes taking many years, and may result in clinical evidence of a deficiency; perhaps in the skin, hair, nails, tongue, or eyes. Often, clinicians do not detect a problem until a deficiency produces outward symptoms, such as pinprick-like sites of bleeding on the skin from a vitamin C deficiency.

■ Overnutrition

Prolonged consumption of more nutrients than the body needs can lead to overnutrition. In the short run (e.g., 1 to 2 weeks), overnutrition may cause only a few symptoms, such as stomach distress from excess iron intake. But if an excess intake continues, some nutrients may accumulate to toxic amounts, which can lead to serious disease. For example, too much vitamin A can have negative effects, particularly during pregnancy.

The most common type of overnutrition in industrialized nations—excess intake of calories—often leads to obesity. In the long run, outcomes of obesity include other serious diseases, such as type 2 diabetes and certain forms of cancer. Use the website shapeup.org to learn more about the importance of lifelong weight control.

For most vitamins and minerals, the gap between desirable intake and overnutrition is wide. Therefore, even if people take a typical balanced multivitamin and mineral supplement daily, they probably won't receive a harmful dose of any nutrient. The difference between optimal intake and overnutrition is smallest for vitamin A, and the minerals calcium, iron, and copper. Thus, if you take nutrient supplements, keep a close eye on your total vitamin and mineral intake from both food and supplements to avoid toxicity (see Chapter 8 for further advice on use of nutrient supplements).

subclinical Stage of a disease or disorder that is present but not severe enough to produce symptoms that can be detected or diagnosed.

symptom A change in health status noted by the person with the problem, such as stomach pain.

How Can Your Nutritional State Be Measured?

To find out how nutritionally fit *you* are, a nutritional assessment—either whole or in part—needs to be performed (Table 2-4). Generally, this is performed by a physician, often with the aid of a registered dietitian.

Analyzing Background Factors

Since family history plays an important role in determining nutritional and health status, it must be carefully recorded and critically analyzed as part of a nutritional assessment. Other related background parameters include: (1) a medical history, especially for any disease states or treatments that could impede nutrient absorptive processes or ultimate use; (2) a list of medications taken; (3) a social history; (4) information about the person's level of education to determine the degree of complexity that can be used in written materials and oral discussions; and (5) economic status to determine the ability of the person to purchase, transport, and cook food.

Evaluating the ABCDEs

In addition to background factors, four nutritional parameters complete the picture of nutritional status. **Anthropometric assessment** measurements of height, weight (and weight changes), skinfolds, and body circumferences provide an outline of the current state of nutrition. Measures of body composition are easy to obtain and are generally reliable. However, an in-depth examination of nutritional health is impossible without the more expensive process of **biochemical assessments**. This involves the measurement of the concentrations of nutrients and nutrient by-products in the blood, urine, and feces and of specific blood enzyme activities.

A **clinical assessment** would follow, during which a health professional would search for any physical evidence (e.g., high blood pressure) of diet-related diseases. Then, a close look at the person's diet **(dietary assessment)**, including a record of at least the previous few days' intake, would look into possible problem areas. Finally, adding the **economic assessment** (from the background analysis), which impacts the ability to purchase and prepare foods needed to maintain health, provides further detail to the picture. Now the true nutritional state of a person emerges. Taken together, these five assessments form the ABCDEs of nutritional assessment: **a**nthropometric, **b**iochemical, **c**linical, **d**ietary, and **e**conomic (Fig. 2-3).

anthropometric assessment Pertaining to the measurement of body weight and the lengths, circumferences, and thicknesses of parts of the body.

biochemical assessment An assessment focusing on biochemical functions (e.g., concentrations of nutrient by-products or enzyme activities in the blood or urine) related to a nutrient's function.

clinical assessment An assessment that focuses on one's general appearance of skin, eyes, and tongue; evidence of rapid hair loss; sense of touch; and ability to cough and walk.

dietary assessment An assessment that focuses on the typical food choices of the person, relying mostly on the recounting of one's usual intake or a record of one's previous days' intake.

economic assessment An assessment that focuses on the ability of the person to purchase, transport, and cook food. The person's weekly budget for food purchases is also a key factor to consider.

Table 2-4 Conducting an Evaluation of Nutritional Health

Parameters	Example
Background	Medical history (e.g., current diseases, past surgeries, current weight, weight history, and current medications)
	Social history (marital status, cooking facilities)
	Family history
	Education attainment
	Economic status
Nutritional	Anthropometric assessment: height, weight, skinfold thickness, arm muscle circumference, and other parameters
	Biochemical (laboratory) assessment of blood and urine: enzyme activities, concentrations of nutrients or their by-products
	Clinical assessment (physical examination): general appearance of skin, eyes, and tongue; rapid hair loss; sense of touch; ability to walk
	Dietary assessment: usual intake or record of previous days' meals

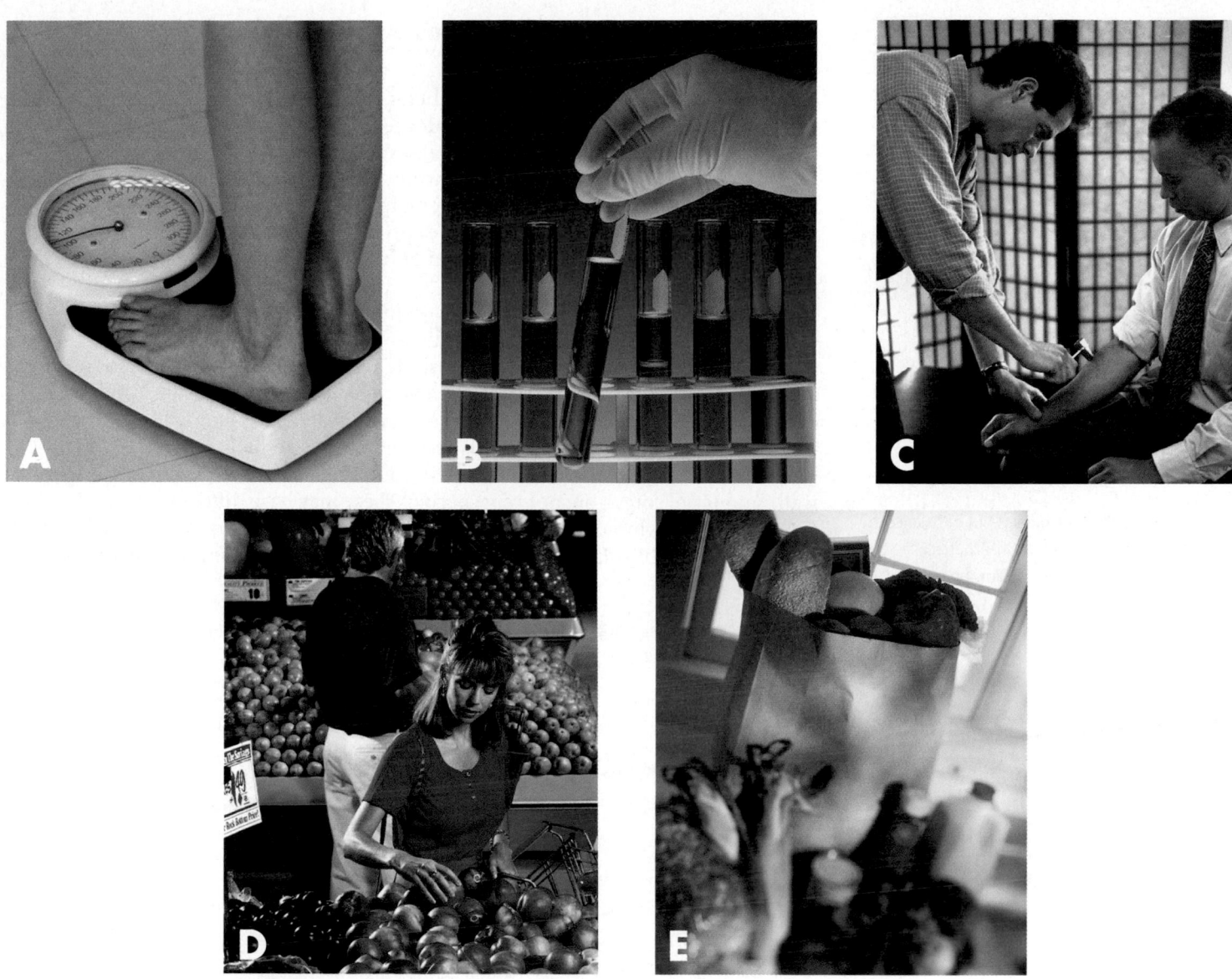

Figure 2-3 (a) Anthropometric, (b) biochemical, (c) clinical, and (d) dietary information helps determine a person's nutritional state. (e) Economic status adds further information, rounding out the ABCDEs of nutritional assessment.

Another Bite

A practical example using the ABCDEs for evaluating nutritional state can be illustrated in a person who chronically abuses alcohol. Upon evaluation, the physician notes:

(a) Low weight-for-height, recent 10 pound weight loss, muscle wasting in the upper body
(b) Low amounts of the vitamins thiamin and folate in the blood
(c) Psychological confusion, facial sores, and uncoordinated movement
(d) Dietary intake of little more than alcohol-fortified wine and hamburgers for the last week
(e) Currently residing in a homeless shelter; $35.00 in wallet; unemployed

Evaluation: This person needs professional attention, including nutrient repletion.

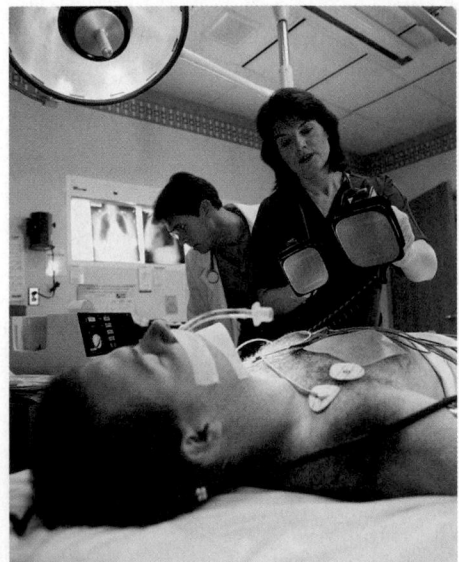

The first evidence that one's diet is out of balance with one's physiology could be a heart attack. About 25% of all heart attack victims do not survive the event.

heart attack Rapid fall in heart function caused by reduced blood flow through the heart's blood vessels. Often part of the heart dies in the process. Technically called a myocardial infarction.

∎ Recognizing the Limitations of Nutritional Assessment

As mentioned, a long time may elapse between the initial development of poor nutritional health and the first clinical evidence of a problem. Recall that a diet high in saturated (typically solid) fat often increases blood cholesterol, but without producing any clinical evidence for years. However, when the blood vessels become sufficiently blocked by cholesterol and other materials, chest pain during physical activity or a **heart attack** may occur. Much of the current nutrition research is designed to develop better methods for early detection of nutrition-related problems such as heart attack risk.

Another example of a serious health condition with delayed symptoms is low bone density resulting from a calcium deficiency—a particularly relevant issue for adolescent females. Many young women consume well below the needed amount of calcium but often suffer no ill effects in their younger years. However, the bone structures of these women with low calcium intakes do not reach full potential during the years of growth, which makes osteoporosis more likely later in life.

Furthermore, clinical symptoms of nutritional deficiencies—diarrhea, an irregular walk, and facial sores—are not very specific. These may have different causes. The long time it takes for symptoms to develop and their potential to be quite vague often make it difficult to establish a link between an individual's current diet and nutritional state.

∎ Concern about the State of Your Nutritional Health Is Important

Table 1-6 in Chapter 1 portrayed the close relationship between nutrition and health. The good news is that people who focus on maintaining nutritional health are apt to enjoy a long, vigorous life. For example, a recent study found that women who observe a healthy lifestyle experienced an 80% reduction in risk for heart attacks compared to women without such healthy practices. The healthy habits included:

- Consumed a healthy diet
  - Varied
  - Rich in fiber
  - Included some fish
  - Low in animal fat and *trans* fat
- Avoided becoming overweight
- Regularly drank a small amount of alcohol
- Exercised for at least 30 minutes daily
- Did not smoke

Should all adults follow this example (with optional use of alcohol)?

Concept Check

A desirable nutritional state results when the body has enough nutrients to function fully and contains stores to use in times of increased needs. When nutrient intake fails to meet body needs, undernutrition develops. Symptoms of such an inadequate nutrient intake can take months or years to develop. Overloading the body with nutrients, leading to overnutrition, is another potential problem to avoid. Nutritional state can be assessed by using anthropometric, biochemical, clinical, dietary, and economic assessments (ABCDEs).

Recommendations for Food Choice

The following sections of Chapter 2 will describe various guidelines for planning healthy diets.

MyPyramid—A Menu-Planning Tool

Since the early twentieth century, researchers have worked to clarify the science of nutrition into practical terms, so that people with no special training could estimate whether their nutritional needs were being met. A seven food-group plan, based on foods traditionally eaten by people in North America, was one of the first formats designed by USDA. Daily food choices had to include items from each group. This plan had been simplified by the mid-1950s to a four food-group plan: a milk group, a meat group, a fruit and vegetable group, and a bread and cereal group. In 1992 this plan was illustrated using a pyramid shape (i.e., Food Guide Pyramid).

In April 2005, USDA unveiled their latest food guide plan, MyPyramid. Entitled "Steps to a Healthier You," MyPyramid provides a more individualized approach to improving diet and lifestyle than previous food guides. Overall, MyPyramid translates the latest nutrition advice into twelve separate pyramids based on calorie needs (1000 to 3200 kcal/day). Its goal is to provide advice that will help us live longer, better, and healthier lives. (MyPyramid replaces the Food Guide Pyramid.)

The MyPyramid symbol represents the recommended proportion of foods from each food group to create a healthy diet. Physical activity is a new element in the pyramid. To get the individualized advice that is the hallmark of the plan, however, consumers need to use the website, **MyPyramid.gov.**

MyPyramid is designed to illustrate (Fig. 2-4):

- **Personalization** demonstrated at the MyPyramid website, MyPyramid.gov.
- **Gradual improvement** encouraged by the statement, "Steps to a Healthier You."
- **Physical activity** represented by the steps and the person climbing them.
- **Variety** symbolized by the six color bands representing the five food groups and oils. Foods from all groups are needed each day for good health. Orange is for grains, green is for vegetables, red is for fruits, yellow is for oils, blue is for milk and milk products, and purple is for meat & beans.
- **Proportionality,** shown by the different widths of the food group bands. The widths suggest how much food a person should choose from each group. The bands are wider for grains, vegetables, and fruits since these groups should form the bulk of one's diet. The narrowest band is for oils, indicating these should be eaten sparingly. The widths are a general guide, however, and not exact proportions. Check MyPyramid.gov for the amount right for you.
- **Moderation,** represented by the narrowing of each food group from bottom to top. The wider base is for foods with little or no solid fats, added sugars or caloric sweeteners, and salt. These should be selected more often to get the most nutrition from calories consumed.

An innovative aspect of MyPyramid is the interactive technology found on MyPyramid.gov. This includes:

MyPyramid Plan—provides a quick estimate of what and how much food the individual should eat from the different food groups based on age, gender, and activity level.

Inside MyPyramid—provides in-depth information for every food group, including recommended daily amounts in commonly used measures, such as cups and ounces, with examples and everyday tips. The section also includes recommendations for choosing healthy oils, **discretionary calories,** and physical activity. (See Another Bite on page 46 for a discussion of the concept of discretionary calories. This refers to the calories allowed from food choices rich in added sugars or solid fat. For most of us very few discretionary calories are available in daily diet planning.)

Appendix B contains the Canadian Food Guide to Healthy Eating.

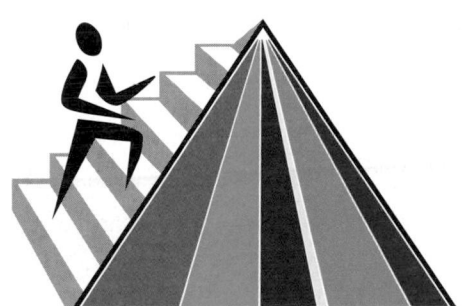

MyPyramid.gov
STEPS TO A HEALTHIER YOU

discretionary calories The calories allowed in a diet after the person has met overall nutrition need. This generally small amount of calories gives individuals the flexibility to consume some foods and beverages that may contain alcohol (e.g., beer and wine), added sugars (e.g., soft drinks, candy, and desserts), or added fats that are part of moderate- or high-fat foods (e.g., many snack foods).

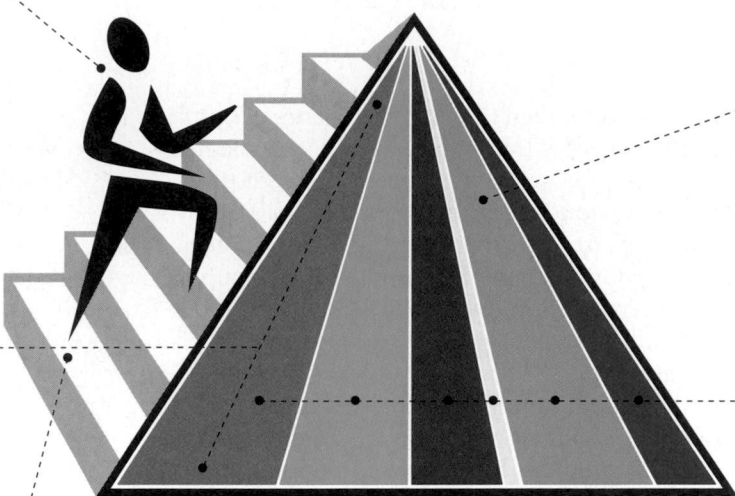

Activity
Activity is represented by the steps and the person climbing them, as a reminder of the importance of daily physical activity.

Moderation
Moderation is represented by the narrowing of each food group from bottom to top. The wider base stands for foods with little or no solid fats or added sugars. These should be selected more often. The narrower top area stands for foods containing more added sugars and solid fats. The more active you are, the more of these foods can fit into your diet.

Personalization
Personalization is shown by the person on the steps, the slogan, and the Web site. Find the kinds and amounts of food to eat each day at MyPyramid.gov.

Proportionality
Proportionality is shown by the different widths of the food group bands. The widths suggest how much food a person should choose from each group. The widths are just a general guide, not exact proportions. Check the Web site for how much is right for you.

Variety
Variety is symbolized by the 6 color bands representing the 5 food groups of the Pyramid and oils. This illustrates that foods from all groups are needed each day for good health.

Gradual Improvement
Gradual improvement is encouraged by the slogan. It suggests that individuals can benefit from taking small steps to improve their diet and lifestyle each day.

MyPyramid.gov
STEPS TO A HEALTHIER YOU

| Grains | Vegetables | Fruits | Oils | Milk | Meat & Beans |

Figure 2-4 The anatomy of MyPyramid. USDA's new MyPyramid symbolizes a personalized approach to healthy eating and physical activity. The symbol has been designed to be simple. It has been developed to remind consumers to make healthy food choices and to be active every day. In this figure, the different parts of the symbol are described.

Another Bite

Discretionary calories are estimated as follows:

Calorie Intake (kcal)	Discretionary Calories (kcal)	Calorie Intake (kcal)	Discretionary Calories (kcal)
1000	165*	2200	290
1200	171*	2400	362
1400	171*	2600	410
1600	132	2800	426
1800	195	3000	512
2000	267	3200	648

The overall intent is not to exceed this discretionary calorie allowance from the combination of foods and beverages with alcohol, added sugars, or added fats.

*The amount of discretionary calories is higher for 1000–1400 kcal diets than for a 1600 kcal diet because these lower calorie diets are intended for children 2–8 years of age. Adult calorie recommendations typically start at 1600 kcal.

MyPyramid Tracker—provides more detailed information on diet quality and physical activity status by comparing a day's worth of foods eaten to the guidance provided by MyPyramid. It allows the user to select from 8,000 foods and 600 activities. Nutrition and physical activity messages are based on the need to maintain current weight or to lose weight.

Start Today—provides tips and resources that include downloadable suggestions on all the food groups and physical activity and a worksheet to track one's diet.

Putting MyPyramid into Action

To put MyPyramid into action, first you need to estimate your calorie needs (the website helps you calculate this). Figure 2-5 provides a rough guide.

Once you have determined the calorie allowance appropriate for you, you can use Table 2.5 to discover how that calorie allowance corresponds to the recommended number of servings from each food group.

■ What Counts as One Serving?

MyPyramid provides serving sizes of foods for the various food groups in household units:

- **Grains:** 1 slice of bread, 1 cup of ready-to-eat breakfast cereal, or ½ cup cooked rice; pasta or cooked cereal counts as a 1-ounce equivalent.
- **Vegetables:** 1 cup of raw or cooked vegetables or vegetable juice or 2 cups of raw leafy greens.
- **Fruits:** 1 cup of fruit or 100% fruit juice or ½ cup of dried fruit.
- **Milk:** 1 cup of milk or yogurt, 1.5 ounces of natural cheese, or 2 ounces of processed cheese.
- **Meat & Beans:** 1 ounce of meat, poultry, or fish; 1 egg; 1 tablespoon of peanut butter; one ¼ cup cooked dry beans, or ½ ounce of nuts or seeds are all 1-ounce equivalents.

What about physical activity as part of MyPyramid? Physical activity is movement of the body that uses energy. Walking, gardening, briskly pushing a baby stroller, climbing the stairs, playing soccer, or dancing the night away are all examples of physical activity. For health benefits, physical activity should be moderate or vigorous and add up to at least 30 minutes on most or all days of the week. For weight loss or preventing weight gain, about 60 minutes a day may be needed. (The same goal applies to children and teenagers.) For maintaining prior weight loss, at least 60 to 90 minutes a day may be required.

	Calorie Range (kcal)		
Children	Sedentary	⟶	Active
2–3 years	1000	⟶	1,400
Females			
4–8 years	1200	⟶	1800
9–13	1600	⟶	2200
14–18	1800	⟶	2400
19–30	2000	⟶	2400
31–50	1800	⟶	2200
51+	1600	⟶	2200
Males			
4–8 years	1400	⟶	2000
9–13	1800	⟶	2600
14–18	2200	⟶	3200
19–30	2400	⟶	3000
31–50	2200	⟶	3000
51+	2000	⟶	2800

Sedentary means a lifestyle that includes only the light physical activity associated with typical day-to-day life.

Active means a lifestyle that includes physical activity equivalent to walking more than 3 miles per day at 3 to 4 miles per hour, in addition to the light physical activity associated with typical day-to-day life.

Figure 2-5 Estimates of calorie needs (kcals) provided by MyPyramid.

Table 2-5 MyPyramid Recommendations for Daily Amounts of Foods to Consume from the Six Food Groups Based on Calorie Needs

Daily Amount of Food From Each Group												
Calorie Level	1,000	1,200	1,400	1,600	1,800	2,000	2,200	2,400	2,600	2,800	3,000	3,200
Fruits	1 cup	1 cup	1.5 cups	1.5 cups	1.5 cups	2 cups	2 cups	2 cups	2 cups	2.5 cups	2.5 cups	2.5 cups
Vegetables[1,2]	1 cup	1.5 cups	1.5 cups	2 cups	2.5 cups	2.5 cups	3 cups	3 cups	3.5 cups	3.5 cups	4 cups	4 cups
Grains[3]	3 oz-eq	4 oz-eq	5 oz-eq	5 oz-eq	6 oz-eq	6 oz-eq	7 oz-eq	8 oz-eq	9 oz-eq	10 oz-eq	10 oz-eq	10 oz-eq
Meat & Beans	2 oz-eq	3 oz-eq	4 oz-eq	5 oz-eq	5 oz-eq	5.5 oz-eq	6 oz-eq	6.5 oz-eq	6.5 oz-eq	7 oz-eq	7 oz-eq	7 oz-eq
Milk[4]	2 cups	2 cups	2 cups	3 cups	3 cups	3 cups	3 cups	3 cups	3 cups	3 cups	3 cups	3 cups
Oils[5]	3 tsp	4 tsp	4 tsp	5 tsp	5 tsp	6 tsp	6 tsp	7 tsp	8 tsp	8 tsp	10 tsp	11 tsp
Discretionary calorie allowance[6]	165	171	171	132	195	267	290	362	410	426	512	648

oz-eq stands for ounce equivalent; tsp stands for teaspoon

[1]Vegetables are divided into five subgroups (dark green, orange, legumes, starchy, and other). Over a week's time, a variety of vegetables should be eaten, especially green and orange vegetables.

[2]Dry beans and peas can be counted *either* as vegetables (dry beans and peas subgroup), *or* in the meat & beans group. Generally, individuals who regularly eat meat, poultry, and fish would count dry beans and peas in the vegetable group. Individuals who seldom eat meat, poultry, or fish (vegetarians) would consume more dry beans and peas and count some of them in the meat & beans group until enough servings from that group are chosen for the day.

[3]At least half of these servings should be whole grain varieties.

[4]Most of these servings should be fat-free or low-fat.

[5]Limit solid fats such as butter, stick margarine, shortening, and meat fat, as well as foods that contain these.

[6]Discretionary calories refers to food choices rich in added sugars or solid fat.

Pay close attention to the stated serving size for each choice when following MyPyramid. This aids in controlling total calorie intake. See Figure 2-6 for a convenient guide to estimating common household measures. Note that serving sizes listed for one serving in a MyPyramid group or on a food label are often less than is typically served in restaurants today.

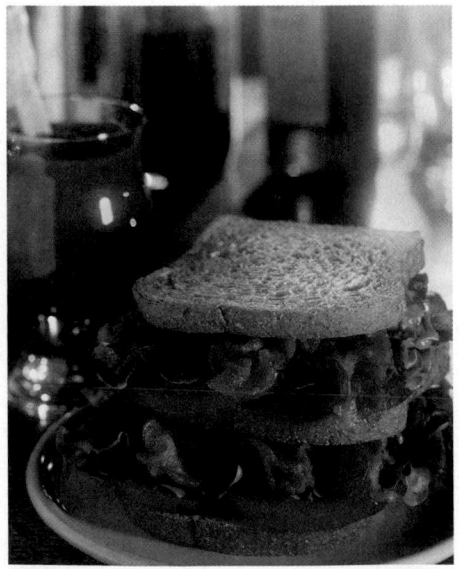

Typical restaurant portions contain numerous servings from the individual groups in MyPyramid.

- **Oils:** A teaspoon of any oil from plants or fish that is liquid at room temperature counts as a serving, as do such servings of foods rich in oils (e.g., mayonnaise and soft margarine).

Menu Planning with MyPyramid

Remember the following points when using MyPyramid to plan your daily menus:

1. The guide does not apply to infants or children under 2 years of age.
2. No one food is absolutely essential to good nutrition. Each food is rich in some nutrients, but deficient in at least one essential nutrient (Table 2-6).
3. No one food group provides all essential nutrients in adequate amounts. Each food group makes an important, distinctive contribution to nutritional intake.
4. Variety is the key to success of MyPyramid and is first guaranteed by choosing foods from all the groups. Furthermore, one should consume a variety of foods within each group, except possibly in the milk, yogurt, and cheese group.
5. The foods within a group may vary widely with respect to nutrients and calories. For example, the calorie content of 3 ounces of baked potato is 98 kcal, whereas that of 3 ounces of potato chips is 470 kcal. Compare an orange and an apple with respect to vitamin C using the food composition table in Appendix J.

Overall, MyPyramid incorporates the foundations of a healthy diet: variety, balance, and moderation. The nutritional adequacy of diets planned using this tool, however, depends on selection of a variety of foods (Table 2-7). In addition, to ensure enough vitamin E, vitamin B-6, magnesium, and zinc—nutrients sometimes low in diets based on this plan—consider the following advice:

1. Choose primarily low-fat and fat-free items from the milk group. By reducing calorie intake in this way, you can select more items from other food groups. If milk causes intestinal gas and bloating, emphasize yogurt and cheese (see Chapter 4 for details on the problem of lactose maldigestion and lactose intolerance).

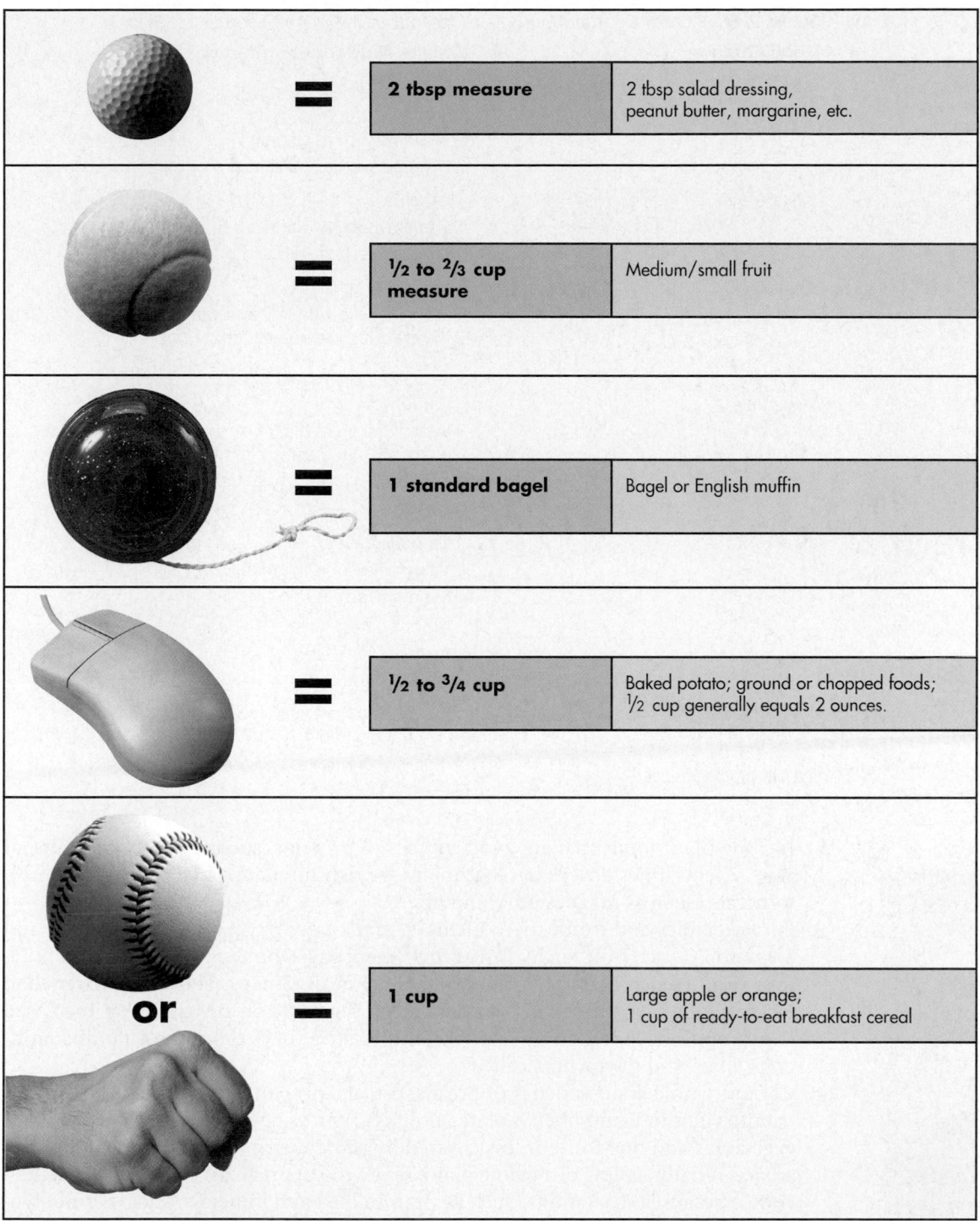

=	**2 tbsp measure**	2 tbsp salad dressing, peanut butter, margarine, etc.
=	**¹/₂ to ²/₃ cup measure**	Medium/small fruit
=	**1 standard bagel**	Bagel or English muffin
=	**¹/₂ to ³/₄ cup**	Baked potato; ground or chopped foods; ¹/₂ cup generally equals 2 ounces.
=	**1 cup**	Large apple or orange; 1 cup of ready-to-eat breakfast cereal

Figure 2-6 A golf ball, tennis ball, small yo-yo, computer mouse, baseball, and fist make convenient guides to judge MyPyramid serving sizes. Additional handy guides include:

thumb = 1 oz of cheese;
4 stacked dice = 1 oz cheese;
thumb tip to first joint = 1 tsp;
matchbox = 1 oz meat;
bar of soap or deck of
  cards = 3 oz meat;

palm of a hand = 3 oz;
1 ice cream scoop = ½ cup;
handful = 1 or 2 oz of a
  snack food; and
ping-pong ball = 2 tbsp.

Table 2-6 Nutrient Contributions of Groups in the MyPyramid Food Guide Plan

Food Category	Major Nutrient Contributions
Milk	Carbohydrate Protein Vitamins such as vitamin D Minerals such as calcium and phosphorus
Meat & Beans	Protein Vitamins such as vitamin B-6 Minerals such as iron and zinc
Fruits	Carbohydrate Vitamins such as folate and vitamin C Minerals such as potassium Fiber
Vegetables	Carbohydrate Vitamins such as plant pigments that form vitamin A Minerals such as magnesium Fiber
Grains	Carbohydrate Vitamins such as thiamin Minerals such as iron Fiber†
Oils	Fat Essential fatty acids Vitamins such as vitamin E

*Whole-grain varieties

2. Include plant foods that are good sources of proteins, such as beans and nuts, at least several times a week because many are rich in vitamins (such as vitamin E), minerals (such as magnesium), and fiber.
3. For vegetables and fruits, try to include a dark green vegetable for vitamin A and a vitamin C–rich fruit, such as an orange, every day. Don't focus primarily on potatoes (e.g., French fries) for your vegetable choices. Surveys show that fewer than 5% of adults eat a full serving of a dark green vegetable on any given day. Increased consumption of these foods is important because they contribute vitamins, minerals, fiber, and phytochemicals.
4. Choose whole-grain varieties of breads, cereals, rice, and pasta because they contribute vitamin E and fiber. A plate about two-thirds covered by grains, fruits, and vegetables and one-third or less covered by protein-rich foods promotes this diet advice. A daily serving of a whole-grain, ready-to-eat breakfast cereal is an excellent choice because the vitamins (such as vitamin B-6) and minerals (such as zinc) typically added to it, along with fiber, help fill in the potential gaps listed earlier.
5. Include some plant oils on a daily basis, such as those in salad dressing, and eat fish at least twice a week. This supplies you with health-promoting essential fatty acids.

How Does Your Current Diet Rate?

Regularly comparing your daily food intake with MyPyramid recommendations for your age, gender, and degree of physical activity, is a relatively simple way to evaluate your overall diet. Strive to meet the recommendations. (The diets of most adults fail in this evaluation, especially with respect to milk, vegetables, fruits, and whole grain breads and cereals.) If that is not possible, identify the nutrients that are low in your diet based on the nutrients found in each food group (review Table 2-6).

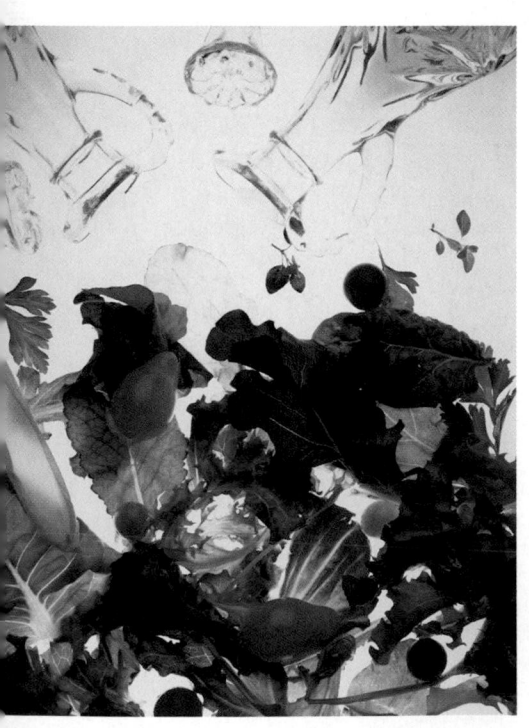

Leafy green vegetables contribute many nutrients to a diet.

Table 2-7 Putting the MyPyramid into Practice

Meal	Food Group
Breakfast	
1 small orange	Fruits
¾ cup Healthy Choice Low-fat Granola	Grains
with ½ cup fat-free milk	Milk
½ toasted, small raisin bagel	Grains
with 1 tsp soft margarine	Oils
Optional: coffee or tea	
Lunch	
Turkey sandwich	
2 slices whole-wheat bread	Grains
2 oz turkey	Meat & Beans
2 tsp mustard	
1 small apple	Fruits
2 oatmeal-raisin cookies (small)	Discretionary calories
Optional: diet soft drink	
3 P.M. Study Break	
6 whole-wheat crackers	Grains
1 tbsp peanut butter	Meat & Beans
½ cup fat-free milk	Milk
Dinner	
Tossed salad	
1 cup romaine lettuce	Vegetables
½ cup sliced tomatoes	Vegetables
1½ tbsp Italian dressing	Oils
½ carrot, grated	Vegetables
3 oz broiled salmon	Meat & Beans
½ cup rice	Grains
½ cup green beans	Vegetables
with 1 tsp soft margarine	Oils
Optional: coffee or tea	
Late-Night Snack	
1 cup "light" fruit yogurt	Milk
Nutrient Breakdown	
1800 kcal	
Carbohydrate	56% of kcal
Protein	18% of kcal
Fat	26% of kcal

This menu meets nutrient needs for all vitamins and minerals for an average adult. For adolescents, teenagers, and older adults add one additional serving of milk or other calcium-rich sources.

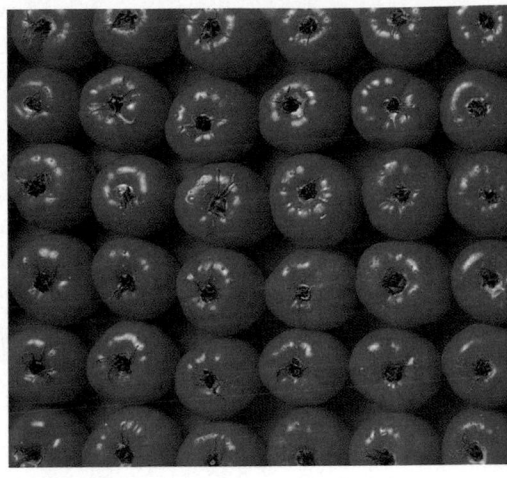

Tomatoes are a rich source of nutrients and phytochemicals.

For example, if you do not consume enough servings from the milk group, your calcium intake is most likely too low. You need to then find foods that you enjoy that supply calcium, such as calcium-fortified orange juice. Customizing MyPyramid to accommodate your food habits may seem a daunting task, but it is not difficult once you gain some additional nutrition knowledge.

Get Going

Start putting MyPyramid into practice and use the MyTracker feature to follow your progress. Implementing even small diet and exercise changes can have positive results. Better health will likely follow as you strive to meet your nutrient needs and balance your physical activity and calorie allowance. In addition, follow the guidance from the **2005 Dietary Guidelines for Americans** regarding alcohol and sodium intake, and safe food preparation.

Dietary Guidelines for Americans
General goals for nutrient intakes and diet composition set by the USDA and the U.S. Department of Health and Human Services.

Concept Check

MyPyramid translates the general needs for carbohydrate, protein, fat, vitamins, and minerals into the recommended number of daily servings from each of five major food groups and oils. It is a convenient and valuable tool for planning daily menus.

Appendix B contains nutrient guidelines for Canadians.

■ Dietary Guidelines—Another Tool for Menu Planning

MyPyramid was designed to help meet nutritional needs for carbohydrate, protein, fat, vitamins, and minerals. However, most of the major chronic "killer" diseases in North America, such as cardiovascular disease, cancer, and alcoholism, are not primarily associated with deficiencies of these nutrients. Deficiency diseases such as scurvy (vitamin C deficiency) and pellagra (niacin deficiency) are no longer common. For many North Americans, the primary dietary culprit is an overconsumption of one or more of the following: calories, saturated fat, cholesterol, *trans* fat, alcohol, and sodium (salt). (Underconsumption of calcium, iron, folate and other B-vitamins, vitamin C, vitamin D, vitamin E, potassium, magnesium, and fiber is also a problem for some people.)

In response to concerns regarding these killer disease patterns, since 1980 the USDA and U.S. Department of Health and Human Services (DHHS) have published Dietary Guidelines for Americans (Dietary Guidelines for short) to aid diet planning.

Compared to past reports, the 2005 Dietary Guidelines for Americans places stronger emphasis on monitoring one's calorie intake and increasing physical activity. This is because more of us are becoming overweight each year.

The report identifies forty-one key recommendations, of which twenty-three are for the general public and eighteen are for special populations. They are grouped into nine general topics:

- Adequate Nutrient Intake Within Calorie Needs
- Weight Management
- Physical Activity
- Specific Food Groups to Encourage
- Fats
- Carbohydrates
- Sodium and Potassium
- Alcoholic Beverages
- Food Safety

Table 2-8 lists the key recommendations within each general topic. The advice provided refers to people two years and older.

- Consume a variety of nutrient-dense foods and beverages within and among the basic food groups of MyPyramid, while choosing foods that limit the intake of saturated and *trans* fats, cholesterol, added sugars, salt, and alcohol (if used). Foods to emphasize are vegetables, fruits, legumes (beans), whole grains, and fat-free or low-fat milk or equivalent milk products.
- Maintain body weight in a healthy range by balancing calorie intake from foods and beverages with calories expended. For the latter, engage in at least 30 minutes of moderate-intensity physical activity, above usual activity, at work or home on most days of the week.
- Practice safe food handling when preparing food. This includes cleaning hands, food contact surfaces, and fruits and vegetables before preparation and cooking foods to a safe temperature to kill microorganisms.

Table 2-8 Key Recommendations Within Each General Topic from the Latest Dietary Guidelines for Americans

Adequate Nutrients Within Calorie Needs

- Consume a variety of nutrient-dense foods and beverages within and among the basic food groups while choosing foods that limit the intake of saturated and *trans* fats, cholesterol, added sugars, salt, and alcohol.
- Meet recommended intakes within calorie needs by adopting a balanced eating pattern, such as MyPyramid.

Key Recommendations for Specific Population Groups

- *People over age 50.* Consume vitamin B-12 in its crystalline form (i.e., fortified foods or supplements).
- *Women of childbearing age who may become pregnant.* Eat foods high in iron from animal products and/or consume iron-rich plant foods or iron-fortified foods with an enhancer of iron absorption, such as vitamin C-rich foods.
- *Women of childbearing age who may become pregnant and those in the first few months of pregnancy.* Consume adequate amount of the synthetic form of the B vitamin folate (called folic acid) daily (from fortified foods or supplements) in addition to food forms of folate found in a varied diet.
- *Older adults, people with dark skin, and people exposed to insufficient ultraviolet band radiation (i.e., sunlight).* Consume extra vitamin D from vitamin D-fortified foods and/or supplements.

Weight Management

- To maintain body weight in a healthy range, balance calorie intake from foods and beverages with calories expended.
- To prevent gradual weight gain over time, make small decreases in calorie intake from food and beverages and increase physical activity.

Key Recommendations for Specific Population Groups

- *Those who need to lose weight.* Aim for a slow, steady weight loss by decreasing calorie intake while maintaining an adequate nutrient intake and increasing physical activity.
- *Overweight children.* Reduce the rate of body weight gain while allowing for growth and development. Consult a healthcare provider before placing a child on a weight-reduction diet.
- *Pregnant women.* Ensure appropriate weight gain as specified by a healthcare provider.
- *Breastfeeding women.* Moderate weight reduction is safe and does not compromise weight gain of the nursing infant.
- *Overweight adults and overweight children with chronic diseases and/or on medication.* Consult a healthcare provider about weight loss strategies prior to starting a weight-reduction program to ensure appropriate management of other health conditions.

Physical Activity

- Engage in regular physical activity and reduce sedentary activities to promote health, psychological well-being, and a healthy body weight.
- To reduce the risk of chronic disease in adulthood, engage in at least 30 minutes of moderate-intensity physical activity, above usual activity, at work or home on most days of the week.
- For most people, greater health benefits can be obtained by engaging in physical activity of more vigorous intensity or longer duration.

(continued)

Table 2-8 (*continued*)

- To help manage body weight and prevent gradual, unhealthy body weight gain in adulthood, engage in approximately 60 minutes of moderate- to vigorous-intensity activity on most days of the week while not exceeding calorie needs.
- To sustain weight loss in adulthood, participate in at least 60 to 90 minutes of daily moderate-intensity physical activity while not exceeding calorie needs. Some people (men over 40 years of age and women over 50 years of age) may need to consult with a healthcare provider before participating in this level of activity.
- Achieve physical fitness by including cardiovascular conditioning, stretching exercises for flexibility, and resistance exercises or calisthenics for muscle strength and endurance.

Key Recommendations for Specific Population Groups

- *Children and adolescents.* Engage in at least 60 minutes of physical activity on most, preferably all, days of the week.
- *Pregnant women.* In the absence of medical complications, incorporate 30 minutes or more of moderate-intensity physical activity on most, if not all, days of the week. Avoid activities with a high risk of falling or abdominal trauma.
- *Breastfeeding women.* Be aware that neither acute nor regular exercise adversely affects the mother's ability to successfully breastfeed.
- *Older adults.* Participate in regular physical activity to reduce functional declines associated with aging and to achieve the other benefits of physical activity identified for all adults.

Food Groups to Encourage

- Consume a sufficient amount of fruits and vegetables while staying within calorie needs. Two cups of fruit and 2 1/2 cups of vegetables per day are recommended for a reference 2,000 kcal intake, with higher or lower amounts depending on one's calorie needs.
- Choose a variety of fruits and vegetables each day. In particular, select from all five vegetable subgroups several times a week.
- Consume three or more ounce-equivalents of whole-grain products per day, with the rest of the recommended grains coming from enriched or whole-grain products. In general, at least half the grains should come from whole grains.
- Consume 3 cups per day of fat-free or low-fat milk or equivalent milk products.

Key Recommendations for Specific Population Groups

- *Children and adolescents.* Consume whole-grain products often; at least half the grains should be whole grains. Children 2 to 8 years should consume 2 cups per day of fat-free or low-fat milk or equivalent milk products. Children 9 years of age and older should consume 3 cups per day of fat-free or low-fat milk or equivalent milk products.

Fats

- Consume less than 10 percent of calorie intake from saturated fatty acids and less than 300 milligrams per day of cholesterol, and keep *trans* fatty acid consumption as low as possible.
- Keep total fat intake between 20 to 35 percent of calorie intake, with most fats coming from sources of polyunsaturated and monosaturated fatty acids, such as fish, nuts, and vegetable oils.
- When selecting and preparing meat, poultry, dry beans, and milk or milk products, make choices that are lean, low-fat, or fat-free.
- Limit intake of fats and oils high in saturated and/or *trans* fatty acids, and choose products low in such fats and oils.

Key Recommendations for Specific Population Groups

- *Children and adolescents.* Keep total fat intake between 30 to 35 percent of calorie intake for children 2 to 3 years of age and between 25 to 35 percent of calorie intake for children and adolescents 4 to 18 years of age, with most fats coming from sources of polyunsaturated and monosaturated fatty acids, such as fish, nuts, and vegetable oils.

Carbohydrates

- Choose fiber-rich fruits, vegetables, and whole grains often.
- Choose and prepare foods and beverages with little added sugars or caloric sweeteners, such as amounts suggested by MyPyramid.
- Reduce the incidence of dental caries by practicing good oral hygiene and consuming sugar- and starch-containing foods and beverages less frequently.

Table 2-8 (continued)

Sodium and Potassium

- Consume less than 2,300 milligrams of sodium per day (approximately 1 tsp of salt).
- Choose and prepare foods with little salt. At the same time, consume potassium-rich foods, such as fruits and vegetables.

Key Recommendations for Specific Population Groups

- *Individuals with hypertension, blacks, and middle-aged and older adults.* Aim to consume no more than 1,500 milligrams of sodium per day, and meet the potassium recommendation (4,700 milligrams per day) with food.

Alcoholic Beverages

- Those who choose to drink alcoholic beverages should do so sensibly and in moderation—up to one drink per day for women and up to two drinks per day for men (12 ounces of a regular beer, 5 ounces of wine or 1-1/2 ounces of 80 proof distilled spirits count as one drink for purposes of explaining moderation.)
- Alcoholic beverages should not be consumed by some individuals, including those who cannot restrict their alcohol intake, women of childbearing age who may become pregnant, pregnant and lactating women, children and adolescents, individuals taking medications that may interact with alcohol, and those with specific medical conditions.
- Alcoholic beverages should be avoided by individuals engaging in activities that require attention; skill; or coordination, such as driving or operating machinery.

Food Safety

To avoid microbial foodborne illness:
- Clean hands, food contact surfaces, and fruits and vegetables. Meat and poultry should *not* be washed or rinsed to avoid spreading bacteria to other foods.
- Separate raw, cooked, and ready-to-eat foods while shopping, preparing, or storing foods.
- Cook foods to a safe temperature to kill microorganisms.
- Refrigerate perishable food promptly and defrost foods properly.
- Avoid unpasteurized milk or any products made from unpasteurized milk, raw or partially cooked eggs or foods containing raw eggs, or raw or undercooked meat and poultry, unpasteurized juices, and raw sprouts.

Key Recommendations for Specific Population Groups

- *Infants and young children, pregnant women, older adults, and those who are immunocompromised.* Do not eat or drink unpasteurized milk or any products made from unpasteurized milk, raw or partially cooked eggs or foods containing raw eggs, raw or undercooked meat and poultry, raw or undercooked fish or shellfish, unpasteurized juices, and raw sprouts.
- *Pregnant women, older adults, and those who are immunocompromised:* Only eat certain deli meats and frankfurters that have been reheated to steaming hot.

A basic premise of the Dietary Guidelines is that nutrient needs should be met primarily through consuming foods. Foods provide an array of nutrients and other compounds that may have beneficial effects on health. Fortified foods and dietary supplements, however, are especially important for people whose typical food choices cannot meet one or more nutrient recommendations, such as for vitamin E or calcium. However, dietary supplements are not a substitute for a healthful diet.

The 2005 Dietary Guidelines for Americans (and the consumer brochure) are available at www.healthierus.gov/dietaryguidelines.

A brochure designed for the public based on the 2005 Dietary Guidelines for Americans is entitled "Finding Your Way to a Healthier You." It communicates the major themes of the *2005 Dietary Guidelines for Americans,* but uses simpler message(s).

Practical Use of the Dietary Guidelines

The Dietary Guidelines are designed to meet nutrient needs while reducing the risk of obesity, hypertension, cardiovascular disease, type 2 diabetes, alcoholism, and foodborne illness.

The Dietary Guidelines are not difficult to implement (Table 2-9). Despite popular misconceptions, this overall diet approach is not especially expensive. Fruits, vegetables, and low-fat and fat-free milk are no more expensive than the chips, cookies, and sugared soft drinks they should in part replace.

Table 2-9 Recommended Diet Changes Based on the Dietary Guidelines

If You Usually Eat This,	Try This Instead	Benefit
White bread	Whole-wheat bread	• Higher nutrient density, due to less processing • More fiber
Sugary breakfast cereal	Low-sugar, high-fiber cereal with fresh fruit	• Higher nutrient density • More fiber • More phytochemicals
Cheeseburger with French fries	Hamburger and baked beans	• Less saturated fat and *trans* fat • Less cholesterol • More fiber • More phytochemicals
Potato salad	Three-bean salad	• More fiber • More phytochemicals
Doughnuts	Bran muffin/bagel with light cream cheese	• More fiber • Less fat
Regular soft drinks	Diet soft drinks	• Fewer calories
Boiled vegetables	Steamed vegetables	• Higher nutrient density, due to reduced loss of water-soluble vitamins
Canned vegetables	Fresh or frozen vegetables	• Higher nutrient density, due to reduced loss of heat-sensitive vitamins • Lower in sodium
Fried meats	Broiled meats	• Less saturated fat
Fatty meats, such as ribs or bacon	Lean meats, such as ground round, chicken, or fish	• Less saturated fat
Whole milk	Low-fat or fat-free milk	• Less saturated fat • Fewer calories • More calcium
Ice cream	Sherbet or frozen yogurt	• Less saturated fat • Fewer calories
Mayonnaise or sour cream salad dressing	Oil and vinegar dressings or light creamy dressings	• Less saturated fat • Less cholesterol • Fewer calories
Cookies	Popcorn (air popped with minimal margarine or butter)	• Fewer calories and *trans* fat
Heavily salted foods	Foods flavored primarily with herbs, spices, lemon juice	• Lower in sodium
Chips	Pretzels	• Less fat

Critical Thinking

Shannon has grown up eating the typical American diet. Having recently read and heard many media reports about the relationship between nutrition and health, she is beginning to look critically at her diet and is considering making changes. However, she doesn't know where to begin. What advice would you give her?

Note also that diet recommendations for adults have been issued by other scientific groups, such as the American Heart Association, U.S. Surgeon General, National Academy of Sciences, American Cancer Society, Canadian Ministries of Health (see Appendix B), and World Health Organization. All are consistent with the spirit of the Dietary Guidelines. These groups encourage people to modify their eating behavior in ways that are both healthful and pleasurable.

The Dietary Guidelines and You

When using the Dietary Guidelines, you should consider your own state of health. Make specific changes and see whether they are effective. Note that results are sometimes disappointing, even when you are following a diet change very closely. Some people can eat a lot of saturated fat and still keep blood cholesterol under control. Other people, unfortunately, have high blood cholesterol even if they eat a diet low in saturated fat. Differences in genetic background are a key cause, as you will learn in Chapter 3. Thus, we have individual nutritional needs and risks of developing certain diseases. One's diet should be planned with this individuality in mind, taking into account when possible, one's current health status and family history for specific diseases. However, tailoring a unique nutrition program for every North American citizen is currently unrealistic. MyPyramid and the 2005 Dietary Guidelines provide typical adults with simple advice, which can be actively practiced by anyone willing to take a step toward good health.

There is no "optimal" diet. Instead, there are numerous healthful diets. Visit the website of the International Food Information Council (*ific.org*). This site is a great resource for current nutrition information.

Advice from the American Dietetic Association suggests five basic principles with regard to diet and health.

- Be realistic, making small changes over time.
- Be adventurous, trying new foods regularly.
- Be flexible, balancing some sweet and fatty foods with physical activity.
- Be sensible, including favorite foods in smaller portions.
- Finally, be active, including physical activity in daily life.

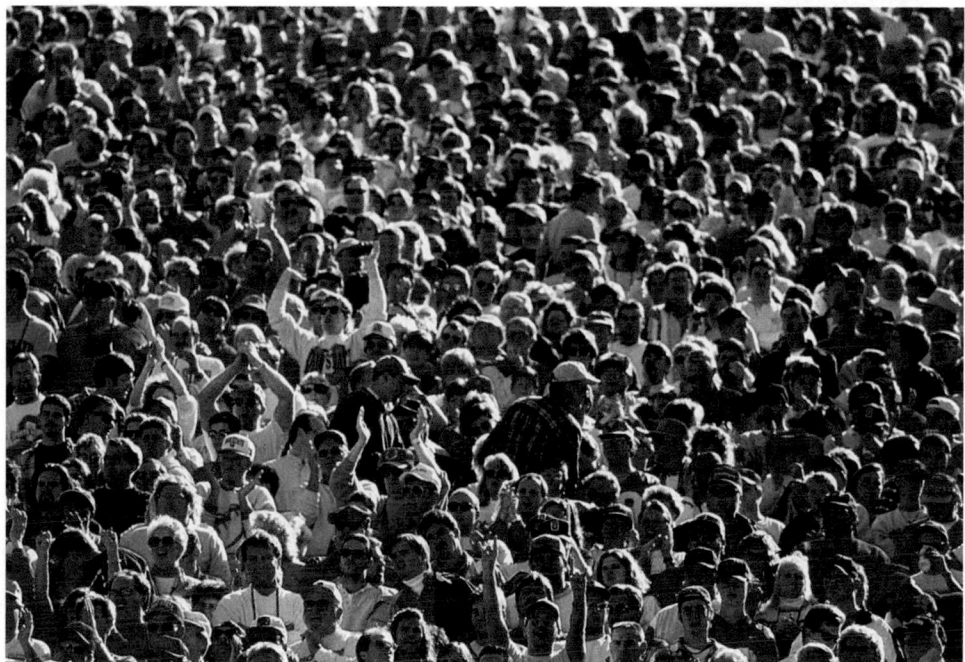

Nutrition recommendations are often made on a population-wide basis. However, in some cases, it would be more appropriate if these were made on an individual basis once a person's particular health status is known.

Concept Check

Dietary Guidelines for Americans have been set by government organizations. These guidelines are designed to reduce the risk of developing obesity, hypertension, type 2 diabetes, cardiovascular disease, alcoholism, and foodborne illness. To do so, they recommend eating a variety of foods, which is fostered by following MyPyramid. They also recommend performing regular physical activity, aiming for a healthy weight, and moderating total fat, saturated fat, *trans* fat, salt, sugar, and alcohol intake, while focusing more on fruits, vegetables, and whole-grain products in daily menu planning. Safe food preparation and storage are also highlighted.

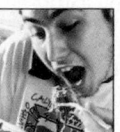

Real Life Scenario Follow-Up

The most positive aspect of Andy's diet is that it contains adequate protein, zinc, and iron because it is rich in animal protein. On the downside, his diet is low in calcium, some B vitamins (such as folate), and vitamin C. This is because it is low in dairy products, fruits, and vegetables. It is also low in many of the phytochemical (plant-based) substances discussed at the beginning of Chapter 2. In addition, his fiber intake is low because fast-food restaurants primarily use refined grain products, rather than whole-grain products. And, since most super-sized options apply to foods rich in fat (French fries) and sugar (soft drinks), his diet is likely excessive in these two components.

He could alternate between tacos and bean burritos to gain the benefits of plant proteins in a diet. He could choose a low-fat granola bar instead of the candy bar for breakfast, or he could take the time to eat a bowl of whole-grain breakfast cereal with low-fat or fat-free milk to increase fiber intake (and calcium intake as well in the latter case). He could also order milk at least half the time at his restaurant visits and substitute diet soft drinks for the regular variety. This would help *moderate* his sugar intake. Overall, Andy could improve his intake of fruits, vegetables, and dairy products if he focused more on variety in food choice and balance among the food groups.

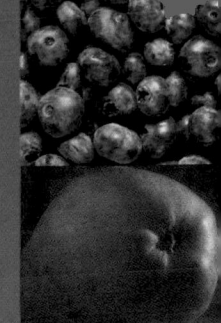
The overarching goal of any healthy diet plan is to meet nutrient needs. To begin, we must determine what amount of each essential nutrient is needed to maintain health. The standards that have been developed for such nutrient needs—DRI, RDA, AI, EER, and UL—can often seem like an alphabet soup of abbreviations. However, you can more easily sift through these nutrient standards if you have a knowledge base about their development and use (Table 2-10).

The ABCs of Nutrient Recommendations

Most of the terms that describe nutrient needs fall under one umbrella term—**Dietary Reference Intakes (DRIs).** The development of DRIs is an ongoing, collaborative effort between Health Canada and the Food and Nutrition Board of the Institute of Medicine in the United States. Included under the DRI umbrella are **Recommended Dietary Allowances (RDAs), Adequate Intakes (AIs), Estimated Energy Requirements (EERs),** and **Tolerable Upper Intake Levels (Upper Levels or ULs).**

■ Recommended Dietary Allowance

A Recommended Dietary Allowance (RDA) is based on meeting the needs of nearly all individuals (about 97%) in a particular age and gender group. A person can compare his or her individual intake of specific nutrients to the RDA. Although an intake slightly above or below the RDA for a particular nutrient is no reason for concern, a significant deviation below (about 70%) or above (about three times or more for some nutrients) the RDA over an extended period of time can eventually result in a deficiency or toxicity of that nutrient, respectively.

A nutrition standard more relevant to everyday life is the Daily Value (DV). This is a generic standard used on food labels. It is applicable to both genders from 4 years of age through adulthood, and is based on a 2000 kcal diet. DVs are mostly set at or close to the highest RDA value or related nutrient standard seen in the various age and gender categories for a specific nutrient (see Appendix A). DVs have been set for vitamins, minerals, protein, and other dietary components. DVs allow consumers to compare their intake from a specific food to desirable (or maximum) intakes.

Table 2-10 Putting the Alphabet Soup of Nutrient Needs to Use

RDA	Recommended Dietary Allowance. Use to evaluate your current intake for a specific nutrient. The further you stray above or below this value, the greater your chances of developing nutritional problems.
AI	Adequate Intake. Use to evaluate your current intake of nutrients, but realize that an AI designation implies that further research is required before scientists can establish a more definitive number.
EER	Estimated Energy Requirement. Use to estimate calorie needs of the average person within a specific height, weight, gender, age, and physical activity pattern.
UL	Upper Level. Use to evaluate the highest amount of daily nutrient intake that is unlikely to cause adverse health effects in the long run in almost all people (97% to 98%) in a population. This number applies to chronic use and is set to protect even very susceptible people in the healthy general population. As intake increases above the Upper Level, the potential for adverse effects generally increases.
DV	Daily Value. Use as a rough guide for comparing the nutrient content of a food to approximate human needs. Typically, the Daily Value used on food labels refers to ages 4 years through adulthood. It is based on a 2000 kcal diet. Some Daily Values also increase slightly with higher calorie intakes (see Fig. 2-8 in the following section on food labeling).

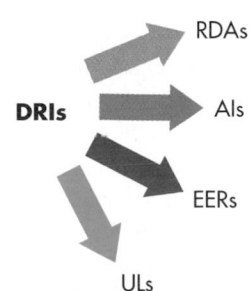

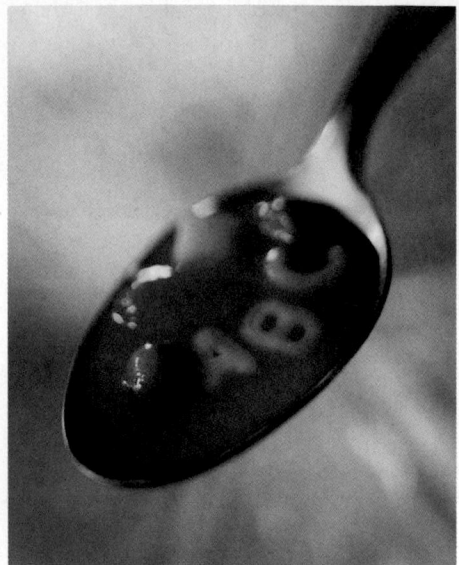

With a little bit of study, you can master the alphabet soup of nutrition.

Figure 2-7 The alphabet soup of dietary standards. Think of the nutrient standards as snapshots along a line. As nutrient intake increases, the Recommended Dietary Allowance (RDA) for the nutrient, if set, is eventually met and a deficient state is no longer present. An individual's needs most likely will be met as RDAs are set high to include almost all people. Related to the RDA concept of meeting an individual's needs are the standards of Adequate Intake (AI) and the Estimated Energy Requirement (EER). These can be used to estimate an individual's needs for some nutrients and calories, respectively. Still, keep in mind that these standards do not share the same degree of accuracy as the RDA. For example, EER may have to be adjusted upward if the individual is very physically active. Finally, as nutrient intake increases above the Upper Level (UL), poor nutritional health is again likely. However, this poor health is due now to the toxic effects of a nutrient, rather than those of a deficiency.

■ Adequate Intake

An RDA can be set for a nutrient only if there is sufficient information on the human needs for that particular nutrient. Today, there is not enough information on some nutrients, such as calcium, to set such a precise standard as an RDA. For this and other nutrients, the DRIs include a category called an Adequate Intake (AI). This standard is derived from the dietary intakes of people that appear to be maintaining nutritional health. That amount of intake is assumed to be adequate, as no evidence of a nutritional deficiency is apparent.

■ Estimated Energy Requirement

Instead of an RDA or AI for calorie needs, we use the Estimated Energy Requirement (EER). As described, the RDAs are set somewhat higher than the average needs for nutrients. This is fine for nutrients rather than calories because a slight excess of vitamins and minerals is not harmful. However, a long-term excess of calories will lead to weight gain. Therefore, the calculation of EER needs to be more specific, taking into account age, gender, height, weight, and physical activity (e.g., sedentary or moderately active). In some cases, the additional calorie needs for growth and lactation are also included (see Chapters 10, 13, and 14 for the specific formulas used). The EER also is based on the "average" person. Thus it can only serve as a starting point for estimating calorie needs.

■ Tolerable Upper Intake Level

A Tolerable Upper Intake Level (Upper Level or UL) has been set for some vitamins and minerals (see the inside cover). The UL is the highest amount of a nutrient that is unlikely to cause adverse health effects in the long run. As intake exceeds the UL, the risk of ill effects increases. These amounts generally should not be exceeded day after day, as toxicity could develop. For people eating a varied diet and/or using a balanced multivitamin and mineral supplement, exceeding the UL is usually not seen. Problems are more likely to arise with diets that promote excessive intakes of a limited variety of foods, or with the use of many fortified foods or excessive doses of individual vitamins or minerals.

How Should These Nutrient Standards Be Used?

To sum up the acronyms described so far, the type of standard that is set for nutrients depends on the quality of available evidence. A nutrient recommendation that is backed by lots of experimental research will have an RDA. For a nutrient that still requires more research, only an AI is presented. We use the EER as a starting point for determining calorie needs. Some nutrients also have a UL if information on toxicity is available. Periodically, new DRIs become available as expert committees review and interpret the available research.

RDAs and related standards are intended mainly for diet planning. Specifically, a diet plan should aim to meet the RDA or AI as appropriate, and not to exceed the UL over the long term (Fig. 2-7). Specific RDA, AI, EER, and UL standards are printed on the inside cover of this book. To learn more about these nutrient standards, visit the link for the Food and Nutrition Board on the Institute of Medicine's web page (www.iom.edu).

Deficient state

Recommended Dietary Allowance (RDA), Adequate Intake (AI), and Estimated Energy Requirement (EER), fall in this range.

Upper Level (UL) met or exceeded

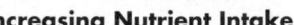

Increasing Nutrient Intake

What Do Food Labels Have to Offer in Diet Planning?

Today, nearly all foods sold in the supermarket must be labeled with the product name, name and address of the manufacturer, amount of product in the package, and ingredients listed in descending order by weight. This food and beverage labeling is monitored in North America by government agencies such as the Food and Drug Administration (FDA) in the United States. The listing of certain food constituents also is required—specifically, on a Nutrition Facts panel (Fig. 2-8). Use this information to learn more about what you eat. The following components must be listed: total calories (kcal), calories from fat, total fat, saturated fat, *trans* fat, cholesterol, sodium, total carbohydrate, fiber, sugars, protein, vitamin A, vitamin C, calcium, and iron. In addition to these required components, manufacturers can choose to list polyunsaturated and monounsaturated fat, potassium, and others. Listing these components is *required*, however, if a claim is made about the health benefits of the specific nutrient (see the upcoming section in Chapter 2 entitled "Health Claims on Food Labels") or if the food is fortified with that nutrient.

The percentage of the Daily Value (% Daily Value) is usually given for each nutrient per serving. It is important to understand that these percentages are based on a 2000 kcal diet. In other words, they are not as applicable to people who require considerably more or less than 2000 kcal per day with respect to fat and carbohydrate intake.

Serving sizes on the Nutrition Facts panel must be consistent among similar foods. This means that all brands of ice cream, for example, must use the same serving size on their label. (These serving sizes may differ from those of MyPyramid since those of food labels are based on typical serving sizes.) In addition, food claims made on packages must follow legal definitions (Table 2-11). For example, if a product claims to be "low sodium," it must have 140 milligrams of sodium or less per serving.

Many manufacturers list the Daily Values set for dietary components such as fat, cholesterol, and carbohydrate on the Nutrition Facts panel. This can be useful as a reference point. As noted before, they are based on 2000 kcal; if the label is large enough, amounts based on 2500 kcal are listed as well for total fat, saturated fat, carbohydrate, and other components.

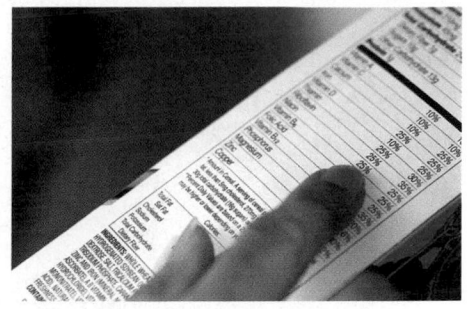

Use the Nutrition Facts label to learn more about the nutrient content of the foods you eat. Nutrient content is expressed as a percent of Daily Value. Canadian food laws and related food labels have a slightly different format (review Appendix B).

Recall from Chapter 1 that the nutrition label uses the term calorie to express energy content in some cases, but kilocalorie (kcal) values are actually listed.

■ Exceptions to Food Labeling

Foods such as fresh fruits and vegetables, fish, meats, and poultry currently are not required to have Nutrition Facts labels. However, many grocers and some meat packers have voluntarily chosen to provide their customers with information about these products. Nutrition Facts labels on meat products will likely be required in the coming years. The next time you are at the grocery store, ask where you might find information on the fresh products that do not have a Nutrition Facts panel. You will likely find a poster or pamphlet near the product; often, these pamphlets contain recipes that use your favorite fruit, vegetable, or cut of meat. They may even assist you in your endeavor to improve your diet.

Because protein deficiency is not a public health concern in the United States, declaration of the % Daily Value for protein is not mandatory on foods for people over 4 years of age. If the % Daily Value is given on a label, FDA requires that the product be analyzed for protein quality. Because this procedure is expensive and time-consuming, many companies opt not to list a % Daily Value for protein rather than undergo the expense. However, labels on food for infants and children under 4 years of age must include the % Daily Value for protein, as must the labels on any food carrying a claim about protein content (see Chapter 14).

Nutrient and herbal supplement labels have a different layout with a "Supplement Facts" heading. Chapters 1 and 8 show examples of these labels.

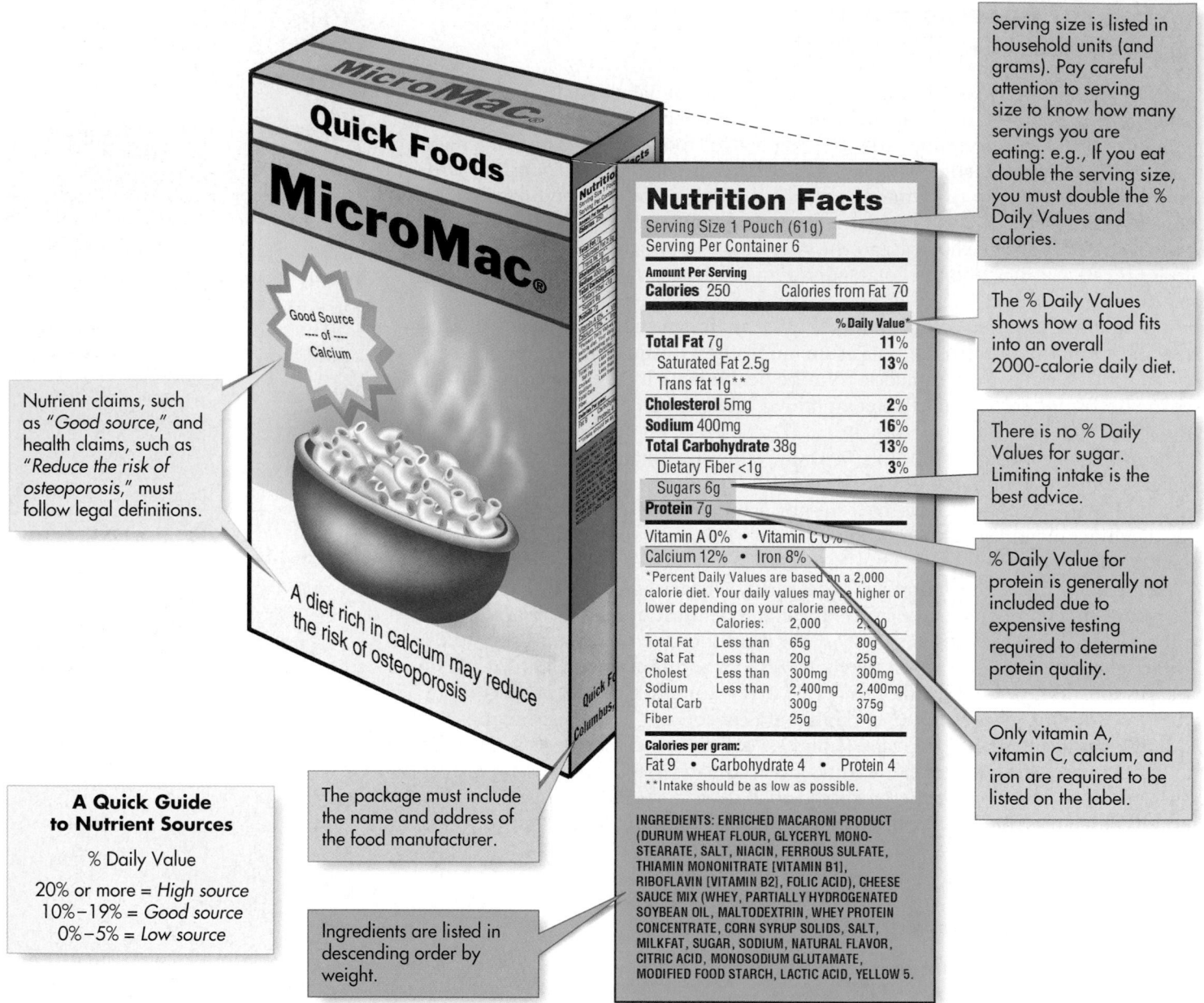

Serving size is listed in household units (and grams). Pay careful attention to serving size to know how many servings you are eating: e.g., If you eat double the serving size, you must double the % Daily Values and calories.

The % Daily Values shows how a food fits into an overall 2000-calorie daily diet.

There is no % Daily Values for sugar. Limiting intake is the best advice.

% Daily Value for protein is generally not included due to expensive testing required to determine protein quality.

Only vitamin A, vitamin C, calcium, and iron are required to be listed on the label.

Nutrient claims, such as "*Good source,*" and health claims, such as "*Reduce the risk of osteoporosis,*" must follow legal definitions.

A Quick Guide to Nutrient Sources

% Daily Value

20% or more = *High source*
10%–19% = *Good source*
0%–5% = *Low source*

The package must include the name and address of the food manufacturer.

Ingredients are listed in descending order by weight.

Nutrition Facts

Serving Size 1 Pouch (61g)
Serving Per Container 6

Amount Per Serving

Calories 250   Calories from Fat 70

	% Daily Value*
Total Fat 7g	**11**%
Saturated Fat 2.5g	**13**%
Trans fat 1g**	
Cholesterol 5mg	**2**%
Sodium 400mg	**16**%
Total Carbohydrate 38g	**13**%
Dietary Fiber <1g	**3**%
Sugars 6g	
Protein 7g	

Vitamin A 0% • Vitamin C 0%
Calcium 12% • Iron 8%

*Percent Daily Values are based on a 2,000 calorie diet. Your daily values may be higher or lower depending on your calorie needs.

		Calories:	2,000	2,500
Total Fat	Less than		65g	80g
Sat Fat	Less than		20g	25g
Cholest	Less than		300mg	300mg
Sodium	Less than		2,400mg	2,400mg
Total Carb			300g	375g
Fiber			25g	30g

Calories per gram:

Fat 9 • Carbohydrate 4 • Protein 4

**Intake should be as low as possible.

INGREDIENTS: ENRICHED MACARONI PRODUCT (DURUM WHEAT FLOUR, GLYCERYL MONO-STEARATE, SALT, NIACIN, FERROUS SULFATE, THIAMIN MONONITRATE [VITAMIN B1], RIBOFLAVIN [VITAMIN B2], FOLIC ACID), CHEESE SAUCE MIX (WHEY, PARTIALLY HYDROGENATED SOYBEAN OIL, MALTODEXTRIN, WHEY PROTEIN CONCENTRATE, CORN SYRUP SOLIDS, SALT, MILKFAT, SUGAR, SODIUM, NATURAL FLAVOR, CITRIC ACID, MONOSODIUM GLUTAMATE, MODIFIED FOOD STARCH, LACTIC ACID, YELLOW 5.

Figure 2-8 The Nutrition Facts panel on a current food label. This nutrition information is required on virtually all processed food products. The % Daily Value listed on the label is the percentage of the generally accepted amount of a nutrient needed daily that is present in 1 serving of the product. You can use the % Daily Values to compare your diet with current nutrition recommendations for certain diet components. Let's consider fiber. Assume that you consume 2000 kcal per day, which is the energy intake for which the % Daily Values listed on labels have been calculated. If the total % Daily Value for dietary fiber in all the foods you eat in one day adds up to 100%, your diet meets the recommendations for fiber. Food labels also contain the name and address of the food manufacturers. This allows consumers to contact the manufacturer if they desire.

∎ Health Claims on Food Labels

As a marketing tool directed toward the health-conscious consumer, food manufacturers like to assert that their products have all sorts of health benefits. After reviewing hundreds of comments on the proposed rule allowing health claims, FDA, which has legal oversight over most food products, has decided to permit some health claims with certain restrictions.

Table 2-11 Definitions for Comparative and Absolute Nutrient Claims on Food Labels

Sugar

- **Sugar free:** less than 0.5 grams (g) per serving.
- **No added sugar; without added sugar; no sugar added:**
  - No sugars were added during processing or packing, including ingredients that contain sugars (for example, fruit juices, applesauce, or jam).
  - Processing does not increase the sugar content above the amount naturally present in the ingredients. (A functionally insignificant increase in sugars is acceptable for processes used for purposes other than increasing sugar content.)
  - The food that it resembles and for which it substitutes normally contains added sugars.
  - If the food doesn't meet the requirements for a low- or reduced-calorie food, the product bears a statement that the food is not low calorie or calorie reduced and directs consumers' attention to the Nutrition Facts panel for further information on sugars and calorie content.
- **Reduced sugar:** at least 25% less sugar per serving than reference food

Calories

- **Calorie free:** fewer than 5 kcal per serving
- **Low calorie:** 40 kcal or less per serving and, if the serving is 30 g or less or 2 tablespoons or less, per 50 g of the food
- **Reduced or fewer calories:** at least 25% fewer kcal per serving than reference food

Fiber

- **High fiber:** 5 g or more per serving. (Foods making high-fiber claims must meet the definition for low fat, or the level of total fat must appear next to the high-fiber claim.)
- **Good source of fiber:** 2.5 to 4.9 g per serving
- **More or added fiber:** at least 2.5 g more per serving than reference food

Fat

- **Fat free:** less than 0.5 g of fat per serving
- **Saturated fat free:** less than 0.5 q per serving, and the level of *trans* fatty acids does not exceed 0.5 g per serving
- **Low fat:** 3 g or less per serving and, if the serving is 30 g or less or 2 tablespoons or less, per 50 g of the food. 2% milk can no longer be labeled low fat, as it exceeds

3 g per serving. *Reduced fat* will be the term used instead.

- **Low saturated fat:** 1 g or less per serving and not more than 15% of kcal from saturated fatty acids
- **Reduced or less fat:** at least 25% less per serving than reference food
- **Reduced or less saturated fat:** at least 25% less per serving than reference food

Cholesterol

- **Cholesterol free:** less than 2 milligrams (mg) of cholesterol and 2 g or less of saturated fat per serving
- **Low cholesterol:** 20 mg or less cholesterol and 2 g or less of saturated fat per serving and, if the serving is 30 g or less or 2 tablespoons or less, per 50 g of the food
- **Reduced or less cholesterol:** at least 25% less cholesterol and 2 g or less of saturated fat per serving than reference food

Sodium

- **Sodium free:** less than 5 mg per serving
- **Very low sodium:** 35 mg or less per serving and, if the serving is 30 g or less or 2 tablespoons or less, per 50 g of the food
- **Low sodium:** 140 mg or less per serving and, if the serving is 30 g or less or 2 tablespoons or less, per 50 g of the food
- **Light in sodium:** at least 50% less per serving than reference food
- **Reduced or less sodium:** at least 25% less per serving than reference food

Other Terms

- **Fortified or enriched:** Vitamins and/or minerals have been added to the product in amounts in excess of at least 10% of that normally present in the usual product. Enriched generally refers to replacing nutrients lost in processing, whereas fortified refers to adding nutrients not originally present in the specific food.
- **Healthy:** An individual food that is low fat and low saturated fat and has no more than 360 to 480 mg of sodium or 60 mg of cholesterol per serving can be labeled "healthy" if it provides at least 10% of the Daily Value for vitamin A, vitamin C, protein, calcium, iron, or fiber.
- **Light or lite:** The descriptor *light* or *lite* can mean two things: first, that a nutritionally altered product contains one-third

fewer kcal or half the fat of reference food (if the food derives 50% or more of its kcal from fat, the reduction must be 50% of the fat) and, second, that the sodium content of a low-calorie, low-fat food has been reduced by 50%. In addition, "light in sodium" may be used for foods in which the sodium content has been reduced by at least 50%. The term *light* may still be used to describe such properties as texture and color, as long as the label explains the intent—for example, "light brown sugar" and "light and fluffy."

- **Diet:** A food may be labeled with terms such as *diet, dietetic, artificially sweetened,* or *sweetened with nonnutritive sweetener* only if the claim is not false or misleading. The food can also be labeled *low calorie* or *reduced calorie.*
- **Good source:** *Good source* means that a serving of the food contains 10% to 19% of the Daily Value for a particular nutrient. If 5% or less it is a **low source.**
- **High:** *High* means that a serving of the food contains 20% or more of the Daily Value for a particular nutrient.

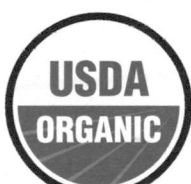

- **Organic:** Federal standards for organic foods allow claims when much of the ingredients do not use chemical fertilizers or pesticides, genetic engineering, sewage sludge, antibiotics, or irradiation in their production. At least 95% of ingredients (by weight) must meet these guidelines to be labeled "organic" on the front of the package. If the front label instead says "made with organic ingredients," only 70% of the ingredients must be organic. For livestock, the animals need to be allowed to graze outdoors and as well be fed organic feed. They also cannot be exposed to large amounts of antibiotics or growth hormones.
- **Natural:** The food must be free of food colors, synthetic flavors, or any other synthetic substance.

The following terms apply only to meat and poultry products regulated by USDA.

- **Extra lean:** less than 5 g of fat, 2 g of saturated fat, and 95 mg of cholesterol per serving (or 100 g of an individual food)
- **Lean:** less than 10 g of fat, 4.5 g of saturated fat, and 95 mg of cholesterol per serving (or 100 g of an individual food)

Many definitions are from FDA's *Dictionary of Terms,* as established in conjunction with the 1990 Nutrition Education and Labeling Act (NELA). g = grams; mg = milligrams

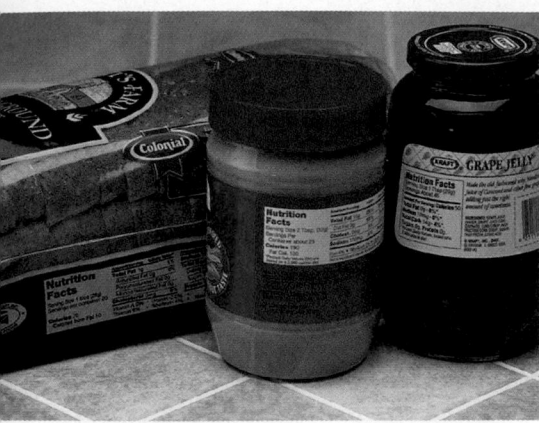

The nutrition information on the food labels on these three products can be combined to indicate nutrient intake for a peanut butter and jelly sandwich.

n addition, the product must meet criteria specific to any health claim being made. For example, a health claim regarding fat and cancer can be made only if the product contains 3 grams or less of fat per serving, which is the standard for low-fat foods.

Currently, FDA limits the use of health messages to specific instances in which there is significant scientific agreement that a relationship exists between a nutrient, food, or food constituent and the disease. The claims allowed at this time may show a link between the following:

- A diet with enough calcium and a reduced risk of osteoporosis
- A diet low in total fat and a reduced risk of some cancers
- A diet low in saturated fat and cholesterol and a reduced risk of cardiovascular disease (typically referred to as heart disease on the label)
- A diet rich in fiber—containing grain products, fruits, and vegetables and a reduced risk of some cancers
- A diet low in sodium and high in potassium and a reduced risk of hypertension and stroke
- A diet rich in fruits and vegetables and a reduced risk of some cancers
- A diet adequate in the synthetic form of the vitamin folate (called folic acid) and a reduced risk of neural tube defects (a type of birth defect)
- Use of sugarless gum and a reduced risk of tooth decay, especially when compared with foods high in sugars and starches
- A diet rich in fruits, vegetables, and grain products that contain fiber and a reduced risk of cardiovascular disease. Oats (oatmeal, oat bran, and oat flour) and psyllium are two fiber-rich ingredients that can be singled out in reducing the risk of cardiovascular disease, as long as the statement also says the diet should also be low in saturated fat and cholesterol.
- A diet rich in whole-grain foods and other plant foods, as well as low in total fat, saturated fat, and cholesterol, and a reduced risk of cardiovascular disease and certain cancers
- A diet low in saturated fat and cholesterol that also includes 25 grams of soy protein and a reduced risk of cardiovascular disease. The statement "one serving of the (name of food) provides _____ grams of soy protein" must also appear as part of the health claim.
- Fatty acids from oils present in fish and a reduced risk of cardiovascular disease
- Margarines containing plant stanols and sterols and a reduced risk of cardiovascular disease (see Chapter 5 for more details on plant stanols and sterols)

A "may" or "might" qualifier must be used in the statement.

In addition, before a health claim can be made for a food product, it must meet two general requirements. First, the food must be a "good source" (before any fortification) of fiber, protein, vitamin A, vitamin C, calcium, or iron. The legal definition of "good source" appears in Table 2-9. Second, a single serving of the food product cannot contain more than 13 grams of fat, 4 grams of saturated fat, 60 milligrams of cholesterol, or 480 milligrams of sodium. If a food exceeds any one of these requirements, no health claim can be made for it, despite its other nutritional qualities. For example, even though whole milk is high in calcium, its label can't make the health claim about calcium and osteoporosis because whole milk contains 5 grams of saturated fat per serving.

Another Bite

n December 2002, FDA created three new preliminary classes of health claims. The agency announced that it would now allow such health claims for foods based on incomplete scientific evidence as long as the label qualified it with a disclaimer such as "this evidence is not conclusive." These preliminary health claims haven't shown up on many foods at this time (fish and nuts such as walnuts have been some of the first examples). These claims also cannot be used on foods considered unhealthy (review Table 2-11 for the definition of healthy with regard to a food).

Overall, claims on foods fall into one of four categories:

- Health claims—closely regulated by FDA
- Preliminary health claims—regulated by FDA but evidence may be scant for the claim
- Nutrient claims—closely regulated by FDA (review Table 2-11)
- Structure/function claims—as discussed in Chapter 1, these are not FDA approved or necessarily valid

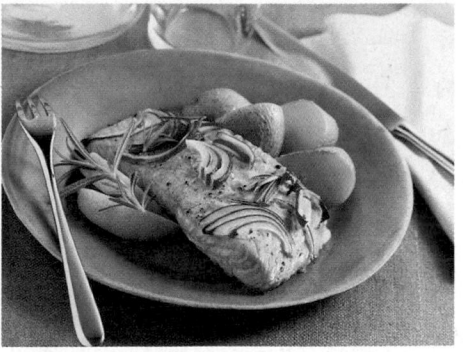

Eating fish at least twice a week contributes to overall health.

Concept Check

The Nutrition Facts panel on a food label provides key information for helping track one's food intake. Nutrient quantities are compared with the Daily Values and expressed on a percentage basis (% Daily Value). This information can be used to either increase or reduce intake of specific nutrients. Health claims on food labels are closely regulated by FDA. Fruits, vegetables, whole-grain breads and cereals, soy, and good sources of calcium are prominent among the foods that can make specific health claims.

Canadian food labels use a slightly different group of health claims and label descriptors (see Appendix B).

Epilogue

The tools discussed in Chapter 2 greatly aid in menu planning. Menu planning can start with MyPyramid. The totality of choices made within the groups can then be evaluated using the Dietary Guidelines. Individual foods that make up a diet can be examined more closely using the Daily Values listed on the Nutrition Facts panel of the product. For the most part, these Daily Values are in line with the Recommended Dietary Allowances and related nutrient standards. The Nutrition Facts panel is especially useful in identifying nutrient-dense foods—foods that are high in a specific nutrient, such as the vitamin folate, but low in comparison with the relative amount of calories provided—as well as foods that fill you up without providing a lot of calories. The latter are described as foods with low energy density. Generally speaking, the more you learn about and use these tools, the more they will benefit your diet.

The **Exchange System** is a final menu-planning tool. This tool organizes foods based on calorie, protein, carbohydrate, and fat content. The result is a manageable framework for designing diets, especially for treatment of diabetes. For more information on the Exchange System see Appendices C and D.

Summary

1. *Variety, balance,* and *moderation* are three watchwords of diet planning.
2. Nutrient density is a useful concept. It reflects the nutrient content of a food in relation to its calorie content. Nutrient-dense foods are relatively rich in nutrients, in comparison with calorie content.
3. Energy density of a food is determined by comparing calorie content with the weight of food. A food that is rich in calories but weighs relatively very little, such as nuts, cookies, fried foods in general, and most snack foods (including fat-free brands), is considered energy dense. Foods with low energy density include fruits, vegetables, and any food that incorporates lots of water during cooking, such as oatmeal.
4. A person's nutritional state can be categorized as *desirable nutrition,* in which the body has adequate stores for times of increased needs; *undernutrition,* which may be present with or without clinical symptoms; and *overnutrition,* which can lead to vitamin and mineral toxicities and various chronic diseases.
5. Evaluation of nutritional state involves analyzing background factors, as well as anthropometric, biochemical, clinical, dietary, and economic assessments. It is not always possible to detect nutritional inadequacies via nutrition assessment since symptoms of deficiencies are often nonspecific and may not appear for many years.
6. MyPyramid is designed to translate nutrient recommendations into a food plan that exhibits variety, balance, and moderation. The best results are obtained by using low-fat or fat-free dairy products; incorporating some vegetable proteins in the diet in addition to animal-protein foods; including citrus fruits and dark green vegetables; and emphasizing whole-grain breads and cereals.
7. Dietary Guidelines for Americans have been issued to help reduce chronic diseases. The guidelines emphasize eating a variety of foods; performing regular physical activity; maintaining or improving weight; moderating consumption of fat, *trans* fat, cholesterol, sugar, salt, and alcohol; eating plenty of whole-grain products, fruits, and vegetables; and safely preparing and storing foods, especially perishable foods.
8. Recommended Dietary Allowances (RDAs) are set for many nutrients. These amounts yield enough of each nutrient to meet the needs of healthy individuals within specific gender and age categories. Adequate Intake (AI) is the standard used when not enough information is available to set a more specific RDA. Estimated Energy Requirements (EERs) set calorie needs for both genders at various ages and physical activity patterns. Tolerable Upper Intake Levels (Upper Levels or ULs) for nutrient intake have been set for some vitamins and minerals. All of the many dietary standards fall under the term *Dietary Reference Intakes (DRIs).* Daily Values are used as a basis for expressing the nutrient content of foods on the Nutrition Facts panel and are based for the most part on the RDAs.
9. Food labels are a useful tool to track your nutrient intake and learn more about the nutritional characteristics of the foods you eat. Any health claims listed must follow criteria set by FDA.

Study Questions

1. Describe the philosophy underlying the creation of MyPyramid. What dietary changes would you need to make to meet the pyramid guidelines on a regular basis?
2. Trace the progression, in terms of physical results, of a person who went from an overnourished to an undernourished state.
3. How could the nutritional state of the person at each state in question 2 be evaluated?
4. Describe the intent of the Dietary Guidelines for Americans. Point out one criticism for its general application to all North American adults.
5. Based on the discussion of the Dietary Guidelines for Americans, suggest two key dietary changes the typical North American adult should consider making.
6. How do RDAs and Adequate Intakes differ from Daily Values in intention and application?
7. How would you explain the concepts of nutrient density and energy density to a fourth grade class?
8. Nutritionists encourage all people to read labels on food packages to learn more about what they eat. What four nutrients could easily be tracked in your diet if you read the Nutrition Facts panels regularly on food products?
9. Explain why consumers can have confidence in FDA-approved health claims on food packages.
10. Relate the importance of variety in a diet, especially with regard to fruit and vegetable choices, to the discovery of various phytochemicals in foods.

Further Readings

1. ADA Reports: Position of the American Dietetic Association: Functional foods. *Journal of the American Dietetic Association* 104:814, 2004.

   Functional foods are foods that have health-promoting properties beyond those provided by nutrient content alone. The many potential benefits of functional foods are described in the article. Still, since foods naturally contain numerous different nutrients and phytochemicals, an important focus is to consider any functional food to be a part of an otherwise healthy diet, especially one rich in fruits and vegetables.

2. Barr SI and others: Planning diets for individuals using the Dietary Reference Intakes. *Nutrition Reviews* 61:352, 2003.

   This article describes appropriate uses of the Recommended Dietary Allowances, Adequate Intakes, and Tolerable Upper Intake Levels. Dietary intakes from individuals is best evaluated with the Recommended Dietary Allowances and Adequate Intakes.

   Upper Levels should not be exceeded on a chronic basis.

3. DeBoer SW and others: Dietary intake of fruits, vegetables, and fat in Olmsted County, Minn. *Mayo Clinic Proceedings* 78:161, 2003.

   Most of the adults in this diet survey consumed less than the recommended amounts of fruits and vegetables and more fat than is recommended. Efforts are needed to convince adults in general to follow a healthier diet.

4. Food and Nutrition Board: *Dietary reference intakes for energy, carbohydrate, fiber, fat, fatty acids, cholesterol, protein, and amino acids.* Washington DC: National Academy Press, 2002.

   This report provides the latest guidance for macronutrient and energy intakes. With regard to calorie intake in adulthood, this should generally match energy output so weight maintenance is achieved.

5. Hasler CM: Functional foods: Benefits, concerns, and challenges—A position paper from the American Council on Science and Health. *Journal of Nutrition* 132:3772, 2002.

   We now know that our diet and its constituents from both plant and animal sources provide more than the essential nutrients such as protein and vitamins, namely a variety of phytochemical and other components that also contribute to health. Foods rich in specific phytochemicals are often termed functional foods. This article lists a variety of phytochemicals under study, as well as current approved health claims for food labels.

6. Is your diet up-to date? *Consumer Reports on Health* 15(1):1, 2003.

   A healthful diet is one that is rich in whole grains, produce, and lean protein sources, as well as low in saturated fat, trans fat, and salt. In addition, plant oils are the preferred source of fat.

7. Kral TVE and others: Combined effects of energy density and portion size on energy intake in women. *American Journal of Clinical Nutrition* 79: 962, 2004.

   The combination of increasing portion size and increasing energy density resulted in a greater food intake in the women in this study. The researchers suggest that both factors may be contributing to the excess calorie intake seen in some adults.

8. Liebman B: Claims crazy: Which ones can you believe? *Nutrition Action Healthletter* 30(5):1, 2003 (June).

   Consumers can rely on the accuracy of the various health claims approved by FDA. Structure/function claims and the forthcoming preliminary health claims (i.e., those that must carry a disclaimer concerning FDA approval) should be viewed cautiously.

9. Liebman B: Bigger meals: smaller waists. *Nutrition Action HeathLetter* p. 1 June 2005.

   The article contains a discussion on energy density and practical applications to a daily diet.

10. Marcus JB: New age foods for disease prevention. *Today's Dietitian*, p. 24, May 2003.

    Fruits, vegetables, nuts, and whole grains are good sources of phytochemicals. Dietary guidance should be based on consuming these foods, and ideally in the whole state.

11. Meadows M: Healthier eating. *FDA Consumer* p. 10 May-June 2005.

    The latest Dietary Guidelines for Americans (2005) are reviewed. The article provides practical advice to put these guidelines into action—a task too few adults are doing well.

12. Mitka M: Government unveils new food pyramid. *Journal of the American Medical Association* 293:2581, 2005.

    Both the pros and cons of MyPyramid are raised by nutrition and medical experts. The biggest criticism is that the tool is practically useless unless a person logs on to the MyPyramid website to find out the details regarding the diet plan.

13. Rebuilding the pyramid. *Tufts University Health & Nutrition Letter* p. 1, June 2005.

    The latest nutrition advice from MyPyramid is discussed. How to apply the recommendations to every day life is highlighted.

14. Reeves MJ and Rafferty AP: Healthy lifestyle characteristics among adults in the United States, 2000. *Archives of Internal Medicine* 165:854, 2005.

    Few adults (about 3% of those in the survey) are following all of the four keys to a healthy lifestyle. The keys are nonsmoking, maintaining healthy weight, consuming at least a combination of at least 5 fruit and vegetable servings per day, and performing at least 30 minutes of physical activity 5 days or more per week.

15. Revised dietary guidelines to help Americans live better lives. *FDA Consumer*, p. 18, March–April 2005.

    The latest Dietary Guidelines for Americans are summarized in simple terms. A figure providing practical advice concerning food choices is included.

16. Rimm EB and Stampfer MJ: Diet, lifestyle and longevity—the next steps. *Journal of the American Medical Association* 292:1490, 2004.

    The authors discuss recent studies that show a benefit on longevity by following a healthy diet. Such a plan is effective in reducing cardiovascular disease and cancer risk—two important diseases that eventually affect many older adults.

17. Stampfer JM and others: Primary prevention of coronary heart disease in women through diet and lifestyle. *The New England Journal of Medicine* 343:16, 2000.

    Women who consume a varied diet (one that is rich in fiber, includes some fish, and is low in fried foods and animal fat), avoid overweight, drink small amounts of alcohol, exercise on a daily basis for about 30 minutes, and avoid smoking reduce their risk of heart attack by over 80%, compared to other women.

18. Uncle Sam's diet book. *Tufts University Health & Nutrition Letter* p. 1, March 2005.

    Implementation of the latest Dietary Guidelines for Americans is discussed. The authors suggest even small changes that conform to this plan provide health benefits.

19. Willett WC: *Eat, drink, and be healthy.* New York: Simon & Schuster, 2001 (or Willett WC, Stampfer MJ: Rebuilding the pyramid. *Scientific American*, p. 64, January 2003).

    The diet plan proposed emphasizes whole grains, plant oils, vegetables eaten daily; fruits at least 2 to 3 times per day; nuts and legumes 1 to 3 times per day; fish, poultry, and eggs eaten 0 to 2 times per day; dairy products or calcium supplements one to two times per day; and little use of red meat, butter, white rice, white bread, potatoes, pasta, and sweets. Regular physical activity and weight control is also recommended, as is alcohol intake in moderation (if of legal age) and a balanced multivitamin and mineral supplement for most people.

I. Does Your Diet Meet Nutrient Needs, MyPyramid Recommendations, and the Dietary Guidelines?

Complete either Part I or Part II. Then complete Parts III, IV, and V. (For help in following the instructions for this activity, see the sample assessment in Appendix E.)

Part I

Manual Diet Analysis

A. Take the information from the 1-day food-intake record you completed in Chapter 1 and record it on the blank form provided in Appendix E or by your instructor. Be sure to record the food or drink ingested and the amount (e.g., weight) consumed. Note: Your instructor may require you to keep the food record for more than 1 day.

B. Review the various nutrient standards on the inside cover of this book and choose the appropriate recommendations for your gender and age. Write the appropriate value for each nutrient on the line on the form labeled "Nutrient Need."

C. Look up the foods and drinks that you listed on the form in the food composition table, Appendix J. Record on the form the amounts of each nutrient and the calorie content, based on the serving size and the number of servings you ate. For example, if you drank 2 cups of milk and the serving size listed in Appendix J is 1 cup, double all nutrient values as you record them. If the food is not listed, choose a substitute, such as cola for root beer.

D. For each food and drink, add the amounts in each column and record the results on the line labeled "Totals."

E. Compare the totals to your nutrient needs. Divide the total for each nutrient by the specific amount and multiply that by 100. Record the result on the line labeled "% of Nutrient Needs."

Part II

NutritionCalc Plus CD Diet Analysis

(See accompanying User's Guide for further details. Also be sure to keep these analysis reports for activities in subsequent chapters.)

1. Open the program and select Create a New Profile, Enter your personal information (e.g., gender, age, weight).

2. View/print your RDAs and related nutrient goals on your Profile screen.

3. Select the Day 1 Intake icon and begin entering foods based upon the 1-day food intake record you compiled in Chapter 1. Be sure to enter each food and drink and the specific amount you consumed.

4. Select the following Report icons to view/print information on your nutrient intake for Day 1;
   a. Bar Graph: displays the nutrient values from your food list as a percentage of the goals defined in your Profile.
   b. Spreadsheet: calculates the total kcals and key nutrients for each food in your intake list by day.

NutritionCalc Plus Online Diet Analysis

(See accompanying User's Guide for further details. Also be sure to keep these analysis reports for activities in subsequent chapters.)

1. Log on to nutritioncalc.mhhe.com, register your passcode (found on inside cover of User's Guide), and select the Profile icon. Enter your personal information (e.g., gender, age, weight).

2. View/print your RDAs and related nutrient goals on your Profile screen.

3. Click on Intake icon, select Day 1, and begin entering foods based upon the 1-day food intake record you compiled in Chapter 1. Be sure to enter each food and drink and the specific amount you consumed.

4. Click on the Reports icon to view/print the following reports from the list on the left:
   a. Bar Graph: displays the nutrient values from your food list as a percentage of the goals defined in your personal Profile.
   b. Spreadsheet: calculates the total kcals and key nutrients for each food in your intake list by day.

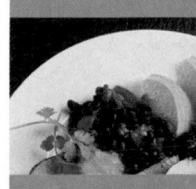

Part III

Evaluation of Nutrient Intakes as a Percentage of Nutrient Needs

Remember that you don't necessarily need to consume your estimated nutrient needs every day. A general standard is meeting needs averaged over 5 to 8 days. It is best not to exceed the Upper Level (if set) over the long term to avoid potential toxic effects for some nutrients.

A. For which nutrients did your intakes fall below estimated nutrient needs (i.e., less than 70% of the RDA/AI)?

B. For which nutrients did you exceed the Upper Level (if set)?

C. What dietary changes could you make to correct or improve your dietary profile? If you're not sure, Chapters 4 through 9 will help guide your decisions.

Part IV

MyPyramid Assessment

Using the same food-intake record used in Part I or II, place each food item in the appropriate group of the MyPyramid chart in Appendix E. Indicate how many servings it contributes to each group based on the amount you ate (see page 47 for serving sizes). Many of your food choices may contribute to more than one group. For example, toast with soft margarine contributes to two categories: (1) grains group; and (2) oils group. After entering all the values, add the number of servings consumed in each group. Finally, compare your total in each food group with the recommended number of servings by www.MyPyramid.gov. Enter a minus sign (−) if your total falls below the recommendation or a plus sign (+) if it equals or exceeds the recommendation.

Part V

Further Diet Evaluation

Do the weaknesses, if any, suggested in your nutrient analysis (see Part III) correspond to missing servings in the MyPyramid food guide? If so, consider changing your food choices based on your MyPyramid to help improve your nutrient profile. If yes, indicate a specific plan to better meet your MyPyramid recommendations. There are many tips provided on the MyPyramid website. You can perform the same diet comparison using MyPyramid Tracker at www.MyPyramid.gov.

- Go to MyPyramid Tracker and scroll down to Access. Select one of the log in links (New User Registration, Existing User Registration, Check It Out-No registration).

- Enter your age, gender, activity, height, and weight.

- Select "Proceed to Food Intake." Enter your food items from your 1-day food record. Select "serving size" and "quantity." Save after each entry is complete. After entering all of your foods and quantities, select "Save and Analyze."

- Choose "MyPyramid Recommendations." For each group, record your "Pyramid Stats," including your equivalent for each group and the recommended equivalent for each group. Also record the percent recommendation for each group from the Percent Table at the bottom.

- Compare your totals in each food group with the recommended number of servings (equivalents). Again, do you need to change your food choices based on this analysis?

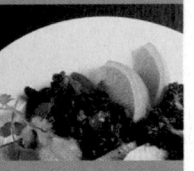

II. Applying the Nutrition Facts Label to Your Daily Food Choices

Imagine that you are at the supermarket looking for a quick meal before a busy evening. In the frozen food section, you find two brands of frozen cheese manicotti (see labels a and b). Which of the two brands would you choose? What information on the Nutrition Facts label in the figure contributed to this decision?

_____

_____

_____

_____

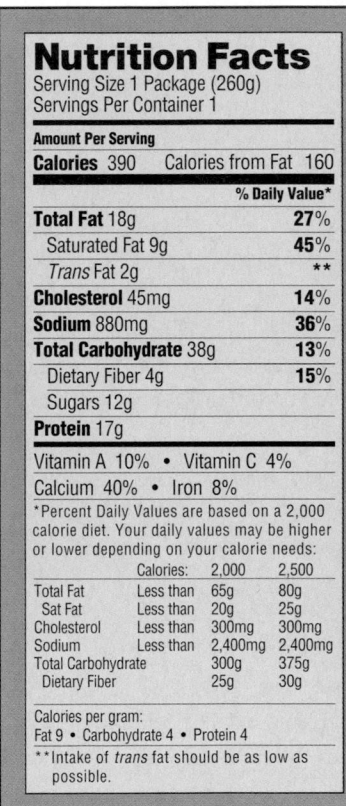

(a)

Nutrition Facts	
Serving Size 1 Package (260g)	
Servings Per Container 1	

Amount Per Serving	
Calories 390	Calories from Fat 160

	% Daily Value*
Total Fat 18g	**27**%
Saturated Fat 9g	**45**%
Trans Fat 2g	**
Cholesterol 45mg	**14**%
Sodium 880mg	**36**%
Total Carbohydrate 38g	**13**%
Dietary Fiber 4g	**15**%
Sugars 12g	
Protein 17g	

Vitamin A 10% • Vitamin C 4%
Calcium 40% • Iron 8%

*Percent Daily Values are based on a 2,000 calorie diet. Your daily values may be higher or lower depending on your calorie needs:

	Calories:	2,000	2,500
Total Fat	Less than	65g	80g
Sat Fat	Less than	20g	25g
Cholesterol	Less than	300mg	300mg
Sodium	Less than	2,400mg	2,400mg
Total Carbohydrate		300g	375g
Dietary Fiber		25g	30g

Calories per gram:
Fat 9 • Carbohydrate 4 • Protein 4

**Intake of _trans_ fat should be as low as possible.

(b)

Nutrition Facts	
Serving Size 1 Package (260g)	
Servings Per Container 1	

Amount Per Serving	
Calories 230	Calories from Fat 35

	% Daily Value*
Total Fat 4g	**6**%
Saturated Fat 2g	**10**%
Trans Fat 1g	**
Cholesterol 15mg	**4**%
Sodium 590mg	**24**%
Total Carbohydrate 28g	**9**%
Dietary Fiber 3g	**12**%
Sugars 10g	
Protein 19g	

Vitamin A 10% • Vitamin C 10%
Calcium 35% • Iron 4%

*Percent Daily Values are based on a 2,000 calorie diet. Your daily values may be higher or lower depending on your calorie needs:

	Calories:	2,000	2,500
Total Fat	Less than	65g	80g
Sat Fat	Less than	20g	25g
Cholesterol	Less than	300mg	300mg
Sodium	Less than	2,400mg	2,400mg
Potassium		3,500mg	3,500mg
Total Carbohydrate		300g	375g
Dietary Fiber		25g	30g

Calories per gram:
Fat 9 • Carbohydrate 4 • Protein 4

**Intake of _trans_ fat should be as low as possible.

The Human Body:

A Nutrition Perspective

3

Real Life Scenario

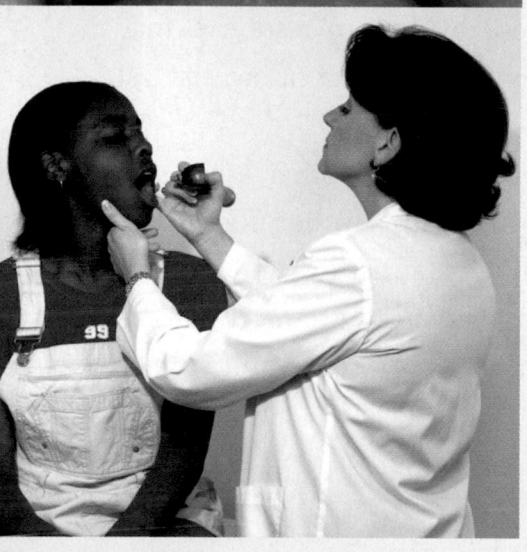

Elise is a 20-year-old college sophomore. Over the last few months, she has been experiencing regular bouts of heartburn. This usually happens after a large lunch or dinner. Occasionally she has even bent down after dinner to pick up something and had some stomach contents travel back up her esophagus and into her mouth. This especially frightened Elise, so she visited the University Health Center.

The nurse practitioner at the Center told Elise it was good that she came in for a checkup. The nurse practitioner suspects Elise has a disease called gastroesophageal reflux disease (GERD). She tells Elise that this can lead to serious problems if not controlled, such as a rare form of cancer. She provides Elise with a pamphlet describing GERD and schedules an appointment with a physician for further evaluation.

What type of dietary habits likely contribute to Elise's symptoms of GERD? What types of medications have been especially useful for treating this problem? Overall, how will Elise cope with this health problem, and will it ever go away?

Chapter 3 Objectives

Chapter 3 is designed to allow you to:

1. Identify the functions of the common cellular components.

2. Define tissue, organ, and organ system.

3. List some basic characteristics of the 12 organ systems and outline a role for each related to nutrition.

4. Understand the role of genetic background in the development of nutrition-related diseases.

5. Outline the overall processes of digestion and absorption in the mouth, stomach, small intestine, and large intestine, as well as the roles played by the liver, gallbladder, and pancreas.

6. Become familiar with some specific enzymes and hormones that act in digestion.

7. Identify the major nutrition-related gastrointestinal health problems and approaches to treatment.

Check out the **Contemporary Nutrition Online Learning Center**
www.mhhe.com/wardlawcont6 *for quizzes, flash cards, other activities, and web links designed to further help you learn about issues surrounding human physiology.*

Chapter 3 Outline

Merely eating food won't nourish you. You must first digest the food—in other words, break it down into usable forms of the essential nutrients that can be absorbed into the bloodstream. Once nutrients are taken up by the bloodstream, they can be distributed to and used by body cells.

We rarely think about, let alone control, digesting and absorbing foods. Except for a few voluntary responses—such as deciding what and when to eat, how well to chew food, and when to eliminate the remains—most digestion and absorption processes control themselves. We don't consciously decide when the pancreas will secrete digestive substances into the small intestine or how quickly foodstuffs will be propelled down the intestinal tract. Various hormones and the nervous system mostly control these functions. Your only awareness of these involuntary responses may be a hunger pang right before lunch or a "full" feeling after eating that last slice of pizza.

Let's examine digestion and absorption as well as other aspects of human physiology that support nutritional health. In the process you will become acquainted with the basic anatomy (structure) and physiology (function) of the circulatory system, nervous system, endocrine system, immune system, digestive system, urinary system, and storage capabilities of the human body.

Refresh Your Memory

As you begin your study of human physiology in Chapter 3, you may want to review:

- The basic chemical composition of carbohydrates, proteins, and lipids (fat) in Chapter 1
- Cell structure and function from previous coursework in university-level biology courses
- Also from any previous biology training, each of the body's organ systems

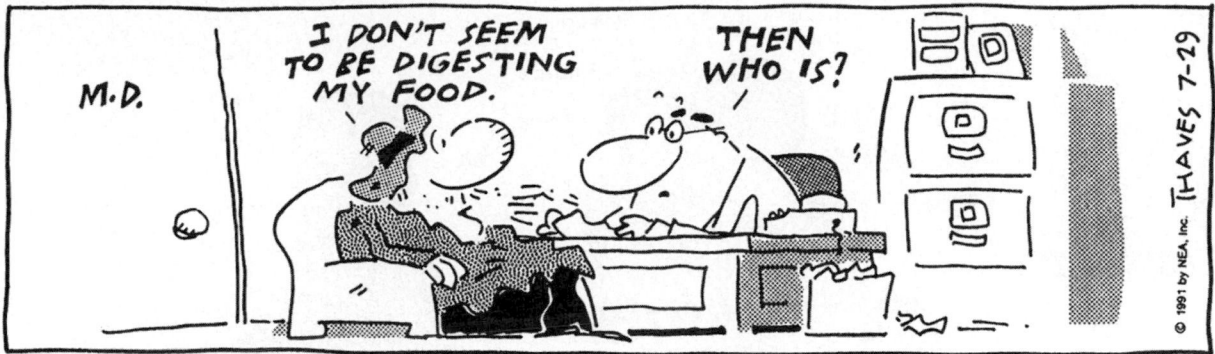

Some popular (fad) diets suggest not combining meat and potatoes in order to improve digestion and that fruit should only be eaten before noon. These diets might also proport that foods get stuck in the body and in turn putrefy and create toxins. Are there any scientific reasons to pay so much attention to food intake in order to help out digestion? Do certain food practices actually improve digestion and subsequent absorption? This chapter provides some answers.

FRANK AND ERNEST reprinted by permission of Newspaper Enterprise Association, Inc.

Human Physiology

The human body is composed of about 100 trillion cells. Each cell is a self-contained, living entity. Cells of the same type normally join together, using intercellular substances to form **tissues,** such as muscle tissue. One, two, or more tissues then combine in a particular way to form more complex structures, called **organs.** All organs contribute to nutritional health, and a person's overall nutritional state determines how well each organ functions. At a still higher level of coordination, several organs can cooperate for a common purpose to form an **organ system,** such as the digestive system. Overall, the human body is a coordinated unit of many highly structured organ systems (Fig. 3-1).

Chemical processes (reactions) occur constantly in every living cell: The production of new substances is balanced by the breaking down of older ones, as exemplified by the constant formation and degradation of bone. For this turnover of substances to occur, cells require a continuous supply of energy in the form of dietary carbohydrate, protein, and/or fat. Cells also need water; building supplies, especially protein and minerals; and chemical regulators, such as the vitamins. Almost all cells also need a steady supply of oxygen. All of these substances enable the tissues, made from individual cells, to function properly.

Getting an adequate supply of all nutrients to the body's cells begins with a healthful diet. To assure optimal use of nutrients, the body's cells, tissues, organs, and organ systems also must work efficiently.

Chapter 3 covers the anatomy and physiology of the cell and major organ systems, especially as they relate to human nutrition. The information you are about to study is limited to the components of the various organ systems that are specifically influenced by the 45-plus essential nutrients discussed in this text.

The Cell: Structure and Function

The cell is the basic structural and functional component of life. Living organisms are made of many different kinds of cells specialized to perform particular functions, and all cells are derived from preexisting cells. In the human body, all cells have certain

tissues Collections of cells adapted to perform a specific function.

organ A group of tissues designed to perform a specific function—for example, the heart, which contains muscle tissue, nerve tissue, and so on.

organ system A collection of organs that work together to perform an overall function.

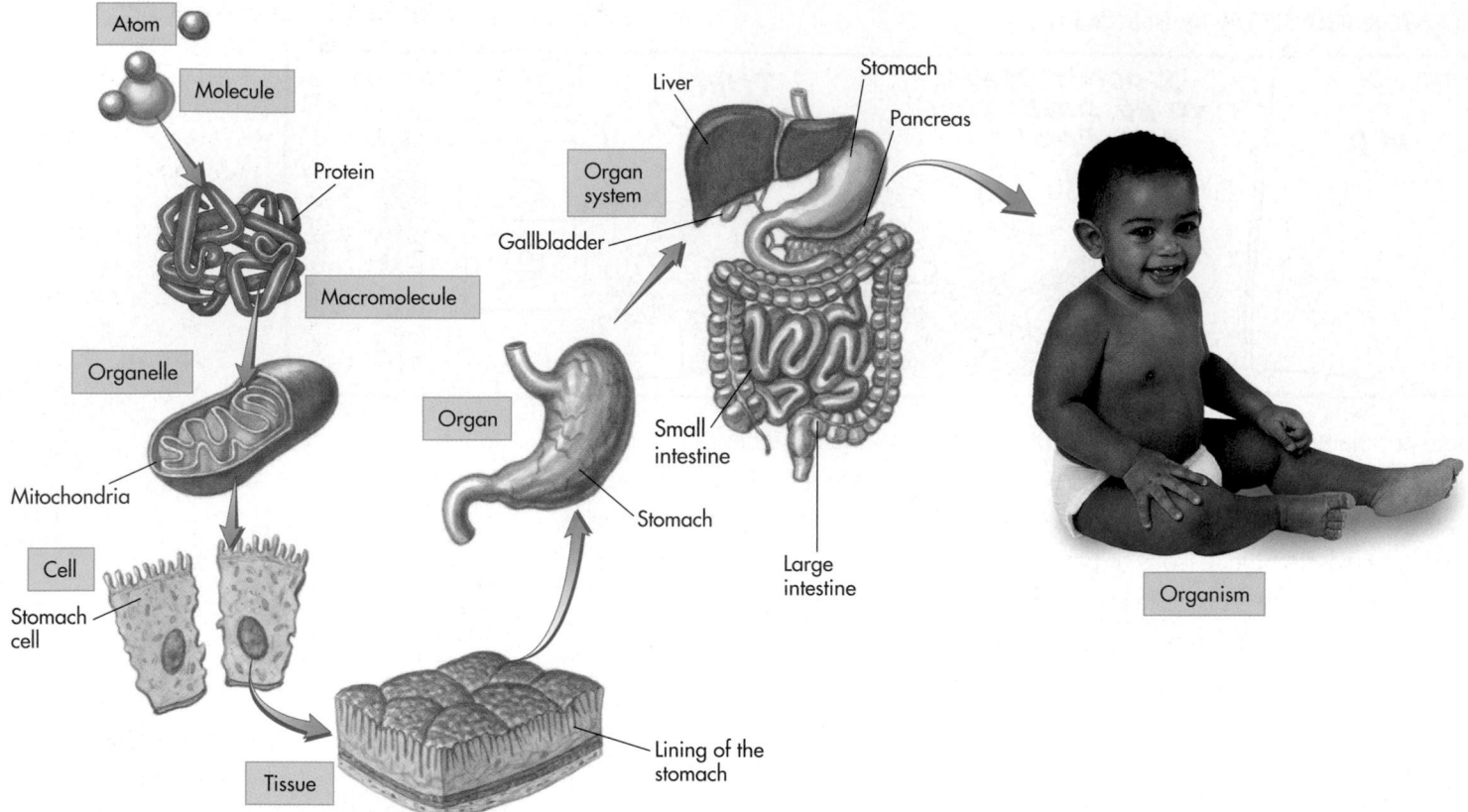

Figure 3-1 Levels of organization of the human body. Each level is more complex than the previous level. The organ system shown is the gastrointestinal (GI) tract.

common features. These cells have compartments, particles, or filaments that perform specialized functions; these structures are called **organelles** (Fig. 3-2). There are at least 15 different organelles, but this section discusses only 8. The numbers following the names of the cell structures correspond to the structures illustrated in Figure 3-2.

■ Cell (Plasma) Membrane 1

There is an outside and inside to every cell, as defined by the cell (plasma) membrane. This membrane holds the cellular contents together and regulates the direction and flow of substances into and out of the cell. Cell-to-cell communication also occurs by way of this membrane.

The cell membrane is a lipid bilayer (or double membrane) of **phospholipids** with their water-soluble heads facing both the interior of the cell and the exterior of the cell. Their water-insoluble tails are tucked into the center portion of the cell membrane.

Cholesterol is a fat-soluble component of the membrane. Since it is fat soluble, it is embedded within the bilayer. This cholesterol provides rigidity and thus stability to the membrane.

There are also various proteins embedded in the cell membrane. Proteins provide structural support, act as transport vehicles, and function as **enzymes** that affect chemical processes within the membrane (see the later section on digestion for more about enzymes). Some proteins form open channels that allow water-soluble substances to pass into and out of the cell. Proteins on the outside surface of the membrane act as receptors, snagging essential substances the cell needs and drawing them into the cell. Other proteins act as gates, opening and closing to control the flow of various particles into and out of the cell.

In addition to the lipid and protein, the membrane also contains carbohydrates that mark the exterior of the cell. These carbohydrates are combined either with protein or fat and provide a delivery service for sending messages to the cell's organelles.

organelles Compartments, particles, or filaments that perform specialized functions within a cell.

phospholipid Any of a class of fat-related substances that contain phosphorus, fatty acids, and a nitrogen-containing component. Phospholipids are an essential part of every cell.

enzyme A compound that speeds the rate of a chemical process but is not altered by that process. Almost all enzymes are proteins.

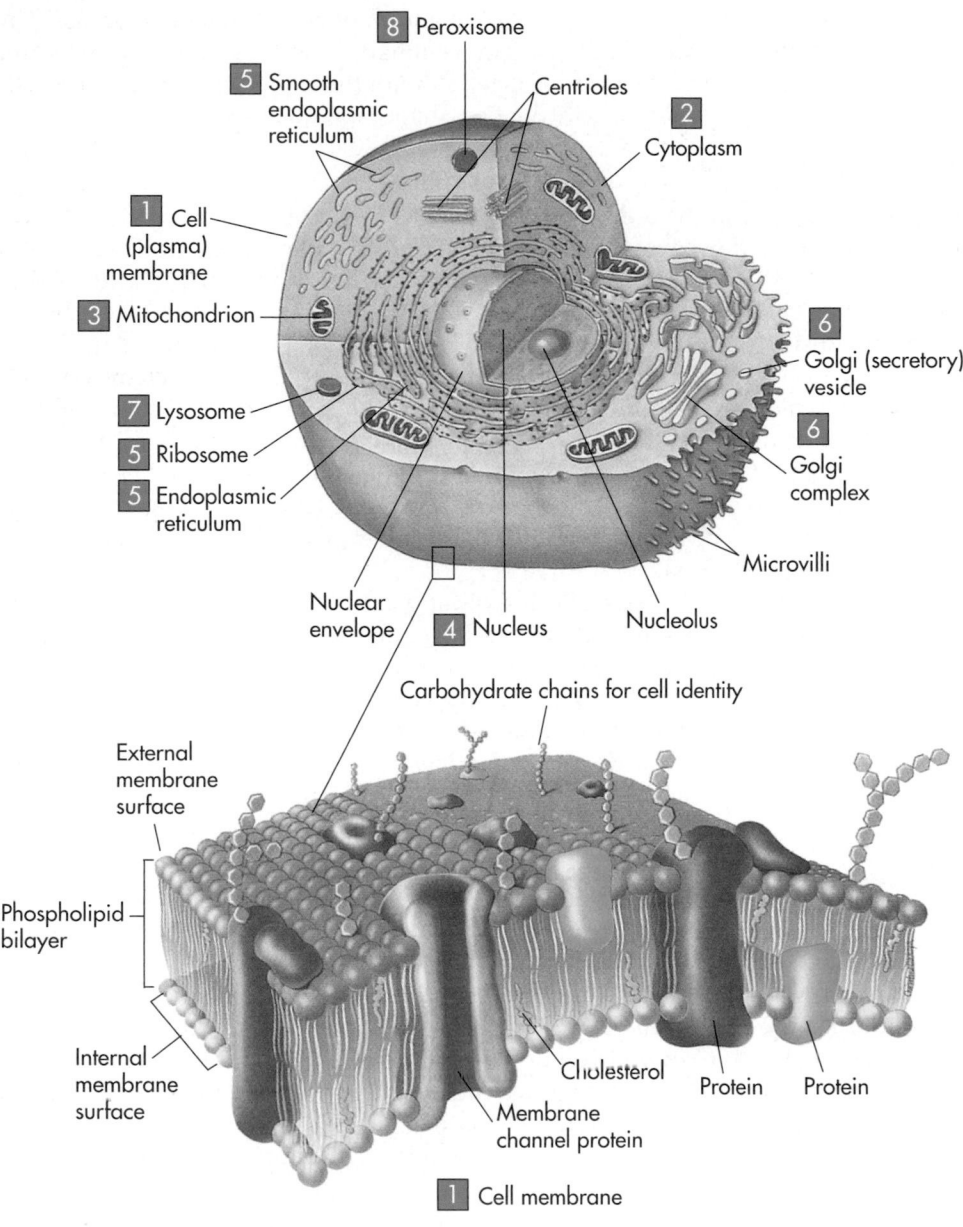

8 Peroxisome

5 Smooth endoplasmic reticulum

Centrioles

2 Cytoplasm

1 Cell (plasma) membrane

3 Mitochondrion

7 Lysosome

5 Ribosome

5 Endoplasmic reticulum

6 Golgi (secretory) vesicle

6 Golgi complex

Microvilli

Nuclear envelope

4 Nucleus

Nucleolus

Carbohydrate chains for cell identity

External membrane surface

Phospholipid bilayer

Internal membrane surface

Cholesterol

Protein

Protein

Membrane channel protein

1 Cell membrane

Figure 3-2 An animal cell. Almost all human cells contain these various organelles. The cell membrane is shown in greater detail. Note: Not all cells have microvilli. Shown here, but not discussed in the text, are the **nucleolus,** nuclear envelope, and centrioles. The nucleolus participates in genetic-related functions. The nuclear envelope encloses the nucleus. The centrioles participate in cell division. The numbers in this Figure correspond to the numbered descriptions in the text.

cytoplasm The fluid and organelles (except the nucleus) in a cell.

anaerobic Not requiring oxygen.

mitochondria The main sites of energy production in a cell. They also contain the pathway for oxidizing fat for fuel, among other metabolic pathways.

These structures also act as identification markers for the cell. In addition, they detect invaders and initiate defensive actions. In sum, these carbohydrates provide tags that are important to cellular identity and interaction.

▪ Cytoplasm 2

The **cytoplasm** is the combination of fluid material and organelles within the cell, not including the nucleus. A small amount of energy for use by the cell can be produced by chemical processes that occur in the cytoplasm. This contributes to the survival of all cells, and is the sole source of energy production in red blood cells. This energy production is called **anaerobic** metabolism because it doesn't require oxygen.

Organelles

Included within the cytoplasm are organelles. They carry out vital roles in cell functions.

▪ Mitochondria 3

Mitochondria are sometimes called the "power plants," or the powerhouse of the cell. These organelles are capable of converting the energy in energy-yielding nutrients

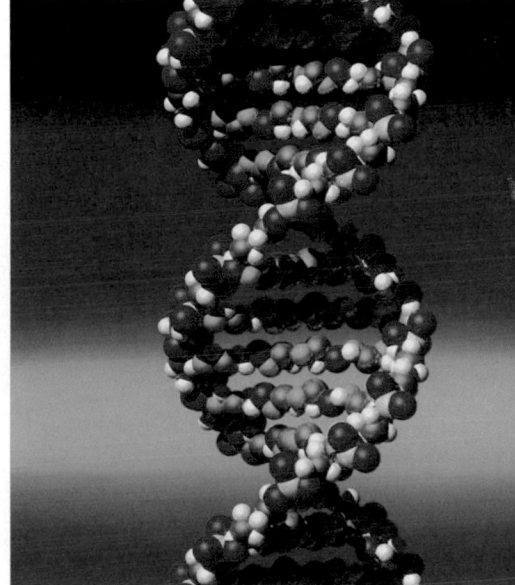

Genes are present on DNA—a double helix. The cell nucleus contains most of the DNA in the body.

aerobic Requiring oxygen.

cell nucleus An organelle bound by its own double membrane and containing chromosomes, the genetic information for cell protein synthesis and cell replication.

deoxyribonucleic acid (DNA) The site of hereditary information in cells; DNA directs the synthesis of cell proteins.

gene A specific segment on a chromosome. Genes provide the blueprint for the production of cell proteins.

chromosome A single, large DNA molecule and its associated proteins; contains many genes to store and transmit genetic information.

ribonucleic acid (RNA) The single-stranded nucleic acid involved in the transcription of genetic information and translation of that information into protein structure.

ribosomes Cytoplasmic particles that mediate the linking together of amino acids to form proteins; may exist freely in the cytoplasm or attached to endoplasmic reticulum.

endoplasmic reticulum (ER) An organelle in the cytoplasm composed of a network of canals running through the cytoplasm. Part of the endoplasmic reticulum contains ribosomes.

Golgi complex The cell organelle near the nucleus that processes newly synthesized protein for secretion or distribution to other organelles.

secretory vesicles Membrane-bound vesicles produced by the Golgi apparatus; contains protein and other compounds to be secreted by the cell.

lysosome A cellular organelle that contains digestive enzymes for use inside the cell for turnover of cell parts.

peroxisome A cell organelle that destroys toxic products within the cell.

hydrogen peroxide Chemically, H_2O_2.

from food (carbohydrate, protein, and fat) to a form of energy that cells can use. This is an **aerobic** process that uses the oxygen we inhale, as well as water, enzymes, and other compounds (see Chapter 11 for details). With the exception of red blood cells, all cells contain mitochondria; only the size, shape, and quantity vary.

■ Cell Nucleus 4

With the exception of the red blood cell, all cells have one or more nuclei. The **cell nucleus** is bounded by its own double membrane. The nucleus controls actions that occur in the cell, using hereditary material called **deoxyribonucleic acid (DNA).** DNA is the "code book" that contains directions for making substances the cell needs. It consists of **genes** on **chromosomes.** This "code book" remains in the nucleus of the cell, but conveys its information to other cell organelles by way of a similar molecule called **ribonucleic acid (RNA).** The RNA has the responsibility of *transcribing* the information on the DNA. It then moves out through pores in the nuclear membrane to the cytoplasm. The RNA then carries the transcribed DNA code to protein-synthesizing sites called **ribosomes.** There, the RNA code is *translated* into a specific protein. This process is also known as **gene expression** (see Chapter 6 for details on protein synthesis).

DNA has the secondary task of cell replication. DNA is a double-stranded molecule, and when the cell begins to divide, each strand is separated and an identical copy of each is made. Thus, each new DNA contains one new strand of DNA and one strand from the original DNA. In this way, the genetic code is preserved from one cell generation to the next. (The mitochondria contain their own DNA, so they reproduce themselves independent of action in the nucleus.)

The transport of proteins, vitamins, and other material from the cytoplasm to the nucleus also occurs through pores in the nuclear membrane as just mentioned (see Fig. 6-1 in Chapter 6). These small molecules serve a variety of functions, including the activation (or inactivation) of certain parts of the DNA in cells.

■ Endoplasmic Reticulum (ER) 5

The outer membrane of the cell nucleus is continuous with a network of tubes called the **endoplasmic reticulum (ER).** Part of the endoplasmic reticulum (termed the rough [as opposed to smooth] endoplasmic reticulum) contains the ribosomes, where proteins are synthesized. Many of these proteins play a central role in human nutrition. Parts of the endoplasmic reticulum also are involved in lipid synthesis, detoxification of toxic substances, and calcium storage and release in the cell.

■ Golgi Complex 6

The **Golgi complex** is a packaging site for proteins that are used in the cytoplasm or exported from the cell. It consists of sacs within the cytoplasm in which proteins are "packaged" as **secretory vesicles** for secretion by the cell.

■ Lysosomes 7

Lysosomes are the cell's digestive system. They are sacs that contain enzymes for the digestion of foreign material. Sometimes known as "suicide bags," they are responsible for digesting worn-out or damaged cell components. Certain cells that are associated with immune functions contain many lysosomes (see the later section on the immune system).

■ Peroxisomes 8

Peroxisomes contain enzymes that detoxify harmful chemicals. **Hydrogen peroxide** (H_2O_2) is formed as a result of such enzyme action. Peroxisomes contain a protective enzyme called *catalase,* which prevents excessive accumulation of hydrogen peroxide in the cell, which would be very damaging. Peroxisomes also play a minor role in metabolizing one possible source of energy for cells—alcohol.

Concept Check

In Chapter 1, you learned that fat (lipids), protein, and carbohydrate function as fuels. Now you recognize that these organic nutrients also serve as structural materials in the cell membrane. This is typical of many nutrients; they can carry out multiple functions. The cell receives nutrients and other substances through the cell membrane by using various transport systems.

The basic structural unit in the body is the cell. Within the cell are a variety of organelles with unique functions to perform. Although there is no typical cell, virtually all cells have the same organelles, each performing the same essential task.

epithelial tissue The surface cells that line the outside of the body and all external passages within it.

connective tissue Protein tissue that holds different structures in the body together. Some structures are made up of connective tissue—notably, **tendons** and **cartilage.** Connective tissue also forms part of bone and the nonmuscular structures of arteries and veins.

muscle tissue A type of tissue adapted to contract in order to cause movement.

nervous tissue Tissue composed of highly branched, elongated cells, which transport nerve impulses from one part of the body to another.

Organization of the Body

As noted earlier, when groups of similar cells work together to accomplish a specialized task, the arrangement is referred to as a tissue. Humans are composed of four primary types of tissue: **epithelial, connective, muscle,** and **nervous.** Epithelial tissue is composed of cells that cover surfaces both inside and outside the body. These cells of epithelial tissue secrete important substances, absorb nutrients, and excrete waste. Connective tissue supports and protects the body, stores fat, and produces blood cells. Muscle tissue is designed for movement. Nervous tissue found in the brain and spinal cord is designed for communication. These four types of tissues then go on to form various organs, and ultimately, organ systems (Table 3-1).

Table 3-1 Organ Systems of the Body

System	Major Components	Functions Related to Nutrition
Cardiovascular	Heart, blood vessels, and blood	Transports nutrients, waste products, gases, and hormones throughout the body and plays a role in the immune response and the regulation of body temperature
Lymphatic	Lymph vessels, lymph nodes, and other lymph organs	Removes foreign substances from the blood and lymph, combats disease, maintains tissue fluid balance, and aids in fat absorption
Nervous	Brain, spinal cord, nerves, and sensory receptors	A major regulatory system: detects sensation, controls movements, and controls physiological and intellectual functions
Endocrine	Endocrine glands, such as the pituitary, thyroid, and adrenal glands	A major regulatory system: participates in the regulation of metabolism, reproduction, and many other functions through the action of hormones
Immune	White blood cells, lymph vessels and nodes, spleen, thymus gland, and other lymph tissues	Provides defense against foreign invaders; formation of white blood cells
Digestive	Mouth, esophagus, stomach, intestines, and accessory structures (liver, gallbladder, and pancreas)	Performs the mechanical and chemical processes of digestion, absorption of nutrients, and elimination of wastes
Urinary	Kidneys, urinary bladder, and the ducts that carry urine	Removes waste products from the circulatory system and regulates the acidity, chemical composition, and water content of the blood
Integumentary	Skin, hair, nails, and sweat glands	Protects the body, regulates temperature, prevents water loss, and produces a substance that converts to vitamin D upon sun exposure
Skeletal	Bones, associated cartilage, and joints	Supports the body, and allows for body movement, produces blood cells, and stores minerals
Muscular	**Smooth, cardiac,** and **skeletal muscle**	Produces body movement, maintains posture, and produces body heat
Respiratory	Lungs and respiratory passages	Exchanges gases (oxygen and carbon dioxide) between the blood and the atmosphere and regulates blood acid-base (pH) balance
Reproductive	Gonads, accessory structures, and genitals of males and females	Performs the processes of reproduction and influences sexual functions and behaviors

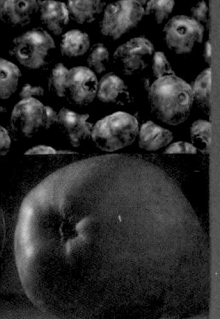
The growth, development, and maintenance of cells, and ultimately of the entire organism, are directed by genes present in the cells. The genes contain the codes that control the expression of individual traits, such as height, eye color, and susceptibility to many diseases. Although it is not the only factor, an individual's genetic risk for a given disease is an important determinant for development of a specific disease.

Each of these genes essentially represents a recipe, noting the ingredients (amino acids) and how those ingredients should be put together (to make proteins). The end products (proteins) of all the recipes in the cookbook (the human genome) would then make up the human organism.

It is likely that soon it will be relatively easy to screen a person's DNA for genes that increase the risk for specific diseases. Genetic screening is a brand new field, but is about to become a significant part of medical practice, as almost every medical condition has a genetic component. Most diseases, however, are not the result of single gene disorders; instead, genetic disease risk arises from alterations in a number of genes.

Each year, new links between specific genes and diseases are reported. It is thought that the recent decoding of the human genome will ultimately allow for early detection of health-related genetic risks (such as a form of breast cancer) as well as tailoring of diets with respect to individual nutrient needs or the individual's response to certain diet patterns. (A genetic test is available for a form of breast cancer [abnormal BRCA genes], but is expensive—$2700.) Another hope is to replace genes that encourage diseases, such as cancer, with those that do not. This practice, known as *gene therapy*, has proven to be effective for a few disorders, but is not widely available at this time.

Nutritional Diseases with a Genetic Link

Studies of families, including those with twins and adopted children, provide strong support for the effects of genetics in various disorders. In fact, family history is considered to be an important risk factor in the development of many nutrition-related diseases.

Cardiovascular Disease

About 1 of every 500 people in North America has a defective gene that greatly delays cholesterol removal from the bloodstream. As you saw in Chapter 1, elevated blood cholesterol is one major risk factor for development of cardiovascular disease. Diet changes can help these people, but medications and even surgery are often needed to address these problems.

Hypertension

An estimated 10% to 15% of the North American population is very sensitive to salt-induced hypertension. Information from the genetic code may one day identify those hypertensive individuals who have this problem. At present, the only way to determine whether individuals with hypertension are salt sensitive is to place them on a salt-restricted diet and see if their blood pressure falls. Note also that many cases of hypertension are not caused primarily by salt sensitivity, but by other factors, such as obesity and inactivity.

■ Obesity

Most obese North Americans have at least one parent who is also obese. This strongly suggests a genetic link. Findings from many human studies suggest that a variety of genes (likely 60 or more) are involved in the regulation of body weight. Little is known, however, about the specific nature of these genes in humans or how the actual changes in body metabolism (such as lower calorie-burning in general or fat use in particular) are produced.

Still, although some individuals may be genetically predisposed to store body fat, whether they actually do so depends on how many calories they consume relative to their needs. A common concept in nutrition is that *nurture*—how people live and the environmental factors that influence them—allows *nature*—each person's genetic potential—to be expressed. Although not every person with a genetic tendency toward obesity becomes obese, those who are genetically predisposed to weight gain have a higher lifetime risk than individuals without a genetic predisposition to obesity.

■ Diabetes

Both of the two common types of diabetes—type 1 and type 2—have genetic links, as revealed by family and twin studies. Only sensitive and expensive testing can determine who is at risk. The most common form of diabetes (90% of all cases), type 2 diabetes, also has a strong link to obesity. Typically a genetic tendency for type 2 diabetes is expressed once a person becomes obese but often not before, again illustrating that nurture affects nature.

■ Cancer

A few types of cancer (e.g., some forms of colon [*colon* is another name for the large intestine] and breast cancer) have a strong genetic link, and genetics may play a role in others, such as **prostate cancer.** Because obesity increases the risk of several forms of cancer, a long-standing excess calorie intake is also a risk factor. Although genes are an important determinant in the development of cancer, environmental and lifestyle factors, such as excessive sun exposure and a poor diet, also contribute significantly to the risk profile.

Your Genetic Profile

From this discussion, you can see that a family history of certain diseases raises your risk of developing those diseases. By recognizing your potential for developing a particular disease, you can avoid behavior that further raises your risk. For example, women with a family history of breast cancer should avoid becoming obese, should minimize alcohol use, and should obtain mammograms regularly. In general, the greater number of your relatives who had a genetically transmitted disease and the closer they are related to you, the greater your risk. One way to assess your risk is to put together a family tree of illnesses and deaths by compiling a few key facts on your primary relatives: siblings, parents, aunts and uncles, and grandparents, as suggested in the Rate Your Plate section.

Figure 3-3 shows an example of a family tree (also called a *genogram*). High-risk conditions include two or more first-degree relatives in a family with a specific disease (first-degree relatives include one's parents, siblings, and offspring). Another sign of risk of inherited disease is development of the disease in a first-degree relative before 50 to 60 years. In the family depicted in Figure 3-3, prostate cancer killed the man's father. Knowing this, the man should be tested regularly for prostate cancer. His sisters should consider frequent mammograms and other preventive practices because their mother died of breast cancer. Because heart attack and stroke are also common in the family, all the children should adopt a lifestyle that minimizes the risk of developing these conditions, such as avoiding excessive

Critical Thinking

Wesley notices that at family gatherings his parents, uncles, aunts, and older siblings typically drink excessive amounts of alcohol. His father has been arrested for driving while intoxicated, as has one of his aunts. Two of his uncles died before the age of 60 from alcohol abuse. As Wesley approaches the age of legal drinking, he wonders if he is destined to fall into the pattern of alcohol abuse. What advice would you give to Wesley concerning his future use of alcohol?

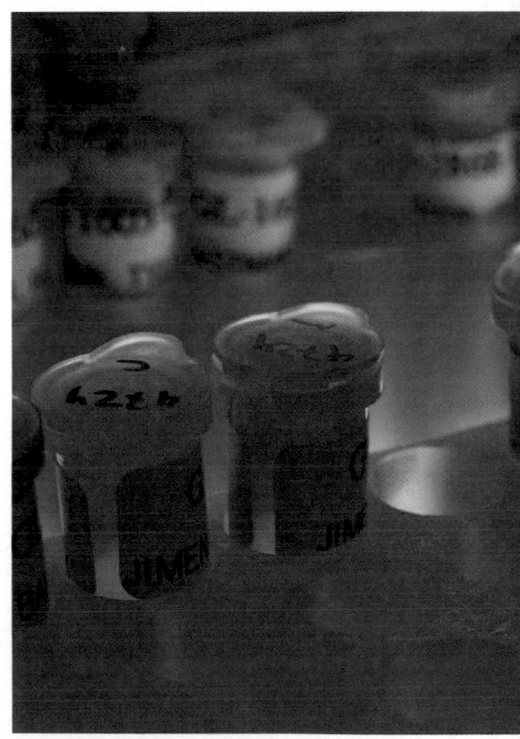

Genetic testing for disease susceptibility will be more common in the future as the genes that increase risk for various diseases are isolated and decoded.

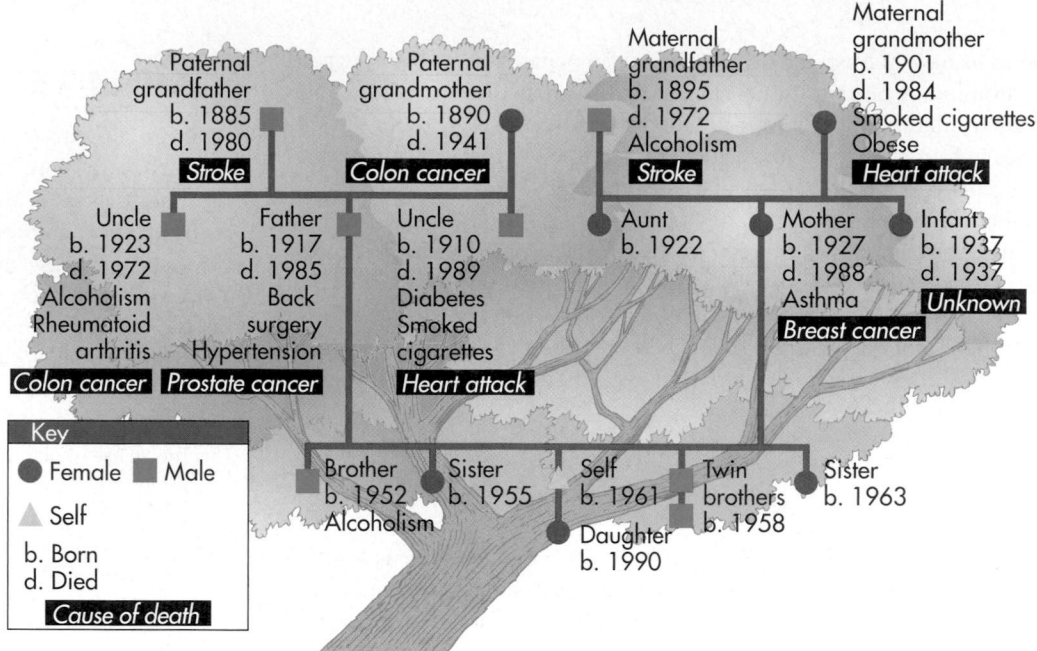

Figure 3-3 Example of a family tree for Eugene, designated as "Self" at the trunk of the tree. The gender of each family member is identified by color (blue squares for males, orange circles for females). Dates of birth (b) and death (d) are listed below each family member. If deceased, the cause of death is highlighted using white text against a black background. In addition to causes of death, medical conditions the family members experienced are noted beneath each name. Create your own family tree of frequent diseases using this figure as a guide. Then show your family tree to your physician to get a more complete picture of what the information means for your health.

animal fat and salt intake. Colon cancer is also evident in the family, so careful screening throughout life is important.

Throughout this book, discussions will point out how you can personalize nutrition advice based on your genetic background. In this way, you can identify and avoid the "controllable" risk factors that would contribute to development of genetically linked diseases present in your family.

The following web links will help you gather more information about genetic conditions and testing:

www.geneticalliance.org Alliance of Genetic Support Groups.

www.kumc.edu/gec/support Information on genetic conditions and rare conditions.

www.cancer.gov/cancertopics/prevention-geneticcauses Genetics information from the National Cancer Institute.

www.nhgri.nih.gov National Human Genome Research Institute (at the National Institutes of Health) home page. Describes the latest research findings, discusses some ethics issues, and provides a talking glossary.

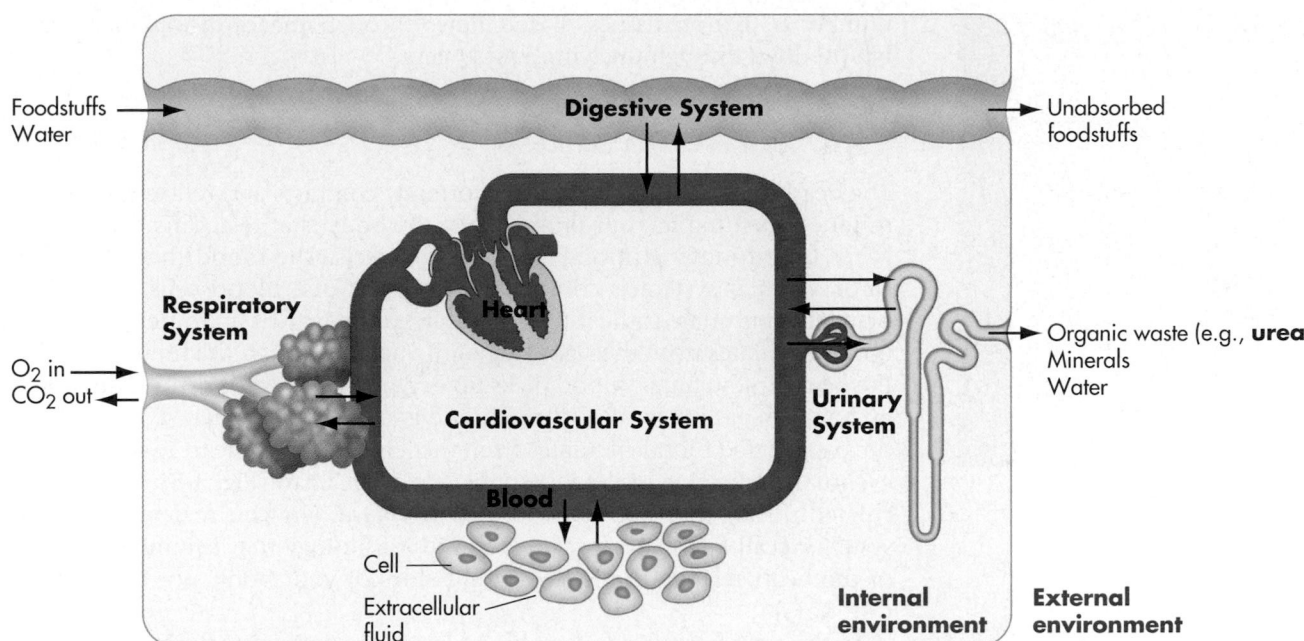

Figure 3-4 Exchanges of nutrients occur between our external environment and the internal environment of the circulatory system via the digestive, respiratory, and urinary systems. Overall, the human body is a combination of 12 systems working together to support cell needs.

We will be particularly concerned in Chapter 3 with the digestive system. The nutrients we consume in food are unavailable until such time as they have been processed by the digestive system. This employs chemical and mechanical means to alter food so that the nutrients can be released and absorbed into the body for distribution to body tissues.

Sometimes organs within a system can serve another system. For example, the basic function of the digestive system is to convert the food we eat into absorbable nutrients. At the same time, the digestive system serves the immune system by preventing dangerous pathogens from invading the body and causing illness. As you study nutrition, you will note the multiple roles played by many organs (Fig. 3-4).

The overriding theme of human nutrition is to understand the actions of nutrients as they affect different cells, tissues, organs, and organ systems. Each type of organ system is impacted by nutrient intake and simultaneously determines how each nutrient is used.

Our task now is to explore the key systems in the body as they specifically relate to the study of human nutrition: circulatory (cardiovascular and lymphatic), nervous, endocrine, immune, digestive, and urinary systems. This part of Chapter 3 will set the stage for a more detailed look at these and other organ systems in later chapters covering various aspects of human nutrition.

Cardiovascular System and Lymphatic System

The body has two separate organ systems that circulate fluids in the body: the **cardiovascular system** and the **lymphatic system.** The cardiovascular system consists of the heart and blood vessels. The lymphatic system consists of lymphatic vessels and a

urea Nitrogenous waste product of protein metabolism; major source of nitrogen in the urine.

cardiovascular system The body system consisting of the heart, blood vessels, and blood. This system transports nutrients, waste products, gases, and hormones throughout the body, and plays an important role in immune responses and regulation of body temperature.

lymphatic system A system of vessels and lymph that accepts fluid surrounding cells and large particles, such as products of fat absorption. Lymph eventually passes into the bloodstream from the lymphatic system.

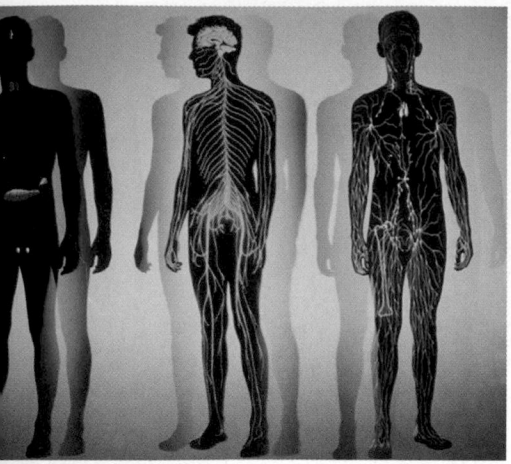

The body is made up of numerous organ systems.

number of lymph tissues. Blood flows through the cardiovascular system, while **lymph** flows through the lymphatic system.

■ Cardiovascular System

The heart is a muscular pump that normally contracts and relaxes 50 to 90 times per minute (resulting in your pulse) when the body is at rest. This continual pumping keeps blood moving through the blood vessels. The blood that flows through the cardiovascular system is composed of **plasma,** red blood cells, white blood cells, platelets, and many other substances. It travels two basic routes. In the first route, blood circulates from the right side of the heart, through the lungs, and then back to the heart. In the lungs, blood picks up oxygen and releases carbon dioxide. After this exchange of gases has taken place, blood is said to be *oxygenated*. In the second route, the oxygenated blood circulates from the left side of the heart to all other body cells, eventually returning back to the right side of the heart (Fig. 3-5). Once blood has circulated throughout the body, it is *deoxygenated*. (As you review the cardiovascular system, recall from your previous studies of biology that *left* and *right* designations of the heart refer to the left and right sides of your body, not of the page in your textbook.)

In the cardiovascular system, blood leaves the heart via **arteries,** which branch into **capillaries,** a network of tiny blood vessels. Exchange of nutrients, oxygen, and waste products between the blood and cells occurs through the minute, weblike pores of the capillaries (Fig. 3-6). Capillaries service every region of the body via individual capillary beds that are only one cell layer thick. The blood then returns to the heart via the **veins.**

The cardiovascular system distributes nutrients derived from food and oxygen from the air to all body cells (review Fig. 3-4). Other functions include delivery of hormones to their target cells, maintenance of a constant body temperature, and dispersal of white blood cells throughout the body to protect against pathogens as part of the immune system (see the later section, Immune system).

Portal Circulation in the Gastrointestinal Tract

Water and nutrients, once absorbed through the stomach or intestinal wall, reach one of two destinations. Some nutrients are taken up by cells in the intestines and portions of the stomach for nourishment of those organs, but most of the nutrients from recently eaten foods are transferred into **portal circulation.** The actual transfer points are the capillary beds in these organs. To enter portal circulation, the nutrients pass from those capillaries into veins that eventually merge into a very large vein called a **portal vein.** Unlike most veins in the body—which carry blood back to the heart—this portal vein leads directly to the liver. This enables the liver to process absorbed nutrients before they enter the general circulation of the bloodstream. Overall, portal circulation represents a special form of circulation in the cardiovascular system.

■ Lymphatic System

The **lymphatic system** is also a circulatory system. It consists of a network of lymphatic vessels and the fluid (**lymph**) that moves through them. Lymph is similar to blood, consisting largely of blood plasma that has found its way out of capillaries and into the spaces between cells. It contains a full array of the various white blood cells which play an important role in the immune system. However, neither red blood cells nor platelets are present. Lymph is collected in tiny lymph vessels all over the body and moves through even larger vessels until it eventually opens into major veins near the heart. This flow is driven by muscle contractions arising from normal body movements.

plasma The fluid, extracellular portion of the circulating blood. This includes the blood serum plus all blood-clotting factors. In contrast, **serum** is the fluid that remains after clotting factors have been removed from plasma.

artery A blood vessel that carries blood away from the heart.

capillary A microscopic blood vessel that connects the smallest arteries and veins; site of nutrient, oxygen, and waste exchange between body cells and the blood.

vein A blood vessel that carries blood to the heart.

portal circulation The portion of the circulatory system that utilizes a large vein (portal vein) to carry nutrient-rich blood from capillaries in the intestines and portions of the stomach to the liver.

lymph A clear fluid that flows through lymph vessels; carries most forms of fat after their absorption by the small intestine.

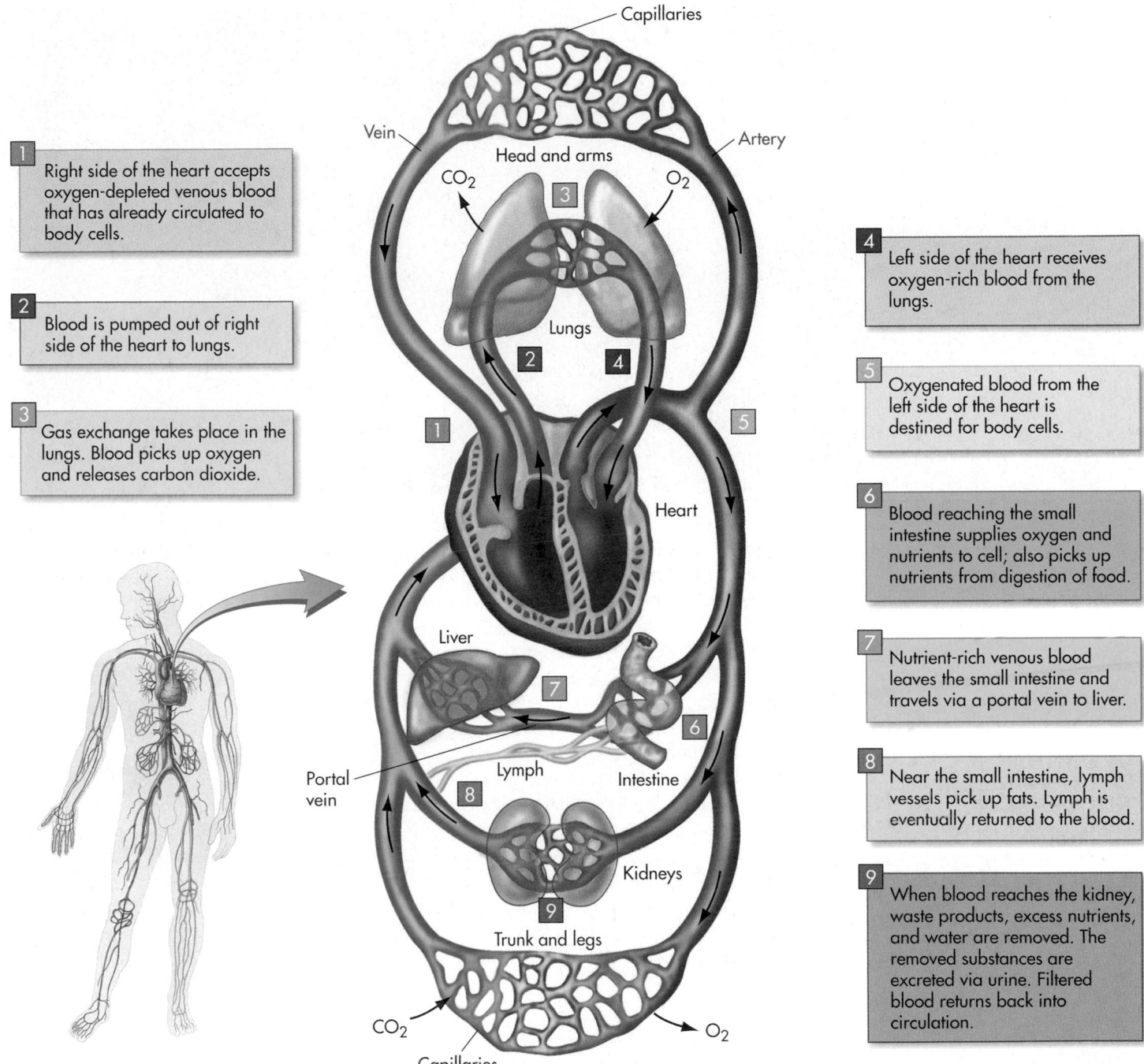

1 Right side of the heart accepts oxygen-depleted venous blood that has already circulated to body cells.

2 Blood is pumped out of right side of the heart to lungs.

3 Gas exchange takes place in the lungs. Blood picks up oxygen and releases carbon dioxide.

4 Left side of the heart receives oxygen-rich blood from the lungs.

5 Oxygenated blood from the left side of the heart is destined for body cells.

6 Blood reaching the small intestine supplies oxygen and nutrients to cell; also picks up nutrients from digestion of food.

7 Nutrient-rich venous blood leaves the small intestine and travels via a portal vein to liver.

8 Near the small intestine, lymph vessels pick up fats. Lymph is eventually returned to the blood.

9 When blood reaches the kidney, waste products, excess nutrients, and water are removed. The removed substances are excreted via urine. Filtered blood returns back into circulation.

Figure 3-5 Blood circulation through the body. This figure shows the paths that blood takes from the heart to the lungs ([1]–[3]), back to the heart ([4]), and through the rest of the body ([5]–[9]). The red color indicates blood that is richer in oxygen; blue is for blood carrying more carbon dioxide. Keep in mind that arteries and veins go to all parts of the body.

Lymphatic Circulation in the Gastrointestinal Tract

Besides contributing to the defense of the body against invading pathogens, lymphatic vessels that serve the small intestine play an important role in nutrition. These vessels pick up and transport the majority of products yielded from fat absorption. These products are too large to enter the bloodstream directly. They are generally emptied into the bloodstream only after passing through the lymphatic system.

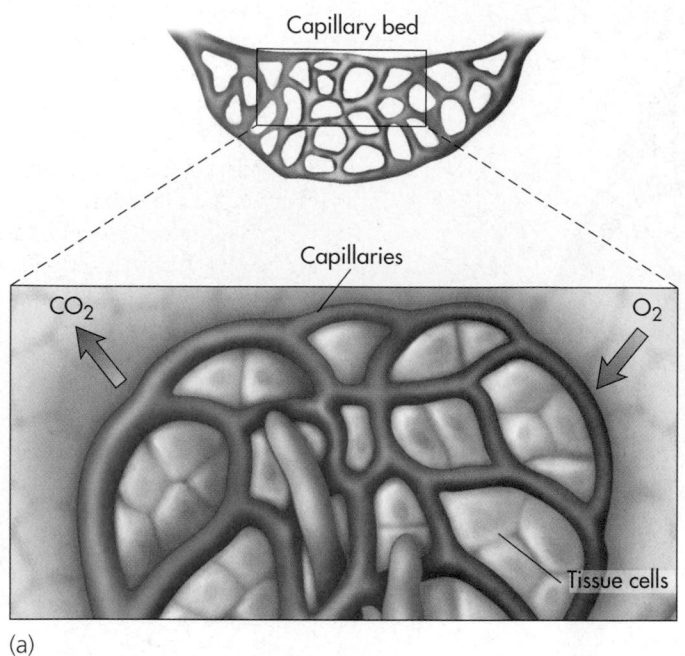

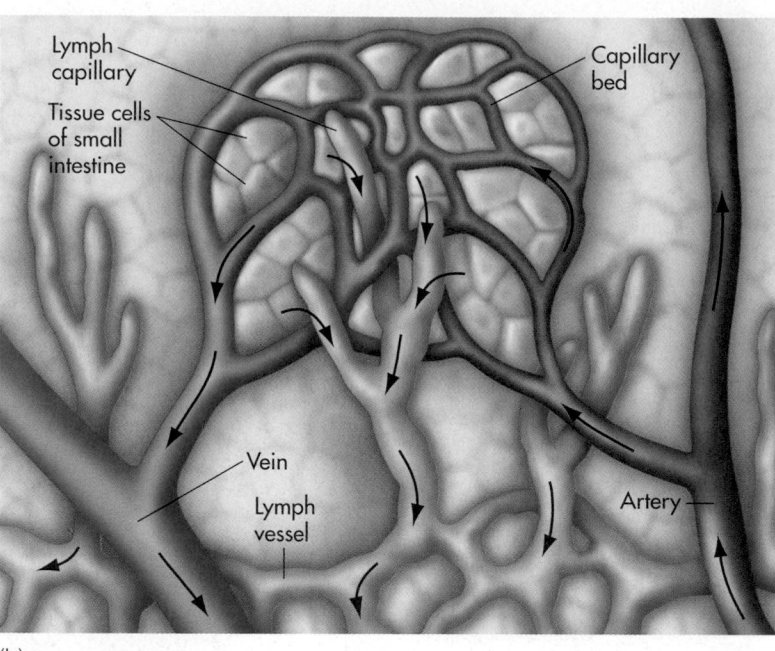

Figure 3-6 Capillary and lymph vessels. (a) Exchange of oxygen and nutrients for carbon dioxide and waste products occurs between the capillaries and the surrounding tissue cells. (b) Lymph vessels are also present in capillary beds, such as in the small intestine. Lymph vessels in the small intestine are also called **lacteals.** Note that the lymph vessels are blind-ended.

Concept Check

Blood is transported from the right side of the heart to the capillaries in the lungs. Carbon dioxide is removed and oxygen is taken up by red blood cells. The oxygenated blood returns to the left side of the heart. Here it is pumped into general circulation. In the capillaries, oxygen is released from the red blood cells and delivered through pores in the capillaries to the surrounding cells. Nutrients also are distributed from the bloodstream via the capillaries. Carbon dioxide released from cells travels through the capillary pores to the blood.

The lymph system serves several purposes: the transport of absorbed dietary lipids, the uptake and return to the bloodstream of excess fluid that collects between cells, and the defense of the body against invading pathogens.

Nervous System

The **nervous system** is a regulatory system that exercises centralized control over most body functions. The nervous system can detect changes occurring in various organs and the external environment and take corrective action when needed to maintain the constancy of the internal environment. The nervous system also regulates activities that change almost instantly, such as muscle contractions and perception of danger. The body has many receptors that receive information about what is happening within the body and in the outside environment. For the most part these receptors are found in our eyes, ears, skin, nose, and stomach. We act on information from these receptors via the nervous system.

The basic structural and functional unit of the nervous system is the **neuron**. These are elongated, highly branched cells. The body contains about 100 billion neurons. Neurons respond to electrical and chemical signals, conduct electrical impulses, and

nervous system The body system consisting of the brain, spinal cord, nerves, and sensory receptors. This system detects sensations, directs movements, and controls physiological and intellectual functions.

neuron The structural and functional unit of the nervous system. Consists of a **cell body, dendrites,** and an **axon.**

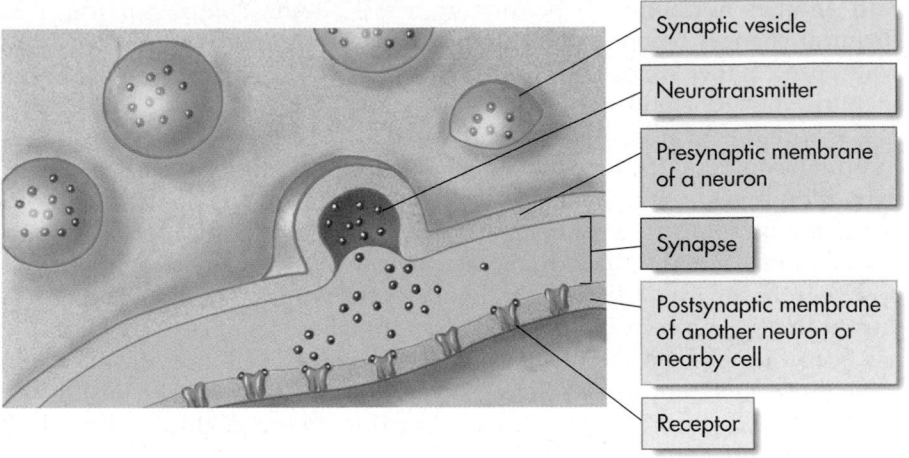

Synaptic vesicle

Neurotransmitter

Presynaptic membrane of a neuron

Synapse

Postsynaptic membrane of another neuron or nearby cell

Receptor

Figure 3-7 Transmission of a message from one neuron to another neuron or to another type of cell that relies on neurotransmitters. Vesicles containing neurotransmitters, formed within the neuron, fuse with the membrane of the neuron and the neurotransmitter is released into the synapse. The neurotransmitter then binds to the receptors on the nearby neuron (or cell). In this way, the message is transmitted from one neuron to another, or to the cell that ultimately performs the action directed by the message.

release chemical regulators. Overall, neurons allow us to perceive what is occurring in our environment, engage in learning, store vital information in memory, and control the body's voluntary (and involuntary) actions.

The brain stores information, reacts to incoming information, solves problems, and generates thoughts. In addition, the brain plans a course of action based on the other sensory inputs. Responses to the stimuli are carried out mostly through the rest of the nervous system.

Simply put, the nervous system receives information through stimulation of various receptors, processes this information, and sends out signals through its various branches for an action that needs to be taken. Actual transmission of the signal utilizes a change in the sodium and potassium concentration in the neuron. There is an influx of sodium and a loss of potassium as the message is sent. Concentrations of these minerals are then restored to normal amounts in the neuron after the signal passes and it is now ready to conduct another message.

When the signal must bridge a gap **(synapse)** between the branches of different neurons, the message is generally converted to a chemical signal called a **neurotransmitter.** The neurotransmitter itself is then released into the gap, and its target may be another neuron or another type of cell, such as a muscle cell (Fig. 3-7). If the signal is sent to another neuron, this allows it to continue on to its final destination. The neurotransmitters used in this process are often made from common nutrients found in foods, such as amino acids. The amino acid tryptophan is converted to the neurotransmitter serotonin, and the amino acid tyrosine is converted to the neurotransmitters **norepinephrine** and **epinephrine** (also called adrenaline).

Other nutrients also play a role in the nervous system. Calcium is needed for the release of neurotransmitters from neurons. Vitamin B-12 plays a role in the formation of the **myelin sheath,** which provides insulation around specific parts of most neurons. Finally, a regular supply of carbohydrate in the form of glucose is important for supplying fuel for the brain. The brain can use other calorie sources, but generally relies on glucose.

synapse The space between one neuron and another neuron (or cell).

neurotransmitter A compound made by a nerve cell that allows for communication between it and other cells.

myelin sheath A lipid and protein combination (lipoprotein) that covers nerve fibers.

endocrine system The body system consisting of the various glands and the hormones these glands secrete. This system has major regulatory functions in the body, such as reproduction and cell metabolism.

endocrine gland A hormone-producing gland.

Endocrine System

The **endocrine system** plays a major role in the regulation of metabolism, reproduction, water balance, and many other functions by producing hormones in the **endocrine glands** of the body and subsequently releasing them into the blood. The term *hormone* comes from the Greek word for "to stir or excite." A true hormone is a regulatory compound that has a specific site of synthesis from which it then enters the bloodstream to reach target cells. Hormones are the messengers of the body. They can be permissive (turn on), antagonistic (turn off), or synergistic (work in cooperation

thyroid hormone Hormones produced by the thyroid gland that among their functions increase the rate of overall metabolism in the body.

receptor A site in a cell at which compounds (such as hormones) bind. Cells that contain receptors for a specific compound are partially controlled by that compound.

with another hormone) in performing a task. Some compounds must undergo chemical changes before they can function as hormones. For example, vitamin D, synthesized in the skin or obtained from food, is converted into an active hormone by chemical changes made in the liver and kidneys.

The hormone **insulin,** which is synthesized in and released from the pancreas, helps control the amount of glucose in the blood. Insulin is mostly produced when glucose in the blood rises to a certain level, usually after a meal. At this point, insulin is released and it travels to the muscle, adipose, and liver cells of the body. Among its many functions, insulin allows for the movement of glucose from the blood into muscle and adipose cells. In the liver cells, insulin stimulates the synthesis of glycogen from glucose, thus promoting an increase in stored glycogen. Once a sufficient amount of glucose has been cleared from the blood, the production of insulin lessens. The hormones epinephrine, norepinephrine, glucagon, and growth hormone have just the opposite effect on blood glucose. They all cause an increase in blood glucose through a variety of actions (Table 3-2). **Thyroid hormones,** which are synthesized in and released from the thyroid gland, help to control the body's rate of metabolism. Other hormones are especially important in regulating digestive processes (see the later section, Digestive system).

Hormones are not available to all cells in the body, but only those with the correct **receptor** protein. These binding sites are highly specific for a certain hormone. They are generally found on the cell membrane. The hormone attaches to its receptor on the cell membrane. This binding activates additional compounds called second messengers within the cell to carry out the assigned task. This is true of insulin. A few hormones can penetrate the cell membrane and eventually bind to receptors on the DNA in the nucleus (e.g., thyroid hormone and estrogen).

■ **Concept Check**

The functional unit of the nervous system is the neuron. Communication between neurons themselves, and other types of cells, is via neurotransmitters released into the synapse between the cells.

In the endocrine system, hormones are produced by glands in response to a change in the internal or external environment of the body. The gland secretes the hormone into the blood, and the blood delivers it to target cells. The hormone either enters the cell and binds to the DNA in the cell to cause changes within the cell, or attaches to receptors in the cell membrane and, through the action of second messengers, causes changes within the cell.

Table 3-2 Some Hormones of the Endocrine System with Nutritional Significance

Hormone	Gland/Organ	Target	Effect	Role in Nutrition
Epinephrine, Norepinephrine	Adrenal glands	Heart, blood vessels, brain, lungs	Increased body metabolism	Release of glucose into the blood, fat mobilization
Thyroid hormones	Thyroid gland	Most organs	Increased oxygen consumption, growth, brain development, development of the nervous system	Protein synthesis, increased body metabolism
Insulin	Pancreas	Adipose (fat) and muscle cells	Decreased blood glucose	Uptake and storage of glucose, fat, and amino acids by cells
Glucagon	Pancreas	Liver	Increased blood glucose	Release of glucose from liver stores, increased fat mobilization
Growth hormone	Pituitary gland	Most cells	Promotion of amino acid uptake by cells, increased blood glucose	Promotion of protein synthesis and growth, increased fat utilization for energy

Immune System

Many types of body cells and body components work in cooperation as part of the **immune system** to maintain a defense against infection (Fig. 3-8). The components that work as part of the immune system include the skin, intestinal cells, and white blood cells. It is easy to demonstrate the importance of nutritional health for immune function. Early humans were plagued by famine; this contributed to infections, often leading to death. Today, largely because of better nutrition, most of the world avoids that cycle.

■ Skin

The skin is a large component of the immune system, forming an almost continuous barrier surrounding the body. Invading microorganisms have difficulty penetrating the skin. However, if the skin is split by lesions, bacteria can easily penetrate this barrier. Skin health is hampered by deficiencies of such nutrients as essential fatty acids, vitamin A, niacin, and zinc. Vitamin A deficiency also decreases gland secretions in the skin that contain the enzyme **lysozyme,** which is capable of killing bacteria. Bacterial eye infections are common in developing countries, often as a result of a vitamin A deficiency.

■ Intestinal Cells

The cells of the intestines form an important barrier to invading microorganisms. Not only are the cells packed closely together, but specialized cells that produce immune factors—such as **immunoglobulins**—are also scattered throughout the intestinal tract. These immune factors bind to the invading microorganisms, preventing them from entering the bloodstream. This process contributes to the **mucosal membrane** aspect of immunity.

immune system The body system consisting of white blood cells, lymph glands and vessels, and various other body tissues. The immune system provides defense against foreign invaders, primarily due to the action of various types of white blood cells.

lysozyme An enzyme produced by a variety of cells; it can destroy bacteria by rupturing their cell membranes.

immunoglobulins Proteins found in the blood that bind to specific **antigens;** also called **antibodies.** The five major classes of immunoglobulins play different roles in antibody-mediated immunity.

antigen Any substance that induces a state of sensitivity and/or resistance to microorganisms or toxic substances after a lag period; foreign substance that stimulates a specific aspect of the immune system.

antibody Blood protein (immunoglobulin) that binds foreign proteins found in the body. This helps to prevent and control infections.

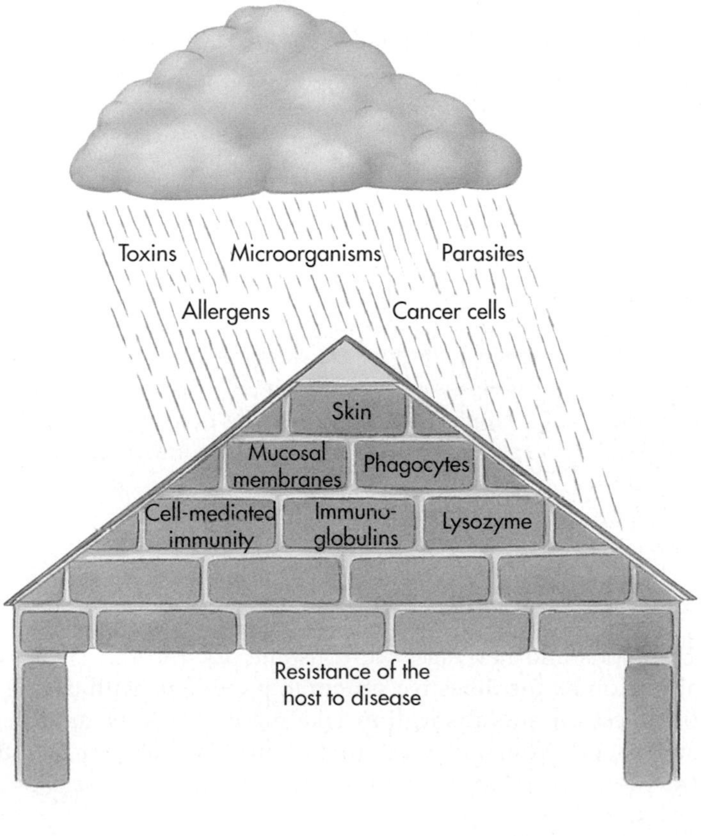

Figure 3-8 Some host protective factors that shelter humans from threats such as diseases and toxins. We are born with most of these aspects of immune function; these are termed **nonspecific** (or innate) since the targets are a variety of microorganisms. In contrast, white blood cells produce immunoglobulins that target specific organisms or foreign proteins, constitute **specific** (or adaptive) immune function. And once exposed, a memory is created such that a second exposure to the substance will produce a more vigorous and rapid attack.

Nutrient deficiencies can cause the intestinal cells to break down so that microorganisms more easily enter the body and cause infections. Thus, two common results of undernutrition are diarrhea and bacterial infections of the bloodstream. To protect the health of the intestinal tract, an adequate nutrient intake is necessary—especially of protein, vitamin A, vitamin B-6, vitamin B-12, vitamin C, folate, and zinc.

Another Bite

Although many studies show that a healthy nutritional state is associated with good immune status, other studies show that an overabundance of certain nutrients can actually harm the immune system. For example, taking too much zinc may decrease immune function (see Chapter 9).

■ White Blood Cells

Once a microorganism enters the bloodstream, **white blood cells** move in to attack it. A variety of types of white blood cells participate in this response and function in unique ways. For example, a class called **phagocytes** circulates throughout the circulatory system and ingests and sometimes digests microorganisms and foreign particles (via lysosomes present in the cells) in a process called **phagocytosis.** Other white blood cells participate in **cell-mediated immunity,** achieved when certain immune cells recognize foreign cells or proteins and directly attack and destroy them. Immunoglobulins in their role as antibodies elicit an antibody-antigen response that binds microorganisms and proteins that are foreign to the body and destroys them, and then creates a template (memory) that allows future recognition of the microorganism or foreign protein. Recognition allows more rapid attacks in the future.

Some white blood cells live only a few days. Their constant resynthesis requires steady nutrient intake. The immune system needs (1) iron to produce an important killing factor, (2) copper for the synthesis of a specific type of white blood cell, and (3) adequate amounts of protein, vitamin B-6, vitamin B-12, vitamin C, and folate for general cell synthesis and, later, cell activity. Zinc and vitamin A are also needed for the overall growth and development of immune cells.

Concept Check

Many types of body cells and body components work in cooperation as part of the immune system to maintain a defense against infection. The skin forms an almost continuous barrier surrounding the body. Cell secretions contain the enzyme lysozyme. Specialized cells in the intestines and certain white blood cells secrete antibodies (immunoglobulins). Phagocytes roam throughout the circulatory system and ingest and sometimes digest microorganisms and foreign particles. Other white blood cells participate in cell-mediated immunity. This occurs when certain immune cells recognize foreign cells and directly attack them. Many nutrients are needed for the overall growth and development of immune cells.

Digestive System

The foods and beverages we consume, for the most part, must undergo extensive alteration by the **digestive system** to provide us with usable nutrients. The processes of **digestion** and **absorption** take place in a long tube that is open at both ends and extends from the mouth to the anus. This tube is called the **gastrointestinal (GI) tract** (Fig. 3-9). Nutrients from the food we eat must pass through the walls of the

---

white blood cells One of the formed elements of the circulating blood system; also called *leukocytes.* White blood cells are able to squeeze through intracellular spaces and migrate. They phagocytize bacteria, fungi, and viruses, as well as detoxify proteins that may result from allergic reactions, cellular injury, and other immune system cells.

phagocytosis A process in which a cell forms an indentation, and particles or fluids entering the indentation are then engulfed by the cell.

cell-mediated immunity A process in which certain white blood cells come in actual contact with the invading cells in order to destroy them.

digestive system The body system consisting of the gastrointestinal tract and accessory structures such as the liver, gallbladder, and pancreas. This system performs the mechanical and chemical processes of digestion, absorption of nutrients, and elimination of wastes.

digestion The process by which large ingested molecules are mechanically and chemically broken down to produce basic nutrients that can be absorbed across the wall of the GI tract.

absorption The process by which substances are taken up from the GI tract and enter the bloodstream or the lymph.

gastrointestinal (GI) tract The main sites in the body used for digestion and absorption of nutrients. It consists of the mouth, esophagus, stomach, small intestine, large intestine, rectum, and anus. Also called the *digestive tract.*

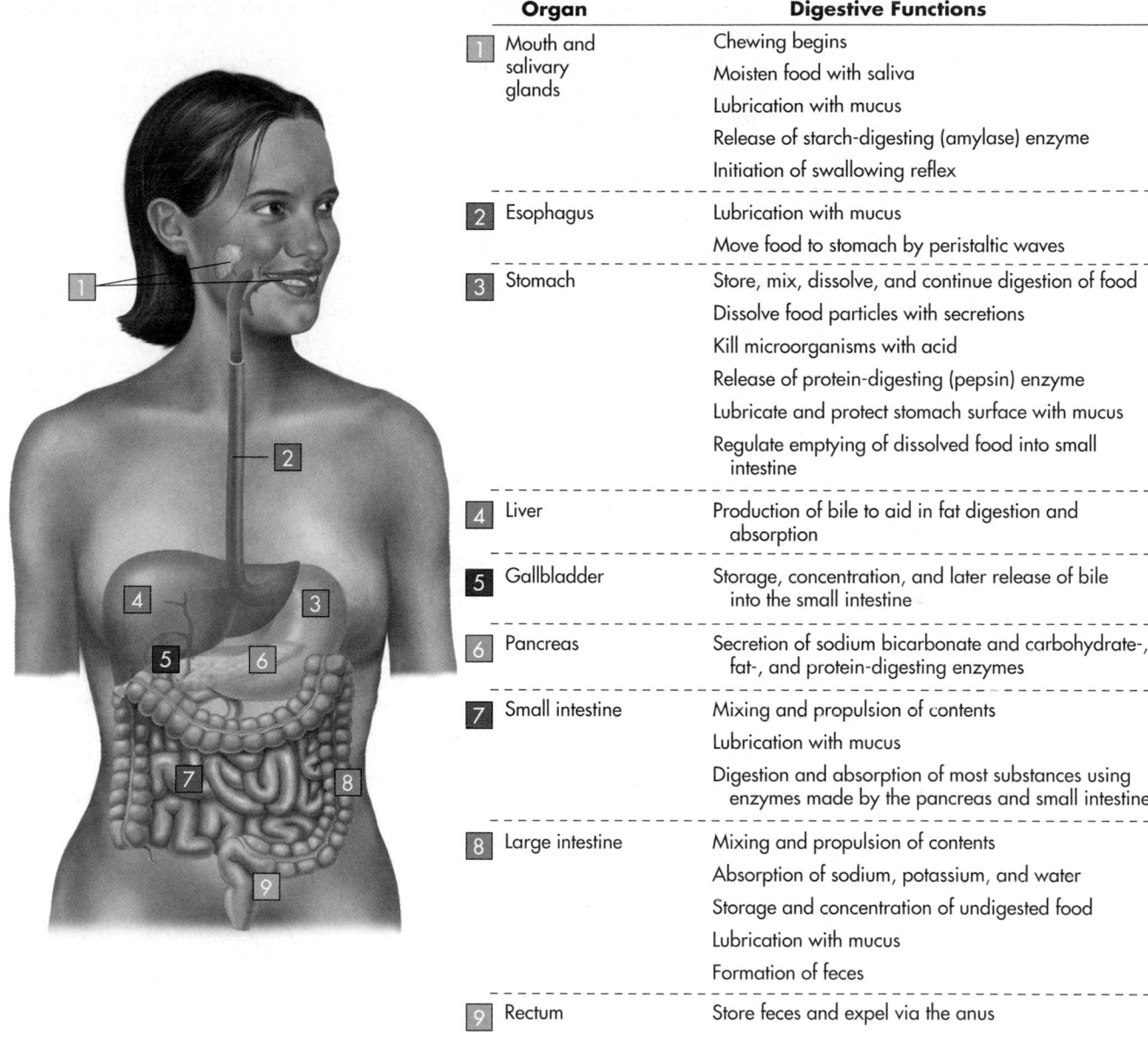

Organ	Digestive Functions
1 Mouth and salivary glands	Chewing begins
	Moisten food with saliva
	Lubrication with mucus
	Release of starch-digesting (amylase) enzyme
	Initiation of swallowing reflex
2 Esophagus	Lubrication with mucus
	Move food to stomach by peristaltic waves
3 Stomach	Store, mix, dissolve, and continue digestion of food
	Dissolve food particles with secretions
	Kill microorganisms with acid
	Release of protein-digesting (pepsin) enzyme
	Lubricate and protect stomach surface with mucus
	Regulate emptying of dissolved food into small intestine
4 Liver	Production of bile to aid in fat digestion and absorption
5 Gallbladder	Storage, concentration, and later release of bile into the small intestine
6 Pancreas	Secretion of sodium bicarbonate and carbohydrate-, fat-, and protein-digesting enzymes
7 Small intestine	Mixing and propulsion of contents
	Lubrication with mucus
	Digestion and absorption of most substances using enzymes made by the pancreas and small intestine
8 Large intestine	Mixing and propulsion of contents
	Absorption of sodium, potassium, and water
	Storage and concentration of undigested food
	Lubrication with mucus
	Formation of feces
9 Rectum	Store feces and expel via the anus

Figure 3-9 Physiology of the GI tract. Many organs cooperate in a regulated fashion to allow digestion and subsequent absorption of nutrients in foods.

GI tract—from the inside to the outside—to be absorbed into the bloodstream. The organs that make up the GI tract, as well as some additional accessory organs located nearby, are collectively known as the digestive system.

In the digestive system, food is broken down mechanically and chemically. Mechanical digestion takes place as soon as you begin chewing your food and continues as muscular contractions simultaneously mix and move food through the length of the GI tract (as part of a process known as **motility**). Chemical digestion refers to the chemical breakdown of foods by substances which are secreted into the GI tract. Finally, the digestive system eliminates wastes. In addition to nutrients that arise from digestion of food, the bacteria that live in the intestine produce vitamin K and the vitamin biotin, some of which we can absorb and use.

Most of the processes of digestion and absorption are under autonomic control; that is, they are involuntary. Almost all of the functions involved in digestion and absorption are controlled by hormones, hormone-like compounds, and nervous system

motility Generally, the ability to move spontaneously. It also refers to movement of food through the GI tract.

GI Tract Flow

Mouth
↓
Esophagus (10 inches long)
↓
Stomach—4-cup (1-liter) capacity. Food remains about 2 to 3 hours, or longer for large meals.
↓
Small intestine—duodenum (10 in long), jejunum (4 ft long), ileum (5 ft long)—about 10 ft (3.1 meters) in total length. Food remains about 3 to 10 hours.
↓
Large intestine (colon)—cecum, ascending colon, transverse colon, descending colon, sigmoid colon—3½ ft (1.1 meters) in total length. Food can remain up to 72 hours.
↓
Rectum
↓
Anus

umami A brothy, meaty, savory flavor in some foods. Monosodium glutamate enhances this flavor when added to foods.

input. Many common ailments arise from problems with the digestive system (see the next Looking Further section).

The digestive system is composed of six separate organs; each organ performs one or more specific job(s). Let's look briefly at the role of each organ. A more complete description of the digestive process will be explained in later chapters as each nutrient is introduced.

■ Mouth

The mouth performs many functions in the digestion of food. Besides chewing food to reduce it to smaller particles, the mouth also senses the taste of the foods we consume. In tasting, the tongue, through the use of its taste buds, identifies foods on the basis of their specific flavor(s). Sweet, sour, salty, bitter, and **umami** comprise the primary taste sensations we experience. Surprisingly, the nose and our sense of smell greatly contribute to our ability to sense the taste of food. When we chew a food, chemicals are released that stimulate the nasal passages. Thus, it makes perfect sense that when we are sick and our noses are stuffed up and congested, even our most favorite foods will not taste as good as they normally do.

The taste of food, or the anticipation of it, signals the rest of the GI tract to prepare for the digestion of food. Once in the mouth, mechanical and chemical digestion begins. Salivary glands produce **saliva,** which functions as a solvent so that food particles can be further separated and tasted. In addition, saliva contains a starch-digesting enzyme, **salivary amylase** (see Chapter 4 for more on starch-digesting enzymes). This and other enzymes are a key part of digestion. Overall, enzymes work to hasten certain events that take place in the body (Fig. 3-10). The pancreas and the small intestine produce the most digestive enzymes; however, the mouth and the stomach also contribute their own enzymes to digestion. **Mucus,** another component of saliva, makes it easy to swallow a mouthful of food (Table 3-3). The food then travels to the esophagus.

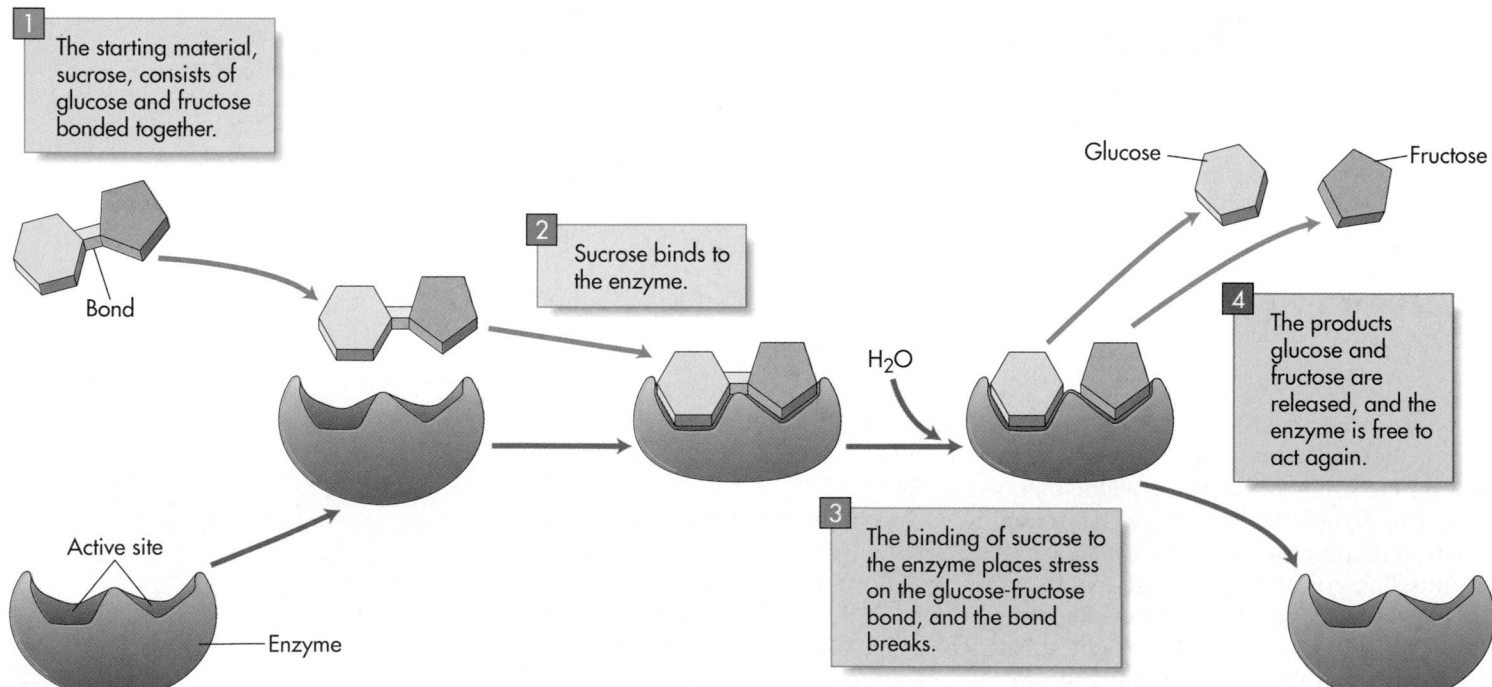

1 The starting material, sucrose, consists of glucose and fructose bonded together.

2 Sucrose binds to the enzyme.

3 The binding of sucrose to the enzyme places stress on the glucose-fructose bond, and the bond breaks.

4 The products glucose and fructose are released, and the enzyme is free to act again.

Bond

Active site

Enzyme

Glucose

Fructose

H_2O

Figure 3-10 A model of enzyme action. Enzymes increase the speed with which chemical reactions occur, but they are not altered themselves as they do so. In the reaction illustrated here, an enzyme is splitting the sugar sucrose into two simpler sugars: glucose and fructose. Only these simpler sugars are absorbed from the small intestine to enter the bloodstream. Note that sometimes energy input is needed to push the reaction along, but not in this case.

Table 3-3 Important Secretions and Products of the Digestive Tract

Secretion	Site of Production	Purpose
Saliva	Mouth	Contributes to starch digestion, utilizing **salivary amylase,** lubrication, swallowing
Mucus	Mouth, stomach, small intestine, large intestine	Protects GI tract cells, lubricates food as it travels through the GI tract
Enzymes	Mouth, stomach, small intestine, pancreas	Promote digestion of foodstuffs into particles small enough for absorption utilizing **amylases, lipases,** and **proteases**
Acid	Stomach	Promotes digestion of protein among other functions
Bile	Liver (stored in gallbladder)	Suspends fat in water utilizing **bile acids, cholesterol,** and **lecithin** to aid fat digestion in the small intestine
Bicarbonate	Pancreas, small intestine	Neutralizes stomach acid when it reaches the small intestine
Hormones	Stomach, small intestine, pancreas	Hormones such as **gastrin, secretin, insulin, cholecystokinin,** and **glucagon** stimulate production and/or release of acid, enzymes, bile, and bicarbonate; help regulate peristalsis and overall GI tract flow

Another Bite

Each enzyme is specific to one type of chemical process. For example, enzymes that recognize and digest table sugar (sucrose) ignore milk sugar (lactose). Besides working on only particular types of chemicals, enzymes are sensitive to acidic and alkaline conditions, temperature, and the types of vitamins and minerals they require. Digestive enzymes that work in the acidic environment of the stomach do not work well in the alkaline environment of the small intestine. The body is also able to increase the production of certain digestive enzymes in response to the type of diet consumed. Because of this fine-tuning, the GI tract can respond to the nutritional makeup and amount of food consumed. Multiple enzymes attack foods consumed to prepare them for absorption. The authors of some popular (fad) diet books contend that eating certain combinations of foods, such as meats and fruits together, hinders the digestive process. This does not make sense in light of our knowledge about GI tract physiology.

■ Esophagus

The **esophagus** is a long tube that connects the **pharynx** with the stomach. Near the pharynx is a flap of tissue (called the **epiglottis**) that prevents the **bolus** of swallowed food from entering the trachea (wind pipe). During swallowing, food lands on the epiglottis, folding it down to cover the opening of the trachea. Breathing also stops automatically. These responses ensure that swallowed food will only travel down the esophagus. If food instead travels down the trachea, choking may occur (the victim will not be able to speak or breathe). A group of techniques to treat such a person are called the Heimlich maneuver (see www.heimlichinstitute.org for details).

At the top of the esophagus, nerve fibers release signals to tell the GI tract that food has been consumed. This results in an increase in gastrointestinal muscle action, called **peristalsis.** Continual waves of muscle contractions, followed by muscle relaxation, force the food down the digestive tract from the esophagus onward (Fig. 3-11).

salivary amylase A starch-digesting enzyme produced by salivary glands.

mucus A thick fluid secreted by many cells throughout the body. It contains a compound that has both carbohydrate and protein parts. It acts as a lubricant and means of protection for cells.

amylase Starch-digesting enzyme produced by the salivary glands and pancreas.

lipase Fat-digesting enzyme produced by the salivary glands, stomach, and pancreas.

protease Protein-digesting enzyme produced by the stomach, small intestine, and pancreas.

esophagus A tube in the GI tract that connects the pharynx with the stomach.

pharynx The organ of the digestive tract and respiratory tract located at the back of the oral and nasal cavities, commonly known as the throat.

epiglottis The flap that folds down over the trachea during swallowing.

bolus A moistened mass of food that is swallowed from the oral cavity into the pharynx.

Figure 3-11 Peristalsis. Peristalsis is a progressive type of movement, propelling material from point to point along the GI tract. To begin this, a ring of contraction occurs where the GI wall is stretched, passing the food mass forward. The moving food mass triggers a ring of contraction in the next region, which pushes the food mass even farther along. The overall result is a ring of contraction that moves like a wave along the GI tract, pushing the food mass down the tract. In a related action, the intestinal muscles contract, causing an alternative forward-and-backward mixing movement. This process, called **segmentation,** results in little net forward movement.

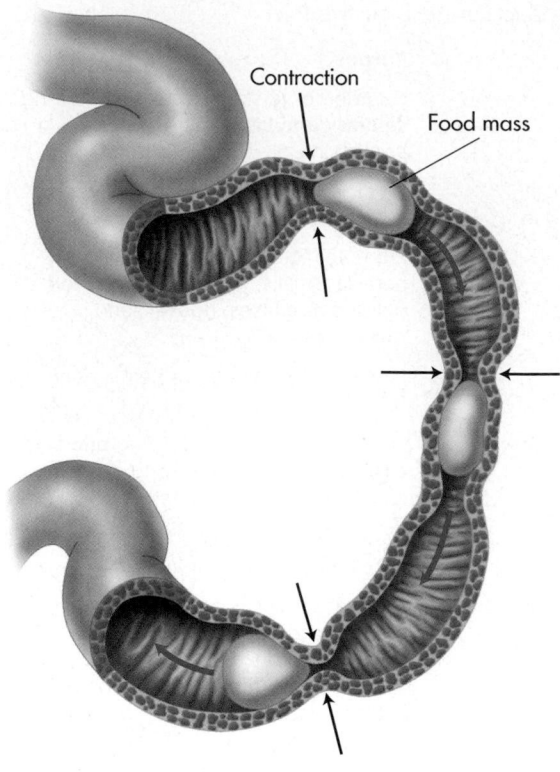

Contraction

Food mass

lower esophageal sphincter A circular muscle that constricts the opening of the esophagus to the stomach. Also called the *gastroesophageal sphincter*.

chyme A mixture of stomach secretions and partially digested food.

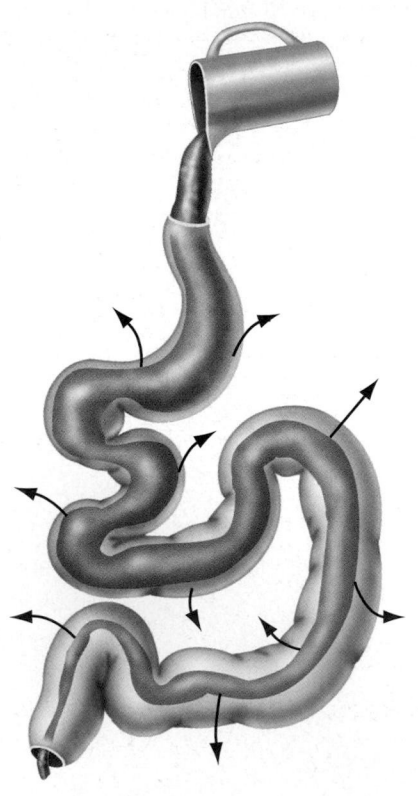

As the intestinal contents pass down the tract, nutrients are absorbed from the internal cavity (called the lumen) of the gastrointestinal tract into the body.

At the end of the esophagus is the **lower esophageal sphincter,** a muscle that constricts (closes) after food enters the stomach (Fig. 3-12). The main function of sphincters is to prevent the backflow of GI tract contents. Sphincters respond to various stimuli, such as signals from the nervous system, hormones, acidic versus alkaline conditions, and pressure that builds up around the sphincter itself. The primary function of the lower esophageal sphincter is to prevent the acidic contents of the stomach from flowing back up into the esophagus—which can cause many health problems (see the next Looking Further section).

■ Stomach

The stomach is a large tank that can hold up to 4 cups of food for several hours until all of the food is able to enter the small intestine. Stomach size varies individually and can be reduced surgically as a radical treatment for obesity (more on this in Chapter 10). While in the stomach, the food is mixed with gastric juice, which contains water, a very strong acid, and enzymes. The acid in the gastric juice maintains the acidity of the stomach, thereby destroying the biological activity of proteins, converting inactive digestive enzymes to their active form, partially digesting food protein, and making dietary minerals soluble so that they can be absorbed. This mixing produces a watery food mixture, called **chyme,** which then leaves the stomach a teaspoon (5 milliliters) at a time and enters the small intestine. Following a meal, the stomach contents are emptied into the small intestine over the course of 1 to 4 hours.

You might wonder how the stomach prevents itself from being digested by the acid and enzymes it produces. First, the stomach has a thick layer of mucus that lines and protects it. The production of acid and enzymes is also tied to the release of a specific hormone (gastrin). This release happens primarily when we are thinking about eating or are actually in the process of eating. Lastly, as the concentration of acid in the stomach increases, acid production tapers off, also because of hormonal control.

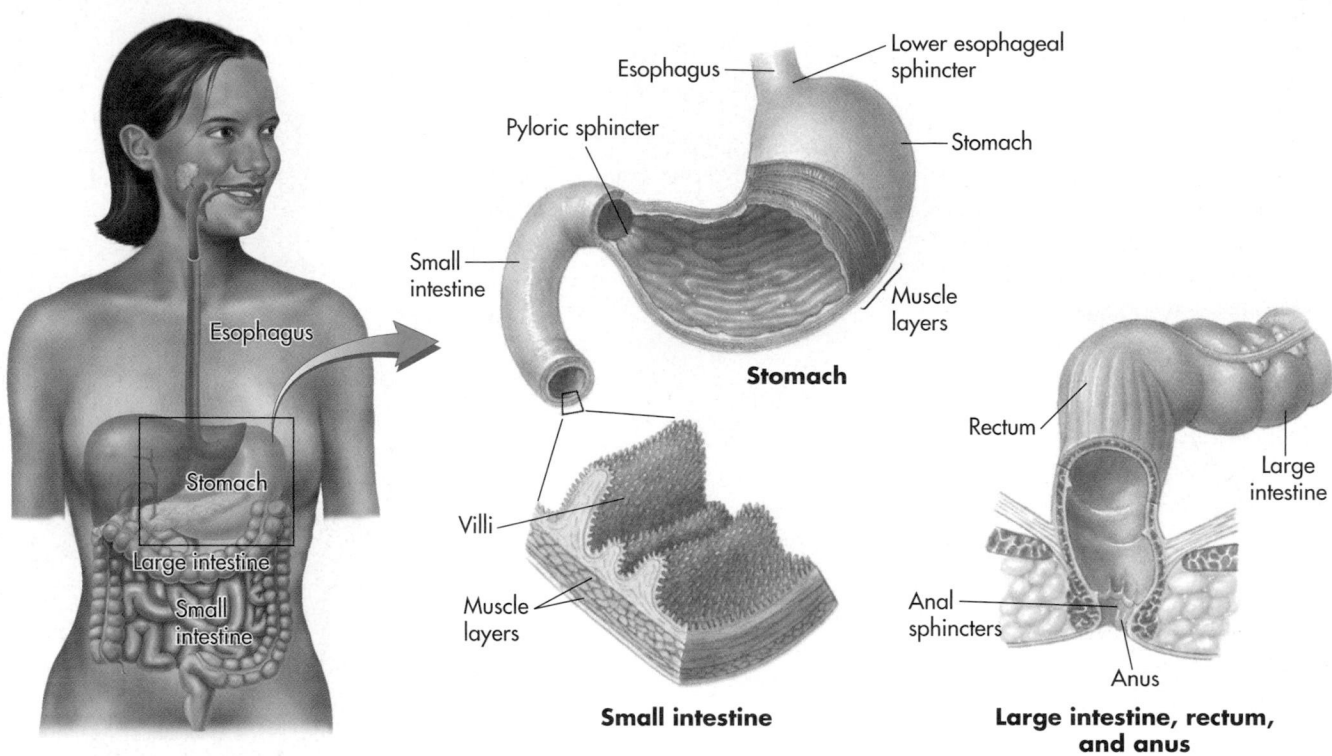

Esophagus

Lower esophageal sphincter

Pyloric sphincter

Stomach

Small intestine

Muscle layers

Stomach

Esophagus

Stomach

Large intestine

Small intestine

Rectum

Large intestine

Villi

Muscle layers

Anal sphincters

Anus

Small intestine

Large intestine, rectum, and anus

Figure 3-12 A close-up view of the muscles, sphincters, and villi of the GI tract. These features of the GI tract perform key roles in digestion, absorption, and elimination.

The **pyloric sphincter,** located at the base of the stomach, controls the rate at which the chyme is released into the small intestine (review Fig. 3-12). There is very little absorption of nutrients from the stomach, except for some alcohol.

One other important function of the stomach is the production of a substance called **intrinsic factor.** This vital material is essential for the absorption of vitamin B-12.

■ Small Intestine

The small intestine is about 10 feet (3 meters) long, beginning at the stomach on the "north" and ending at the large intestine (colon) on the "south." The small intestine is considered "small" because of its narrow (1 inch [2.5 centimeters]) diameter. Most of the digestion and absorption of food occurs in the small intestine. The chyme secreted from the stomach is moved through the small intestine by peristaltic contractions so that it can be well mixed with the digestive juices of the small intestine. These juices contain many enzymes that function in the breakdown of carbohydrates, protein, and fat, as well as in the preparation of vitamins and minerals for absorption.

The physical structure of the small intestine is very important to the body's ability to digest and absorb the nutrients it needs. The lining of the small intestine is folded many times; within these folds are fingerlike projections called **villi.** These "fingers" are constantly moving, which helps them trap food to enhance absorption. Each individual villus (singular) is made up of many absorptive cells, and each of these cells has a highly folded cap. The combined folds, villi, and caps in the small intestine increase its surface area 600 times beyond that of a simple tube (Fig. 3-13).

New **absorptive cells** are constantly produced and appear daily along the surface of each villus "finger." This is probably because absorptive cells are subjected to a harsh environment, so renewal of the intestinal lining is necessary. This rapid cell turnover leads to high nutrient needs for the small intestine. Fortunately, many of the old cells can be broken down and have their component parts reused. The health of

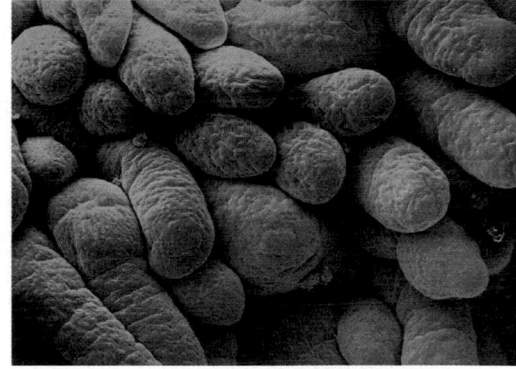

A close-up view of the finger-like projections of the intestinal villi.

pyloric sphincter The ring of smooth muscle between the stomach and the small intestine.

villi (singular, **villus**) The fingerlike protrusions into the small intestine that participate in digestion and absorption of food.

absorptive cells A class of cells that line the villi; these cells participate in nutrient absorption.

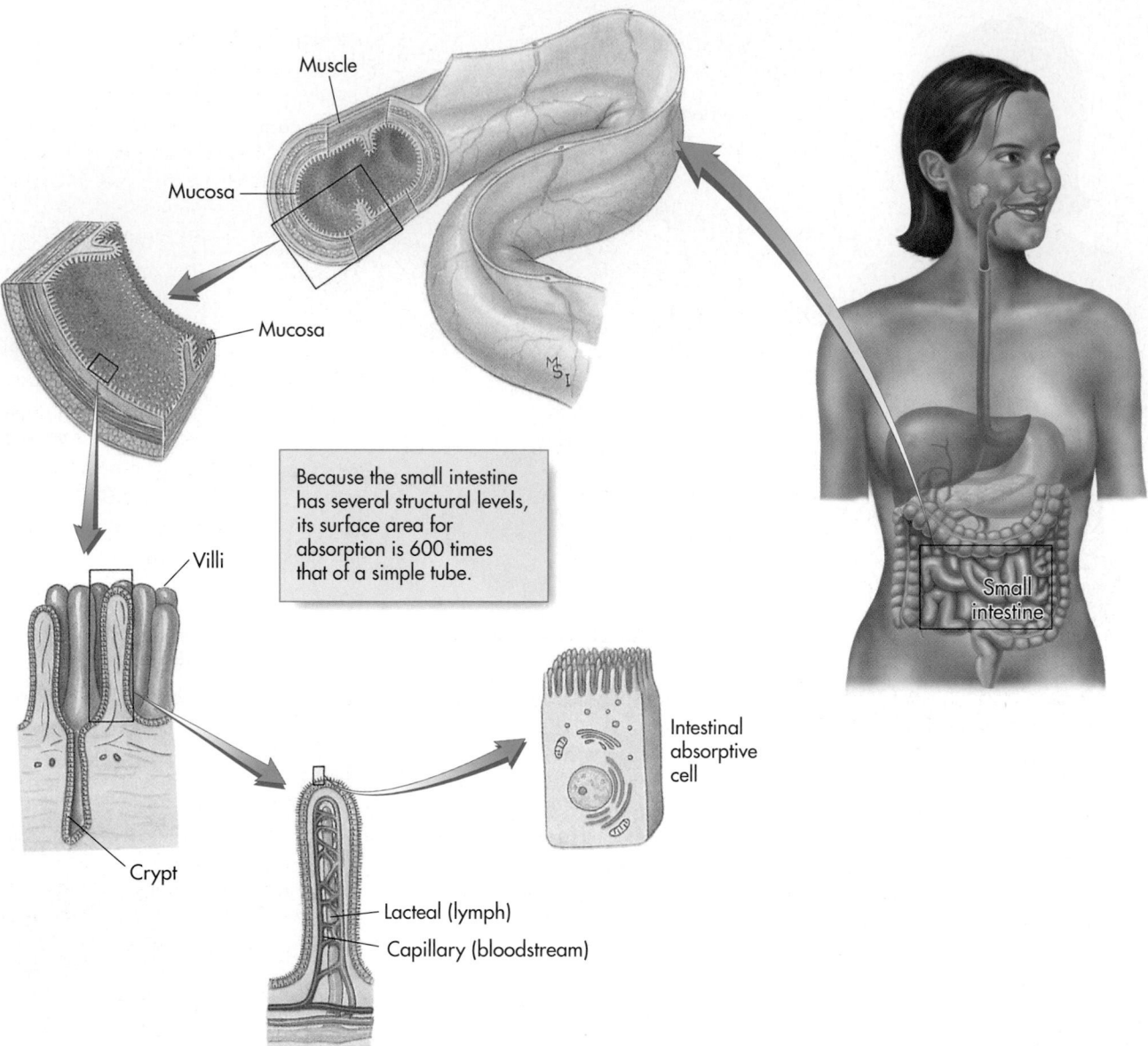

Figure 3-13 Organization of the small intestine. The small intestine has several structural levels, which increase the surface area for absorption up to 600 times that of a simple tube.

the cells is further enhanced by various hormones and other substances that participate in or are produced as part of the digestive process.

The small intestine absorbs nutrients through the intestinal wall through various means and processes, as illustrated in Figure 3-14:

- **Passive diffusion:** When the nutrient concentration is higher in the cavity (lumen) of the small intestine than in the absorptive cells, the difference in nutrient concentration drives the nutrient into the absorptive cells by diffusion. Passive diffusion allows for the absorption of fats, water, and some minerals.
- **Facilitated diffusion:** For some compounds, passive diffusion is not sufficient to drive absorption. In those cases, facilitated diffusion, which uses a carrier protein, can drive certain nutrients into absorptive cells. Fructose is one example of a compound that makes use of such a carrier to allow for facilitated diffusion.
- **Active absorption:** In addition to the need for a carrier protein, some nutrients also require energy input to move from the lumen of the small intestine into the

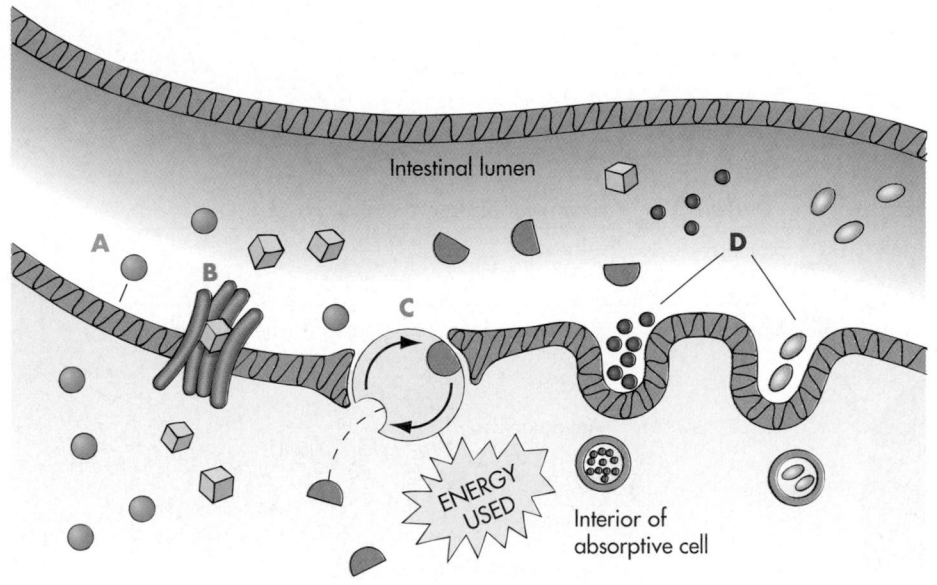

Intestinal lumen

ENERGY USED

Interior of absorptive cell

Figure 3-14 Nutrient absorption relies on four major absorptive processes. (A) ● Passive diffusion is simple diffusion of nutrients across the absorptive cell membranes. (B) ■ Facilitated diffusion uses a carrier protein to move nutrients down a concentration gradient. (C) ◗ Active absorption involves a carrier protein as well as energy to move nutrients (against a concentration gradient) into absorptive cells. (D) ● Pinocytosis and ◖ phagocytosis are forms of active absorption in which the absorptive cell membrane engulfs a nutrient to bring it into the cell.

In **cystic fibrosis**—an inherited disease of infants, children, and sometimes adults—the pancreas often develops thick mucus that blocks its ducts, and active cells then die. As a result, the pancreas is not able to effectively deliver its digestive enzymes into the small intestine. Digestion of carbohydrate, protein, and—most notably—fat then is impaired. Often the missing enzymes must be ingested in capsule form with meals to aid in digestion. Another intestinal problem gaining attention is **celiac disease.** People with this disease experience an allergic reaction to the protein gluten in certain cereals, such as wheat and rye. This reaction damages the absorptive cells, resulting in a much reduced surface area due to flattening of the villi. Elimination of wheat, rye, and certain other grains from the diet typically cures the problem.

absorptive cells. This mechanism makes it possible for cells to take up nutrients even when they are consumed in low concentrations. Some sugars, such as glucose, are actively absorbed, as are amino acids.

- **Phagocytosis and pinocytosis:** In a further means of active absorption, absorptive cells literally engulf compounds (phagocytosis) or liquids (pinocytosis). As described earlier, a cell membrane can form an indentation of itself so that when particles or fluids move into the indentation, the cell membrane surrounds and engulfs them. This process is used when an infant absorbs immune substances from human milk (see Chapter 13).

ileocecal sphincter The ring of smooth muscle between the end of the small intestine and the large intestine.

Once absorbed, water-soluble compounds such as glucose and amino acids go to the capillaries and then on to a portal vein. Recall that the liver is the end point of this process. Most fats eventually go into the lymph vessels. In doing so, they can eventually enter the bloodstream (see the earlier section on the circulatory system for details; and review Figs. 3-5 and 3-6).

Any undigested food that reaches the end of the small intestine must pass through the **ileocecal sphincter** on the way to the large intestine. This sphincter prevents the contents of the large intestine from reentering the small intestine.

■ Large Intestine

When the contents of the small intestine enter the large intestine, the material that is left bears little resemblance to the food that was eaten originally. Under normal circumstances, only a minor amount (5%) of carbohydrate, protein, and fat escape absorption to reach the large intestine (Fig. 3-15).

Physiologically, the large intestine differs from the small intestine in that there are no villi or digestive enzymes. The absence of villi means that little absorption takes place in the large intestine in comparison to the small intestine. Nutrients that are

Foods containing certain microorganisms such as lactobacilli are getting a lot of attention these days. The term **probiotic** is used for these microorganisms because once consumed, they take up residence in the large intestine and lead to some health benefits, such as improving intestinal tract health. You can find these probiotic microorganisms in certain forms of fluid milk, fermented milk, and yogurt. They can even be found in pill form. A related term is **prebiotic.** These are substances that increase growth of probiotic microorganisms. One example is fructooligosaccharides (see Table 2-1 in Chapter 2 for dietary sources).

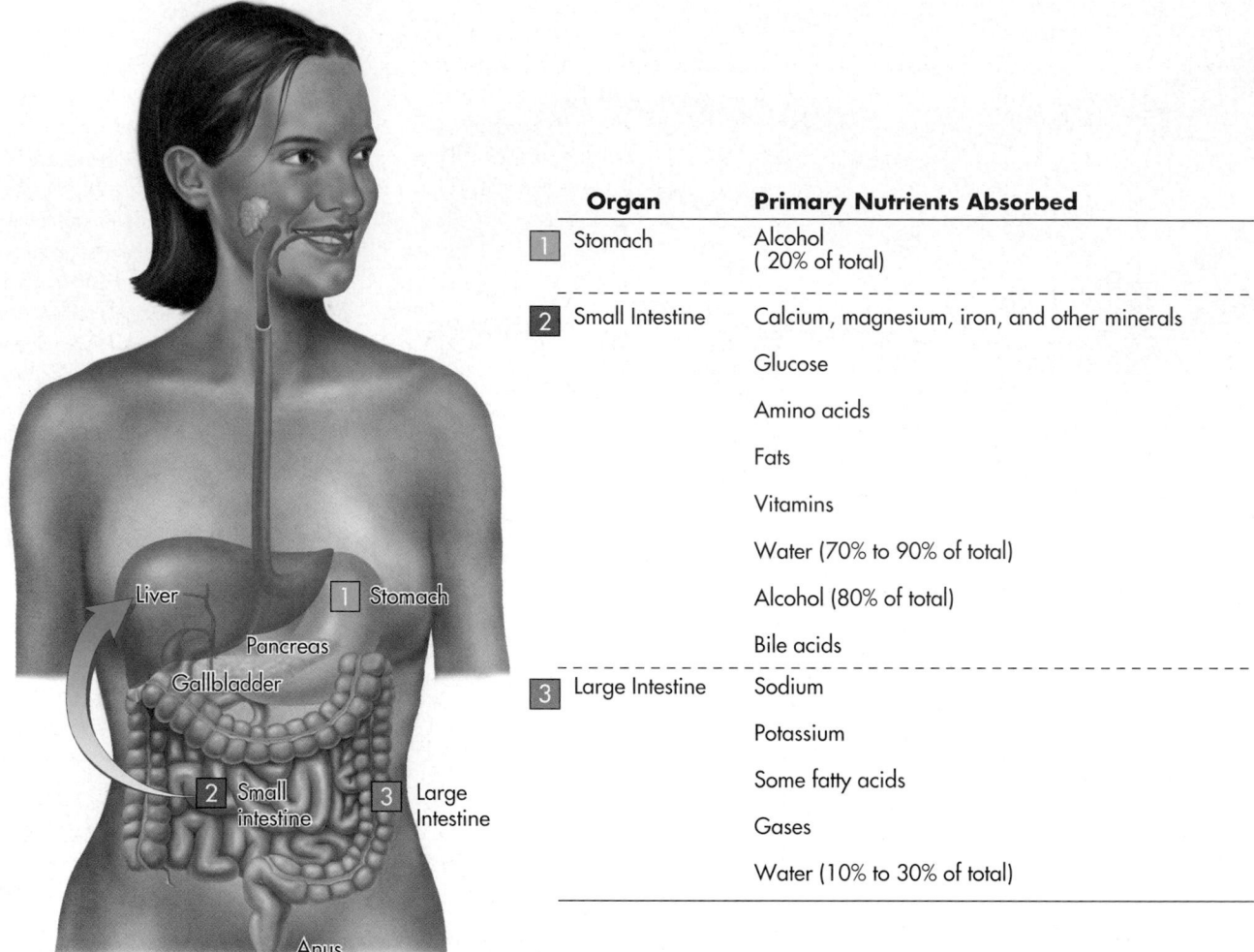

Organ	Primary Nutrients Absorbed
1 Stomach	Alcohol (20% of total)
2 Small Intestine	Calcium, magnesium, iron, and other minerals
	Glucose
	Amino acids
	Fats
	Vitamins
	Water (70% to 90% of total)
	Alcohol (80% of total)
	Bile acids
3 Large Intestine	Sodium
	Potassium
	Some fatty acids
	Gases
	Water (10% to 30% of total)

Figure 3-15 Major sites of absorption along the GI tract. Note that some absorption of vitamin K and biotin takes place in the large intestine. All nutrients except most of those that are fat soluble travel through the portal vein to the liver after their absorption.

Critical Thinking

The medical history of a young girl who is greatly underweight shows that she had three-quarters of her small intestine removed after she was injured in a car accident. Explain how this accounts for her underweight condition, even though her medical chart shows that she eats well.

absorbed from the large intestine include water, some vitamins, some fatty acids, and the minerals sodium and potassium. Unlike the small intestine, the large intestine has a number of mucus-producing cells. The mucus secreted by these cells functions to hold the feces together and to protect the large intestine from ongoing bacterial activity within it. The large intestine is home to a large population of bacteria (over 500 different species). Note that these bacteria are able to break down some of the remaining food products that enter the large intestine, such as the milk sugar lactose (in people who are lactose intolerant), and some components of fiber. The products of bacterial metabolism in the large intestine, which include various acids, can then be absorbed (Chapter 4 will discuss this further).

Some water remains in the material that enters the large intestine because the small intestine absorbs only 70% to 90% of the fluid it receives, which included large amounts of GI-tract secretions produced during digestion. The remnants of a meal also contain some minerals and some fiber. And because water is removed, the contents of the large intestine become semisolid by the time they have passed through the first two-thirds of it. What remains in the **feces,** besides water and undigested fiber, is tough connective tissues (from animal foods), bacteria from the large intestine, and some body wastes, such as parts of dead intestinal cells.

■ Rectum

The stool remains in the last portion of the large intestine, the **rectum**, until muscular movements push it into the **anus** to be eliminated. The presence of feces in the rectum stimulates elimination. The anus contains two **anal sphincters** (internal and external), one of which is under voluntary control (external sphincter). Once children are toilet trained, they can generally control when the external anal sphincter will relax and when it will stay rigid. Relaxation of this sphincter allows for elimination.

■ Accessory Organs

Accessory organs are not part of the GI tract through which food passes, but they play necessary roles in the process of digestion. These organs secrete digestive fluids into the GI tract and enable the process of converting food into absorbable nutrients. The **liver, gallbladder,** and **pancreas** work with the GI tract and are considered accessory organs to the process of digestion (review Fig. 3-9).

The liver produces a substance called **bile.** The bile is stored and concentrated in the gallbladder until it receives a hormonal "release" signal, which is induced by the presence of fat in the small intestine. Once this hormonal signal is received by the gallbladder, bile is released and delivered to the small intestine via a tube called the bile duct.

In action, bile is very much like soap. Constituents in the bile take large portions of fat and break them into smaller bits so that they can be suspended in water (Chapter 5 will cover this process in detail). Interestingly, some of the bile constituents can be "recycled" in a process known as **enterohepatic circulation.** These components of bile are reabsorbed from the small intestine, returned to the liver via a portal vein, and reused.

In addition to bile, the liver releases a number of other substances that travel with the bile to the gallbladder and eventually end up in the small intestine. The liver functions in this manner to remove unwanted substances from the blood. (Other byproducts are excreted via the urine; see the next section, Urinary system.)

The pancreas manufactures hormones and pancreatic juice. The hormones include glucagon and insulin, which as noted earlier function in glucose regulation. Pancreatic juice contains water, bicarbonate, and a variety of digestive enzymes capable of breaking apart carbohydrates, proteins, and fats into small fragments. Bicarbonate is a base that neutralizes the acidity of chyme as it moves from the stomach into the small intestine. Recall that the stomach produces a thick layer of mucus to protect itself from the acid of gastric secretions. The small intestine, however, does not have a protective layer of mucus, because mucus would impede nutrient absorption. Instead, the neutralizing capacity of bicarbonate from the pancreas protects the walls of the small intestine from erosion by acid, which would otherwise lead to formation of an ulcer (see the following Looking Further section).

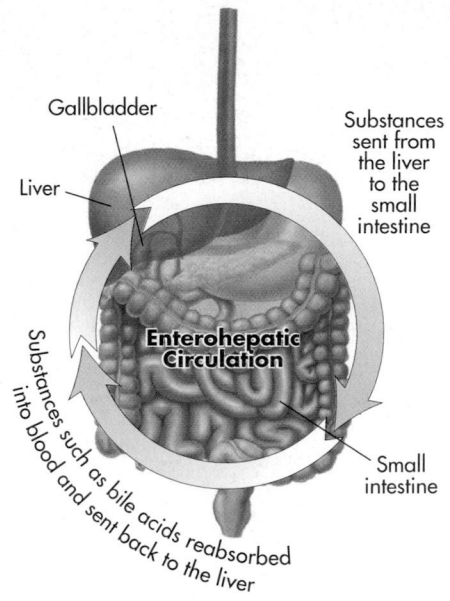

gallbladder An organ attached to the underside of the liver; site of bile storage, concentration, and eventual secretion.

bile A liver secretion that is stored in the gallbladder and released through the common bile duct into the first segment of the small intestine. It is essential for the absorption of fat.

enterohepatic circulation A continual recycling of compounds between the small intestine and the liver; bile acids are one example of a recycled compound.

Concept Check

Digestion is a mechanical and chemical process mediated by enzymes and coordinated by hormones and nerves. Whereas swallowing and ultimate elimination of feces from the anus are voluntary, the majority of the digestive processes are involuntary. The stomach initiates the process of digestion by mixing food with gastric juice and converting this partially digested food into chyme. The end products of digestion are molecules of the original food or beverage small enough to be absorbed into the villi of the small intestine and transferred to the blood or lymph. For the most part, nutrients are absorbed in the small intestine; only a few are absorbed in the large intestine. Any dietary component that escapes digestion by human or bacterial enzymes exits the body as feces.

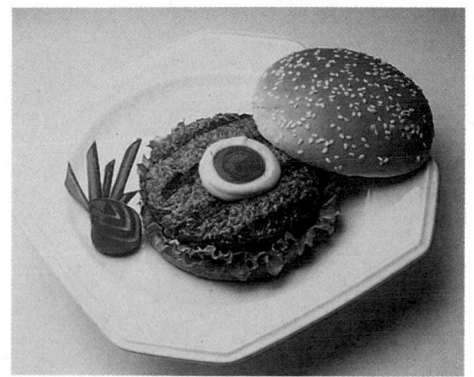

The body digests the foods presented—the order in which foods are eaten plays no role in digestion.

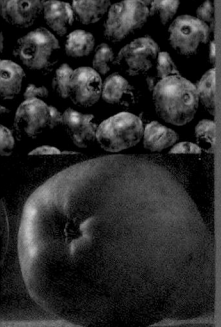

Looking Further

Two other common GI tract-related problems are diverticulosis and lactose maldigestion and intolerance. These disorders will be discussed in Chapter 4 after you learn more about carbohydrates.

The fine-tuned organ system we call the digestive system can develop problems. Knowing about these common problems can help you avoid or lessen them.

Ulcers

Millions of North Americans develop **ulcers** during their lifetimes. The principal causes are an acid-resistant bacterial infection *(Helicobacter pylori [H. pylori])*, the heavy use of aspirin and related medications, and disorders that cause excessive acid production in the stomach (Fig. 3-16). And, after being out of favor for some years, stress is again regarded as a predisposing factor for ulcers, especially if the person is infected with *H. pylori* or has certain anxiety disorders.

As the stomach lining deteriorates in ulcer development and loses its mucus layer protection, the acid further erodes the stomach tissue. Acid can also erode the tissue lining of the first part of the small intestine. *Peptic ulcer* is the general term for both types of ulcers. Most ulcers in young people occur in the small intestine; in older people they occur primarily in the stomach.

The typical symptom of an ulcer is pain about 2 hours after eating. Stomach acid acting on a meal irritates the ulcer after most of the meal has moved from the site of the ulcer.

ulcer Erosion of the tissue lining, usually in the stomach or the upper small intestine. As a group these are generally referred to as *peptic ulcers.*

NSAIDs Nonsteroidal anti-inflamatory drugs; includes aspirin, ibuprofen (Advil®), and naproxen (Aleve®).

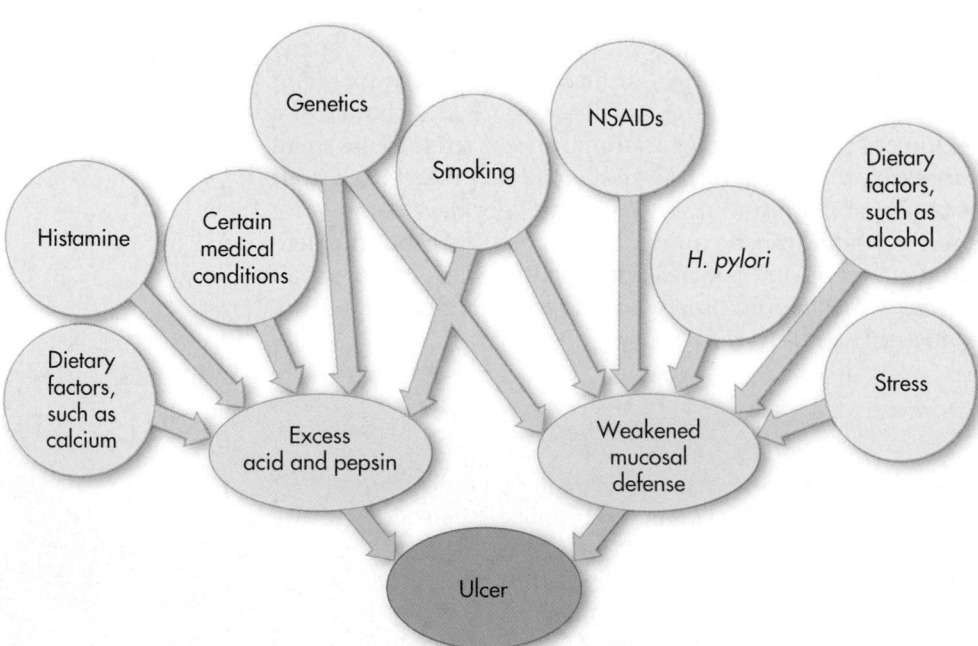

Figure 3-16 Development of a peptic ulcer. *H. pylori* bacteria and **NSAIDs** (e.g., aspirin) cause ulcers by impairing mucosal defense, especially in the stomach. In the same way, smoking, genetics, and stress can impair mucosal defense, as well as cause an increase in the release of pepsin and stomach acid. All of these factors can contribute to ulcers.

Table 3-4 Recommendations to Prevent Ulcers and Heartburn from Occurring or Recurring

Ulcers

1. Stop smoking if you are now a smoker.
2. Avoid large doses of aspirin, ibuprofen, and other NSAID compounds unless a physician advises otherwise. For people who must use these medications, FDA has approved an NSAID combined with a medication to reduce gastric damage. The medication reduces gastric acid production and enhances mucus secretion.
3. Limit consumption of coffee, tea, and alcohol (especially wine), if this helps.
4. Limit consumption of pepper, chili powder, and other strong spices, if this helps.
5. Eat nutritious meals on a regular schedule; include enough fiber (see Chapter 4 for sources of fiber).
6. Chew foods well.
7. Lose weight if you are currently overweight.

Heartburn

1. Observe the recommendations for ulcer prevention.
2. Wait about 2 hours after a meal before lying down.
3. Don't overeat at mealtime. Smaller meals that are low in fat are advised.
4. Try elevating the head of the bed (6-inch blocks).

The primary risk associated with an ulcer is the possibility that it will erode entirely through the stomach or intestinal wall. The GI contents could then spill into the body cavities, causing a massive infection. In addition, an ulcer may erode a blood vessel, leading to substantial blood loss. For these reasons, it is important not to ignore the early warning signs of ulcer development.

In the past, milk and cream therapy—the Sippy diet—was used to help cure ulcers. Clinicians now know that milk and cream are two of the worst foods for an ulcer. The calcium in these foods stimulates stomach acid secretion and actually inhibits ulcer healing.

Today, a combination of approaches is used for ulcer therapy. People infected with *H. pylori* are given antibiotics as well as stomach acid-blocking medications called **proton pump inhibitors** (e.g., omeprazole [Prilosec]) and possibly bismuth. (Note that proton is another term for the hydrogen ion that creates acidity.) In many cases, there is a 90% cure rate for *H. pylori* infections in the first week of this treatment. Recurrence is unlikely if the infection is cured, but an incomplete cure almost certainly leads to repeated ulcer formation.

Antacid medications may also be part of ulcer care, as is a class of medicines called **H₂ blockers.** These include cimetidine (Tagamet), ranitidine (Zantac), and famotidine (Pepcid), all of which prevent **histamine**-related acid secretion in the stomach. Medications that coat the ulcer, such as sucralfate (Carafate), are also commonly used.

People with ulcers should refrain from smoking and minimize the use of aspirin and related NSAIDs. These practices reduce the mucus secreted by the stomach. Medications that are used to treat arthritis pain, called "Cox-2 inhibitors" (e.g., celecoxib [Celebrex]), are less likely to cause stomach ulcers and, so, have been used as a replacement for NSAIDs. They do offer some advantages over NSAIDS, but they may not be totally safe for some people, such as people with a history of cardiovascular disease or strokes. Overall, a combination of lifestyle therapy and medical treatment has so revolutionized ulcer therapy that dietary changes are of minor importance today. Current diet-therapy approaches recommend simply avoiding foods that increase ulcer symptoms (Table 3-4).

proton pump inhibitor A medication that inhibits the ability of gastric cells to secrete hydrogen ions. Examples are esomeprazole (Nexium) and lansoprazole (Prevacid). Low doses of this class of medications are also availbale without prescription (e.g., omeprazole Prilosec).

histamine A breakdown product of the amino acid histidine that stimulates acid secretion by the stomach and has other effects on the body, such as contraction of smooth muscles, increased nasal secretions, relaxation of blood vessels, and changes in relaxation of airways.

Heartburn

About half of North American adults experience occassional **heartburn.** This gnawing pain in the upper chest is caused by the movement of acid from the stomach into the esophagus. The more serious form of the problem is called **gastroesophageal reflux disease (GERD).** Unlike

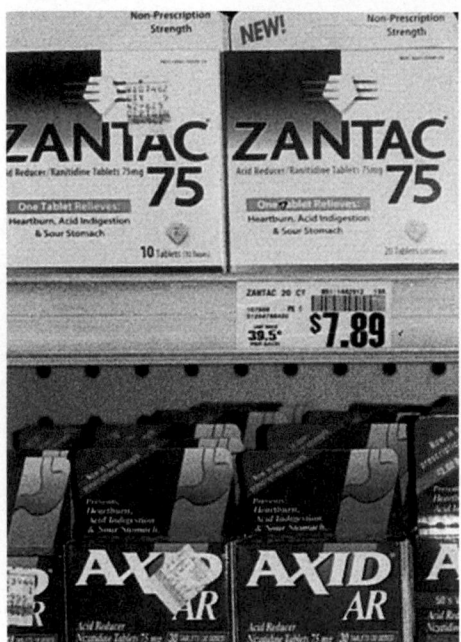

A number of over-the-counter medications are marketed for heartburn including H₂ blockers as well as proton pump inhibitors. Attention to diet and lifestyle, however, is generally a more important measure to take.

the stomach, the esophagus has very little mucus lining to protect it, so acid quickly erodes the lining of the esophagus, causing pain. Symptoms may also include nausea, gagging, cough, or hoarseness. GERD is characterized by such symptoms of acid reflux two or more times per week. People who have GERD experience occasional relaxation of the sphincter. Typically it should be relaxed only during swallowing, but in individuals with GERD it is relaxed at other times as well.

Certain physical conditions can lead to heartburn. For example, both pregnancy and obesity result in increased production of estrogen and progesterone. These hormones relax the lower esophageal sphincter, making heartburn more likely. In the case of obesity, adipose tissue turns certain circulating hormones into estrogen; thus, the more adipose tissue, one has, the more estrogen produced.

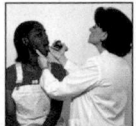

Real Life Scenario Follow-Up

Elise's GERD can be treated, but currently most likely will be a lifelong condition. Typical dietary advice includes consuming smaller, more frequent meals that are low in fat, not overeating at mealtimes, waiting about 2 hours after meals before lying down, and elevating the head of the bed about 6 inches (review Table 3-4). All of these recommendations reduce the risk of stomach contents forcing their way back up the esophagus. Other helpful advice includes stopping smoking if practiced, losing excess weight if overweight, and limiting intake of chili powder, onions, garlic, peppermint, caffeine, alcohol, and chocolate. All of these factors encourage relaxation of the sphincter and/or irritate the esophagus. If this advice doesn't control symptoms, the primary medications used to control GERD inhibit acid production in the stomach (see the earlier discussion on the ulcer medication omeprazole (Prilosec)). If this and other medical therapy fails to control the problem, surgery to strengthen the lower esophageal sphincter is possible, but generally will not cure the problem. Currently, lifetime diet and lifestyle management, and most likely medications, will still be needed to manage the problem. Such management is important since long-standing GERD increases the risk of esophageal cancer.

▌ Constipation and Laxatives

Constipation, which is difficult or infrequent evacuation of the bowels, is commonly reported by adults. Slow movement of fecal material through the large intestine causes constipation. As fluid is increasingly absorbed during the extended time the feces stay in the large intestine, they become dry and hard.

Constipation can result when people regularly inhibit their normal bowel reflexes for long periods. People may ignore normal urges when it is inconvenient to interrupt occupational or social activities. Muscle spasms of an irritated large intestine can also slow the movement of feces and contribute to constipation. Medications such as antacids and calcium and iron supplements can also cause constipation.

Eating foods with plenty of fiber, such as whole-grain breads and cereals, along with drinking more fluid to avoid dehydration, is the best method for treating mild cases of constipation. Fiber stimulates peristalsis by drawing water into the large intestine and helping form a bulky, soft fecal output. Eating dried fruits can also help stimulate the bowel. In addition, people with constipation may need to develop more regular bowel habits; allowing the same time each day for a bowel movement can help train the large intestine to respond routinely. Finally, relaxation facilitates regular bowel movements, as does regular physical activity.

constipation A condition characterized by infrequent bowel movements.

Laxatives can also lessen constipation, as well as various other medications. Laxatives work by irritating the intestinal nerve junctions to stimulate the peristaltic muscles, or by drawing water into the intestine (by means of bulk-forming fiber) to enlarge fecal output. The larger output stretches the peristaltic muscles, making them rebound and then constrict. Regular use of laxatives, however, should be supervised by a physician. Overall the bulk-forming fiber laxatives are the safest to use.

laxative A medication or other substance that stimulates evacuation of the intestinal tract.

Hemorrhoids

Hemorrhoids, also called *piles,* are swollen veins of the rectum and anus. The blood vessels in this area are subject to intense pressure, especially during bowel movements. Added stress to the vessels from pregnancy, obesity, prolonged sitting, violent coughing or sneezing, or straining during bowel movements, particularly with constipation, can lead to a hemorrhoid. Hemorrhoids can develop unnoticed until a strained bowel movement precipitates symptoms, which may include pain, itching, and bleeding.

Itching, caused by moisture in the anal canal, swelling, or other irritation, is perhaps the most common symptom. Pain, if present, is usually aching and steady. Bleeding may result from a hemorrhoid and appear in the toilet as a bright red streak in the feces. The sensation of a mass in the anal canal after a bowel movement is symptomatic of an internal hemorrhoid that protrudes through the anus.

Anyone can develop a hemorrhoid, and about half of adults over age 50 do. Pressure from prolonged sitting or exertion is often enough to bring on symptoms, although diet, lifestyle, and possibly heredity play a role. For example, a low-fiber diet can lead to hemorrhoids as a result of straining during bowel movements. If you think you have a hemorrhoid, you should consult your physician. Rectal bleeding, although usually caused by hemorrhoids, may also indicate other problems, such as cancer.

A physician may suggest a variety of self-care measures for hemorrhoids. Pain can be lessened by applying warm, soft compresses or sitting in a tub of warm water for 15 to 20 minutes. Dietary recommendations are the same as those for treating constipation, emphasizing the need to consume adequate fiber and fluid. Over-the-counter remedies, such as Preparation H, can also offer relief of symptoms.

Perhaps you have heard that taking laxatives after overeating prevents deposition of body fat from excess calorie intake. This erroneous and dangerous premise has gained popularity among followers of numerous fad diets. You may temporarily feel less full after using a laxative because laxatives hasten emptying of the large intestine and increase fluid loss. Most laxatives, however, do not speed the passage of food through the small intestine, where digestion and most nutrient absorption take place. As a result, you can't count on laxatives to prevent fat gain from excess calorie intake.

Irritable Bowel Syndrome

Many adults (25 million or more in the United States alone) have irritable bowel syndrome, noted as a combination of cramps, gassiness, bloating, and irregular bowel function (diarrhea, constipation, or alternating episodes of both). It is more common in younger women than in younger men. In older adults the ratio is closer to 50:50. The disease leads to about 3.5 million visits to physicians in the United States each year.

Symptoms associated with irritable bowel syndrome include visible abdominal distension, pain relief after a bowel movement, increased stool frequency, and loose stools with pain onset, mucus in stool, and a feeling of incomplete elimination even after a bowel movement.

The cause is thought to be altered intestinal peristalsis coupled with a decreased pain threshold for abdominal distension—in other words, a minor amount of abdominal bloating causes pain that the average person would not sense. It is also noteworthy that up to 50% of sufferers report a history of verbal or sexual abuse.

Therapy is individualized and can include a trial of high-fiber foods or elimination diets that focus on avoiding dairy products and gas-forming foods, such as legumes, certain vegetables (cabbage, beans, and broccoli), and some fruits (grapes, raisins, cherries, and cantaloupe). This is especially helpful in mild cases of irritable bowel syndrome. The patient should have only moderate caffeine intake or eliminate caffeine-containing foods/beverages altogether. Low-fat and more frequent, small meals may help the patient because large meals can trigger contractions of the large intestine. Other strategies include a reduction in stress, psychological counseling, and certain antidepressant and other medications.

Referral to a registered dietitian can be beneficial, as many patients experience improvement with the elimination of specific problem foods. A good patient/physician relationship is also necessary for the treatment of irritable bowel syndrome; however, before any single treatment is applauded, it is important to note that response to placebos alone has been as high as 70% in this population. Although irritable bowel syndrome can be uncomfortable and upsetting, it is harmless as it carries no risk for cancer or other serious digestive problems. The website www.ibsgroup.org provides further information.

Diarrhea

Diarrhea, a GI tract disease that generally lasts only a few days, is defined as increased fluidity, frequency, or amount of bowel movements compared to a person's usual pattern. Most cases of diarrhea result from infections in the intestines, with bacteria and viruses the usual offending agents. They produce substances that cause the intestinal cells to secrete fluid rather than absorb fluid. Another form of diarrhea can be caused by consumption of substances that are not readily absorbed, such as the sugar alcohol sorbitol found in sugarless gum (see Chapter 4). When consumed in large amounts the unabsorbed substance draws much water into the intestines, in turn leading to diarrhea. Treatment of diarrhea generally requires drinking lots of fluid during the affected stage; reduced intake of the poorly absorbed substance also is important if that is a cause. Prompt treatment—within 24 to 48 hours—is especially important for infants and older people, as they are more susceptible to the effects of dehydration associated with diarrhea (see Chapters 14 and 15). Diarrhea that lasts more than 7 days in adults should be investigated by a physician as it can be a symptom of more serious intestinal disease, especially if there is also blood in the stool.

Gallstones

Gallstones are a major cause of illness and surgery, affecting 10 percent to 20 percent of U.S. adults. Gallstones are pieces of solid material that develop in the gallbladder when substances in the bile—primarily cholesterol (80% of gallstones)—form crystal-like particles. They may be as small as a grain of sand or as large as a golf ball. These stones are caused by a combination of factors, with excess weight being the primary modifiable factor, especially in women 20 to 60 years old. Other factors include generic background (e.g., Native Americans), advanced age (> 60 years for both women and men), reduced activity of the gallbladder (contracts less than normal), altered bile composition (e.g., too much cholesterol or not enough bile salts), diabetes, and diet (e.g., low-fiber diets). In addition, gallstones may develop during rapid weight loss or prolonged fasting (as the liver metabolizes more fat, it secretes more cholesterol into the bile).

Attacks due to gallstones include intermittent pain in the upper right abdomen, gas and bloating, nausea or vomiting, or other health problems. Surgical removal of the gallbladder is the most common method for treating gallstones (500,000 surgeries per year in the United States).

Prevention of gallstones revolves around avoiding becoming overweight, especially for women. Avoiding rapid weight loss (> 3 lbs. per week), limiting animal protein and focusing more on plant protein intake (especially some nut intake), and following a high-fiber diet can help as well. Regular physical activity is also recommended, as is moderate to no caffeine and alcohol intake.

Overall, typical medical disorders of the GI tract arise from differences in anatomical features and lifestyle habits among individuals. Because of the importance of various nutrition and lifestyle habits, such as adequate fiber and fluid intake, as well as not smoking or abusing NSAID medications, nutrition and lifestyle therapy is often effective in helping treat GI tract disorders.

Urinary System

The **urinary system** is composed of two kidneys, one on each side of the spinal column. Each kidney is connected to the bladder by a **ureter.** The bladder is emptied by way of the **urethra** (Fig. 3-17). The main function of the kidneys is to remove waste from the body. The kidneys are constantly filtering blood to control its composition. This results in the formation of urine, which is mostly water; however, it does contain dissolved substances such as urea, and excess and unneeded water-soluble vitamins and various minerals.

Together with the lungs, the kidneys also maintain the acid-base balance **(pH)** of the blood. The kidneys also convert a form of vitamin D into its active hormone form, and produce a hormone that stimulates red blood cell synthesis (**erythropoietin;** see Chapter 11 for information on misuse of this hormone by some athletes). During times of fasting, the kidneys even produce glucose from certain amino acids. Thus, the kidneys perform many important functions and are a vital component of the body.

The proper function of the kidneys is closely tied to the strength of the cardiovascular system (i.e., adequate blood pressure) and the consumption of sufficient fluid. Uncontrolled diabetes, hypertension, and drug abuse are very harmful to the kidneys.

urinary system The body system consisting of the kidneys, urinary bladder, and the ducts that carry urine. This system removes waste products from the circulatory system and regulates blood acid-base balance, overall chemical balance, and water balance in the body.

pH A measure of relative acidity or alkalinity of a solution. The pH scale is 0 to 14. A pH below 7 is acidic; a pH above 7 is alkaline.

erythropoietin A hormone secreted mostly by the kidneys that enhances red blood cell synthesis and stimulates red blood cell release from bone marrow.

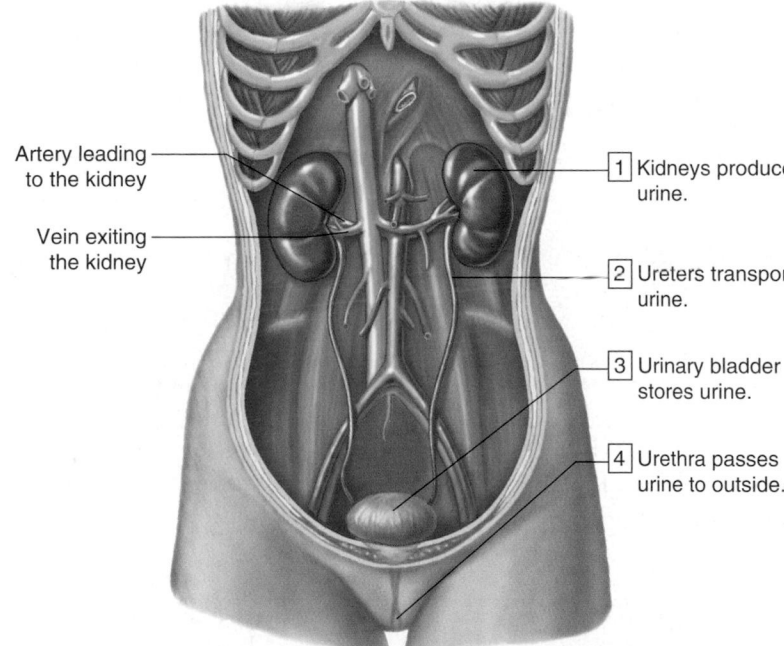

Artery leading to the kidney

Vein exiting the kidney

1 Kidneys produce urine.

2 Ureters transport urine.

3 Urinary bladder stores urine.

4 Urethra passes urine to outside.

Figure 3-17 Organs of the urinary system. 1 The kidneys, bean-shaped organs located on either side of the spinal column, filter waste from the blood, which is then 2 transported to the bladder by the ureters and 3 stored in the bladder as urine. 4 The urethra transports the urine to outside the body. The urinary system of the female is shown. The male's urinary system is the same, except that the urethra extends through the penis.

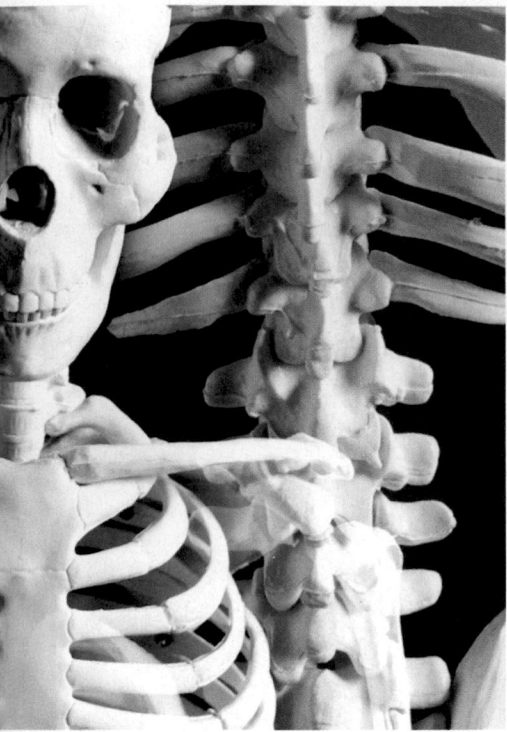

The skeletal system provides a reserve of calcium for day-to-day needs when dietary intake is inadequate. Long-term use of this reserve, however, reduces bone strength.

Storage Capabilities

The human body must maintain reserves of nutrients, otherwise we would need to eat continuously. Storage capacity varies for each different nutrient. Most fat is stored at sites designed specifically for this—adipose tissue. Short-term storage of carbohydrate occurs in muscle and liver, and the blood maintains a small reserve of glucose and amino acids. Many vitamins and minerals are stored in the liver, while other nutrient stores are found in other sites in the body.

When people do not meet certain nutrient needs, these nutrients are obtained by breaking down a tissue that contains high concentrations of the nutrient. Calcium is taken from bone and protein is taken from muscle. In cases of long-term deficiency, these nutrient losses weaken and harm these tissues.

Many people believe that if too much of a nutrient is obtained—for example, from a vitamin or mineral supplement—only what is needed is stored and the rest is excreted by the body. Though true for some nutrients, as with vitamin C, the large dosages of other nutrients frequently found in supplements, such as vitamin A and iron can cause harmful side effects because these are not readily excreted. This is one reason why obtaining your nutrients primarily (or exclusively) from a balanced diet is the safest means to acquire the building blocks you need to maintain the good health of all organ systems.

This review of human anatomy and physiology from a nutrition perspective sets the stage for developing a more detailed understanding of the nutrients. Chapters 4, 5, and 6 will build on this information.

Concept Check

The urinary system removes the wastes that are produced by the body and many nutrients that are ingested in excess of storage capacity and need. The kidneys maintain the chemical composition and acidity of the blood. In addition, the kidneys help convert vitamin D to its active form and participate in red blood cell synthesis.

In well-nourished individuals, nutrients are constantly present in the blood for immediate use and are stored in the body tissues for later use when sufficient amounts from food intake are unavailable. However, when the body suffers a nutrient deficiency caused by an inadequate diet, it breaks down vital tissues for their nutrients, which can lead to ill health. Additionally, too much of any nutrient can be detrimental, and with some more than others. It's best to focus primarily (or exclusively) on obtaining all essential nutrients from a balanced diet rather than mostly from dietary supplements.

Summary

1. The basic structural unit of the human body is the cell. Although almost all cells contain the same collection of organelles (nucleus, mitochondria, endoplasmic reticulum, lysosomes, peroxisomes, and cytoplasm), cell structure varies according to the type of job they must perform.

2. Cells join together to make up tissues, tissues unite to form organs, and organs work together as an organ system.

3. Genetic background influences the risk for many health-related diseases. Examining one's family tree provides clues for an individual to such risks. Preventative measures are then important to implement, especially with respect to diet.

4. Blood is pumped from the heart to the lungs, picking up oxygen. Then, the blood delivers essential nutrients, oxygen, and water to all body cells. Nutrients and wastes are exchanged between the blood and cells across the cell membrane. This exchange occurs in the capillaries.

5. Water-soluble compounds absorbed by the small intestine cells enter a portal vein and travel to the liver. Fat-soluble compounds enter the lymphatic system, which eventually connects to the bloodstream.

6. The nervous system's neurons are the body's communication network. They control and manage all other organ systems of the

body. Neurotransmitters are used to carry the message from one neuron to another (or to another cell).

7. The endocrine system produces hormones, which chemically regulate almost all other cells.

8. The immune system is responsible for protecting the body from invading pathogens. We activate immunity, such as production of antibodies (immunoglobulins), when we come in contact with a pathogen.

9. The gastrointestinal (GI) tract consists of the mouth, esophagus, stomach, small intestine, large intestine (colon), rectum, and anus.

10. Spaced along the GI tract are ringlike valves (sphincters) that regulate the flow of foodstuffs. Muscular contractions, called *peristalsis,* move the foodstuffs down the GI tract. A variety of nerves, hormones, and other substances control the activity of sphincters and peristaltic muscles.

11. Digestive enzymes are secreted by the mouth, stomach, wall of the small intestine, and pancreas. The presence of food in the small intestine stimulates the release of pancreatic enzymes.

12. The major absorptive sites consist of fingerlike projections called *villi,* located in the small intestine. Absorptive cells cover the villi. This intestinal lining is continually renewed. Absorptive cells can perform various forms of passive diffusion and active absorption.

13. Little digestion and absorption occur in the stomach or large intestine, but some protein is digested in the stomach. Some constituents of fiber and undigested starch are broken down by bacteria in the large intestine and some of the products are absorbed; any undigested fiber that remains is eliminated in the feces.

14. Final water and mineral absorption takes place in the large intestine. Products from bacterial breakdown of some fibers and other substances are also absorbed here. The presence of feces in the rectum provides the impetus for elimination.

15. The liver, gallbladder, and pancreas participate in digestion and absorption. Products from these organs, such as enzymes and bile, enter the small intestine and play important roles in digesting protein, fat, and carbohydrate.

16. Common GI-tract diseases, such as heartburn, constipation, and irritable bowel syndrome, can be treated with diet changes. These can include increasing fiber intake and avoiding large meals high in fat. Medications are also very helpful in many cases.

17. The urinary system, including the kidneys, is responsible for filtering the blood, removing body wastes, and maintaining the chemical composition of the blood.

18. Limited stores of nutrients are present in the blood for immediate use and stored to a greater or lesser extent in body tissues for later use when sufficient food is unavailable. When the body suffers a nutrient deficiency caused by a poor diet, it breaks down vital tissues for their nutrients, which can lead to ill health. Additionally, too much of any nutrient can be detrimental.

Study Questions

1. Identify at least one contribution to overall nutrition status provided by each of the 12 organ systems of the body.

2. Draw and label parts of the cell, and explain the function of each organelle discussed in the text as it relates to human nutrition.

3. What is the difference between nature and nurture? Relate these terms to the attempt to prevent three common chronic diseases.

4. Trace the flow of blood from the right side of the heart around the body and back to the same site. How is blood routed through the small intestine? Which class of nutrients enters the body via the blood? Via the lymph?

5. Explain why the small intestine is better suited than the other GI tract organs to carry out the absorptive process.

6. Identify the four basic tastes. Give an example of one food that exemplifies each of these basic taste sensations. Why can't you taste food when you have a cold? What is umami?

7. What is one role of acid in the process of digestion? Where is it secreted?

8. Contrast the processes of active absorption and passive diffusion of nutrients.

9. Identify the two accessory organs that empty their contents into the small intestine. How do the digestive substances secreted by these organs contribute to the digestion of food?

10. In which organ systems would the following substances be found?
chyme
plasma
lymph
urine

Further Readings

1. Against the grain: Who needs to avoid wheat? *Consumer Reports on Health* p. 10 July 2005.

   Although a high fiber diet leads to many health benefits, using wheat products to achieve such a goal is harmful for people with celiac disease. It is especially important that people who experience flushing, itching, hives, vomitting, or breathing difficulties within two hours of eating wheat be tested for the disease. The article discusses methods of diagnosis and treatment for celiac disease.

2. Answering your questions about immunity. *UC Berkeley Wellness Letter,* p. 4, May 2001.

   An adequate diet helps maintain the immune system. Nutrients such as protein, essential fatty acids, and certain vitamins and minerals play key roles. Moderate exercise and adequate sleep also improve immune function. Severely malnourished people are particularly vulnerable to immune dysfunction. Since many older people may not consume much food, there is evidence that they stay healthier if they take a multivitamin and mineral supplement. Still, megadoses of certain nutrients, such as zinc, can significantly harm some immune responses.

3. Baum C and others: Gastrointestinal disease. In Bowman BA, Russell RM (eds.): *Present knowledge in nutrition.* 8th ed. Washington, DC. ISLI Press, 2001.

   Disruption in any number of the steps in the digestive process can lead to malabsorption and in turn to protein, energy, and micronutrient deficiencies. Just as the GI tract is essential for nutrient utilization, ingested nutrients also play an active role in maintaining gastrointestinal health and function.

4. Bender DA, Mayes PA: Nutrition, digestion and absorption. In Murray RK and others (eds.): *Harper's illustrated biochemistry.* 26th ed. New York: Lange Medical Books/McGraw-Hill, 2003.

Most foodstuffs ingested are initially unavailable to humans; they cannot be absorbed by the digestive system until broken down into smaller molecules. This chapter provides a clear step-by-step description of this digestion, and subsequent absorption.

5. Clayton EW: Ethical, legal, and social implications of genomic medicine. *The New England Journal of Medicine* 349:562, 2003.

   The expanding use of genetic testing is raising many questions regarding protection of the person's rights of privacy and future ability to purchase health and life insurance. Further efforts to determine when genetic tests are reliable and useful in clinical practice are needed.

6. Devault KR: Gastroesophageal reflux: medical and surgical options. *American Family Physician* 68:1271, 2003.

   Medications such as proton pump inhibitors are helpful in treating gastroesopageal reflux disease. The surgical treatments are much more risky, and so use must be carefully considered.

7. Gropper SS and others: *Advanced nutrition and human metabolism*, 4th edition, Thomson Wadsworth, Belmont CA 2005.

   Chapter 2 of this textbook provides a detailed description of the digestive processes of the human body. Students seeking more details about digestion and absorption will find this chapter helpful.

8. Heidelbaugh JJ and others: Management of gastroesophageal reflux disease. *American Family Physician* 68:1311, 2003.

   It is important to treat recurring heartburn as it can lead to a form of esophageal cancer. Reducing the size of meals and elevating the head of the bed are two lifestyle considerations. Acid-blocking medications are very helpful; types and use of such medications are summarized in the article.

9. Keku TO and others: Gene testing: what the health professional needs to know. *Journal of Nutrition* 133:3754S, 2003.

   Genetic testing for some diseases is now available, such as for some forms of breast cancer. Still, there are risks of such testing that need to be considered, such as discrimination by insurance companies, and so any application of this technology needs to be carefully considered.

10. Le Coutre J: Taste: the metabolic sense. *Food Technology* 57(8):34, 2003.

The primary taste sensations are sweet, salt, sour, and bitter. Umami rounds out the list. Research into the use of this knowledge of taste perception to improve the taste of some foods is ongoing.

11. Liebman B: Who you gonna call? Gasbusters. *Nutrition Action Healthletter*, p. 1, May 2003.

    This article focuses on an interview with Dr. Michael Levitt, a noted expert on intestinal gas. Causes and treatment for uncomfortable cases are reviewed, such as the possible link to lactose maldigestion, sorbitol intake, and consumption of beans and various vegetables. Some people are bothered more by this gas production than others; some people experience little or no symptoms from daily gas production.

12. Mertz HR: Irritable bowel disease. *The New England Journal of Medicine* 349:2136, 2003.

    The most common symptoms of irritable bowel syndrome include a change in the appearance or frequency of stools, and abdominal pain that is relieved by defecation. Affected people should especially seek medical help if weight loss, GI tract bleeding, fever, or frequent nighttime symptoms are present. In some cases increasing fiber intake is helpful. Regular yogurt consumption may also be helpful as this can increase the concentration of beneficial types of bacteria that reside in the large intestine.

13. Meurer LN, Bower DJ: Management of Helicobacter pylori infection. *American Family Physician* 65:1327, 2002.

    Helicobacter pylori is the cause of most peptic ulcer disease and is also a risk factor for gastric cancer. Eradication of this organism is important for ulcer healing and reducing the risk of ulcer reoccurrence. Generally a two-week period of antibiotics and acid suppression is employed. Follow-up testing with analysis of breath or fecal samples is recommended for people who do not respond to therapy.

14. Muller-Lisser and others: Myths and misconceptions about constipation. *American Journal of Gastroenterology* 100:232, 2005.

    Increasing fiber intake and avoiding dehydration often helps in mild cases of constipation. More difficult cases require a careful physician evaluation and likely the use of laxative and other medications. Often the latter are very helpful, and are reviewed in the article.

15. Nilsson M and others: Obesity and estrogen as risk factors for gastroesophageal reflux symptoms. *Journal of the American Medical Association* 290:66, 2003.

    Obesity is a major risk factor for gastrointestinal reflux disease. Production of estrogen by adipose tissue is one likely reason for the relationship. Weight loss reverses the course of the disease and so is very beneficial to these persons.

16. Sanders ME: Probiotics: Considerations for human health. *Nutrition Reviews* 61 (3):91, 2003.

    Probiotic microorganisms may play an important role in helping the body protect itself from infection, especially that which arises along the interior surfaces of the gastrointestinal tract. In North America foods currently containing probiotics are exclusively dairy products, such as yogurt, some forms of milk, some forms of cottage cheese, and a few other products.

17. Schardt D: Not everybody must get stones. *Nutrition Action Healthletter*, p. 89, November 2004.

    Excess body weight is the primary modifiable risk factor for developing gallbladder stones. Low fiber diets are also implicated.

18. Seeley RR and others: *Anatomy and physiology.* 7th ed. Boston: McGraw-Hill, 2006.

    This text provides comprehensive coverage of the anatomy and physiology of the gastrointestinal tract, as well as other related body systems.

19. Smith L: Updated ACG guidelines for diagnosis and treatment of GERD. *American Family Physician* 71:2376, 2005.

    The article outlines the diagnosis and treatment of GERD. The authors suggest that simple diet and lifestyle changes, such as avoiding high fat meals and not lying down immediatley after a meal, can help treat the disease in many cases.

20. The low-down on hemorrhoids. *UC Berkeley Wellness Letter*, p. 4, July, 2004.

    Hemorrhoids are commonly experienced by many adults during one's lifetime. Measures to reduce such risk and as well treat the problem are discussed, such as an adequate fluid and fiber intake. Fortunately hemorrhoids rarely lead to serious health problems.

I. Are You Taking Care of Your Digestive Tract?

People need to think about the health of their digestive tracts. There are symptoms we need to notice, as well as habits we need to practice in order to protect it. The following assessment is designed to help you examine your habits and symptoms associated with the health of your digestive tract. The second Looking Further section explained why these habits are important to examine. Put a *Y* in the blank to the left of the question to indicate yes and an *N* to indicate no.

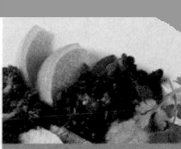

_____ 1.   Are you currently experiencing greater than normal stress and tension?

_____ 2.   Do you have a family history of digestive tract problems (e.g., ulcers, hemorrhoids, recurrent heartburn, constipation)?

_____ 3.   Do you experience pain in your stomach region about 2 hours after you eat?

_____ 4.   Do you smoke cigarettes?

_____ 5.   Do you take aspirin frequently?

_____ 6.   Do you have heartburn at least once per week?

_____ 7.   Do you commonly lie down after eating a large meal?

_____ 8.   Do you drink alcoholic beverages more than two or three times per day?

_____ 9.   Do you experience abdominal pain, bloating, and gas about 30 minutes to 2 hours after consuming milk products?

_____ 10.   Do you often have to strain while having a bowel movement?

_____ 11.   Do you consume less than 9 (women) or 13 (men) cups of a combination of water and other fluids per day?

_____ 12.   Do you perform physical activity for less than 60 minutes or more on most or all days of the week (e.g., jog, swim, walk briskly, row, stair climb).

_____ 13.   Do you eat a diet relatively low in fiber (recall that significant fiber is found in whole fruits, vegetables, legumes, nuts and seeds, whole-grain breads, and whole-grain cereals)?

_____ 14.   Do you frequently have diarrhea?

_____ 15.   Do you frequently use laxatives or antacids?

Interpretation

Add up the number of yes answers you gave and record the total in the blank to the right.   _____

If your score is from 8 to 15, your habits and symptoms put you at risk for experiencing future digestive tract problems. Take particular note of the habits to which you answered yes. Consider trying to cooperate more with your digestive tract.

II. Create Your Family Tree for Health-Related Concerns

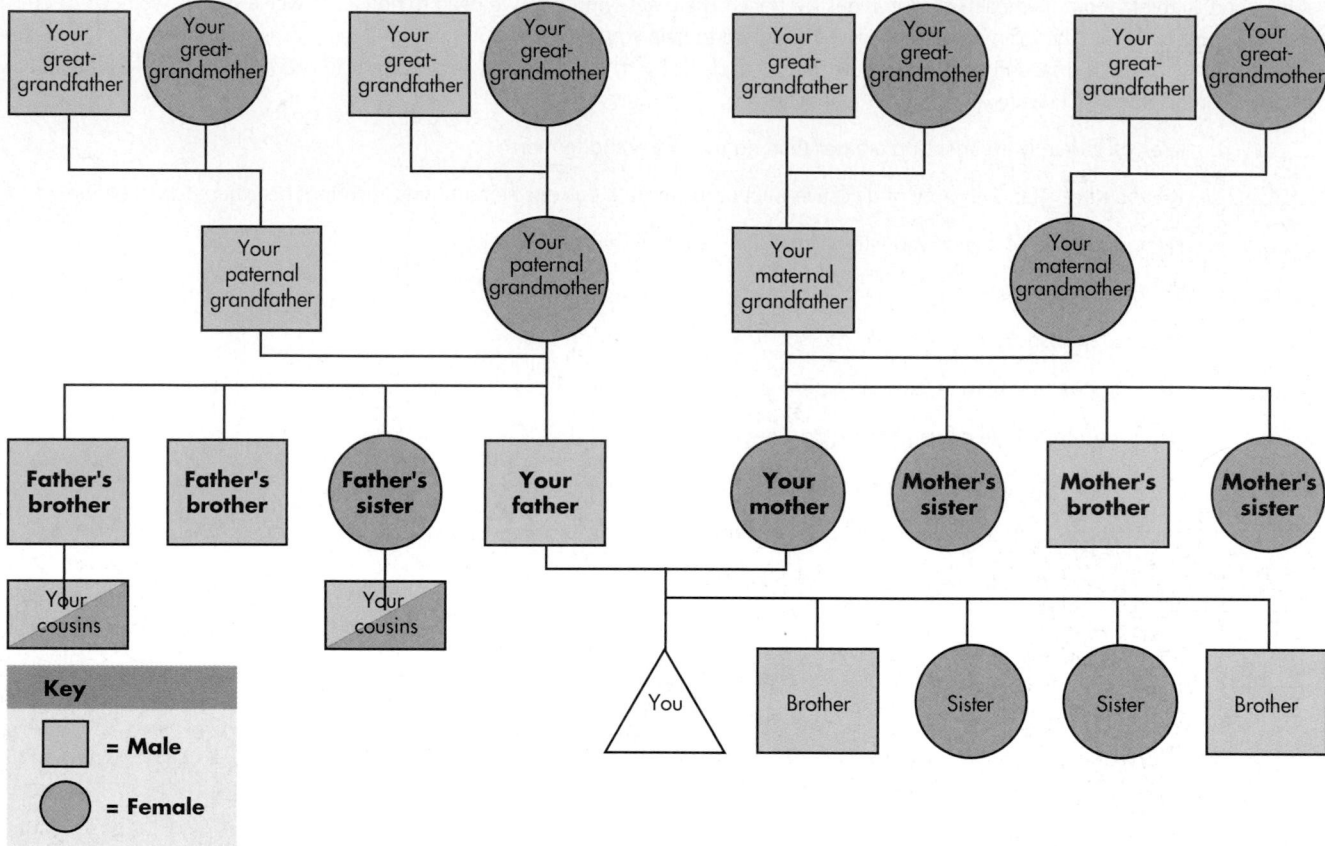

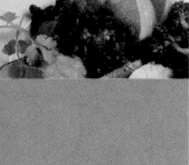

Adapt this diagram to your own family tree. Under each heading, list year born, year died (if applicable), major diseases that developed during the person's lifetime, and cause of death (if applicable). Figure 3-3 provides one such example.

Note that you are likely to be at risk for any diseases listed. Creating a plan for preventing such diseases when possible, especially those that developed in your family members before age 50 to 60 years, is advised. Speak with your physician about any concerns arising from this exercise.

Carbohydrates

4

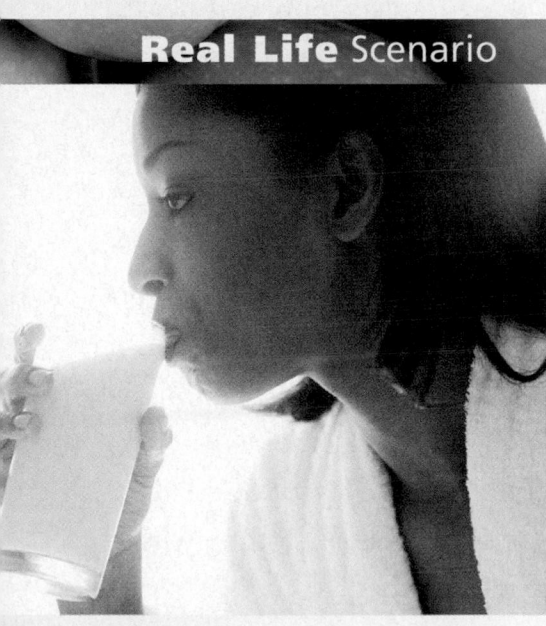

Myeshia is a 19-year-old African-American female who recently read about the health benefits of calcium and decided to increase her intake of dairy products. To start, she drank a cup of 1% milk at lunch. Not long afterward, she experienced bloating, cramping, and increased gas production. She suspected that the culprit of this pain was the milk she consumed, especially since her parents and her sister complain of the same problem. She wanted to determine if other milk products were, in fact, the cause of her discomfort so the next day she substituted a cup of yogurt for the glass of milk at lunch. Subsequently, she did not have any pain.

What has Myeshia discovered? What component of milk is likely causing the problem?

Chapter 4 Objectives

Chapter 4 is designed to allow you to:

1. Identify the basic structures and food sources of the major carbohydrates—monosaccharides, disaccharides, polysaccharides (e.g., starches), and fiber.

2. Describe food sources of carbohydrate and list some alternative sweeteners.

3. List the functions of carbohydrate in the body and the problems that result from not eating enough carbohydrate.

4. Describe the regulation of blood glucose and the nutrients that can become blood glucose.

5. Outline the beneficial effects of fiber on the body.

6. State the RDA for carbohydrate and various guidelines for carbohydrate intake.

7. Identify the consequences of lactose maldigestion and diabetes, and explain appropriate dietary measures that will reduce the adverse effects of these health problems.

Check out the **Contemporary Nutrition Online Learning Center**
www.mhhe.com/wardlawcont6 for quizzes, flash cards, other activities, and web links designed to further help you learn about carbohydrates.

What did you eat to obtain the calories you are using right now? Chapters 4, 5, and 6 will examine this question by focusing on the main nutrients the human body uses for fuel. These nutrients are carbohydrates (on average, 4 kcal per gram) and fats and oils (on average, 9 kcal per gram). Although protein (on average, 4 kcal per gram) *can* be used for energy needs, the body typically reserves this nutrient for other processes. Most people know that potatoes are rich in carbohydrates and steak contains mostly fat and protein, but many people do not know how to use this information.

It is likely that you have recently consumed fruits, vegetables, dairy products, cereal, breads, and pasta. All of these foods supply carbohydrates. Unfortunately, the benefits of these foods are often misunderstood. Many people think carbohydrate-rich foods are fattening—they are not. Pound for pound, carbohydrates are much less fattening than fats and oils. Furthermore, high-carbohydrate foods, especially fiber-rich foods such as fruits, vegetables, whole-grain breads and cereals, and legumes, are promoted by many experts for the important health benefits they supply. Some people think sugars cause hyperactivity in children—not so, according to well-designed scientific investigations. Almost all carbohydrate-rich foods, except pure sugars, provide essential nutrients and should generally constitute 45% to 65% of our daily calorie intake. Let's take a closer look at carbohydrates, including why the current craze of carbohydrate-bashing is misguided.

Refresh Your Memory

As you begin your study of carbohydrates in Chapter 4, you may want to review:

- The concept of energy density and the health claims for various carbohydrates in Chapter 2
- The processes of digestion and absorption in Chapter 3
- The hormones that regulate blood glucose in Chapter 3

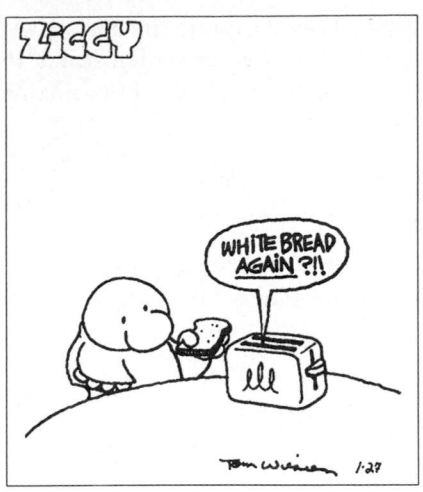

The class of carbohydrate that has gained the most attention recently is fiber. Why is this so? Which health problems typically result from a limited intake of fiber? Which health problems can be prevented by an adequate intake? How much fiber is enough? Too much? Chapter 4 provides some answers.

Carbohydrates—An Introduction

Carbohydrates are a main fuel source for some cells, especially those in the brain, nervous system, and red blood cells. Muscles also rely on a dependable supply of carbohydrate to fuel intense physical activity. Yielding on average 4 kcal per gram, carbohydrates are a readily available fuel for all cells, both in the form of blood glucose and that stored in the liver and muscles as **glycogen.** The glycogen stored in the liver can be used to maintain blood glucose availability in times when the diet does not supply enough carbohydrate. Regular intake of carbohydrate is important, because liver glycogen stores are depleted in about 18 hours if no carbohydrate is consumed. After that point, the body is forced to produce carbohydrate, much of which comes from breakdown of proteins in the body. This eventually leads to health problems.

We humans have sensors on our tongues that recognize sweet carbohydrates. Researchers surmise that this sweetness indicated a safe energy source to early humans, and so it became an important energy source. The returning Crusaders brought **sugar** from the Holy Land to Europe. Columbus introduced sugarcane to the Americas. The French later exploited sugar beets as a source of sugar.

Despite their important role as a calorie source, some forms of carbohydrate promote health more than others. As you will see in Chapter 4, whole-grain breads and cereals have greater health benefits than refined and processed forms of carbohydrate. Choosing predominantly the healthiest carbohydrate sources, while moderating intake of those that are less healthful, contributes to a healthy diet. It is difficult to eat so little carbohydrate that body needs are not met, but it is easy to overconsume the carbohydrates that can contribute to health problems. Let's explore this concept further as we look at carbohydrates in detail.

Forms of Simple Carbohydrates

As the name suggests, most carbohydrate molecules are composed of carbon, hydrogen, and oxygen atoms. Simple forms of carbohydrates are called *sugars.* Larger, more complex forms are primarily called either **starches** or **fibers,** depending on their digestibility by human GI tract enzymes. Starches are the digestible form.

glycogen A carbohydrate made of multiple units of glucose with a highly branched structure; sometimes known as *animal starch.* It is the storage form of glucose in humans and is synthesized (and stored) in the liver and muscles.

sugar A simple carbohydrate with the chemical composition $(CH_2O)_n$. Most sugars form a ringed structure when in solution. The primary sugar in the diet is sucrose, which is made up of glucose and fructose.

starch A carbohydrate made of multiple units of glucose attached together in a form the body can digest; also known as *complex carbohydrate.*

fiber Substances in plant foods that are not digested by the processes that take place in the stomach or small intestine. These add bulk to feces. Fibers naturally found in foods are also called dietary fiber.

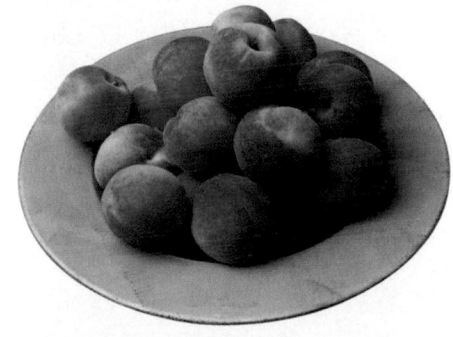

Fruits such as peaches are an excellent source of carbohydrate for your diet.

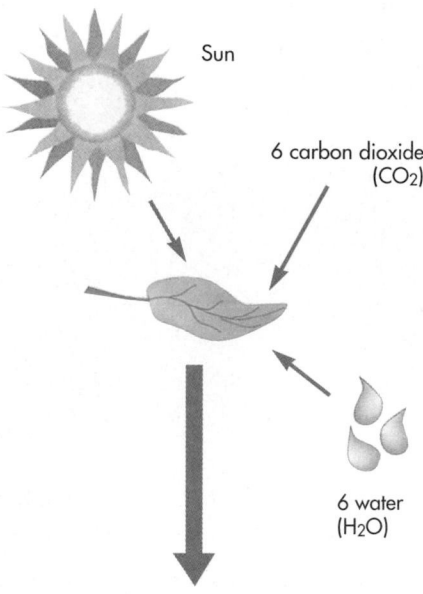

Sun

6 carbon dioxide
(CO₂)

6 water
(H₂O)

Glucose (C₆H₁₂O₆) + 6 oxygen (O₂)

A summary of photosynthesis. Glucose is stored in the leaf, but can also undergo further metabolism.

Green plants create the carbohydrates in our foods. Leaves capture the sun's solar energy in their cells and transform it to chemical energy. This energy is then stored in the chemical bonds of the carbohydrate glucose as it is produced from carbon dioxide and water. This complex process is called **photosynthesis.**

$$6 \text{ carbon dioxide} + 6 \text{ water} \rightarrow \text{glucose} + 6 \text{ oxygen}$$
$$(CO_2) \qquad (H_2O) \quad (C_6H_{12}O_6) \quad (O_2)$$

Translated into English, this reads: 6 molecules of carbon dioxide combine with 6 molecules of water to form one molecule of **glucose.** Trapping solar energy and converting this into chemical bonds in the sugar is a key part of the process. Six molecules of oxygen are then released into the air.

■ Monosaccharides—Glucose, Fructose, and Galactose

Monosaccharides are the simple sugar units (*mono* means one) that serve as the basic unit of all sugar structures. The most common monosaccharides in foods are glucose, fructose, and galactose (Fig. 4-1).

Glucose is the major monosaccharide found in the body. Glucose is also known as *dextrose*, and glucose in the bloodstream may be called blood sugar. Glucose is an important source of energy for human cells, although foods contain little of this single sugar form. Most glucose comes from the breakdown of starches and **sucrose** (common table sugar). The latter is made up of the monosaccharides glucose and fructose. For the most part, sugars and other carbohydrates in foods are eventually converted to glucose in the liver. This glucose then goes on to serve as a source of fuel for cells.

Fructose, also called *fruit sugar,* is another common monosaccharide. After it is consumed, fructose is absorbed by the small intestine and then transported to the liver, where it is quickly metabolized. Much is converted to glucose, and the rest goes on to form other compounds, such as fat, if fructose is consumed in very high amounts. Most of the fructose as such in our diets comes from the use of **high-fructose corn syrup** in food production (see the later discussion on nutritive sweeteners). Fructose also is found in fruits, and forms half of sucrose, as previously noted.

The sugar **galactose** has nearly the same structure as glucose. Large quantities of pure galactose do not exist in nature. Instead, galactose is usually found bonded to glucose in **lactose,** a sugar found in milk and other milk products. After it is absorbed, galactose arrives in the liver. There it is either transformed into glucose or further metabolized into glycogen.

photosynthesis Process by which plants use energy from the sun to synthesize energy-yielding compounds, such as glucose.

glucose A six-carbon monosaccharide that usually exists in a ring form; found as such in blood, and in table sugar bonded to fructose; also known as *dextrose*.

sucrose Fructose bonded to glucose; table sugar.

fructose A six-carbon monosaccharide that usually exists in a ring form; found in fruits and honey; also known as *fruit sugar*.

galactose A six-carbon monosaccharide that usually exists in a ring form; closely related to glucose.

lactose Glucose bonded to galactose; also known as *milk sugar.*

Monosaccharides

Glucose

Fructose

Galactose

Figure 4-1 Chemical Forms of the Important Monosaccharides.

Another Bite

Now is a good time to begin emphasizing a key concept in nutrition: the difference between *intake* of a substance and the body's *use* of that substance. The body often does not use all nutrients in their original states. Some of these substances are broken down and later reassembled into the same or a different substance when and where necessary. For example, much of the galactose in the diet is metabolized to glucose. When later required, as in the mammary gland of a lactating female, galactose is resynthesized to help form the milk sugar lactose.

■ Disaccharides—Sucrose, Lactose, and Maltose

Disaccharides are formed when two monosaccharides combine (*di* means two). The disaccharides in food are sucrose, lactose, and **maltose.** All contain glucose (Fig. 4-2).

Sucrose forms when the two sugars glucose and fructose bond together. Sucrose is found naturally in sugarcane, sugar beets, honey, and maple sugar. These products are processed to varying degrees to make brown, white, and powdered sugars. Animals do not produce sucrose, or typically much of any carbohydrate for that matter (glycogen is an exception).

Lactose forms when glucose bonds with galactose. Again, our major food source for lactose is milk products. A later section on lactose maldigestion and lactose intolerance discusses the problems that result when a person can't readily digest lactose.

Maltose results when starch is broken down to just two glucose molecules bonded together. Maltose has a role in the beer and liquor industry. In the production of alcoholic beverages, starches in various cereal grains are first converted to simpler carbohydrates by enzymes present in the grains. The end products of this step—maltose, glucose, and other sugars—are then mixed with yeast cells in the absence of oxygen. The yeast cells convert most of the sugars to alcohol (ethanol) and carbon dioxide, a process called **fermentation.** Little maltose remains in the final product. Few other food products and beverages contain maltose. In fact, most maltose that we ultimately digest in the small intestine is produced during the digestion of starch.

Monosaccharides and disaccharides are often referred to as **simple sugars** because they contain only one or two sugar units. Food labels lump all of these sugars under one category, listing them as "sugars."

maltose Glucose bonded to glucose.

fermentation The conversion of carbohydrates to alcohols, acids, and carbon dioxide without the use of oxygen.

polysaccharides Carbohydrates containing many glucose units, from 10 to 1000 or more.

Simple	Monosaccharides
	Glucose, fructose, galactose
	Disaccharides
	Sucrose, lactose, maltose
	Polysaccharides
	Starches (amylose and
	amylopectin), glycogen
Complex	Most fibers

Forms of the More Complex Carbohydrates

In many foods, single-sugar units are bonded together to form a chain, known as a polysaccharide (*poly* means many). **Polysaccharides,** also called *complex carbohydrates* or *starch,* may contain 1000 or more glucose units, and are found chiefly in grains,

Disaccharides

Sucrose: glucose + fructose
Lactose: glucose + galactose
Maltose: glucose + glucose

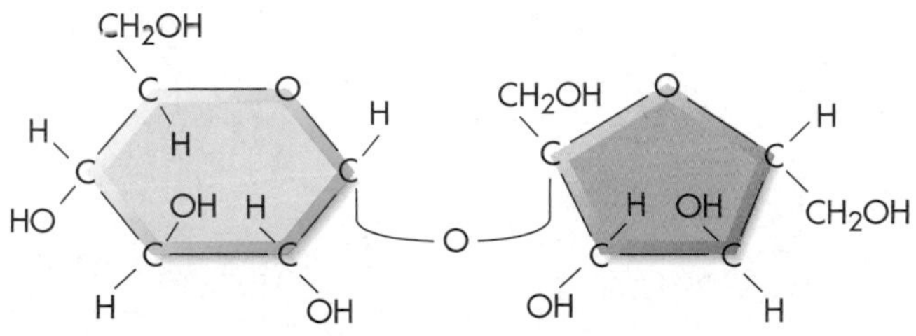

Sucrose

Figure 4-2 Chemical Form of the Disaccharide Sucrose.

amylose A digestible straight-chain type of starch composed of glucose units.

amylopectin A digestible branched-chain type of starch composed of glucose units.

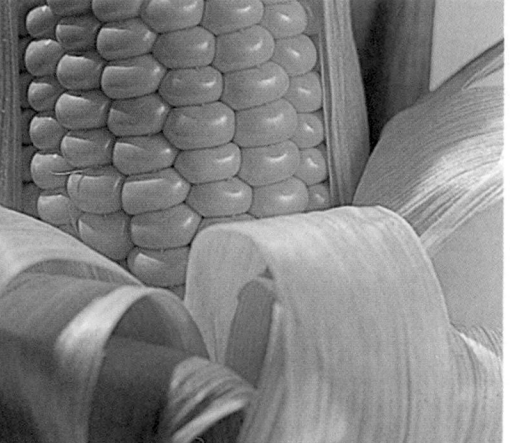

As plants mature, some sugars are turned into starch.

vegetables, and fruits. When food labels list "Other Carbohydrates," this primarily refers to starch content.

Plants store carbohydrate in two forms that are digestible by humans: **amylose** and **amylopectin.** Amylose, a long, straight chain of glucose units, comprises about 20% of the digestible starch found in vegetables, beans, breads, pasta, and rice. Amylopectin makes up the rest of digestible starch. Whereas amylose is a straight chain, the structure of amylopectin is highly branched (Fig. 4-3). Cellulose (a fiber) is another complex carbohydrate in plants. Although similar to amylose, it cannot be digested by humans, as discussed in the next section.

The enzymes that break down starches to glucose and other related sugars act only at the end of a glucose chain. Amylopectin, since it is branched, provides many more sites (ends) for enzyme action. Therefore, amylopectin raises blood glucose much more readily than amylose (see the discussion of glycemic load in a later section of Chapter 4).

As noted earlier, animals—including humans—store glucose in the form of glycogen. Glycogen consists of a chain of glucose units with many branches, providing even more sites for enzyme action than amylopectin (review Fig. 4-3). Because of its branched structure that can be quickly broken down, glycogen is an ideal form for carbohydrate storage in the body.

The liver and muscles are the major storage sites for glycogen. Because only about 120 kcal of glucose are immediately available as such in body fluids, these storage sites for carbohydrate energy as glycogen—amounting to about 1800 kcal—are extremely important. Of this 1800 kcal, liver glycogen (about 400 kcal) can readily contribute to blood glucose. Muscle glycogen stores (about 1400 kcal) cannot raise blood glucose, but instead supply glucose for muscle use, especially during high-intensity and endurance exercise (see Chapter 11 for a detailed discussion of carbohydrate use in exercise).

If animals store glycogen in their muscles, are meats, fish, and poultry a good source of carbohydrates? No—animal products are not good food sources of this (or any other) carbohydrate because glycogen stores quickly degrade after the animal dies.

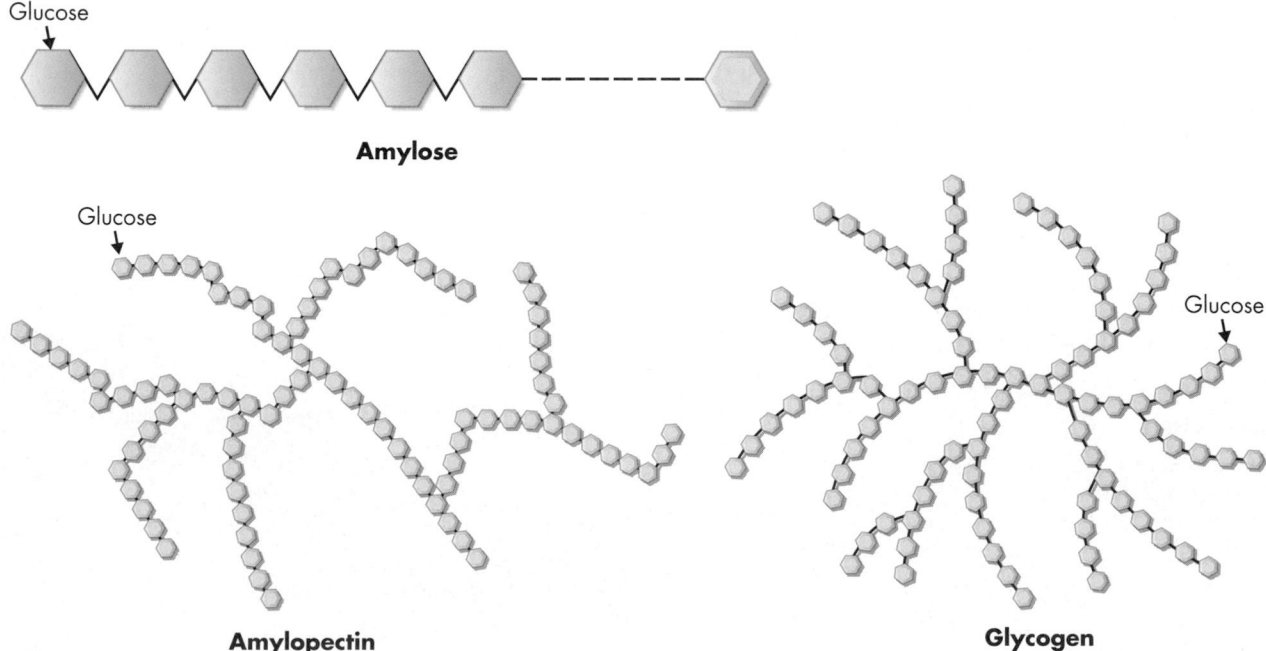

Figure 4-3 Some Common Starches. We consume essentially no glycogen. All glycogen found in the body is made by our cells, primarily in the liver and muscles.

Forms of Fiber

Fiber as a class is mostly made up of polysaccharides, but they differ from starches insofar as the chemical links that join the individual sugar units cannot be digested by human enzymes in the GI tract. This prevents the small intestine from absorbing the sugars that make up the various fibers. Fiber is not a single substance, but a group of substances with similar characteristics (Table 4-1). The group is comprised of the carbohydrates **cellulose, hemicelluloses, pectins, gums,** and **mucilages,** as well as the noncarbohydrate, **lignin.** In total, these constitute all the nonstarch polysaccharides in foods. Note that Nutrition Facts labels generally do not list these individual forms of fiber, but instead lump them together under the term **dietary fiber.**

Cellulose, hemicelluloses, and lignin form the structural parts of plants. Bran fiber is rich in hemicelluloses and lignin. (The woody fibers in broccoli are partly lignin.) Bran layers form the outer covering of all grains, so **whole grains** (i.e., unrefined) are good sources of this fiber (Fig. 4-4). Because the majority of these fibers neither readily dissolve in water nor are easily metabolized by intestinal bacteria, they are called **insoluble** (or **poorly fermented**) **fibers.**

Pectins, gums, and mucilages are contained around and inside plant cells. These fibers either dissolve or swell when put into water and are therefore called **soluble** (or **viscous**) **fibers.** They also are readily fermented by bacteria in the large intestine. These fibers are found in salad dressings, some frozen desserts, jams, and jellies as gum arabic, guar gum, locust bean gum, and various pectin forms. Some forms of hemicelluloses also fall into the soluble category.

Most foods contain mixtures of soluble and insoluble fibers, but food labels do not generally distinguish between the two types. Still, manufacturers have the option to do so. Often times, if food is listed as a good source of one type of fiber, it usually contains some of the other type of fiber as well.

Another Bite

The definition of fiber has recently been expanded to include both the dietary fiber that is found naturally in foods, and other forms of fiber that may be added to foods. This second category is called **functional fiber;** a fiber of this type must show beneficial effects in humans to be included in the category. **Total fiber** (or just the term *fiber*) is then the combination of dietary fiber and functional fiber in the food product. Currently the Nutrition Facts label only includes the category dietary fiber; the label has yet to be updated to reflect the latest definition of fiber.

cellulose An insoluble straight-chain polysaccharide made of glucose molecules that is undigestible.

hemicellulose An insoluble fiber containing xylose, galactose, glucose, and other monosaccharides bonded together.

pectin A soluble fiber containing chains of galacturonic acid and other monosaccharides; characteristically found between plant cell walls.

gums A soluble fiber containing chains of galactose, glucuronic acid, and other monosaccharides; characteristically found in exudates from plant stems.

mucilages A soluble fiber consisting of chains of galactose, mannose, and other monosaccharides; characteristically found in seaweed.

lignins An insoluble fiber made up of a multiringed alcohol (noncarbohydrate) structure.

dietary fiber Fiber found in food.

whole grains Grains containing the entire seed of the plant, including the bran, germ, and endosperm (starchy interior). Examples are whole wheat and brown rice.

functional fiber Fiber added to foods that has shown to provide health benefits.

total fiber Combination of dietary fiber and functional fiber in a food. Also just called *fiber.*

Table 4-1 Classification of Fibers

Type	Component(s)	Examples	Physiological Effects	Major Food Sources
Insoluble (poorly fermented)				
Noncarbohydrate form	Lignin	Wheat bran	Increases fecal bulk	Whole grains
Carbohydrate form	Cellulose, hemicelluloses	Wheat products Brown rice	Increases fecal bulk Decreases intestinal transit time	All plants Wheat, rye, rice, vegetables
Soluble (viscous)				
Carbohydrate form	Pectins, gums, mucilages, some hemi-celluloses	Apples Bananas Oranges Carrots Barley Oats Kidney beans	Delays stomach emptying; slows glucose absorption; can lower blood cholesterol	Citrus fruits, oat products, beans, thickeners added to foods

Figure 4-4 Soluble and Insoluble Fiber. (a) The skin of an apple consists of the insoluble fiber cellulose, which provides structure for the fruit. The soluble fiber pectin "glues" the fruit cells together. (b) The outside layer of a wheat kernel is made of layers of bran—primarily hemicellulose, an insoluble fiber—making this whole grain a good source of fiber. Overall, fruits, vegetables, whole-grain breads and cereals, and beans are rich in fiber.

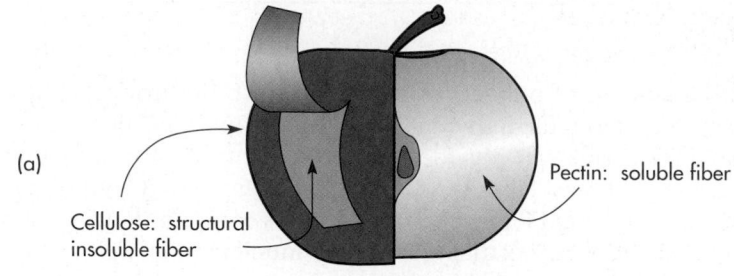

(a)

Cellulose: structural insoluble fiber

Pectin: soluble fiber

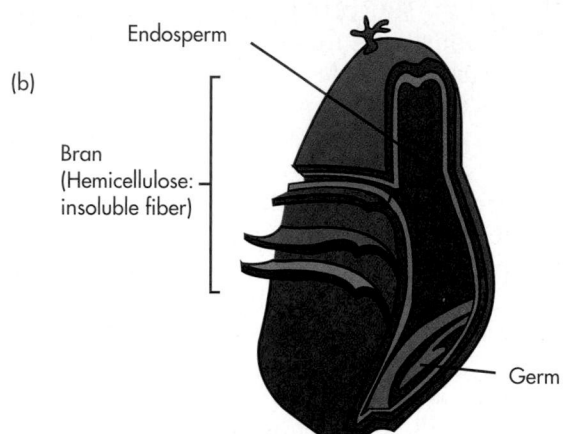

(b)

Endosperm

Bran (Hemicellulose: insoluble fiber)

Germ

Food Sources of Carbohydrate

Food item	Carbohydrate (grams)	Calories from carbo- hydrate (%)
Baked potato (1 each)	51	91
Cola drink (12 fluid oz)	39	100
Plain M&M's (1.5 oz)	30	58
Banana (1 each)	28	96
Cooked rice (½ cup)	22	90
Cooked corn (½ cup)	21	81
Light yogurt (1 cup)	19	77
Kidney beans (½ cup)	19	72
Spaghetti noodles (½ cup)	19	87
Orange (1 each)	16	94
Seven grain bread (1 slice)	12	75
Fat-free milk (1 cup)	12	56
Pineapple chunks (½ cup)	10	89
Cooked carrots (½ cup)	8	87
Peanuts (1 oz)	6	7

Concept Check

Important monosaccharides in nutrition are glucose, fructose, and galactose. Glucose is a primary energy source for body cells. Disaccharides form when two monosaccharides bond together. Important disaccharides in nutrition are sucrose (glucose + fructose), maltose (glucose + glucose), and lactose (glucose + galactose). Once digested into monosaccharide forms and absorbed, most carbohydrates are transformed into glucose by the liver.

Amylose, amylopectin, and glycogen are all storage forms of glucose, called polysaccharides. The major digestible plant polysaccharides—amylose and amylopectin—contain multiple glucose units bonded together. Glycogen is a storage form of glucose in our liver and muscle cells.

Fiber is essentially the portion of ingested food that remains undigested as it enters the large intestine. Fiber components include cellulose, hemicelluloses, lignins, pectins, gums, and mucilages. There are two general classes of fiber: insoluble and soluble. Insoluble fibers (or poorly fermented fibers) are mostly made up of cellulose, hemicelluloses, and lignins. Soluble fibers (or viscous fibers) are made up mostly of pectins, gums, and mucilages. Both insoluble and soluble fibers are resistant to human digestive enzymes, but bacteria in the large intestine can break down soluble fibers.

Carbohydrates in Foods

The food components that yield the highest percentage of calories from carbohydrates are table sugar, honey, jam, jelly, fruit, and plain baked potatoes. These items are the richest sources of carbohydrate; carbohydrates deliver most of their calories. Corn flakes, rice, bread, and noodles all contain at least 75% of calories as carbohydrates.

Foods with moderate amounts of carbohydrate calories are peas, broccoli, oatmeal, dry beans and other legumes, cream pies, French fries, and fat-free milk. In these foods, the carbohydrate content is diluted either by protein, as in the case of fat-free milk, or by fat, as in the case of a cream pie. Foods with essentially no carbohydrates include beef, eggs, chicken, fish, vegetable oils, butter, and margarine.

The percentage of calories from carbohydrate is more important than the total amount of carbohydrate in a food when planning a healthy high-carbohydrate diet. Figure 4-5 shows that, in planning such a high-carbohydrate diet, you need to emphasize grains, pasta, fruits, and vegetables. On the other hand, you can't create a diet high in carbohydrate calories from chocolate, potato chips, and French fries because these foods contain too much fat. Currently, the top five carbohydrate sources for U.S. adults are white bread, soft drinks, cookies and cakes (including doughnuts), sugars/syrups/jams, and potatoes. Clearly many North Americans (teenagers included) should take a closer look at their main carbohydrate sources and strive to improve them from a nutritional standpoint by including more whole grains, fruits, and vegetables.

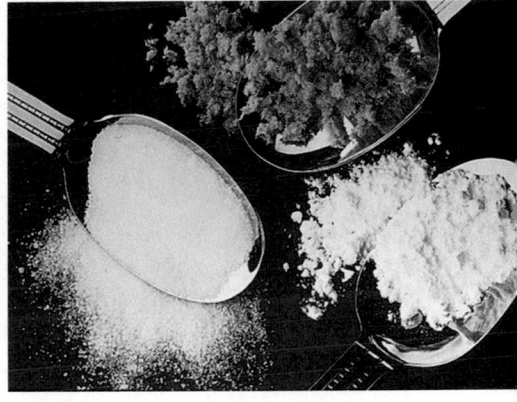

There are many forms of sugar on the market. Used in many foods, together they contribute to our daily intake of approximately 82 grams (16 teaspoons) of sugars in our diets.

■ A Closer Look at Sweeteners

The various substances that impart sweetness to foods fall into two broad classes: nutritive sweeteners, which can provide calories for the body; and alternative sweeteners, which, for the most part provide no calories. As shown in Table 4-2, the alternative sweeteners are much sweeter on a per-gram basis than the nutritive sweeteners.

Nutritive Sweeteners

Both sugars and sugar alcohols provide calories along with sweetness. Sugars are found in many different food products, whereas sugar alcohols have rather limited uses.

Grains	Vegetables	Fruits	Oils	Milk	Meat & Beans
• All varieties	• All varieties	• All varieties	• None	• Milk • Yogurt	• Beans • Nuts

Figure 4-5 Sources of Carbohydrates from the MyPyramid. The height of the background color (none, 1/3, 2/3 or completely covered) within each group in the pyramid indicates the average nutrient density for carbohydrate in that group. Overall, the grain group, vegetable group, fruit group, and milk group contain many foods that are nutrient-dense sources of carbohydrate. Based on serving sizes for MyPyramid, milk and yogurt contain about 12 grams, beans (legumes) about 10 grams, nuts about 4 grams, fruits about 18 grams, grains about 15 grams, and vegetables about 5 grams of carbohydrates per serving. With regard to physical activity, carbohydrates are a key fuel in most endeavors.

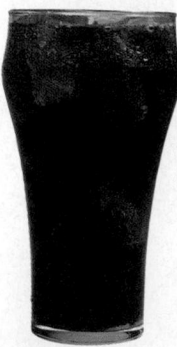

Soft drinks are typical sources of either sugars or alternative sweeteners, depending on the type of soft drink chosen.

Cyclamate is not available in the United States, but is so in Canada.

Table 4-2 The Sweetness of Sugars (Nutritive) and Alternative Sweeteners

Type of Sweetener	Relative Sweetness* (Sucrose = 1)	Typical Sources
Sugars		
Lactose	0.2	Dairy products
Maltose	0.4	Sprouted seeds
Glucose	0.7	Corn syrup
Sucrose	1.0	Table sugar, most sweets
Invert sugar†	1.3	Some candies, honey
Fructose	1.2–1.8	Fruit, honey, some soft drinks
Sugar Alcohols		
Sorbitol	0.6	Dietetic candies, sugarless gum
Mannitol	0.7	Dietetic candies
Xylitol	0.9	Sugarless gum
Maltitol	0.9	Baked goods, chocolate, candies
Alternative Sweeteners		
Tagatose	0.9	Ready-to-eat breakfast cereals, diet soft drinks, meal replacement bars, frozen desserts, candy, and frosting
Cyclamate‡	30	Tabletop sweetener, medicines
Aspartame (Equal®)	180	Diet soft drinks, diet fruit drinks, sugarless gum, powdered diet sweetener
Acesulfame-K (Sunette)	200	Sugarless gum, diet drink mixes, powdered diet sweeteners, puddings, gelatin desserts
Saccharin (sodium salt) (Sweet'N Low)	300	Diet soft drinks, powdered diet sweetener
Sucralose (Splenda)	600	Diet soft drinks, powdered diet sweetener, sugarless gums, jams, frozen desserts
Neotame	7000 to 13,000	Powdered diet sweetener, baked goods, frozen desserts, and jams

*On a per gram basis. †Sucrose broken down into glucose and fructose.
‡Not available in the United States, but available in Canada.
From the American Dietetic Association, 2004, and other sources.

Sugars　All of the monosaccharides (glucose, fructose, and galactose) and disaccharides (sucrose, lactose, and maltose) discussed earlier are designated *nutritive sweeteners* (Table 4-3). The taste and sweetness of sucrose make it the benchmark against which all other sweeteners are measured. Sucrose is obtained from sugar cane and sugar beet plants.

High-fructose corn syrup, which is generally 55% fructose, is used extensively in the food industry today. High-fructose corn syrup is made by treating cornstarch with

Table 4-3 Names of Sugars Used in Foods

Sugar	Invert sugar	Honey	Maple syrup
Sucrose	Glucose	Corn syrup or sweeteners	Dextrose
Brown sugar	Sorbitol		Fructose
Confectioner's sugar (powdered sugar)	Levulose	High-fructose corn syrup	Maltodextrins
	Polydextrose	Molasses	Caramel
Turbinado sugar	Lactose	Date sugar	Fruit sugar

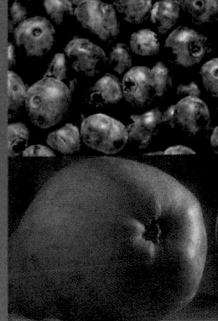
Food manufacturers and consumers have numerous options for obtaining sweetness while consuming less sugar and calories.

Sugar Alcohols

Sugar alcohols such as **sorbitol** and **xylitol** are used as nutritive sweeteners. Sugar alcohols contribute fewer calories than sugars (about 2.6 kcal per gram). They also are absorbed and metabolized to glucose more slowly than are simple sugars. Because of this in large quantities, they can cause diarrhea. In fact, any products whose foreseeable consumption may result in a daily ingestion of 50 grams of sugar alcohols must bear this labeling statement: "Excess consumption may have a laxative effect."

Sugar alcohols are used in sugarless gum, breath mints, and candy. Unlike sucrose, these are not readily metabolized by bacteria to acids in the mouth and thus do not promote tooth decay (see the later section on problems linked to carbohydrate intake).

Sugar alcohols must be listed on labels, and if only one sugar alcohol is used in a product, it must be distinguished; however, if two or more are used in one product, they are grouped together under the heading "sugar alcohols." The actual caloric value is calculated, taking in account each sugar alcohol, so that when one reads the total amount of calories a product provides, it includes the sugar alcohols in the overall amount.

Sugar alcohols as a class are also called polyols.

Alternative Sweeteners

Often called artificial sweeteners, alternative sweeteners include **saccharin,** cyclamate, **aspartame, neotame, acesulfame-K,** and **sucralose.** Unlike sugar alcohols, alternative sweeteners yield little or no calories when consumed in amounts typically used in food products. Five are currently available in the United States: saccharin, aspartame, neotame, acesulfame-K, and sucralose. Cyclamate was banned for use in the United States in 1970, although it has never been conclusively proven to cause health problems when used appropriately. Cyclamate is used in Canada as a sweetener in medicines and as a tabletop sweetener.

Saccharin

The oldest alternative sweetener, saccharin, was first produced in 1879 and is currently approved for use in more than 90 countries. It represents about half of the alternative sweetener market in North America (typically packaged in pink packets). Saccharin was once thought to pose a risk of bladder cancer based on laboratory animal studies, but it is no longer listed as a potential cause of cancer in humans.

Aspartame

In 1981, the alternative sweetener aspartame became available. Its trade name is Equal® when sold as a powder. Aspartame is in widespread use throughout the world. It has been approved for use by more than 90 countries, and its use has been endorsed by the World Health Organization, the American Medical Association, the American Diabetes Association, and the American Academy of Pediatrics Committee on Nutrition.

> ### Sugarless Gum
>
> Ingredients: Sorbitol, gum base, mannitol, glycerol, hydrogenated glucose syrup, xylitol, artificial and natural flavors, aspartame, red 40, yellow 6 and BHT (to maintain freshness). Phenylketonurics: contains phenylalanine.

Sugar alcohols can be found in sugarless gum. Aspartame is also used to sweeten this product. *Note the warning for people with PKU that this product with aspartame contains phenylalanine* (discussed further on next page).

Persons with an uncommon disease called **phenylketonuria (PKU),** which interferes with the metabolism of phenylalanine, should avoid aspartame because of its high phenylalanine content. A warning label for people with PKU that a product with aspartame contains phenylalanine is required.

The components of aspartame are the amino acids phenylalanine and aspartic acid, along with methanol. Recall that amino acids are the building blocks of proteins, so aspartame is more of a protein than a carbohydrate. Aspartame yields about 4 kcal per gram, but it is about 200 times sweeter than sucrose. Thus, only a small amount of aspartame is needed to obtain the desired sweetness, so the amount of calories added is insignificant unless the product is consumed in unusually high amounts. Aspartame is used in beverages, gelatin desserts, chewing gum, toppings and fillings in precooked bakery goods, and cookies. Aspartame does not cause tooth decay. Like other proteins, however, aspartame is damaged when heated for a long time and thus would lose its sweetness if used in products requiring cooking.

Some complaints have been filed with FDA by people claiming to have had adverse reactions to aspartame: headaches, dizziness, seizures, nausea, and other side effects. It is important for people who are sensitive to aspartame to avoid it, but the percentage of sensitive people is likely to be extremely small.

The acceptable daily intake of aspartame set by FDA is 50 milligrams per kilogram of body weight. This is equivalent to about 14 cans of diet soft drink for an adult or about 80 packets of Equal®. Aspartame appears to be safe for pregnant women and children, but some scientists suggest cautious use by these groups, especially young children, who need ample calories to grow.

■ Neotame

Stevia comes from a South American shrub; it is 100 to 300 times sweeter than sucrose and provides zero calories. This is a sweetener that has been used in small amounts by the Japanese since the 1970s. FDA has not approved the use of stevia in foods, but stevia can be purchased at natural- and health-food stores as a dietary supplement.

Neotame was recently approved by FDA for use as a general-purpose sweetener in a wide variety of food products, other than meat and poultry. Neotame is a nonnutritive, high-intensity sweetener that, depending on its food application, is approximately 7,000 to 13,000 times sweeter than table sugar. It has a chemical structure similar to aspartame. Neotame is heat stable and can be used as a tabletop sweetener as well as in cooking applications. Examples of uses for which it has been approved include baked goods, nonalcoholic beverages (including soft drinks), chewing gum, confections and frostings, frozen desserts, gelatins and puddings, jams and jellies, processed fruits and fruit juices, toppings and syrups. Neotame is safe for use by the general population, including children, pregnant and lactating women, and people with diabetes. In addition, no special labeling for people with phenylketonuria is needed since neotame is not broken down in the body to its amino acid components.

■ Acesulfame-K

The alternative sweetener acesulfame-K (Sunette; the *K* stands for potassium) was approved by FDA in July 1988. It is approved for use in more than 40 countries and has been in use in Europe since 1983. Acesulfame-K is 200 times sweeter than sucrose. It contributes no calories to the diet because it is not digested by the body, and it does not cause dental caries.

Unlike aspartame, acesulfame-K can be used in baking because it does not lose its sweetness when heated. In the United States, it is currently approved for use in chewing gum, powdered drink mixes, gelatins, puddings, baked goods, tabletop sweeteners, candy, throat lozenges, yogurt, and nondairy creamers; additional uses may soon be approved. One recent trend is to combine it with aspartame in soft drinks.

■ Sucralose

Tagatose is a slightly altered form of the simple sugar fructose. It was approved for use in 2003 for ready-to-eat breakfast cereals, diet soft drinks, meal replacement bars, frozen desserts, candy, frosting, and chewing gum. Because tagatose is poorly absorbed, it yields only 1.5 kcal per gram to the body. Use also does not raise the risk for dental caries, nor does it increase blood glucose. Eventual fermentation in the large intestine may even lead to a beneficial effect on that organ (i.e., a probiotic effect, covered in Chapter 3).

Sucralose (Splenda) is 600 times sweeter than sucrose. It is made by putting three chlorines on sucrose. FDA approved use of sucralose in 1998 as an additive to foods such as soda, gum, baked goods, syrups, gelatins, frozen dairy desserts such as ice cream, jams, and processed fruits and fruit juices, and for tabletop use. Sucralose doesn't break down under high heat conditions and can be used in cooking and baking. It is also excreted as such in the feces. The little that is absorbed is excreted in the urine.

Overall, sugar alcohols and alternative sweeteners enable people with diabetes to enjoy the flavor of sweetness while controlling sugars in their diets; they also provide noncaloric or very-low-calorie sugar substitutes for persons trying to lose (or control) body weight.

acid and enzymes. This treatment breaks down much of the starch into glucose. Then some of the glucose is converted by enzymes into fructose. The final syrup is usually as sweet as sucrose. Its major advantage is that it is cheaper than sucrose. Also, it doesn't form crystals and it has better freezing properties. High-fructose corn syrups are used in soft drinks, candies, jam, jelly, other fruit products, and desserts (e.g., packaged cookies).

In addition to sucrose and high-fructose corn syrup, brown sugar, turbinado sugar (sold as raw sugar), honey, maple syrup, and other sugars are also added to foods. Turbinado sugar, a partially refined version of raw sucrose, has a slight molasses flavor. Brown sugar is essentially sucrose containing some molasses; either the molasses is not totally removed from the sucrose during processing or it is added to the sucrose crystals.

Maple syrup is made by boiling down and concentrating the sap that runs during the late winter in sugar maple trees. Most pancake syrup sold in supermarkets is not pure maple syrup, which is quite expensive. Instead, it is primarily corn syrup and high-fructose corn syrup with maple flavor added.

Honey is a product of plant nectar that has been altered by bee enzymes. The enzymes break down much of the nectar's sucrose into fructose and glucose. Honey offers essentially the same nutritional value as other simple sugars—a source of energy and little else. However, honey is not safe to feed to infants because it can contain spores of the bacterium *Clostridium botulinum*. These spores can become the bacteria that cause fatal foodborne illness. Honey does not pose the same threat to adults because the acidic environment of an adult's stomach inhibits the growth of the bacteria. An infant's stomach, however, does not produce much acid, making infants susceptible to the threat that this bacterium poses.

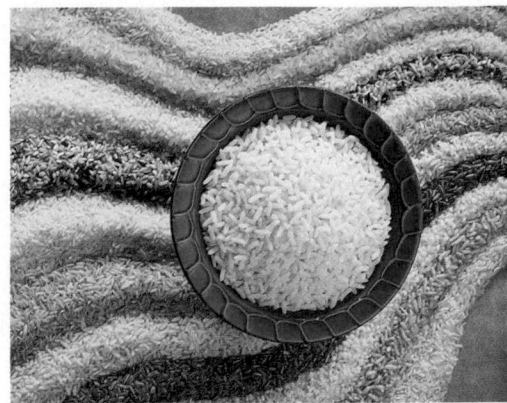

Rice is a rich source of carbohydrates.

Concept Check

Table sugar, honey, jam, fruit, and plain baked potatoes contain the highest percentage of calories from carbohydrates. Foods such as cream pies, potato chips, whole milk, and oatmeal contain moderate amounts of carbohydrate. Common nutritive sweeteners added to foods include sucrose, maple sugar, honey, brown sugar, and high-fructose corn syrup. For people who want to limit sugar intake, other sweeteners are available and include the sugar alcohols, saccharin, aspartame, neotame, acesulfame-K, and sucralose. Of these, aspartame is the most common alternative sweetener in use.

Making Carbohydrates Available for Body Use

As discussed in Chapter 3, simply eating a food does not supply nutrients to body cells. Digestion and absorption must occur first.

▌Digestion

Food preparation can be viewed as the start of carbohydrate digestion because cooking softens tough connective structures in the fibrous parts of plants, such as broccoli stalks. When starches are heated, the starch granules swell as they soak up water, making them much easier to digest. All of these effects of cooking generally make carbohydrate-containing foods easier to chew, swallow, and break down during digestion.

The enzymatic digestion of starch begins in the mouth, when the saliva, which contains an enzyme called salivary **amylase,** mixes with the starchy products during the chewing of the food. This amylase breaks down starch into many smaller units

amylase Starch-digesting enzyme from the salivary glands or pancreas.

(e.g., disaccharides, such as maltose) (Fig. 4-6). You can observe this conversion while chewing a saltine cracker. Prolonged chewing of the cracker causes it to taste sweeter as some starch breaks down into the sweeter sugars, such as maltose. Still, food is in the mouth for such a short amount of time that this phase of digestion is negligible. In addition, once the food moves down the esophagus and reaches the stomach, the acidic environment inactivates salivary amylase.

After the carbohydrates have reached the small intestine—which has a more alkaline environment and thus is better suited for further carbohydrate digestion—the pancreas releases enzymes, such as pancreatic amylase. This is the last stage of starch digestion. After amylase action, the original carbohydrates in a food are now present in the small intestine as monosaccharides (glucose and fructose present as such in food) and disaccharides (maltose from starch breakdown, lactose mainly from dairy products, and sucrose from food and that added at the table).

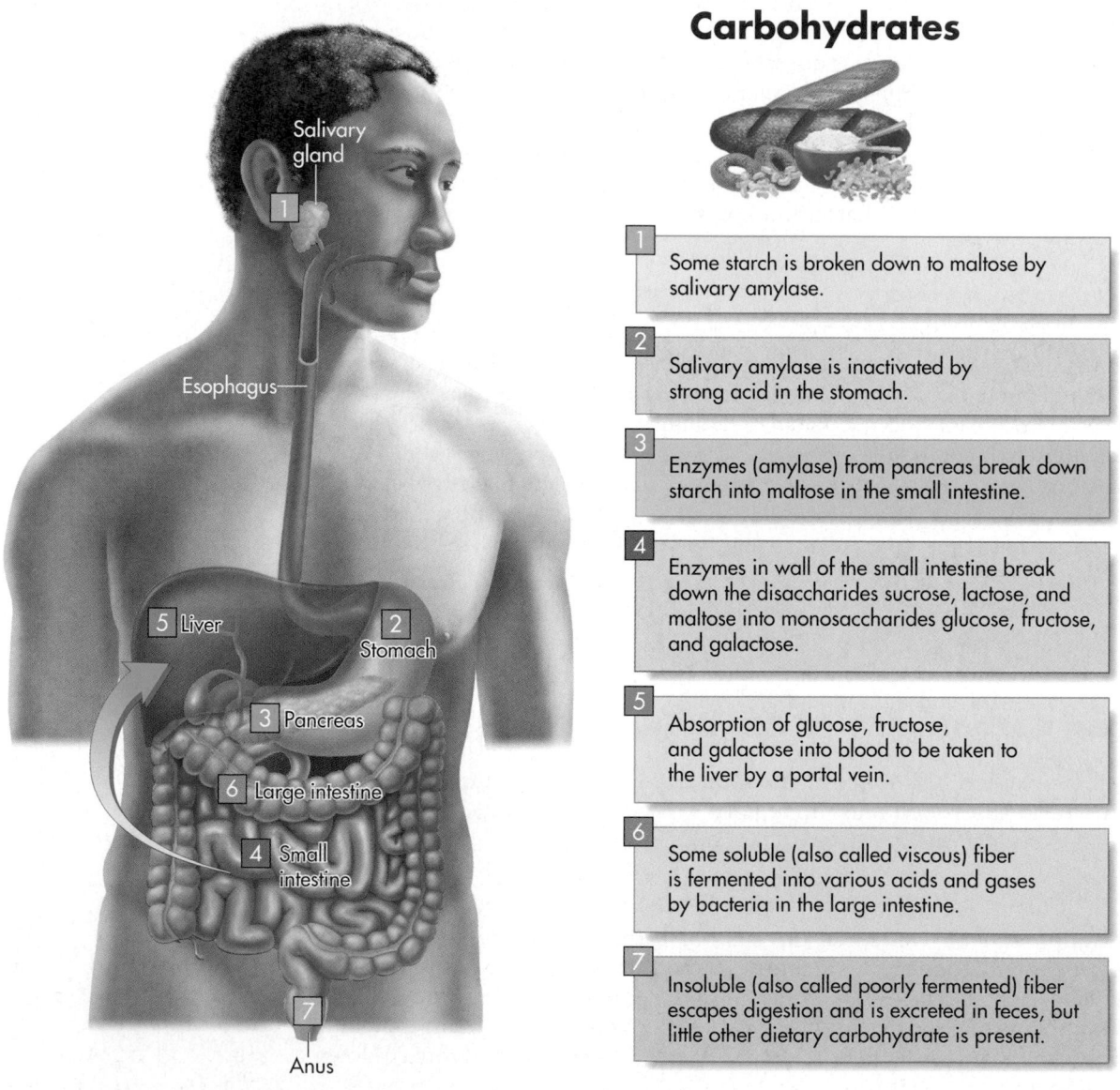

Carbohydrates

1. Some starch is broken down to maltose by salivary amylase.

2. Salivary amylase is inactivated by strong acid in the stomach.

3. Enzymes (amylase) from pancreas break down starch into maltose in the small intestine.

4. Enzymes in wall of the small intestine break down the disaccharides sucrose, lactose, and maltose into monosaccharides glucose, fructose, and galactose.

5. Absorption of glucose, fructose, and galactose into blood to be taken to the liver by a portal vein.

6. Some soluble (also called viscous) fiber is fermented into various acids and gases by bacteria in the large intestine.

7. Insoluble (also called poorly fermented) fiber escapes digestion and is excreted in feces, but little other dietary carbohydrate is present.

Figure 4-6 Carbohydrate Digestion and Absorption. Enzymes made by the mouth, pancreas, and small intestine participate in the process of digestion. Most carbohydrate digestion and absorption takes place in the small intestine. Note that Chapter 3 covered the physiology of digestion and absorption in detail.

The disaccharides are digested to their monosaccharide units once they reach the wall of the small intestine, where the specialized enzymes on the absorptive cells digest each disaccharide into monosaccharides. The enzyme **maltase** acts on maltose to produce two glucose molecules. **Sucrase** acts on sucrose to produce glucose and fructose. **Lactase** acts on lactose to produce glucose and galactose.

■ Absorption

Single sugars found naturally in foods and those formed as by-products of earlier starch digestion in the mouth and small intestine generally follow an active absorption process. Recall from Chapter 3 that this is a process that requires a specific carrier and energy input in order for the substance to be taken up by the absorptive cells in the small intestine. Glucose and its close relative, galactose, undergo active absorption. They are pumped into the absorptive cells along with sodium.

Another Bite

Fructose is taken up by the absorptive cells via facilitated diffusion. In this case, a carrier is used, but no energy input is needed. This absorptive process is thus slower than that seen with glucose or galactose. So, large doses of fructose are not readily absorbed and can contribute to diarrhea as this remains in the small intestine and attracts water.

Once glucose, galactose, and fructose enter the absorptive cells, some fructose is metabolized into glucose. The single sugars in the absorptive cells are then transferred to the portal vein that goes directly to the liver. The liver then metabolizes those sugars by transforming the monosaccharides into glucose and:

- Releasing it directly into the bloodstream for transport to organs such as the brain, muscles, kidneys, and adipose tissues
- Producing glycogen for storage of carbohydrate
- Producing fat (minor amount, if any)

Of these three options, producing fat is the least likely, except when carbohydrates are consumed in high amounts and overall calorie needs are exceeded.

Unless an individual has a disease that causes malabsorption, or an intolerance to a carbohydrate such as lactose (or fructose), only a minor amount of some sugars (about 10%) escapes digestion. The undigested carbohydrate travels to the large intestine and is fermented there by bacteria. The acids and gases produced by bacterial metabolism of the undigested carbohydrate are absorbed into the bloodstream. Scientists suspect that some of these products of bacterial metabolism actually promote the health of the large intestine by providing it with a source of calories.

Concept Check

Carbohydrate digestion is the process of breaking down larger carbohydrates into smaller units, and eventually to monosaccharide forms. The enzymatic digestion of starches in the body begins in the mouth with salivary amylase. Enzymes made by the pancreas and small intestine complete the digestion of carbohydrates to single sugars in the small intestine. Following primarily an active absorption process, the single sugars (glucose and galactose)—either resulting from the digestive process or present in the meal—are taken up by absorptive cells in the intestine. Fructose undergoes facilitated absorption. All of the monosaccharides then enter the portal vein that goes directly to the liver. The liver finally exercises its metabolic options, producing glucose, glycogen, and even fat if carbohydrates are consumed in great excess and overall calorie needs are exceeded.

maltase An enzyme made by absorptive cells of the small intestine; this enzyme digests maltose to two glucoses.

sucrase An enzyme made by absorptive cells of the small intestine; this enzyme digests sucrose to glucose and fructose.

lactase An enzyme made by absorptive cells of the small intestine; this enzyme digests lactose to glucose and galactose.

Bacteria in the large intestine ferment soluble fibers into such products as acids and gases. The acids, once absorbed, also provide calories for the body. In this way, soluble fibers provide about 1.5 to 2.5 kcal per gram. Although the intestinal gas (flatulence) produced by this bacterial fermentation is not harmful, it can be painful and sometimes embarrassing. Over time, however, the body tends to adapt to a high-fiber intake, eventually producing less gas.

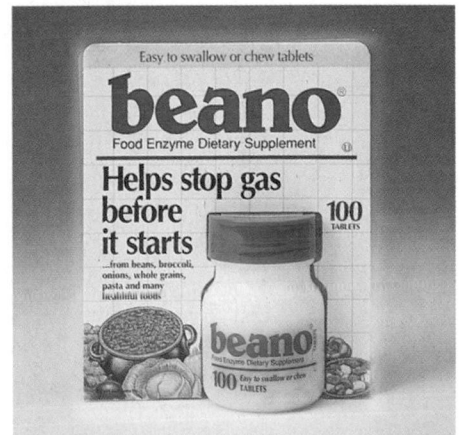

Beano® is a dietary supplement that contains natural digestive enzymes. It can be used to reduce intestinal gas produced by bacterial metabolism of undigested sugars in beans and some vegetables in the large intestine.

Putting Simple Carbohydrates to Work in the Body

The functions of glucose in the body start with supplying calories to fuel the body. Because the other sugars can generally be converted to glucose and starches are broken down to yield glucose, the functions described here apply to most carbohydrates.

■ Yielding Energy

The main function of glucose is to supply calories for use by the body. Certain tissues in the body, such as red blood cells, can use only glucose and other simple carbohydrate forms for fuel. Most parts of the brain and central nervous system also derive energy only from glucose, unless the diet contains almost none. In that case, much of the brain can use partial breakdown products of fat—called **ketone bodies**—for energy needs. Simple carbohydrates can also fuel muscle cells and other body cells, but many of these cells can also use fat for energy needs.

■ Sparing Protein from Use as an Energy Source and Preventing Ketosis

A diet that supplies enough digestible carbohydrates to prevent breakdown of proteins for energy needs is considered *protein sparing*. Under normal circumstances, digestible carbohydrates in the diet mostly end up as blood glucose, and protein is reserved for functions such as building and maintaining muscles and vital organs. However, if you don't eat enough carbohydrates, your body is forced to make glucose from body proteins, draining the pool of amino acids available in cells for other critical functions. During long-term starvation, the continuous withdrawal of proteins from the muscles, heart, liver, kidneys, and other vital organs can result in weakness, poor function, and even failure of body systems.

In addition to the loss of protein, when you don't eat enough carbohydrates, the metabolism of fats is inefficient. In the absence of adequate carbohydrate, fats don't break down completely in metabolism and instead form ketone bodies. This condition, known as **ketosis,** should be avoided because it disturbs the body's normal acid-base balance and leads to other health problems. This is another good reason to question the long-term safety of the low-carbohydrate diets that are so popular today.

ketone bodies Products of incomplete breakdown of fat containing three or four carbons.

ketosis The condition of having a high concentration of ketone bodies and related breakdown products in the bloodstream and tissues.

Another Bite

The life-threatening wasting of protein that occurs during long-term fasting has prompted companies that produce medical products for rapid weight loss to include sufficient carbohydrate in the formulation to decrease protein breakdown and thereby help to protect vital tissues and organs, including the heart. Most of these products are powders that can be mixed with different kinds of fluids, are consumed five or six times per day, and are very low in calories.

Regulating This Energy Source

Under normal circumstances, a person's blood glucose concentration is regulated within a very narrow range. Recall from Chapter 3 that when carbohydrates are digested and taken up by the absorptive cells of the small intestine, the resulting monosaccharides are transported directly to the liver. One of the liver's roles, then, is to guard against excess glucose entering the bloodstream after a meal. The liver works in concert with the pancreas to regulate blood glucose.

When the supply of glucose in the blood is high, such as during and immediately after a meal, the pancreas releases the hormone **insulin** into the bloodstream. Insulin delivers two different messages to various body cells to cause the level of glucose in the blood to fall. First, insulin directs the liver to store the glucose as glycogen. Second, insulin directs muscle, adipose, and other cells to remove glucose from the bloodstream by taking it into those cells. By triggering both glycogen synthesis in the liver and glucose movement out of the bloodstream into certain cells, insulin keeps the concentration of glucose from rising too high in the blood (Fig. 4-7).

On the other hand, when a person has not eaten for a few hours and blood glucose begins to fall, the pancreas releases the hormone **glucagon.** This hormone has the opposite effect of insulin. It prompts the breakdown of glycogen from the liver into glucose, which is then released into the bloodstream. In this way, glucagon keeps blood glucose from falling too low.

A different mechanism increases blood glucose during times of stress. **Epinephrine** (adrenaline) is the hormone responsible for the "flight or fight" reaction. Epinephrine and a related compound are released in large amounts from the adrenal glands (located on each kidney) and various nerve endings in response to a perceived threat, such as a car approaching head-on. These hormones cause glycogen in the liver to be quickly broken down into glucose. The resulting rapid flood of glucose from the liver into the bloodstream helps promote quick mental and physical reactions.

In essence, the actions of insulin on blood glucose are balanced by the actions of glucagon, epinephrine, and other hormones. If hormonal balance is not maintained, such as during over- or underproduction of insulin or glucagon, major changes in blood glucose concentrations occur. To maintain blood glucose within an acceptable range, the body relies on a complex regulatory system. This provides a safeguard against extremely high blood glucose (**hyperglycemia**) or low blood glucose (**hypoglycemia**).

insulin A hormone produced by the pancreas. Among other processes, insulin increases the synthesis of glycogen in the liver and the movement of glucose from the bloodstream into body cells.

glucagon A hormone made by the pancreas that stimulates the breakdown of glycogen in the liver into glucose; this ends up increasing blood glucose. Glucagon also performs other functions.

epinephrine A hormone also known as *adrenaline;* it is released by the adrenal glands (located on each kidney) and various nerve endings in the body. It acts to increase glycogen breakdown in the liver, among other functions.

hyperglycemia High blood glucose, above 125 milligrams per 100 milliliters of blood.

hypoglycemia Low blood glucose, below 40 to 50 milligrams per 100 milliliters of blood.

Figure 4-7 Regulation of Blood Glucose. Insulin and glucagon are key hormones in controlling blood glucose concentration. Other hormones, such as epinephrine, also contribute to blood glucose regulation. When we eat a meal, insulin is released to promote glucose uptake by cells, thus reversing the increase in blood glucose that results from absorption of various sugars after a meal, and in turn restoring the balance. When fasting, blood glucose falls. Glucagon is released to promote glucose release from liver stores (initially present in the form of glycogen). This raises blood glucose, again restoring the balance.

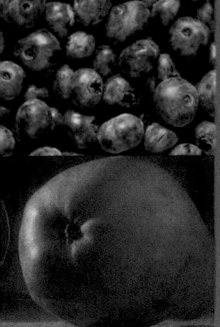

When Blood Glucose Regulation Fails

Improper regulation of blood glucose results in either hyperglycemia (high blood glucose) or hypoglycemia (low blood glucose) as noted in Chapter 4. High blood glucose is most commonly associated with diabetes (technically, *diabetes mellitus*), a disease that affects 6% of the North American population. Of these, it is estimated one-third to one-half of these people do not know that they have the disease. Diabetes leads to about 200,000 deaths each year in North America. Note that diabetes is currently increasing in epidemic proportions in North America. New recommendations promote testing fasting blood glucose in adults over age 45 every 3 years to help diagnose the problem. Diabetes is diagnosed when one's fasting blood glucose is 126 milligrams per 100 milliliters of blood or greater. In contrast, low blood glucose is a much rarer condition.

Diabetes

type 1 diabetes A form of diabetes prone to ketosis and that requires insulin therapy.

type 2 diabetes A form of diabetes in which ketosis is not commonly seen. Insulin therapy can be used but is often not required. This form of the disease is often associated with obesity.

There are two major forms of diabetes: **type 1** (formerly called insulin-dependent or juvenile-onset diabetes), and **type 2** (formerly called non–insulin-dependent or adult-onset **diabetes**) (Table 4-4). The change in names to type 1 and type 2 diabetes stems from the fact that many type 2 diabetics eventually must also rely on insulin injections as a part of their treatment. In addition, many children today have type 2 diabetes. A third form, called gestational diabetes, occurs in some pregnant women (see Chapter 13). It is usually treated with an insulin regimen

Traditional symptoms of diabetes are excessive urination, excessive thirst, and excessive hunger. No one symptom is diagnostic of diabetes, and other symptoms—such as unexplained weight loss, exhaustion, blurred vision, tingling in hands and feet, frequent infections, poor wound healing, and impotence—often accompany traditional symptoms.

Table 4-4 Comparing and Contrasting Type 1 and Type 2 Diabetes

	Type 1 Diabetes	Type 2 Diabetes
Occurrence	5%–10% of cases of diabetes	90% of cases of diabetes
Cause	Immune System attack of the pancreas	Insulin resistance
Risk Factors	Moderate genetic predisposition	Strong genetic predisposition Obesity Sedentary lifestyle Ethnicity
Characteristics	Distinct symptoms (frequent thirst, hunger, and urination) Ketosis	Mild symptoms, especially in early phases of the disease (fatigue and nighttime urination)
Cell Response to Insulin	Normal	Resistant
Treatment	Diet Exercise Insulin Aspirin Medications to lower blood cholesterol	Diet Exercise Oral medications Insulin (in advanced cases) Aspirin Medications to lower blood cholesterol
Complications*	Cardiovascular disease Kidney disease Nerve damage Blindness	Cardiovascular disease Kidney disease Nerve damage Blindness

*In both cases maintaining a healthy blood lipid profile and normal blood pressure is vital to avoid these complications (see Chapters 5 and 9 for strategies).

and diet, and resolves after delivery of the baby. However, women who have gestational diabetes during pregnancy are at high risk for developing type 2 diabetes later in life.

■ Type 1 Diabetes

Type 1 diabetes often begins in late childhood, around the age of 8 to 12 years, but can occur at any age. The disease runs in certain families, indicating a clear genetic link. Children usually are admitted to the hospital with abnormally high blood glucose after eating, as well as evidence of ketosis.

The onset of type 1 diabetes is generally associated with decreased release of insulin from the pancreas. As insulin in the blood declines, blood glucose increases, especially after eating. Figure 4-8 shows a typical glucose tolerance curve observed in a patient with this form of diabetes after consuming a load of glucose (about 50 grams). When blood glucose exceeds the kidney's threshold, excess glucose spills over into the urine.

Most cases of type 1 diabetes begin with an immune system disorder, which causes destruction of the insulin-producing cells in the pancreas. Most likely, a virus or protein foreign to the body sets off the destruction. In response to their damage, the affected pancreatic cells release other proteins, which stimulate a more furious attack. Eventually, the pancreas loses its ability to synthesize insulin, and the clinical stage of the disease begins. Consequently, early treatment to stop the immune-linked destruction in children may be important. Research into this area is ongoing.

Type 1 diabetes is treated primarily by insulin therapy, either with injections two to six times per day or with an insulin pump. The pump dispenses insulin at a steady rate into the body, with greater amounts delivered after each meal. Dietary therapy includes three regular meals and one or more snacks (including one at bedtime), having a regulated ratio of carbohydrate:protein:fat to maximize insulin action and minimize swings in blood glucose. If one does not eat often enough, the injected insulin can cause severe hypoglycemia, since it acts on whatever glucose is available. The diet should include ample fiber and polyunsaturated fat, supply an amount of calories in balance with needs, and be low in both animal and *trans* fats, include fish twice a week, as well as moderate in simple carbohydrates. Meeting magnesium needs is also helpful.

If a high carbohydrate intake raises triglycerides and cholesterol in the blood beyond desired ranges, carbohydrate intake can be reduced and replaced with unsaturated fat. This change tends to reduce blood triglycerides and cholesterol. Chapter 5 discusses how to implement such

A common clinical method to determine a person's success in controlling blood glucose is to measure glycated (also termed glycosylated) hemoglobin (hemoglobin A1c). Over time, blood glucose attaches to (glycates) hemoglobin in red blood cells, and more so when blood glucose remains elevated. A hemoglobin A1c value of over 7% indicates poor blood glucose control. An acceptable value is 6% of less. Elevated blood glucose also leads to glycation of various proteins and fats in the body, forming what are called advanced glycation endproducts. These have been shown to be toxic to cells, especially those of immune system and kidneys. (Cigarette smoke is also a source.)

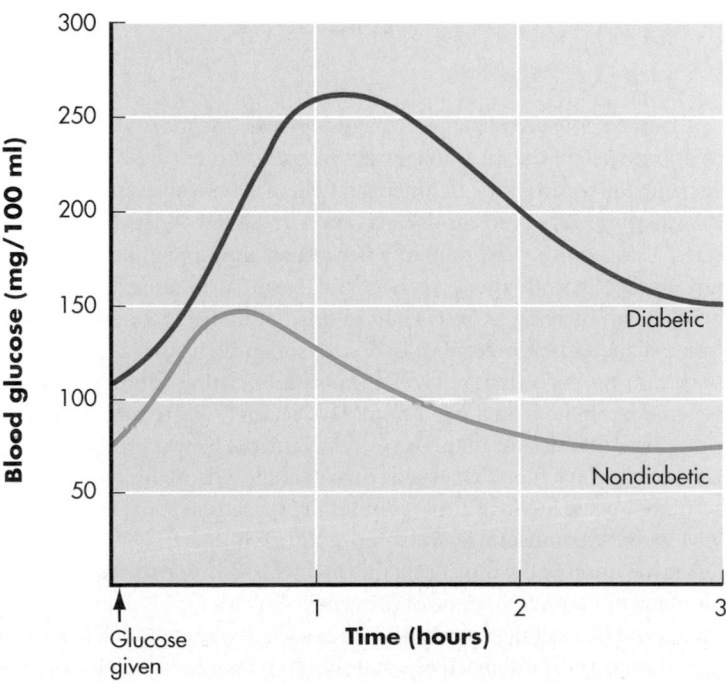

Figure 4-8 Glucose Tolerance Test. A comparison of blood glucose concentrations in untreated diabetic and healthy (normal) persons after consuming a load of glucose (about 50 grams).

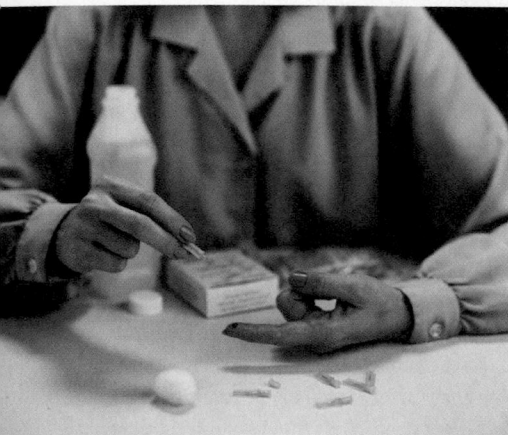

Regularly checking blood glucose is part of diabetes therapy today.

Recently people with diabetes have been cautioned not to cook foods at high temperatures for prolonged periods of time. This lead to deliterious advanced glycation end products forming in food, especially during frying and broiling. Use of a lower power setting with a microwave oven, lower oven temperatures, and minimal use of prolonged broiling and prolonged frying is advised. Colas and coffee are also sources of these substances, so moderate consumption is also advised. Foods low in advanced glycation end points are those high in carbohydrate (e.g., starches, fruits, vegetables, and milk).

a diet (as well as when certain related medications may be beneficial). Some consumption of sugars with meals is fine, as long as blood glucose regulation is preserved and the sugars replace other carbohydrates in the meal, so that undesirable weight gain does not take place.

The latest evidence suggests that diabetes essentially guarantees development of cardiovascular disease. Because people with diabetes (type 1, as well as type 2) are at a high risk for cardiovascular disease and related heart attacks, they should take an aspirin each day (generally 80 to 160 milligrams per day) if their physicians find no reason not to do so. Blood cholesterol lowering medications also may be prescribed. As discussed in Chapter 5, these practices reduce the risk of heart attack.

The hormone imbalances that occur in people with untreated type 1 diabetes—chiefly, not enough insulin—lead to mobilization of body fat, which is taken up by liver cells. Ketosis is the result because the fat is mostly converted to ketone bodies. Ketone bodies can rise excessively in the blood, eventually forcing ketone bodies into the urine. These pull sodium and potassium ions with them into the urine. This series of events can contribute to a chain reaction which eventually leads to dehydration, ion imbalance, coma, and even death, especially in patients with poorly controlled type 1 diabetes. Treatment includes insulin, fluids, and minerals such as sodium and potassium.

In addition to cardiovascular disease, other degenerative complications that result from poor blood glucose regulation include blindness, kidney disease, and deterioration of nerves. When improper nerve stimulation occurs in the intestinal tract, intermittent diarrhea and constipation result. Because of nerve deterioration in the extremities, many people with diabetes lose the sensation of pain associated with injuries or infections. Not having as much pain, they often delay treatment of hand or foot problems. This delay, combined with a rich environment for bacterial growth (bacteria thrive on glucose) sets the stage for damage and death of tissues in the extremities, sometimes leading to the need for amputation of feet and legs.

Current research, such as the Diabetes Control and Complications Trial (DCCT), has shown that the development of blood vessel and nerve complications of diabetes can be slowed with aggressive treatment directed at keeping blood glucose within the normal range. The therapy poses some risks of its own, such as hypoglycemia, so it must be implemented under the close supervision of a physician.

A person with diabetes generally must work closely with a physician and registered dietitian to make the correct alterations in diet and medications and to perform physical activity safely. Physical activity enhances glucose uptake by muscles independent of insulin action, which in turn can lower blood glucose. This outcome is beneficial, but people with type 1 diabetes need to be aware of their own blood glucose response to physical activity and compensate appropriately.

▪ Type 2 Diabetes

Type 2 diabetes usually begins after age 40. This is the most common type of diabetes, accounting for about 90% of the cases diagnosed in North America. Minority populations such as Latino/Hispanic Americans, African Americans, Asian Americans, Native Americans, and those from Pacific Islands are at particular risk. As noted in the introduction, the overall number of people affected also is on the rise, primarily because of widespread inactivity and obesity in our population. In fact, recently there has been a substantial increase in type 2 diabetes in children, due mostly to an increase in overweight in this population (coupled with limited physical activity). Type 2 diabetes is also genetically linked, so family history is a very important risk factor. However, the initial problem is not with the insulin-secreting cells of the pancreas. Instead, it arises with the insulin receptors on the cell surfaces of certain body tissues, especially when muscle tissue becomes insulin resistant. In this case, blood glucose is not readily transferred into cells, so the person develops high blood glucose as a result of the glucose remaining in the bloodstream. The pancreas attempts to increase insulin output to compensate, but there is a limit to its ability to do this. Thus, rather than insufficient insulin production, there is an abundance of insulin, particularly during the onset of the disease. As the disease develops, pancreatic function can fail, leading to reduced insulin output. Because of the genetic link for type 2 diabetes, those who have a family history should be careful to avoid risk factors such as obesity, a diet rich in animal and *trans* fats, simple carbohydrates, and inactivity, and should schedule regular blood glucose tests.

Many cases of type 2 diabetes (about 80%) are associated with obesity (especially fat located in the abdominal region), but high blood glucose is not directly caused by the obesity. In fact, some lean people also develop this type of diabetes. Obesity associated with oversized adipose cells simply increases the risk for insulin resistance by the body as weight is gained.

Type 2 diabetes linked to obesity often disappears if the obesity is corrected. Achieving a healthy weight therefore should be a primary goal of treatment, but even limited weight loss can lead to better blood glucose regulation. Certain oral medications can also help control blood glucose. Adequate chromium intake is also important for blood glucose regulation (see Chapter 9).

Sometimes it may be necessary to provide insulin injections in type 2 diabetes because nothing else is able to control the disease. (This eventually becomes the case in about half of all cases of type 2 diabetes.) Regular physical activity also helps the muscles take up more glucose. And regular meal patterns, with an emphasis on control of calorie intake and consumption of mostly fiber-rich carbohydrates, as well as regular fish intake, is important therapy. Note that nuts help fulfill the fiber goal. (An almost daily intake of nuts was even shown to reduce the risk of developing type 2 diabetes in one recent study.) Some intake of sugars is fine with meals, but again these must be substituted for other carbohydrates, not simply added to the meal plan. Distributing carbohydrates throughout the day is also important, as this helps minimize the high and low swings in blood glucose concentrations. Moderate alcohol use is acceptable (1 serving per day). Studies have shown that this practice substantially reduces heart attack risk in people with type 2 diabetes. Still, the person must be warned that alcohol can lead to hypoglycemia and that the person must test him- or herself regularly for this possibility. And, as mentioned before, meeting magnesium needs is also helpful.

People with type 2 diabetes who have high blood triglycerides should moderate their carbohydrate intake and increase their intake of unsaturated fat and fiber, as noted earlier for people with type 1 diabetes.

Although many cases of type 2 diabetes can be relieved by reducing excess adipose tissue stores, many people are not able to lose weight. They remain affected with diabetes and may experience the degenerative complications seen in the type 1 form of the disease. Ketosis, however, is not usually seen in type 2 diabetes.

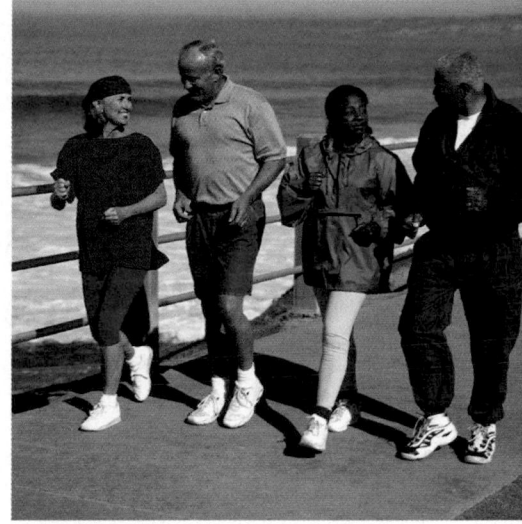

Development of type 2 diabetes in those at risk and progression of type 1 diabetes can both be decreased almost 60% by participating in regular exercise and controlling body weight.

For more information on diabetes, consult the following websites: www.diabetes.org and ndep.nih.gov. Also, see the latest guidelines for diets in diabetes treatment in the January 2002 issue of the *Journal of the American Dietetic Association*.

Hypoglycemia

As noted earlier, people with diabetes who are taking insulin sometimes have hypoglycemia if they don't eat frequently enough. Hypoglycemia can also develop in nondiabetic individuals. The two common forms of nondiabetic hypoglycemia are termed *reactive* and *fasting*.

Reactive hypoglycemia is described as irritability, nervousness, headache, sweating, and confusion 2 to 4 hours after eating a meal, especially a meal high in simple sugars. The cause of reactive hypoglycemia is unclear, but it may be overproduction of insulin by the pancreas in response to rising blood glucose. **Fasting hypoglycemia** usually is caused by pancreatic cancer, which may lead to excessive insulin secretion. In this case, blood glucose falls to low concentrations after fasting for about 8 hours to 1 day. This form of hypoglycemia is rare.

The diagnosis of hypoglycemia requires the simultaneous presence of low blood glucose and the typical hypoglycemic symptoms. Blood glucose of 40 to 50 milligrams per 100 milliliters is suggestive, but just having low blood glucose after eating is not enough evidence to make the diagnosis of hypoglycemia. Although many people think they have hypoglycemia, few actually do.

It is normal for healthy people to have some hypoglycemic symptoms, such as irritability, headache, and shakiness, if they have not eaten for a prolonged period of time. Although not diagnostic of hypoglycemia, if you sometimes have symptoms of hypoglycemia, the standard nutrition therapy is one we all could follow. You need to eat regular meals, make sure you have some protein and fat in each meal, and eat complex carbohydrates with ample soluble fiber. Avoid meals or snacks that contain little more than simple carbohydrates. If symptoms continue, try small protein-containing snacks between meals or fruits and juice. Fat, protein, and soluble fiber in the diet tend to moderate swings in blood glucose. Last, moderate caffeine and alcohol intake.

reactive hypoglycemia Low blood glucose that follows a meal high in simple sugars, with corresponding symptoms of irritability, headache, nervousness, sweating, and confusion; also called *postprandial hypoglycemia*.

fasting hypoglycemia Low blood glucose that follows about a day of fasting.

Concept Check

Carbohydrates provide glucose for the energy needs of red blood cells and parts of the brain and nervous system. Eating too little carbohydrates forces the body to make glucose using primarily amino acids from proteins found in muscles and other vital organs. A low glucose supply in cells also inhibits efficient metabolism of fats. Ketosis can then result.

Blood glucose concentration is maintained within a very narrow range. When blood glucose rises after a meal, the hormone insulin is released in great amounts from the pancreas. Insulin acts to lower blood glucose by increasing glucose storage in the liver and glucose uptake by other body cells. If blood glucose falls during fasting, glucagon and other hormones increase the liver's release of glucose into the bloodstream to restore normal blood glucose concentrations. In a similar way, the hormone epinephrine can make more glucose available in response to stress. This balance in hormone activity helps maintain blood glucose within a healthy range.

Putting Fiber to Work

Fiber supplies mass to the feces, making elimination much easier. This is especially true for insoluble fibers. When enough fiber is consumed, the stool is large and soft because many types of plant fibers attract water. The larger size stimulates the intestinal muscles to contract, which aids elimination. Consequently, less pressure is necessary to expel the stool.

When too little fiber is eaten, the opposite can occur: very little water is present in the feces, making it small and hard. Constipation may result, which forces one to exert excessive pressure in the large intestine during defecation. This high pressure can force parts of the large intestine (colon) wall out from between the surrounding bands of muscle, forming small pouches called **diverticula.** Multiple diverticula are normally present in this condition (Fig. 4-9). **Hemorrhoids** may also result from excessive straining during defecation (review Chapter 3).

Diverticula are asymptomatic in about 80% of affected people; that is, they are not noticeable. The asymptomatic form of this disease is called **diverticulosis.** If the diverticula become filled with food particles, such as hulls and seeds, they may eventually become inflamed, a condition known as **diverticulitis.** Intake of fiber then should be reduced to limit further bacterial activity. Once the inflammation subsides, a high-fiber diet is resumed to ease stool elimination and reduce the risk of a future attack.

Additional health benefits can result from the consumption of fiber. A diet high in fiber likely controls weight and reduces the risk of developing obesity. The bulky nature of high-fiber foods takes time to chew and fills us up without yielding many calories. Increasing intake of foods rich in fiber is one strategy for remaining satisfied after a meal (review the discussion of energy density in Chapter 2). This is still another reason to question the low-carbohydrate craze—where is the whole-grain fiber going to come from?

Over the past 30 years, many population studies have shown a link between increased fiber intake and a decrease in colon cancer development. However, some recent research has refuted the relationship between intake of fiber and colon cancer development, while others have been supportive. Currently, most of the research on colon cancer is focusing on the potential preventive effects of fruits, vegetables, whole-grain breads and cereals, and bean intakes (rather than fiber per se); regular exercise; the use of aspirin and related pain medications; and meeting vitamin D, folate, selenium, and calcium needs. Smoking, obesity in men, excessive alcohol use, starch- and sugar-rich foods, and processed meat intake are under study as potential causes. Overall, the

diverticula Pouches that protrude through the exterior wall of the large intestine.

hemorrhoid A pronounced swelling of a large vein, particularly veins found in the anal region.

diverticulosis The condition of having many diverticula in the large intestine.

diverticulitis An inflammation of the diverticula caused by acids produced by bacterial metabolism inside the diverticula.

Figure 4-9 Diverticula in the Colon. A diet low in fiber increases the risk for their development. The disease is commonly seen in older people in Western societies.

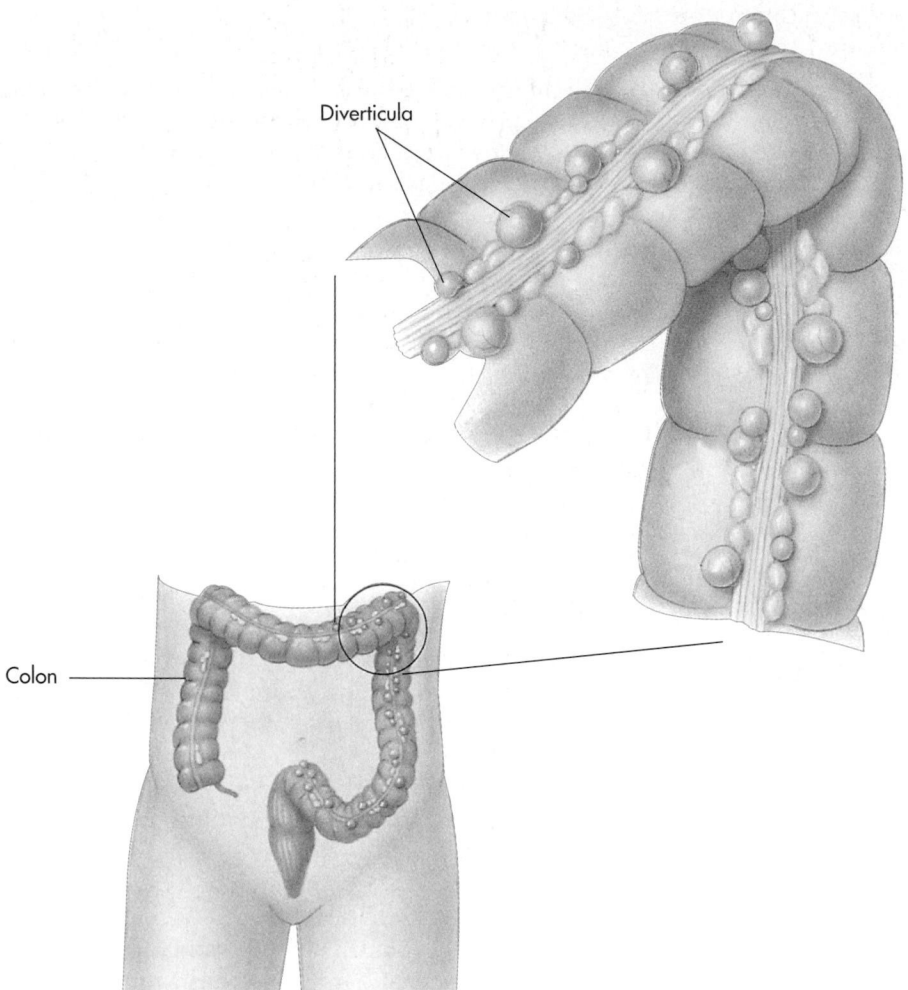

Diverticula

Colon

Recall from Chapter 2 that FDA has approved the following claim: "Diets rich in whole-grain foods and other plant foods and low in total fat, saturated fat, and cholesterol may decrease the risk for cardiovascular (heart) disease and certain cancers."

health benefits to the colon that stem from a high-fiber diet are at least in part due to the nutrients that are commonly part of high-fiber foods, such as vitamins, minerals, phytochemicals, and in some cases essential fatty acids. Thus it is more advisable to increase fiber intake using fiber-rich foods, rather than mostly relying on fiber supplements.

When consumed in large amounts, soluble fibers slow glucose absorption from the small intestine, and so contribute to better blood glucose regulation. This effect can be helpful in the treatment of diabetes. In fact, adults whose main carbohydrate source is low-fiber foods are much more likely to develop diabetes than those who have high-fiber diets.

A high intake of soluble fiber also inhibits absorption of cholesterol and cholesterol-rich bile acids from the small intestine, thereby reducing blood cholesterol and possibly reducing the risk of cardiovascular disease and gallstones. Certain fatty acids resulting from bacterial degradation of soluble fiber probably also reduce cholesterol synthesis in the liver. In addition, the slower glucose absorption that occurs with diets high in soluble fiber is linked to a decrease in insulin release. Since one of the effects of insulin is to stimulate cholesterol synthesis in the liver, this reduction in insulin may contribute to the ability of soluble fiber to lower blood cholesterol. Overall, a fiber-rich diet containing fruits, vegetables, beans, and whole-grain breads and cereals (including whole-grain breakfast cereals) is advocated as part of a strategy to reduce cardiovascular disease (coronary heart disease and stroke) risk. And again, this is something that a low-carbohydrate diet can't promise.

Critical Thinking

Karla has a family history of colon cancer, and at age 20 she is curious about the lifestyle factors she can employ to prevent developing the disease. What advice would you provide her?

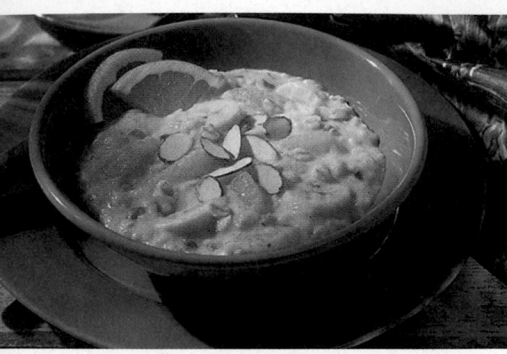

Oatmeal is a rich source of soluble (also called viscous) fiber. FDA allows a health claim for the benefits of oatmeal to lower blood cholesterol that arise from the effects of this soluble fiber.

The 2005 Dietary Guidelines for Americans provide the following advice regarding carbohydrate intake:

- Choose fiber-rich fruits, vegetables, and whole grains often. (In general, at least half of one's intake of grains [3 ounces or more] should come from whole grains.)
- Choose and prepare foods and beverages with little added sugars or caloric sweeteners, such as in amounts suggested by MyPyramid.
- Reduce the incidence of dental caries by practicing good oral hygiene and consuming sugar- and starch-containing foods and beverages less frequently.

Concept Check

Fiber forms a vital part of the diet by adding mass to the stool, which eases elimination. Fiber-rich foods also help in weight control and reduce the risk of developing obesity and cardiovascular disease, and possibly colon cancer. Soluble fiber can also be useful for controlling blood glucose in patients with diabetes and in lowering blood cholesterol. Whole-grain breads and cereals, vegetables, beans, and fruits are excellent sources of fiber.

Carbohydrate Needs

The RDA for carbohydrates is 130 grams per day for adults. This is based on the amount needed to supply adequate glucose for the brain and nervous system, without having to rely on partial replacement of glucose by ketone bodies for such a calorie source. Exceeding this amount somewhat is fine; the Food and Nutrition Board recommends that carbohydrate intake should range from 45% to 65% of total calorie intake. North Americans consume about 180 to 330 grams of carbohydrates per day.

In North America, carbohydrates supply about 50% of calorie intake for adults. Worldwide, however, carbohydrates account for about 70% of all calories consumed. In some countries, carbohydrates account for up to 80% of the calories consumed.

Currently, recommendations for carbohydrate intake vary widely in the scientific literature and popular press. Aside from the low-carbohydrate intakes used to induce ketosis as part of a plan for quick weight loss (note that this diet is not recommended for long-term use; see Chapter 10), recommendations vary from the 45% to 65% of calorie intake by the Food and Nutrition Board to more than 70% in the *Pritikin Program* and *Eat More, Weigh Less* plan. The Nutrition Facts panel on food labels uses 60% of calorie intake as the standard for recommended carbohydrate intake. In addition, one recommendation on which almost all experts agree is that one's carbohydrate intake should be based primarily on fruits, vegetables, whole-grain breads and cereals, and beans, not mostly on refined grains, potatoes, and sugar.

■ How Much Fiber Do We Need?

The Adequate Intake for fiber for adults is 25 grams per day for women and 38 grams per day for men. This is based on a goal of 14 grams per 1000 kcal in a diet. After age 50 the Adequate Intake falls to 21 grams per day and 30 grams per day, respectively. The rationale for the Adequate Intake is the ability of fiber to reduce risk of cardiovascular disease (and likely many cases of diabetes). The Daily Value used for fiber on food and supplement labels is 25 grams for a 2000 kcal diet. In North America, the average whole-grain intake is less than one serving per day. Fiber intake averages 13 grams per day for women and 17 grams per day for men. This low intake is attributed to the lack of knowledge on the benefits of whole grains, as well as the lack of ability to recognize whole-grain products at the time of purchase. Thus, most of us should increase our fiber intake. At least three servings of whole grains per day is recommended. Eating a high-fiber cereal (at least 3 grams of fiber per serving) for breakfast is one easy way to increase fiber intake (Fig. 4-10).

Table 4-5 shows a diet containing 25 or 38 grams of fiber within very moderate calorie intakes. Diets to meet the fiber recommendations are possible and enjoyable if you incorporate plenty of whole-wheat bread, fruits, vegetables, and beans. Use Table 4-6 to estimate the fiber content of your diet. What is *your* fiber score?

Nutrition Facts

Serving Size 1 cup (55g/2.0 oz.)
Servings Per Container 10

Amount Per Serving	Cereal	Cereal with ½ Cup Vitamins A & D Skim Milk
Calories	170	210
Calories from Fat	10	10
	% Daily Value**	
Total Fat 1.0g*	**2%**	**2%**
Sat. Fat 0g	**0%**	**0%**
Trans Fat 0g		*
Cholesterol 0mg	**0%**	**0%**
Sodium 300mg	**13%**	**15%**
Potassium 340mg	**10%**	**16%**
Total Carbohydrate 43g	**14%**	**16%**
Dietary Fiber 7g	**28%**	**28%**
Sugars 16g		
Other Carbohydrate 20g		
Protein 4g		
Vitamin A	15%	20%
Vitamin C	20%	22%
Calcium	2%	15%
Iron	65%	65%
Vitamin D	10%	25%
Thiamin	25%	30%
Riboflavin	25%	35%
Niacin	25%	25%
Vitamin B$_6$	25%	25%
Folic acid	30%	30%
Vitamin B$_{12}$	25%	35%
Phosphorus	20%	30%
Magnesium	20%	25%
Zinc	25%	25%
Copper	10%	10%

*Amount in cereal. One half cup skim milk contributes an additional 40 calories, 65mg sodium, 6g total carbohydrate (6g sugars), and 4g protein.
**Percent Daily Values are based on a 2,000 calorie diet. Your daily values may be higher or lower depending on your calorie needs:

	Calories:	2,000	2,500
Total Fat	Less than	65g	80g
Sat Fat	Less than	20g	25g
Cholesterol	Less than	300mg	300mg
Sodium	Less than	2,400mg	2,400mg
Potassium		3,500mg	3,500mg
Total Carbohydrate		300g	375g
Dietary Fiber		25g	30g

Calories per gram:
Fat 9 • Carbohydrate 4 • Protein 4

*Intake of *trans* fat should be as low as possible.

Ingredients: Wheat bran with other parts of wheat, raisins, sugar, corn syrup, salt, malt flavoring, glycerin, iron, niacinamide, zinc oxide, pyridoxine hydrochloride (vitamin B$_6$), riboflavin (vitamin B$_2$), vitamin A palmitate, thiamin hydrochloride (vitamin B$_1$), folic acid, vitamin B$_{12}$, and vitamin D.

Nutrition Facts

Serving Size: ¾ Cup (30g)
Servings Per Package: About 17

Amount Per Serving	1 Cup Cereal	Cereal With ½ Cup Skim Milk
Calories	170	200
Calories from Fat	0	5
	%Daily Value**	
Total Fat 0g*	**0%**	**1%**
Saturated Fat 0g	**0%**	**1%**
Trans Fat 0g		*
Cholesterol 0mg	**0%**	**1%**
Sodium 60mg	**2%**	**4%**
Potassium 80mg	**2%**	**8%**
Total Carbohydrate 35g	**9%**	**11%**
Dietary Fiber 1g	**4%**	**4%**
Sugars 20g		
Other Carbohydrate 13g		
Protein 3g		
Vitamin A	25%	30%
Vitamin C	0%	2%
Calcium	0%	15%
Iron	10%	10%
Vitamin D	10%	20%
Thiamin	25%	25%
Riboflavin	25%	35%
Niacin	25%	25%
Vitamin B$_6$	25%	25%
Folic acid	25%	25%
Vitamin B$_{12}$	25%	30%
Phosphorus	4%	15%
Magnesium	4%	8%
Zinc	10%	10%
Copper	2%	2%

*Amount in Cereal. One-half cup skim milk contributes an additional 65mg sodium, 6g total carbohydrate (6g sugars), and 4g protein.
**Percent Daily Values are based on a 2,000 calorie diet. Your daily values may be higher or lower depending on your calorie needs:

	Calories:	2,000	2,500
Total Fat	Less than	65g	80g
Sat. Fat	Less than	20g	25g
Cholesterol	Less than	300mg	300mg
Sodium	Less than	2,400mg	2,400mg
Potassium		3,500mg	3,500mg
Total Carbohydrate		300g	375g
Dietary Fiber		25g	30g

Calories per gram:
Fat 9 • Carbohydrate 4 • Protein 4

*Intake of *trans* fat should be as low as possible.

Ingredients: Wheat, Sugar, Corn Syrup, Honey, Caramel Color, Partially Hydrogenated Soybean Oil, Salt, Ferric Phosphate, Niacinamide (Niacin), Zinc Oxide, Vitamin A (Palmitate), Pyridoxine Hydrochloride (Vitamin B6), Riboflavin, Thiamin Mononitrate, Folic Acid (Folate), Vitamin B12 and Vitamin D.

Figure 4-10 Reading the Nutrition Facts on food labels helps us choose more nutritious foods. Based on the information from these nutrition labels, which cereal is the better choice for breakfast? Consider the amount of fiber in each cereal. Did the ingredient lists give you any clues? (Note: Ingredients are always listed in descending order by weight on a label.) When choosing a breakfast cereal, it is generally wise to focus on those that are rich sources of fiber. Sugar content can also be used for evaluation. However, sometimes this number does not reflect added sugar but simply the addition of fruits, such as raisins, complicating the evaluation.

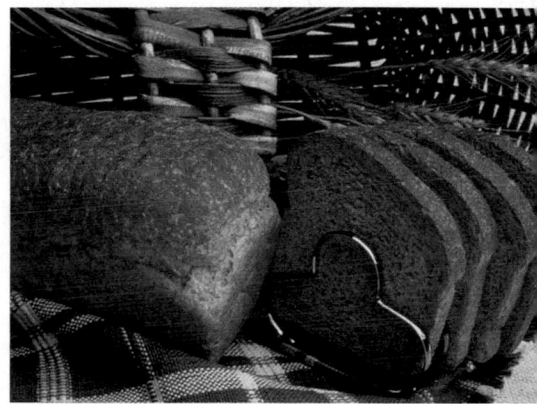

Whole-grain breads are an excellent source of fiber.

Table 4-5 Sample of Menus Containing 1600 kcal and 25 grams of Fiber, and 2000 kcal and 38 grams of Fiber*

Menu	25 grams Fiber			38 grams Fiber		
	Serving Size	Carbohydrate Content (grams)	Fiber Content (grams)	Serving Size	Carbohydrate Content (grams)	Fiber Content (grams)
Breakfast						
Orange juice (with pulp)	1 cup	28	0.5	1 cup	28	0.5
Wheaties	¾ cup	17	2	¾ cup	17	2
2% fat-reduced milk	½ cup	6	—	½ cup	6	—
Whole-wheat toast	1 slice	13	2	1 slice	13	2
Margarine	1 tsp	—	—	1 tsp	—	—
Coffee		1	—		1	—
Lunch						
Lean ham	2 oz	—	—	2 oz	—	—
Whole-wheat bread	2 slices	26	4	2 slices	26	4
Mayonnaise	2 tsp	2	—	2 tsp	2	—
Lettuce	¼ cup	—	0.2	¼ cup	—	0.2
Cooked white beans	⅓ cup	15	4	1 cup	45	12
Pear (with skin)	½	12	2	1	25	4
1% low-fat milk	½ cup	6	—	½ cup	6	—
Snack						
Carrot (as carrot sticks)	1	8	2	1	8	2
Dinner						
Broiled chicken (no skin)	3 oz	—	—	3 oz	—	—
Baked potato (large, with skin)	½	15	1.5	1	30	3
Margarine	1½ tsp	—	—	1½ tsp	—	—
Cooked green beans	1 cup	10	4	1 cup	10	4
Margarine	½ tsp	—	—	½ tsp	—	—
1% low-fat milk	1 cup	12	—	1 cup	12	—
Apple (with peel)	½	16	1.8	1	32	3.7
Snack						
Raisin bagel	1	39	1.2	1	39	1.2
Total		226 grams	25 grams		300 grams	38 grams

*The overall diet pattern is based on the MyPyramid. Breakdown of approximate calorie content: carbohydrate, 55%; protein, 20%; fat, 25%.

Another Bite

Note that manufacturers list enriched white (refined) flour as wheat flour on food labels. Most people think that if "wheat bread" is on the label, they are buying a whole-wheat product. Not so. If the label does not list "whole-wheat flour" first, then the product is not primarily a whole-wheat bread and thus does not contain as much fiber as it could. Careful reading of labels is important in the search for more fiber—look especially for whole grains.

In the final analysis, keep in mind that any nutrient can lead to health problems when consumed in excess. High carbohydrate, high fiber, and low fat does not mean zero calories. Carbohydrates help moderate calorie intake in comparison with fats, but the contribution of high-carbohydrate foods to total calorie intake still has to be accounted for.

Table 4-6 Estimate Your Fiber Intake

To roughly estimate your daily fiber consumption, determine the number of servings that you consumed yesterday from each food category listed below. Multiply the serving amount by the value listed and then add up the total amount of fiber. How does your total fiber intake for yesterday compare with the general recommendation of 25 to 38 grams of fiber per day for women and men, respectively?

Food	Servings	Grams
Vegetables (serving size: 1 cup raw leafy greens or ½ cup other vegetables)	_____ × 2	_____
Fruits (serving size: 1 whole fruit; ½ grapefruit; ½ cup berries or cubed fruit; ¼ cup dried fruit)	_____ × 2.5	_____
Beans, lentils, split peas (serving size: ½ cup cooked)	_____ × 7	_____
Nuts, seeds (serving size: ¼ cup; 2 tbsp peanut butter)	_____ × 2.5	_____
Whole grains (serving size: 1 slice whole-wheat bread; ½ cup whole-wheat pasta, brown rice, or other whole grain; ½ each bran or whole-grain bagel or muffin)	_____ × 2.5	_____
Refined grains (serving size: 1 slice bread, ½ cup pasta, rice, or other processed grains; and ½ each refined bagels or muffins)	_____ × 1	_____
Breakfast cereals (serving size: check package for serving size and amount of fiber per serving)	_____ × grams fiber per serving	_____
Total Grams of Fiber =		_____

Adapted from Fiber: Strands of protection. *Consumer Reports on Health,* p. 1, August 1999.

Health Concerns Related to Carbohydrate Intake

Aside from the health risks related to ketosis, both excessive fiber and sugar intakes can pose health problems. Too much lactose in the diet is also a problem for some people.

Problems with High-Fiber Diets

Very high intakes of fiber—for example, 60 grams per day—can pose some health risks and therefore should be followed only under the guidance of a physician. Increased fluid intake is extremely important with a high-fiber diet. Inadequate fluid intake can leave the stool very hard and painful to eliminate. In more severe cases, the combination of excess fiber and insufficient fluid may contribute to blockages in the intestine, which may require surgery.

Aside from problems with the passage of materials through the GI tract, a high-fiber diet may also decrease the availability of nutrients. Certain components of fiber may bind to essential minerals, keeping them from being absorbed. For example, when fiber is consumed in large amounts, zinc and iron absorption may be hindered. In children, a very high fiber intake may reduce overall calorie intake, since fiber can quickly fill a child's small stomach before food intake meets energy needs.

Problems with High-Sugar Diets

The main problem with consuming an overabundant amount of sugar is that it provides empty calories and increases the risk for dental decay.

There is a widespread notion that high sugar intake by children causes hyperactivity, typically part of the syndrome called *attention deficit hyperactive disorder (ADHD)*. However, most researchers find that sucrose may actually have the opposite effect. A high-carbohydrate meal, if also low in protein and fat, has a calming effect and induces sleep; this effect may be linked to changes in the synthesis of certain neurotransmitters in the brain, such as serotonin. If there is a problem, it is probably the excitement or tension in situations in which high sugar-rich foods are served, such as at birthday parties and on Halloween.

An excess intake of sugared soft drinks has recently been linked to a risk for both weight gain and type 2 diabetes in adults.

dental caries Erosions in the surface of a tooth caused by acids made by bacteria as they metabolize sugars.

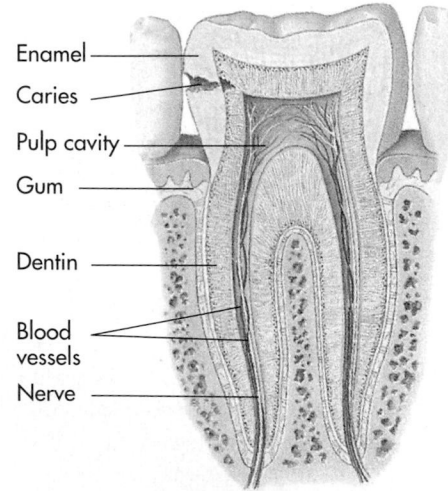

Enamel
Caries
Pulp cavity
Gum
Dentin
Blood vessels
Nerve

Figure 4-11 Dental Caries.
Bacteria can collect in various areas on a tooth. Using simple sugars such as sucrose, bacteria then create acids that can dissolve tooth enamel, leading to caries. If the caries process progresses and enters the pulp cavity, damage to the nerve and resulting pain are likely. The bacteria also produce plaque whereby they adhere to the tooth surface.

Diet Quality Declines When Sugar Intake Is Excessive

Overcrowding the diet with sweet treats can leave little room for important, nutrient-dense foods, such as fruits and vegetables. Children and teenagers are at the highest risk for overconsuming empty calories in place of nutrients that are essential for growth. Many children and teenagers are drinking an excess of sugared soft drinks and other sugar-containing beverages and much less milk than ever before. Milk contains calcium and vitamin D, both of which are essential for bone health; therefore, this exchange of soft drinks for milk can compromise bone health.

Supersizing sugar-rich beverages is also a growing problem; for example, in the 1950s a typical serving size of a soft drink was a 6½ ounce bottle, and now a 20 ounce plastic bottle is a typical serving. This one change in serving size contributes 170 extra kcal of sugars to the diet. Most convenience stores now offer cups that will hold 64 ounces of soft drinks. Filling up on sugared soft drinks in place of foods is not a healthy practice, but enjoying an occasional soft drink or limiting intake to one 12 ounce serving a day is generally fine. Switching to diet soft drinks would spare the simple sugar calories, but still lacks in nutritional value, except for the fluid.

The sugar found in cakes, cookies, and ice cream supplies many extra calories that promote weight gain, unless an individual is physically active. Today's low-fat and fat-free snack products usually contain lots of added sugar to produce a product with an acceptable taste. The result is to produce a high-calorie food that is equal to or greater in calorie content than the high-fat food product it was designed to replace.

With regard to sugar intake, the World Health Organization suggests that sugars added to foods during processing and preparation ("added sugars") should provide no more than about 10% of total daily calorie intake; an upper limit of 25% has been set by the Food and Nutrition Board. Diets that go beyond this upper limit become scarce in more healthy foods.

A moderate intake of about 10% of calorie intake corresponds to a maximum of approximately 50 grams (or 12 tsp) of sugars per day, based on a 2000 kcal diet. Most of the sugars we eat come from foods and beverages to which sugar has been added during processing and/or manufacture. On average, North Americans eat about 82 grams of added sugars daily, amounting to about 16% of calorie intake. Major sources of added sugars include soft drinks, cakes, cookies, fruit punch, and dairy desserts, such as ice cream. Following the recommendation of having no more than 10% of added calories from sugars is easier if sweet desserts such as cakes, cookies, and ice cream (full and reduced fat) are consumed sparingly (Table 4-7).

Dental Caries

Sugars in the diet (and starches that are readily fermented in the mouth, such as crackers and white bread) also increase the risk of developing **dental caries.** Recall that caries, also known as cavities, are formed when sugars and other carbohydrates are metabolized into acids by bacteria that live in the mouth (Fig. 4-11). These acids dissolve the tooth enamel and underlying structure. Bacteria also use the sugars to make plaque, a sticky substance that both adheres acid-producing bacteria to teeth and diminishes the acid-neutralizing effect of saliva.

The worst offenders in terms of promoting dental caries are sticky and gummy foods high in sugars, such as caramel, because they stick to the teeth and supply the bacteria with a long-lived carbohydrate source. Although liquid sugar sources (e.g., fruit juices) are not as potent at causing dental caries as sticky and gummy foods, they still warrant consideration.

Snacking regularly on sugary foods is also likely to cause caries because it gives the bacteria on the teeth a steady source of carbohydrate from which to continually make acid. Sugared gum chewed between meals is a prime example of a poor dental habit. Still, sugar-containing foods are not the only foods that promote acid production by

Table 4-7 Suggestions for Reducing Simple-Sugar Intake

At the Supermarket

- Read ingredient labels. Identify all the added sugars in a product. Select items lower in total sugar when possible.
- Buy fresh fruits or fruits packed in water, juice, or light syrup, rather than those packed in heavy syrup.
- Buy fewer foods that are high in sugar, such as prepared baked goods, candies, sugared cereals, sweet desserts, soft drinks, and fruit-flavored punches. Substitute vanilla wafers, graham crackers, bagels, English muffins, and diet soft drinks, for example.
- Buy reduced fat microwave popcorn to replace candy for snacks.

In the Kitchen

- Reduce the sugar in foods prepared at home. Try new low-sugar recipes or adjust your own. Start by reducing the sugar gradually until you've decreased it by one-third or more. Consider using splenda to substitute for some sugar.
- Experiment with spices such as cinnamon, cardamom, coriander, nutmeg, ginger, and mace to enhance the flavor of foods.
- Use home-prepared items (with less sugar) instead of commercially prepared ones that are higher in sugar.

At the Table

- Use less of all sugars. This includes white and brown sugars, honey, molasses, syrups, jams, and jellies.
- Choose fewer foods high in sugar, such as prepared baked goods, candies, and sweet desserts.
- Reach for fresh fruit instead of cookies or candy for dessert or between-meal snacks.
- Add less sugar to foods—coffee, tea, cereal, and fruit. Get used to using half as much; then see if you can cut back even more.
- Cut back on the number of sugared soft drinks, punches, and fruit juices you drink. Substitute water, diet soft drinks, and whole fruits rather than fruit juice.

Modified from USDA *Home and Garden Bulletin* No. 232-5, 1986.

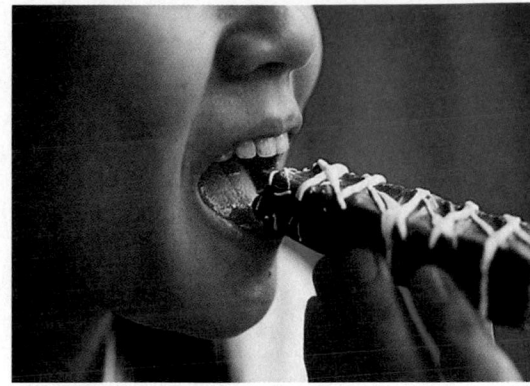

Many foods we enjoy are sweet. These should be eaten in moderation.

bacteria in mouth. As mentioned, if starch-containing foods (e.g., crackers and bread) are held in the mouth for a long time, they can be acted on by enzymes in the mouth that break down the starch to sugars; bacteria can then produce acid from these sugars. Overall, the sugar and starch content of a food and its ability to remain in the mouth largely determine its potential to cause caries.

Fluoridated water and toothpaste have contributed to fewer dental caries in North American children over the past 20 years due to fluoride's tooth-strengthening effect (see Chapter 9). Research has also indicated that certain foods—such as cheese, peanuts, and sugar-free chewing gum—can actually help reduce the amount of acid on teeth. In addition, rinsing the mouth after meals and snacks reduces the acidity in the mouth. Certainly, good nutrition, habits that do not present an overwhelming challenge to oral health (e.g., chewing sugar-free gum), and routine visits to the dentist all contribute to improved dental health.

High Glycemic Index and Glycemic Load Also Deserve Consideration

Our bodies react uniquely to different sources of carbohydrates, such that a serving of a high-fiber food, such as baked beans, results in lower blood glucose levels compared to the same size serving of mashed potatoes. Researchers have developed two tools that are useful in predicting the blood sugar response to various foods and for planning a diet to avoid hyperglycemia.

The first of these tools is **glycemic index (GI)**. Glycemic index is a ratio of the blood glucose response to a given food compared to a standard (typically, glucose

Critical Thinking

John and Mike are identical twins who like the same games, sports, and foods. However, John likes to chew sugar-free gum and Mike doesn't. At their last dental visit, John had no cavities, but Mike had two. Mike wants to know why John, who chews gum after eating, doesn't have cavities and he does. How would you explain this to him?

glycemic index (GI) The blood glucose response of a given food, compared to a standard (typically, glucose or white bread). Glycemic index is influenced by starch structure, fiber content, food processing, physical structure, and macronutrients in the meal, such as fat.

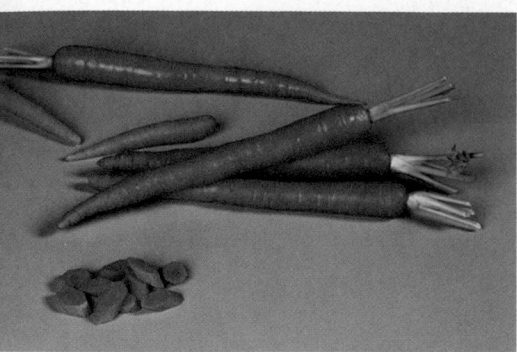

Carrots, criticized in the popular press for having a high glycemic index (which isn't even true), actually contribute a low glycemic load to a diet.

Y ou might wonder why the glycemic index and glycemic load of white bread and whole wheat are similar. This is because whole-wheat flour is typically so finely ground that it is quickly digested. Thus the effect of fiber in slowing diges- tion and related absorption of glucose is no longer present. Some experts suggest we focus more on minimally processed (e.g., coarsely ground, steel cut, or rolled) grains, such as with whole-wheat flour and oatmeal, to get the full benefits of these fiber sources.

Table 4-8 Glycemic Index (GI) and Glycemic Load (GL) of Common Foods

Reference food glucose = 100
Low GI foods—below 55
Intermediate GI foods—between 55 and 70
High GI foods—more than 70

Low GL foods—below 15
Intermediate GL foods—between 15 and 20
High GL foods—more than 20

	Serving Size (grams)	Glycemic Index (GI)	Carbohydrate (grams)	Glycemic Load (GL)
Pastas/Grains				
Brown rice	1 cup	55	46	25
White, long grain	1 cup	56	45	25
White, short grain	1 cup	72	53	38
Spaghetti	1 cup	41	40	16
Vegetables				
Carrots, boiled	1 cup	49	16	8
Sweet corn	1 cup	55	39	21
Potato, baked	1 cup	85	57	48
New (red) potato, boiled	1 cup	62	29	18
Dairy Foods				
Milk, whole	1 cup	27	11	3
Milk, skim	1 cup	32	12	4
Yogurt, low-fat	1 cup	33	17	6
Ice cream	1 cup	61	31	19
Legumes				
Baked beans	1 cup	48	54	26
Kidney beans	1 cup	27	38	10
Lentils	1 cup	30	40	12
Navy beans	1 cup	38	54	21
Sugars				
Honey	1 tsp	73	6	4
Sucrose	1 tsp	65	5	3
Fructose	1 tsp	23	5	1
Lactose	1 tsp	46	5	2
Breads and Muffins				
Bagel	1 small	72	30	22
Whole-wheat bread	1 slice	69	13	9
White bread	1 slice	70	10	7
Croissant	1 small	67	26	17
Fruits				
Apple	1 medium	38	22	8
Banana	1 medium	55	29	16
Grapefruit	1 medium	25	32	8
Orange	1 medium	44	15	7
Beverages				
Apple juice	1 cup	40	29	12
Orange juice	1 cup	46	26	13
Gatorade	1 cup	78	15	12
Coca-Cola	1 cup	63	26	16
Snack Foods				
Potato chips	1 oz	54	15	8
Vanilla wafers	5 cookies	77	15	12
Chocolate	1 oz	49	18	9
Jelly beans	1 oz	80	26	21

Source: Foster-Powell K and others: International table of glycemic index and glycemic load. *American Journal of Clinical Nutrition* 76:5, 2002.

or white bread) (Table 4-8). Glycemic index is influenced by starch structure, fiber content, food processing, physical structure, and other macronutrients in the meal, such as fat. Foods with particularly high glycemic index values are potatoes, especially baking potatoes (due to higher amylopectin content compared to red potatoes), mashed potatoes (due to greater surface area exposed), short grain white rice, honey, and jelly beans. A major shortcoming of glycemic index is that the number is based on a serving of food that would provide 50 grams of carbohydrate. As you can imagine, this amount of food may not reflect the amount typically consumed.

Another way of describing how different foods affect blood glucose (and insulin) levels is **glycemic load (GL).** The glycemic load takes into account the glycemic index and the amount of carbohydrate consumed, and therefore actually better reflects a food's effect on one's blood glucose than either number alone. To calculate the glycemic load of a food, the grams of carbohydrate in a serving of the food are multiplied by the glycemic index of that food, and then divided by 100 (since glycemic index is actually a percentage). For example, vanilla wafers have a glycemic index of 77, and a small serving contains 15 grams of carbohydrate:

$$(77 \times 15) \div 100 = 12$$

Even though the glycemic index of vanilla wafers is considered high, the glycemic load calculation shows that the impact of this food on blood glucose levels is fairly low (review Table 4-8).

Why are we concerned with the effects of various foods on blood glucose? Foods that have a high glycemic load elicit a large release of insulin from the pancreas. Chronically high insulin output leads to many deleterious effects on the body: high blood triglycerides, increased fat deposition in the adipose tissue, increased tendency for blood to clot, increased fat synthesis in the liver, and a more rapid return of hunger after a meal (insulin rapidly lowers the macronutrients in the blood as it stimulates their storage, signaling hunger). Over time, this increase in insulin output may actually cause the muscles to become resistant to the action of insulin, and eventually lead to type 2 diabetes in some people.

There are many ways to address this problem of high glycemic load foods. The most important is to not overeat these foods at any one meal. This greatly minimizes their effects on blood glucose and the related increased insulin release. Consider substituting at least once per meal a food which has a low glycemic load for one with a higher value, such as long grain rice or spaghetti for short grain white rice. Combining a low glycemic load food, such as an apple, kidney beans, milk, or salad with dressing, with a high glycemic load food also reduces the effect on blood glucose. In addition, maintaining a healthy body weight and performing regular physical activity further reduces the effects of a high glycemic load diet.

A focus on low glycemic load carbohydrates can help in the treatment of diabetes; Chapter 11 discusses the use of foods with different glycemic load values in planning diets for athletes.

■ Contributing to the Metabolic Syndrome

Despite the current trend to "demonize" carbohydrates, the only time a carbohydrate-rich diet may not be recommended is when a person's blood triglycerides are high, in turn contributing to the **metabolic syndrome.** (This syndrome will be covered further in Chapter 5.) Note that about 25% of North American adults have this condition. Actually, the chief culprits contributing to high blood triglycerides are not often carbohydrates as a class of nutrients but excessively large meals full of foods both rich in simple sugars and refined starches and low in fiber, coupled with little physical activity. These practices should not form the basis of daily habits, but unfortunately, they do for many adults.

A term you might see on food labels is "net carbs." This has no legal FDA definition as of yet. It is used to describe the content of carbohydrates that increase blood glucose. Fiber and sugar alcohol content are substracted from total carbohydrate content to yield "net carbs," as these have a negligible effect on blood glucose. Still, sugar alcohols and some fibers do yield calories.

glycemic load (GL) The amount of carbohydrate in a food multiplied by the glycemic index of that carbohydrate. The result is then divided by 100.

metabolic syndrome A condition in which the person has poor blood glucose regulation, hypertension, increased blood triglycerides, and other health problems. This condition is usually accompanied by obesity, lack of physical activity, and a diet high in refined carbohydrates. Also called Syndrome X.

lactose maldigestion (primary and secondary) Primary lactose maldigestion occurs when production of the enzyme lactase declines for no apparent reason. Secondary lactose maldigestion occurs when a specific cause, such as long-standing diarrhea, results in a decline in lactase production. When significant symptoms develop after lactose intake, it is then called lactose intolerance.

It is hypothesized that approximately 3000 to 5000 years ago, a genetic mutation occurred in regions that relied on milk and dairy foods as a main food source, allowing those individuals (mostly in northern Europe, pastoral tribes in Africa, and the Middle East) to retain the ability to maintain high lactase output for their entire lifetime. This was not seen in other populations in the world, and so such digestive capability was not retained in those areas of the world.

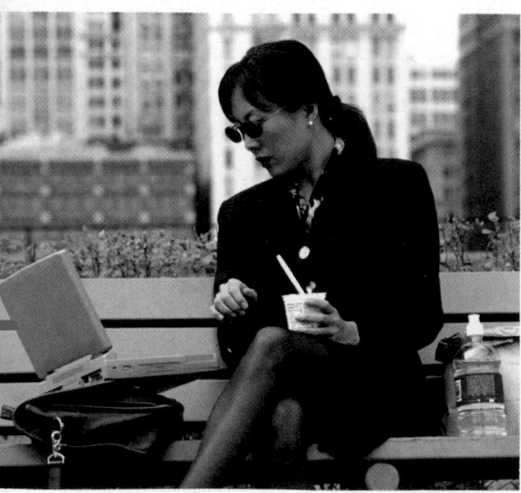

Use of yogurt helps lactose maldigesters meet calcium needs.

■ Moderation in Lactose Intake Is Important for Some People

Lactose maldigestion is a normal pattern of physiology that often begins to develop after early childhood, at about ages 3 to 5 years. It can lead to symptoms of abdominal pain, gas, and diarrhea after consuming lactose, generally when eaten in large amounts. This *primary* form of lactose maldigestion is estimated to be present in about 75% of the world's population, although not all of these individuals experience symptoms. (When significant symptoms develop after lactose intake it is then called lactose intolerance.) Another form of the problem, *secondary* lactose maldigestion, is a temporary condition in which lactase production is decreased in response to an underlying disease, such as intestinal diarrhea. The symptoms of lactose intolerance include gas, abdominal bloating, cramps, and diarrhea. The bloating and gas are caused by bacterial fermentation of lactose in the large intestine. The diarrhea is caused by undigested lactose in the large intestine as it draws water from the circulatory system into the large intestine.

In North America, approximately 25% of adults show signs of decreased lactose digestion in the small intestine. Many lactose maldigesters are Asian Americans, African Americans, and Latio/Hispanic Americans, and the occurrence increases as people age. Still, many of these individuals can consume moderate amounts of lactose with minimal or no gastrointestinal discomfort because of eventual lactose breakdown by bacteria in the large intestine. Thus, it is unnecessary for these people to greatly restrict their intake of lactose-containing foods, such as milk and milk products. These calcium-rich food products are important for maintaining bone health. Obtaining enough calcium and vitamin D from the diet is much easier if milk and milk products are included in a diet.

Recent studies have shown that nearly all individuals with decreased lactase production can tolerate ½ to 1 cup of milk with meals, and that most individuals adapt to intestinal gas production resulting from the fermentation of lactose by bacteria in the large intestine. Combining lactose-containing foods with other foods also helps because certain properties of foods can have positive effects on rates of digestion. For example, fat in a meal slows digestion, leaving more time for lactase action. Hard cheese and yogurt also are more easily tolerated than milk. Much of the lactose is lost in the production of cheese, and the active bacteria cultures in yogurt digest the lactose when these bacteria are broken apart in the small intestine and release their lactase. In addition, an array of products, such as low-lactose milk and lactase pills, are available to assist lactose maldigesters when needed.

Concept Check

The RDA for carbohydrate is 130 grams per day. The typical North American diet provides 180 to 330 grams per day. A reasonable goal is to have about half of our calorie intake coming from starch and our total carbohydrate intake making up about 60% of our calorie intake, with a range of 45% to 65%. This should allow for the recommended intake of 25 to 38 grams of fiber per day for women and men, respectively. High-fiber diets must be accompanied by adequate fluid intakes to avoid constipation and should be followed only under a physician's guidance.

North Americans eat about 82 grams of sugars added to foods each day. Most of these sugars are added to foods and beverages in processing. To reduce consumption of sugars, one must reduce consumption of items with added sugars, such as some baked goods, sweetened beverages, and presweetened ready-to-eat breakfast cereals. This is one practice that can help reduce the development of dental caries and likely improve diet quality and various aspects of health. Lactose maldigestion is a condition that results when cells of the intestine do not make sufficient lactase, the enzyme necessary to digest lactose, resulting in symptoms such as abdominal gas, pain, and diarrhea. Most people with lactose maldigestion can tolerate cheeses and yogurt, as well as moderate amounts of milk. When significant symptoms develop after lactose intake, it is called lactose intolerance.

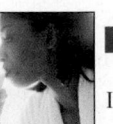

Real Life Scenario Follow-Up

In the Real Life Scenario, Myeshia suspected she was sensitive to milk because, when she consumed it during one meal, she developed bloating and gas. She tried to reproduce these symptoms by eating yogurt, but was not successful. As you just learned, yogurt is tolerated better than milk by people with lactose maldigestion because the bacteria that are present in yogurt digest much of the lactose. Note, however, many people with lactose maldigestion can consume moderate amounts of milk with few or no symptoms from the lactose present.

Summary

1. The common monosaccharides in food are glucose, fructose, and galactose. Once these are absorbed from the small intestine and delivered to the liver, much of the fructose and galactose is converted to glucose.

2. The major disaccharides are sucrose (glucose + fructose), maltose (glucose + glucose), and lactose (glucose + galactose). When digested, these yield their component monosaccharides.

3. One major group of polysaccharides consists of storage forms of glucose: starches in plants and glycogen in humans. These can be broken down by human digestive enzymes, releasing the glucose units. The main plant starches—straight-chain amylose and branched-chain amylopectin—are digested by enzymes in the mouth and small intestine. In humans, glycogen is synthesized in the liver and muscle tissue from glucose. Under the influence of hormones, liver glycogen is readily broken down to glucose, which can enter the bloodstream.

4. Fiber is composed primarily of the polysaccharides cellulose, hemicellulose, pectin, gum, and mucilage, as well as the noncarbohydrate lignins. These substances are not broken down by human digestive enzymes. However, soluble (also called viscous) fiber is fermented by bacteria in the large intestine.

5. Table sugar, honey, jelly, fruit, and plain baked potatoes are some of the most concentrated sources of carbohydrates. Other high-carbohydrate foods, such as pie and fat-free milk, are diluted by either fat or protein. Nutritive sweeteners in food include sucrose, high-fructose corn syrup, brown sugar, and maple syrup.

6. Some starch digestion occurs in the mouth. Carbohydrate digestion is completed in the small intestine. Some plant fibers are digested by the bacteria present in the large intestine; undigested plant fibers become part of the feces. Monosaccharides in the intestinal contents mostly follow an active absorption process. They are then transported via the portal vein that leads directly to the liver.

7. Carbohydrates provide calories (on average, 4 kcal per gram), protect against wasteful breakdown of food and body protein, and prevent ketosis. The RDA for carbohydrate is 130 grams per day. If carbohydrate intake is inadequate for the body's needs, protein is metabolized to provide glucose for energy needs. However, the price is loss of body protein, ketosis, and eventually a general body weakening. For this reason, low-carbohydrate diets are not recommended for extended periods.

8. Diabetes is characterized by a persistent high blood glucose concentration. A healthy diet and regular physical activity is helpful in treating both type 1 and type 2 diabetes. Insulin is the main medication employed—it is required in type 1 diabetes and may be used in type 2 diabetes.

9. Insoluble (also called poorly fermented) fiber provides mass to the feces, thus easing elimination. In high doses, soluble fiber can help control blood glucose in diabetic people and lower blood cholesterol.

10. Diets high in complex carbohydrates are encouraged as a replacement for high-fat diets. A goal of about half of calories as complex carbohydrates is a good one, with about 45% to 65% of total calories coming from carbohydrates in general. Foods to consume are whole-grain cereal products, pasta, legumes, fruits, and vegetables. Many of these foods are rich in fiber.

11. Moderating sugar intake, especially between meals, reduces the risk of dental caries. Alternative sweeteners, such as aspartame, aid in reducing intake of sugars.

12. The ability to digest large amounts of lactose often diminishes with age. People in some ethnic groups are especially affected. This condition often develops early in childhood and is referred to as *lactose maldigestion*. Undigested lactose travels to the large intestine, resulting in such symptoms as abdominal gas, pain, and diarrhea. Most people with lactose maldigestion can tolerate cheese, yogurt, and moderate amounts of milk.

Study Questions

1. Outline the basic steps in blood glucose regulation, including the roles of insulin and glucagon.

2. What are the three major monosaccharides and the three major disaccharides? Describe how each plays a part in the human diet.

3. Why are some foods that are high in carbohydrates, such as cookies and fat-free milk, not considered to be concentrated sources of carbohydrates?

4. Describe the digestion of the various types of carbohydrates in the body.

5. Describe the reason why some people are unable to tolerate high intakes of milk.

6. What are the important roles that fiber plays in the diet?

7. What, if any, are the proven ill effects of sugar in the diet?

8. Why do we need carbohydrates in the diet?

9. Summarize current carbohydrate intake recommendations.

10. List three alternatives to simple sugars for adding sweetness to the diet.

Further Readings

1. ADA Reports: Position of the American Dietetic Association: Health implications of dietary fiber. *Journal of the American Dietetic Association* 102:993, 2002.

   It is preferable that fiber be obtained from foods as opposed to fiber supplements. This paper discusses the possible health benefits of fiber, as well as some of the potential negative effects of excessive fiber intake.

2. ADA Reports: Position of the American Dietetic Association: Use of nutritive and nonnutritive sweeteners. *Journal of the American Dietetic Association* 104:225, 2004.

   When currently recommended diet practices are met, such as the Dietary Guidelines for Americans, use of some nutritive and nonnutritive sweeteners is acceptable. The text of the article explores in detail both classes of sweeteners, in turn supporting this overall conclusion.

3. American Diabetes Association: Standards of care in diabetes. *Diabetes Care* 28:S36, 2005.

   This article provides a comprehensive look at the treatment of diabetes. Goals for therapy and medical tools to help reach those goals are highlighted.

4. Aderson JW and others: Carbohydrate and fiber recommendations for individuals with diabetes. *Journal of the American College of Nutrition* 23(1):5, 2004.

   The carbohydrate : protein : fat calorie ratio in a diabetic diet should be 55% or more : 12% to 15% : less than 30%. The diet should provide 25–50 grams of fiber per day, and low glycemic load foods should form the bulk of daily food choices.

5. Bingham SA and others: Dietary fibre in food and protection against colorectal cancer in the European Prospective Investigation into Cancer and Nutrition (EPIC): An observational study. *The Lancet* 361:1496, 2003.

   A diet rich in high-fiber foods is associated with a 40% reduction in colorectal cancer risk—especially in the colon—compared to a diet low in fiber. It is not known if fiber per se, or something in the high-fiber foods (e.g., phytochemicals), is the reason for the effect. Thus, one's focus should be on a diet rich in high-fiber foods, not fiber supplements.

6. Brand-Miller J: Glycemic load and chronic disease. *Nutrition Reviews* 61(5):S49, 2003.

   A diet rich in high glycemic load carbohydrates increases the risk of developing cardiovascular disease and type 2 diabetes. Such a diet may also contribute to obesity, colon cancer, and breast cancer. Following a diet rich in low glycemic load carbohydrates is on the other hand beneficial in these regards, especially if one is sedentary or obese.

7. Diabetes. *Mayo Clinic Health Letter* (Suppl.) February 2004.

   Excellent summary of diabetes—from causes to treatments. Weight control, a healthy diet, and regular exercise are an important part of the latter.

8. Diverticular disease : The importance of getting enough fiber. *Mayo Clinic Health Letter* 23(2): 1, 2005.

   Meeting one's fiber needs is very important for preventing diverticular disease. To do so, eat plenty of fruits, vegetables, and whole grain products. Regular physical activity also helps prevent the problem.

9. Deen D: Metabolic syndrome: Time for action. *American Family Physician* 69(12):2875, 2004.

   The metabolic syndrome leads to many deleterious effects on the body. Weight control and regular physical activity are key parts of a plan for the prevention and treatment of the metabolic syndrome.

10. Food and Nutrition Board: *Dietary reference intakes for energy, carbohydrate, fiber, fat, fatty acids, cholesterol, protein, and amino acids.* Washington, DC: National Academy Press, 2002.

    This report provides the latest guidance for macronutrient intakes. With regard to carbohydrate, the RDA has been set at 130 grams per day. Carbohydrate intake should range from 45 to 65% of calorie intake. Sugars added to foods should constitute no more than 25% of calorie intake.

11. Hu G and others: Physical activity, body mass index, and risk of type 2 diabetes in patients with normal or impaired glucose regulation. *Archives of Internal Medicine* 164(8):892, 2004.

    Increasing physical activity can reduce the risk of developing type 2 diabetes. Weight control is also important; this weight control advice includes people who already have poor glucose control and are overweight.

12. Klein S and others: Weight management through lifestyle modification for the prevention and management of type 2 diabetes. *American Journal of Clinical Nutrition* 80:257, 2004.

    Overweight and obesity are important causes of type 2 diabetes. Moderate weight loss and increased physical activity can both forestall and improve poor blood glucose regulation.

13. Montonen J and others: Whole-grain and fiber intake and the incidence of type 2 diabetes. *American Journal of Clinical Nutrition* 77:622, 2003.

    Regular intake of whole-grain foods reduces the risk of developing type 2 diabetes. The effect was especially linked to the cereal fiber portion of a diet. Other components in foods rich in cereal fiber, such as certain phytochemicals, may also be part of the protective effect.

14. Schulze MB and others: Glycemic index, glycemic load, and dietary fiber intake and incidence of type 2 diabetes in younger and middle-aged women. *American Journal of Clinical Nutrition* 80:348, 2004.

    A diet rich in rapidly-absorbed carbohydrates and low in cereal fiber is associated with an increased risk of developing type 2 diabetes. Thus the types of carbohydrates chosen for a diet are important to consider.

15. Swagerty D and others: Lactose intolerance. *American Family Physician* 65:1845, 2002.

    Lactose maldigestion and intolerance result from a deficiency in the lactose-digesting enzyme, lactase. This is present in up to 15% of Northern Europeans, 22% of American Whites, 70% of Indians, 80% of Blacks and Hispanics, and 100% of Native Americans and Asians. Most individuals with lactose maldigestion and intolerance can consume small amounts of dairy products without experiencing symptoms, and yogurts with live cultures tend to be especially well tolerated.

16. Sweeteners can sour your health. *Consumer Reports on Health* p.8, January 2005.

    Limiting simple sugars in a diet is important in order to lessen the risk of developing obesity, diabetes, and dental caries, as well as increasing diet quality. Moderate use of the alternative sweeteners listed in the article helps one meet that goal.

17. The whole grain story. *Tufts University Health & Nutrition Letter* p.4 July 2005.

    Regular whole grain consumption may help prevent cardiovascular disease, unnecessary weight gain, and the metabolic syndrome. This is easier to do so today because many whole grain products are now available.

18. Wang Y and others: Comparison of abdominal adiposity and overall obesity in predicting risk of type 2 diabetes in men. *American Journal of Clinical Nutrition* 81:555, 2005.

    Obesity and excess upper body fat stores are both risk factors for developing type 2 diabetes. Avoiding both conditions is important, especially excess upper body fat distribution.

19. Warshaw HS: FAQs about polyols. *Today's Dietitian* p.37 April 2004.

    Polyols (ie sugar alcohols) yields from 0.2–3.0 kcal per gram, so still need to be considered when calculating the calorie content of a diet. A major attribute of these products is that they do not increase the risk for dental caries.

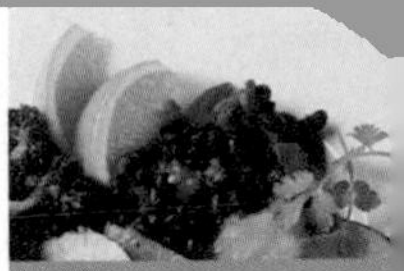

I. How Does Your Diet Rate for Carbohydrate and Fiber?

Let's reevaluate the nutritional assessment you completed at the end of Chapter 2. Here are your tasks:

1. Look at your analysis (NutritionCalc Plus Bar Graph report) and find the total number of grams of carbohydrate you ate.

   TOTAL GRAMS OF CARBOHYDRATE _____

   A. Did you consume at least the RDA of 130 grams? Yes _____ No _____
   B. Now calculate the percentage of calories in your diet from carbohydrate. You will need the total grams of carbohydrate from your assessment, as well as the total kcals you ate. Use this formula to calculate it:

   $$\frac{\text{Total grams of carbohydrate} \times 4}{\text{Total kcals consumed}} \times 100 = \% \text{ of calorie intake from carbohydrate}$$

   ANSWER: _____

   Was about 60% of your total calorie intake from carbohydrate? Yes _____ No _____

   If not, list several ways you could increase your carbohydrate intake.

   _____

   _____

   _____

2. Look again at the list of foods you ate, including the amounts, and determine the total amount of fiber you consumed. Refer to either the Bar Graph or Single Nutrient (dietary fiber) report from your NutritionCalc Plus analysis to determine your fiber intake. Otherwise, look up the fiber content of each food you ate in the food composition table in Appendix J; then calculate your total intake, taking into account the amount of each food you ate.

   TOTAL AMOUNT OF FIBER CONSUMED _____ grams

   A. Did you consume the 25 to 38 grams suggested for women and men, respectively, in this chapter? Yes _____ No _____
   B. If not, what could you do to increase your fiber intake? What foods could you substitute for some of the foods you ate?

   _____

   _____

   _____

3. Finally, use Table 4-7 as a guide if you need to reduce your intake of added sugars, especially if you need to watch your total calorie intake to maintain an appropriate weight. What three foods might you limit in the future?

   _____

   _____

   _____

II. Can You Choose the Sandwich with the Most Fiber?

Assume the sandwiches on the blackboard below are available at your local deli and sandwich shop. All of the sandwiches provide about 350 kcal. The fiber content ranges from about 1 gram to about 7.5 grams. Rank the sandwiches from highest amount of fiber to lowest amount; then check your answers at the bottom of the page.

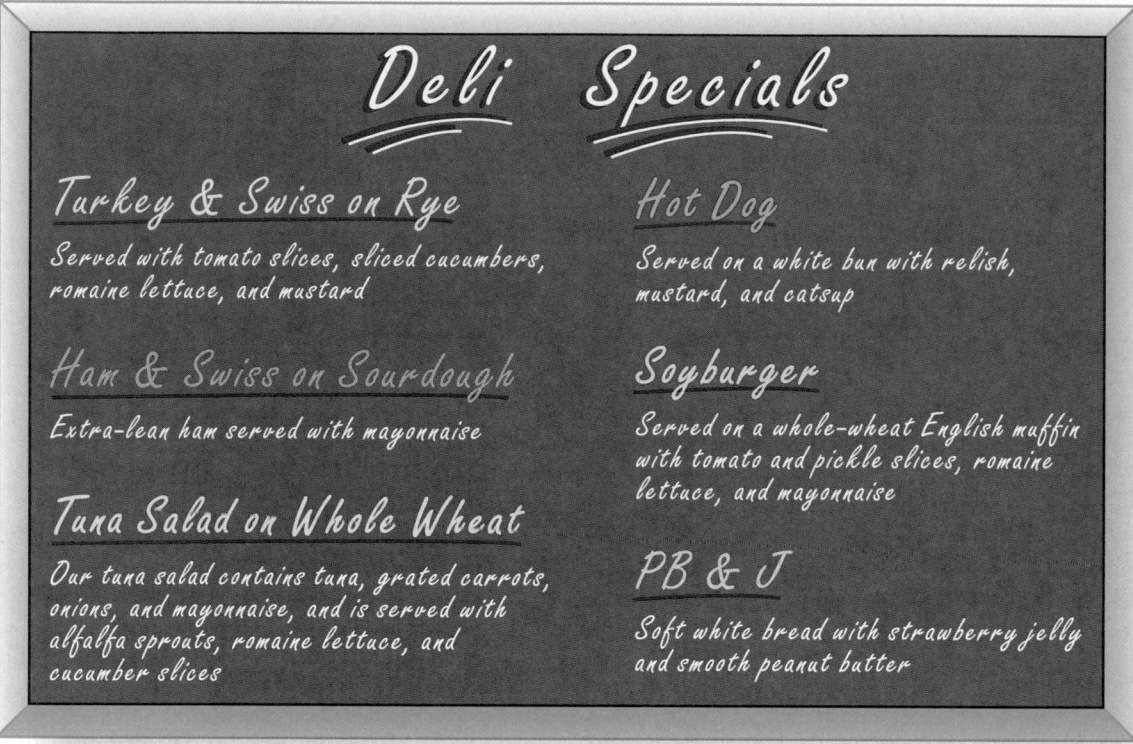

Deli Specials

Turkey & Swiss on Rye

Served with tomato slices, sliced cucumbers, romaine lettuce, and mustard

Ham & Swiss on Sourdough

Extra-lean ham served with mayonnaise

Tuna Salad on Whole Wheat

Our tuna salad contains tuna, grated carrots, onions, and mayonnaise, and is served with alfalfa sprouts, romaine lettuce, and cucumber slices

Hot Dog

Served on a white bun with relish, mustard, and catsup

Soyburger

Served on a whole-wheat English muffin with tomato and pickle slices, romaine lettuce, and mayonnaise

PB & J

Soft white bread with strawberry jelly and smooth peanut butter

Answer Key:
1. Soyburger: 7.5 grams, 2. Tuna Salad on Whole Wheat: 7 grams, 3. Turkey & Swiss on Rye: 4 grams, 4. PB&J: 3 grams, 5. Ham & Swiss on Sourdough: 1.5 grams, 6. Hot Dog: 1 gram.

Lipids

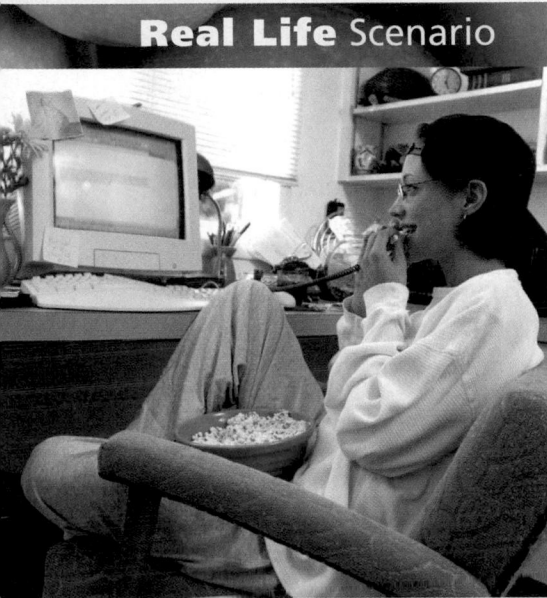

Jackie is a 21-year-old health-conscious individual majoring in business. She recently learned that a diet high in saturated fat can contribute to high blood cholesterol and that exercise is beneficial for the heart. Jackie now takes a brisk 30-minute walk each morning before going to class, and she has started to cut as much fat out of her diet as she can, replacing it mostly with carbohydrates. A typical day for Jackie now begins with a bowl of Fruity Pebbles with 1 cup of skim milk and ½ cup of apple juice. For lunch, she might pack a turkey sandwich on white bread with lettuce, tomato, and mustard; a small package of fat-free pretzels; and a handful of reduced-fat vanilla wafers. Dinner could be a large portion of pasta with some olive oil and garlic mixed in, and a small iceberg lettuce salad with lemon juice squeezed over it. Her snacks are usually baked chips, low-fat cookies, fat-free frozen yogurt, or fat-free pretzels. She drinks diet soft drinks throughout the day as her main beverage.

Do you think this is a healthy way for Jackie to reduce fat in her diet? Point out some positive practices. What would you suggest changing in her diet to make it more heart healthy?

Chapter 5 Objectives

Chapter 5 is designed to allow you to:

1. List four classes of lipids (fats) and the role of each in nutritional health.
2. Distinguish between fatty acids and triglycerides.
3. Differentiate among saturated, monounsaturated, and polyunsaturated fatty acids in terms of structure and food sources.
4. Name the two essential fatty acids and explain why they are called "essential."
5. Name the classes of lipoproteins and classify them according to their functions.
6. Characterize the symptoms of cardiovascular disease and highlight some known risk factors.
7. Discuss the implications of various fats, including omega-3 fatty acids, with respect to cardiovascular disease.

Check out the **Contemporary Nutrition Online Learning Center**
www.mhhe.com/wardlawcont6 *for quizzes, flash cards, other activities, and web links designed to further help you learn about dietary lipids.*

Your bill from a medical laboratory reads "Blood lipid profile—$55." Your doctor informs you that your "triglycerides are too high." A health-food advertisement suggests using Benecol margarine to lower blood cholesterol. Advertisers plug foods "lowest in saturated fat." All of these substances—triglycerides, saturated fat, and cholesterol—are lipids, a collective term referring to fats and oils.

Lipids contain more than twice the calories per gram (on average, 9 kcal) as proteins and carbohydrates (on average, 4 kcal each). Consumption of common saturated fatty acids also contributes to the risk of cardiovascular disease. For these reasons, some concern about certain lipids is warranted, but lipids also play vital roles both in the body and in foods. Their presence in the diet is essential to good health, and in general, lipids such as those found in vegetable oils should comprise 20% to 35% of an adult's total calorie intake.

Let's look at lipids in detail—their forms, functions, metabolism, and food sources. Chapter 5 will also look at the link between various lipids and the major "killer" disease in North America: cardiovascular disease, which involves the heart, including the coronary arteries (coronary heart disease), as well as other arteries in the body.

Refresh Your Memory

As you begin your study of lipids in Chapter 5, you may want to review:

- Legal definitions for various labeled descriptors, such as low-fat and fat-free in Chapter 2
- The concept of energy density in Chapter 2
- The processes of digestion and absorption in Chapter 3
- The glycemic load of foods in Chapter 4

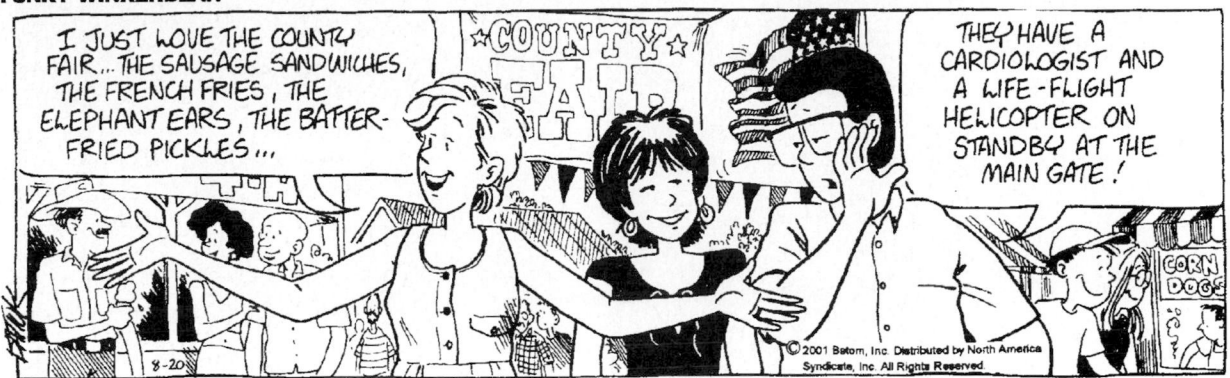

High fat, low fat, no fat—which is best? And why is there such a debate? Would it be easier just to avoid fat altogether? Doesn't a high-fat diet lead to obesity? To cardio-vascular disease? Overall, which are the "best" fats, and why are French fries, dough-nuts, stick margarine, and crackers getting such a bad rap? Chapter 5 provides some answers.

Lipids: Common Properties and Main Types

Humans need very little fat in their diet to maintain health. In fact, daily consumption of 2 to 4 tablespoons or so of plant oil incorporated into foods and at least twice weekly consumption of fatty fish such as salmon or tuna meet the body's need for the essential fatty acids. If fish is not consumed, the essential fatty acids in canola oil, soybean oil, and walnuts contribute much of the same health benefit as those found in fish. Thus, one could follow a purely vegetarian diet containing about 10% of calories from fat and still maintain health. However, as long as saturated fat, cholesterol, and partially-hydrogenated fat (typically called *trans* fat) is minimized, fat intake can safely be higher than that 10% allotment. The Food and Nutrition Board suggests that fat intake can be as high as 35% of calories consumed, for an adult. Some experts suggest that an intake as high as 40% of calories is appropriate. After learning more about lipids—fats, oils, and related compounds—in Chapter 5, you can decide for yourself how much fat you want to consume, as well as how to track your daily intake.

Lipids are a diverse group of chemical compounds. They share one main characteristic: They do not readily dissolve in water. Think of an oil and vinegar salad dressing. The oil is not soluble in the water-based vinegar; on standing, the two separate into distinct layers, with oil on top and vinegar on the bottom.

The diversity of lipids is evident when you compare the structures of two common examples: a **triglyceride** versus **cholesterol**, shown in Figure 5-1a. Triglycerides are the most common type of lipid found in the body and in foods. Each triglyceride molecule consists of three fatty acids bonded to **glycerol**. **Phospholipids** (Fig. 5-1b) and **sterols** (Fig. 5-1c) are also classified as lipids, although their structures can be quite different from the structure of triglycerides. All of these lipid compounds are described in Chapter 5.

As noted in Chapter 1, lipids that are solid at room temperature are called *fats*, and lipids that are liquid are called *oils*. Most people use the word *fat* to refer to all lipids because they don't realize there is a difference. As already covered, however, *lipid* is a generic term that includes triglycerides and many other substances. To simplify our discussion, Chapter 5 primarily uses the term *fat*; however, as you will see later, not all the substances we call fats truly are fats. When necessary for clarity, the name of a

triglyceride The major form of lipid in the body and in food. It is composed of three fatty acids bonded to glycerol, an alcohol.

cholesterol A waxy lipid found in all body cells. It has a structure containing multiple chemical rings that is found only in foods that contain animal products.

glycerol A three-carbon alcohol used to form triglycerides.

phospholipid Any of a class of fat-related substances that contain phosphorus, fatty acids, and a nitrogen-containing base. The phospholipids are an essential part of every cell.

sterol A compound containing a multi-ring (steroid) structure and a hydroxyl group (–OH). Cholesterol is a typical example.

Figure 5-1 Chemical forms of common lipids: (a) triglyceride, (b) phospholipid (in this case, lecithin), and (c) sterol (in this case, cholesterol).

Triglyceride

(a)

Lecithin—A Phospholipid

(b)

Cholesterol—A Sterol

(c)

specific lipid, such as cholesterol, will be used. This word usage is consistent with the way many people use these terms.

■ Fatty Acids: The Simplest Form of Lipids

Fatty acids are found in the lipids that exist in the body and in foods. A fatty acid is basically a long chain of carbons bonded together and flanked by hydrogens. At one end of the molecule (the alpha end), is an acid group. At the other end (the omega end), is a methyl group (Fig. 5-2).

Fats in foods are not composed of a single type of fatty acid. Rather, each dietary fat is a complex mixture of many different fatty acids, the combination of which provides each food its unique taste and smell.

Recall from Chapter 1 that fatty acids can be saturated or unsaturated. Chemically speaking, a carbon atom can form four bonds. Within the carbon skeleton of a fatty acid, the carbons bond to other carbons and to hydrogens. The carbons that make up the skeleton of a **saturated fatty acid** are all connected by single bonds. This allows for a maximum number of bonds to hydrogens. Just as a sponge can be saturated (full) with water, a saturated fatty acid such as stearic acid is saturated with hydrogen (Fig. 5-2a).

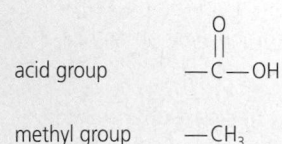

acid group

methyl group   —CH₃

saturated fatty acid A fatty acid containing no carbon-carbon double bonds.

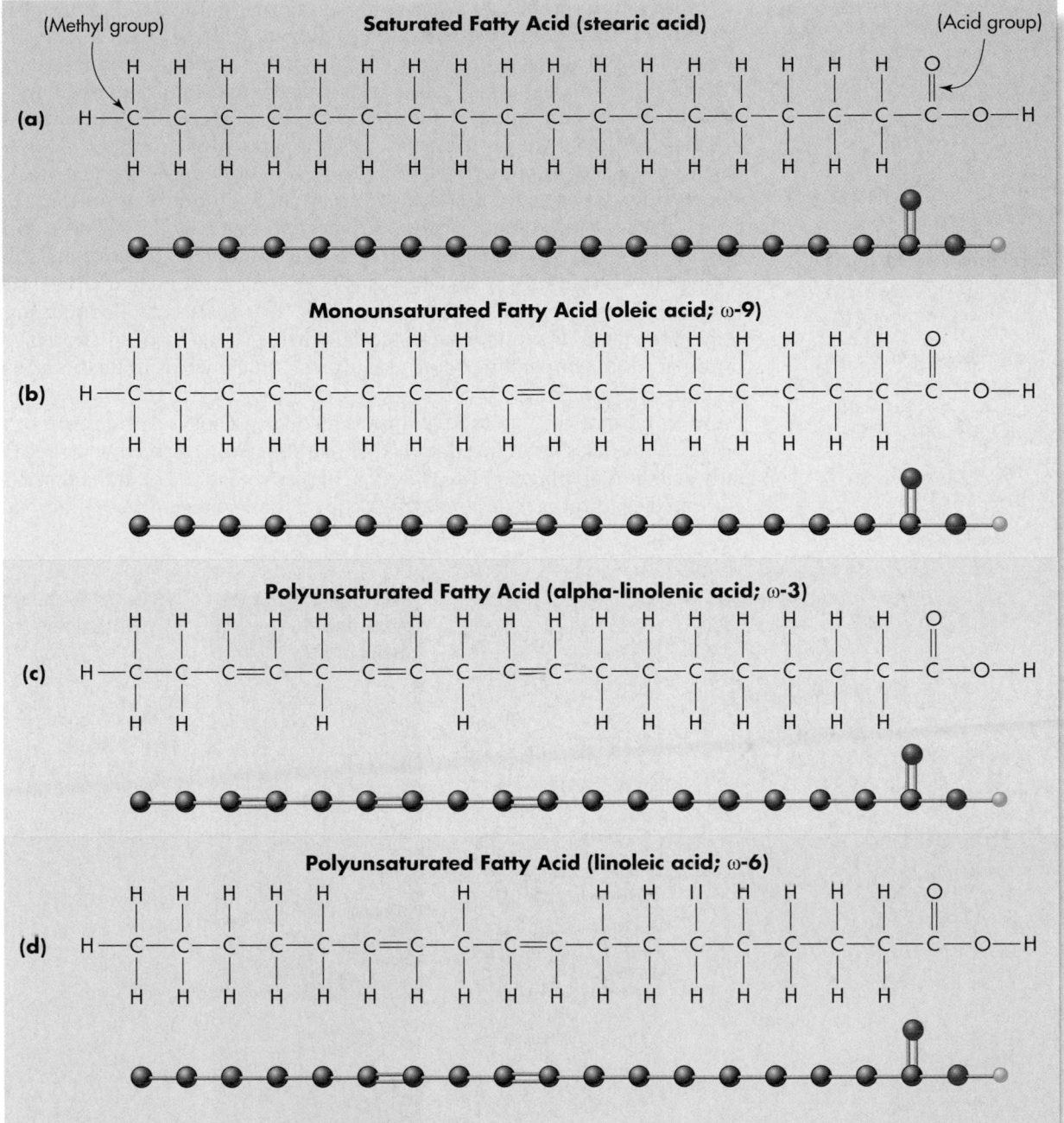

Figure 5-2 Chemical forms of saturated, monounsaturated, and polyunsaturated fatty acids. Each of the depicted fatty acids contains 18 carbons, but they differ from each other in the number and location of double bonds. The linear shape of saturated fatty acids, as shown in (a), allows them to pack tightly together and so form a solid at room temperature. In contrast, unsaturated fatty acids have "kinks" where double bonds interrupt the carbon chain (see Fig. 5-4). Thus, unsaturated fatty acids pack together only loosely, and are usually liquid at room temperature. Note that in the simplified structure shown for each fatty acid, the black balls represent carbon atoms (with the maximum number of hydrogen atoms attached), while the red balls represent oxygen and the blue balls hydrogen.

As noted earlier, most fats high in saturated fatty acids, such as animal fats, remain solid at room temperature. A good example is the solid fat surrounding a piece of uncooked steak. Chicken fat, semisolid at room temperature, contains less saturated fat than beef fat. Note, however, that in some foods, such as whole milk, saturated fats are suspended in liquid, so the solid nature of these fats at room temperature is less apparent.

monounsaturated fatty acid A fatty acid containing one carbon-carbon double bond.

polyunsaturated fatty acid A fatty acid containing two or more carbon-carbon double bonds.

long-chain fatty acid A fatty acid that contains 12 or more carbons.

omega-3 (ω-3) fatty acid An unsaturated fatty acid with the first double bond on the third carbon from the methyl end (—CH₃).

omega-6 (ω-6) fatty acid An unsaturated fatty acid with the first double bond on the sixth carbon from the methyl end (—CH₃).

If the carbon skeleton of a fatty acid contains a double bond, those carbons in the chain have fewer bonds to share with hydrogen, and the chain is said to be *unsaturated*. A fatty acid with only one double bond is **monounsaturated** (Fig. 5-2b). Canola and olive oils contain a high percentage of monounsaturated fatty acids. Likewise, if two or more bonds between the carbons are double bonds, the fatty acid is even less saturated with hydrogens, and so it is **polyunsaturated** (Fig. 5-2c,d). Corn, soybean, sunflower, and safflower oils are rich in polyunsaturated fatty acids.

Overall, a fat or an oil is classified as saturated, monounsaturated, or polyunsaturated based on the nature of the fatty acids present in the greatest concentration (Fig. 5-3). Fats in foods that contain primarily saturated fatty acids are solid at room temperature, especially if the fatty acids have long carbon chains (i.e., a **long-chain fatty acid**), as opposed to shorter versions. In contrast, fats containing primarily polyunsaturated or monounsaturated fatty acids (long chain or shorter) are usually liquid at room temperature. Note that almost all fatty acids in the body and in foods are long-chain varieties.

An important characteristic of unsaturated fatty acids is the location of the double bonds. If the first double bond starts three carbons from the methyl (omega) end of the fatty acid, it is an **omega-3 (ω-3) fatty acid** (review Fig. 5-2c). If the first double bond is located six carbons from the omega end, it is an **omega-6 (ω-6) fatty acid** (review

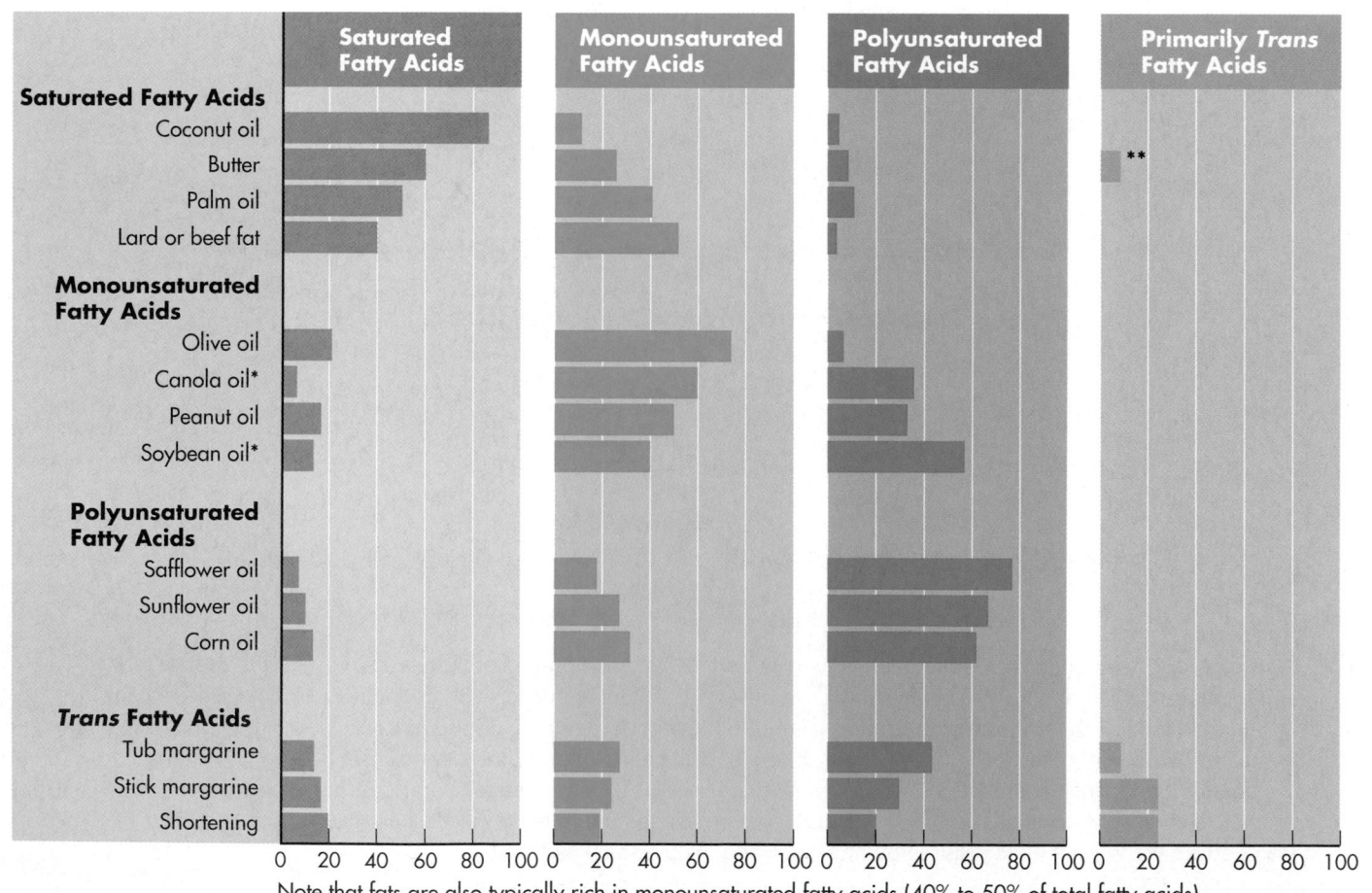

Note that fats are also typically rich in monounsaturated fatty acids (40% to 50% of total fatty acids).
*Rich source of the omega-3 fatty acid alpha-linolenic acid (7% and 12% of total fatty acid for soybean oil and canola oil, respectively).
**The natural *trans* fatty acids in butter are not harmful, and may even have health-promoting properties, such as preventing certain forms of cancer.

Figure 5-3 Saturated, monounsaturated, polyunsaturated, and *trans* fatty acid composition of common fats and oils (expressed as % of all fatty acids in the product).

Fig. 5-2d). Following this scheme, an omega-9 fatty acid has its first double bond starting at the ninth carbon from the methyl end (review Fig. 5-2b). In foods, **alpha-linolenic acid** is the major omega-3 fatty acid; **linoleic acid** is the major omega-6 fatty acid. These are also the **essential fatty acids** we need to consume (more on this in the later section on putting lipids to work in the body). **Oleic acid** is the major omega-9 fatty acid.

Another Bite

The form of fatty acids known as *trans* fatty acids was briefly described in Chapter 1. In their natural form, monounsaturated and polyunsaturated fatty acids usually are in the *cis* form (Fig. 5-4). By definition, the resulting *cis* fatty acid has the hydrogens on the same side of the carbon-carbon double bond. During certain types of food processing (discussed later in this chapter), some hydrogens are transferred to opposite sides of the carbon-carbon double bond, creating the *trans* form, or a *trans* fatty acid. As seen in Figure 5-4, the *cis* bond causes the fatty acid backbone to bend, whereas the *trans* bond allows the backbone to remain straighter. This makes it similar to the shape of a saturated fatty acid. The Food and Nutrition Board suggests limiting intake of *trans* fatty acids in processed foods (also referred to as *trans* fats) as much as possible. Later you will see why.

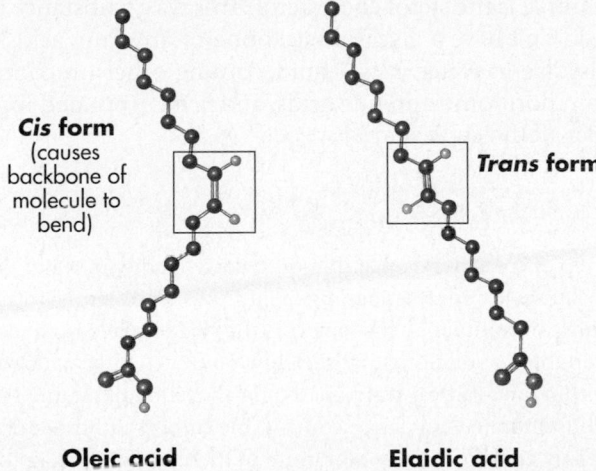

Figure 5-4 *Cis* and *trans* fatty acids. In the *cis* form at carbon-carbon double bonds in a fatty acid, the hydrogens (in blue) lie on the same side of the double bond. This causes a "kink" at that point in the fatty acid, which is typical of unsaturated fatty acids in nature. In contrast, in the *trans* form at carbon-carbon double bonds in a fatty acid, the hydrogens lie across from each other at the double bond. This causes the fatty acid to exist in a linear form, like a saturated fatty acid. *Cis* fatty acids are much more common in foods than *trans* fatty acids. The latter are primarily found in foods containing partially-hydrogenated fats, notably stick margarine, shortening, and deep-fat fried foods.

■ Triglycerides

Fats and oils in foods are mostly in the form of triglycerides. The same is true for fats found in body structures. Some fatty acids are transported in the bloodstream attached to proteins. However, most fatty acids do not exist in the body as such. Instead, they are formed into triglycerides by cells in the body.

As noted before, triglycerides contain a simple three-carbon alcohol, glycerol, which serves as a backbone for the three attached fatty acids (review Fig. 5-1). Removing one fatty acid from a triglyceride forms a **diglyceride.** Removing two fatty acids from a triglyceride forms a **monoglyceride.** Later you will see that before most

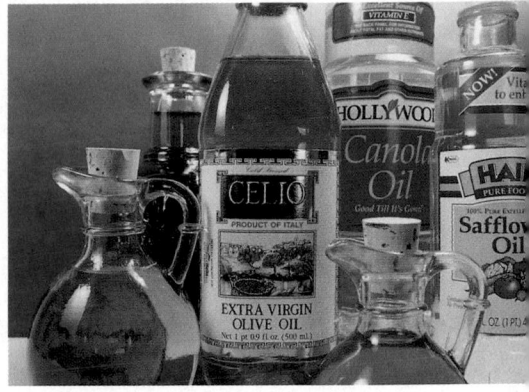

Plant oils vary in their content of specific fatty acids. Oils that are similar in appearance may vary significantly in fatty acid composition. Olive and canola oils are rich in monounsaturated fat; olive oil has been awarded much attention in recent years. Canola oil, however, is a much less expensive choice of mono-unsaturated fat. Safflower oil is rich in polyunsaturated fat.

alpha-linolenic acid An essential omega-3 fatty acid with 18 carbons and three double bonds.

linoleic acid An essential omega-6 fatty acid with 18 carbons and two double bonds.

essential fatty acids Fatty acids that must be supplied by the diet to maintain health. Currently, only linoleic acid and alpha-linolenic acid are classified as essential.

oleic acid An omega-9 fatty acid with 18 carbons and one double bond.

cis fatty acid A form of an unsaturated fatty acid that has the hydrogens lying on the same side of the carbon-carbon double bond.

trans fatty acid A form of an unsaturated fatty acid, usually a monounsaturated one when found in food, in which the hydrogens on both carbons forming the double bond lie on opposite sides of that bond.

diglyceride A breakdown product of a triglyceride consisting of two fatty acids bonded to a glycerol backbone.

monoglyceride A breakdown product of a triglyceride consisting of one fatty acid attached to a glycerol backbone.

dietary fats are absorbed in the small intestine, the two outer fatty acids are typically removed from the triglyceride. This produces a mixture of fatty acids and monoglycerides, which are absorbed into the intestinal cells. After absorption the fatty acids and monoglycerides are mostly re-formed into triglycerides.

■ Phospholipids

Phospholipids are another class of lipid. Like triglycerides, they are built on a backbone of glycerol. However, at least one fatty acid is replaced with a compound containing phosphorus (and often other elements, such as nitrogen) (review Fig. 5-1b). Many types of phospholipids exist in the body, especially in the brain. They form important parts of cell membranes. **Lecithin** is a common example of a phospholipid. Various forms are found in body cells and they participate in fat digestion in the small intestine. The body is able to produce all the phospholipids it needs. Even though lecithin is sold as a dietary supplement and is present as an additive in many foods, phospholipids such as this one are not essential components of the diet.

lecithin A group of compounds that are major components of cell membranes.

■ Sterols

Sterols are the last class of lipids Chapter 5 covers. Their characteristic multi-ringed structure makes them different from the other lipids already discussed (review Fig. 5-1c). One example is the sterol cholesterol. This waxy substance doesn't look like a triglyceride—it doesn't have a glycerol backbone or any fatty acids. Still, because it doesn't readily dissolve in water, it is a lipid. Among other functions, cholesterol is used to form certain hormones and bile acids, and is incorporated into cell structures. The body can make all the cholesterol it needs.

Concept Check

Lipids are a group of compounds that do not dissolve readily in water. Included in this group are fatty acids, triglycerides, phospholipids, and sterols. Fatty acids can be distinguished from one another by the length of the carbon skeleton and the number and position of double bonds along that skeleton. Saturated fatty acids contain no double bonds within their carbon skeleton; that is, they are fully saturated with hydrogens. Monounsaturated fatty acids contain one carbon-carbon double bond, and polyunsaturated fatty acids contain two or more of these bonds. Certain omega-3 and omega-6 fatty acids are essential in the human diet.

Triglycerides are the major form of fat in the body and in foods. These consist of three fatty acids bonded to a glycerol backbone. Phospholipids are similar to triglycerides in structure, but at least one fatty acid is replaced by another compound. Phospholipids play an important structural role in cell membranes. Sterols, another class of lipids, do not resemble either triglycerides or phospholipids, but instead have a multi-ringed structure. Cholesterol, one example of a sterol, forms parts of cells, some hormones, and bile acids. Whereas certain essential fatty acids (as components of triglycerides) are needed in the diet, the body produces all the triglycerides, phospholipids and cholesterol it needs.

Fats and Oils in Foods

The foods that are highest in fat (and are therefore energy dense) include salad oils, butter, margarine, and mayonnaise (Fig. 5-5). All of these foods contain close to 100% of calories as fat. In reduced-fat margarines, water replaces some of the fat. Typical margarines are 80% fat by weight (11 grams per tablespoon). Some reduced-fat margarines are as low as 30% fat by weight (4 grams per tablespoon). When used in recipes, the extra water added to these margarines can cause texture and volume changes in the

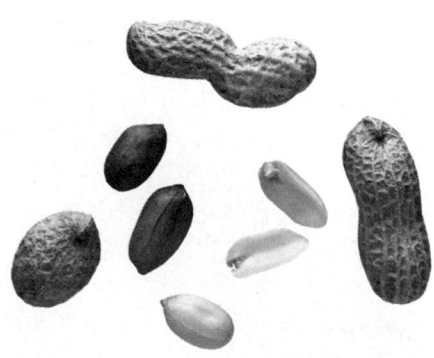

Peanuts are a source of lecithins, as are wheat germ and egg yolks.

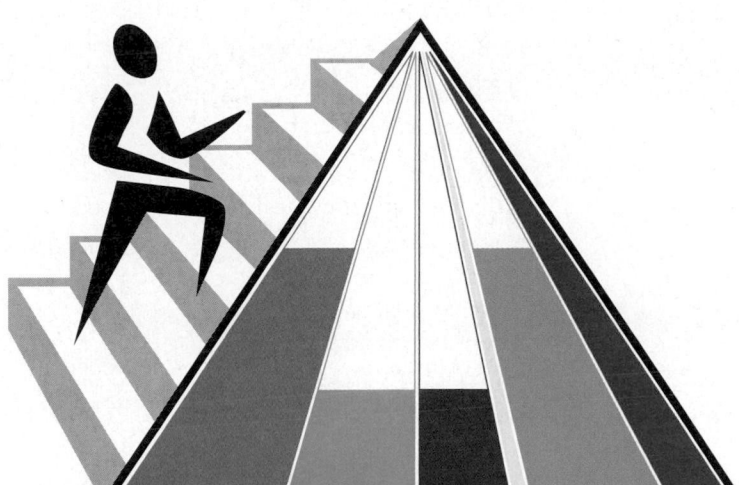

Figure 5-5 Sources of fats from MyPyramid. The height of the background color (none, 1/3, 2/3 or completely covered) within each group in the pyramid indicates the average nutrient density for fat in that group. The fruit group and vegetable groups are generally low in fat. In the other groups, both high-fat and low-fat choices are available. Careful reading of food labels can help you choose lower-fat versions of some foods. In general, any type of frying adds significant amounts of fat to a product, as with French fries and fried chicken. With regard to physical activity, fats are a key fuel in events that are prolonged, such as long-distance cycling, long-distance running, and prolonged slow to brisk walking.

Grains	Vegetables	Fruits	Oils	Milk	Meat & Beans
• Crackers • Pasta dishes with added fat	• French fried potatoes	• Fruit pies • Avocados	• All	• Whole milk • Some yogurts • Many cheeses • Premium ice cream	• Marbled meat • Bacon • Poultry (skin) • Deep-fat fried meat • Nuts

finished product. Cookbooks can provide guidance for appropriate use of these products by suggesting alterations in recipes to compensate for the increased water content.

Lipids in the form of triglycerides are abundant in the North American diet. Nuts, bologna, avocados, and bacon have about 80% of calories as fat. Peanut butter and cheddar cheese have about 75%. Marbled steak and hamburgers (ground chuck) have about 60%, and chocolate bars, ice cream, doughnuts, and whole milk have about 50% of calories as fat. Eggs, pumpkin pie, and cupcakes have 35%, as do lean cuts of meat, such as top round (and ground round) and sirloin. Bread contains about 15%. Cornflakes, sugar, and fat-free milk have essentially no fat. Careful label reading is necessary to determine the true fat content of food—these are only rough guidelines.

Animal fats are the chief contributors of saturated fatty acids to the North American diet, with about 40% to 60% of its total fat in the form of saturated fatty acids. In contrast, plant oils contain mostly unsaturated fatty acids, ranging from 73% to 94% of total fat. A moderate to high proportion of total fat (49% to 77%) is supplied by monounsaturated fatty acids in canola oil, olive oil, and peanut oil. Some animal fats are also good sources of monounsaturated fatty acids (30% to 47%) (review Fig. 5-3). Corn, cottonseed, sunflower, soybean, and safflower oils contain mostly polyunsaturated fatty acids (54% to 77%). These plant oils supply the majority of the linoleic and alpha-linolenic acid in the North American food supply.

Wheat germ, peanuts, egg yolk, soy beans, and organ meats are rich sources of phospholipids. Phospholipids such as lecithin, a component of egg yolks, are often added to salad dressing. Lecithin is used in these and other products because of its ability to keep mixtures of lipids and water from separating (see Fig. 5-12).

Cholesterol is found only in animal foods (Table 5-1). An egg yolk contains about 210 milligrams of cholesterol. This is our main dietary source of cholesterol, along with meats and whole milk. Manufacturers who advertise their brand of peanut butter, vegetable shortening, margarines, and vegetable oils as "cholesterol-free" are taking advantage of uninformed consumers—all of these products are naturally

Food Sources of Fat

Food item	Fat (grams)	Calories from Fat (%)
T-bone steak (3 oz)	17	66%
Mixed nuts (1 oz)	16	78%
Canola oil (1 tbsp)	14	100%
Hamburger with bun (1 each)	12	39%
Margarine (1 tbsp)	12	100%
Avocado (1/2 cup)	11	86%
Cheddar cheese (1 oz)	10	74%
Whole milk (1 cup)	8	49%
Chicken breast with skin (3 oz)	7	36%
Whole milk yogurt (8 oz)	7	28%
Snack crackers (1 oz)	7	45%
Baked beans (1/2 cup)	7	31%
M&M chocolate candies (1 oz)	6	39%
Flax seeds (1 tbsp)	3	62%
Fig Newton cookies (2 each)	3	23%

Table 5-1 Cholesterol Content of Selected Foods in Ascending Order

Food	Amount	Cholesterol in Milligrams	Food	Amount	Cholesterol in Milligrams
Skim milk	1 cup	4	Oysters, salmon	3 ounces	40
Mayonnaise	1 tablespoon	10	Clams, halibut, tuna	3 ounces	55
Butter	1 pat	11	Chicken, turkey* (white meat)	3 ounces	70
Lard	1 tablespoon	12	Beef,* pork	3 ounces	75
Cottage cheese	½ cup	15	Lamb, crab	3 ounces	85
Low-fat milk (2%)	1 cup	22	Shrimp, lobster	3 ounces	110
Half-and-half	¼ cup	23	Heart (beef)	3 ounces	165
Hot dog*	1	29	Egg (egg yolk)*†	1	210
Ice cream, ~10% fat	½ cup	30	Liver (beef)	3 ounces	410
Cheese, cheddar	1 ounce	30	Kidney	3 ounces	540
Whole milk	1 cup	34	Brains	3 ounces	2640

*Leading contributors of cholesterol to the North American diet.
†Egg whites are cholesterol-free.

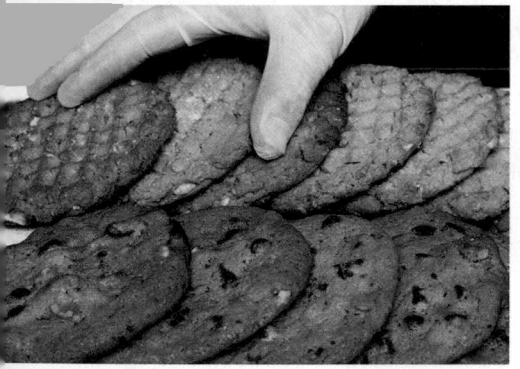

The North American diet contains many high-fat foods—including typical cookie choices. Portion control with these foods is thus important, especially if one is trying to control calorie intake.

When many North Americans think of a low-fat diet, they include reduced-fat versions of pastries, cookies, and cakes. When health professionals refer to a low-fat diet, they often have a very different plan in mind: focusing primarily on fruits, vegetables, and whole-grain breads and cereals.

cholesterol-free. Some plants contain other sterols that are similar to cholesterol, but they do not pose the heart health risks associated with cholesterol. In fact, some plant sterols have blood cholesterol-lowering properties (see the later section on medical interventions to lower blood lipids).

■ Fat Is Hidden in Some Foods

Some fat discussed so far is obvious: butter on bread, mayonnaise in potato salad, and marbling in raw meat. Fat is harder to detect in other foods that also contribute significant amounts of fat to our diets. Fat is hidden in whole milk, pastries, cookies, cake, cheese, hot dogs, crackers, French fries, and ice cream. When we try to cut down on fat intake, hidden fats need to be considered, along with the more obvious sources.

A place to begin searching for hidden fat is on the Nutrition Facts labels of foods you buy. Some signals from the ingredient list that can alert you to the presence of fat are animal fats, such as bacon, beef, ham, lamb, pork, chicken, and turkey fats; lard; vegetable oils; nuts; dairy fats, such as butter and cream; egg and egg-yolk solids; and partially-hydrogenated shortening or vegetable oil. Conveniently, the label lists ingredients by order of weight in the product. If fat is one of the first ingredients listed, you are probably looking at a high-fat product. Use food labels to learn more about the fat content of the foods you eat (Fig. 5-6).

Table 2-11 in Chapter 2 listed the definitions for various fat descriptors on food labels, such as "low-fat," "fat-free," and "reduced-fat." Recall that "low-fat" indicates, in most cases, that a product contains no more than 3 grams of fat per serving. Products that are marketed as "fat-free" must have less than one-half of a gram of fat per serving. A claim of "reduced-fat" means the product has at least 25% less fat than is usually found in that food. When there is no Nutrition Facts label to inspect, controlling portion size is a good way to control fat intake.

Whether or not to choose a fat-rich food should depend on how much fat you have eaten or will eat for that particular day. So, if you plan to eat high-fat foods at your evening meal, you could reduce your fat intake at a previous meal in order to balance overall fat intake for the day.

■ Wise Use of Reduced-Fat Foods Is Important

In recent years, manufacturers have introduced reduced-fat versions of numerous food products. The fat content of these alternatives ranges from 0% in fat-free Fig

Nutrition Facts

Serving Size 1 Link (45g)
Servings Per Container 10

Amount Per Serving

Calories 140   Calories from Fat 120

	% Daily Value*
Total Fat 13g	**20**%
Saturated Fat 5g	**23**%
Trans Fat 0g	**
Cholesterol 20mg	**7**%
Sodium 420mg	**17**%
Total Carbohydrate 2g	**1**%
Dietary Fiber 0g	**0**%
Sugars 1g	
Protein 5g	

Vitamin A 0% • Vitamin C 0%

Calcium 0% • Iron 2%

*Percent Daily Values are based on a 2,000 calorie diet.
**Intake of *trans* fat should be as low as possible.

Wiley's Our Best WIENERS

INGREDIENTS: PORK, WATER, BEEF, SALT, FLAVORINGS, CORN SYRUP SOLIDS, DEXTROSE, HYDROLYZED SOY AND POTATO PROTEIN, SODIUM PHOSPHATES, EXTRACT OF PAPRIKA, SODIUM ERYTHORBATE, SODIUM NITRITE.

KEEP REFRIGERATED

NET WT. 16 OZ.
(1 LB.) 454g.

U.S. INSPECTED AND PASSED BY DEPARTMENT OF AGRICULTURE EST. 575

Figure 5-6 Reading labels helps locate hidden fat. Who would think that wieners (hot dogs) can contain about 85% of food calories as fat? Looking at the hot dog itself does not suggest that almost all of its food calories comes from fat, but the label shows otherwise. Let's do the math: (13 grams × 9 kcal per gram)/140 kcal = 0.84, or 84%.

Newtons to about 75% of the original fat content in other products. However, the total calorie content of most fat-reduced products is not substantially lower than that of their conventional versions. Generally, when fat is removed from a product, something must be added—commonly, sugars—in its place. It is very difficult to reduce both the fat and sugar contents of a product at the same time. For this reason, many reduced-fat products (e.g., cakes and cookies) are still very energy dense. Use the Nutrition Facts label to guide the portion size you choose.

■ Fat Replacement Strategies for Foods

Currently, five types of fat replacements are available to food manufacturers. Addition of these substances during manufacturing yields products that, to varying degrees, satisfy consumers' desire for reduced-fat products that are still tasty.

Water, Starch Derivatives, and Fibers

The first and simplest fat replacement is water. The addition of water yields a product, such as diet margarine, with less fat per serving than the normal product. Starch derivatives that bind water form a second type of fat replacement. The resulting gel replaces some of the mouth feel lost by the removal of fat. Z-trim is one example. It is made from the hulls or bran of various plants, including oats, peas, soybeans, rice, corn, and wheat. Other starch derivatives commonly used by food manufacturers include the fiber cellulose, Maltrin, Stellar, and Oatrim. These substances are used in a variety of foods, including luncheon meats, salad dressings, frozen desserts, table spreads, dips, baked goods, and candies. Most starch derivatives contain some calories, but at least half the amount that is in fat. Note that these starch derivatives cannot be used in fried foods.

Gum fiber extracted from plants can also be used to replace fat. This thickens a product and replaces some of the body that fat provides. Diet salad dressings and fat-reduced ice cream have gums added for this reason.

Protein-Derived Fat Replacements

Still another type of fat replacement on the market consists of proteins that have been treated to produce microscopic, mistlike protein globules. Both egg and milk proteins can be used. When these substances replace fat in a food product, they feel like fat in the mouth, although the product does not contain any fatty acids. One example is

Critical Thinking

Allison has decided to start eating a low-fat diet. Allison has mentioned to you that all she needs to do is add less butter, oil, or margarine to her foods and she will dramatically lower her fat intake. How can you explain to Allison that she needs to be aware of the hidden fats in her diet as well?

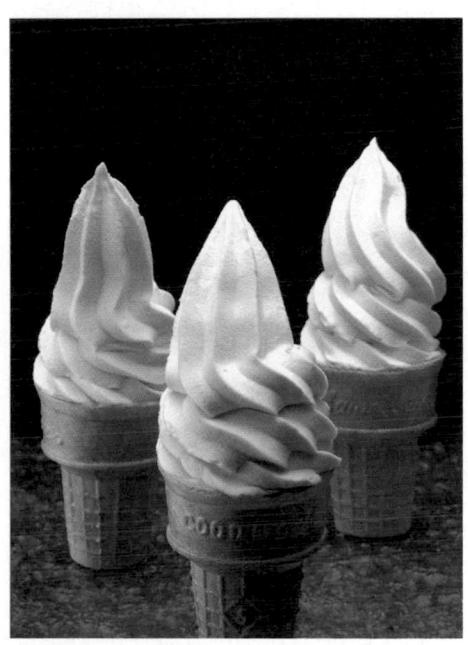

Fat replacements such as gum fiber are typically seen in soft serve ice cream.

Dairy-Lo, which is used in milk and other dairy products, baked goods, frostings, salad dressings, and mayonnaise-type products. Such fat replacements yield some calories—but only about 1 to 2 kcal per gram. They have this low-calorie value for two reasons: Proteins contain only 4 kcal per gram and the products have a high water content.

Engineered Fats and Related Products

The last form of fat replacement is engineered fat. This type of product is synthesized in the laboratory from various food constituents. Olestra (Olean) is a good example. It is made by chemically bonding fatty acids to sucrose (table sugar). The resulting product cannot be digested by either the human digestive enzymes or bacteria that live in the intestinal tract. Therefore, olestra is not absorbed and so provides no calories for the body.

Olestra can replace much of the fat in salad dressing and cakes and was the first fat replacement that could be used in fried foods. Olestra was approved by FDA in 1996 for use in fried snack foods, such as potato chips.

The major problem associated with the use of olestra is that it binds the fat-soluble vitamins A, D, E, and K, thus reducing their absorption. To compensate, the manufacturer adds these vitamins to food products containing olestra. Other suspected problems, such as GI tract discomfort, have not been supported by careful research. Thus, warnings about use of olestra and GI tract disturbances, which used to be required on labels for olestra-containing foods, are no longer mandatory.

Food manufacturers are working on other types of engineered fats, which either wholly or partially escape absorption by the body. One example is salatrim, which is marketed under the name Benefat and yields only about 5 kcal per gram. It is composed of some saturated fatty acids that are poorly absorbed by the body. This product has been used in reduced-fat chocolate.

Canada has not approved the use of olestra in food products; the United States is the sole country that permits the use of this fat substitute in foods.

Another Bite

So far, fat replacements have had little impact on our diets, partly because the currently approved forms either are not very versatile or have not been used extensively by manufacturers. The public, in fact, has shown very little interest in the use of fat replacers, such as olestra. In addition, fat replacements are not practical to use in the foods that contribute the greatest quantity of fat to our diets—beef, cheese, whole and reduced-fat milk, and pastries.

The main benefit of fat replacements will be in helping us cut some fat and calories from our diets. The reduction in overall calorie intake, however, will probably be small because we tend to compensate for the fewer calories per serving by simply eating more servings.

Concept Check

Fat-dense foods—those with more than 60% of total calories as fat—include plant oils, butter, margarine, mayonnaise, nuts, bacon, avocados, peanut butter, cheddar cheese, steak, and hamburger. Of the foods we typically eat, cholesterol is found naturally only in those of animal origin, with eggs being a primary source. Fat is often hidden in foods such as whole milk, pastries, cookies, cake, cheese, hot dogs, crackers, French fries, and ice cream. Fat free doesn't mean calorie free; moderation in the use of reduced-fat products is still important.

Making Lipids Available for Body Use

lipase Fat-digesting enzyme produced by the salivary glands, stomach, and pancreas.

It's no secret that fats and oils make foods more appealing. Their presence in foods adds flavor, lubrication, and texture. What happens to lipids once they are eaten? Let's take a closer look at the digestion, absorption, and physiological roles of lipids in the body.

■ Digestion

In the first phase of fat digestion, the stomach (and salivary glands to some extent) secretes **lipase.** This enzyme acts primarily on triglycerides that have fatty acids with chain lengths shorter than typical fatty acids, such as those found in butterfat. The action of this enzyme, however, is usually dwarfed by that of a lipase enzyme released from the pancreas and active in the small intestine. Triglycerides and other lipids found in common vegetable oils and meats have longer chain lengths and are generally not digested until they reach the small intestine (Fig. 5-7).

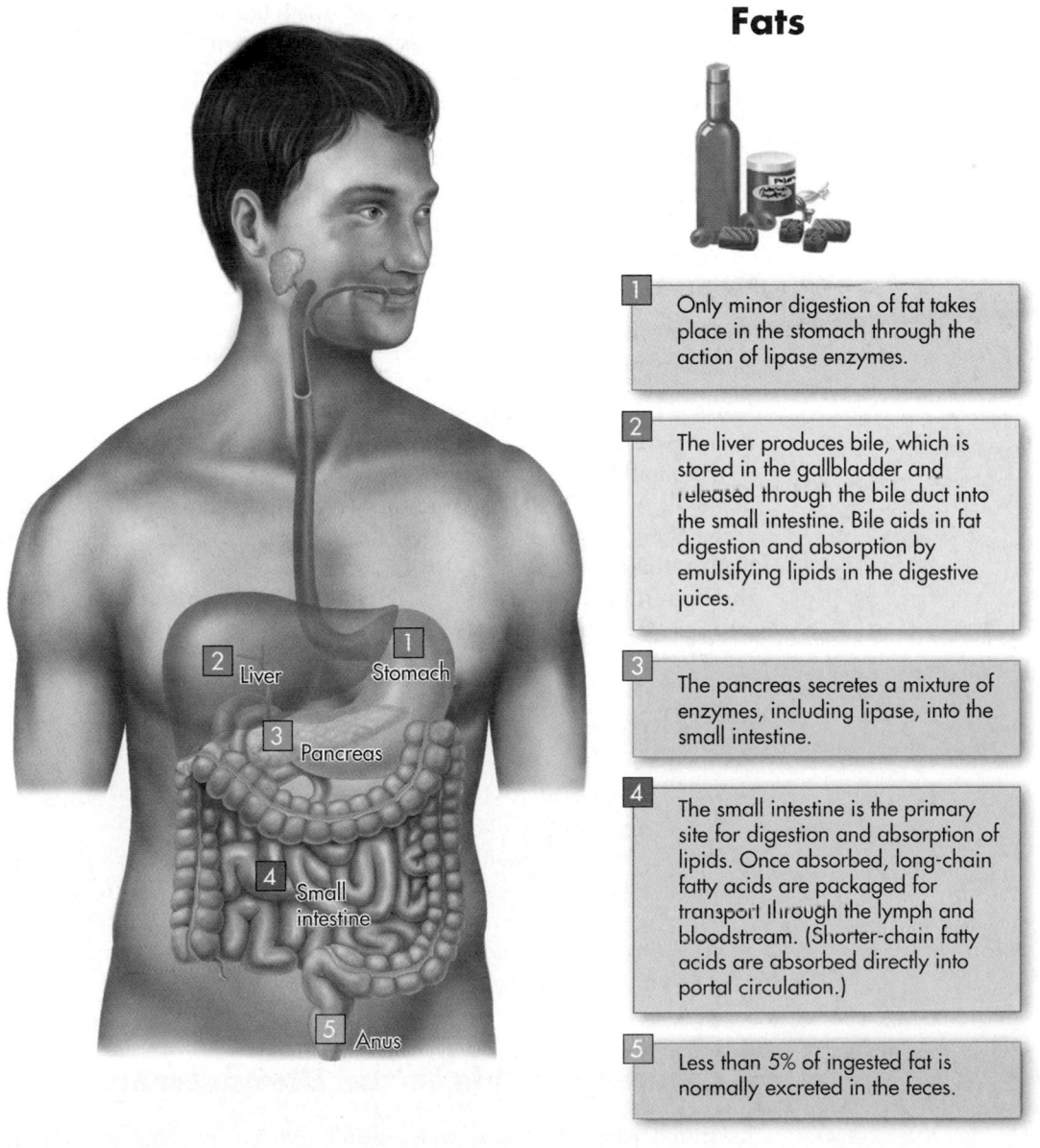

Fats

1. Only minor digestion of fat takes place in the stomach through the action of lipase enzymes.

2. The liver produces bile, which is stored in the gallbladder and released through the bile duct into the small intestine. Bile aids in fat digestion and absorption by emulsifying lipids in the digestive juices.

3. The pancreas secretes a mixture of enzymes, including lipase, into the small intestine.

4. The small intestine is the primary site for digestion and absorption of lipids. Once absorbed, long-chain fatty acids are packaged for transport through the lymph and bloodstream. (Shorter-chain fatty acids are absorbed directly into portal circulation.)

5. Less than 5% of ingested fat is normally excreted in the feces.

Figure 5-7 A summary of fat digestion and absorption. Chapter 3 covered general aspects of this process.

In the small intestine, triglycerides break down into smaller products, namely monoglycerides (glycerol backbones with a single fatty acid attached) and fatty acids. Under the right circumstances, digestion is very rapid and thorough. The "right" circumstances include the presence of bile from the gallbladder. Bile acids present in the bile act as an emulsifier on the digestive products of lipase action, suspending the monoglycerides and fatty acids in the watery digestive juices. This emulsification improves digestion and absorption because as large fat globules are broken down into smaller ones, the total surface area for lipase action increases.

With regard to phospholipid digestion, certain enzymes from the pancreas and cells in the wall of the small intestine digest phospholipids. The eventual products are glycerol, fatty acids, and remaining parts. With regard to cholesterol digestion, any cholesterol with a fatty acid attached is broken down to free cholesterol and fatty acids by certain enzymes released from the pancreas.

Another Bite

During meals, bile acids circulate in a path that begins in the liver, goes on to the gallbladder, and then moves to the small intestine. After participating in fat digestion, most bile acids are absorbed and end up back at the liver. Approximately 98% of the bile acids are recycled. Only 1% to 2% ends up in the large intestine to be eliminated in the feces. Using medicines that block some of this reabsorption of bile acids is one way to treat high blood cholesterol. The liver takes cholesterol from the bloodstream to form replacement bile acids. Soluble fiber in the diet can also bind to bile acids to produce the same effect (see a later section on medical interventions related to cardiovascular disease for details).

■ Absorption

Most products of fat digestion have by now been reduced to mere fatty acids and monoglycerides in the small intestine. These diffuse as such into the absorptive cells of the small intestine. In this way about 95% of dietary fat is absorbed. One key characteristic of fatty acids and monoglycerides affects their ultimate fate after absorption. If the chain length of a fatty acid is less than 12 carbon atoms, it is water soluble and will therefore probably travel as such through the portal vein that connects directly to the liver. If the fatty acid is a more typical long-chain variety, it must be reformed into a triglyceride and eventually enter circulation via the lymphatic system (review Chapter 3 for an overview of this process).

Concept Check

In the small intestine, a lipase enzyme released from the pancreas digests dietary triglycerides into monoglycerides (glycerol backbones with single fatty acids attached) and fatty acids. These breakdown products then diffuse into the absorptive cells of the small intestine. Long-chain fatty acids are transported through the lymphatic system, whereas fatty acids with shorter carbon chains are absorbed directly into the portal vein that connects directly to the liver. Other lipids are prepared for absorption by different enzymes.

lipoprotein A compound found in the bloodstream containing a core of lipids with a shell composed of protein, phospholipid, and cholesterol.

Carrying Lipids in the Bloodstream

As noted earlier, fat and water don't mix easily. This incompatibility presents a challenge for the transport of fats through the watery media of the blood and lymph. **Lipoproteins**—including chylomicrons, VLDL, LDL, and HDL—serve as

Table 5-2 Composition and Roles of the Major Lipoproteins in the Blood

Lipoprotein	Primary Component	Key Role
Chylomicron	Triglyceride	Carries dietary fat from the small intestine to cells
VLDL	Triglyceride	Carries lipids made and taken up by the liver to cells
LDL	Cholesterol	Carries cholesterol made by the liver and from other sources to cells
HDL	Protein	Contributes to cholesterol removal from cells and, in turn, excretion of it from the body

vehicles for transport of lipids from the small intestine and liver to the body tissues (Table 5-2).

Lipoproteins are classified based on their densities. Lipids are less dense than proteins. Therefore, lipoproteins that contain a large percentage of lipids in comparison to protein are less dense than those that are depleted of lipids.

■ Dietary Fats Are Carried by Chylomicrons

As you learned in the previous section, digestion of dietary fats results in a mixture of glycerol, monoglycerides, and fatty acids. Once these products are absorbed by the cells of the small intestine, they are reassembled into triglycerides. Then, the intestinal cells package the triglycerides into **chylomicrons,** which enter the lymphatic system and eventually the bloodstream (review Fig. 3-5 in Chapter 3 for a depiction of lymphatic circulation). Chylomicrons originate only from the intestinal cells. Like the other lipoproteins described in the next section, chylomicrons are composed of large droplets of lipid surrounded by a thin shell of phospholipids, cholesterol, and protein (Fig. 5-8). The water-soluble shell around a chylomicron allows the lipid to float freely in the water-based blood. Some of the proteins present may also help other cells identify the lipoprotein as a chylomicron.

Once a chylomicron enters the bloodstream, the triglycerides in its core are broken down into fatty acids and glycerol by an enzyme called **lipoprotein lipase,** which is attached to the inside walls of the blood vessels (Fig. 5-9). As soon as they are available, the fatty acids are absorbed by cells in the vicinity, while much of the glycerol circulates back to the liver. Muscle cells can immediately use the absorbed fatty acids

chylomicron Lipoprotein made of dietary fats surrounded by a shell of cholesterol, phospholipids, and protein. Chylomicrons are formed in the absorptive cells of the small intestine after fat absorption and travel through the lymphatic system to the bloodstream.

lipoprotein lipase An enzyme attached to the cells that form the inner lining of blood vessels; it breaks down triglycerides into free fatty acids and glycerol.

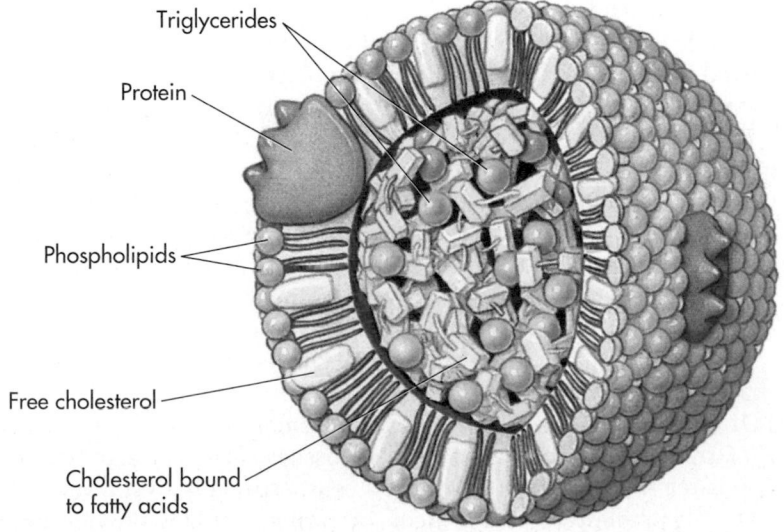

Triglycerides

Protein

Phospholipids

Free cholesterol

Cholesterol bound to fatty acids

Figure 5-8 The structure of a lipoprotein, in this case an LDL. This structure allows fats to circulate in the water-based bloodstream. Various lipoproteins are found in the bloodstream.

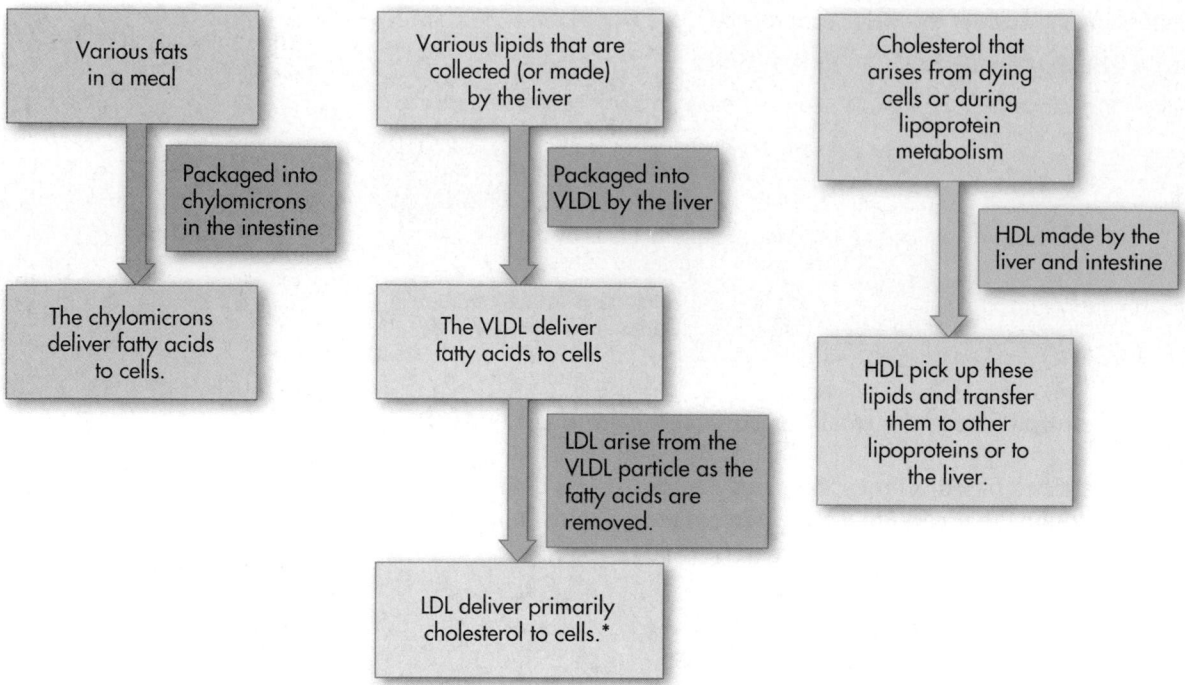

* Cholesterol not taken up by body cells can be taken up by scavenger cells in the arteries. The eventual cholesterol buildup leads to atherosclerosis.

Figure 5-9 Lipoprotein interactions. Chylomicrons carry absorbed fat to body cells. VLDL carries fat taken up from the bloodstream by the liver, as well as any fat made by the liver, to body cells. LDL arises from VLDL and carries mostly cholesterol to cells. HDL arises mostly from the liver and intestine. HDL carries cholesterol from cells to other lipoproteins and to the liver for excretion.

for fuel. Adipose cells, on the other hand, tend to re-form the fatty acids into triglycerides for storage. After triglycerides have been removed, a chylomicron remnant remains. Chylomicron remnants are removed from circulation by the liver and their components are recycled to make other lipoproteins and bile acids.

■ Other Lipoproteins Transport Lipids from the Liver to the Body Cells

The liver takes up various lipids from the blood. The liver also is the manufacturing site for lipids and cholesterol. The raw materials for lipid and cholesterol synthesis include free fatty acids taken up from the bloodstream, as well as carbon and hydrogen derived from carbohydrates, protein, and alcohol. The liver then must package these synthesized lipids as lipoproteins for transport in the blood to body tissues.

First in our discussion of lipoproteins made by the liver are **very-low-density lipoproteins (VLDL).** These particles are composed of cholesterol and triglycerides surrounded by a water-soluble shell. VLDLs are rich in triglycerides and thus are very low in density. Once in the bloodstream, lipoprotein lipase on the inner surface of the blood vessels breaks down the triglyceride in the VLDL into fatty acids and glycerol. Fatty acids and glycerol are released into the bloodstream and taken up by the body cells.

As its triglycerides are released, the VLDL becomes proportionately denser. Much of what eventually remains of the VLDL fraction is then called **low-density lipoprotein (LDL);** this is composed primarily of the remaining cholesterol. The primary function of LDL is to transport cholesterol to tissues. LDL particles are taken up from the bloodstream by specific receptors on cells, especially liver cells, and are then broken down. The cholesterol and protein components of LDL provide some of the building

very-low-density lipoprotein (VLDL) The lipoprotein created in the liver that carries cholesterol and lipids both taken up (and newly synthesized) by the liver.

low-density lipoprotein (LDL) The lipoprotein in the blood containing primarily cholesterol; elevated LDL is strongly linked to cardiovascular disease risk.

blocks necessary for cell growth and development, such as synthesis of cell membranes and hormones.

A critical and beneficial participant in this process of lipid transport is **high-density lipoprotein (HDL)**. Its high proportion of protein makes it the densest lipoprotein. The liver and intestine produce most of the HDL in the blood. It roams the bloodstream, picking up cholesterol from dying cells and other sources. HDL donates the cholesterol primarily to other lipoproteins for transport back to the liver to be excreted. Some HDL travels directly back to the liver.

▪ "Good" and "Bad" Cholesterol in the Bloodstream

You may have heard of these various lipoproteins described as "good" and "bad" cholesterol. So which is which? Many studies demonstrate that the amount of HDL in the bloodstream can closely predict the risk for cardiovascular disease. Risk increases with low HDL because little cholesterol is transported back to the liver and excreted. Women tend to have high amounts of HDL, especially before **menopause**, compared to men. Because high amounts of HDL slow the development of cardiovascular disease, any cholesterol carried by HDL can be considered "good" cholesterol.

On the other hand, LDL is sometimes considered "bad" cholesterol. In our discussion of LDL, you learned that LDL is taken up by receptors on various cells. If LDL is not readily cleared from the bloodstream, **scavenger cells** in the arteries take up the lipoprotein, leading to a buildup of cholesterol in the blood vessels. This buildup, known as **atherosclerosis**, greatly increases the risk for cardiovascular disease (see the following Looking Further section). Still, LDL is only a problem when it is too high in the bloodstream; low amounts are needed as part of routine body functions.

high-density lipoprotein (HDL) The lipoprotein in the blood that picks up cholesterol from dying cells and other sources and transfers it to the other lipoproteins in the bloodstream, as well as directly to the liver; low HDL increases the risk for cardiovascular disease.

menopause (MEN-oh-paws) The cessation of menses in women, usually beginning at about 50 years of age.

scavenger cells Specific form of white blood cells that can bury themselves in the artery wall and accumulate LDL. As these cells take up LDL, they contribute to the development of atherosclerosis.

atherosclerosis A buildup of fatty material (plaque) in the arteries, including those surrounding the heart.

Another Bite

The cholesterol in foods is not designated as "good" or "bad." It is only after cholesterol has been made or processed by the liver that it shows up in the bloodstream as LDL or HDL. Dietary patterns can affect the metabolism of cholesterol, however. Diets that are low in saturated fat, *trans* fat, and cholesterol encourage the uptake of LDL by the liver, thereby removing LDL from the bloodstream and decreasing the ability of scavenger cells to form atherosclerosis in the blood vessels. Likewise, diets high in saturated fat, *trans* fat, and cholesterol reduce the uptake of LDL by the liver, increasing cholesterol in the blood and the risk for cardiovascular disease.

It appears that saturated fatty acids promote an increase in the amount of free cholesterol (not attached to fatty acids) in the liver, whereas unsaturated fatty acids do the opposite. As free cholesterol in the liver increases, it causes the liver to reduce cholesterol uptake from the bloodstream, contributing to elevated LDL in the blood. (*Trans* fatty acids are thought to act in the same ways as saturated fatty acids.)

Concept Check

Lipids generally move through the bloodstream as part of lipoproteins. Dietary fats absorbed from the small intestine are packaged and transported as chylomicrons, whereas lipids that are synthesized in the liver are packaged as very-low-density lipoproteins (VLDL). Lipoprotein lipase removes triglycerides from the interiors of both chylomicrons and VLDL, breaking the triglycerides down into glycerol and fatty acids, which are taken up by tissues for energy needs or storage. What remains after the action of lipoprotein lipase are chylomicron remnants, the components of which are recycled by the liver, or low-density lipoproteins (LDL), which are rich in cholesterol. LDL is picked up by receptors on body cells, especially liver cells. Scavenger cells in the arteries may do the same, speeding the development of atherosclerosis. High-density lipoprotein (HDL), also produced in part by the liver, picks up cholesterol from cells and transports it primarily to other lipoproteins for eventual transport back to the liver. Risk factors for cardiovascular disease include an elevated level of LDL and/or low amounts of HDL in the blood.

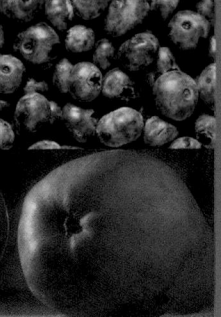

Lipoproteins and Cardiovascular Disease

Cardiovascular disease typically involves the coronary arteries and, thus, frequently the term coronary heart disease (CHD) or coronary artery disease (CAD) is used.

A heart attack can strike with the sudden force of a sledgehammer, with pain radiating up the neck or down the arm. It can sneak up at night, masquerading as indigestion, with slight pain or pressure in the chest. Many times, the symptoms are so subtle in women that it often is too late once she or the health professional realizes that a heart attack is taking place. If there is any suspicion at all that a heart attack is taking place, the person should first chew an aspirin (325 milligrams) thoroughly and then call 911. Aspirin helps reduce the blood clotting that leads to a heart attack. Typical warning signs are:

- Intense, prolonged chest pain or pressure, sometimes radiating to other parts of the upper body (men and women)
- Shortness of breath (men and women)
- Sweating (men and women)
- Nausea and vomiting (especially women)
- Dizziness (especially women)
- Weakness (men and women)
- Jaw, neck, and shoulder pain (especially women)
- Irregular heartbeat (men and women)

Cardiovascular disease is the major killer of North Americans. Each year about 500,000 people die of coronary heart disease in the United States alone, about 60% more than die of cancer. The figure rises to almost 1 million if strokes and other circulatory diseases are included in the global term *cardiovascular disease*. About 1.5 million people in the United States each year have a heart attack. The overall male-to-female ratio for cardiovascular disease is about 2:1. Women generally lag about 10 years behind men in developing the disease. Still, it eventually kills more women than any other disease—twice as many as does cancer. And, for each person in North America who dies of cardiovascular disease, 20 more (over 13 million people) have symptoms of the disease.

Healthy People 2010 has set a goal of reducing death from coronary heart disease by 30%, compared with today's incidence.

Development of Cardiovascular Disease

The symptoms of cardiovascular disease develop over many years and often do not become obvious until old age. Nonetheless, autopsies of young adults under 20 years of age have shown that many of them had atherosclerotic **plaque** in their arteries (Fig. 5-10). This finding indicates that plaque buildup can begin in childhood and continue throughout life, although it usually goes undetected for quite some time.

The typical forms of cardiovascular disease—coronary heart disease and strokes—are associated with inadequate blood circulation in the heart and brain related to buildup of this plaque. Blood supplies the heart muscle, brain, and other body organs with oxygen and nutrients. When blood flow via the coronary arteries surrounding the heart is interrupted, the heart muscle can be damaged. A heart attack, or **myocardial infarction,** may result (review Fig. 5-10). This may cause the heart to beat irregularly or to stop altogether. About 25% of people do not survive their first heart attack. If blood flow to parts of the brain is interrupted long enough, part of the brain dies, causing a **cerebrovascular accident,** or stroke.

Continuous formation and breakdown of blood clots in the blood vessels is a normal process. However, in areas where plaques build up, blood clots are more likely to remain as such and then lead to a blockage, cutting off or diminishing the supply of blood to the heart

plaque A cholesterol-rich substance deposited in the blood vessels; it contains various white blood cells, smooth muscle cells, various proteins, cholesterol and other lipids, and eventually calcium.

myocardial infarction Death of part of the heart muscle. Also termed a *heart attack*.

cerebrovascular accident (CVA) Death of part of the brain tissue due typically to a blood clot. Also termed a *stroke*.

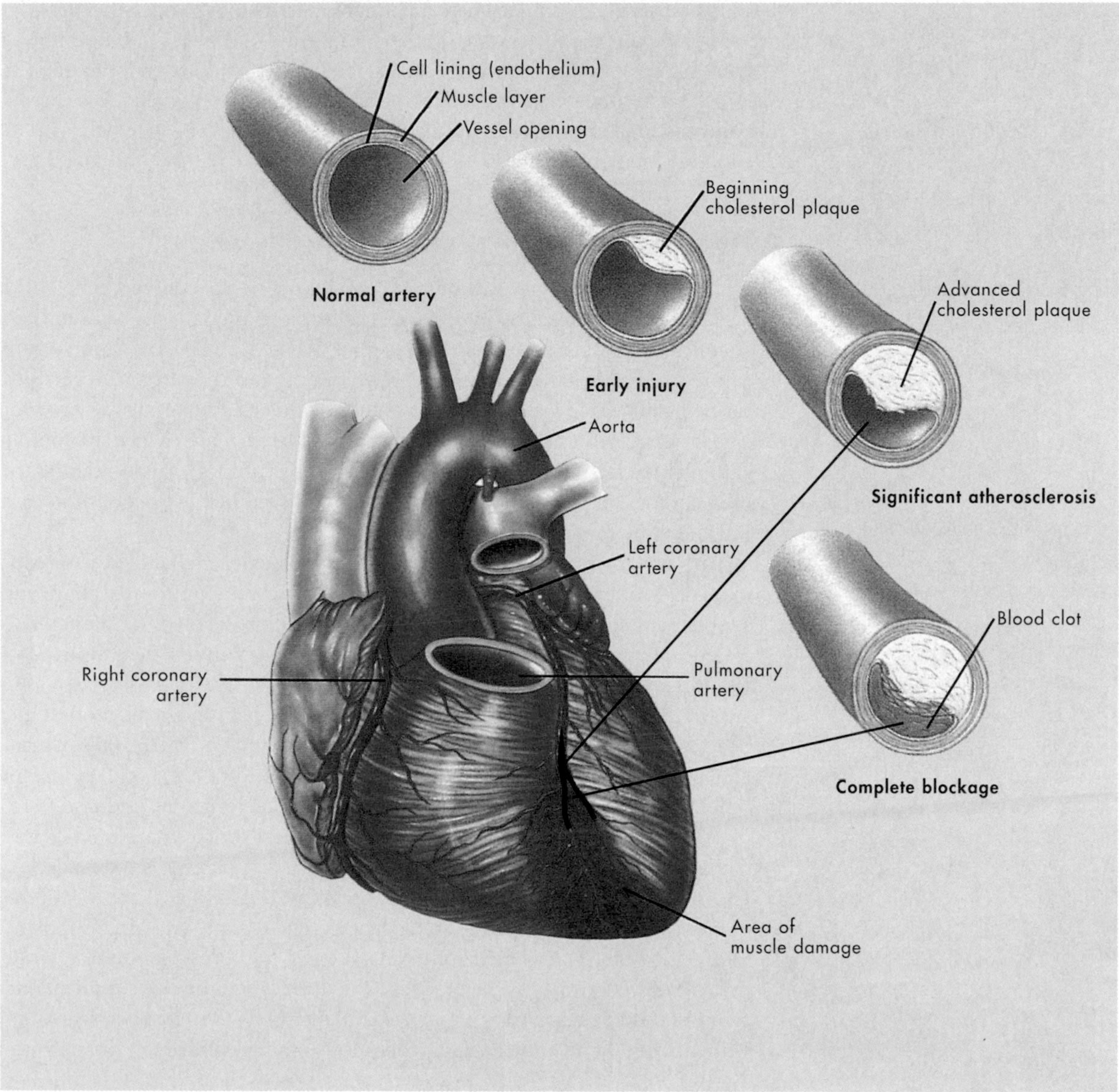

Figure 5-10 The road to a heart attack. Injury to an artery wall begins the process. This is followed by a progressive buildup of plaque in the artery walls. The heart attack represents the final phase of the process. Blockage of the left coronary artery by a blood clot is evident. The point where arteries such as these branch into small arteries is the typical site of major blockage. The heart muscle that is served by the portion of the coronary artery beyond the point of blockage lacks oxygen and nutrients, leading to damage and possible death of heart tissue. This can lead to a significant drop in heart function and often total heart failure.

(coronary arteries) or brain (carotid arteries). More than 95% of all heart attacks are caused by such blood clots. In essence, heart attacks generally are caused not by total blockage of the coronary arteries by plaque but by disruption of a partial blockage, leading to eventual clot formation.

Atherosclerosis probably first develops to repair damage in a vessel lining. The damage that starts this process can be caused by smoking, diabetes, hypertension, **homocysteine** (likely, but not a major factor), LDL, and viral and bacterial infection. Ongoing blood vessel inflammation is also implicated. (A laboratory test for c-reactive protein in the blood is used to assess if inflammation is present.) Atherosclerosis can be seen in arteries throughout the body. The damage

homocysteine An amino acid not used in protein synthesis, but instead arises during metabolism of the amino acid methionine. Homocysteine is likely toxic to many cells, such as those lining the blood vessels.

oxidize In the most basic sense, the loss of an electron or gain of an oxygen by a chemical substance. This change typically alters the shape and/or function of the substance.

antioxidant Generally a compound that stops the damaging effects of reactive substances seeking an electron (i.e., oxidizing agents). This prevents breakdown (oxidizing) of substances in foods or the body, particularly lipids.

For more information on cardiovascular disease, see the website of the American Heart Association at www.americanheart.org or the heart disease section of Healthfinder at www.healthfinder.gov/tours/heart.htm. This is a site created by the U.S. government for consumers. In addition, visit the website www.nhlbi.nih.gov/.

develops especially at points where an artery branches into two smaller vessels. A great deal of stress is placed on the vessel walls at these points due to changes in blood flow.

Once blood vessel damage has occurred, the next step in the development of atherosclerosis is the progression phase. This step is characterized by deposition of plaque at the site of initial damage. The rate of plaque buildup during the progression phase is directly related to the amount of LDL in the blood. As plaque accumulates, arteries harden, narrow, and lose their elasticity.

Another Bite

The form of LDL that contributes to atherosclerosis is **oxidized** LDL. This form is preferentially taken up by scavenger cells in the arterial wall. Nutrients and phytochemicals that have **antioxidant** properties may reduce LDL oxidation. Fruits and vegetables are particularly rich in these compounds. Eating fruits and vegetables regularly is one positive step we can make to reduce plaque buildup and slow the progression of cardiovascular disease. Some fruits and vegetables that are particularly helpful in this regard include legumes (beans), nuts, dried plums (prunes), raisins, berries, plums, apples, cherries, oranges, grapes, spinach, broccoli, red bell peppers, potatoes, and onions. Tea and coffee are also sources.

Are large doses of antioxidant vitamin supplements a reliable way to reduce LDL oxidation, and thereby prevent cardiovascular disease? Controversy about such dietary supplementation exists among the experts, as will be detailed in Chapter 8. Currently the American Heart Association does not support use of antioxidant supplements (such as vitamin E) to reduce cardiovascular disease risk. This is because large-scale studies have shown no benefit from such use, and a recent trial even showed a modest increase for heart failure in people with diabetes or otherwise at high risk for cardiovascular disease. However, further trials of antioxidant supplementation (e.g., 600 IU of vitamin E every other day) for prevention of heart disease in men are ongoing, and results are expected by 2007. (With regard to women, 600 IU of natural-source vitamin E taken every other day provided no overall benefit for major cardiovascular events (or cancer). More research is warranted, however, as a decrease in sudden cardiac death was seen in a subset of older women in this study.) Some experts suggest daily vitamin E supplementation (100 IU to 400 IU) may be helpful for *preventing* cardiovascular disease, while other experts recommend against the practice. One thing is certain: any supplementation of vitamin E should be taken only under the guidance of a physician, because of interactions with vitamin K and anti-clotting medications (and possibly high-dose aspirin use).

Affected arteries become further damaged as blood pumps through them and pressure increases. Finally, in the terminal phase, a clot or spasm in a plaque-clogged artery leads to a heart attack.

Factors that typically bring on a heart attack in a person at risk include dehydration, acute emotional stress (such as firing an employee), strenuous physical activity when not otherwise physically fit (shoveling snow, for example), waking during the night or getting up in the morning (linked to an abrupt increase in stress), and consuming large, high-fat meals (increases blood clotting).

Risk Factors for Cardiovascular Disease

Many of us are free of the risk factors that contribute to rapid development of atherosclerosis. If so, the advice of health experts is to simply consume a balanced diet, perform regular physical activity, have a complete fasting lipoprotein analysis performed at age 20 or beyond, and reevaluate risk factors every 5 years.

For most people, however, the most likely risk factors are:

- **Total blood cholesterol over 200 milligrams per 100 milliliters of blood** (mg/dl; dl is short for deciliter or 100 milliliters). Risk is especially high when total cholesterol is at or over 240 mg/dl and coupled with LDL-cholesterol readings over 130 to 160 mg/dl. (The terms

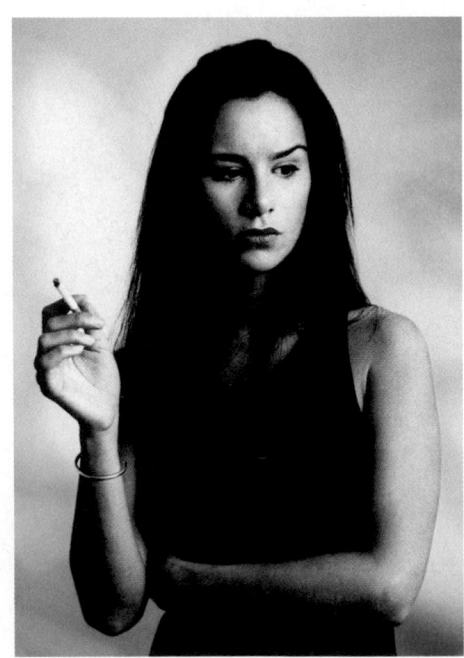

Smoking is one of the four major risk factors for developing cardiovascular disease.

LDL-cholesterol and HDL-cholesterol are used when expressing the blood concentration since it is the cholesterol content of these lipoproteins that is actually measured.)

- **Smoking.** This generally negates the female advantage of later occurrence of the disease and is the main cause of about 20% of cardiovascular disease deaths. A combination of smoking and oral contraceptive use worsens matters even more. Smoking greatly increases the ultimate expression of a person's genetically linked risk for cardiovascular disease and even increases risk if one's blood lipids are low. Smoking also makes blood more likely to clot. Even secondhand smoke has been implicated as a risk factor.
- **Hypertension. Systolic blood pressure** over 139 (millimeters of mercury) and **diastolic blood pressure** over 89 indicate hypertension. More healthy blood pressure values are less than 120 and 80, respectively. (Treatment of hypertension is reviewed in Chapter 9.)
- **Diabetes.** This disease negates any female advantage. Insulin increases cholesterol synthesis in the liver, in turn increasing LDL in the bloodstream. Diabetes virtually guarantees development of cardiovascular disease, and so puts such a person in the high-risk group.

Together the previous four risk factors explain most cases of cardiovascular disease.

Other risk factors to consider:

- HDL-cholesterol under 40 mg/dl, especially when the ratio of total cholesterol to HDL-cholesterol is greater than 4:1 (3.5:1 or less is optimal). Women often have high values for HDL-cholesterol and therefore it is important for this to be measured in women to establish cardiovascular disease risk. A value of 60 mg/dl or more is especially protective.
- Age. Men over 45 years and women over 55 years.
- Family history of cardiovascular disease, especially before age 50.
- Blood triglycerides 200 mg/dl or greater in the fasting state (less than 100 mg/dl is optimal).
- Obesity (especially fat accumulation in the waist). Typical weight gain seen in adults is a chief contributor to the increase in LDL seen with aging. Obesity also typically leads to insulin resistance, creating a diabetes-like state, and ultimately the disease itself. It also increases overall inflamation throughout the body.
- Inactivity. Exercise conditions the arteries to adapt to physical stress. Regular exercise also improves insulin action in the body. The corresponding reduction in insulin output leads to a reduction in lipoprotein synthesis in the liver. Both regular aerobic exercise and resistance exercise are recommended. A person with existing cardiovascular disease should seek physician approval before starting such a program, as should older adults.

Researchers are currently trying to unravel and quantify numerous other factors that may be linked to premature cardiovascular disease, such as the connection between inadequate intake of vitamin B-6, folate, and vitamin B-12, which can lead to increased homocysteine in the blood. As noted, homocysteine may damage the cells lining the blood vessels, in turn promoting atherosclerosis. Elevated blood homocysteine is likely the cause in about 10% of cases, especially if the person has evidence of cardiovascular disease.

The term *risk factor* is not intended to mean causality; nevertheless, the more of these risk factors one has, the greater the chances of ultimately developing cardiovascular disease. A good example is the **metabolic syndrome** (also called *Syndrome X*). A person with the metabolic syndrome would have abdominal obesity, high blood triglycerides, low HDL-cholesterol, hypertension, poor blood glucose regulation (i.e., high fasting blood glucose), and increased blood clotting. This profile raises the risk for cardiovascular disease considerably. On a positive note, cardiovascular disease is rare in populations who have low LDL-cholesterol, normal blood pressure, and do not smoke or have diabetes. By minimizing these risk factors, along with following the dietary recommendations of the American Heart Association on pages 172–173 and staying physically active, one will most likely reduce many of the other controllable risk factors listed. In other words, develop and follow a total lifestyle plan. Medications may also be added to lower blood lipids, as discussed later in this chapter. Finally, if a person has a family history of cardiovascular disease but the usual risk factors aren't present, a rarer defect might be the cause. In this case, having a detailed physical examination for other potential causes is advised.

systolic blood pressure The pressure in the arterial blood vessels associated with the pumping of blood from the heart.

diastolic blood pressure The pressure in the arterial blood vessels when the heart is between beats.

Healthy People 2010 has set a goal of reducing total blood cholesterol among adults from an average of 206 mg/dl to 199 mg/dl, as well as a reduction in the percentage of adults with high blood cholesterol from 21% to 17%.

metabolic syndrome A condition in which the person has poor blood glucose regulation, hypertension, increased blood triglycerides, and other health problems. This condition is usually accompanied by obesity, lack of physical activity, and a diet high in refined carbohydrates. Also called *Syndrome X.*

Two approaches have been shown to cause reversal of atherosclerosis in the body. One employs a vegan diet and other lifestyle changes that are part of the Dr. Dean Ornish program. The other employs aggressive LDL-lowering with medications.

eicosapentaenoic acid (EPA) An omega-3 fatty acid with 20 carbons and five carbon-carbon double bonds. It is present in large amounts in fatty fish and is slowly synthesized in the body from alpha-linolenic acid.

docosahexaenoic acid (DHA) An omega-3 fatty acid with 22 carbons and six carbon-carbon double bonds. It is present in large amounts in fatty fish and is slowly synthesized in the body from alpha-linolenic acid. DHA is especially present in the retina and brain.

Omega-3 Fatty Acids in Fish (grams per 3 ounce serving)	
Atlantic salmon	1.8
Anchovy	1.7
Sardines	1.4
Rainbow trout	1.0
Coho salmon	0.9
Bluefish	0.8
Striped bass	0.8
Tuna, white, canned	0.7
Halibut	0.4
Catfish, channel	0.2

Essential Functions of Fatty Acids

The various classes of lipids have diverse functions in the body. All are necessary for health, but, as mentioned earlier, not all are needed in our diet. Of all the classes of lipids, only certain polyunsaturated fatty acids are essential parts of a diet.

▪ The Essential Fatty Acids

Because we must obtain linoleic acid (omega-6) and alpha-linolenic acid (omega-3) from foods in order to maintain health, they are called *essential* fatty acids (Fig. 5-11). These omega-3 and omega-6 fatty acids form parts of vital body structures, perform important roles in immune system function and vision, help form cell membranes, and produce hormone-like compounds. Omega-6 and omega-3 fatty acids must be obtained through the diet because human cells lack the enzymes needed to produce these fatty acids. Other fatty acids, such as omega-9 fatty acids, can be synthesized in the body, and therefore are not essential components of the diet.

Still, we need to consume only about 5% of our total calories from essential fatty acids. That corresponds to about 2 to 4 tablespoons of plant oil each day. We can easily get that much—from mayonnaise, salad dressings, and other foods—without much effort. Regular consumption of whole-grain breads and cereals and vegetables also helps to supply enough essential fatty acids.

Current research also suggests that we should not only include a regular intake of alpha-linolenic acid, but also its related omega-3 fatty acids, **eicosapentaenoic acid (EPA)** and **docosahexaenoic acid (DHA).** This would almost certainly require consumption of fatty fish—salmon, tuna, sardines, anchovies, striped bass, catfish, herring, mackerel, trout, or halibut—at least twice a week. Additional sources of omega-3 fatty acids include canola and soybean oils, walnuts, flax seeds, mussels, crab, and shrimp.

Another Bite

Some fish can be a source of mercury, which is toxic in high amounts, especially swordfish, shark, king mackerel, and tile fish (see Chapter 16). Albacore tuna also is a potential source, while other forms of tuna are much lower in mercury. Those fish low in mercury are salmon, sardines, bluefish, and herring. Shrimp is also low in mercury. For others, varying your choices rather than always eating the same species of fish and limiting overall intake to 12 ounces per week (on average 2 to 3 meals of fish or shellfish per week) is recommended to reduce mercury exposure, especially for pregnant women and children.

Figure 5-11 The essential fatty acid (EFA) family. All these fatty acids are available from dietary sources; linoleic acid and alpha-linolenic acid must be consumed as body synthesis does not take place. These are the essential fatty acids. The other fatty acids in this figure can be synthesized from the essential fatty acids.

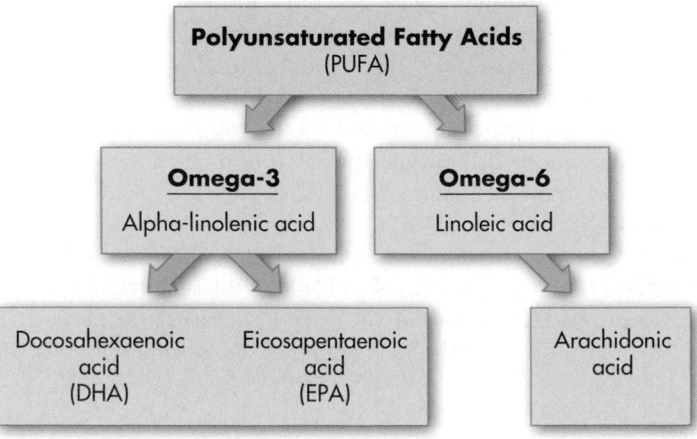

This recommendation for consuming omega-3 fatty acids stems from the observation that compounds made from omega-3 fatty acids tend to decrease blood clotting and inflammatory processes in the body, whereas the omega-6 fatty acids (notably **arachidonic acid;** this is made from linoleic acid) generally increase these processes. (Satured fatty acids also increase blood clotting.)

Some studies show that people who eat fish at least twice a week (total weekly intake: 8 ounces [240 grams]) run lower risks for heart attack than do people who rarely eat fish. In these cases, the omega-3 fatty acids in fish oil are probably acting to reduce blood clotting. As was covered in detail in the Looking Further section, blood clots are part of the heart attack process. In addition, these omega-3 fatty acids have a favorable effect on heart rhythm. Consequently, the risk of heart attack decreases, especially for people already at high risk.

We need to remember, however, that blood clotting is a normal body process. Certain groups of people, such as Eskimos in Greenland, eat so much seafood that their normal blood-clotting ability can be impaired. An excess of omega-3 fatty acid intake can allow uncontrolled bleeding and may cause **hemorrhagic stroke.** However, no increase in risk of stroke has been observed in studies using moderate amounts of omega-3 fatty acids.

Studies also have shown that large amounts of omega-3 fatty acids from fish (2 to 4 grams per day) can lower blood triglycerides in people with high triglyceride concentrations. In addition, these omega-3 fatty acids are suspected to be helpful in managing the pain of inflammation associated with rheumatoid arthritis (by suppressing immune system responses) and may help with certain behavioral disorders and cases of mild depression.

In some instances, fish oil capsules can be safely substituted for fish consumption if a person does not like fish. Generally, about 1 gram of omega-3 fatty acids (about three capsules) from fish oil per day is recommended, especially for people with evidence of cardiovascular disease. (Note that freezing fish oil capsules before consumption will reduce the fishy aftertaste.) The American Heart Association also recently suggested that fish oil supplements (providing 2 to 4 grams of omega-3 fatty acids per day) could be employed to treat elevated blood triglycerides, as previously noted. However, for individuals who have bleeding disorders, take anticoagulant medications, or anticipate surgery, fish oil capsules may increase risk of uncontrollable bleeding and hemorrhagic stroke. Thus for fish oil capsules, as well as other dietary supplements, it is important to follow a physician's recommendations.

Another Bite

Flax seeds are getting attention today because they are a rich vegetable source of the omega-3 alpha-linolenic acid. About 2 tablespoons per day is typically recommended if used as an omega-3 fatty acid source. Flax seeds can be purchased in many natural food stores rather inexpensively. These need to be chewed thoroughly or they will pass through the GI tract undigested. Many people find it easier to grind them in a coffee grinder before eating them. Flax seed oil is also available, but it turns **rancid** very quickly, especially if not refrigerated.

■ Effects of a Deficiency of Essential Fatty Acids

If humans fail to consume enough essential fatty acids, their skin becomes flaky and itchy, and diarrhea and other symptoms such as infections often are seen. Growth and wound healing may be restricted. These signs of deficiency have been seen in people fed **total parenteral nutrition** solutions containing little or no fat for 2 to 3 weeks, as well as in infants receiving formulas low in fat. However, because our bodies need the equivalent of only about 2 to 4 tablespoons of plant oils a day, even a low-fat diet will provide enough essential fatty acids if it follows a balanced plan such as MyPyramid and includes a serving of fatty fish at least twice a week.

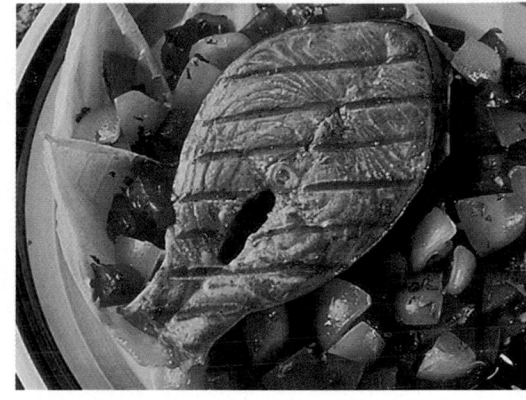

The American Heart Association recommends eating fatty fish such as salmon at least twice a week. As a source of omega-3 fatty acids, fish is a heart-healthy alternative to other animal sources of protein, which can be high in saturated fat and cholesterol.

Critical Thinking

Advertisements often claim that fats are bad. Your classmate Mike asks, "If fats are so bad for us, why do we need to have any in our diets?" How would you answer him?

arachidonic acid An omega-6 fatty acid made from linoleic acid with 20 carbon atoms and 4 carbon-carbon double bonds.

hemorrhagic stroke Damage to part of the brain resulting from rupture of a blood vessel and subsequent bleeding within or over the internal surface of the brain.

rancid Containing products of decomposed fatty acids that have an unpleasant flavor and odor.

total parenteral nutrition The intravenous feeding of all necessary nutrients, including the most basic forms of protein, carbohydrates, lipids, vitamins, minerals, and electrolytes.

Concept Check

Because humans can't make either omega-3 or omega-6 fatty acids, which perform vital functions in the body, they are essential parts of a diet and therefore called essential fatty acids. Plant oils are generally rich in omega-6 fatty acids. Eating fatty fish at least twice a week is a good way to meet omega-3 fatty acid needs. Fish oil supplementation (about 1 gram per day of the related omega-3 fatty acids) is generally acceptable under a physician's guidance if a person does not like fish; however, people with certain medical conditions (e.g., taking anticoagulant medications) should be cautious with use of fish oil supplements due to increased risk of hemorrhagic stroke. Essential fatty acid deficiency can occur after 2 to 3 weeks if fat is omitted from total parenteral nutrition solutions, which in turn can lead to skin disorders, diarrhea, and other health problems.

Broader Roles for Fatty Acids and Triglycerides in the Body

Many key functions of fat in the body require the use of fatty acids in the form of triglycerides. Triglycerides are used for energy storage, insulation, and transportation of fat-soluble vitamins.

■ Providing Energy

Triglycerides contained in the diet and stored in adipose tissue provide the fatty acids that are the main fuel for muscles while at rest and during light activity. Only in endurance exercise, such as long-distance running and cycling, or in short bursts of intense activity, such as a 200-meter run, do muscles use a lot of carbohydrate in addition to fatty acids supplied by triglycerides for fuel. Other body tissues also use fatty acids for energy needs. Overall, about half of the energy used by the entire body at rest and during light activity comes from fatty acids. On a whole-body basis, the use of fatty acids by skeletal and heart muscle is balanced by the use of glucose by the nervous system and red blood cells. Recall from Chapter 4 that cells also need carbohydrate to efficiently process fatty acids for fuel.

■ Storing Energy for Later Use

We store energy mainly in the form of triglycerides. The body's ability to store fat is essentially limitless. Its fat storage sites, adipose cells, can increase about 50 times in weight. If the amount of fat to be stored exceeds the ability of the cells to expand, the body can form new adipose cells.

An important advantage of using triglycerides to store energy in the body is that they are energy dense. Recall that these yield, on average, 9 kcal per gram, whereas proteins and carbohydrates yield only about 4 kcal per gram. In addition, triglycerides are chemically very stable, so they are not likely to react with other cell constituents, making them a safe form for storing energy. Finally, when we store triglycerides in adipose cells, we store little else, notably water. Adipose cells contain about 80% lipid and only 20% water and protein. In contrast, imagine if we were to store energy as muscle tissue, which is about 73% water. Body weight linked to energy storage would increase dramatically. The same would be true if we stored energy primarily as glycogen, as about 3 grams of water are stored for every gram of glycogen.

■ Insulating and Protecting the Body

The insulating layer of fat just beneath the skin is made mostly of triglycerides. Fat tissue also surrounds and protects some organs—kidneys, for example—from injury.

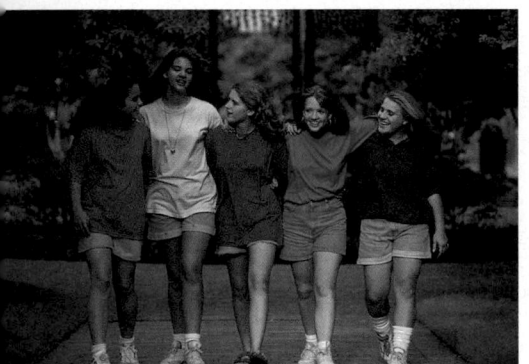

When at rest or during light activity, the body uses mostly fatty acids for fuel.

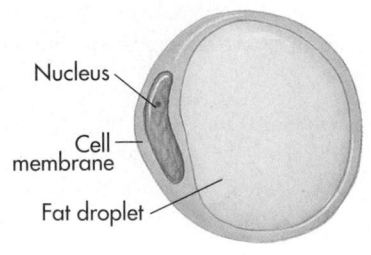

Nucleus

Cell membrane

Fat droplet

Adipose cell.

We usually don't notice the important insulating function of fat tissue, because we wear clothes and add more as needed. A layer of insulating fat is very important in animals living in cold climates. Polar bears, walruses, and whales all build a thick layer of fat tissue around themselves to insulate against cold-weather environments. The extra fat also provides energy storage for times when food is scarce.

■ Transporting Fat-Soluble Vitamins

Triglycerides and other fats in food carry fat-soluble vitamins to the small intestine and aid their absorption. People who absorb fat poorly, such as those with the disease cystic fibrosis, are at risk for deficiencies of fat-soluble vitamins, especially vitamin K. A similar risk comes from taking mineral oil as a laxative at mealtimes. Because the body cannot digest or absorb mineral oil, the undigested oil carries the fat-soluble vitamins from the meal into the feces, where they are eliminated.

Unabsorbed fatty acids can bind minerals, such as calcium and magnesium, and draw them into the stool for elimination. This can harm mineral status (see Chapter 9).

Phospholipids in the Body

Many types of phospholipids exist in the body, especially in the brain. They form important parts of cell membranes. Phospholipids are found in body cells, and they participate in fat digestion in the intestine. Recall that the various forms of lecithin (discussed earlier) are common examples of phospholipids (review Fig. 5-1b).

Cell membranes are composed primarily of phospholipids. A cell membrane looks much like a sea of phospholipids with protein "islands" (review Fig. 3-2). The proteins form receptors for hormones, function as enzymes, and act as transporters for nutrients. The fatty acids on the phospholipids serve as a source of essential fatty acids for the cell. Some cholesterol is also present in the membrane.

Some phospholipids allow fat and water to mix by functioning as **emulsifiers** (as covered earlier). By breaking fat globules into small droplets, emulsifiers enable a fat to be suspended in water. In essence, they act as bridges between the oil and water that in turn lead to the formation of tiny oil droplets surrounded by thin shells of water. In an emulsified solution, millions of tiny oil droplets are separated by shells of water (Fig. 5-12).

emulsifier A compound that can suspend fat in water by isolating individual fat droplets, using a shell of water molecules or other substances to prevent the fat from coalescing.

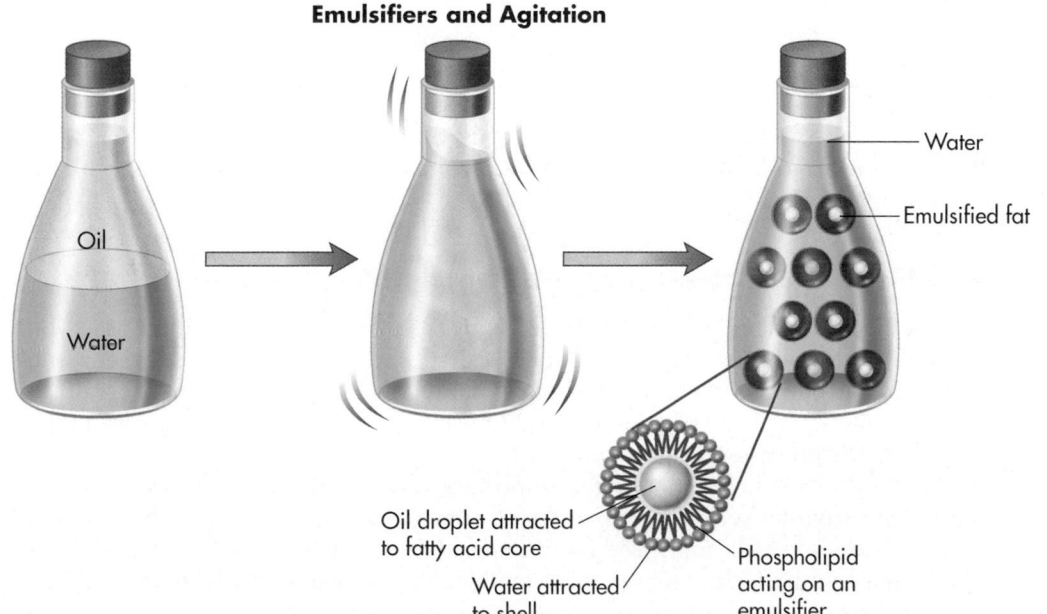

Emulsifiers and Agitation

Water

Emulsified fat

Oil

Water

Oil droplet attracted to fatty acid core

Water attracted to shell

Phospholipid acting on an emulsifier

Figure 5-12 Emulsifiers in action. Emulsifiers prevent many brands of salad dressings and other condiments from separating into layers of water and fat. Emulsifiers attract fatty acids inside and have a water-attracting group on the outside. Add them to salad dressing, shake well, and they hold the oil in the dressing away from the water. Emulsification is important in both food production and fat digestion/absorption.

The body's main emulsifiers are the lecithins and bile acids, which are produced by the liver and released into the small intestine via the gallbladder during digestion.

Cholesterol in the Body

Cholesterol forms part of some important hormones, such as estrogen, testosterone, and a form of the active vitamin D hormone. Cholesterol is also the building block of bile acids, which are needed for fat digestion. Finally, cholesterol is an essential structural component of cells and the outer layer of particles that transport lipids in the blood. The cholesterol content of the heart, liver, kidney, and brain is quite high, reflecting its critical role in these organs.

About two-thirds of the cholesterol circulating through your body is made by body cells; the remaining one-third is consumed in the diet. Each day, our cells produce approximately 875 milligrams of cholesterol. Of the 875 milligrams of cholesterol made by the body, about 400 milligrams are used to make new bile acids to replenish those lost in the feces, and about 50 milligrams are used to make hormones. In addition to all the cholesterol cells make, we consume about 180 to 325 milligrams of cholesterol per day from animal-derived food products, with men consuming the higher amount compared to women. Absorption of cholesterol from food ranges from about 40% to 65%.

Concept Check

Triglycerides are the major form of fat in the body. They are used for and stored as energy, they insulate and protect body organs, and they transport fat-soluble vitamins. Phospholipids are emulsifiers—compounds that can suspend fat in water. Phospholipids also form parts of cell membranes and various compounds in the body. Cholesterol, a sterol, forms part of cell membranes, hormones, and bile acids. If sufficient amounts are not consumed, the body makes what phospholipids and cholesterol it needs.

Exploring Another Dimension of Fat—Properties in Foods

Since various fats play important roles in foods, much ingenuity must go into the production of reduced-fat products to preserve flavor and texture. In some cases, "fat-free" also means tasteless.

Fat in Food Provides Some Satiety, Flavor, and Texture

Fat in foods has generally been considered to be the most satiating of all the macronutrients. However, this assumption has been called into question because recent studies show that protein and carbohydrate probably lead to the most satiety (gram for gram). High-fat meals do provide satiety, but primarily because one consumes a lot of calories in the process. A high-fat meal is likely to be a high-calorie meal.

Fat components in foods provide important textures and carry flavors. If you've ever eaten a high-fat yellow cheese or cream cheese, you probably agree that fat melting on the tongue feels good. The fat in reduced-fat and whole milk also gives body, which fat-free milk lacks, and the most tender cuts of meat are high in fat, visible as the marbling of meat. In addition, many flavorings dissolve in fat. Heating spices in

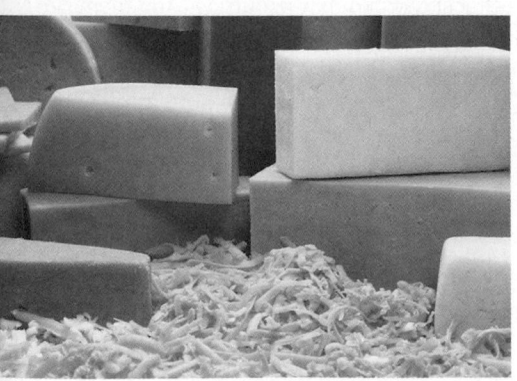

Fat is an important component of the flavor and overall appeal of cheese.

oil intensifies the flavors of an Indian curry or a Mexican dish which are carried to the sensory cells that discriminate taste and smell in the mouth.

Another Bite

A person who has been following a typical North American diet will probably need some time to adjust to the taste of a lower-fat diet. For example, if one changes from the regular use of whole milk to 1% low-fat milk but then after a few weeks switches back to the whole milk, it will taste more like cream than milk. One has thus adjusted to the flavor of the low-fat milk and will likely now find the whole milk to be not as palatable. Emphasizing flavorful fruits, vegetables, and whole grains also helps one to adapt to a low-fat diet. Thus, it is possible to make the change from a higher-fat diet to a lower-fat diet, but it takes some effort.

■ Hydrogenation of Fatty Acids in Food Production Increases Trans Fatty Acid Content

As mentioned previously, most fats with long-chain saturated fatty acids are solid at room temperature, and those with unsaturated fatty acids are liquid at room temperature. In some kinds of food production, solid fats work better than liquid oils. In pie crust, for example, solid fats yield a flaky product, whereas crusts made with liquid oils tend to be greasy and more crumbly. If they are used to replace solid fats, oils with unsaturated fatty acids often must be made more saturated (with hydrogen), as this solidifies the vegetable oils into shortenings and margarines. Hydrogen is added by bubbling hydrogen gas under pressure into liquid vegetable oils in a process called **hydrogenation** (Fig. 5-13). The fatty acids aren't fully hydrogenated

hydrogenation The addition of hydrogen to a carbon-carbon double bond, producing a single carbon-carbon bond with two hydrogens attached to each carbon. Because hydrogenation of unsaturated fatty acids in a vegetable oil increases its hardness, this process is used to convert liquid oils into more solid fats, which are used in making margarine and shortening. *Trans* fatty acids are a by-product of hydrogenation of vegetable oils.

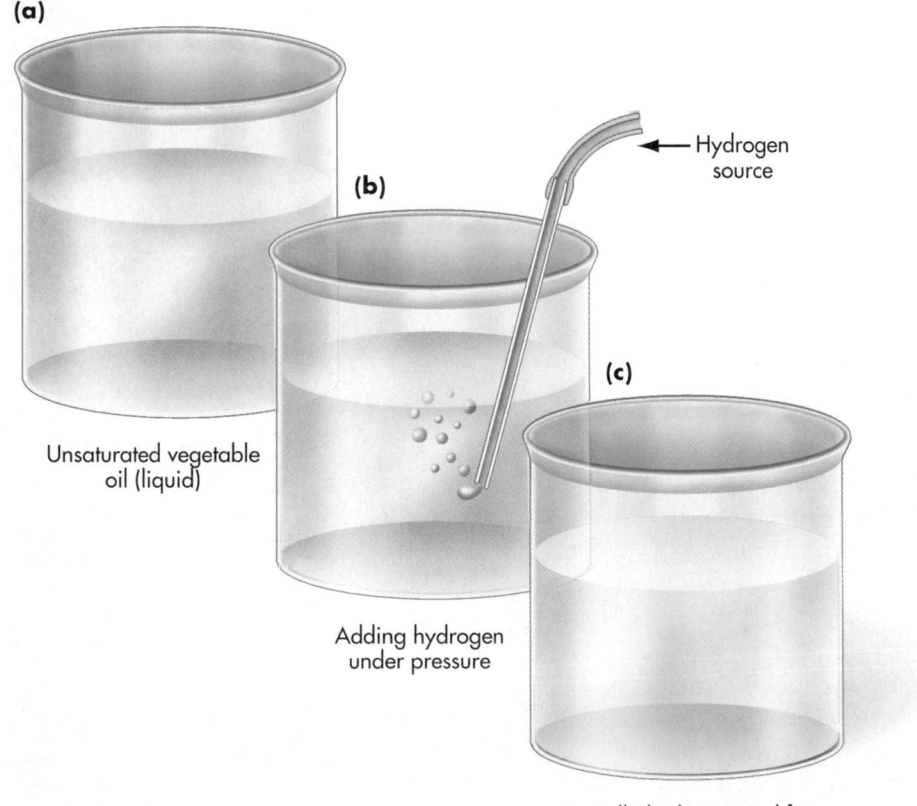

(a)

Unsaturated vegetable oil (liquid)

(b)

← Hydrogen source

Adding hydrogen under pressure

(c)

Partially-hydrogenated fat (semisolid)

Figure 5-13 How liquid oils become solid fats. (a) Unsaturated fatty acids are present in liquid form. (b) Hydrogens are added (hydrogenation), changing some carbon-carbon double bonds to single bonds and producing some *trans* fatty acids. (c) The partially-hydrogenated product is likely to be used in margarine, shortening, or for deep-fat frying.

You may be surprised to learn that some *trans* fatty acids occur naturally. The bacteria that live in the rumens of some animals (cows, sheep, and goats, for example) produce *trans* fatty acids that eventually appear in foods such as beef, milk, and butter. These naturally occurring *trans* fats are currently under study for possible health benefits, including prevention of cancer. About 20% of *trans* fatty acids in our diets come from this source.

Recent studies also indicate that *trans* fats increase overall inflammation in the body, which is not healthful.

to the saturated fatty acid form, as this would make the product too hard and brittle. Partial hydrogenation—leaving some monounsaturated fatty acids—creates a semisolid product.

The process of hydrogenation produces *trans* fatty acids as was described earlier in this chapter. Most natural monounsaturated and polyunsaturated fatty acids exist in the *cis* form, causing a bend in the carbon chain, whereas the straighter carbon forms of *trans* fat more closely resemble saturated fatty acids. This may be the mechanism whereby *trans* fat increase(s) LDL. In addition, *trans* fat also lower(s) HDL. Thus, people with elevated LDL especially should limit intake of partially-hydrogenated fat and thus *trans* fat. This may not be such a concern for the average person, as long as *trans* fat intake is not excessive and the diet is adequate in polyunsaturated fat. However, since *trans* fatty acids serve no particular role in maintaining body health, the latest Dietary Guidelines for Americans, the American Heart Association, and the Food and Nutrition Board each recommend minimal *trans* fat intake.

As public pressure has persuaded manufacturers to eliminate the tropical oils rich in saturated fat (palm, palm olein, and coconut) from food processing, partially-hydrogenated soybean oil—rich in *trans* fat—has become the major replacement. Currently, *trans* fat intake in North America is estimated to contribute about 3% to 4% of total calories, amounting to 10 grams per day, on average. Table 5-3 lists typical sources.

FDA is now requiring the *trans* fat content in foods on food labels (review Fig 5-6). The food labels in Canada also must list *trans* fat content. FDA hopes to make consumers more aware of the amounts of *trans* fat in foods as well as the negative health consequences associated with their excessive consumption. North American companies are already responding to this issue by creating products that are free of *trans* fat. For example, Promise, Smart Beat, and some Fleischmann's margarines are lower in or free of *trans* fat (less than 0.5 grams per serving) compared to typical margarines.

This addition of the *trans* fat listing on labels helps consumers at the supermarket, but when dining out, consumers are "left in the dark" as to which foods contain *trans* fat. Knowing which foods are low in *trans* fat when ordering at a restaurant is difficult because information about preparation methods and precise fat composition is rarely

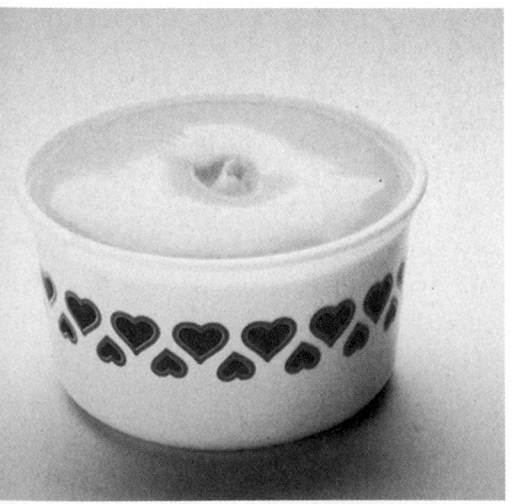

Tub margarine is much lower in *trans* fat than stick margarine or shortenings. Some newer brands of tub margarines are even free of *trans* fatty acids.

Table 5-3 Total Fat, Saturated Fat, and *Trans* Fat Content of Typical Sources of *Trans* Fat

Food Item	Serving Size	Fat (grams)	Saturated Fat (grams)	*Trans* Fat (grams)
French fried potatoes (fast-food variety)	Medium size	26.9	6.7	7.8
Butter	1 tbsp	10.8	7.2	0.3
Margarine, stick	1 tbsp	11.0	2.1	2.8
Margarine, tub	1 tbsp	6.7	1.2	0.6
Mayonnaise (soybean oil)	1 tbsp	10.8	1.6	0
Shortening	1 tbsp	13.0	3.4	4.2
Potato Chips	Small bag	11.2	1.9	3.2
Milk, whole	1 cup	6.6	4.3	0.2
Doughnut	1	18.2	4.7	5.0
Cookies (cream filled)	3	6.1	1.2	1.9
Cake, pound	1 slice	16.4	3.4	4.3

Source: http://www.cfsan.fda.gov/~dms/qatrans2.html

available. To minimize *trans* fat intake, a general guideline is to limit consumption of fried (especially deep-fat fried) food items, any pastries or flaky bread products (such as pie crusts, crackers, croissants, and biscuits), and cookies.

Until all foods are labeled with *trans* fat content, consumers can also make educated guesses on the *trans* fat content of foods by examining the list of ingredients on the food label. If partially-hydrogenated vegetable oil is one of the first three ingredients on the label, you can assume there is a significant amount of *trans* fat in the product.

Limiting *trans* fat at home is a much easier task. Most importantly, use little or no stick margarine or shortening. Instead, substitute vegetable oils and softer tub margarines (whose labels list vegetable oil or water as the first ingredient). Avoid deep-fat frying any food in shortening. Substitute baking, panfrying, broiling, steaming, grilling, or deep-fat frying in unhydrogenated vegetable oils. Replace nondairy creamers with reduced-fat or fat-free milk, since most nondairy creamers are rich in partially-hydrogenated vegetable oils. Finally, read the ingredients on food labels, using the tips above to estimate *trans* fat content.

■ Fat Rancidity Limits Shelf Life of Foods

Decomposing oils emit a disagreeable odor and taste sour and stale. Stale potato chips are a good example. The double bonds in unsaturated fatty acids break down, producing rancid by-products. Ultraviolet light, oxygen, and certain procedures can break double bonds and, in turn, destroy the structure of polyunsaturated fatty acids. Saturated fats and *trans* fats can much more readily resist these effects because they contain fewer carbon-carbon double bonds.

Rancidity is not a major problem for consumers because, although eating rancid oils can cause sickness, the odor and taste generally discourage us from eating enough to become sick. However, rancidity is a problem for manufacturers because it reduces a product's shelf life. To increase shelf life, manufacturers often add partially-hydrogenated plant oils to products. Foods most likely to become rancid are deep-fried foods and foods with a large amount of exposed surface (such as powdered eggs or powdered milk). The fat in fish is also very susceptible to rancidity because it is highly polyunsaturated.

Antioxidants such as vitamin E help protect foods against rancidity. Antioxidants guard against the fat breakdown caused by various agents, such as metals found as impurities in vegetable oils. The vitamin E in plant oils reduces the breakdown of double bonds in fatty acids. (The role of vitamin E is explained more fully in Chapter 8.) When food manufacturers want to prevent rancidity in polyunsaturated fats, they often add the synthetic antioxidants **BHA** and **BHT**. (Chapter 16 discusses the safety of these and other food additives.) Look for these food additives in salad dressings, cake mixes, and other products that contain fat. They can even be added to a food's paper packaging. Vitamin C may also be added for the same reason. Manufacturers also tightly seal products and use other methods to reduce oxygen levels inside packages.

■ Emulsifiers Improve Many Food Products

Food manufacturers add emulsifiers in the preparation of many food products, primarily to improve texture. For example, lecithins, monoglycerides and diglycerides, polysorbate 60, and other emulsifiers are added to salad dressings to keep the vegetable oil suspended in water (review Fig. 5-12). Eggs added to cake batters likewise emulsify the fat with the milk. Monoglycerides and related compounds are also good emulsifiers and, for that reason, are sometimes used in cake mixes and salad dressings. Over the next few days, examine the labels of salad dressings and cake mixes, and see how many emulsifiers are listed.

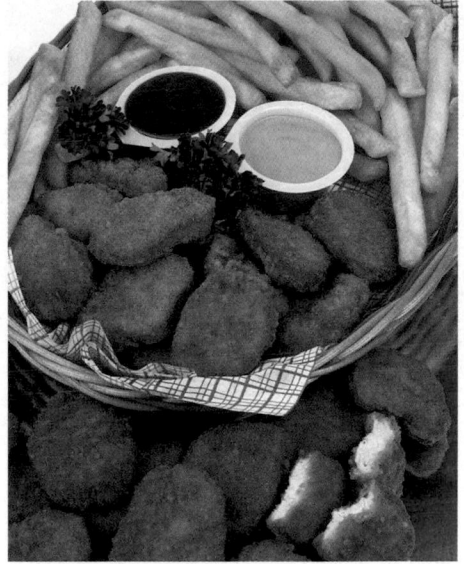

French fries and other fried foods are a common source of fat and *trans* fatty acids for many adults. For those who choose to consume these products on a regular basis a small serving size is recommended, especially if a person has elevated blood lipids.

BHA, BHT Butylated hydroxyanisole and butylated hydroxytoluene—two common synthetic antioxidants added to foods.

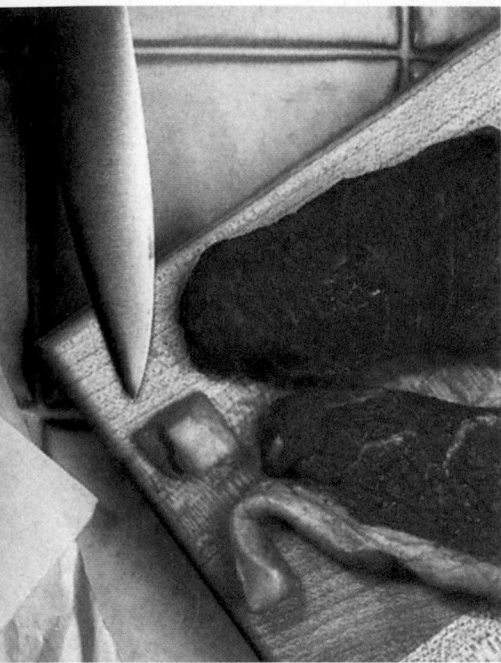

Trim the fat from meats before cooking to help reduce your saturated fat intake. Also, limit use of meat that is highly marbled with fat (seen as streaks of fat).

Moderating alcohol and sugar intake, avoiding overeating and obesity, consuming fish on a regular basis, not smoking, and performing regular physical activity are the primary lifestyle interventions to lower blood triglycerides.

One goal of *Healthy People 2010* is to increase the proportion of persons age 2 years and older who consume less than 10% of calorie intake from saturated fat.

Concept Check

Fat has a variety of roles in foods, including that of contributing to flavor and texture. Fat also provides the pleasurable mouth feel of many of our favorite foods, intensifies the taste of many spices, and tenderizes many popular cuts of meat.

Hydrogenation of unsaturated fatty acids is the process of adding hydrogen to carbon-carbon double bonds to produce single bonds. This results in the creation of some *trans* fatty acids. Hydrogenation changes vegetable oil to solid fat. It is wise to monitor *trans* fat intake, as this form of fat raises LDL and lowers HDL.

The carbon-carbon double bonds in polyunsaturated fatty acids are easily broken, yielding products responsible for rancidity. The presence of antioxidants, such as vitamin E in oils, naturally protects unsaturated fatty acids against oxidative destruction. Manufacturers can use hydrogenated fats and add natural or synthetic antioxidants to reduce the likelihood of rancidity.

Emulsifiers, such as lecithins, monoglycerides and diglycerides, and polysorbate 60 are added to salad dressings and other fat-rich products to keep the vegetable oils and other fats suspended in the water.

Recommendations for Fat Intake

There is no RDA for total fat intake for adults, although there is an Adequate Intake set for total fat for infants (see Chapter 14). The most specific recommendations for fat intake come from the American Heart Association (AHA). Because many North Americans are at risk for developing cardiovascular disease, AHA promotes dietary and lifestyle goals aimed at reducing this risk. The AHA recommendations for the general public are presented in Table 5-4. In Table 5-5, a more detailed list of recommendations is provided for those who currently are at high risk or have cardiovascular disease.

To reduce risk for cardiovascular disease, the AHA recommends that total fat intake should not exceed 20% to 30% of total calories, which equates to 47 to 70 grams per day for a person who consumes 2100 kcal daily. Within that fat allowance, no more than 7% to 10% of total calories should come from saturated fat and *trans* fat combined. These are the primary fatty acids that raise LDL. In addition, cholesterol should amount to a maximum of 200 to 300 mg per day. This often goes along with the reduction in saturated fat and *trans* fat intake. Table 5-6 is an example of a diet that adheres to these guidelines. Compare these recommendations to the actual dietary intake patterns of these fats currently by North Americans: 33% of calories from total fat, about 13% of calories from saturated fat, and 180 to 320 milligrams of cholesterol each day.

Table 5-4 Current Dietary Guidance for the General Population (2 Years of Age and Older) from the American Heart Association

Population Goals	Major Guidelines
Overall healthy eating pattern	Include a variety of fruits, vegetables, grains, low-fat or fat-free dairy products, fish, legumes, poultry, lean meats.
Appropriate body weight	Match calorie intake to overall needs, with appropriate changes to achieve weight loss when indicated.
Desirable blood cholesterol profile	Limit foods high in saturated fat and cholesterol; and substitute unsaturated fat from vegetables, fish, legumes, nuts.
Desirable blood pressure	Limit salt and alcohol (see Table 5-5); maintain a healthy body weight; and follow a diet with emphasis on vegetables, fruits, and fat-free or fat-free dairy products.

Table 5-5 Specific Dietary Recommendations from American Heart Association, Especially for Those People at High Risk or Who Currently Have Cardiovascular Disease

Diet	**Consume at least:**
	5 servings of fruits and vegetables each day. Up to 9 servings per day is advised if the person has hypertension.
	6 servings of grains, including some whole grains, each day.
	At least 2 (3 ounce) servings of fish per week (or 1 gram of a combination of omega-3 fatty acids from fish oil supplements per day).
	25 grams of fiber each day, including some sources of soluble fiber.†
	Consume no more than:
	30% of calories from total fat or 20% if blood lipids are still too high.
	10% of calories as saturated fat, or 7% if blood lipids are still too high, as well as limit *trans* fat intake (included in saturated fat gram allowance).
	300 milligrams of cholesterol per day (on average), or 200 milligrams per day if blood lipids are still too high or the person has diabetes or cardiovascular disease.
	6 grams of salt each day (6 grams equals 2400 milligrams of sodium).
	2 alcoholic drinks per day for men or one drink for women or anyone age 65 and older.
	Additional advice includes:
	Specifically meeting vitamin B-6, folate, vitamin B-12, and potassium needs, limiting sugar intake, and possible use of soy protein and stanol/sterol-containing margarines. Megadose vitamin E supplements are not recommended at this time, and vitamin C and beta-carotene supplements provide no benefit.
Body weight	Maintain a **body mass index** between 18.5 and 25. Waist circumference should not exceed 40 inches (102 centimeters) in men or 35 inches (88 centimeters) in women.
Physical activity	30 to 60 minutes of brisk activity on most, if not all, days of the week.

These specific recommendations apply to individuals 2 years of age and older. The latest guidelines from the National Cholesterol Education Program in the United States also concur with this advice for high-risk individuals, except that fat could be as high as 35% of total calories if saturated fat intake is 7% of calories or less and cholesterol intake does not exceed 200 milligrams per day.

†Note that the latest guidance for fiber from the Food and Nutrition Board is that men consume 38 grams per day, while 25 grams per day is fine for women.

For raising HDL, exercising for at least 45 minutes four times a week can increase it by about 5 mg/dl. Losing excess weight (especially around the waist) and avoiding smoking and overeating also help maintain or raise HDL, as does moderate alcohol consumption.

body mass index Weight (in kilograms) divided by height squared (in meters). A healthy value is 18.5 to 24.9. A value of 25 or greater indicates a risk for body weight-related health disorders. 1 BMI unit equals 6 to 7 pounds.

Both the National Cholesterol Education Program (NCEP) and the Food and Nutrition Board are in agreement with the advice of the AHA. One exception in the latest guidelines from the NCEP is that fat intake could be as high as 35% of total calories as long as intakes of saturated fat, cholesterol, and *trans* fat are minimized. The Food and Nutrition Board combines the AHA and NCEP recommendations, suggesting that fat provide a range of 20% to 35% of calories. (The 2005 Dietary Guidelines also support this advice.) It is important to note that in addition to fat intake, controlling total calorie intake is also significant, as weight control is a vital component of cardiovascular disease prevention.

Regarding essential fatty acids, the Food and Nutrition Board has issued recommendations for both omega-6 and omega-3 fatty acids. The amounts listed below work out to about 5% of calorie intake for the total of both essential fatty acids. Infants and children have lower needs (again, see Chapter 14). Consumption of fish at least twice a week is one step toward meeting requirements for essential fatty acids.

Meeting calcium needs is also important as studies show calcium in the intestinal tract can find saturated fatty acids and inhibit their absorption.

	Men (grams per day)	Women (grams per day)
Linoleic acid (omega-6)	17	12
Alpha-linolenic acid (omega-3)	1.6	1.1

Table 5-6 Daily Menu Examples Containing 2,000 kcal and 30% or 20% of Calories as Fat

30% of Calories as Fat		20% of Calories as Fat	
Food	Fat (grams)	Food	Fat (grams)
Breakfast			
Orange juice, 1 cup	0.5	Same	0.5
Shredded wheat, ¾ cup	0.5	Shredded wheat, 1 cup	0.7
Toasted bagel	1.1	Same	1.1
Tub margarine, 3 teaspoons	11.4	Tub margarine, 2 teaspoons	7.6
1% low-fat milk, 1 cup	2.5	Fat-free milk, 1 cup	0.6
Lunch			
Whole-wheat bread, 2 slices	2.4	Same	2.4
Roast beef, 2 ounces	4.9	Light turkey roll, 2 ounces	0.9
Mayonnaise, 3 teaspoons	11.0	Mayonnaise, 2 teaspoons	7.3
Lettuce	—	Same	—
Tomato	—	Same	—
Oatmeal cookie, 1	3.3	Oatmeal cookie, 2	6.6
Snack			
Apple	—	Same	—
Dinner			
Chicken tenders frozen meal	18.0	Fat-free chicken tenders	—
Dinner roll, 1	2.0	Same	2.0
Margarine, 1 teaspoon	3.8	Same	3.8
Banana	0.6	Same	0.6
1% low-fat milk, 1 cup	2.5	Fat-free milk, 1 cup	0.6
Snack			
Raisins, 2 teaspoons	—	Raisins, ½ cup	—
Air-popped popcorn, 3 cups	1.0	Air-popped popcorn, 6 cups	2.0
Margarine, 2 teaspoons	7.6	Same	7.6
Totals	**73.1**		**44.3**

Some advice regarding fat intake from the 2005 Dietary Guidelines:

- Limit intake of fats and oils high in saturated and/or *trans* fatty acids, and choose products low in such fats and oils.
- Consume fats high in polyunsaturated and monounsaturated fatty acids, such as from fish, nuts, and vegetable oils.
- When selecting and preparing meat, poultry, dry beans, and milk or milk products, make choices that are lean, low-fat, or fat-free.

vegan A person who eats only plant foods.

The typical North American diet derives about 7% of calories from polyunsaturated fatty acids, and thus meets essential fatty acid needs. An upper limit of 10% of calorie intake as polyunsaturated fatty acids is often recommended, in part because the breakdown (oxidation) of those present in lipoproteins is linked to increased cholesterol deposition in the arteries (review the Looking Further section in this chapter). Depression of immune function is also suspected to be caused by an excessive intake of polyunsaturated fatty acids.

Major sources of fat in the typical North American diet include animal flesh, whole milk, pastries, cheese, margarine, and mayonnaise. In contrast, the major sources of fat in the Mediterranean diet include liberal amounts of olive oil and the fat found in the small amounts of animal flesh and dairy products in the diet. The main sources of fat in Dr. Dean Ornish's purely vegetarian (**vegan**) diet plan are a scant amount of vegetable oil used in cooking and the small amounts found in various plant foods.

Monitoring by a physician is important if fat is restricted to 20% of calories, as the resulting increase in carbohydrate intake can increase blood triglycerides in some people, which is not a healthful change. Over time, however, the initial problem of high blood triglycerides on a low-fat diet may self-correct, as has been shown in people following the Dr. Dean Ornish vegan diet for a year or more. Their blood triglycerides increased initially on the diet but, within a year, fell to normal values as long as they emphasized carbohydrate sources high in fiber, controlled (or improved) body weight, and followed a regular exercise program.

Another Bite

The advice to consume 20% to 30% of calories as fat does not apply to infants and toddlers below the age of 2 years. These youngsters are forming new tissue that requires fat, especially in the brain, so their intake of fat and cholesterol should not be greatly restricted.

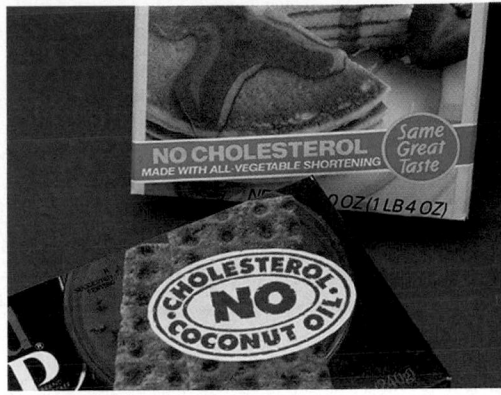

Manufacturers now offer a variety of low-cholesterol foods.

Recently some researchers have proposed that fat may comprise as much as 40% of total calorie intake, as long as saturated fat and *trans* fat intake is minimal and body weight is maintained (or improved). This change in advice is discussed in the book by Dr. Walter C. Willett, entitled *Eat, Drink, and Be Healthy* (2001). The diet plan in the book emphasizes whole grains, plant oils, abundant vegetables, at least 2 to 3 servings of fruit per day, nuts and legumes one to three times per day, fish, poultry, and eggs zero to two times per day, good sources of calcium one to two times per day, and little use of red meat, butter, white rice, white bread, potatoes, pasta, and sweets. Overall, this diet especially avoids simple sugars and refined carbohydrates because diets high in these constituents tend to raise blood triglycerides in some people. Diets high in these carbohydrates are discouraged, especially if a person is overweight (and therefore potentially insulin-resistant) and performs little physical activity (regular physical activity increases carbohydrate use). Table 5-7 shows a diet that contains 40% calories as fat and follows the plan promoted by Dr. Willett. This type of diet is also advocated for people who have the metabolic syndrome (also called *Syndrome X*). Note that about 25% of North American adults are so affected. Still, neither the American Heart Association nor the Food and Nutrition Board endorses such a high fat intake.

Most people probably have no idea how much of the calories in their diets comes from fat. You've already tracked your food intake for one day. A Rate Your Plate exercise at the end of this chapter asks you to compare your fat intake with current guidelines. Using the information on food labels and recording and analyzing daily food intake also allow you to track fat intake.

Table 5-7 A Sample Menu That Follows Dr. Willett's Proposed Diet Plan from *Eat, Drink, and Be Healthy*

Food
Breakfast
¾ cup fresh orange juice
1 whole-grain bagel
2 teaspoons soft *trans* fat-free margarine
Snack
1 cup raw carrots
2 celery stalks
3 tablespoons smooth *trans* fat-free peanut butter
Lunch
¾ cup apple juice
Sandwich:
2 slices whole-wheat bread, 2 teaspoons mayonnaise, 2 ounces light meat turkey, 2 pieces of lettuce, and 1 slice of tomato
Salad:
1½ cups tossed salad greens, 3 tablespoons Italian salad dressing, 2 teaspoons dry sunflower seeds, 1 ounce low-fat cheddar cheese, ¼ cup green pepper slices, and 3 baby carrots
Snack
1 cup fresh strawberries
½ cup plain fat-free yogurt

(Continued)

Table 5-7 (Continued)

Dinner
1 cup V8 juice
3.5 ounces broiled chicken breast
⅛ cup Italian dressing (marinade)
⅔ cup brown rice
2 teaspoons soft *trans* fat-free margarine
½ cup green beans
2 teaspoons soft *trans* fat-free margarine
1 cup grapes

Snack
3 cups air-popped popcorn

This diet provides 2,400 kcal. Although this diet supplies 40% (107 grams) of these calories as fat, saturated fat is limited to 7% (19 grams) of total calorie intake. Whether monounsaturated fat or polyunsaturated fat would dominate depends on the type of oil used for salad dressings, such as canola oil for monounsaturated fat versus corn oil for polyunsaturated fat. Use of a vegetable oil rich in monounsaturated fat is preferable. The cholesterol content is 180 milligrams. The *trans* fat content is less than 1% of the calories.

In summary, the general consensus among nutrition experts suggests that limitation of saturated fat, cholesterol, and *trans* fat intake should be the primary focus, and that the diet needs to contain some omega-3 and omega-6 fatty acids (Table 5-8). Furthermore, if fat intake exceeds 30% of total calories, the extra fat should come from monounsaturated fat.

Table 5-8 Tips for Avoiding Too Much Fat, Saturated Fat, Cholesterol, and *Trans* Fat

	Eat Less of These Foods	Eat More of These Foods
Grains, cereals, rice, & pasta	• Pasta dishes with cheese or cream sauces • Croissants • Pie crust	• Whole-grain breads • Whole-grain pasta • Brown rice
Vegetables	• French fries • Vegetables cooked in butter, cheese, or cream sauces	• Fresh, frozen, baked, or steamed vegetables
Fruit	• Fruit pies	• Fresh, frozen, or canned fruits
Milk, yogurt, and cheese	• Whole milk • High-fat cheese	• Fat-free and reduced-fat milk • Reduced-fat/part-skim cheese
Meats, poultry, fish, dry beans, eggs, and nuts	• Bacon • Sausage • Organ meats (e.g., liver) • Egg yolks	• Fish • Skinless poultry • Lean cuts of meat (with fat trimmed away) • Soy products • Egg whites/egg substitutes
Fats, oils, and sweets	• Butter and stick margarine • Cheesecake • Pastries • Doughnuts • Ice cream • Potato chips	• Angel food cake • Fig bars • Animal or graham crackers • Air-popped popcorn • Low-fat frozen desserts (e.g., yogurt, sherbet, ice milk) • Canola oil or olive oil • Tub or liquid margarine (in small amounts)

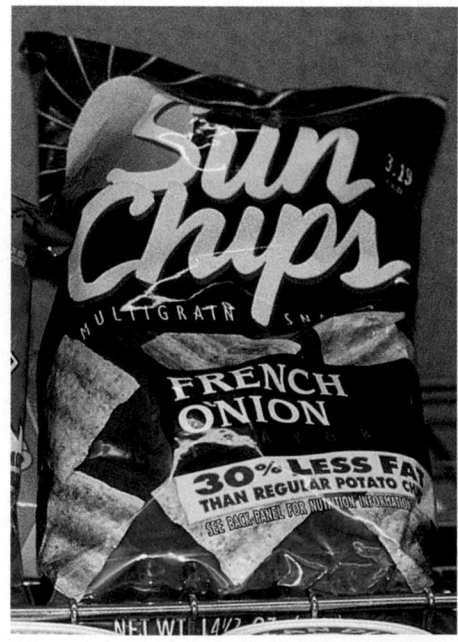

Many manufacturers offer products that are lower in fat than the traditional product. Even though these products are lower in fat, portion size and the total calories supplied still must be considered.

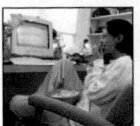

Real Life Scenario Follow-Up

Jackie's approach to lowering blood cholesterol does not incorporate the best choices; she has excluded a great deal of fat in her diet by merely replacing it with refined carbohydrates. To make a shift to a more heart-healthy diet, Jackie would need to include at least 2 cups of fruit and 3 cups of vegetables a day, along with more whole-grain products (such as whole-wheat bread and a breakfast cereal that has at least 3 grams of fiber per serving). Lowering fat as drastically as she has is not really necessary, especially for a 21-year-old female who is physically active. Jackie could allow a more liberal amount of fat in her diet by including more monounsaturated fats (canola oil and olive oil, as well as fats found in nuts and avocados). These do not increase blood cholesterol. In addition to allowing more liberal fat intake from monounsaturated oils and including more fruits, vegetables, and whole grains, Jackie would benefit from including good sources of omega-3 fatty acids (fatty fish, flaxseeds, walnuts, or soybean and canola oil). One option is to use a canola oil-and-vinegar dressing on her salad, rather than lemon juice.

Medical Interventions to Lower Blood Lipids

Some people need even more aggressive therapy added to their regimen of a diet and lifestyle overhaul to treat elevated blood lipids. The clearest indication for this more aggressive approach is in people who already have had a heart attack or have cardiovascular disease symptoms or diabetes.

Medications are the cornerstone of this more aggressive therapy. The National Cholesterol Education Program in the United States has developed a formula based on age, total blood cholesterol, HDL-cholesterol, smoking history, and blood pressure to determine who needs such medications. Check out this formula at www.nhlbi.nih.gov/atpiii/calculator.asp?usertype=pvb. This formula provides an estimate for having a heart attack in the next 10 years. Currently, medications work to lower LDL in one of two ways. Some reduce cholesterol synthesis in the liver. Such medicines are known as "statins" (e.g., atorvistatin [Lipitor]). The cost of treatment with one of these drugs ranges from $600 to $3,000 per year, depending on the dose needed. These medications lead to problems in some people, and so require physician monitoring. The other group of medications binds bile acids or the cholesterol that is part of bile secreted into the small intestine. This binding leads to their elimination in the feces and so requires the liver to synthesize new bile acids and/or cholesterol. The liver removes LDL from the blood to do this. Some of these medications taste gritty and therefore are not very popular. Use of one or both of these classes of medications should ideally drive LDL down to less than 70 mg/dl—the current therapeutic goal for people with (or at high risk for) cardiovascular disease (Table 5-9).

A third group of drugs can be used to lower blood triglycerides by decreasing the triglyceride production of the liver. These include gemfibrozil (Lopid) and megadoses of the vitamin nicotinic acid. The use of nicotinic acid does result in pesky side effects, however, but these are typically manageable.

■ Other Possible Medical Therapies for Cardiovascular Disease

FDA has approved two margarines that have positive effects on blood cholesterol levels—Benecol and Take Control. These margarines contain plant stanols/sterols. The plant stanols/sterols work by reducing cholesterol absorption in the small intestine and lowering its return to the liver. The liver responds by taking up more cholesterol from the blood so it can continue to make bile acids. The studies done on the

As noted earlier, aspirin in small doses reduces blood clotting. It is often used under a physician's guidance to treat people at risk for heart attack or stroke, especially if one has already occurred. About 80 to 160 milligrams per day is needed for such benefits. Individuals who may especially benefit from aspirin therapy are men over 40, smokers, postmenopausal women, and people with diabetes, hypertension, or a family history of cardiovascular disease.

Table 5-9 Sorting out one's goals for cardiovascular disease prevention/treatment

Risk Class	This is you if . . .	Your LDL (mg/dl) goal
Very high	You have cardiovascular disease *and* other risk factors such as diabetes, obesity, smoking	Below 70
High	You have cardiovascular disease *or* diabetes *or* two or more risk factors for cardiovascular disease (e.g., smoking, hypertension)	Below 100
Moderately high	You have cardiovascular disease risks and an increased 10-year risk of developing a heart attack	100–130
Moderate	You have 2 or more risk factors and a marginal chance of developing cardiovascular disease in the next 10 years.	Below 130
Low	You have few or no cardiovascular disease risk factors	Below 160

The two most common surgical treatments for coronary artery blockage are percutaneous transluminal coronary angioplasty (PTCA) and coronary artery bypass graft (CABG). PTCA involves the insertion of a balloon catheter into an artery. Once it is advanced to the area of the lesion, the balloon is expanded to crush the lesion. This method works best when only one vessel is blocked, and it may be held open with metal mesh, called a stent. CABG involves the removal and use of a saphenous vein from the leg or use of a mammary artery. The saphenous vein is sewn to the main heart vessel (aorta) and then used to by-pass the blocked artery, as is the mammary artery. The procedure can be performed on one or more blockages.

cholesterol-lowering effect of these margarines have found that 2 to 5 grams of plant stanols/sterols per day reduces total blood cholesterol by 8% to 10% and LDL-cholesterol by 9% to 14% (similar to what is seen with some cholesterol-lowering drugs).

Benecol is made from plant stanols which are extracted from wood pulp. This product is sold as margarine and has been added to salad dressings. Take Control is made from plant sterols which are isolated from soybeans. The recommended amount for both is about 2 to 3 grams per day as part of at least two meals; this works out to about 2 tablespoons of Take Control or 1 tablespoon of Benecol per day. Use would cost about $1.00 per day, as these margarines are more expensive than regular margarines.

In people who have borderline high total blood cholesterol (between 200 and 239 mg/dl), these margarines can be helpful in avoiding future drug therapy. Recently plant stanols/sterols have been made available in pill form as well.

Concept Check

There is no RDA for fat. We need about 5% of total calorie intake from plant oils to obtain the needed essential fatty acids. Eating fatty fish at least twice a week is also advised to supply omega-3 fatty acids. Many health-related agencies recommend a diet containing no more than 35% of calorie intake as fat, with no more than 7% to 10% of calorie intake as a combination of saturated fat and *trans* fat for the general public. Cholesterol intake should be limited to 200 to 300 milligrams per day. These practices help maintain a normal LDL value in the blood. Medications such as "statins" may be added to lower LDL even more. The current North American diet contains about 33% of calories as fat, with about 13% of calories as saturated fat and about 3% as *trans* fatty acids. Cholesterol intake varies from about 200 to 400 milligrams per day.

Summary

1. Compared with carbohydrates and proteins, lipids are a group of relatively oxygen-poor compounds that do not dissolve in water. Saturated fatty acids contain no carbon-carbon double bonds, monounsaturated fatty acids contain one carbon-carbon double bond, and polyunsaturated fatty acids contain two or more carbon-carbon double bonds in the carbon chain.

2. In omega-3 polyunsaturated fatty acids, the first of the carbon-carbon double bonds is located three carbons from the methyl end of the carbon chain. In omega-6 polyunsaturated fatty acids, the first carbon-carbon double bond counting from the methyl end occurs at the sixth carbon. Both omega-3 and omega-6 fatty acids are essential fatty acids; these must be included in the diet to maintain health.

3. Triglycerides are formed from a glycerol backbone with three fatty acids. Triglycerides rich in long-chain saturated fatty acids tend to be solid at room temperature, whereas those rich in

monounsaturated and polyunsaturated fatty acids are liquid at room temperature. Triglyceride is the major form of fat in both food and the body. It allows for efficient energy storage, protects certain organs, transports fat-soluble vitamins, and helps insulate the body.

4. Phospholipids are derivatives of triglycerides in which one or two of the fatty acids are replaced by phosphorus-containing compounds. Phospholipids are important parts of cell membranes, and some act as efficient emulsifiers.

5. Cholesterol forms vital biological compounds, such as hormones, components of cell membranes, and bile acids. Cells in the body make cholesterol whether we eat it or not. It is not a necessary part of an adult's diet.

6. Body cells can synthesize hormone-like compounds from both omega-3 and omega-6 fatty acids. These compounds produced from omega-3 fatty acids tend to reduce blood clotting, blood pressure, and inflammatory responses in the body. Those produced from omega-6 fatty acids tend to increase blood clotting.

7. Foods rich in fat include salad oils, butter, margarine, and mayonnaise. Nuts, bologna, avocados, and bacon are also high in fat, as are peanut butter and cheddar cheese. Steak and hamburger are moderate in fat content, as is whole milk. Many grain products, and fruits and vegetables in general, are very low in fat.

8. Fat digestion takes place primarily in the small intestine. Lipase enzyme released from the pancreas digests long-chain triglycerides into smaller breakdown products—namely, monoglycerides (glycerol backbones with single fatty acids attached) and fatty acids. The breakdown products are then taken up by the absorptive cells of the small intestine. These products are mostly remade into triglycerides and eventually enter the lymphatic system, in turn passing into the bloodstream.

9. Lipids are carried in the bloodstream by various lipoproteins, which consist of a central triglyceride core encased in a shell of protein, cholesterol, and phospholipid. Chylomicrons are released from intestinal cells and carry lipids arising from dietary intake. Very-low-density lipoprotein (VLDL) and low-density lipoprotein (LDL) carry lipids both taken up by and synthesized in the liver. High-density lipoprotein (HDL) picks up cholesterol from cells and acts in allowing transport of it back to the liver.

10. In the blood, elevated amounts of LDL and low amounts of HDL are strong predictors of the risk for cardiovascular disease. Additional risk factors for the disease are smoking, hypertension, diabetes, obesity, and inactivity.

11. Fats and oils have several functions as components of foods. Fats add flavor and texture to foods and provide some satiety after meals. Some phospholipids are used in foods as emulsifiers, which suspend fat in water. When fatty acids break down, food becomes rancid, resulting in a foul odor and unpleasant flavor.

12. Hydrogenation is the process of converting carbon-carbon double bonds into single bonds by adding hydrogen at the point of unsaturation. The partial-hydrogenation of fatty acids in vegetable oils changes the oils to semisolid fats and helps in food formulation and reduces rancidity. Hydrogenation also increases *trans* fatty acid content. High amounts of *trans* fat in the diet are discouraged, as these increase LDL and reduce HDL.

13. There is currently no RDA for fat for adults. Plant oils should contribute about 5% of total calories to achieve the Adequate Intakes proposed for essential fatty acids (linoleic acid and alpha-linolenic acid). Fatty fish are a rich source of omega-3 fatty acids and should be consumed at least twice a week.

14. Many health agencies and scientific groups suggest a fat intake of no more than 30% to 35% of total calories. Some health experts advocate an even further reduction to 20% of calorie intake for some people to maintain a normal LDL value, but such a diet requires professional guidance. Medications such as "statins" may be added also to lower LDL. If fat intake exceeds 30% of total calories, the diet should emphasize monounsaturated fat. The typical North American diet contains about 33% of total calories as fat.

Study Questions

1. Describe the chemical structures of saturated and polyunsaturated fatty acids and their different effects in both food and the human body.

2. Relate the need for omega-3 fatty acids in the diet to the recommendation to consume fatty fish at least twice a week.

3. Describe the structures, origins, and roles of the four major blood lipoproteins.

4. What are the recommendations from various health-care organizations regarding fat intake? What does this mean in terms of actual food choices?

5. What are two important attributes of fat in food? How are these different from the general functions of lipids in the human body?

6. Describe the significance of and possible uses for reduced-fat foods.

7. Does the total cholesterol concentration in the bloodstream tell the whole story with respect to cardiovascular disease risk?

8. List the four main risk factors for the development of cardiovascular disease.

9. What three lifestyle factors decrease the risk of cardiovascular disease development?

10. When are medications most needed in cardiovascular disease therapy, and how in general do the various classes of medications operate to reduce risk?

Further Readings

1. ADA Reports: Position of the American Dietetic Association: Fat replacers. *Journal of the American Dietetic Association* 105:266, 2005.

   The majority of fat replacers, when used in moderation by adults, can be safe and useful adjuncts to lowering the fat content of foods, and may play a role in decreasing total calorie and fat intake. Still, consumers should not be led to believe that fat and calorie-reduced products can be consumed in unlimited amounts

2. Cholesterol: How low should you go? *Consumer Reports on Health*, p. 8, March 2004.

   Good review of the diet and medication regimens used to lower blood cholesterol. Despite the power of medications to lower blood cholesterol, lifestyle changes are also needed to get the full effect of the medications.

3. Coronary bypass: *Mayo Clinic Health Letter* 22(4):1, 2004.

   Complete description of coronary bypass surgery is provided. This will help you learn more about this common procedure to treat cardiovascular disease.

4. Covington MB: Omega-3 fatty acids. *American Family Physician* 70(1):133, 2004.

   Omega-3 fatty acids can reduce the risk of sudden cardiac death in people with cardiovascular disease. These fatty acids also have anti-inflammatory effects. Fatty fish such as salmon are rich in omega-3 fatty acids.

5. Coulston AM and Peragallo-Ditto KV: Insulin resistance syndrome: A potent culprit in cardiovascular disease. *Journal of the American Dietetic Association* 104(2):176, 2004.

   Insulin resistance as evidenced by mild increases in fasting blood glucose leads to many deleterious effects on the body. Weight loss (when needed) along with regular physical activity and a diet rich in whole grains, fruits, vegetables, and low-fat dairy products helps treat the condition.

6. Djousse L and others: Fruit and vegetable consumption and LDL cholesterol. *American Journal of Clinical Nutrition* 79:213, 2004.

   Regular fruit and vegetable intake can reduce LDL cholesterol. It is important to put his recommendation into practice.

7. Food and Nutrition Board: *Dietary reference intakes for energy, carbohydrate, fiber, fat, fatty acids, cholesterol, protein, and amino acids.* Washington DC: The National Academy Press, 2002.

   This report provides the latest guidance for macronutrient intakes. With regard to fat intake, Adequate Intakes were set for omega-6 and omega-3 fatty acids. Intake of total fat can range from 20% to 35% of total calorie intake. Intake of saturated fat, cholesterol, and trans fat should be minimal as these dietary constituents are not essential nutrients, and are associated with increasing risk for cardiovascular disease.

8. Ford ES and others: Sedentary behavior, physical activity, and the metabolic syndrome among U.S. adults. *Obesity Research* 13(3):608, 2005.

   Sedentary behavior is an important potential determinant of the presence of metabolic syndrome. Efforts to lessen the amount of time that U.S. adults spend watching television or videos or using a computer, especially if coupled with increases in physical activity, could result in substantial decreases in the prevalence of metabolic syndrome.

9. Greenland P and others: Major risk factors as antecedents of fatal and nonfatal coronary heart disease events. *Journal of the American Medical Association* 290:891, 2003.

   Cardiovascular disease deaths predominate in people with four major factors: elevated total cholesterol, elevated blood pressure, cigarette smoking, and diabetes. Presence of one or more of these risk factors predicted such deaths in almost 90% of all cases, emphasizing the importance of considering all these major risk factors.

10. Grundy SM and others: Implications of recent clinical trials for the National Cholesterol Education Program Adult Treatment Panel III Guidelines. *Circulation* 110:227, 2004.

    This report outlines the goals for LDL cholesterol for people at various risk classifications for developing cardiovascular disease. The newest guideline is to lower LDL cholesterol to less than 70 mg/dl for those at high risk for or have cardiovascular disease.

11. Grundy, SM and others: Diagnosis and Management of the Metabolic Syndrome. *Circulation* 112: 1350, 2005

    The constellation of metabolic risk factors known as metabolic syndrome consists of many factors, including elevated blood triglycerides, low HDL cholesterol concentrations, elevated blood pressure, elevated blood glucose, increased blood clotting, and an inflammatory state in the body. The most important of these underlying risk factors are abdominal obesity and insulin resistance. Other associated conditions include physical inactivity, aging, hormonal imbalance, and genetic or ethnic predisposition.

12. Hansson, GK: Inflammation, atherosclerosis, and coronary artery disease. *The New England Journal of Medicine* 352:1685, 2005.

    Excellent review of the role of inflammation in causing cardiovascular disease. Identifying atherosclerosis as an inflammatory disease offers new opportunities for the prevention and treatment of coronary artery disease.

13. Jensen MK and others: Intakes of whole grains, bran, and germ and the risk of coronary heart disease in men. *American Journal of Clinical Nutrition* 80:1492, 2004.

    This study supports the reported beneficial association of whole-grain intake with coronary heart disease and suggests that the bran component of whole grains could be a key factor in this relation.

14. Krauss RM and others: AHA Dietary Guidelines: Revision 2000: A statement for healthcare professionals from the Nutrition Committee of the American Heart Association. *Circulation* 102:2284, 2000.

    This report contains the latest advice for the public regarding diet and cardiovascular disease from the American Heart Association. The revised guidelines place an increased emphasis on the need for weight control and a heart-healthy diet. See also in the same journal 109:672, 2004 for further advice regarding cardiovascular disease prevention in women and 109:551, 2004 for treatment of the metabolic syndrome. The general advice provided is similar to that provided in Chapter 5.

15. Kris-Etherton PM and others: Fish consumption, fish oil, omega-3 fatty acids, and cardiovascular disease. *Circulation* 106:2747, 2002.

    Omega-3 fatty acids can reduce cardiac events (e.g., death) and decrease progression of atherosclerosis. A food-based approach to increasing omega-3 fatty acid intake is preferable. A dose of omega-3 fatty acids from fish oils (1 gram per day) is also appropriate if done in consultation with a physician. Such supplements also could be a component of the medical management of high blood triglycerides; doses of 2 to 4 grams per day are required.

16. Kris-Etherton PM and others: Antioxidant vitamin supplements and cardiovascular disease. *Circulation* 110:637, 2004.

    There is no scientific data to clearly justify the use of antioxidant supplements such as vitamin E for the prevention of cardiovascular disease. It is much more important to focus on a healthy diet, regular physical activity, and control of blood pressure.

17. Lau, VWY and others: Plant sterols are efficacious in lowering plasma LDL and non-HDL cholesterol in hypercholesterolemic type 2 diabetic and nondiabetic persons. *American Journal of Clinical Nutrition* 81:1351, 2005.

    Incorporation of plant sterols into a low-saturated-fat and low-cholesterol diet for persons at increased risk of CVD mortality could have a positive effect on reducing the mortality rate, including in those people with type 2 diabetes.

18. Lee I and others: Vitamin E in the primary prevention of cardiovascular disease and cancer: the women's health study: a randomized controlled trial. *Journal of the American Medical Association* 294:56, 2005.

    The data from this large trial indicated that 600 IU of natural-source vitamin E taken every other day provided no overall benefit for major cardiovascular events or cancer. These data do not support recommending vitamin E supplementation for cardiovascular disease or cancer prevention among healthy women, but more research is warranted, as a decrease in sudden cardiac death was seen in a subset of older women in this study.

19. Lonn E and others: Effects of long-term vitamin E supplementation on cardiovascular events and cancer: a randomized controlled trial. *Journal of the American Medical Association* 293:1338, 2005.

    No significant differences were noted between the vitamin E supplementation group and the control group in the incidence of cancer or deaths related to cancer. There also were no differences in the main composite of cardiovascular outcomes including death or rehospitalization. A significant increased risk in heart failure and related complications occurred in the vitamin E group.

20. Meisinger C and others: Plasma oxidized low-density lipoprotein, a strong predictor for acute coronary heart disease events in apparently healthy, middle-aged men from the general population. *Circulation* 112:651, 2005.

    Elevated concentrations of oxidized low-density lipoprotein are predictive of future coronary heart disease events in apparently healthy men. Thus, oxidized LDL may represent a promising risk marker for clinical coronary heart disease complications and should be evaluated in further studies.

I. Are You Eating a Diet That Includes Many Saturated Fat and Trans Fatty Acid Sources?

Instructions: In each row of the following list, circle your typical food selection from either column A or B.

Column A		**Column B**
Bacon and eggs	*or*	Ready-to-eat whole-grain breakfast cereal
Doughnut or sweet roll	*or*	Whole-wheat roll, bagel, or bread
Breakfast sausage	*or*	Fruit
Whole milk	*or*	Reduced-fat, low-fat, or fat-free milk
Cheeseburger	*or*	Turkey sandwich, no cheese
French fries	*or*	Plain baked potato with salsa
Ground chuck	*or*	Ground round
Soup with cream base	*or*	Soup with broth base
Macaroni and cheese	*or*	Macaroni with marinara sauce
Cream/fruit pie	*or*	Graham crackers
Ice cream	*or*	Frozen yogurt, sherbet, or reduced-fat ice cream
Butter or stick margarine	*or*	Vegetable oils or soft margarine in a tub

Interpretation

The foods listed in column A tend to be high in saturated fat, *trans* fatty acids, cholesterol, and total fat. Those in column B generally are low in these dietary components. If you want to help reduce your risk of cardiovascular disease, choose more foods from column B and fewer from column A.

II. What Is Your Current Fat and Cholesterol Intake?

How do your food practices compare with general guidelines suggested for fat, saturated fat, and cholesterol intake? Refer to the nutritional assessment you completed at the end of Chapter 2, and compare it with the following guidelines, issued by the American Heart Association and the Food and Nutrition Board. The American Heart Association Guidelines pertain to people at high risk for developing cardiovascular disease.

- Limit or reduce total fat intake to 20% to 35% of total calories.

- Reduce saturated fat intake to 7% to 10% of calorie intake or less.

- Limit cholesterol to 200 to 300 milligrams per day.

To compare your nutritional assessment with these guidelines, first fill in the values for your intakes of the following. (Refer to the Bar Graph report from NutritionCalc Plus for this information.)

TOTAL ENERGY: _____ kcal   **TOTAL FAT:** _____ grams

SATURATED FAT: _____ grams   **CHOLESTEROL:** _____ milligrams

Now complete the following steps:

1. Multiply your total grams of fat by 9 (kcal per grams of fat). Then divide the result by your total calorie intake. Next multiply this number by 100. This will give you the percentage of calories you consumed from fat.

    % OF CALORIES FROM FAT _____ IS IT WITHIN THE RANGE OF 20% TO 35% OF TOTAL CALORIE INTAKE? YES _____ NO _____

    Compare your answer with the Calories from Fat value on the Bar Graph report (NutritionCalc Plus).

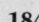

2. Multiply your grams of saturated fat by 9 (kcal per grams of fat). Divide the result by your total energy intake. Now multiply this number by 100. This will give you the percentage of energy you consumed from saturated fat.

   % OF CALORIES FROM SATURATED FAT _____ IS IT 7% to 10% OF CALORIE INTAKE OR LESS? YES _____ NO _____

   Compare your answer with the Source of Fat percentage (saurated fat) from the Ratios report (NutritionCalc Plus).

3. Look at your milligrams of cholesterol. (For NutritionCalc Plus analysis, look at the cholesterol value on the Bar Graph report.)

   IS YOUR INTAKE LESS THAN 200 to 300 milligrams? YES _____ NO _____

4. Look back at the foods you ate (NutritionCalc Plus Spreadsheet report) and notice the foods that contributed the most fat, saturated fat, and cholesterol. If you didn't meet one or more of the guidelines and had elevated LDL (putting you at high risk for developing cardiovascular disease), how could you change what you ate that day to improve your diet?

5. Now take the next step. Do you know your blood lipid values? If not, have them checked soon. All adults should know whether these values are in the abnormal ranges.

6. Finally, fill in the following assessment of your risk for developing cardiovascular disease. Decide today how you could modify your diet and lifestyle, if necessary, to reduce your risk.

Do you have:	YES	NO		YES	NO
A history of smoking?	_____	_____	Diabetes?	_____	_____
Hypertension?	_____	_____	A history of physical inactivity?	_____	_____
High LDL?	_____	_____	A family history of cardiovascular disease?	_____	_____
Low HDL?	_____	_____	A history of obesity?	_____	_____
			A diet that lacks sufficient B vitamins, such as B-6, folate, and B-12?	_____	_____

Other factors also could be considered, as discussed in the Looking Further section of this chapter, but this provides a good start for assessing your risk.

Proteins

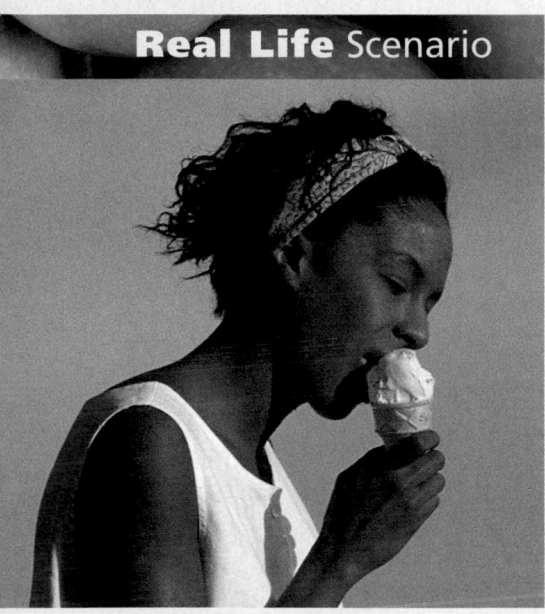

Shannon is a freshman in college. She lives in a campus residence hall and teaches aerobics in the afternoon. She eats two or three meals a day at the residence hall cafeteria and snacks between meals. Shannon and her roommate both decided to become vegetarians because they recently read a magazine article describing the health benefits of a vegetarian diet. Yesterday her vegetarian diet consisted of a danish pastry for breakfast and a tomato-rice dish (no meat) with pretzels and a diet soft drink for lunch. In the afternoon, after her aerobics class, she had an ice cream cone and two cookies. At dinnertime, she had a vegetarian sub sandwich consisting of lettuce, sprouts, tomatoes, cucumbers, and cheese, with two glasses of fruit punch. In the evening, she had a bowl of popcorn.

What is missing from this current diet plan in terms of foods that should be emphasized in a vegetarian diet? How could she improve her new diet to meet her nutritional needs?

Chapter 6 Objectives

Chapter 6 is designed to allow you to:

1. Describe how amino acids make up proteins.

2. Distinguish between essential and nonessential amino acids.

3. Explain why adequate amounts of each of the essential amino acids are required for protein synthesis.

4. List the primary functions of protein in the body.

5. Calculate the RDA for protein for an adult when a healthy weight is given.

6. Describe what is meant by positive protein balance, negative protein balance, and protein equilibrium.

7. Distinguish between high-quality and low-quality proteins, identify examples of each, and describe the concept of complementary proteins.

8. Describe how protein-calorie malnutrition eventually can lead to disease in the body.

9. Develop vegetarian diet plans that meet the body's nutritional needs.

Check out the **Contemporary Nutrition Online Learning Center**

www.mhhe.com/wardlawcont6 for quizzes, flash cards, other activities, and web links designed to further help you learn about proteins.

Chapter 6 Outline

onsuming enough protein is vital for maintaining health. Proteins form important structures in the body, make up a key part of the blood, help regulate many body functions, and can fuel body cells.

North Americans generally eat more protein than is needed to maintain health. Our daily protein intake comes mostly from animal sources such as meat, poultry, fish, eggs, milk, and cheese. In contrast, our Stone Age ancestors obtained a greater percentage of their protein from vegetables. They primarily picked and gathered their dietary protein from plant sources, rather than hunted it in the form of animals. Not until the appearance of *Homo erectus*, our immediate ancestors, about 1 million years ago did meat displace other foods in a primarily vegetarian diet. Diets that are mostly vegetarian still predominate in much of Asia and areas of Africa, and some North Americans are currently adopting the practice.

Few of us wish to exchange our comfortable modern lifestyles with those of our Stone-Age ancestors, yet we could benefit from eating more plant sources of proteins. It is possible—and desirable—to incorporate the most nutritious practices of both eras and enjoy the benefits of animal and plant protein as we meet the goal of consuming 10% to 35% of total calories as protein. Let's see why a detailed study of protein is worth your attention.

Refresh Your Memory

As you begin your study of proteins in Chapter 6, you may want to review:

- Organization of the cell in Chapter 3
- The process of digestion and absorption in Chapter 3
- The nervous system and immune system in Chapter 3
- The role of carbohydrates in preventing ketosis in Chapter 4

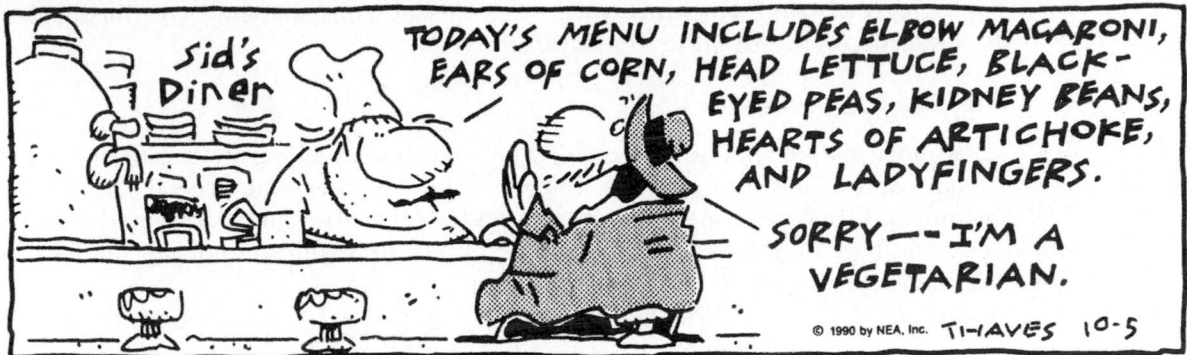

Can a vegetarian diet provide enough protein? What is prompting the growing interest in various forms of vegetarian diets? Why are plant protein *sources*, especially soy and nuts, gaining more attention? Should meat-eaters abandon that dietary practice? Chapter 6 provides some answers.

Protein—An Introduction

The term *protein* comes from the Greek word *protos*, which means "to come first." In the developing world, it is important to focus on protein in diet planning because diets in those areas of the world can be deficient in protein. In contrast, diets in the developed world are generally rich in protein, and therefore a specific focus on eating enough protein is, for the most part, not needed.

High-protein diets have come and gone over the past 30 years. Recently, they have re-emerged as weight-loss diets. The latest advice from the Food and Nutrition Board allows for up to 35% of total calorie intake to be supplied by protein, so in general these diets are appropriate if otherwise nutritionally sound, such as has enough fiber (i.e., follow MyPyramid). Still, as discussed in Chapter 10, these types of diets are hardly a magic wand for weight loss.

Proteins—Vital to Life

Thousands of substances in the body are made of proteins. Aside from water, proteins form the major part of lean body tissue, totaling about 17% of body weight. Amino acids—the building blocks for proteins—contain a special form of nitrogen: essentially, nitrogen bonded to carbon. Plants combine nitrogen from the soil with carbon and other elements to form amino acids. They then link these amino acids together to make proteins. We get the nitrogen we need by consuming dietary proteins. Proteins are thus an essential part of a diet because they supply nitrogen in a form we can readily use—namely, amino acids. Directly using simpler forms of nitrogen is, for the most part, impossible for humans.

Proteins are crucial to the regulation and maintenance of the body. Body functions such as blood clotting, fluid balance, hormone and enzyme production, visual processes, transport of many substances in the bloodstream, and cell repair require specific proteins. The body makes proteins in many configurations and sizes so that they can serve these greatly varied functions. Formation of these many body proteins begins with amino acids from both the protein-containing foods we eat and those that are synthesized from other compounds within the body. Proteins can also be broken down to supply energy for the body—on average, 4 kcal per gram.

If you fail to consume an adequate amount of protein for weeks at a time, many metabolic processes slow down. This is because the body does not have enough

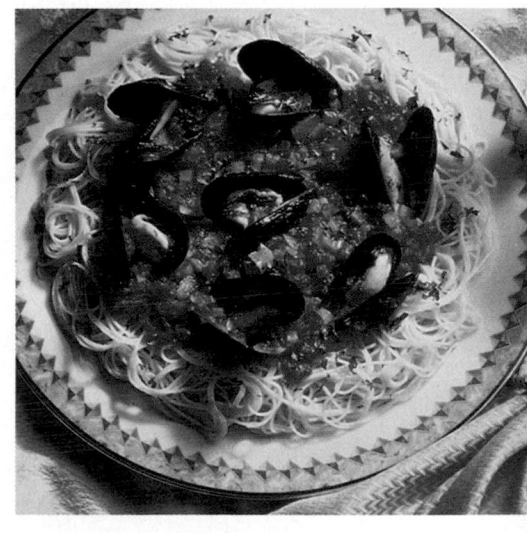

Small amounts of animal protein in a meal easily add up to meet daily protein needs.

amino acids available to build the proteins it needs. For example, the immune system no longer functions efficiently when it lacks key proteins, thereby increasing the risk of infections, disease, and eventually death.

■ Amino Acids

Amino acids—the building blocks of proteins—are formed mostly of carbon, hydrogen, oxygen, and nitrogen. The following diagram shows the general form of an amino acid and what one of the amino acids looks like. The amino acids used to make protein have different chemical makeups, but all are slight variations of the generic amino acid pictured (see Appendix F).

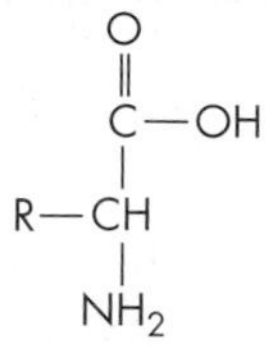

Generic" amino acid. The R signifies another chemical group that would be present.

One example of an R group

Part of generic amino acid foundation

Glutamic acid

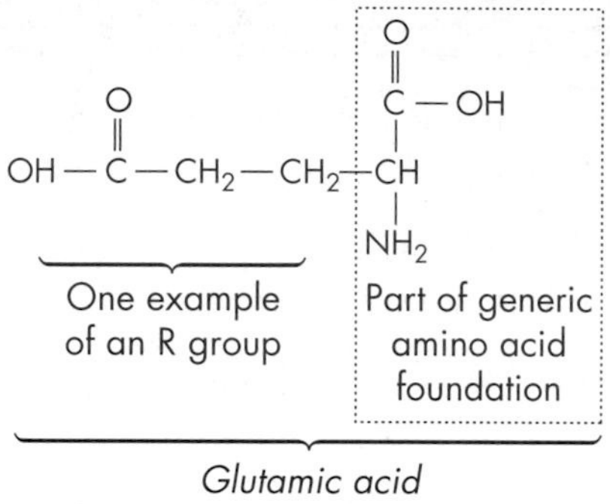

Another Bite

The R group on some amino acids has a branched shape, like a tree. These so-called **branched-chain amino acids** are leucine, isoleucine, and valine (see Appendix F for the chemical structures of the amino acids). The branched-chain amino acids are the primary amino acids used by muscles for energy needs. This is one reason why proteins from milk (e.g. whey proteins) are a current rage in strength-training athletes (see Chapter 11 for details).

Your body needs to use 20 different types of amino acids to function (Table 6-1). Although all these commonly found amino acids are important, 11 are considered **nonessential** (also called *dispensable*) with respect to our diets. Human cells can produce these certain amino acids as long as the right ingredients are present—the key

branched-chain amino acids Amino acids with a branching carbon backbone, these are leucine, isoleucine, and valine. All are essential amino acids.

nonessential amino acids Amino acids that can be synthesized by a healthy body in sufficient amounts; there are 11 nonessential amino acids. These are also called *dispensable amino acids.*

semiessential amino acids Amino acids that, when consumed, spare the need to use an essential amino acid for their synthesis. Tyrosine in the diet, for example, spares the need to use phenylalanine for tyrosine synthesis. Also called *conditionally essential amino acids.*

Table 6-1 Classification of Amino Acids

Essential Amino Acids	Nonessential Amino Acids
Histidine	Alanine
Isoleucine*	Arginine[†]
Leucine*	Asparagine
Lysine	Aspartic acid
Methionine	Cysteine[†]
Phenylalanine	Glutamic acid
Threonine	Glutamine[†]
Tryptophan	Glycine[†]
Valine*	Proline[†]
	Serine
	Tyrosine[†]

*A branched-chain amino acid

[†]These amino acids are also classed as **semiessential** (or conditionally essential). This means they must be made from essential amino acids if insufficient amounts are eaten. When that occurs, the body's supply of certain essential amino acids is depleted.

factor being nitrogen that is already part of another amino acid. Therefore it is not essential that these amino acids be in our diet.

The nine amino acids the body cannot make in sufficient amounts or at all are known as **essential** (also called *indispensable*)—they must be obtained from foods. This is because body cells either cannot make the needed carbon-based foundation of the amino acid, cannot put a nitrogen group on the needed carbon-based foundation, or just cannot do the whole process fast enough to meet body needs.

Both nonessential and essential amino acids are present in foods that contain protein. If you don't eat enough essential amino acids, your body first struggles to conserve what essential amino acids it can. However, eventually your body progressively slows production of new proteins until at some point you will break protein down faster than you can make it. When that happens, health deteriorates.

■ Putting Essential and Nonessential Amino Acids into Perspective

Eating a balanced diet can supply us with both the essential and nonessential amino-acid building blocks needed to maintain good health. Let's now take a more detailed look at the relationship between essential and nonessential amino acids.

Physiological Aspects

The disease phenylketonuria (PKU) illustrates the importance of one essential amino acid. Recall from Chapter 4 that a person with PKU has a limited ability to metabolize the essential amino acid phenylalanine. Normally, the body uses an enzyme to convert much of our dietary phenylalanine intake into the nonessential amino acid tyrosine.

In PKU-diagnosed persons, the enzyme activity may be grossly or mildly insufficient due to the insertion of an incorrect amino acid into the enzyme used in processing phenylalanine to tyrosine. When the enzymes cannot synthesize enough tyrosine, both amino acids must be derived from foods. The key point here is that both amino acids become *essential* in terms of dietary needs because the body can't produce enough tyrosine from phenylalanine. PKU is treated by controlling the consumption of phenylalanine with a special diet (ideally throughout life) so that phenylalanine and its by-products do not rise to toxic concentrations in the body and cause the severe mental retardation seen in untreated PKU cases.

Dietary Considerations—Protein Quality

Animal and plant proteins can differ greatly in their proportions of essential and nonessential amino acids. Animal proteins contain ample amounts of all nine essential amino acids. (Gelatin—made from the animal protein collagen—is an exception because it loses one essential amino acid during processing and is low in other essential amino acids.) With the exception of soy protein, plant proteins don't match our need for essential amino acids as precisely as animal proteins. Many plant proteins, especially those found in grains, are low in one or more of the nine essential amino acids.

As you might expect, human tissue composition resembles animal tissue more than it does plant tissue. The similarities enable us to use proteins from any single animal source more efficiently to support human growth and maintenance than we do those from any single plant source. For this reason, animal proteins, except gelatin, are considered **high-quality** (also called **complete**) **proteins**, which contain the nine essential amino acids we need in sufficient amounts. Individual plant sources of proteins, except for soy beans, are considered **lower-quality** (also called **incomplete**) **proteins** because their amino-acid patterns can be quite different from ours. Thus a single plant protein source, such as corn alone, cannot easily support body growth and maintenance. To obtain a sufficient amount of essential amino acids, a variety of plant proteins need to be consumed because each plant protein lacks adequate amounts of one or more essential amino acids.

essential amino acids The amino acids that cannot be synthesized by humans in sufficient amounts or at all and therefore must be included in the diet; there are nine essential amino acids. These are also called *indispensable amino acids.*

Critical Thinking

Rina is 7 months pregnant and has read about various tests that her baby will undergo when he or she is born. How can you explain to Rina the purpose and significance of one of those tests, the one that screens for PKU?

high-quality (complete) proteins Dietary proteins that contain ample amounts of all nine essential amino acids.

lower-quality (incomplete) proteins Dietary proteins that are low in or lack one or more essential amino acids.

limiting amino acid The essential amino acid in lowest concentration in a food or diet relative to body needs.

complementary proteins Two food protein sources that make up for each other's inadequate supply of specific essential amino acids; together they yield a sufficient amount of all nine and, so, provide high-quality (complete) protein for the diet.

When only lower-quality protein foods are consumed, enough of the essential amino acids needed for protein synthesis may not be obtained. Therefore, when compared to high-quality proteins, a greater amount of lower-quality protein is needed to meet the needs of protein synthesis. Moreover, once any of the nine essential amino acids in the plant protein we have eaten is used up, further protein synthesis becomes impossible. Because the depletion of just one of the essential amino acids prevents protein synthesis, the process illustrates the *all-or-none principle:* Either all essential amino acids are available or none can be used. The remaining amino acids would then be used for energy needs, or converted to carbohydrate or fat.

The essential amino acid in smallest supply in a food or diet in relation to body needs becomes the limiting factor (called the **limiting amino acid**) because it limits the amount of protein the body can synthesize. For example, assume the letters of the alphabet represent the 20 or so different amino acids we consume. If *A* represents an essential amino acid, we need three of these letters to spell the hypothetical protein *BANANA*. If the body had a *B*, two *N*s, but only two *A*s, the "synthesis" of *BANANA* would not be possible. *A* would then be seen as the limiting amino acid.

When two or more proteins combine to compensate for deficiencies in essential amino acid content in each protein, the proteins are called **complementary proteins** (Table 6-2). Mixed diets generally provide high-quality protein because a complementary protein pattern results. Therefore, healthy adults should have little concern about balancing foods to yield the proteins needed to obtain enough of all nine essential amino acids. Even on plant-based diets, complementary proteins need not be consumed at the same meal by adults. Meeting amino-acid needs over the course of a day is a reasonable goal because there is a ready supply of amino acids from those present in body cells and in the blood (see Fig. 6-8 on page 199). In addition, adults need only about 11% of their total protein requirement to be supplied by essential amino acids. Typical diets supply an average of 50% of protein as essential amino acids.

The estimated needs for essential amino acids for infants and preschool children are 40% of total protein intake; however, in later childhood the need drops to 20%. Diets designed for infants and young children need to take this into account to make sure enough proteins are present to yield a high-quality protein intake. Including some animal products in the diet, such as human milk or formula for infants, or cow's milk for children, helps ensure this. Otherwise, complementary amino acids from

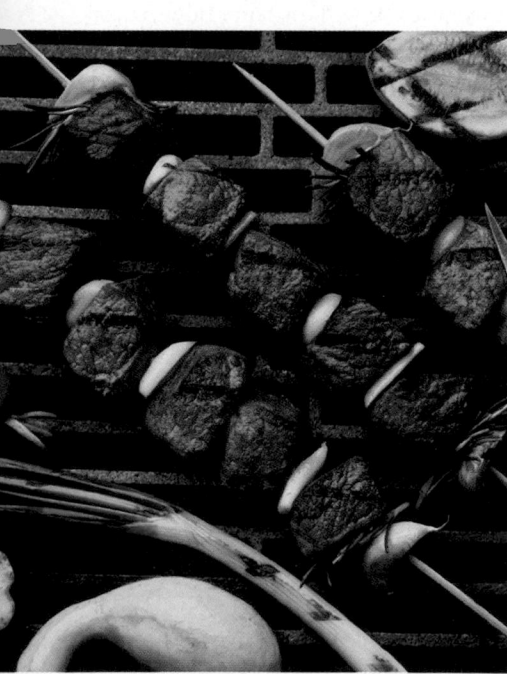

When combined with vegetables, high-protein foods such as meats also help balance the amino acid content of the diet.

Table 6-2 Limiting Amino Acids in Plant Foods

Food	Limiting Amino Acids	Possible Plant Source of the Limiting Amino Acids*	Traditional Food Combinations in Which the Proteins Complement Each Other in a Meal
Legumes (beans)	Methionine	Grains, nuts, seeds	Red beans and rice
Grains	Lysine, threonine, tryptophan	Legumes	Rice and red beans; lentil curry and rice; corn tortillas and beans
Nuts and seeds	Lysine	Legumes	Soybeans and ground sesame seeds (miso); peanuts, rice, and black-eyed peas; green peas and sunflower seeds
Vegetables	Methionine	Grains, nuts, seeds	Green beans and almonds

Note: As you might suspect from the information in Table 6-2, the amino acids most likely to be low in a diet are lysine, methionine, threonine, and tryptophan. If a diet is low in an amino acid, nutrition experts recommend finding a good food source to supply it. Finding the right combinations of amino acids, such as a dish of rice and beans, is recommended. Forget about amino-acid supplements—they can lead to problems, such as decreased absorption of other, similar amino acids. Amino acids as such also have a disagreeable odor and flavor and are also much more expensive than food protein.

*Animal products in the diet serve the same purpose, such as when fish is consumed with rice, or cheese with macaroni.

plant proteins should be consumed in each meal or within two subsequent meals. A major health risk for infants and children occurs in famine situations in which only one type of cereal grain is available, increasing the probability that one or more of the nine essential amino acids is lacking in the total diet. This is discussed further in a later section on protein-calorie malnutrition.

Concept Check

The human body uses 20 different amino acids from protein-containing foods. Because a healthy body can synthesize 11 of the amino acids, it is not necessary to obtain all amino acids from foods—only nine of these must come from the diet and are therefore termed *essential (indispensable) amino acids.* Foods that contain all nine essential amino acids in about the proportions we need are considered high-quality (complete) protein foods. Those low in one or more essential amino acids are lower-quality (incomplete) protein foods. When different lower-quality protein foods are eaten together, the total intake of amino acids generally makes up for the shortcomings of each individual food to yield a high-quality protein meal.

Proteins—Amino Acids Bonded Together

Amino acids are linked together by chemical bonds—technically called **peptide bonds**—to form proteins. Although these bonds are difficult to break, acids, enzymes, and other agents are able to do so—for example, during digestion.

The body can synthesize many different proteins by linking together the 20 common types of amino acids with such peptide bonds.

■ Protein Synthesis

To begin a discussion of protein synthesis, we need to focus on DNA, which is present in the nucleus of the cell. Recall from Chapter 3 that DNA is a double-stranded molecule. DNA contains coded instructions for protein synthesis (i.e., which specific amino acids are to be placed in a protein and in which order).

Protein synthesis in a cell, however, takes place in the cytoplasm, not in the nucleus. Thus, the DNA code used for synthesis of a specific protein must be transferred from the nucleus to the cytoplasm to allow for such synthesis. This transfer is the job of messenger RNA (mRNA). Enzymes in the nucleus read the code on one strand of the DNA and *transcribe* that into a single-stranded mRNA molecule (Fig. 6-1). The segment that is read is the gene. This mRNA undergoes processing and then it is ready to leave the nucleus.

Once in the cytoplasm, mRNA travels to the ribosomes. The ribosomes read the mRNA code and *translate* those instructions to produce a specific protein. Amino acids are added one at a time to the growing **polypeptide** chain as directed by the instructions on the mRNA. Another key participant in protein synthesis, transfer RNA (tRNA), is responsible for bringing specific amino acids to the ribosomes as needed during protein synthesis (review Fig. 6-1). Energy input is required to add each amino acid to the chain, making protein synthesis very "costly" to the body.

Once synthesis of a polypeptide is complete, it twists and folds into the appropriate three-dimensional structure of the intended protein due to interactions between the amino acids that make up the polypeptide chain (see the next section on protein organization for details). Some polypeptides, such as the hormone insulin, also undergo further metabolism in the cell before they are functional.

The important message in this discussion is the relationship between DNA and the proteins eventually produced by a cell. If the DNA contains errors, an incorrect mRNA

Critical Thinking

Leon, a vegetarian, has heard of the "all-or-none principle" of protein synthesis but doesn't understand how this principle applies to protein synthesis in the body. He asks you, "How important is this nutritional concept for diet planning?" How would you answer his question?

peptide bond A chemical bond formed between amino acids in a protein.

polypeptide A group of amino acids bonded together, from 50 to 2000 or more.

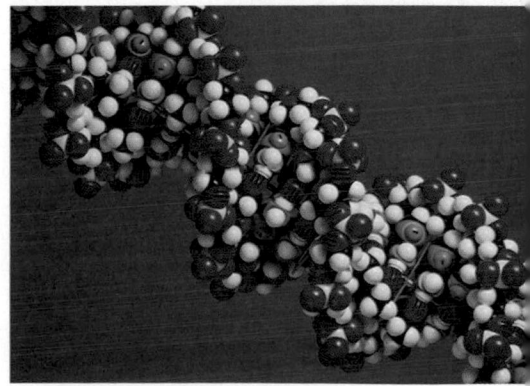

Genes are present on DNA—a double-stranded helix. The cell nucleus contains most of the DNA in the body.

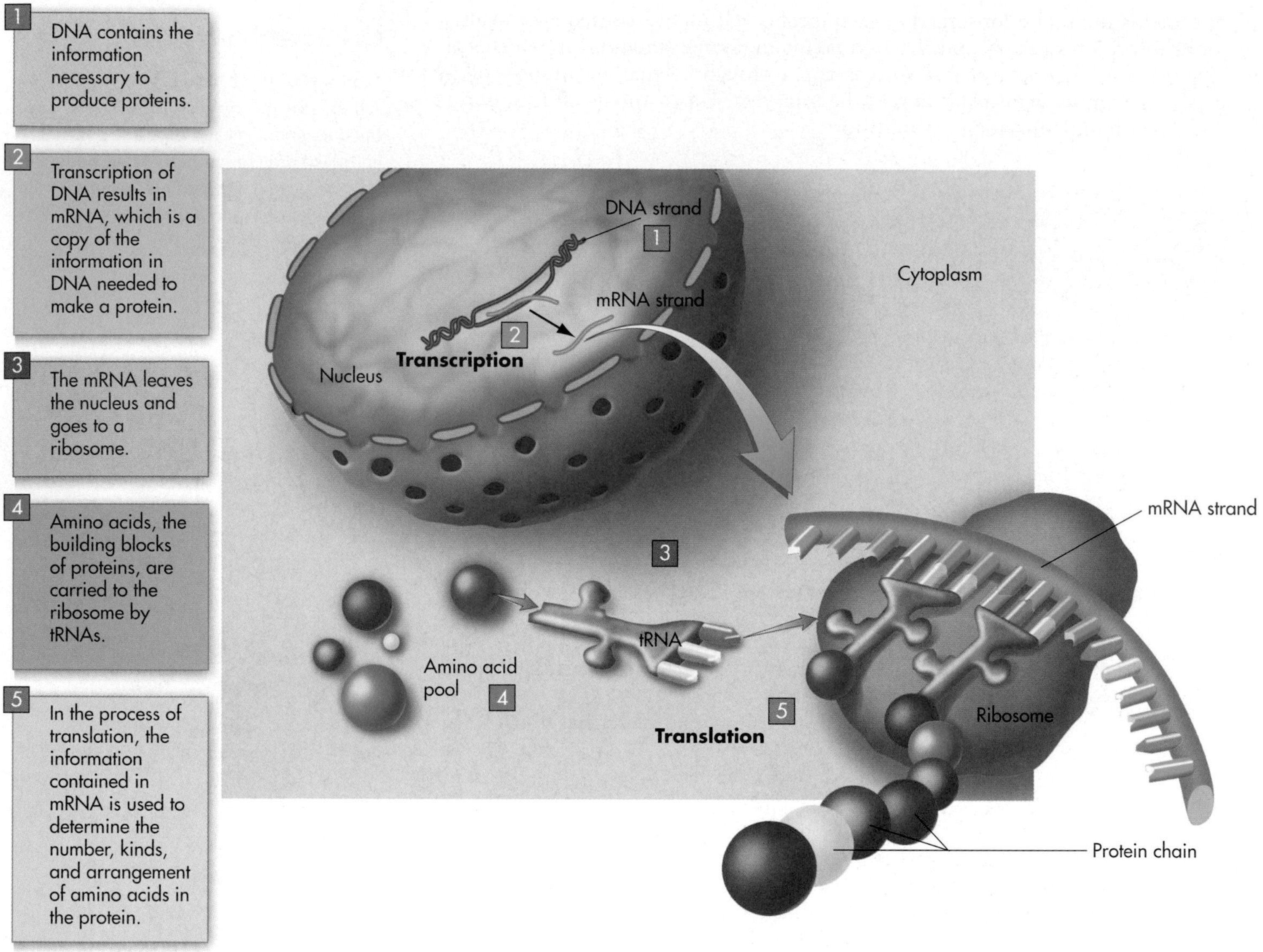

1 DNA contains the information necessary to produce proteins.

2 Transcription of DNA results in mRNA, which is a copy of the information in DNA needed to make a protein.

3 The mRNA leaves the nucleus and goes to a ribosome.

4 Amino acids, the building blocks of proteins, are carried to the ribosome by tRNAs.

5 In the process of translation, the information contained in mRNA is used to determine the number, kinds, and arrangement of amino acids in the protein.

DNA strand

1

mRNA strand

Cytoplasm

2

Transcription

Nucleus

3

mRNA strand

Amino acid pool

4

tRNA

5

Translation

Ribosome

Protein chain

Figure 6-1 Protein synthesis (simplified). Note that once the mRNA is fully read, the polypeptide is released into the cytoplasm. It generally is then processed further to become a cell protein.

will be produced. The ribosomes will then read this incorrect message and produce an incorrect polypeptide chain. As discussed in Chapter 3, ultimately we may be able to correct many gene defects in humans, by placing the correct DNA code in the nucleus, so that the correct protein can be made by the ribosomes.

■ Protein Organization

As noted before, by bonding together various combinations of the 20 common types of amino acids, the body synthesizes thousands of different proteins. The sequential order of the amino acids then ultimately determines the protein's shape. The main point is that only correctly positioned amino acids can interact and fold properly to form the intended shape for the protein. The resulting unique, three-dimensional form goes on to dictate the function of each particular protein (Fig. 6-2). If it lacks the appropriate configuration, a protein cannot function.

Sickle cell disease (also called **sickle cell anemia**) is one example of what happens when amino acids are out of order on a protein. North Americans of African descent

sickle cell disease (sickle cell anemia) An illness that results from a malformation of the red blood cell because of an incorrect structure in part of its hemoglobin protein chains. The disease can lead to episodes of severe bone and joint pain, abdominal pain, headache, convulsions, paralysis, and even death.

are especially prone to this genetic disease. It originates in defective production of the protein chains of hemoglobin, a protein that carries oxygen in red blood cells. In two of its four protein chains, an error in the amino-acid order occurs. This error produces a profound change in hemoglobin structure. It can no longer form the shape needed to carry oxygen efficiently inside the red blood cell. Instead of forming normal circular disks, the red blood cells collapse into crescent (or sickle) shapes (Fig. 6-3). Health deteriorates, and eventually episodes of severe bone and joint pain, abdominal pain, headache, convulsions, and paralysis may occur.

These life-threatening symptoms are caused by a minute, but critical, error in the hemoglobin amino-acid order. Why does this error happen? It results from a defect in a person's genetic blueprint, DNA, which is inherited through one's parents. A defect in the DNA can dictate that a wrong amino acid will be built into the sequence of the body proteins. Many diseases stem from incorrect DNA information passed on in the body, such as cancer (see Chapter 15).

■ Denaturation of Proteins

Exposure to acid or alkaline substances, heat, or agitation can alter a protein's structure, leaving it unraveled or otherwise deformed. This process of altering the three-dimensional structure of a protein is called **denaturation** (Fig. 6-4). Changing a protein's shape often destroys its ability to function normally, such that it loses its biological activity.

Denaturation of proteins is useful for some body processes, especially digestion. The heat produced during cooking denatures some proteins. For example, a protein in raw eggs (avidin) binds to the vitamin biotin so that it cannot be absorbed, but cooking denatures avidin, thus preventing a potential decrease in biotin availability. After food is ingested, the secretion of stomach acid denatures some bacterial proteins, plant hormones, many active enzymes, and other forms of proteins in foods, making it safer to eat. Digestion is also enhanced by denaturation because the unraveling increases exposure of the polypeptide chain to digestive enzymes. Denaturing proteins in some foods can also reduce their tendencies to cause allergic reactions.

Recall that we need the essential amino acids that the proteins in the diet supply—not the proteins themselves. We dismantle ingested dietary proteins and use the amino acid building blocks to assemble the proteins we need.

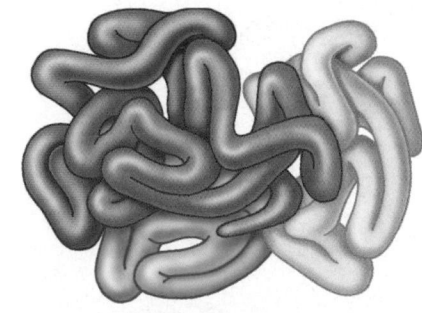

Figure 6-2 Protein organization. Proteins often form a coiled shape, as shown by this drawing of the blood protein hemoglobin. This shape is dictated by the order of the amino acids in the protein chain. To get an idea of its size, consider that each teaspoon (5 milliliters) of blood contains about 10^{18} hemoglobin molecules. Note that 1 billion is 10^9.

denaturation Alteration of a protein's three-dimensional structure, usually because of treatment by heat, enzymes, acid or alkaline solutions, or agitation.

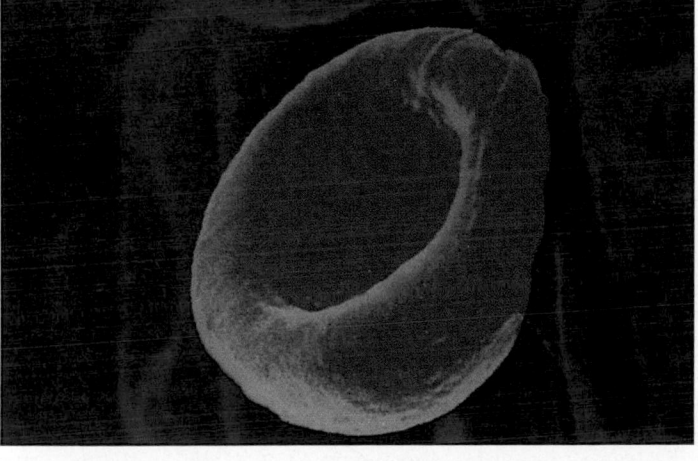

(a)

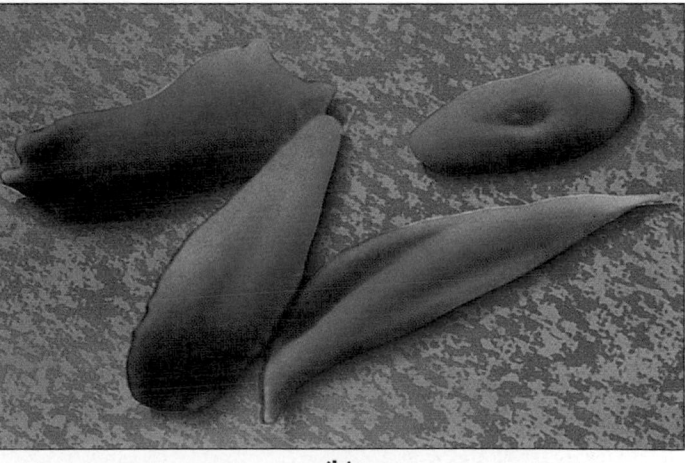

(b)

Figure 6-3 An example of the consequences of errors in DNA coding of proteins. (a) Normal red cell, (b) red blood cells from a person with sickle cell disease. Note the abnormal crescent (sicklelike) shape of the red blood cell near the center.

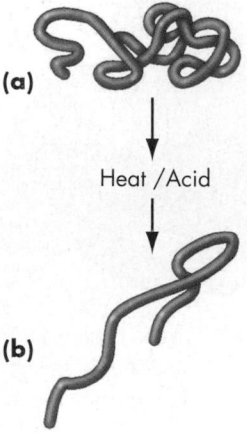

(a)

Heat /Acid

(b)

Figure 6-4 Denaturation. (a) Protein showing typical coiled state. (b) Protein is now partly uncoiled. This uncoiling can reduce biological activity.

> ### Concept Check
>
> Amino acids are bonded together in specific sequences to form distinct proteins. DNA provides the directions for synthesizing these new proteins. Specifically, DNA directs the order of the amino acids on the protein. The amino acid order within a protein determines its ultimate shape and function. Destroying the shape of a protein denatures it. Acid conditions present during the body's digestive processes, heat, and other factors can denature proteins, causing them to lose their biological activity.

■ Protein in Foods

Of the typical foods we eat, about 70% of our protein comes from animal sources (Fig. 6-5). The most nutrient-dense source of protein is water-packed tuna, which has 87% of calories as protein. The top five contributors of protein to the North American diet are beef, poultry, milk, white bread, and cheese. In North America, meat and poultry consumption amounts to about 150 pounds per person per year. Worldwide, 35% of protein comes from animal sources. In Africa and East Asia, only about 20% of the protein eaten comes from animal sources.

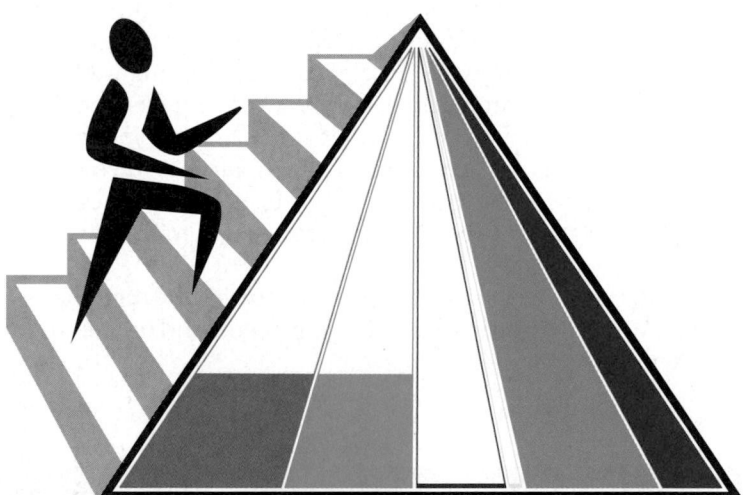

Grains	Vegetables	Fruits	Oils	Milk	Meat & Beans
• Bread • Breakfast cereals • Rice • Noodles	• Carrots • Corn • Broccoli	• Apples • Oranges • Bananas	• None	• Milk • Yogurt • Cheese	• Meat • Eggs • Fish • Dry beans • Nuts

Figure 6-5 Sources of protein from MyPyramid. The height of the background color (none, 1/3, 2/3 or completely covered) within each group in the pyramid indicates the average nutrient density for protein in that group. Overall, the milk group and the meat & beans group contain many foods that are nutrient-dense sources of protein. Based on serving sizes listed for MyPyramid, the fruits group and oils group provide little or no protein (less than 1 gram per serving). Food choices from the vegetables group and grains group provide moderate amounts of protein (2 to 3 grams per serving). The milk group provides much protein (8 to 10 grams per serving), as does the meat & beans group (7 grams per serving). With regard to physical activity, proteins are a minor source of fuel for most endeavors, but can become somewhat important during endurance activities.

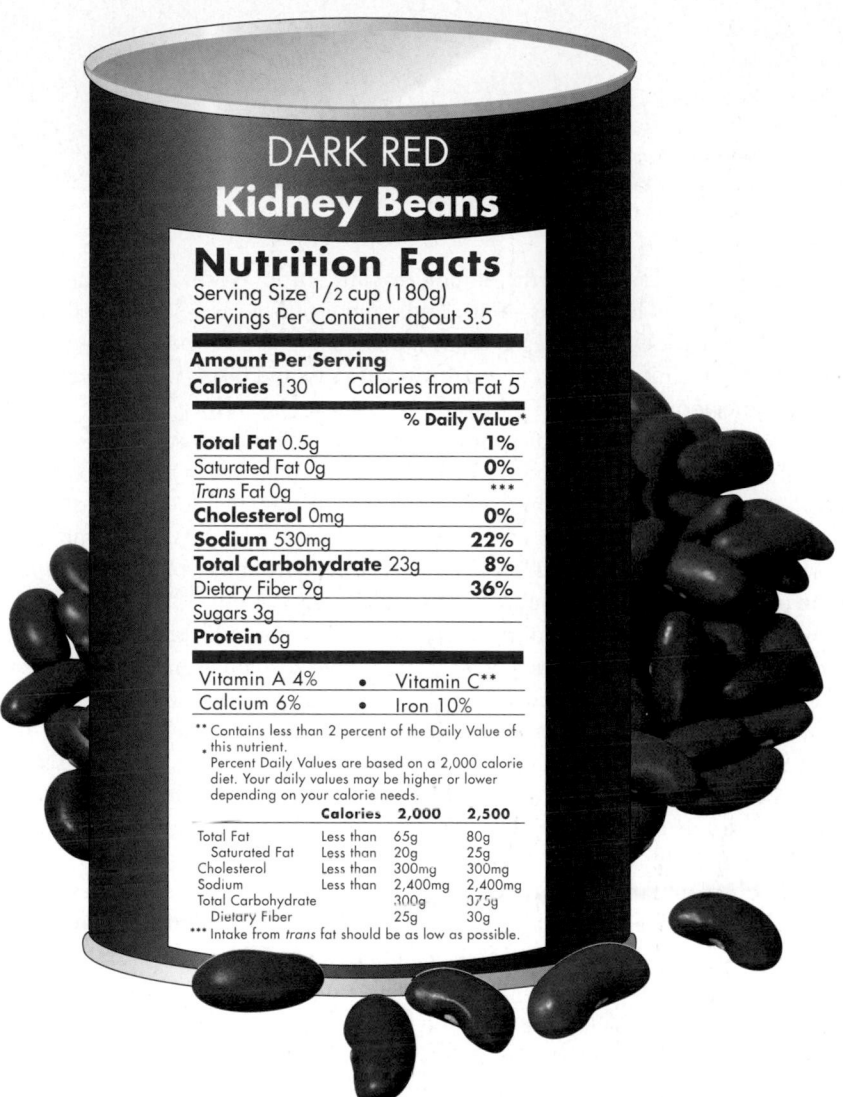

Food Sources of Protein		
Food Item and Amount	Protein (grams)	Calories from Protein (%)
Canned tuna, 3 oz	21.6	87
Broiled chicken, 3 oz	21.3	40
Beef chuck, 3 oz	15.3	30
Yogurt, 1 cup	10.6	35
Kidney beans, ½ cup	8.1	29
1% low-fat milk, 1 cup	8.0	31
Peanuts, 1 oz	7.3	18
Cheddar cheese, 1 oz	7.0	25
Egg, 1	5.5	32
Cooked corn, ½ cup	2.7	12
Seven grain bread, 1 slice	2.6	16
White rice, ½ cup	2.1	8
Pasta, 1 oz	1.2	16
Banana, 1	1.2	4

Figure 6-6 Legumes are rich sources of protein. One-half cup meets about 10% of protein needs, and at a cost of only about 5% of calorie needs.

In general, plant sources of protein deserve more attention and use than they currently receive from many North Americans. Plant foods contribute fewer calories to the diet than most animal products and they supply an ample amount of protein, plus magnesium, plenty of fiber, and several other nutritional benefits (Fig. 6-6). The vegetable proteins we eat are a heart-healthy alternative to animal proteins since they contain no cholesterol and little saturated fat, aside from that added during processing or cooking. Legumes and nut sources of protein especially have received a lot of recent attention. The first Looking Further section reviews some of the many benefits of plant proteins.

Another Bite

A relatively new source of protein comes from fermented fungus, and is called quorn. It is mixed with other food products to form various low-fat meat substitutes. Consumers can decide if these products fit into their diets; FDA has approved quorn for human use, but sales have been quite poor to date.

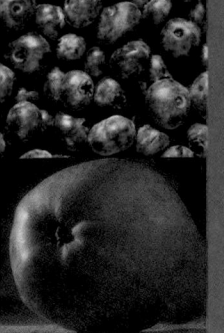

Plant sources of protein are worthy of more attention from North Americans. In the early 1900s, plant sources of proteins—nuts, seeds, and legumes—were consumed just as often as animal proteins. Over the years, though, plant proteins have been sidelined by meats. During this time, nuts have been viewed as high-fat foods, and beans have gotten the inferior reputation of "the poor man's meat."

Note that processing and cooking are crucial points at which the healthiness of foods are affected. For example, canned beans may be high in added salt, but by purchasing those labeled "low-sodium," or rinsing canned beans with cool water before cooking, you can reduce the salt content. Likewise, cooking in butter or adding cheese will increase the saturated fat and cholesterol content of legumes.

Contrary to these popular misconceptions, sources of plant proteins offer a wealth of nutritional benefits—from lowering blood cholesterol to preventing certain forms of cancer. In proportion to the amount of calories they supply, plant foods provide not only protein, but also magnesium, fiber, folate, vitamin E, iron (absorption is increased by the vitamin C also present), zinc, and some calcium. In addition, phytochemicals from these foods are implicated in prevention of a wide variety of chronic diseases.

Nuts have a hard shell surrounding an edible kernel. Almonds, pistachios, walnuts, and pecans are some common examples. The defining characteristic of a nut is that it grows on a tree. (Peanuts, because they grow underground, are actually legumes.) Seeds (such as pumpkin, sesame, and sunflower seeds) differ from nuts in that seeds grow on vegetable or flowering plants, but they are similar to nuts in nutrient composition. In general, nuts and seeds supply 160 to 190 kcal, 6 to 10 grams of protein, and 14 to 19 grams of fat per 1 ounce serving. Although they are a dense source of calories, you will learn that nuts and seeds make a powerful contribution to health when consumed in moderation.

Legumes are a plant family with pods that contain a single row of seeds. Besides peanuts, examples include garden and black-eyed peas, kidney beans, great northern beans, lentils, soy beans, and soy products. Dried varieties of the mature legume seeds—what we know as beans—also make an impressive contribution to the protein, vitamin, mineral, and fiber content of a meal. A one-half cup serving of legumes provides 100 to 150 kcal, 5 to 10 grams of protein, less than one gram of fat, and about 5 grams of fiber.

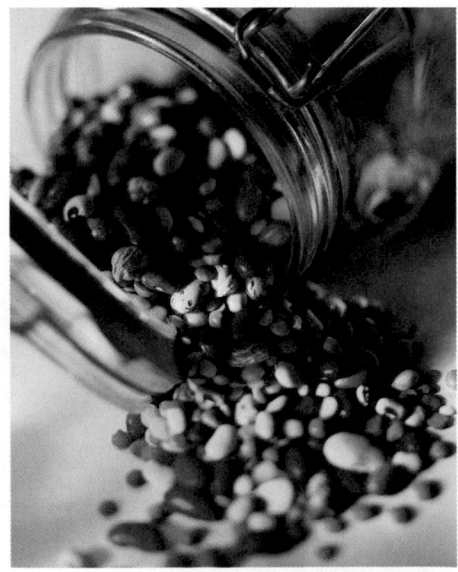

Rich sources of plant proteins add much nutritional value to a diet.

Good for Your Heart

Plant sources of proteins can positively impact heart health in several ways. First, the plant foods we eat contain no cholesterol nor *trans* fat and little saturated fat. The major type of fats in plant foods are monounsaturated and polyunsaturated fats. Nuts in particular are high in monounsaturated fat, which helps to keep blood cholesterol low.

Beans and nuts contain soluble fiber, which binds to cholesterol in the small intestine and prevents it from being absorbed by the body. Also, due to the activity of some phytochemicals, foods made from soy beans can lower production of cholesterol by the body. The effect is modest (about a 2% to 6% drop). In 1999, the Food and Drug Administration allowed health claims for the cholesterol-lowering properties of soy foods, and in 2000, the American Heart Association recommended inclusion of some soy protein in the diets of people with high blood cholesterol. As noted in Chapter 2, a food product must have at least 6.25 grams of soy protein and less than 3 grams of fat, 1 gram of saturated fat, and 20 milligrams of cholesterol per serving to list a health claim for soy on the label.

There are several other compounds in plant foods that are under study for their heart-protective roles. Some of the phytochemicals may help to prevent blood clots and relax the blood vessels. Nuts are an especially good source of nutrients that are implicated in heart health, including vitamin E, folate, magnesium, and copper. Frequent consumption of nuts (about 1 ounce of nuts five times per week) is associated with a decreased risk of cardiovascular disease. Recall from Chapter 2 that FDA also allows a provisional health claim to link nuts with a reduced risk of developing cardiovascular disease.

Cancer-Fighting Agents

The numerous phytochemicals in plant foods may help prevent cancer. Many of the proposed anti-cancer effects of foods containing plant protein are through antioxidant mechanisms. Plant sources of proteins are primarily thought to aid in preventing cancers of the breast, prostate, and colon.

Another Bite

Much of the excitement surrounding the ability of soy intake to combat a host of medical problems has waned as study-after-study has shown little benefit in preventing many forms of cancer, contributing to bone maintenance after menopause in women, and treating menopausal symtpoms in women.

Topics for Future Research

Consumption of plant sources of proteins can aid in prevention of cardiovascular disease and cancer, but there are also other areas for future study. Some studies show that replacing animal proteins with plant proteins is beneficial for kidney health. However, since plant foods such as soy are high in oxalates, people with a history of kidney stones should probably limit intake of soy (see Chapter 9 for more about oxalates). Plants may be particularly good sources of protein for people with diabetes or impaired glucose tolerance because they lead to a slower increase in blood glucose (review Chapter 4 for a discussion of glycemic load). Frequent nut consumption may even reduce the risk of developing gallstones; a reduced risk for obesity and type 2 diabetes is also likely.

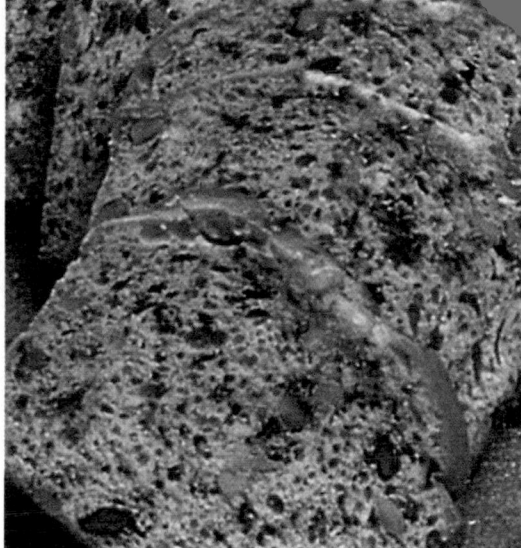

Plant proteins, like those in walnuts, can be incorporated into one's diet in numerous ways, such as adding them to banana bread.

From Theory to Practice

Now that you've seen how much you can benefit from including plant proteins in your diet, here are some suggestions for putting the theory onto your plate:

* At your next cookout, try a veggie burger instead of a hamburger. These are usually made from beans and are available in the frozen foods section of the grocery store and come in a variety of delicious flavors. Many restaurants have added veggie burgers to their menus.
* Sprinkle sunflower seeds or chopped almonds on top of your salad to add taste and texture.
* Mix chopped walnuts into the batter of your banana bread to boost your intake of monounsaturated fats.
* Eat soy nuts (oil-roasted soy beans) as a great snack.
* Spread some peanut butter on your bagel instead of butter or cream cheese.
* Instead of having beef or chicken tacos for dinner, heat up a can of great northern beans in your skillet with one half of a packet of taco seasoning and chopped tomatoes. Use this as a filling in a tortilla shell.
* Consider using soy milk, especially if you have lactose malabsorption or lactose intolerance. Look for varieties that are fortified with calcium.

Still, for some of us, food allergies from soy, peanuts and tree nuts (e.g., almonds and walnuts), and wheat are a concern. Overall, food allergies in general occur in up to 8% of children

Recall from Chapter 4 that consumption of beans can lead to intestinal gas because our bodies lack the enzymes to break down certain carbohydrates that beans contain. An over-the counter preparation called Beano® can greatly lessen symptoms if taken right before the meal. It is also helpful to soak dry beans in water, which leaches the indigestible carbohydrates into the water so they can be disposed. However, intestinal gas is not harmful. In fact, fermentation products of ingestible carbohydrates promote the health of your colon (review Chapter 3 for more information on probiotics and prebiotics).

4 years of age or younger, and in up to 2% of adults. Eight foods account for 90% of all food-related allergies; soy, peanuts, tree nuts, and wheat are four of these foods. (The other foods are milk, egg, fish, and shellfish.) The allergic reactions can range from a mild intolerance to fatal allergic rections (see Chapter 14 for details). Curent guidelines regarding plant sources of allergens advise that infants not be fed wheat products before 6 months of age. Children less than 3 years of age should not eat peanuts or tree nuts. In addition, any of the plant sources of allergens need to be avoided in children and adults who continue to experience such allergies.

In sum, plant proteins are a nutritious alternative to animal proteins. They are inexpensive, versatile, tasty, add color to your plate, and benefit health beyond their contribution of protein to the diet. Simply adding these foods to your diet can lead to weight gain, but learning to substitute plant proteins in place of other, less healthy foods is one way to reduce your risk for many diseases. Keep an eye out for news about additional research progress into this area.

Protein Digestion and Absorption

As with carbohydrates, cooking food can be viewed as a first step in protein digestion. Cooking unfolds (denatures) proteins and softens tough connective tissue in meat. Cooking also makes many protein-rich foods easier to chew, swallow, and break down during later digestion and absorption. As you will see in Chapter 16, cooking also makes many protein-rich foods, such as meats, eggs, fish, and poultry, much safer to eat.

Digestion

The enzymatic digestion of protein begins in the stomach (Fig. 6-7). Proteins are first denatured by stomach acid, then **pepsin,** a major enzyme for digesting proteins, goes to work on the unraveled polypeptide chains. Pepsin attacks these and breaks them down into shorter chains of amino acids. Pepsin does not completely separate proteins into amino acids because it can break only a few of the many peptide bonds found in these large molecules.

The release of pepsin is controlled by the hormone gastrin. Thinking about food or chewing food stimulates gastrin release in the stomach. Gastrin also strongly stimulates the stomach to produce acid.

The partially-digested proteins move with the rest of the nutrients and other substances in a meal (chyme) from the stomach into the small intestine. Once in the small intestine, the partially-digested proteins (and any fats accompanying them) trigger the release of the hormone cholecystokinin (CCK) from the walls of the small intestine. CCK, in turn, travels through the bloodstream to the pancreas. Its arrival causes the pancreas to release protein-splitting enzymes, such as **trypsin.** These digestive enzymes further divide the partially-digested proteins into segments of two to three amino acids and some individual amino acids. Eventually, digestion of this mixture into amino acids occurs, using other enzymes secreted into the intestine by glands located in the lining of the small intestine, as well as enzymes present in the absorptive cells themselves.

pepsin A protein-digesting enzyme produced by the stomach.

trypsin A protein-digesting enzyme secreted by the pancreas to act in the small intestine.

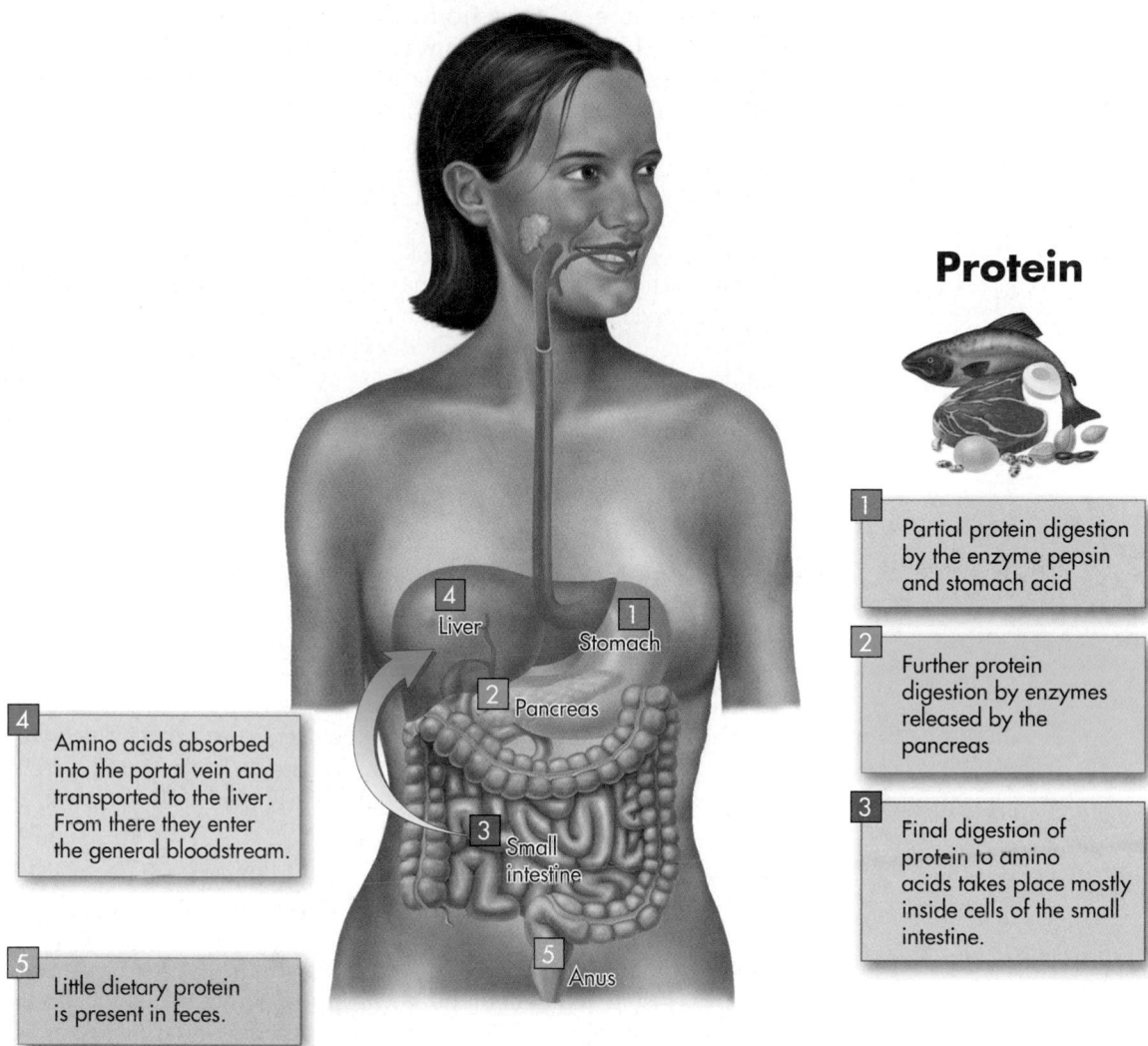

Protein

1 Partial protein digestion by the enzyme pepsin and stomach acid

2 Further protein digestion by enzymes released by the pancreas

3 Final digestion of protein to amino acids takes place mostly inside cells of the small intestine.

4 Liver

1 Stomach

2 Pancreas

4 Amino acids absorbed into the portal vein and transported to the liver. From there they enter the general bloodstream.

3 Small intestine

5 Anus

5 Little dietary protein is present in feces.

Figure 6-7 A summary of protein digestion and absorption. Enzymatic protein digestion begins in the stomach and ends in the absorptive cells of the small intestine, where any remaining short groupings of amino acids are broken down into single amino acids. Stomach acid and enzymes contribute to protein digestion. Absorption from the intestinal lumen into the absorptive cells requires energy input.

■ Absorption

The short chains of amino acids and any individual amino acids in the small intestine are taken up by active transport into the absorptive cells lining the small intestine. Any remaining peptide bonds are broken down to yield individual amino acids inside the intestinal cells. Since they are water-soluble, the amino acids travel to the liver via the portal vein which drains absorbed nutrients from the intestinal tract. In the liver, individual amino acids can undergo several modifications, depending on the requirements of the body. Individual amino acids may be combined into the proteins needed by the body, broken down for energy needs, released into the bloodstream, or converted to nonessential amino acids, glucose, or fat. With excess protein intake, conversion of amino acids to fat comes last.

Except during infancy, it is uncommon for intact proteins to be absorbed from the digestive tract. In the period of infancy (up to 4 to 5 months of age), the gastrointestinal tract is somewhat permeable to small proteins, so some whole proteins can be absorbed. Because proteins from some foods (e.g., cow's registered milk and egg whites) may predispose an infant to food allergies, pediatricians and dietitians recommend waiting until an infant is at least 6 to 12 months of age before introducing commonly allergenic foods (see Chapter 14 for details).

Concept Check

Protein digestion begins with cooking, as proteins are denatured by heat. Once protein reaches the stomach, enzymes cleave proteins into smaller segments of amino acids. As food travels through the small intestine, protein breakdown products formed in the stomach are broken down further to individual amino acids or short segments of amino acids, and taken up into the absorptive cells of the small intestine lining where final breakdown into amino acids occurs. The amino acids then travel via the portal vein that connects to the liver.

Putting Proteins to Work in the Body

As you have learned, proteins function in many crucial ways in human metabolism and in the formation of body structures. We rely on foods to supply the amino acids needed to form these proteins. Note, however, that only when we also eat enough carbohydrate and fat can food proteins be used most efficiently. If we don't consume enough calories to meet needs, some amino acids from proteins are broken down to produce energy, rendering them unavailable to build body proteins.

▌Producing Vital Body Structures

Every cell contains protein. Muscles, connective tissue, mucus, blood-clotting factors, transport proteins in the bloodstream, lipoproteins, enzymes, immune bodies, some hormones, visual pigments, and the support structure inside bones are primarily made of protein (Fig. 6-8). Excess protein in the diet doesn't enhance the synthesis of these body components, but eating too little can impede it.

Most vital body proteins are in a constant state of breakdown, rebuilding, and repair. For example, the intestinal tract lining is constantly sloughed off. The digestive tract treats sloughed cells just like food particles, digesting them and absorbing their amino acids. In fact, most of the amino acids released throughout the body can be recycled to become part of the pool of amino acids available for synthesis of future proteins. Overall, **protein turnover** is a process by which a cell can respond to its changing environment by producing proteins that are needed and disassembling proteins that are not needed.

During any day, an adult makes and degrades about 250 grams of protein, recycling many of the amino acids. Relative to the 65 to 100 grams of protein typically consumed by adults in North America, recycled amino acids make an important contribution to total protein metabolism.

If a person's diet is low in protein for a long period of time, the processes of rebuilding and repairing body proteins slow. Over time, skeletal muscles, blood proteins, and vital organs, such as the heart and liver, will decrease in size or volume. Only the brain resists protein breakdown.

▌Maintaining Fluid Balance

Blood proteins maintain body fluid balance. Normal blood pressure in the arteries forces blood into capillary beds. The blood fluid then moves from the **capillary beds** into the spaces between nearby cells **(extracellular spaces)** to provide nutrients to

protein turnover The process of breaking down proteins and then resynthesizing new proteins by cells. In this way the cell will have the proteins it needs to function at that time.

capillary bed Network of one-cell thick vessels that create a junction between arterial and venous circulation. It is here that gas and nutrient exchange occurs between body cells and the blood.

extracellular space The space outside cells; represents one-third of all body fluid.

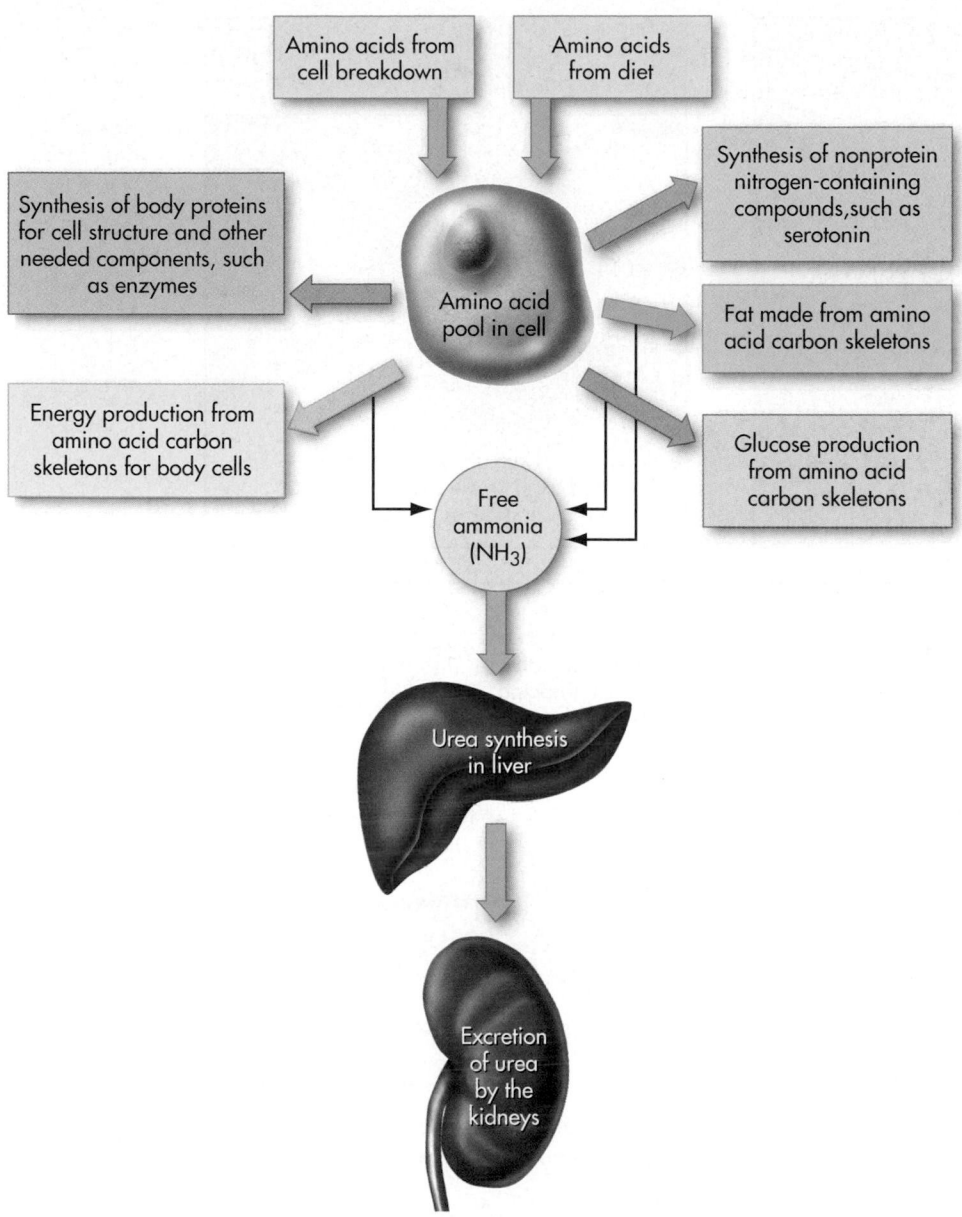

Figure 6-8 Amino acid metabolism. The amino acid **pool** in a cell can be used to form body proteins, as well as a variety of other possible products—from fat and glucose from amino acid **carbon skeletons** to **urea.** The urea is a waste product made from the nitrogen-containing ammonia (NH_3) released during amino acid breakdown. It is excreted in the urine.

those cells (Fig. 6-9). Proteins in the bloodstream are too large however, to move out of the capillary beds into the tissues. The presence of these proteins in the capillary beds attracts the proper amount of fluid back to the blood, partially counteracting the force of blood pressure.

With an inadequate consumption of protein, the concentration of proteins in the bloodstream drops below normal. Excessive fluid then builds up in the surrounding tissues because the counteracting force produced by the smaller amount of blood proteins is too weak to pull enough of the fluid back from the tissues into the bloodstream. As fluids accumulate in the tissues, the tissues swell, causing **edema.** Because edema may be a symptom of a variety of medical problems, the cause must be identified. An important step in diagnosing the cause is to measure the concentration of blood proteins.

■ Contributing to Acid-Base Balance

Proteins help regulate acid-base balance in the blood. Proteins located in cell membranes pump chemical ions in and out of cells. The ion concentration that results from the pumping action, among other factors, keeps the blood slightly alkaline. In

pool The amount of a nutrient stored within the body that can be mobilized when needed.

carbon skeleton Amino acid structure that remains after the amino group (—NH_2) has been removed.

urea Nitrogenous waste product of protein metabolism; major source of nitrogen in the urine, chemically NH_2—$\overset{\overset{\text{O}}{||}}{C}$—$NH_2$.

edema The buildup of excess fluid in extracellular spaces.

(a)

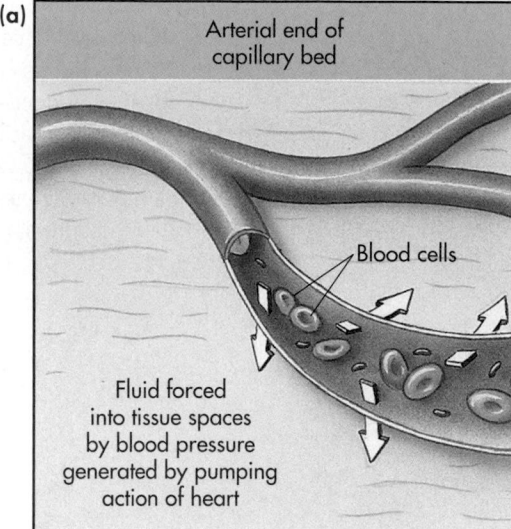

Arterial end of capillary bed

Blood cells

Fluid forced into tissue spaces by blood pressure generated by pumping action of heart

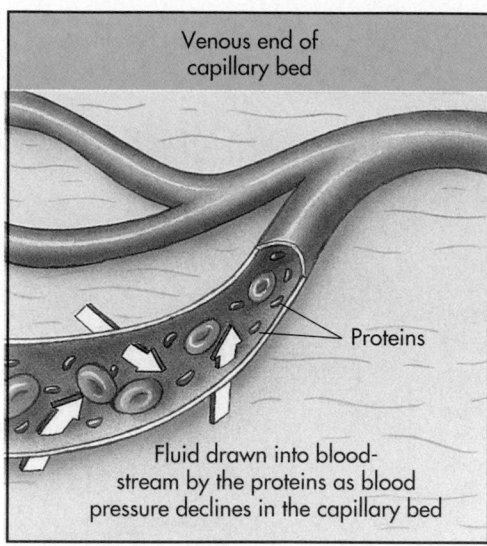

Venous end of capillary bed

Proteins

Fluid drawn into bloodstream by the proteins as blood pressure declines in the capillary bed

(b)

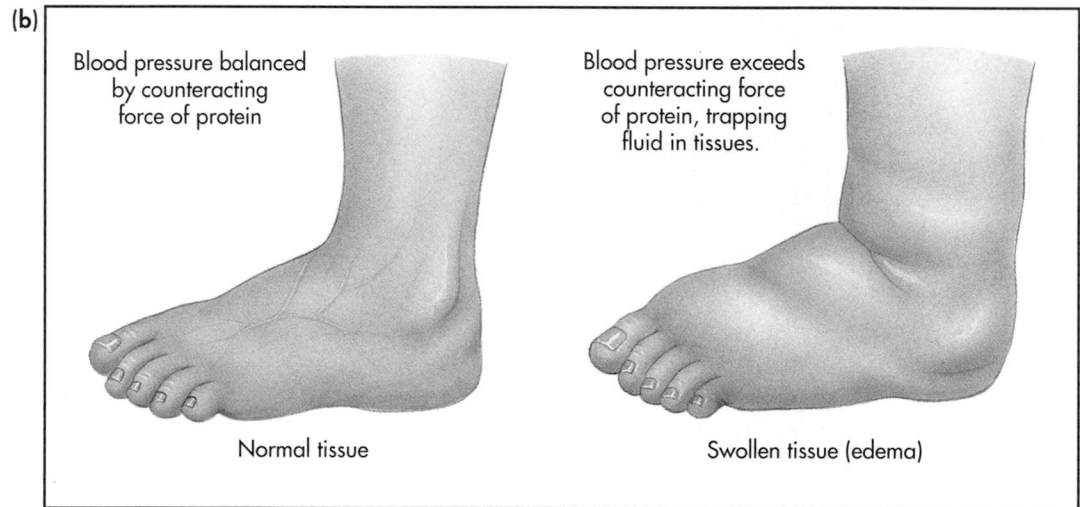

Blood pressure balanced by counteracting force of protein

Blood pressure exceeds counteracting force of protein, trapping fluid in tissues.

Normal tissue

Swollen tissue (edema)

Figure 6-9 Blood proteins in relation to fluid balance. (a) Blood proteins are important for maintaining the body's fluid balance. (b) Without sufficient protein in the bloodstream, edema develops.

buffers Compounds that cause a solution to resist changes in acid-base conditions.

addition, some blood proteins are especially good **buffers** for the body. Buffers are compounds that maintain acid-base conditions within a narrow range.

■ Forming Hormones and Enzymes

Amino acids are required for the synthesis of many hormones—our internal body messengers. Some hormones, such as the thyroid hormones, are made from only one type of amino acid, tyrosine. Insulin, on the other hand, is composed of 51 total amino acids. Almost all enzymes also are proteins or have a protein component.

■ Contributing to Immune Function

Neurotransmitters, released by nerve endings, are often derivatives of amino acids. This is true for dopamine (synthesized from the amino acid tyrosine), norepinephrine (synthesized from the amino acid tyrosine), and serotonin (synthesized from the amino acid tryptophan).

Proteins are a key component of the cells used by the immune system. Also, the antibodies produced by one type of white blood cell are proteins. These antibodies can bind to foreign proteins in the body, an important step in removing invaders from the body. Without sufficient dietary protein, the immune system lacks the materials needed to function properly. For example, a compromised protein status can turn measles into a fatal disease for a malnourished child.

■ Forming Glucose

In Chapter 4 you learned that the body must maintain a fairly constant concentration of blood glucose to supply energy for the brain, red blood cells, and nervous tissue. At rest, the brain uses about 19% of the body's energy requirements, and it gets most of that energy from glucose. If you don't consume enough carbohydrate to supply the glucose, your liver (and kidneys, to a lesser extent) will be forced to make glucose from amino acids present in body tissues (review Fig. 6-8).

Making some glucose from amino acids is normal. For example, when you skip breakfast and haven't eaten since 7 P.M. the preceding evening, glucose must be manufactured. In an extreme situation, however, such as in starvation, the conversion of amino acids into glucose wastes much muscle tissue and can produce edema.

■ Providing Energy

Proteins supply very little energy for a weight-stable person. Two situations in which a person does use protein to meet energy needs are during prolonged exercise (see Chapter 11 for information about the use of amino acids for energy needs during exercise) and during calorie restriction, as with a weight-loss diet. In these cases, the amino group ($-NH_2$) from the amino acid is removed and the remaining carbon skeleton is metabolized for energy needs (review Fig. 6-8). Still, under most conditions, cells primarily use fats and carbohydrates for energy needs. Although proteins contain the same amount of calories (on average, 4 kcal per gram) as carbohydrates, proteins are a very costly source of calories, considering the amount of processing the liver and kidneys must perform to use this calorie source.

Concept Check

Vital body constituents—such as muscle, connective tissue, blood transport proteins, enzymes, hormones, buffers, and immune factors—are mainly proteins. The degradation of existing proteins and synthesis of new proteins takes place constantly, amounting to a turnover rate of about 250 grams a day for the entire human body. Proteins can also be used for glucose and other fuel production.

■ Protein Needs

How much protein (actually, amino acids) do we need to eat each day? People who aren't growing need to eat only enough protein to match whatever they lose daily from protein breakdown. The amount of breakdown can be determined by measuring the amount of urea and other nitrogen-containing compounds in the urine, as well as losses of protein from feces, skin, hair, nails, and so on. In short, people need to balance protein intake with such losses to maintain a state of **protein equilibrium,** also called *protein balance* (Figs. 6-10 and 6-11).

When a body is growing or recovering from an illness or injury, it needs a **positive protein balance** to supply the raw materials required to build new tissues. To achieve this, a person must eat more protein daily than he or she loses. In addition, the hormones insulin, growth hormone, and testosterone all stimulate positive protein balance. Resistance exercise (weight training) also enhances positive protein balance. Consuming less protein than needed leads to **negative protein balance,** such as when acute illness reduces the desire to eat and so one loses more protein than consumed.

For healthy people, the amount of dietary protein needed to maintain protein equilibrium (wherein intake equals losses) can be determined by increasing protein intake until it equals losses of protein and its related breakdown products (e.g., urea). Calorie needs must also be met so that amino acids are not diverted for such use.

Today, the best estimate for the amount of protein required for nearly all adults to maintain protein equilibrium is 0.8 grams of protein per kilogram of healthy body

The vitamin niacin can be made from the amino acid tryptophan, illustrating another role of proteins.

Recent studies have shown that gram for gram, protein is the macronutrient with the highest satiety value. Thus it is important not to skimp on protein when planning meals.

protein equilibrium A state in which protein intake is equal to related protein losses; the person is said to be in protein balance.

positive protein balance A state in which protein intake exceeds related protein losses, such as during times of growth.

negative protein balance A state in which protein intake is less than related protein losses, such as often seen during acute illness.

The RDA for protein translates into about 10% of total calories. Many experts recommend up to 15% of total calories to provide more flexibility in diet planning, in turn allowing for the variety of protein-rich foods North Americans typically consume. As noted earlier, the Food and Nutrition Board has set an upper range for protein intake at 35% of calories consumed.

(a)

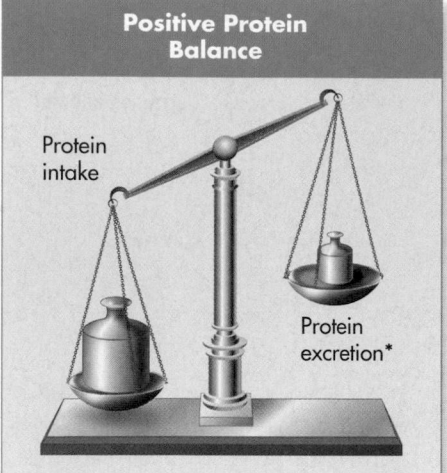

Positive Protein Balance

Protein intake

Protein excretion*

Situations in which protein balance is positive:

Growth
Pregnancy
Recovery stage after illness, injury
Athletic training**
Increased secretion of certain hormones, such as insulin, growth hormone, and testosterone

(b)

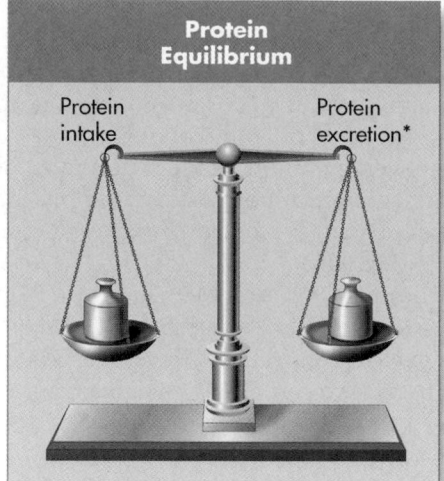

Protein Equilibrium

Protein intake

Protein excretion*

(c)

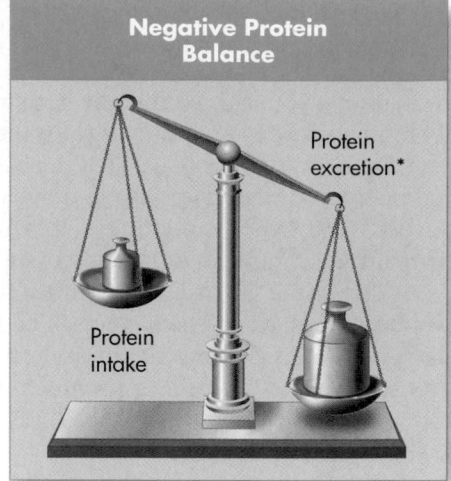

Negative Protein Balance

Protein excretion*

Protein intake

Situations in which protein balance is negative:

Inadequate intake of protein (fasting, intestinal tract diseases)
Inadequate calorie intake
Conditions such as fevers, burns, and infections
Bed rest (for serveral days)
Deficiency of essential amino acids (e.g., poor-quality protein comsumed)
Increased protein loss (as in some forms of kidney disease)
Increased secretion of certain hormones, such as thyroid hormone and cortisol

---

*Based on losses of urea and other nitrogen-containing compounds in the urine, as well as protein itself lost from feces, skin, hair, nails, and other minor routes.

**Only when additional lean body mass is being gained. Nevertheless, the athlete is probably already eating enough protein to support this extra protein synthesis; protein supplements are not needed.

Figure 6-10 Protein balance in practical terms: (a) positive protein balance; (b) protein equilibrium; (c) negative protein balance.

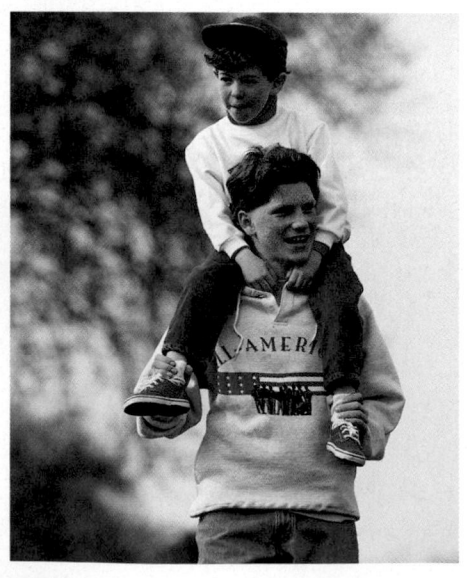

(a)

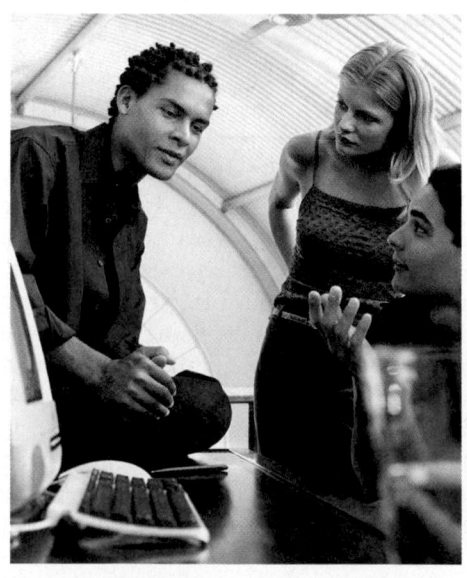

(b)

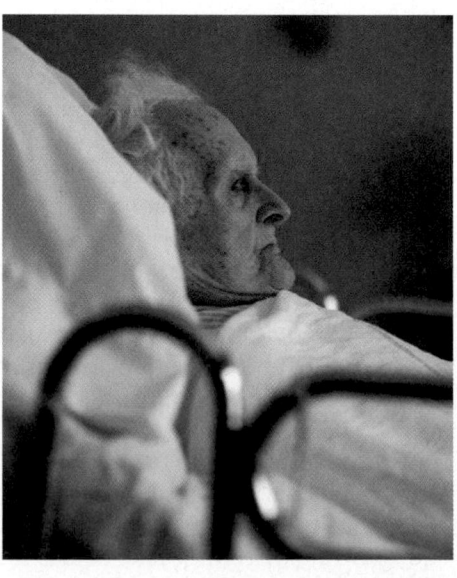

(c)

Figure 6-11 Protein balance throughout the lifecycle. (a) Growing children will be in positive protein balance. (b) Adults generally are in protein equilibrium. (c) Illness, particularly in one's older years, typically leads to negative protein balance.

weight. This is the RDA for protein. Requirements are higher during periods of growth, such as infancy and pregnancy (see Chapters 13 and 14 for specific values for infants, children, and pregnant women). Healthy weight is used as a reference in the determination of protein needs because excess fat storage doesn't contribute much to protein needs (see Chapter 10 for insight into the concept of healthy weight). Calculations using this RDA are shown in the margin and estimate a requirement of about 56 grams of protein daily for a typical 70-kilogram (154-pound) man and about 46 grams of protein daily for a typical 57-kilogram (125-pound) woman.

It is easy to meet currently suggested daily protein needs (Table 6-3). On a daily basis, typical North American protein intakes are about 100 grams of protein for men and 65 grams for women. Thus, most of us consume much more protein than the RDA recommends because we like many high-protein foods and can afford to buy them. Our bodies cannot store excess protein once it is consumed, so the carbon skeletons are turned into glucose or fat and then stored as fat or metabolized for energy needs (review Fig. 6-8).

Note that mental stress, physical labor, and recreational weekend sports activities do not require an increase in the protein RDA. For some highly trained athletes, such as those participating in endurance or strength training, protein consumption may need to exceed the RDA. This is an area of debate in sports nutrition: the Food and Nutrition Board does not support an increased need, but some experts suggest an increase to about 1.7 grams per kilogram. Many North Americans already consume that much protein, especially men.

Convert weight from pounds to kilograms:

$$\frac{154 \text{ pounds}}{2.2 \text{ pounds/kilogram}}$$

$$= 70 \text{ kilograms}$$

$$\frac{125 \text{ pounds}}{2.2 \text{ pounds/kilogram}}$$

$$= 57 \text{ kilograms}$$

Calculate protein RDA:

$$70 \text{ kilograms} \times \frac{0.8 \text{ grams protein}}{\text{kilogram body weight}}$$

$$= 56 \text{ grams}$$

$$57 \text{ kilograms} \times \frac{0.8 \text{ grams protein}}{\text{kilogram body weight}}$$

$$= 46 \text{ grams}$$

Table 6-3 The Protein Contents of a 1600 kcal Diet and a 2400 kcal Diet*

1600 kcal Diet	Protein (grams)	2400 kcal Diet	Protein (grams)
Breakfast			
1% milk, 1 cup	8	2% reduced-fat milk, 1 cup	8
Cheerios, 1 cup	2	Cheerios, 1 cup	2
Orange	1	Eggs, soft cooked, 2	12
		Orange	1
Lunch			
Whole-wheat bread, 2 slices	5	Whole-wheat bread, 2 slices	5
Chicken breast, 2 ounces	17	Chicken breast, 2 ounces	17
Mayonnaise, 1 teaspoon	—	Provolone cheese, 2 ounces	15
Tomato slices, 2	—	Tomato slices, 2	—
Carrot sticks, 1 cup	1	Mayonnaise, 1 teaspoon	—
Oatmeal raisin cookie, 1	2		
Fig, 1 large	0.5	Oatmeal-raisin cookies, 2	4
Diet soft drink	—	Figs, 2	1
		Diet soft drink	
Dinner			
Mixed green salad, 1 cup	—	Mixed green salad, ½ cup	—
Italian dressing, 2 teaspoons	—	Italian dressing, 2 teaspoons	—
Beef tenderloin, 3 ounces	21	Beef tenderloin, 4 ounces	28
Spinach pasta, 1 cup, with garlic butter, 1 teaspoon	7	Spinach pasta, 1 cup, with garlic butter, 1 teaspoon	7
Zucchini, ½ cup, sauteed in oil, 1 teaspoon	0.5	Zucchini, ½ cup, sauteed in oil, 1 teaspoon	0.5
1% milk, 1 cup	8	Carrot sticks, ½ cup	0.5
		2% reduced-fat milk, 1 cup	8
Snack		**Snack**	
Bagel, toasted, ½ of a 3½-inch bagel	4	Bagel, toasted, ½ of 3½-inch bagel	4
Jam, 2 teaspoons	—	Jam, 2 teaspoons	—
Fruited yogurt, 1 cup	10	Fruited yogurt, 1 cup	10
TOTAL	87		124

*This table illustrates how few calories need be consumed while still meeting the RDA for protein. It also shows how much protein we eat when we consume typical calorie intakes.

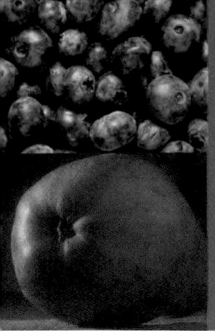

Vegetarianism has evolved over the centuries from a necessity into an option. Historically, vegetarianism was linked with specific philosophies and religions or with science. Today, about 1 in 40 adults in the United States (and about 1 in 25 in Canada) is a vegetarian. Over the past decades, vegetarian diets have evolved to include such new products as soy-based sloppy joes, chili, tacos, burgers, and more. In addition, cookbooks that feature the use of a variety of fruits, vegetables, and seasonings are enhancing food selection for vegetarians of all degrees.

Vegetarianism is popular among college students. Fifteen percent of college students in one survey said they select vegetarian options at lunch or dinner on any given day. In response, dining services offer vegetarian options at every meal, such as pastas with meatless sauce and pizza. Many teenagers are also turning to vegetarianism. In addition, a survey by the National Restaurant Association found that 20% of its customers want a vegetarian option when they eat out. Many customers cite health and taste as reasons for choosing vegetarian meals.

As nutrition science has grown, new information has enabled the design of nutritionally adequate vegetarian diets. It is important for vegetarians to take advantage of this information because a diet of only plant-based foods has the potential to promote various nutrient deficiencies and substantial growth retardation in infants and children. People who choose a vegetarian diet can meet their nutritional needs by following a few basic rules and knowledgeably planning their diets.

Studies show that death rates from some chronic diseases, such as certain forms of cardiovascular disease, hypertention, many forms of cancer, type 2 diabetes, and obesity, are lower for vegetarians than for nonvegetarians. These individuals also often live longer, as has been shown in religious groups that practice vegetarianism. However, healthful lifestyles (not smoking, abstaining from alcohol and drugs, and regular physical activity) and social class bias probably partially account for these findings.

As you learned in Chapter 2, MyPyramid and the 2005 Dietary Guidelines for Americans emphasize a plant-based diet of whole-grain breads and cereals, fruits, and vegetables. In addition the American Institute for Cancer Research promotes "The New American Plate" with plant-based foods covering two-thirds (or more) of the plate and meat, fish, poultry, or low-fat dairy covering one-third (or less) of the plate. Although these recommendations do allow the inclusion of animal products, they are definitely more "vegetarian-like" than typical North American diets.

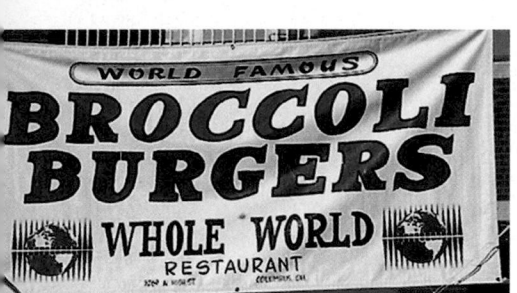

Vegetarian adaptations of traditional foods are a growing trend in our society.

Why Do People Become Vegetarians?

People choose vegetarianism for a variety of reasons. Some believe that killing animals for food is unethical. Hindus and Trappist monks eat vegetarian meals as a practice of their religion. In North America, many Seventh Day Adventists base their practice of vegetarianism on biblical texts and believe it is a more healthful way to live.

Some advocates of vegetarianism base their food preference upon the inefficient use of animals as a source of protein. Note that 40% of the world's grain production is used to raise meat-producing animals. Although animals that humans eat sometimes eat grasses that humans cannot digest, many also eat grains that humans can eat.

People might also practice vegetarianism because while encouraging a high intake of complex carbohydrates, vitamins A, E, and C, carotenoids, magnesium, and fiber, it limits saturated fat and cholesterol intake.

Food Planning for Vegetarians

There are a variety of vegetarian diet styles. **Vegans,** or "total vegetarians," eat only plant foods (and do not use animal products for other purposes, such as leather shoes or feather pillows). **Fruitarians** primarily eat fruits, nuts, honey, and vegetable oils. This plan is not recommended because it can lead to nutrient deficiencies in people of all ages. **Lactovegetarians** modify vegetarianism a bit—they include dairy products and plant foods. **Lactoovovegetarians** modify the diet even further and eat dairy products and eggs, as well as plant foods. Including these animal products makes food planning easier because they are rich in some nutrients that are missing or minimal in plants, such as vitamin B-12 and calcium. The more variety in the diet, the easier it is to meet nutritional needs. Thus, the practice of eating no animal sources of food significantly separates the vegans and fruitarians from all other semivegetarian styles.

Most people who call themselves vegetarians consume at least some dairy products, if not all dairy products and eggs. A food-group plan has been developed for lactovegetarians and vegans (Table 6-4). This plan includes servings of nuts, grains, legumes, and seeds to help meet protein needs. There is also a vegetable group, a fruit group, and a milk group.

Vegan Diet Planning

Planning a vegan diet requires knowledge and creativity to yield high-quality protein and other key nutrients without animal products. Earlier in this chapter, you learned about complementing proteins, whereby the essential amino acids deficient in one protein source are supplied by those of another consumed at the same meal or the next. Recall that many legumes are deficient in the essential amino acid methionine, while cereals are limited in lysine. Eating a combination of legumes and cereals, such as beans and rice, will supply the body with adequate amounts

vegan A person who eats only plant foods.

fruitarian A person who primarily eats fruits, nuts, honey, and vegetable oils.

lactovegetarian A person who consumes plant products and dairy products.

lactoovovegetarian A person who consumes plant products, dairy products, and eggs.

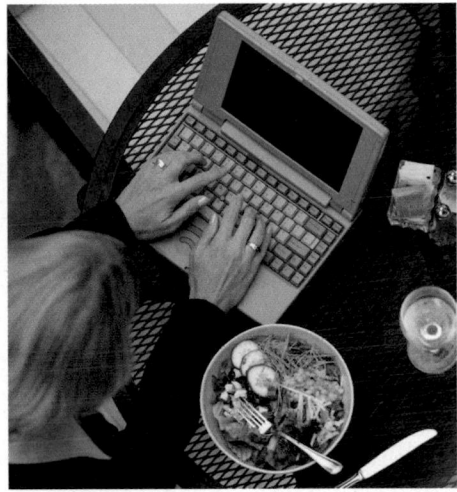

A salad containing numerous types of vegetables and legumes is a healthy vegetarian choice.

Table 6-4 Food-Group Plan for Lactovegetarians and Vegans Which Also Follows MyPyramid§

| Group† | Servings | | Key Nutrients Supplied |
	Lactovegetarian‡	Vegan§ǁ	
Grains¶	6–11	8–11	Protein, thiamin, niacin, folate, vitamin E, zinc, phosphorus, magnesium, iron, and fiber
Legumes	2–3	3	Protein, vitamin B-6, zinc, phosphorus, magnesium, and fiber
Nuts, seeds	2–3	3	Protein, vitamin E, and magnesium
Vegetables	3–5 (include one dark green or leafy variety daily)	4–6 (include one dark green or leafy variety daily)	Vitamin A, vitamin C, and folate
Fruits	2–4	4	Vitamin A, vitamin C, and folate
Milk	3	—	Protein, riboflavin, vitamin D, vitamin B-12, and calcium and phosphorus

†Base serving size on those listed for MyPyramid (see Chapter 2). This plan yields about 1600 to 1800 kcal. Increase the number of servings, or add other foods to meet higher calorie needs.
‡Contains about 75 grams of protein in 1650 kcal.
§A calcium-fortified food, such as orange juice or soy milk, is needed unless a calcium supplement is used. In addition, use of or foods fortified with vitamin B-12 a supplemental source of vitamin B-12 is a must. Use of iodized salt is also important.
ǁContains about 79 grams of protein in 1800 kcal.
¶One serving of vitamin- and mineral-enriched breakfast cereal is recommended. Alternately, a balanced multivitamin and mineral supplement can be used to help close possible nutrient gaps.

Table 6-2, earlier in Chapter 6, lists traditional dishes in which vegetable proteins combine to provide high-quality (complete) protein in the meal.

As noted in Chapter 5, a vegan diet coupled with regular exercise and other lifestyle changes can lead to a reversal of atherosclerotic plaque in various arteries in the body.

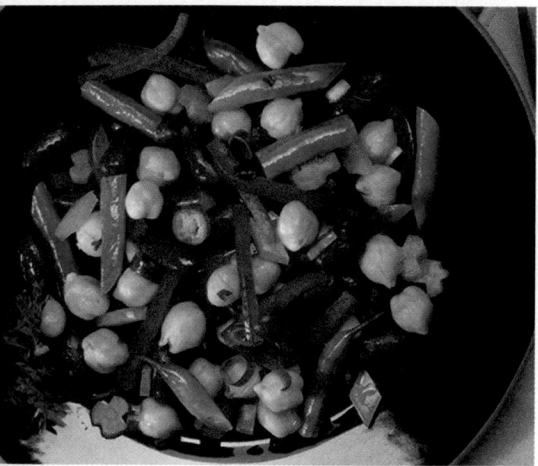

Keep in mind that amino acids in vegetables are best used when a combination of sources is consumed.

Consuming adequate quantities of omega-3 fatty acids is yet another nutritional concern for vegetarians, especially vegans. Fish and fish oils, which are abundant sources of these heart-healthy fats, are omitted from many types of vegetarian diets. Alternative plant sources of omega-3 fatty acids include canola oil, soybean oil, seaweed, microalgae, flax seeds, and walnuts.

of all essential amino acids. As for any diet, variety is an especially important characteristic of a nutritious vegan diet.

Aside from amino acids, low intakes of certain micronutrients can be a problem for the vegan. At the forefront of nutritional concerns are riboflavin, vitamins D and B-12, iron, zinc, iodide, and calcium. The following dietary advice should be implemented. In addition, use of a balanced multivitamin and mineral supplement can help as well.

Riboflavin can be obtained from green leafy vegetables, whole grains, yeast, and legumes—components of most vegan diets. Alternate sources of vitamin D include fortified foods (e.g., margarine), as well as regular sun exposure (see Chapter 8).

Vitamin B-12 only occurs naturally in animal foods. Plants can contain soil or microbial contaminants that provide trace amounts of vitamin B-12, but these are negligible sources of the vitamin. Because the body can store vitamin B-12 for about 4 years, it may take a long time after removal of animal foods from the diet for a vitamin B-12 deficiency to surface. If dietary B-12 inadequacy persists, deficiency can lead to a form of anemia, nerve damage, and mental dysfunction. These dire deficiency consequences have been noted in the infants of vegetarian mothers whose breast milk was low in vitamin B-12. Chronically low vitamin B-12 consumption may also result in excess blood concentration of homocysteine, which likely is a risk factor for cardiovascular disease. As you can see, vegans need to be careful to prevent a vitamin B-12 deficiency. This can be achieved by finding a reliable source of vitamin B-12, such as fortified soybean milk, ready-to-eat breakfast cereals, and special yeast grown on media rich in vitamin B-12.

For iron, the vegan can consume whole grains (especially ready-to-eat breakfast cereals), dried fruits and nuts, and legumes. Note that the iron in these foods is not absorbed as well as iron in animal foods, but a good source of vitamin C taken with these foods helps with the absorption. Thus, a recommended strategy is to consume vitamin C with every meal that contains iron-rich plant foods. Cooking in iron pots and skillets can also add iron to the diet (see Chapter 9).

The vegan can find zinc in whole grains (especially ready-to-eat breakfast cereals), nuts, and legumes, but phytic acid and other substances in these foods limit zinc absorption. Grains are most nutritious when either fortified with zinc or consumed as breads. The latter is because the leavening process (rising of the bread dough) reduces the influence of phytic acid. Iodized salt is a reliable source of iodide. It should be used instead of plain salt, both of which are found in U.S. supermarkets.

Of all nutrients, calcium is the most difficult to consume in sufficient quantities for vegans. Fortified foods are the vegan's best option for obtaining calcium. These include fortified soy milk, fortified orange juice, calcium-rich tofu (check the label), as well as certain ready-to-eat breakfast cereals and snacks. Green leafy vegetables and nuts also contain calcium, but the mineral is either not well absorbed or not very plentiful from these sources. Calcium supplements are another option (see Chapter 9). Special diet planning is always required, because even a multivitamin and mineral supplement will not supply enough calcium to meet the needs of the body.

Special Concerns for Infants and Children

The populations at highest risk for nutrient deficiencies as a result of improperly planned vegetarian and vegan diets are infants and children, who are notoriously picky eaters in the first place. With the use of complementary proteins and good sources of problem nutrients just discussed, the calorie, protein, vitamin, and mineral needs of vegetarian and vegan infants and children can be met. The most common nutritional concerns for infants and children following vegetarian and vegan diets are deficiencies of iron, vitamin B-12, vitamin D, and calcium.

Vegetarian and vegan diets tend to be high in bulky, high-fiber, low-calorie foods that cause a feeling of fullness. While this is a welcome advantage for adults, children have small stomach volume and relatively high nutrient needs compared to their size, and therefore may feel full before their calorie needs are met. For this reason, the fiber content of a child's diet may need to be decreased by replacing high-fiber sources with some refined grain products, fruit juices, and peeled fruit. Other concentrated sources of calories for vegetarian and vegan children include fortified soy milk, nuts, dried fruits, avocados, and cookies made with vegetable oils or tub margarine.

Overall, vegetarian and vegan diets can be appropriate during infancy and childhood, but these diets must be implemented with knowledge and, ideally, professional guidance. An especially informative website on vegetarianism in general is www.ivu.org, supported by the International Vegetarian Union. See also www.vrg.org and www.vegetariannutrition.net.

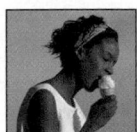

Real Life Scenario Follow-Up

Shannon's dietary intake for this day, although vegetarian, is not as healthy as it could be since it does not come close to following the recommendations provided in the Looking Further section on vegetarian diets. Many components of a healthy vegetarian diet—whole grains, nuts, soy products, beans, two to four servings of fruits, and three to five servings of vegetables per day—are missing. With so few fruits and vegetables, her diet is also low in the many phytochemicals that are under study for numerous health benefits. It is apparent that she has not yet learned to implement the concept of complementary proteins, so the quality of protein in her diet is low. Unless she makes a more informed effort at diet planning, Shannon will not reap the health benefits she had hoped for when she chose to follow a vegetarian diet.

Does Eating a High-Protein Diet Harm You?

People frequently ask about the potential harm of protein intakes in excess of the RDA. The extra vitamin B-6, iron, and zinc that accompany protein-rich foods are often beneficial. However, diets that are high in protein foods typically rely on animal sources of protein and may be simultaneously low in plant sources, and therefore low in fiber, some vitamins (e.g., folate), some minerals (e.g., magnesium), as well as phytochemicals. Additionally, high-protein foods from animals are rich in saturated fat and cholesterol, and thus do not follow the recommendations of the Dietary Guidelines for Americans or the Food and Nutrition Board in terms of reducing risk for cardiovascular disease.

Some, but not all, studies show that high-protein diets can increase calcium losses in urine. Certain types of amino acids—especially those that are predominant in animal proteins—produce this effect. Still, when seen, it is typically minimal. For people with adequate calcium intakes, little concern about this relationship is warranted, but keep in mind that calcium is commonly deficient in North American diets.

Meat is one of the richest sources of protein. Excessive intake of red meat, however, especially processed forms, is linked to colon cancer in population studies. There are several possible explanations for this connection. The curing agents used to process meats such as ham and salami may cause cancer. Substances that form during cooking of red meat at high temperatures may also cause cancer (for a discussion of heterocyclic amines (HCAs), see the Looking Further section in Chapter 15). The excessive fat or low-fiber contents of diets rich in red meat may also be a contributing factor. Because of these concerns, some nutrition experts suggest we focus more on poultry, fish, nuts, legumes, and seeds to meet protein needs. In addition, any red or other type of meat should be trimmed of all visible fat before grilling.

Some researchers have expressed concern that a high-protein intake may overburden the kidneys by forcing them to excrete the extra nitrogen as urea. Additionally, animal proteins may contribute to kidney stone formation in certain individuals. To

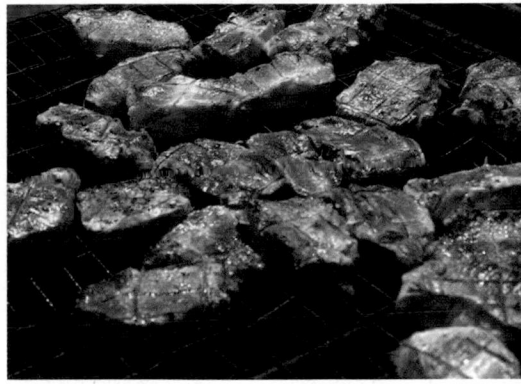

Animal protein foods are typically our main sources of protein in the North American diet.

High-protein diets increase urine output, in turn posing a risk for dehydration. This is a special concern for athletes (see Chapter 11).

prevent these problems, there is some support for limiting protein intake. For instance, for people in the early stages of kidney disease, low-protein diets somewhat slow the decline in kidney function. Also, laboratory animal studies show that protein intakes that just meet nutritional needs preserve kidney function over time better than high-protein diets. Because preserving kidney function is especially important for those who have diabetes, early signs of kidney disease, or only one functioning kidney, a high-protein diet is not recommended for these people. For individuals without diabetes or kidney disease, the risk of suffering kidney failure is minimal; thus, the risk of kidney disease (aside from kidney stones) as a by-product of a high-protein diet is low.

Another Bite

Earlier in this chapter, you learned that the body is designed to handle whole proteins as a dietary source of amino acids. When individual amino acid supplements are taken, they can overwhelm the absorptive mechanisms in the small intestine, triggering amino acid imbalances in the body. Imbalances occur because groups of chemically similar amino acids compete for absorption sites in the absorptive cells. For example, lysine and arginine are absorbed by the same transporter, so an excess of lysine can impair absorption of arginine. The amino acids most likely to cause toxicity when consumed in large amounts are methionine, cysteine, and histidine. Due to the potential for imbalances and toxicities of individual amino acids, the best advice to ensure adequacy is to stick to whole foods rather than supplements as sources of amino acids.

Concept Check

The Recommended Dietary Allowance (RDA) for adults is 0.8 grams of protein per kilogram of healthy body weight. This is approximately 56 grams of protein daily for a 70-kilogram (156-pound) person. The average North American man consumes about 100 grams of protein daily, and a woman consumes about 65 grams. Thus, typically we eat more than enough protein to meet our needs. This even includes well-balanced vegetarian diets. Diets high in protein can compromise kidney health in people with diabetes and those with kidney disease, and animal protein sources likely increase cardiovascular disease and kidney stone risk when consumed in high amounts.

protein-calorie malnutrition (PCM) A condition resulting from regularly consuming insufficient amounts of calories and protein. The deficiency eventually results in body wasting, primarily of lean tissue, and an increased susceptibility to infections.

marasmus A disease resulting from consuming a grossly insufficient amount of protein and calories; one of the diseases classed as protein-calorie malnutrition. Victims have little or no fat stores, little muscle mass, and poor strength. Death from infections is common.

kwashiorkor A disease occurring primarily in young children who have an existing disease and consume a marginal amount of calories and insufficient protein in relation to needs. The child generally suffers from infections and exhibits edema, poor growth, weakness, and an increased susceptibility to further illness.

Protein-Calorie Malnutrition

Protein deficiency is rarely an isolated condition and usually accompanies a deficiency of calories and other nutrients resulting from insufficient food intake. In developing areas of the world, people often have diets low in calories and also in protein. This state of undernutrition stunts the growth of children and makes them more susceptible to disease throughout life. (Note that undernutrition is a main focus of Chapter 17.) People who consume too little protein calories can eventually develop **protein-calorie malnutrition (PCM)**, also referred to as *protein-energy malnutrition (PEM)*. In its milder form, it is difficult to tell if a person with PCM is consuming too little calories or protein, or both. But if the nutrient deficiency—especially for calories—becomes quite severe, a deficiency disease called **marasmus** can result. When an inadequate intake of nutrients, including protein, is combined with an already existing disease, a form of malnutrition called **kwashiorkor** can develop. Both

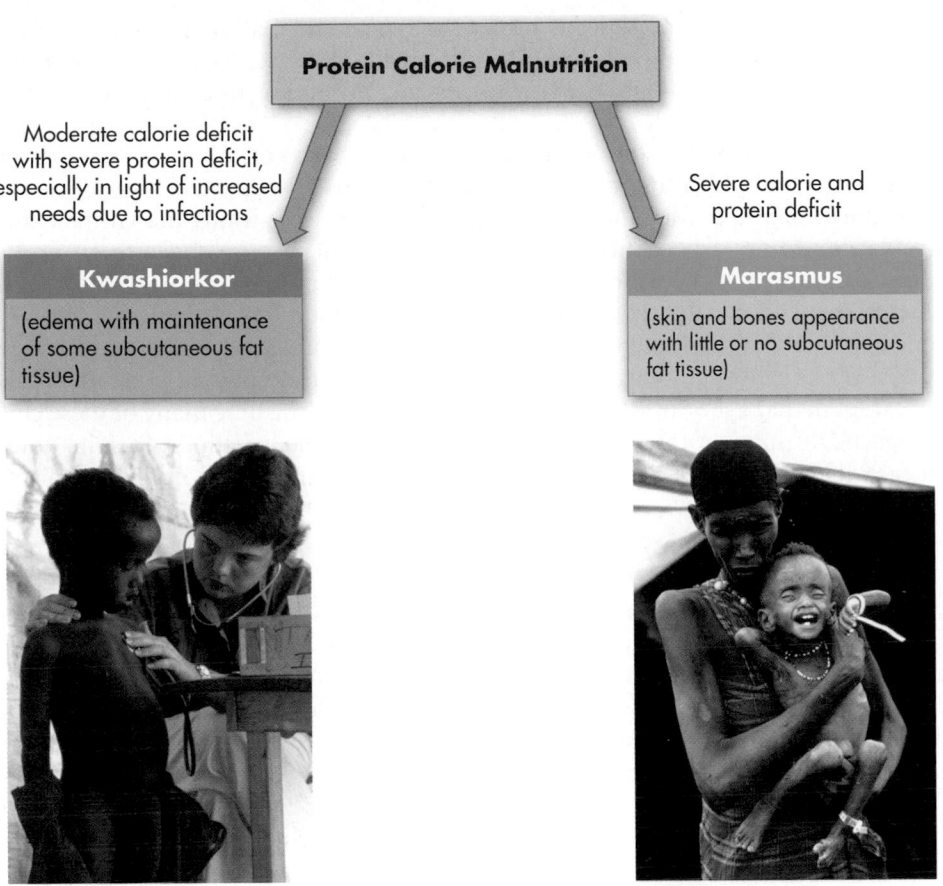

Figure 6-12 Schema for classifying undernutrition in children. The presence of subcutaneous fat (directly underneath the skin) is a diagnostic key for distinguishing kwashiorkor from marasmus.

conditions are seen primarily in children, but also may develop in adults, even in those hospitalized in North America. These two conditions form the tip of the iceberg with respect to states of undernutrition, and symptoms of these two conditions can even be present in the same person (Fig. 6-12).

Toxic products in moldy grains may also contribute to kwashiorkor.

■ Kwashiorkor

Kwashiorkor is a word from Ghana that means "the disease that the first child gets when the new child comes." From birth, an infant in developing areas of the world is usually breastfed. Often by the time the child reaches 1 to 1.5 years of age, the mother is pregnant or has already given birth again, and the new child gets preference for breast-feeding. The older child's diet then abruptly changes from nutritious human milk to starchy roots and **gruels.** These foods have low-protein densities, compared with total energy. Additionally, the foods are usually full of plant fibers, which are often bulky, making it difficult for the child to consume enough to meet calorie needs. The child generally also has infections, which acutely raise calorie and protein needs. For these reasons, calorie needs of these children are met just barely, at best, and their protein consumption is grossly inadequate, especially in view of the increased amount needed to combat infections. Many vitamin and mineral needs are also far from being ful-filled. Famine victims face similar problems.

gruels A thin mixture of grains or legumes in milk or water.

The major symptoms of kwashiorkor are apathy, diarrhea, listlessness, failure to grow and gain weight, and withdrawal from the environment. These symptoms complicate other diseases present. For example, a condition such as measles, a dis-ease that normally makes a healthy child ill for only a week or so, can become se-verely debilitating and even fatal. Further symptoms of kwashiorkor are changes in hair color, potassium deficiency, flaky skin, fatty liver, reduced muscle mass, and massive edema in the abdomen and legs. The presence of edema in a child who has some subcutaneous fat (i.e., directly under the skin) is the hallmark of kwashiorkor (review Fig. 6-12). In addition, these children seldom move. If you pick them up, they don't cry. When you hold them, you feel the plumpness of edema, not muscle and fat tissue.

Many symptoms of kwashiorkor can be explained based on what we know about proteins. Proteins play important roles in fluid balance, lipoprotein transport, immune function, and production of tissues, such as skin, cells lining the GI tract, and hair. We should not expect children with an insufficient protein intake to grow and mature normally, and they don't.

If children with kwashiorkor are helped in time—if infections are treated and a diet ample in protein, calories, and other essential nutrients is provided—the disease process reverses. They begin to grow again and may even show no signs of their previous condition, except perhaps shortness of stature. Unfortunately, by the time many of these children reach a hospital or care center, they already have severe infections. In spite of the best care, they still die. Or, if they survive, they return home only to become ill again.

■ Marasmus

Marasmus typically occurs as an infant slowly starves to death. It is caused by diets containing minimal amounts of calories, as well as too little protein and other nutrients. As previously noted, the condition is also commonly referred to as *protein-calorie malnutrition*, especially when experienced by older children and adults. The word *marasmus* means "to waste away," in Greek. Victims have a "skin-and-bones" appearance, with little or no subcutaneous fat (review Fig. 6-12).

Marasmus commonly develops in infants who either are not breastfed or have stopped breastfeeding in the early months. Often the weaning formula used is improperly prepared because of unsafe water and because the parents cannot afford sufficient infant formula for the child's needs. The latter problem may lead the parents to dilute the formula to provide more feedings, not realizing that this provides only more water for the infant.

Marasmus in infants commonly occurs in the large cities of poverty-stricken countries. When people are poor and sanitation is lacking, bottle feeding often leads to marasmus. In the cities, bottle feeding is often necessary because the infant must be cared for by others when the mother is working or away from home. An infant with marasmus requires large amounts of calories and protein—like a **preterm** infant—and, unless the child receives them, full recovery from the disease may never occur. The majority of brain growth occurs between conception and the child's first birthday. In fact, the brain is growing at its highest rate after birth. If the diet does not support brain growth during the first months of life, the brain may not grow to its full adult size. This reduced or retarded brain growth may lead to diminished intellectual function. Both kwashiorkor and marasmus plague infants and children; mortality rates in developing countries are often 10 to 20 times higher than in North America.

preterm An infant born before 37 weeks of gestation; also referred to as premature.

Concept Check

Most undernutrition consists of mild deficits in calories, protein, and often other nutrients. If a person needs more nutrients because of disease and infection but does not consume enough calories and protein, a condition known as kwashiorkor can develop. The person suffers from edema and weakness. Children around age 2 are especially susceptible to kwashiorkor, particularly if they already have other diseases. Famine situations in which only starchy root products are available to eat contribute to this problem. Marasmus is a condition wherein people—infants, especially—starve to death. Symptoms include muscle wasting, absence of fat stores, and weakness. Both an adequate diet and the treatment of concurrent diseases must be promoted to regain and then maintain nutritional health.

Summary

1. Amino acids, the building blocks of proteins, contain a very usable form of nitrogen for humans. Of the 20 common types of amino acids found in food, 9 must be consumed as food (essential) and the rest can be synthesized by the body (nonessential).

2. High-quality (complete) protein foods contain ample amounts of all nine essential amino acids. Furthermore, foods derived from animal sources provide high biological value protein. Lower-quality (incomplete) protein foods lack sufficient amounts of one or more essential amino acids. This is typical of plant foods, especially cereal grains. Different types of plant foods eaten together often complement each other's amino-acid deficits, thereby providing high-quality protein in the diet.

3. Individual amino acids are bonded together to form proteins. The sequential order of amino acids determines the protein's ultimate shape and function. This order is directed by DNA in the cell nucleus. Diseases such as sickle cell anemia can occur if the amino acids are incorrect on a polypeptide chain. When the three-dimensional shape of a protein is unfolded—denatured—by treatment with heat, acid or alkaline solutions, or other processes, the protein also loses its biological activity.

4. Almost all animal products are nutrient-dense sources of protein. The high quality of these proteins means that they can be easily converted into body proteins. Rich plant sources of protein, are also available, such as beans.

5. Protein digestion begins in the stomach, dividing the proteins into breakdown products containing shorter polypeptide chains of amino acids. In the small intestine, these polypeptide chains eventually separate into amino acids in the absorptive cells. The free amino acids then travel via the portal vein that connects to the liver. Some then enter the bloodstream.

6. Important body components—such as muscles, connective tissue, transport proteins in the bloodstream, visual pigments, enzymes, some hormones, and immune bodies—are made of proteins. These proteins are in a state of constant turnover. The carbon chains of proteins may be used to produce glucose when necessary.

7. The protein RDA for adults is 0.8 grams per kilogram of healthy body weight. For a typical 70-kilogram (154-pound) person, this corresponds to 56 grams of protein daily; for a 57-kilogram (125-pound) person, this corresponds to 46 grams per day. The North American diet generally supplies plenty of protein. Men typically consume about 100 grams of protein daily, and women consume closer to 65 grams. These usual protein intakes are also of sufficient quality to support body functions. This is even true for well-balanced vegetarian diets.

8. Undernutrition can lead to protein-calorie malnutrition in the form of kwashiorkor or marasmus. Kwashiorkor results primarily from an inadequate calorie and protein intake in comparison with body needs, which often increase with concurrent disease and infection. Kwashiorkor often occurs when a child is weaned from human milk and fed mostly starchy gruels. Marasmus results from extreme starvation—a negligible intake of both protein and calories. Marasmus commonly occurs during famine, especially in infants.

Study Questions

1. Discuss the relative importance of essential and nonessential amino acids in the diet. Why is it important for essential amino acids lost from the body to be replaced in the diet?

2. Describe the concept of complementary proteins.

3. What is a limiting amino acid? Explain why this concept is a concern in a vegetarian diet. How can a vegetarian compensate for limiting amino acids in specific foods?

4. Briefly describe the organization of proteins. How can this organization be altered or damaged? What might be a result of damaged protein organization?

5. Describe four functions of proteins. Provide an example of how the structure of a protein relates to its function.

6. How are DNA and protein synthesis related?

7. What would be one health benefit of reducing high-protein intake(s) to RDA amounts for some people?

8. What characteristics of vegetable proteins could improve the North American diet? What foods would you include to provide a diet that has ample protein from both plant and animal sources but is moderate in fat?

9. Outline the major differences between kwashiorkor and marasmus.

10. What are the possible long-term effects of an inadequate intake of dietary protein among children between the ages of 6 months and 4 years?

Further Readings

1. ADA Reports: Position of the American Dietetic Association and Dietitians of Canada: vegetarian diets. *Journal of the American Dietetic Association* 103:748, 2003.

   It is the position of the American Dietetic Association and Dietitians of Canada that appropriately planned vegetarian diets are healthful, nutritionally adequate, and provide health benefits in the prevention and treatment of certain diseases. In some cases, however, use of fortified foods or a multivitamin and mineral supplement may be needed to meet recommendations for individual nutrients.

2. Antony AC: Vegetarianism and vitamin B-12 (colbalamin) deficiency. *American Journal of Clinical Nutrition* 78:3, 2003.

   It is vital that a vegetarian focus on meeting vitamin B-12 needs. Use of vitamin B-12-fortified foods or a vitamin and mineral supplement are two options.

3. Aronson D: Vegetarian nutrition. *Today's Dietitian* p. 3, March 2005.

   This article summarizes the possible nutrient deficiencies that can result from a vegetarian diet. Plant food sources to counteract these risks are reviewed, such as rich sources of calcium.

4. Berkow SE, Barnard ND: Blood pressure regulation and vegetarian diets. *Nutrition Reviews* 63: 1, 2005.

   Vegetarian diets are associated with lower blood pressure. It is likely that the fruit, vegetables, legumes, and nuts in such a diet lead to this health benefit.

5. Borghi L and others: Comparison of two diets for the prevention of recurrent stones in idiopathic hypercalciuria. *The New England Journal of Medicine* 346:77, 2002.

In men with a history of calcium oxalate stones and exhibiting increased calcium in the urine, restricted intakes of animal protein and salt, combined with normal calcium intakes, provided protection against recurrence of such stones.

6. Chao A and others: Meat consumption and colorectal cancer. *Journal of the American Medical Association* 293: 172, 2005.

Diets rich in red meat, especially processed meat, increase the risk of colon cancer. Protein from poultry and fish, in contrast, does not pose the same risk.

7. Davis BC, Kris-Etherton PM: Achieving optimal essential fatty acid status in vegetarians: Current knowledge and practical implications. *American Journal of Clinical Nutrition* 78(suppl): 640S, 2003.

Most of the fat in a vegetarian diet should come from nuts, seeds, olives, avocados, soy foods, and monounsaturated-rich oils, such as canola oil, olive oil, and nut oils. This practice provides a sufficient amount of essential fatty acids. Seaweed and microalge are two possible sources for vegans of the very-long-chain omega-3 fatty acids found in fish.

8. Dawson-Hughes B: Interaction of dietary calcium and protein in bone health in humans. *Journal of Nutrition* 133:852S, 2003.

It is important to meet calcium needs to offset any possible protein-related calcium loss in the urine. In this way the combination of meeting protein and calcium needs can be beneficial to bone health.

9. Eating a high protein diet may accelerate kidney problems. *Today's Dietitian* p. 26, April 2004.

High-protein diets may accelerate kidney disease in people who show evidence of the disease. Note that the National Kidney Foundation suggests one in nine North American adults show evidence of at least mild kidney disease.

10. Food and Nutrition Board: *Dietary reference intakes for energy, carbohydrate, fiber, fat, fatty acids, cholesterol, protein, and amino acids.* Washington DC: The National Academy Press, 2002.

This report provides the latest guidance for macronutrient intakes. With regard to protein intake, the RDA has been set at 0.8 grams per kilogram per day. Protein intake can range from 10% to 35% of calorie intake. The 10% allotment approximates the RDA, based on typical calorie intakes.

11. Garlick PJ: The nature of human hazards associated with excessive intakes of amino acids. *Journal of Nutrition* 134: 1633S, 2004.

The most toxic amino acids are methionine, cysteine, and histidine. Possible health risks from excessive intakes of other amino acids are also reviewed. These risks are seen with amino acid supplements, not whole food sources.

12. Gardner CD and others: The effect of a plant-based diet on plasma lipids in hypercholesterolemic adults. *Annals of Internal Medicine* 142: 725, 2005.

Adding plant proteins to a diet already low in saturated fat and cholesterol provides additional benefits regarding lowering blood cholesterol. The authors emphasize the importance of including fruits, vegetables, legumes, and whole grains in a diet.

13. Hu F: Plant-based foods and prevention of cardiovascular disease: An overview. *American Journal of Clinical Nutrition* 78(suppl):544S, 2003.

Plant-based diets provide numerous factors that reduce cardiovascular disease risk, such as unsaturated fats, phytochemicals, and fiber. The whole-grain breads and cereals, fruits, and vegetables in such a diet are the primary source of these factors. If desired, some lean/low-fat animal products can be added to round out a plant-based diet without decreasing its benefits.

14. Leitzmann C: Vegetarian diets: What are the advantages? *Forum of Nutrition* 57: 147, 2005.

The benefits of a vegetarian diet are a lower intake saturated fat, cholesterol, and animal protein, as well as a higher intakes of complex carbohydrates, fiber, magnesium, folate, vitamin C, vitamin E, carotenoids, and other phytochemicals. Well-balanced vegetarian diets are appropriate for all stages of the lifecycle. The article provides evidence to support these statements, as well as reviews other possible health benefits.

15. Lejeune MP and others: Additional protein intake limits weight regain after weight loss in humans. *British Journal of Nutrition* 93: 281, 2005.

Adding 30 g of protein per day to their usual diets helped people in this study limit weight regain after weight loss. The diet ended up 18% of calorie intake as protein, compared to 15% in the control group. This protein intake in the experimental would not be considered excessive given an upper limit of 35% of calorie intake set by the Food and Nutrition Board.

16. Newby PK: Risk of overweight and obesity among semivegetarian, lactovegetarian, and vegan women. *American Journal of Clinical Nutrition* 81: 1267, 2005.

Semivegetarian women in this study were less likely to be overweight and obese compared to omnivorous women. Consuming more plant foods and less animal products may help individuals control their weight.

17. Nuts are on a roll. *UC Berkeley Wellness Letter,* p. 1, May 2003.

Nuts are a rich source of many nutrients and fiber, but also are very energy-dense. Thus it is best to substitute nuts for other protein sources, especially those rich in saturated fat.

18. Sabate J: The contribution of vegetarian diets to human health. *Forums of Nutrition* 56: 218, 2005.

Components of a healthy vegetarian diet include a variety of vegetables, fruits, whole grain breads and cereals, legumes, and nuts. Such a diet contributes to overall health and increased longevity when these foods are emphasized.

19. "Vegging out" for better health? *HealthNews,* p. 8, November 2003.

Well-balanced plant-based diets can lead to numerous health benefits. One benefit may be a longer life.

20. Weiss R and others; Severe vitamin B-12 deficiency in an infant associated with a maternal deficiency and a strict vegetarian diet. *Journal of Pediatric Hematology and Oncology* 26:270, 2004.

A pregnant women needs to be sure to meet vitamin B-12 needs when following a vegetarian diet. This article describes what happens when a vitamin B-12 deficient pregnant women goes on to breastfeed her infant, notably development of severe anemia and nerve degeneration in the infant.

I. Is Your Protein Intake Sufficient to Meet Your Needs?

1. How much protein do you eat in a typical day? Look at the nutrition assessment you completed at the end of Chapter 2. Review it closely (NutritionCalc Plus Bar Graph report). Find the figure indicating the amount of protein you consumed on that day, and write it in the following space:

TOTAL PROTEIN _____ grams per day

Compare your protein intake with your RDA for protein. Find your healthy weight for height in pounds using Table 10-1 in Chapter 10. Choose a midrange value. Divide this number by 2.2 to reveal your healthy weight in kilograms. Next, multiply this weight (or your current body weight if the numbers are close) by 0.8 grams per kilogram. This will indicate the RDA for protein for your weight and gender. (Your RDA for protein can also be found on your NutritionCalc Plus Profile Recommendations.) Write it in the following space:

RDA FOR PROTEIN _____ grams per day

How does your consumption compare with your RDA for protein? _____

_____

If you consumed either more or less than the RDA, what foods could you add, delete, or eat more or less of? (Look at the foods you ate.)

_____

_____

Was most of your protein from animal or plant sources? _____

_____

If your protein intake was primarily from plants, did this come from a wide variety to encourage protein complementarity for the day?

_____

_____

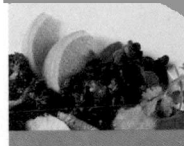

II. Protein and the Vegetarian

Alana is excited about all the health benefits that might accompany a vegetarian diet. However, she is concerned that she will not consume enough protein to meet her needs. She is also concerned about possible vitamin and mineral deficiencies. Use NutritionCalc Plus or Appendix J to calculate her protein intake and see if her concerns are valid.

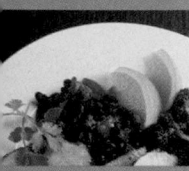

Breakfast

Calcium fortified orange juice, 1 cup

Skim milk, ¾ cup

Raisin bran cereal, 1 cup

Banana, medium

Snack

Calcium-enriched oat bagel

Fat-free blueberry yogurt, 1 ¼ cups

Lunch

Garden Burger, 4 ounces

Whole-wheat bun

Mustard, 1 tablespoon

Soy cottage cheese, 1 ounce

Apple, large

Red leaf lettuce, 1 ounce

Peanuts, salted, 1 ounce

Dry-roasted sunflower seeds, unsalted, ¼ cup

Tomato slices, 2

Mushrooms, 3

Yogurt salad dressing, 2 tablepoons

Iced tea, 8 fluid ounces

Dinner

Kidney beans, ½ cup

Brown rice, ¾ cup

Soft margarine, 1 tablespoon

Mixed vegetables, ¼ cup

Hot tea, 6 fluid ounces

Dessert

Strawberries, ½ cup

Angel food cake, 1 slice

Soy milk, 1 cup

Alana's diet contained 2275 kcal, with _____ grams (you fill in) of protein (is this plenty for her?), 363 grams of carbohydrate, 59 grams of total dietary fat (only 9 grams of which came from saturated fat), and 42 grams of fiber. Her vitamin and mineral intake with respect to those of concern to vegetarians—such as vitamin B-12, vitamin D, calcium, iron, and zinc—met her needs.

Alcohol

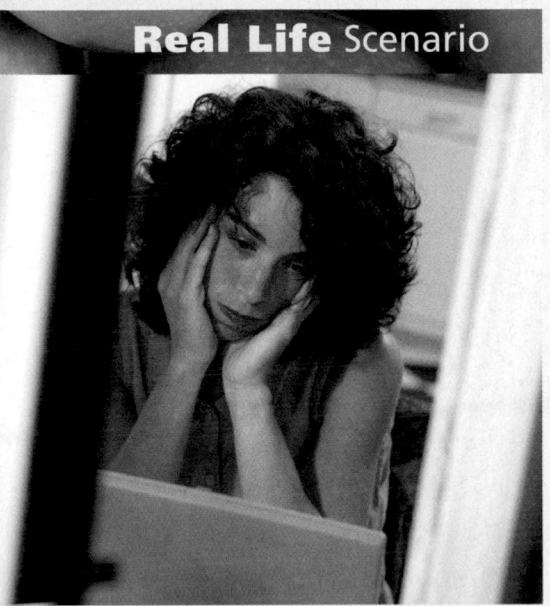

Real Life Scenario

Alyssa and Todd are college juniors. Todd was a very serious student in high school and achieved excellent grades, but as a college student he has begun binge drinking. As a result, his grades have fallen sharply and he is becoming socially isolated. He has been arrested once for drunk driving.

Last night, Todd had eight beers and three shots of whiskey at an off-campus party he attended with Alyssa. Unfortunately, everyone who knows Todd says he tends to get angry and say things he doesn't mean when he drinks too much. He also has been involved in several fights.

As the party began to die down, Alyssa tried to get Todd to leave. He responded rudely and forcefully grabbed her arm, shaking her. She became frightened by his aggressive behavior and left without him.

The next morning, Alyssa awoke early, still thinking about the hurtful events of the previous night. She decided to e-mail Todd, expressing her anxiety about his alcohol abuse. She did not want to see all of Todd's hard work and ambitions ruined by alcohol.

What should Alyssa say in the e-mail about alcohol and how it affects various organs in the body? What long-term problems are associated with such alcohol abuse? Is Alyssa correct in taking the initiative to communicate her concerns about this drinking problem to Todd?

Chapter 7 Objectives

Chapter 7 is designed to allow you to:

1. Describe the process of alcohol metabolism.
2. Describe some benefits of moderate alcohol consumption and define "moderate drinking."
3. List some nutrients that are most likely to be deficient in the diet of a person who abuses alcohol.
4. Explain how alcohol abuse damages body organs, such as the liver, heart, brain, and kidneys.
5. Identify body organs most likely to develop cancer because of alcohol abuse.
6. Outline the methods used to diagnose alcohol abuse.
7. Describe the risks of binge drinking and the corresponding amount of alcohol this represents.
8. List the typical strategies used in treating alcoholism, including the typical medications employed.

Check out the **Contemporary Nutrition Online Learning Center**

www.mhhe.com/wardlawcont6 *for quizzes, flash cards, other activities, and web links designed to further help you learn about issues surrounding alcohol use and abuse.*

217

Chapter 7 Outline

Although not a nutrient per se, alcohol is a source of calories for about half of all adults, constituting about 3% of total calories in the North American diet when averaged across the population. Moderate consumption of alcohol by a person of legal age is an acceptable practice and has some health benefits. However, excessive alcohol consumption has many unfortunate consequences. Currently, only about half of all alcohol consumed is done so in moderate amounts. By far the most commonly abused drug, alcohol can destroy families and friendships; lead to motor vehicle and boating accidents; spur deadly behaviors such as suicide, rape, and violence; and affect abusers with consequences of jail or prison terms.

Nearly 14 million people in the United States alone suffer from alcoholism, and another 31.9 million engage in binge drinking. Approximately 11 million young people under the legal age of 21 are drinking alcohol, and even more serious alcohol abuse is seen in adults beyond this age. From teenage years through later years in life, excess alcohol intake has damaging effects on one's nutritional status and overall health. Alcohol abuse is also a major problem in Canada.

The American Medical Association defines alcoholism as an illness characterized by significant impairment directly related to persistent and excessive use of alcohol. Impairment can involve psychological and social dysfunction, and for psychological, social, and genetic reasons, some people are more vulnerable to this disorder than others. Alcohol abuse touches many of our lives, so let's examine this substance in detail.

Refresh Your Memory

As you begin your study of alcohol in Chapter 7, you may want to review:

- The role of the GI tract, liver, and pancreas in digestion and absorption in Chapter 3
- The process of fermentation in Chapter 4
- Protein-calorie malnutrition in Chapter 6

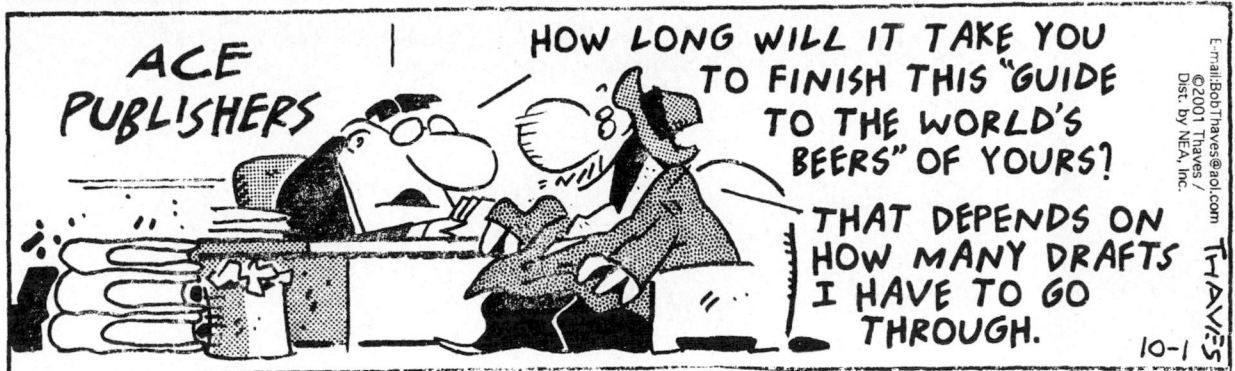

What are the pluses and minuses of alcohol use? And what constitutes alcoholism? Are some of us more susceptible to this chronic illness than others? How is it treated? Based on the relationship between alcohol use and health, should all adults of legal drinking age be abstainers? Chapter 7 provides some answers.

FRANK & ERNEST © United Features Syndicate. Reprinted by Permission.

Alcohol—An Introduction

Given the wide spectrum of alcohol use and **alcohol abuse**—often starting in teenage and college years—knowledge of alcohol consumption and its relationship to overall health is essential to the study of nutrition. Alcoholic beverages contain the chemical form of alcohol known as **ethanol**. Alcohol contributes calories to the diet (about 7 kcal per gram) (Table 7-1). Due to its lowering effect on inhibitions, alcohol commonly is used in social settings. Also, alcohol can be used as a safe alternative to polluted water (such as water containing various microorganisms) or as an analgesic to treat aches and pains.

Alcohol requires no digestion. It is absorbed rapidly from the GI tract by simple diffusion—no specific transport mechanisms are required for alcohol to enter a cell—so it is the most efficiently absorbed of all calorie sources. Different parts of the GI tract absorb alcohol at different rates. The upper parts of the small intestine absorb alcohol fastest, depending on how quickly the stomach empties, which in turn depends on the kinds of foods consumed along with the alcohol. Alcohol then goes on to affect various organs.

When alcohol is consumed in low amounts, it is perceived by the person as a stimulant because of its suppression of inhibitions. But alcohol actually acts as a depressant in the body, especially as the amount in the blood increases, resulting in sedation, reduced physical coordination, and psychological impairment.

How Alcoholic Beverages Are Produced

Any number of natural foods can be fermented. Recall from Chapter 4 that fermentation represents the breakdown of carbohydrates without the use of oxygen. Alcohol, carbon dioxide (CO_2), and various acids are formed. Production temperatures and composition of the food itself determine the characteristics of the final product. High-carbohydrate foods especially encourage the growth of yeast, the microorganism responsible for alcohol production. Brewer's yeast is one source of the enzyme that is necessary to make alcohol production possible.

alcohol abuse Excessive alcohol consumption that leads to severe alcohol-related health and other problems, such as recurrent sickness, inability to fulfill major obligations, use in hazardous situations (e.g., driving), related legal problems, or use despite social and interpersonal difficulties.

ethanol Chemical term for the form of alcohol found in alcoholic beverages.

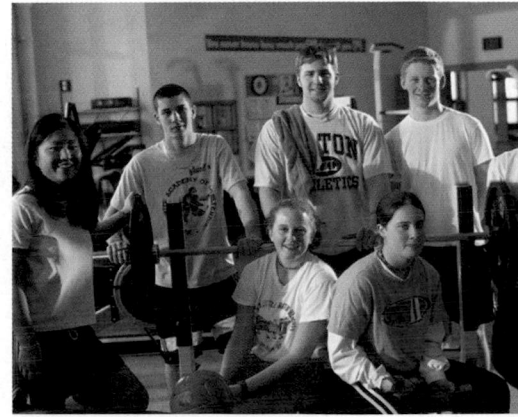

Young people benefit most from a healthy diet and exercise to decrease future risk of disease. There is no disease-related benefit at this age for alcohol use.

219

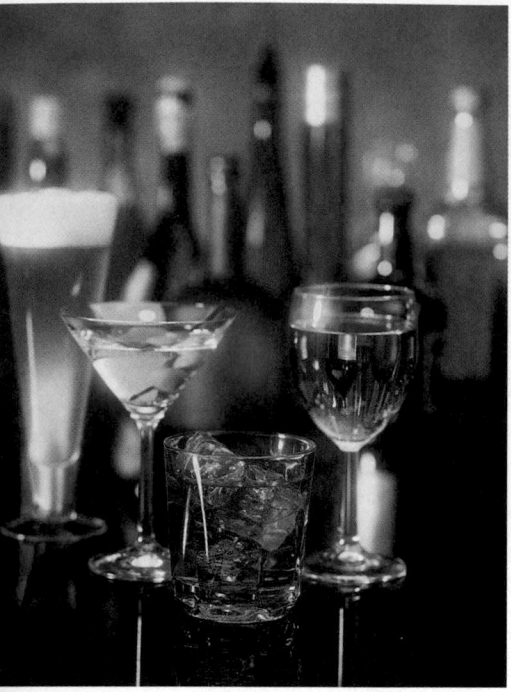

The following servings of each type of alcoholic beverage provide the same amount of alcohol (about 15 grams): wine—5 ounces, hard liquor—1.5 ounces, beer or wine cooler—12 ounces. In determining a safe level of intake, it is important to observe these serving sizes.

Table 7-1 Alcohol, Carbohydrate, and Calorie Content of Alcoholic Beverages*

Beverage	Amount (fluid ounce)	Alcohol (grams)	Carbohydrates (grams)	Calories (kcal)
Beer				
Regular	12.0	13	13	146
Light	12.0	11	5	99
Distilled Spirits				
Gin, rum, vodka, bourbon, whiskey (80 proof)	1.5	14	—	96
Brandy, cognac	1.5	14	—	96
Wine				
Red	5	14	2	102
White	5	14	1	100
Dessert, sweet	5	23	17	225
Rosé	5	14	2	100
Mixed Drinks				
Manhattan	3.0	26	3	191
Martini	3.0	27	—	189
Bourbon and soda	3.0	11	—	78
Whiskey sour	3.0	14	113	144

*There is little to no fat or protein contribution to calorie content.
Source: USDA.

The overall reaction for alcohol production is:

$$C_6H_{12}O_6 \rightarrow 2\ C_2H_5OH + 2\ CO_2 + 2\ H_2O$$

Glucose   Alcohol (ethanol)

The carbohydrate must be a simple sugar, such as maltose or glucose, in order for the yeast to use it as food. If the carbohydrate is a starch, such as that found in cereal grains, it must be broken down to these smaller forms, or "malted." During malting, the cereal grain seeds are allowed to sprout to produce the enzymes that break down the starches to simple sugars. The sprouting is then stopped by heating, and the yeast cells and water are added to the malt. The yeast grows using the sugars for energy needs. When the oxygen in the vat (the mixture of water, yeast, and malt) is used up, the yeast ferments the remaining sugar to produce alcohol and carbon dioxide. After fermentation has ceased, the product is finished in a variety of ways. In some cases, the alcohol itself is recovered from the product.

Beer is made from malted cereal grain, such as barley; it is flavored with hops and brewed by slow fermentation. The carbon dioxide released is collected and used to carbonate the beer, thus producing the desirable fizz associated with a quality beverage.

Wine is the fermented juice of grapes. Climate, geographic region, and variety of grape determine the quality of the wine. After fermentation, wines are typically aged in oak barrels to decrease the acidity and remove undesirable impurities.

Distilled spirits are made from the **distillation** of the alcohol after fermentation. The difference between the boiling point of water and the boiling point of alcohol allows these two liquids to be separated by distillation and the alcohol to be recovered. Any number of fruits, vegetables, and grains can be fermented and the resulting mash distilled. Some distilled spirits are marketed "unaged." Vodka and gin are examples of

distillation A physical method used to separate liquids based on their boiling points.

unaged beverages. Other spirits, such as whiskeys, rums, and brandies, are aged in oak barrels, some for more than 20 years.

Alcohol proof represents twice the volume of alcohol in percentage terms. Thus, 80 proof vodka is 40% alcohol.

Alcohol Metabolism

After a person drinks an alcoholic beverage, his or her blood concentration of alcohol rises rapidly. This happens because alcohol is readily absorbed into the blood from different segments of the GI tract by simple diffusion. You've probably been warned, with good reason, not to drink alcohol on an empty stomach. Alcohol absorption depends partly on the rate of stomach emptying. Food slows the stomach's emptying rate and stimulates secretions, such as gastric acid, which dilute the alcohol and slow its absorption into the bloodstream. Certain drugs also control stomach-emptying time and, thus, overall absorption.

Alcohol is readily distributed into all the fluid compartments within the body because alcohol is found wherever water is distributed in the body. Alcohol moves easily through the cell membranes; however, as it does, it damages proteins in the membranes. Most of alcohol's damaging effects are concentrated in the liver because this is the first organ that is exposed to alcohol after absorption. The liver is also the chief site for alcohol metabolism. Although it is true that cells of the GI tract are in contact with alcohol, they are constantly being replaced because of their naturally short life span. Thus, they are not subject to the same degree of damage as liver cells, which have a much longer life span.

Metabolism of alcohol is dependent on numerous factors, such as gender, race, size, physical condition, what is eaten, the alcohol content of the beverage, and even how much sleep one has had. The ability to produce the enzyme **alcohol dehydrogenase** is the key to alcohol metabolism, as it acts on about 90% of the dose consumed. Women absorb and metabolize alcohol differently than men do. A woman cannot metabolize much alcohol in the cells that line her stomach because of low activity of alcohol dehydrogenase. Women also have less body water in which to dilute the alcohol than do men. So, when a man and a woman of similar size drink equal amounts of alcohol, a larger proportion of the alcohol reaches and remains in the woman's bloodstream. While men can metabolize about 30% of ingested alcohol by enzymes of the stomach lining before it reaches the bloodstream, women only metabolize 10% of ingested alcohol in this manner. Overall, women develop alcohol-related ailments, such as **cirrhosis** of the liver, more rapidly than men do with the same alcohol-consumption habits. Also, certain drugs used to treat ulcers and heartburn inhibit alcohol dehydrogenase activity in the stomach, as does chronic alcohol abuse and aging.

Once acted on by alcohol dehydrogenase, alcohol turns into acetaldehyde. Eventually, this goes on to form carbon dioxide and water:

Alcohol dehydrogenase

$$\text{Alcohol} \longrightarrow \text{Acetaldehyde} \rightarrow \rightarrow \rightarrow CO_2 + H_2O$$

Only a small percentage of alcohol intake is excreted as such through the lungs, urine, and sweat. (Since the alcohol content of expired air maintains a constant relationship to the blood alcohol concentration in the lungs, it is used as the basis of the breathalyzer test.) As one continues to drink, one's blood alcohol concentration (BAC) continues to rise (Fig. 7-1). A social drinker who weighs 150 pounds and has normal liver function metabolizes about 5 to 7 grams of alcohol per hour. This is about one half of a beer or one fourth of an ordinary-sized drink. When the rate of alcohol consumption exceeds the liver's metabolic capacity, blood alcohol rises and symptoms of intoxication appear as the brain begins to be exposed to alcohol (Table 7-2).

alcohol dehydrogenase An enzyme used in alcohol (ethanol) metabolism.

cirrhosis A loss of functioning liver cells, which are replaced by nonfunctioning connective tissue. Any substance that poisons liver cells can lead to cirrhosis. The most common cause is a chronic, excessive alcohol intake. Exposure to certain industrial chemicals also can lead to cirrhosis.

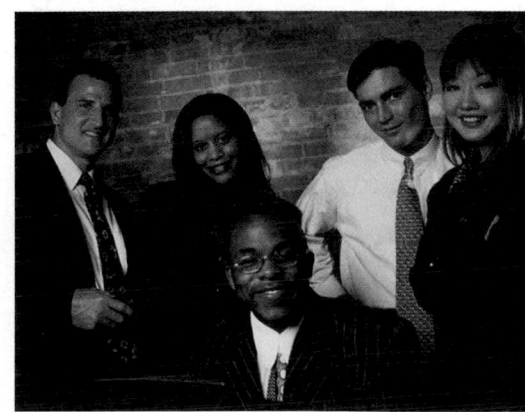

Compared with Caucasians, most Asians and Native Americans have a limited ability to metabolize alcohol, and are therefore more likely to experience intoxication more rapidly.

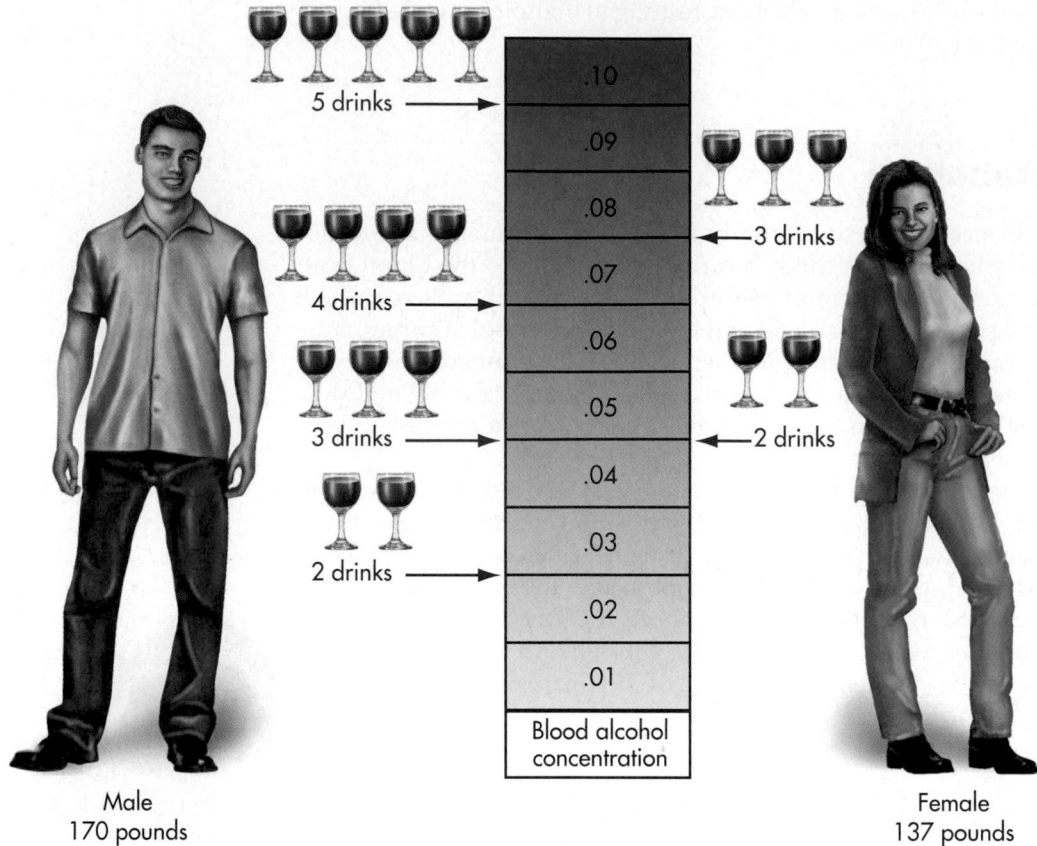

Figure 7-1 Approximate relationship between alcohol consumption and blood alcohol concentration (BAC; units are % or milligrams of alcohol per 100 milliliters of blood). Note that effects can vary among people and whether food is also consumed. A BAC of 0.02 begins to impair driving. One is legally intoxicated at a BAC of 0.08 in the United States and throughout Canada.

Table 7-2 Blood Alcohol Concentration and Symptoms

Concentration*	Sporadic Drinker	Chronic Drinker	Hours for Alcohol to Be Metabolized**
50 (party high) (0.05%)	Congenial euphoria; decreased tension; noticeable impairment in driving and coordination	No observable effect	2–3
75 (0.075%)	Gregarious	Often no effect	3–4
80 to 100 (0.08%–0.1%)	Uncoordinated; 0.08% is legally drunk (as in drunk driving) in the United States and Canada.	Minimal signs	4–6
125–150 (0.125%–0.15%)	Unrestrained behavior; episodic uncontrolled behavior	Pleasurable euphoria or beginning of uncoordination	6–10
200–250 (0.2%–0.25%)	Alertness lost; lethargic	Effort is required to maintain emotional and motor control	10–24
300–350 (0.3%–0.35%)	Stupor to coma	Drowsy and slow	10–24
>500 (>0.5%)	Some will die	Coma	>24

*Milligrams of alcohol per 100 milliliters of blood.

**Social drinker. Alcohol metabolism is somewhat faster in chronic alcohol abusers.

Modified from Wyngaarder JB, Smith LH: *Cecil Textbook of Medicine*, fourth edition, Philadelphia, 1988, WB Saunders. Used with permission.

Because alcohol cannot be stored in the body, it has absolute priority in metabolism as a fuel source, taking precedence over energy sources, such as fat.

Another Bite

In addition to the alcohol dehydrogenase system, two other enzyme systems in body cells also metabolize alcohol, especially when it is consumed in high amounts. Increased activity of these alternate enzyme systems is the key reason for development of tolerance to the effects of alcohol—more rapid alcohol metabolism than seen in Table 7-2 means more alcohol is now needed to achieve desired effects of alcohol use.

Excessive alcohol consumption and use of an alternate pathway for the needed alcohol metabolism also increase the potential for a drug overdose. While enzymes are engaged in metabolism of alcohol in the liver, the capacity of the liver to break down other drugs—such as many sedatives (barbiturates)—is reduced, due to enzyme competition. If large amounts of alcohol and sedatives are consumed simultaneously, the alcohol gets preferential treatment. This means that due to decreased availability of certain enzymes, the liver is not able to break down the sedatives fast enough, therefore the user may lapse into a coma and even die from the effects of the sedatives. Alcohol itself is toxic in high quantities, and mixture of alcohol with sedatives is an extremely lethal combination.

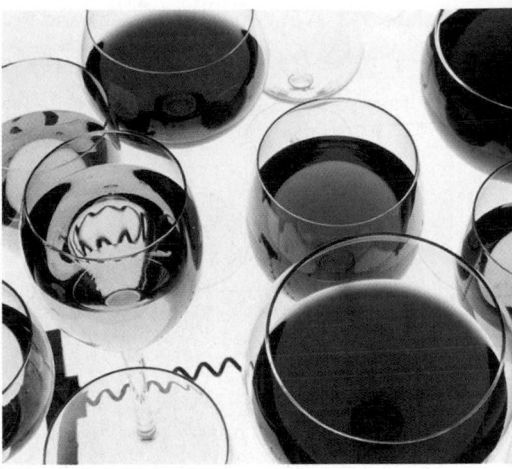

Of all the alcohol sources, red wine in moderation is often singled out as the best choice because of the added bonus of the many phytochemicals present (e.g., resveratrol). These are leached out from the grape skins as the red wine is fermented. Dark beer is also a source of phytochemicals.

Concept Check

Alcohol is not an essential nutrient, but does supply calories for the body. It requires no digestion, and alcohol metabolism takes precedence over metabolism of the other energy-yielding nutrients. Alcohol is metabolized in the liver and other tissues. Metabolism mostly depends on the enzyme alcohol dehydrogenase. A number of individual factors, such as gender, race, and body composition, determine how a person reacts to alcohol.

Benefits of Moderate Alcohol Use

ischemic stroke A stroke caused by the absence of blood flow to a part of the brain.

The benefits of alcohol use are linked to specific intakes of about one drink a day for men and slightly less than one for women. One standard drink is universally defined as one 12-ounce bottle of beer or wine cooler, one 5-ounce glass of wine, 3 ounces of sherry or liqueur, or 1.5 ounces of 80-proof distilled spirits. The actual type of alcoholic drink consumed does not significantly affect the benefits. Note that beer varies considerably in its alcohol content, with malt liquor being higher in alcohol than most other forms of beer.

The benefit of moderate alcohol consumption begins with the many pleasurable and social aspects of its use. People enjoy meeting a friend over a beer or settling down to a glass of wine in the evening with dinner. These behaviors are not considered excessive, as long as they are practiced by people of legal drinking age, remain under control, and cause no obvious harm. The risk of developing cardiovascular diseases, such as coronary heart disease, is lower in middle-aged and older adults who consume moderate amounts of alcohol. **Ischemic stroke** risk also is decreased in light-to-moderate drinkers as opposed to those who abstain from alcoholic beverages. Other potential health benefits are listed in Table 7-3.

Many of the benefits of moderate alcohol use are effective only in the short term. Previous consumers of alcohol no longer experience the benefits of alcohol when consumption ceases.

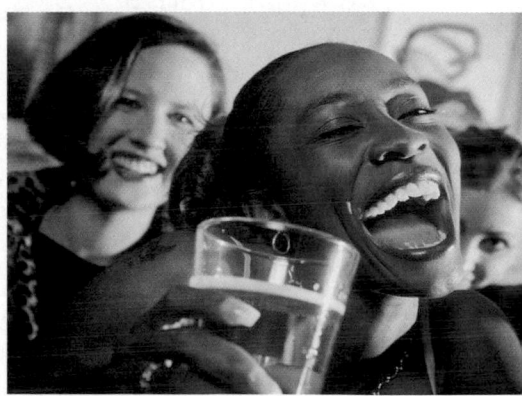

The pleasurable and social aspects of alcohol use are two reasons for its popularity.

Table 7-3 A Summary of Benefits and Risks of Alcohol Use

	Moderate Use*	Alcohol Abuse**
Coronary heart disease	Decreased risk of death in those at high risk for coronary heart disease-related death, primarily by increasing HDL-cholesterol in some people, decreasing blood clotting, and relaxing blood vessels	Heart rhythm disturbances, heart muscle damage, increased blood triglycerides, and increased blood clotting
Hypertension and stroke	Mild decrease in blood pressure; less ischemic stroke in people with normal blood pressure	Increased blood pressure (hypertension); more ischemic and hemorrhagic stroke
Peripheral vascular disease	Decreased risk due to reduced blood clotting	No benefit
Blood glucose regulation and type 2 diabetes	Decreased risk of death from cardiovascular disease	Hypoglycemia; reduced insulin sensitivity; damage to pancreas (site of insulin production)
Bone and joint health	Some increase in bone mineral content in women, linked to estrogen output	Loss of active bone-forming cells and eventual osteoporosis (many nutrient deficiencies also contribute to this problem); increased risk of gout
Brain function	Enhanced brain function and decreased risk of dementia by increasing blood circulation in the brain	Brain tissue damage and decreased memory
Skeletal muscle health	No benefit	Skeletal muscle damage
Cancer	No benefit	Increased risk of oral, esophageal, stomach, liver, lung, colorectal, and breast cancer, to name a few (especially if the diet is deficient in the vitamin folate)
Liver function	No benefit	Fat infiltration and eventual liver cirrhosis, especially if a person is also infected with hepatitis C; iron toxicity
GI tract disease	Decreased risk of certain bacterial infections in the stomach	Inflammation of the stomach (and pancreas); absorptive cell damage leading to malabsorption of nutrients
Immune system function	No benefit	Reduced function and increased infections
Nervous system function	No benefit	Loss of nerve sensation and nervous system control of muscles
Sleep disturbances	Some relaxation	Fragmented sleep patterns; worsens sleep apnea
Impotence and decreased libido	No benefit	Contributes to the problem in both men and women
Drug overdose	No benefit	Contributes to the problem, especially in combination with sedatives
Obesity	No benefit	Increased abdominal fat deposition, contributes to weight gain as calories from alcoholic beverages quickly add up
Nutrient intake	May supply some B vitamins and iron	Leads to numerous nutrient deficiencies: protein, vitamins, and minerals
Alcoholism	No benefit	Increased risk of developing alcoholism, including the teenage and young adult years
Fetal health	No benefit	Variety of toxic effects on the fetus when alcohol is consumed by pregnant women (see Chapter 13)
Socialization and relaxation	Provides some benefit to socialization and leads to relaxation by increasing brain neurotransmitter activity	Contributes to violent behavior and agitation
Traffic deaths and other violent deaths	No benefit	Contributes to both traffic death and violent death

*About one drink a day for men and slightly less than one for women.

**The risks from alcohol abuse begin at an intake of more than two to three drinks per day for men or one to two drinks per day for women and all adults age 65 and older. Binge drinking (more than four drinks in a row for women or more than five drinks for men) can be especially harmful (see Looking Further, p. 228). The Swiss chemist Paracelsus (1493–1541) made the observation that "the dose determines the poison." This is especially true for alcohol, as alcohol abuse typically reduces a person's life expectancy by 15 years.

Health Problems from Alcohol Abuse

Despite the few benefits of regular, moderate alcohol use, the risks of abuse are more numerous and harmful. Alcoholism, in and of itself, is one of the most preventable health problems in North America. Excessive consumption of alcohol contributes significantly to 5 of the 10 leading causes of death in North America—heart failure, certain forms of cancer, cirrhosis of the liver, motor vehicle and other accidents, and suicides (review Table 7-3). Tobacco, often used simultaneously, interacts with alcohol in a way that reinforces its effects and causes esophageal and oral cancer. In addition, excessive alcohol drinking increases the risk of heart rhythm disturbances, hypertension, hemorrhagic stroke, osteoporosis, brain damage, colorectal and breast cancer, inflammation of the stomach lining, suppression of the immune system (and, thus, an increased risk of infections), sleep disturbances, impotence, hypoglycemia, and high blood triglycerides. Figure 7-2 illustrates many of these risks. Alcohol ingestion also reduces use of fat by body cells and promotes a positive energy balance, thus contributing to the risk for obesity, especially abdominal obesity. Finally, by reducing the action of antidiuretic hormone, alcohol increases urination. Death from alcohol abuse usually results from respiratory failure or inhalation of vomit (the latter if the blood alcohol concentration is somewhat lower).

As a nutrient source, alcohol has little nutritional value and, thus, nutrient deficiencies are also a common result of alcoholism. The protein and vitamin content is extremely low, except in beer, where it is marginal. Iron content varies from drink to drink, with red wine ranking especially high in iron. Excess use of some alcoholic beverages can even lead to iron toxicity, and in rare cases, lead or cobalt toxicity as well.

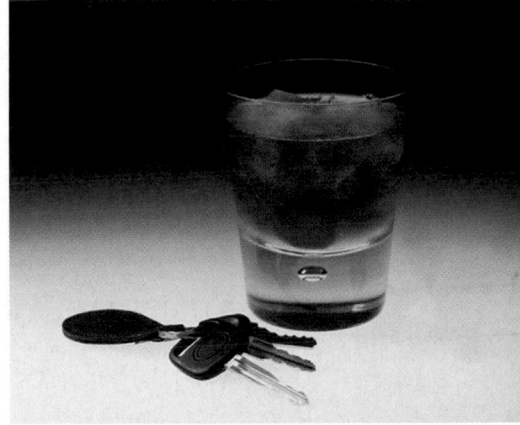

Drinking and driving should never be combined. The consequences are dangerous and possibly deadly.

Critical Thinking

For many people, drinking and smoking go hand-in-hand. What risks and diseases could correlate with the combination of these behaviors with excessive alcohol use?

Another Bite

Typical deficiencies seen in alcoholism include those of the fat-soluble vitamins—vitamin A, vitamin D, vitamin E, and vitamin K—as well as the water-soluble vitamins—thiamin, niacin, vitamin B-6, folate, vitamin B-12, and vitamin C. Mineral deficiencies of calcium, phosphorus, potassium, magnesium, zinc, and iron are possible. These arise mostly due to poor nutrient intakes, but fat malabsorption linked to poor pancreatic function and increased urinary losses are also important in some cases. On the other hand, vitamin and mineral toxicity is also of concern, particularly with vitamin A and iron. In both cases, damage to the GI tract and liver enhance the potential for toxicity from these nutrients. The immediate aim in nutritional treatment of alcoholism is eliminating alcohol intake. Then attention turns to replenishing nutrient stores, generally with nutrient supplements.

■ A Closer Look at Cirrhosis

Long-term alcohol use causes fatty liver, inflammation of the liver (alcoholic hepatitis), and eventually cirrhosis (Fig. 7-3). Cirrhosis is a chronic and usually relentlessly progressive disease characterized by fatty infiltration of the liver. Fatty liver occurs in response to increased synthesis of fat and decreased use of it for energy by the liver. Eventually, the enlarged fat deposits choke off the blood supply, depriving the liver cells of oxygen and nutrients. Liver cells can accumulate so much fat that they burst and die and are replaced by connective (scar) tissue. This scarring process is called *cirrhosis*. When too many liver cells die, the liver dies, and the alcoholic patient dies. In North America, most cases of cirrhosis are caused by alcohol consumption.

Cirrhosis develops in about 15% to 20% of cases of alcoholism and affects about 2 million people in the United States alone. It is the second leading reason for the need for liver transplants. In addition to the amount and duration of alcohol consumption,

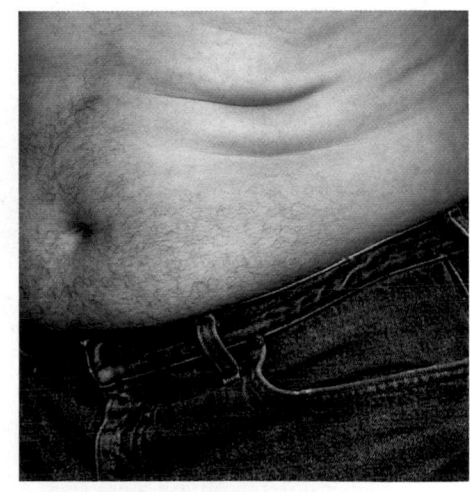

Excessive alcohol intake, notably binge drinking, encourages fat deposition, especially in the abdominal region.

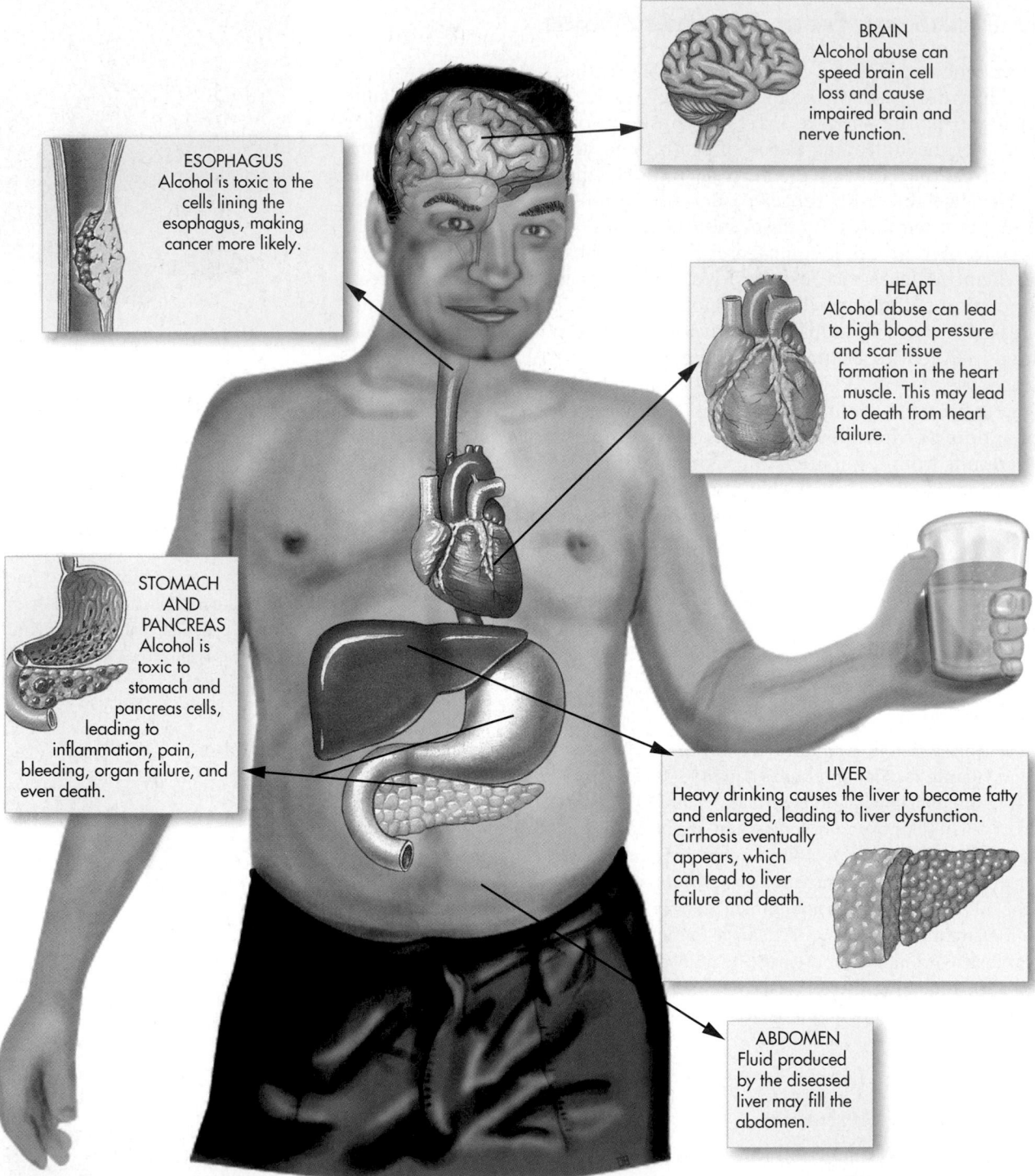

Figure 7-2 Some effects of alcohol abuse on the body. As a drug, alcohol has a **narcotic** effect. The mind-altering effects of alcohol begin soon after it enters the bloodstream. Virtually every organ system is affected by alcohol. Within minutes, alcohol inhibits nerve cells in the brain. The heart muscle strains to cope with alcohol's depressive action. If drinking continues, rising blood alcohol impairs speech, vision, balance, and judgment. With an extremely high blood alcohol content, respiratory failure is possible. Over time, alcohol abuse increases the risk of liver and pancreas failure and certain forms of heart damage and cancer, among other disorders. Table 7-3 summarized the negative effects of excessive alcohol use on physical health, including toxic effects on the fetus if a pregnant woman consumes alcohol.

genetic factors and individual differences, such as obesity, determine one's risk for the disease. Exposure to hepatotoxins (e.g., acetaminophen [Tylenol]) and infections with hepatitis C are also contributors. Once a person has cirrhosis, there is a 50% chance of death within 4 years, a far worse prognosis than many forms of cancer. Most of the deaths from alcoholic cirrhosis occur in people between the ages of 40 and 65 years. The actual death rate in the United States is 8.8 per 100,000 people.

A number of possible mechanisms underlie the liver damage from alcohol abuse. In chronic alcoholism, acetaldehyde concentration increases in the liver, and is thought to be the underlying cause of the toxic effects of alcohol. Another cause of liver damage is the production of **free radicals** from alcohol metabolism. These highly reactive molecules destroy cell membranes and DNA. Inflammation, which results from free radical damage, can destroy healthy liver tissue.

No specific amount of alcohol consumption guarantees cirrhosis. One perceptible pattern is that cirrhosis commonly results from a 10-year or longer consumption of approximately 80 grams of alcohol (the equivalent of six beers) per day. Some evidence suggests that damage is caused by a dose as low as 40 grams per day for men (3 beers) and 20 grams per day for women (1½ beers). Early stages of alcoholic liver injury are reversible, but advanced stages are not. If a person is terminally ill, a liver transplant is necessary for survival.

A nutritious diet helps prevent some complications associated with alcoholism, but usually alcoholism brings about serious destruction of vital tissues regardless of the quality of the food consumed. Laboratory animal studies show clearly that, even when a nutritious diet is consumed, alcohol abuse can lead to cirrhosis. Still, deficient nutritional status compounds the problem of cirrhosis, as it makes the liver more vulnerable to toxic substances, including free radicals, by depleting supplies of antioxidants, such as vitamin E. If present in adequate amounts, this vitamin reduces free radical damage to the liver. A deficiency of the vitamin folate also compounds the damage.

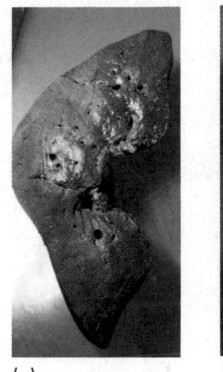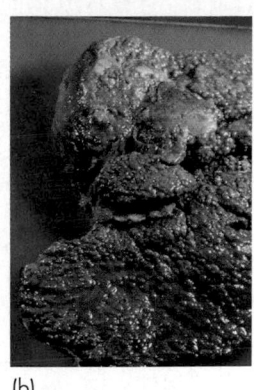

(a)   (b)

Figure 7-3 Alcohol is particularly damaging to the liver. Pictured are (a) healthy liver (b) liver with cirrhosis. Note there is no cure for this disease except a liver transplant.

narcotic An agent that reduces sensations or consciousness.

free radicals Short-lived forms of compounds that exist with an unpaired electron, causing it to seek an electron from another compound. Free radicals can be very destructive to electron-dense cell components, such as DNA and cell membranes.

Concept Check

Excessive alcohol use can result in an array of medical problems. It increases the risk of developing hypertension, certain forms of strokes and heart damage, birth defects, inflammation of the pancreas, damage to the brain, and malnutrition, to name a few. Furthermore, alcoholism interferes with all aspects of family, professional, and social life.

Alcohol exposure also is extremely toxic to the fetus (see Chapter 13 for details on fetal alcohol syndrome).

Guidance Regarding Alcohol Use

The U.S. Surgeon General's office, the National Academy of Science, and the USDA/DHHS do not specifically recommend drinking alcohol. The 2005 Dietary Guidelines for Americans provides the following advice regarding use of alcoholic beverages:

- Those who choose to drink alcoholic beverages should do so sensibly and in moderation—defined as the consumption of up to one drink per day for women and up to two drinks per day for men.
- Alcoholic beverages should not be consumed by some individuals, including those who cannot restrict their alcohol intake, women of childbearing age who may become pregnant, pregnant and lactating women, children and adolescents, individuals taking medications that can interact with alcohol, and those with specific medical conditions.
- Alcoholic beverages should be avoided by individuals engaging in activities that require attention, skill, or coordination, such as driving or operating machinery.

Healthy People 2010 set an important goal regarding alcohol use: Reduce by 25% the proportion of adults who exceed the guidelines for appropriate alcohol use (currently, 73% of those who consume alcohol).

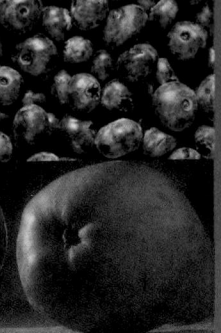

Binge Drinking

College students are drinking more heavily and more frequently than ever before. Excessive alcohol consumption is an even bigger problem than illicit drug use on college campuses today (Table 7-4). Many college students consider drinking alcohol to be a "rite of passage" into adulthood. The largest drinking population in North America consists of young, Caucasian college students. Bars near campus typically promote heavy drinking. Alcohol producers frequently target college students with advertising and other marketing efforts. Adding to the overall problem is the fact that approximately half of all college students are not yet of legal drinking age. In fact, the annual overall cost related to underage alcohol use is estimated at more than $58 billion. This figure includes costs associated with violent crime, traffic accidents, treatment, and alcohol poisonings.

Table 7-4 Sobering Statistics on the Impact of Binge Drinking on College Campuses

Death: 1400 college students between the ages of 18 and 24 die each year from alcohol-related unintentional injuries, including motor vehicle crashes.

Injury: 500,000 students between the ages of 18 and 24 are unintentionally injured each year under the influence of alcohol.

Assault: More than 600,000 students between the ages of 18 and 24 are assaulted each year by another student who has been drinking.

Sexual abuse: More than 70,000 students between the ages of 18 and 24 are victims of alcohol-related sexual assault or date rape each year.

Unsafe sex: Each year about 400,000 students between the ages of 18 and 24 have unprotected sex and more than 100,000 students between the ages of 18 and 24 have been too intoxicated to know if they consented to having sex.

Academic problems: About 25% of college students report academic consequences of their drinking, including missing class, falling behind, doing poorly on exams or papers, and receiving lower grades overall.

Health problems/Suicide attempts: More than 150,000 students develop an alcohol-related health problem and between 1.2% and 1.5% of students indicate that they tried to commit suicide within the past year due to drinking or drug use.

Drunk driving: 2.1 million students between the ages of 18 and 24 drive under the influence of alcohol each year.

Vandalism: About 11% of college student drinkers report that they have damaged property while under the influence of alcohol.

Property damage: More than 25% of administrators from schools with relatively low drinking levels and over 50% from schools with high drinking levels say their campuses have a "moderate" or "major" problem with alcohol-related property damage.

Police involvement: About 5% of 4-year college students are involved with the police or campus security as a result of their drinking and an estimated 110,000 students between the ages of 18 and 24 are arrested for an alcohol-related violation, such as public drunkenness or driving under the influence.

Alcohol abuse and dependence: 31% of college students met criteria for a diagnosis of alcohol abuse and 6% for a diagnosis of alcohol dependence in the past 12 months, according to questionnaire-based self-reports about their drinking.

The consequences of excessive and underage drinking affect virtually all college campuses, college communities, and college students, whether they choose to drink or not.

Source: www.collegedrinkingprevention.gov/facts/snapshot.aspx

Binge drinking—having four or more drinks in a row for women, or five or more for men—is common among college students. Only a minority of drinking by this group is done so in moderation, and the main reported purpose of drinking is "to get drunk." About 50% of college students engage in binge drinking. **Acute alcohol intoxication,** which can result from such rapid consumption of a large quantity of alcohol, is a major cause of suicide and hazing deaths related to binge drinking.

> **acute alcohol intoxication** A temporary deterioration in mental function, accompanied by lack of coordination and partial paralysis, arising from drinking alcoholic beverages too rapidly.

Another Bite

In 2000, a student at the University of Michigan rapidly drank 20 shots to celebrate his 21st birthday and died shortly afterward, with a blood alcohol concentration of 0.39 percent. A student at Old Dominion University choked to death on his own vomit during a pledge-week drinking binge. Two women attending universities in Colorado died of alcohol poisoning in the fall of 2004. A student on the diving team at Ohio State University became so intoxicated that he dove headfirst while "mud-diving." He is lucky to be alive, but is paralyzed from the neck down. Other students have drowned while intoxicated, despite knowing how to swim.

Binge drinking has a variety of contraindications. It can lead to unplanned sexual activity, injury to oneself or others, and even death. Death due to alcohol misuse can result, for example, from inhalation of vomit. In other cases, the body systems slowly shut down due to alcohol's overpowering depressant effect (Table 7-5). Other injuries can occur, resulting in paralysis or other lifelong medical problems.

Problems associated with binge drinking can affect all aspects of life. Regular binge drinking can lead to academic failure, as binge drinkers are more likely to miss class than are students who are light drinkers or abstainers. Property damage, as a result of vandalism and accidents, can be another consequence of binge drinking. Students that live around binge drinkers experience more unwanted sexual advances, assaults, and insults/humiliations. Despite the array of negative outcomes, binge drinkers often do not think they have a problem, because their behavior has become so acceptable on college campuses.

According to U.S. law in all 50 states, one must be 21 years old to drink. In Canada, the legal age is 18 or 19, depending on the province. However, alcohol use often begins in adolescence. For example, 31% of twelfth-graders in the United States reported frequent drinking during 1999, and about 11% of all alcohol is consumed by those under age 21. Influences on premature alcohol use are often seen in conjunction with athletics, if older, highly visible role models advertise products or are seen consuming alcohol. Peer pressure at school and on sports teams can cause many adolescents to drink. Dangerous habits become deadly when young adults choose to drive drunk or ride with friends who are intoxicated. Drinking habits created in youth may continue and worsen over time. Education and prevention strategies should focus on behavioral and psychosocial consequences because athletic performance typically does not suffer initially.

Overall, it is important that binge drinkers be aware that these habits can cause lifelong problems, especially when drinking becomes habitual.

> *Healthy People 2010* includes an important goal regarding binge drinking: Reduce by at least one-half the number of high school and college students engaging in binge drinking (currently estimated at 32% and 40%, respectively).

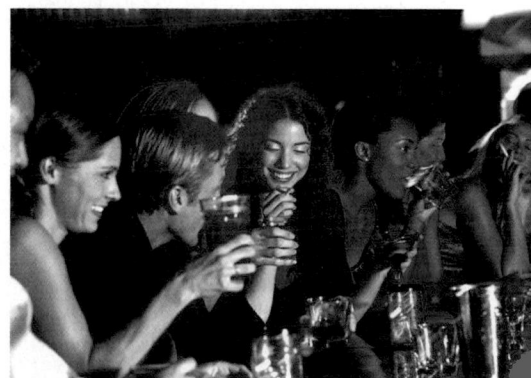

Alcohol use and abuse often begin in young adulthood and are carried into later years.

Table 7-5 Signs and Symptoms of Alcohol Poisoning

Being aware of the warning signs and dangers of alcohol poisoning is important. It could help save the life of someone you love. The warning signs and symptoms include the following:
• Semiconsciousness or unconsciousness
• Slow respiration of eight or fewer breaths per minute or lapses between breaths of more than 8 seconds
• Cold, clammy, pale, or bluish skin
• Strong odor of alcohol, which usually accompanies these symptoms

Note: Although these are obvious warning signs of alcohol poisoning, the list is certainly not all inclusive.

As the understanding of the relationship between drinking alcohol and health grows, registered dietitians and other health professionals can promote healthy lifestyles—not by encouraging indiscriminate drinking—but rather by reassuring adults that moderate alcohol consumption may have beneficial health outcomes.

There is no recommendation for a nondrinker to start consuming alcohol for health benefits, but people of legal age who have one drink or so each day, and are not prone to abuse, should know there's nothing wrong with moderate drinking (as long as they are not putting others at risk). In fact, as shown in Table 7-3, many studies have shown that moderate alcohol consumption has a protective effect against ischemic stroke, coronary heart disease, and type 2 diabetes.

Alcohol Dependency and Abuse

Many factors influence a person's chances of developing **alcohol dependence.** Studies have shown links tying gender, genetics, ethnicity, parental influence, nurture, and depression to alcohol dependency and abuse. For some people, alcohol can be addictive and dangerous, and can eventually lead to alcohol abuse. In Western countries, this is true for about 10% to 15% of men and 5% of women who drink alcohol.

Studies suggest that about 40% of a person's risk for alcoholism comes from genetic factors, although the gene or genes have not been identified. The genetic influence on alcohol dependency and abuse has been indicated by a number of studies, including twin and adoption research. Twins and first-degree relatives share a tendency toward alcohol addiction. This suggests that anyone with a family history of alcohol abuse should be especially aware of their alcohol consumption.

Children of alcoholics have a fourfold-increased risk of developing alcoholism, especially if they live with alcohol abusers. It is recommended that children with a family history of alcoholism be warned of the dangers of drinking by the age of 10. At this age, they are old enough to understand the consequences of alcoholism but are not yet under the strong influence of their peers.

Tolerance to alcohol may be genetic. If this is the case, greater amounts of alcohol are required to produce the desired effects on mood and behavior. Other studies question the relative importance of the genetic component. These note that any one of us can become addicted if we drink long enough and consume ever-increasing quantities of alcohol.

Many ethnic distinctions play an important role in the probability of alcohol dependency and abuse. Compared with Caucasians, Asians and Native Americans are very susceptible to the damaging effects of alcohol for reasons discussed earlier. The major cause of alcohol-related death among Native Americans is unintentional injuries related to alcohol use, especially high rates of motor vehicle accidents. Other alcohol-related mortality statistics confronting Native Americans are suicide, homicide, and domestic abuse. African-American alcoholics are at greater risk than other racial groups for tuberculosis, hepatitis C, HIV/AIDS, and other infectious diseases. Hispanic Americans are at particular risk for cirrhosis-related death.

Depression and alcohol abuse often go hand-in-hand. Researchers have discovered that the risk for heavy drinking is higher among women with a history of depression than among women with no such history. This finding holds up even when other factors that increase the risk of heavy drinking, such as age, family history of drinking, and personality disorder, are accounted for. The more symptoms of depression women report, the more likely they are to drink heavily. There may be several reasons for this association. One reason is self-medication with alcohol is to relieve the symptoms of depression, possibly by increasing **serotonin** and **dopamine** action in the brain. Research has shown that, although alcohol may alleviate depression in the short term, it tends to increase depression over time. A second reason is that women who are more depressed

alcohol dependence The person experiences repeated alcohol-related difficulties, such as an inability to control use, spending a great deal of time associated with alcohol use, continued use of alcohol despite physical or psychological consequences, persistent desire or unsuccessful efforts to cut down or control alcohol use, and withdrawal symptoms. Tolerance is also seen.

Ability to "hold one's liquor" compared to the average person is a strong indicator of genetic risk.

serotonin A neurotransmitter synthesized from the amino acid tryptophan that affects mood (sense of calmness), behavior and appetite, and induces sleep.

dopamine A type of neurotransmitter in the central nervous system that leads to feelings of euphoria, among other functions; it is also used to form norepinephrine, another neurotransmitter molecule.

may not pay attention to their drinking and may not be concerned about the effects it can have on their health and behavior. More research is needed to determine if there are genetic or environmental factors that link depression and heavy drinking.

Alcohol dependence is the most common psychiatric disorder, affecting 13% of the North American population. In the United States alone, about $185 billion is spent annually in terms of lost productivity, premature deaths, direct treatment expenses, and legal fees associated with alcoholism. A liver transplant costs about $150,000 and is needed in cases of excessive alcohol use. On the positive side, with a typical counseling program it costs only about $5000 to treat a person who is abusing alcohol. Identifying alcoholism early can be a way to control and decrease the health care costs of this disease.

■ Alcoholism Diagnosis

Alcoholism is often considered a two-phase problem. Initially, it begins as problem drinking. This includes the repetitive use of alcohol, often in an attempt to alleviate anxiety or solve other emotional problems. Alcohol addiction, the second phase, is defined as a true addiction following the repeated use of alcohol.

The diagnosis of alcoholism is based on a list of major criteria. Alcoholics may exhibit some or all of the following criteria:

- Physiologic dependence on alcohol with evidence of withdrawal symptoms when intake is interrupted
- Tolerance to the effects of alcohol, prompting greater alcohol intake to achieve the desired effect
- Evidence of alcohol-associated illnesses such as alcoholic liver disease or irreversible brain damage exhibited by memory loss, inability to concentrate, and decline in intellectual functions
- Continued drinking in defiance of strong medical and social contraindications and disruptions in normal life
- Depression and blackouts, as well as impairment in social and occupational functioning

Other signs of alcoholism include the basic alcohol stigmas: alcohol odor on the breath, flushed face and reddened skin (the latter due to breakage of small blood vessels, which allows blood to seep under the skin), and nervous system disorders, such as tremors. Unexplained work absences, frequent accidents, and falls or injuries of vague origin may all lead a clinician to consider the possibility of alcoholism. Laboratory tests are also helpful. These tests include measures of impaired liver function, enlarged red blood cell size (to check for a folate deficiency), and a high triglyceride concentration in the blood.

■ Do You Have a Problem with Alcohol?

Asking a person about the quantity and frequency of alcohol consumption is an important means of detecting abuse and dependence. The CAGE questionnaire is commonly used in routine health care.

C: Have you ever felt you ought to *cut* down on drinking?
A: Have people *annoyed* you by criticizing your drinking?
G: Have you ever felt bad or *guilty* about your drinking?
E: Have you ever had a drink first thing in the morning to steady your nerves or get rid of a hangover (*eye-opener*)?

More than one positive response to the CAGE questionnaire suggests an alcohol problem. Another key point to probe is tolerance. Does it take more to make you inebriated than it did in the past?

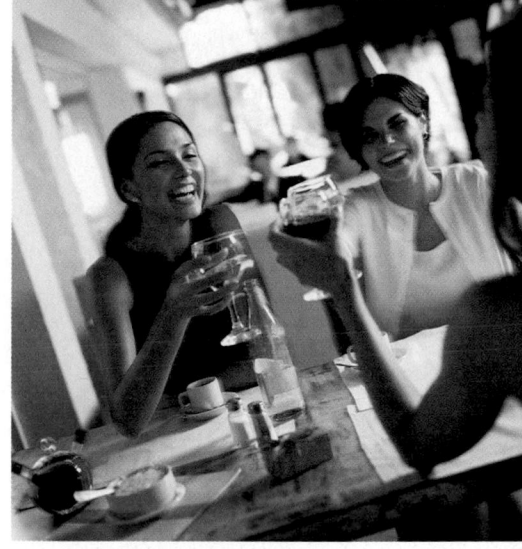

Compared to men, women more readily develop alcohol-related health problems.

Alcohol addiction is seen frequently among homeless individuals.

Critical Thinking

Jose is a well-liked 17-year-old. It always seems as if everything is going his way—an A on a test, a scholarship to his dream school, you name it. Lately, however, Jose has experienced some disappointments. His grandfather has just passed away, and he and his girlfriend of 6 months have broken up. When he arrived home late with the smell of alcohol on his breath, his parents started to worry. They talked to his school counselor, who suggested they look for certain signs that could indicate depression and/or alcohol dependence. What might those signs be?

Another common screening tool is the Michigan Alcohol Screening Test (MAST). It contains 22 questions. Briefer versions are also available. Check out these and still other screening tools at the National Institute on Alcohol Abuse and Alcoholism Web site: http://www.niaaa.nih.gov/publications/niaaa-guide.

Other questions to ask along with the CAGE questionnaire are:

1. Have you had memory lapses or blackouts due to drinking?
2. Do you continue to drink even though you have health problems caused by alcohol?
3. Do you get withdrawal symptoms, such as headaches, chills, shakes, and a strong craving for alcohol, and, as a result, drink more to get rid of these symptoms?
4. Do you take part in high-risk behaviors, such as having unsafe sex in a non-monogamous relationship or driving a car or boat while under the influence of alcohol?
5. Has drinking caused trouble at home, at work, or in relationships with others?
6. Do you have to drink alcohol for any of the following reasons?
   a. To get through the day or unwind at the end of the day
   b. To cope with stressful life events
   c. To escape from ongoing problems

Answering yes to any of these questions should prompt the respondent to consult a family physician or a certified counselor for help.

Treatment of Alcoholism

Once a diagnosis of alcohol abuse or dependence is established, one should seek the guidance of a physician to arrange appropriate treatment and counseling for the person and family. An important goal of counseling is to identify ways to compensate for the loss of pleasure from drinking. This helps the drinker confront the immediate problem of how to stop drinking. Total abstinence must be the ultimate objective. For alcoholics, there is no such thing as controlled drinking. A problem drinker cannot return safely to social drinking.

The person should enter an Alcoholics Anonymous (AA) 12-step program (Al-Anon for the spouse), or another reputable therapy program for people with alcoholism. Check with a local mental health treatment center to find programs available in the community or call 800-245-4656. Substance Abuse and Mental Health Services can be reached at 800-729-6686 or www.health.org for alcohol and drug information. Other helpful websites are www.adultchildren.org, www.nacoa.org, and www.niaaa.nih.gov. In addition, one may visit the Alcoholics Anonymous web page at www.alcoholics-anonymous.org or contact AA at:

AA World Services, Inc.
P.O. Box 459
New York, NY 10163
212-870-3400

To learn more about alcoholism, visit these websites:
www.niaaa.nih.gov
www.asam.org
www.mentalhelp.net/selfhelp.

According to AA's literature, "AA is a fellowship of men and women who share their experience, strength, and hope with each other that they may solve their common problem and help others recover from alcoholism." As an informal society chartered in 1935, Alcoholics Anonymous includes more than 2 million recovered alcoholics. The only requirement for membership is the desire to stop drinking. There are no rules, regulations, dues, or fees. In addition, the group is not a political or formal organization.

It is helpful for the spouse to join the treatment program as well. AA has two types of meetings—open and closed. Alcoholics and their families and friends are invited to the open meetings, whereas the closed meetings are reserved for alcoholics only.

Current research does not support the generally negative public opinion about the prognosis for alcoholism. In most job-related alcoholism treatment programs, wherein workers are socially stable and—because of the risk to jobs and pensions—well motivated, recovery is possible, especially with early detection. Once a person moves from problem drinking to an early identification and intervention remain the most important steps in the treatment of alcoholism. Success is usually proportional to participation in AA, other social agencies' programs, and religious counseling. About two years of treatment should be expected.

Three medications are available to treat alcoholism. The medication naltrexone (ReVia) blocks the craving for alcohol and the pleasure of intoxication. It has shown to be effective for some people, but up to 40% of those treated do not respond to the therapy. (Genetic differences are implicated.) Disulfiram (Antabuse) causes physical reactions, such as vomiting, when drinking alcohol. It does so by blocking acetaldehyde metabolism. However, Antabuse is rarely used today. Finally, acamprosate (Campral) may be useful. It is thought to decrease alcohol cravings by altering neurotransmitter function in the brain.

Concept Check

Treatment of alcoholism often includes the use of medicine, counseling, and social support. The clinicians involved must treat the entire person. Alcoholics Anonymous and other support groups are very helpful. Naltrexone or acamprosate can be prescribed to decrease alcohol intake. Another option is disulfiram, which produces an ill feeling when the patient consumes alcohol with the medication. With all of the treatments for alcoholism, it is important to find the one that works best for the individual concerned.

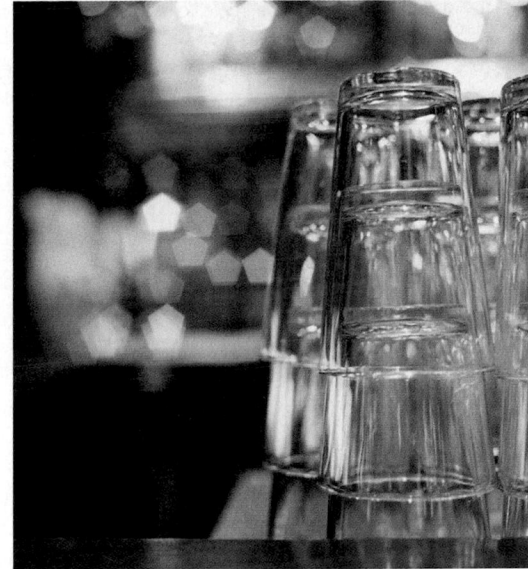

There is no such thing as controlled drinking once a person has alcoholism. Total abstinence is mandatory for recovery.

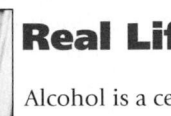

Real Life Scenario Follow-Up

Alcohol is a central nervous system depressant that affects both respiration and heart rate. In large quantities, alcohol can depress both systems to the point of terminating respiration and cardiac function. Obviously, this is fatal. Alcohol abuse is a common problem, and continued alcohol abuse can lead to dependence problems, although alcohol abuse and dependence are different.

As a close friend, Alyssa has a responsibility to hold Todd accountable for his actions. Sometimes it is difficult to realize that one has a drinking problem, although it may be obvious to others. Alyssa should talk privately with Todd about the most recent incident when he is sober and calm. It is important to deal with situations such as these very carefully, as the problem drinker will probably respond defensively. She could explain how his drinking is causing problems for both of them, she could tell him about the harmful consequences of his drinking, and she could refuse to go with him to any alcohol-related events. But she must be prepared to carry out the threat. This is especially important for her as she does not want to risk further physical harm from Todd. Alyssa could talk with a counselor, who may help her learn ways to approach Todd effectively. Offering to go with Todd to a treatment program or an AA meeting to get help is one idea. There is strength in numbers, so other members of Todd's family or close friends also should be enlisted to help, under the guidance of a therapist trained in treating alcoholics.

Summary

1. Alcohol use is a complex issue because it involves psychological, social, economic, health, legal, and family issues.
2. Alcohol is metabolized in the liver and other tissues. Metabolism depends on the enzyme alcohol dehydrogenase. A number of factors, such as gender, race, and body composition, determine how a person reacts to alcohol.
3. The benefits of alcohol use are associated with low to moderate alcohol consumption. These benefits include the pleasurable and social aspects of alcohol use, a reduction in various forms of cardiovascular disease, increase in insulin sensitivity, and protection against some harmful stomach bacteria.
4. Alcohol has the potential to worsen health as well. Excessive consumption of alcohol contributes significantly to 5 of the 10 leading causes of death in North America. Alcohol increases the risk of developing certain forms of heart damage, inflammation of the pancreas, GI tract damage, vitamin and mineral deficiencies,

cirrhosis of the liver, certain forms of cancer, hypertension, and hemmorhagic stroke—to name a few.

5. If alcohol is consumed, it should be consumed in moderation with meals. Women are advised to drink no more than one drink per day, as are adults 65 years and older; men are advised to limit intake to two drinks a day.

6. Gender, genetics, ethnic background, and ongoing depression all play a role in a person's chances of becoming alcohol dependent.

7. Early detection of alcoholism is key to successful treatment and a reduction of health care costs. The CAGE questionnaire can help a person determine whether or not he or she has an alcohol problem.

8. Many methods are available to treat alcoholism. Alcoholics Anonymous and the medication ReVia are among the typical approaches.

Study Questions

1. Where in the body does most of the metabolism of alcohol take place? What is a by-product of alcohol metabolism?

2. Why does it take a woman longer than a man to metabolize alcohol?

3. List two potential health benefits of alcohol use.

4. List four problems associated with alcohol abuse.

5. Which two nutrient deficiencies are common in alcoholism? Why?

6. Define the term *one drink*. How much alcohol use is considered to be moderate for men? for women?

7. Why can some ethnic groups "hold their liquor" better than others can?

8. Name four criteria that might indicate someone has a problem with alcohol. What is this group of criteria called?

9. What is binge drinking? Within which segment of the population is this increasing in popularity?

10. Describe a method used in treating alcoholism. List a pro and con.

Further Readings

1. Alcohol and health: The pros and cons. *Mayo Clinic Health Letter*, p. 4, November 2003.

   The pros and cons of alcohol use are reviewed. Although there are health benefits from alcohol use, moderation is a key theme, and there is no recommendation to start drinking merely to gain the health benefits.

2. Alcohol-attributable deaths and years of potential life lost. *Journal of the American Medical Association* 292: 2831, 2004.

   Excessive alcohol consumption is the third leading cause of preventable death in the United States. These deaths include liver cirrhosis, various cancers, unintentional injuries, and violence

3. Alcohol-an important women's health issue. *Alcohol Alert* 62: 1, 2004.

   When a woman drinks alcohol, the alcohol in her bloodstream typically reaches a higher amount than in a man even if they are drinking the same amount. This is because women have less body water than men. As a result women are very susceptible to alcohol-related organ damage.

4. Dorn JM and others: Alcohol drinking patterns differentially affect central adiposity as measured by abdominal height in women and men. *Journal of Nutrition* 133:2665, 2003.

   Alcohol use increases the risk for abdominal fat deposition. Binge drinking especially was found to be a risk factor.

5. Hanson GR, Li TK: Public health implications of excessive alcohol intake. *Journal of the American Medical Association* 289:1031, 2003.

   Abuse of alcohol is one of the most serious public health problems in our society. Underage drinking is a specific concern, especially because it is also associated with tobacco and illicit drug use.

6. Klatsky AL: Drink to your health? *Scientific American*, p. 75, February 2003.

   Moderate alcohol use provides some health benefits, but alcohol abuse poses many health risks. In light of current knowledge, a person with an established moderate drinking pattern should generally not be advised to abstain from alcohol. However, non-drinkers should not be advised to start drinking for health reasons.

7. McDonough KH: Antioxidant nutrients and alcohol. *Toxicology* 189:89, 2003.

   Oxidant damage is part of the reason alcohol abuse leads to cirrhosis of the liver. An inadequate diet makes this even more likely.

8. Mukamal KJ and others: Roles of drinking pattern and type of alcohol consumed in coronary heart disease in men. *The New England Journal of Medicine* 348:109, 2003.

   Men who drank alcohol at least three to four times per week had a reduced risk of heart attack. The association was strongest with beer and liquor, the predominant types of beverage consumed by this population.

9. Mukamal KJ and others: Alcohol and risk for ischemic stroke in men: the role of drinking pattern and usual beverages. *Annals of Internal Medicine* 142:11, 2005.

   Intake of more than two drinks a day increases the risk of ischemic stroke. In contrast lesser amounts of alcohol, specifically red wine, is associated with a reduced risk of ischemic stroke.

10. Saitz R: Unhealthy alcohol use. *The New England Journal of Medicine* 352: 596, 2005.

    A case study of a man who is abusing alcohol is presented. Both diagnosis and treatment of alcoholism are reviewed in the process.

11. Stampfer MJ and others: Effects of moderate alcohol consumption on cognitive function in women. *The New England Journal of Medicine* 352: 245, 2005.

    Up to one drink per day may increase cognitive function in women. An intake of more than that is not protective, and even has the opposite effect.

12. Underage drinking. *Alcohol Alert* 59:1 (April), 2003.

    Underage drinking may lead to a host of health problems, including traffic accidents and suicide. Early intervention to curb underage drinking is essential to prevent these and other health problems.

13. US Preventative Services Task Force: Screening and behavioral counseling interventions in primary care to reduce alcohol misuse: Recommendation statement. *American Family Physician* 70: 353, 2004.

    The US Preventative Services Task Force recommends screening and behavioral counseling to reduce alcohol misuse. The CAGE questionnaire is one tool discussed that can be used for screening purposes. Other tools are also presented.

14. Wannamethee SG, Shaper AG: Alcohol, body weight, and weight gain in middle-aged men. *American Journal of Clinical Nutrition* 77:1312, 2003.

    Heavy alcohol use contributes to weight gain and obesity. All types of alcoholic beverages are implicated with respect to this effect.

15. Wannamethee SG and others: Alcohol drinking patterns and risk of type 2 diabetes mellitus among younger women. *Archives of Internal Medicine* 163: 1329, 2003.

    Light to moderate alcohol consumption may be associated with a lower risk of type 2 diabetes among women. Intakes in excess of this are not more protective, however, and actually increased such risk.

I. Could You or Someone You Know Have a Problem with Alcohol?

Problem drinking often has its seeds in the teen years. Significant health consequences typically arise in adulthood. It is a contributor to 5 of the 10 leading causes of death in North America. The social consequences of alcohol dependency include divorce, unemployment, and poverty. The following questionnaire was developed by the National Council on Alcoholism. With this assessment, you can determine whether you or someone you know might need help. Answer the following questions by placing an "X" in the appropriate blank.

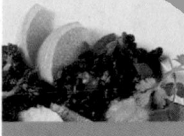

	Yes	No
1. Do you occasionally drink heavily after disappointment, after a quarrel, or when someone gives you a hard time?	____	____
2. When you have trouble or feel under pressure, do you drink more heavily than usual?	____	____
3. Have you ever noticed that you're able to handle liquor better than you did when you first started drinking?	____	____
4. Do you ever wake up the morning after you've been drinking and discover that you can't remember part of the evening before, even though your friends tell you that you didn't pass out?	____	____
5. When drinking with other people, do you try to have a few extra drinks when others won't know it?	____	____
6. Are there certain occasions when you feel uncomfortable if alcohol isn't available?	____	____
7. Have you recently noticed that when you begin drinking, you're in more of a hurry to get the first drink than you used to be?	____	____
8. Do you sometimes feel a little guilty about your drinking?	____	____
9. Are you secretly irritated when your family or friends discuss your drinking?	____	____
10. Have you recently noticed an increase in the frequency of memory blackouts?	____	____
11. Do you often find that you wish to continue drinking after your friends say they've had enough?	____	____
12. Do you usually have a reason for the occasions when you drink heavily?	____	____
13. When you're sober, do you often regret things you have done or said while drinking?	____	____
14. Have you tried switching brands or following different plans to control your drinking?	____	____
15. Have you often failed to keep promises you've made to yourself about controlling or stopping your drinking?	____	____
16. Have you ever tried to control your drinking by changing jobs or moving to a new location?	____	____
17. Do you try to avoid family or close friends while you're drinking?	____	____
18. Are you having an increasing number of financial and work problems?	____	____
19. Do more people seem to be treating you unfairly without good reason?	____	____
20. Do you eat very little or irregularly when you're drinking?	____	____
21. Do you sometimes have the "shakes" in the morning and find that it helps to have a little drink?	____	____
22. Have you recently noticed that you can't drink as much as you once did?	____	____
23. Do you sometimes stay drunk for several days at a time?	____	____
24. Do you sometimes feel very depressed and wonder whether life is worth living?	____	____
25. Sometimes after periods of drinking do you see or hear things that aren't there?	____	____
26. Do you get terribly frightened after you have been drinking heavily?	____	____

Interpretation

These are all symptoms that may indicate alcoholism. "Yes" answers to several of the questions indicate the following stages of alcoholism:

Questions 1–8:   Potential drinking problem
Questions 9–21:   Drinking problem likely
Questions 22–26: Definite drinking problem

It is vital that people assess themselves honestly. If you or someone you know demonstrates some or a number of these symptoms, it is important that help be sought. If there is even a question in your mind, go talk to a professional about it. Alcohol abuse is one of many problems that adults, including older people, face.

II. *Investigate the Calorie Cost of Alcohol Use*

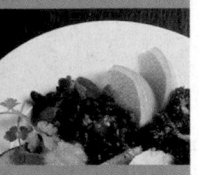

On an upcoming weekend (Friday night through Sunday night) have a few friends keep a log of their alcoholic beverage intake. Include males and females. Then use Table 7-1 or your NutritionCalc Plus analysis to calculate the amount of calories provided by alcoholic beverages over that time period. Assuming that an active man needs about 2800 kcal per day and an active woman needs about 2200 kcal per day, is the amount of calories provided by alcoholic beverages large (i.e., 25% or more of calorie needs) or small (i.e., 10% or less of calorie needs)?

Vitamins

8

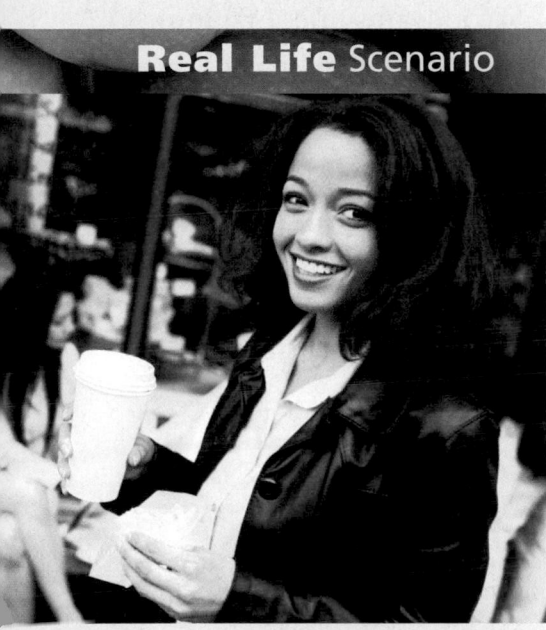

Kristen works nights at a local package distribution center to make some extra money. The combination of taking a full course load at college and working nights has created a lot of stress for her. Kristen's many commitments also make it important that she not become ill. On a recent coffee break at her job, a co-worker suggested she take *Nutramega* supplements to help prevent colds, flu, and other illnesses. The product's label suggests that *Nutramega* helps prevent such problems, especially those associated with the changing of seasons. The label recommends taking two to three tablets every 3 hours at the first sign of feeling ill, and two to three tablets daily for health maintenance. Kristen looks at the Supplement Facts label on the bottle and finds that each tablet contains (as percent of the Daily Value): 33% for vitamin A (three-quarters of which is preformed vitamin A), 700% for vitamin C, 50% for zinc, and 10% for selenium. A month's supply also costs about $50.

Should Kristen use this product? Are there health risks associated with this product, especially considering the dosage recommended on the label?

Chapter 8 Objectives

Chapter 8 is designed to allow you to:

1. Define the term *vitamin*.
2. Classify the vitamins according to whether they are fat soluble or water soluble.
3. List the major functions and deficiency symptoms for each vitamin.
4. List three important food sources for each vitamin.
5. Describe toxicity symptoms from excess consumption of certain vitamins.
6. Evaluate the use of vitamin supplements with respect to their potential benefits and hazards to the body.

Check out the **Contemporary Nutrition Online Learning Center** www.mhhe.com/wardlawcont6 *for quizzes, flash cards, other activities, and web links designed to further help you learn about vitamins.*

When it comes to vitamins, we often hear, "If a little is good, then more must be better." Some people believe that consuming vitamins far in excess of their needs provides them with extra energy, protection from disease, and prolonged youth. About 40% of adults in the United States take vitamin and/or mineral supplements on a regular basis, some at unsafe levels. They are spending about $17 billion annually on supplements. The health-related value of this practice is hotly debated.

Our total vitamin needs to prevent deficiency are actually quite small. In general, humans require a total of about 1 ounce (28 grams) of vitamins for every 150 pounds (70 kilograms) of food consumed. Vitamins are found in plants and animals. Plants synthesize all the vitamins they need. Animals vary in their ability to synthesize vitamins. For example, guinea pigs and humans are two of the very few organisms that are unable to make their own supply of vitamin C.

Chapter 8 reviews some general properties of vitamins. These vital nutrients are divided into two groups: the fat-soluble vitamins and the water-soluble vitamins. Attention focuses on the functions and sources of each vitamin and human needs for them. The current controversy over vitamin and mineral supplement use is also explored.

Refresh Your Memory

As you begin your study of vitamins in Chapter 8, you may want to review:

- Implications of the Dietary Supplement Health and Education Act (DSHEA) in Chapter 1
- The gastrointestinal system for the digestion and absorption of nutrients and the urinary system for vitamin D activation in Chapter 3
- The digestion and absorption of dietary lipids, the formation of lipoproteins, and the definition of antioxidants in Chapter 5
- Amino acid metabolism, protein synthesis, and protein-calorie malnutrition in Chapter 6

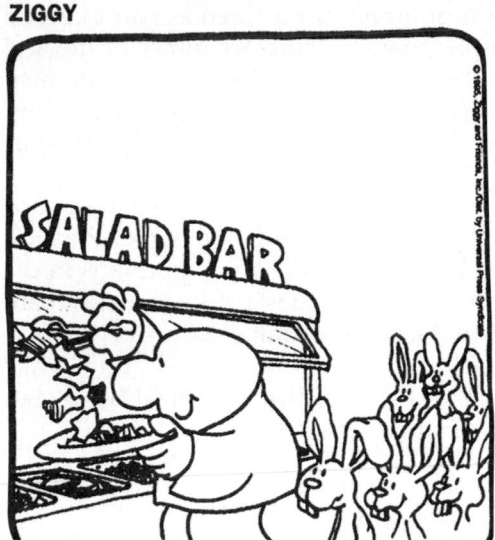

Much attention has been given to vegetable intake in recent years. Which vitamins are especially found in salad greens and other vegetables? What are some other health-related attributes of vegetables in general? Which chronic diseases are associated with a poor intake of vegetables? How can we minimize vitamin losses when cooking vegetables? Chapter 8 provides some answers.

Vitamins: Vital Dietary Components

By definition, **vitamins** are essential organic (carbon-containing) substances needed in small amounts in the diet for normal function, growth, and maintenance of the body. Although vitamins themselves yield no energy to the body, they often participate in energy-yielding reactions. Vitamins A, D, E, and K are **fat soluble,** whereas the B vitamins and vitamin C are **water soluble.** In addition, the B vitamins and vitamin K function as parts of **coenzymes** (that is, compounds that help enzymes function) (Fig. 8-1).

Vitamins are generally indispensable in human diets because they can't be synthesized in the human body, or because their synthesis can be decreased by environmental factors. Notable exceptions to having a strict dietary need for a vitamin are vitamin A, which can be synthesized from certain pigments in plants; vitamin D, which is synthesized by the skin in the presence of adequate sunlight; niacin, which is synthesized from the amino acid tryptophan; and vitamin K and biotin, which are synthesized to some extent by bacteria in the intestinal tract.

To be classified as a vitamin, a compound must meet the criteria to be an essential nutrient: (1) the body is unable to synthesize enough of the compound to maintain health; and (2) absence of the compound from the diet for a defined period of time produces deficiency symptoms that, if caught in time, are quickly cured when the substance is resupplied. A substance does not qualify as a vitamin merely because the body can't make it. Evidence must suggest that health declines when the substance is not consumed.

As scientists began to identify various vitamins, related deficiency diseases such as scurvy, beriberi, pellagra, and rickets were dramatically cured. For the most part, as the vitamins were discovered, they were named alphabetically: A, B, C, D, E, and so on. Later, many substances originally classified as vitamins were found not to be essential for humans and were dropped from the list, such as vitamin P. Other vitamins, thought at first to be only one chemical turned out to be several chemicals, so the alphabetical names had to be broken down by numbers (B-6, B-12, and so on).

In addition to their use in correcting deficiency diseases, a few vitamins have also proved useful in treating several nondeficiency diseases. These medical applications require administration of **megadoses,** well above typical human needs for the

vitamin Compound needed in very small amounts in the diet to help regulate and support chemical reactions and processes in the body.

fat-soluble vitamins Vitamins that dissolve in fat and such substances as ether and benzene but not readily in water. These vitamins are A, D, E, and K.

water-soluble vitamins Vitamins that dissolve in water. These vitamins are the B vitamins and vitamin C.

coenzyme A compound that combines with an inactive enzyme to form a catalytically active form. In this manner, coenzymes aid in enzyme function.

megadose Intake of a nutrient beyond estimates of needs to prevent a deficiency, or what would be found in a balanced diet; 2 to 10 times human needs is a starting point for such a dosage.

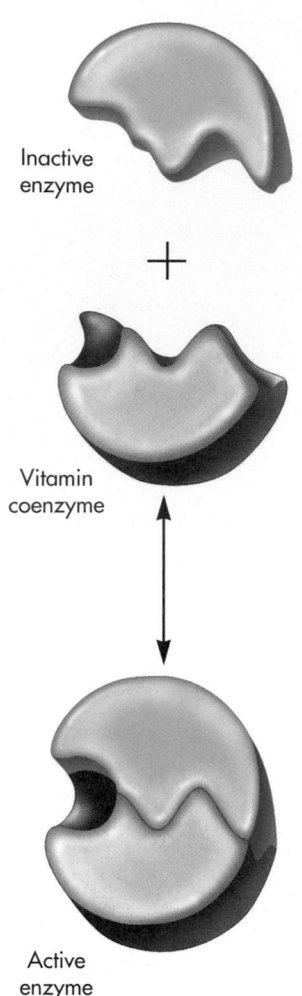

Inactive
enzyme

+

Vitamin
coenzyme

Active
enzyme

Figure 8-1 Coenzymes, such as those formed from B vitamins, aid in the function of various enzymes. Without the coenzyme, the enzyme cannot function, and deficiency symptoms associated with the missing vitamin eventually appear. Note that health-food stores sell the coenzyme forms of some vitamins. These more expensive forms of vitamins are unnecessary. The body makes all the coenzymes it needs from vitamin precursors.

vitamins. For example, megadoses of a form of niacin can be used as part of blood cholesterol–lowering treatment for certain individuals. Other examples of medical use include forms of vitamin D in the treatment of psoriasis. This chapter will mention others as well. Still, any claimed benefits from use of vitamin supplements, especially intakes in excess of the Upper Level (if set), should be viewed critically because unproven claims are common.

Both plant and animal foods supply vitamins in the human diet. Whether isolated from foods or synthesized in the laboratory, vitamins are the same chemical compounds and generally work equally well in the body. Contrary to claims in the health-food literature, "natural" vitamins isolated from foods are, for the most part, no more healthful than those synthesized in a laboratory, but there are exceptions. Vitamin E is much more potent in its natural form than in its synthetic form, while synthetic folic acid, the form of the vitamin added to ready-to-eat breakfast cereals and flour, is 1.7 times more potent than the natural vitamin form.

■ Have Scientists Found All the Vitamins?

You may wonder whether there are vitamins in foods that have yet to be discovered. After all, the first chemical formula of a vitamin (thiamin) was not determined until 1937, and the last structure was characterized in 1948 (vitamin B-12). Although some optimistic researchers hope to discover that one or more additional compounds (e.g., choline; see p. 271) are vitamins, most scientists are confident that all compounds that meet the criteria for classification as a vitamin have been discovered. Evidence supports this assumption. For example, people have lived well for years when receiving only intravenous administration of solutions that consist of protein, carbohydrate, fat, all the known vitamins, and the essential minerals. With appropriate medical monitoring, these people not only continue to live, but also build new body tissues, heal wounds, fight existing diseases, and even have babies.

■ Storage of Vitamins in the Body

Except for vitamin K, the fat-soluble vitamins are not readily excreted from the body. In contrast, excess amounts of the water-soluble vitamins are generally lost from the body quite rapidly, partly because the water in cells dissolves these vitamins and excretes them out of the body via the kidneys. Water-soluble vitamin B-6 and vitamin B-12 are exceptions; these are stored much more readily than the other water-soluble vitamins.

Because of the limited storage of many vitamins, they should be consumed in the diet daily, although an occasional lapse in the intake of even water-soluble vitamins generally causes no harm. Symptoms of a vitamin deficiency occur only when that vitamin is lacking in the diet and body stores are essentially exhausted. For example, an average person must consume no thiamin for 10 days or no vitamin C for 20 to 40 days before developing the first symptoms of deficiency of these vitamins (Fig. 8-2 shows effects of a vitamin C deficiency, as well as other vitamin deficiencies).

■ Vitamin Toxicity

Because fat-soluble vitamins are not readily excreted, some can easily accumulate in the body and cause toxic effects. And, although a toxic effect from an excessive intake of any vitamin is theoretically possible, toxicities of the fat-soluble vitamin A is the most frequently observed. Vitamin E and the water-soluble vitamins niacin, vitamin B-6, and vitamin C can also cause toxic effects, but only when consumed in very large amounts (15 to 100 times human needs or more). These five vitamins are unlikely to cause toxic effects unless taken in supplement (pill) form. Note that vitamin A even causes toxicity with long-term intake as little as three times human needs.

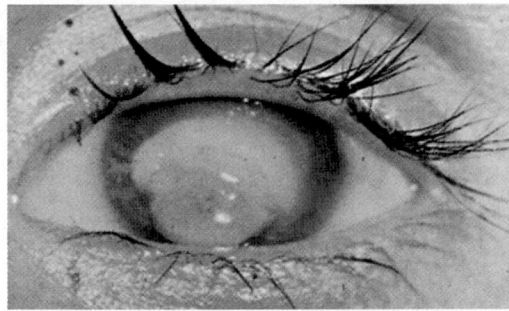

a. Vitamin A deficiency that eventually led to blindness. Note the severe effects on this eye. This problem is commonly seen today in southeast Asia.

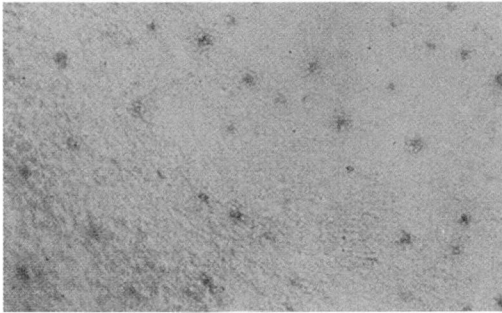

b. Pinpoint hemorrhages of the skin—an early symptom of vitamin C deficiency and **scurvy.** The spots on the skin are caused by slight bleeding into hair follicles. Vitamin C deficiency also slows wound healing.

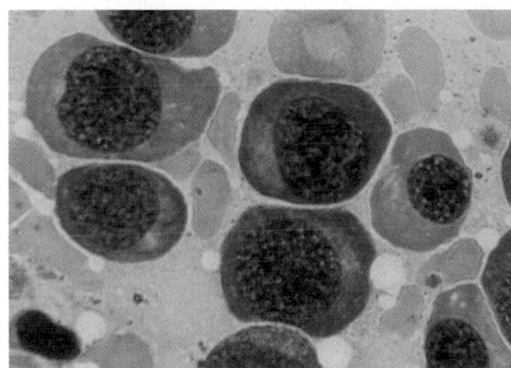

c. Enlarged blood cells seen here in the bone marrow are arrested at an immature stage of development. A folate or vitamin B-12 deficiency could be the cause. The cells still have their nuclei and are slightly larger than normal red blood cells.

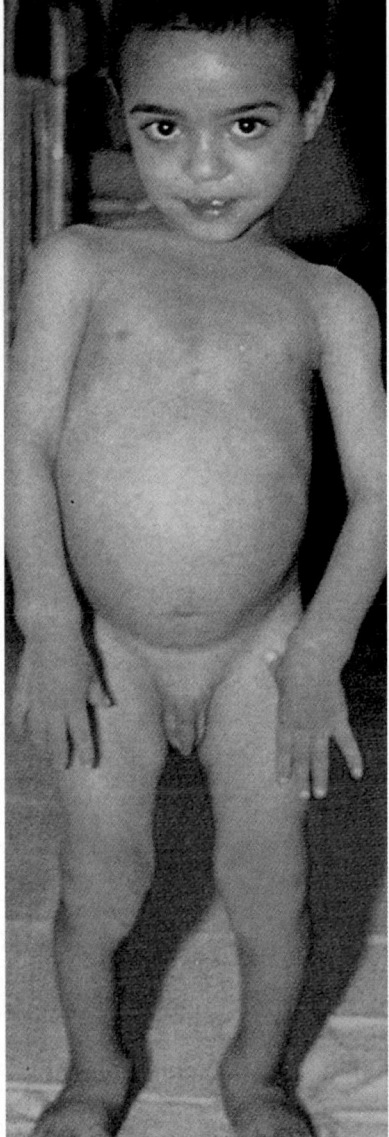

d. The bowed legs of rickets, a vitamin D deficiency disease.

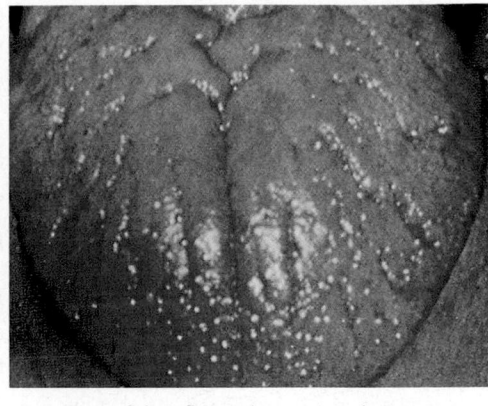

e. A painful, inflamed tongue (glossitis) can signal a deficiency of niacin, vitamin B-6, riboflavin, folate, or vitamin B-12. Often more than one deficiency is the cause.

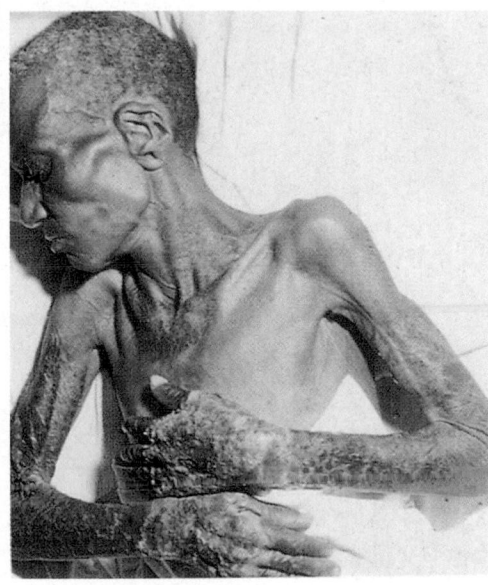

f. The **dermatitis** of a niacin deficiency called pellegra. Dermatitis on both sides of the body (bilateral) is a typical symptom. Sun exposure worsens the condition.

Figure 8-2 Clinical evidence of selected vitamin deficiencies.

Because a "one-a-day" type of multivitamin and mineral supplement usually contains less than two times the Daily Values of the components, regular use of these products is unlikely to cause toxic effects in men and nonpregnant women. But consuming many vitamin pills, especially highly potent sources of vitamin A, can cause problems. Today, concentrated vitamin A supplements are widely available in

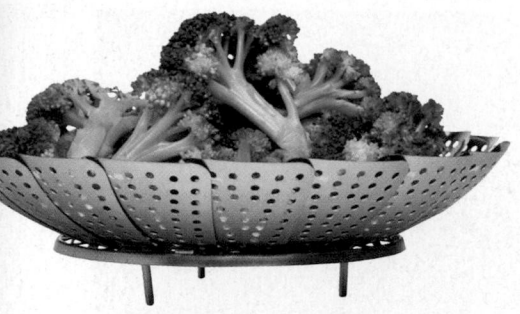

Rapid cooking of vegetables in minimal fluids aids in preserving vitamin content. Steaming is one effective method.

grocery, drug, and health-food stores and pose risks for toxicity when used inappropriately. See the later Looking Further section to find out more about whether you should take a multivitamin and mineral supplement and, if so, how to do it safely.

■ Preservation of Vitamins in Foods

Substantial amounts of vitamins can be lost from the time a fruit or vegetable is picked until it is eaten. The water-soluble vitamins—particularly thiamin, vitamin C, and folate—can be destroyed with improper storage and excessive cooking. Heat, light, exposure to the air, cooking in water, and alkalinity are all factors that can destroy vitamins. The sooner a food is eaten after harvest, the less chance of nutrient loss.

In general, if the food is not eaten within a few days, freezing is the best preservation method to retain nutrients. In fact, frozen vegetables and fruits are often as nutrient-rich as freshly picked ones. Fruits and vegetables are often frozen immediately after harvesting. As part of the freezing process, vegetables are quickly blanched in boiling water. This destroys the enzymes that would otherwise degrade the vitamins. Table 8-1 provides some tips to aid in preserving the vitamins in food.

Concept Check

In general, the fat-soluble vitamins—A, D, E, and K—are less readily excreted than are the water-soluble B vitamins and vitamin C. Regular consumption of foods rich in both water-soluble and fat-soluble vitamins is important for health. However, the occasional inadequate consumption of any one vitamin is of little health concern, because even water-soluble vitamins persist in the body to some extent. For example, when a person ingests a vitamin-free diet, the first deficiency signs (due to lack of thiamin) will not appear for about 10 days. When taken in supplement form, the fat-soluble vitamin A poses the greatest risk of toxicity. For the most part, there is little risk of toxicity when vitamins are obtained from foods.

Table 8-1 Tips for Preserving the Vitamin Content of Foods

What to Do	Why
Keep fruits and vegetables cool.	Enzymes in food begin to degrade vitamins once the fruit or vegetable is picked. Chilling reduces this process. Refrigerate fresh produce (except for potatoes, tomatoes, onions, and bananas) until they are consumed.
Refrigerate foods in moisture-proof air-tight containers.	Nutrients keep best at temperatures near freezing, at high humidity, and away from air.
Trim, peel, and cut fruits and vegetables minimally—just enough to remove rotten or inedible parts.	Oxygen breaks down vitamins faster when more surface is exposed. Outer leaves of lettuce and other greens have higher values of vitamins and minerals than the inner, tender leaves or stems. Potato skins and apple skins are higher in vitamins and minerals than the inner parts.
Microwave, steam, or use a pan or wok with very small amounts of fat and a tight-fitting lid to cook vegetables.	More nutrients are retained when there is less contact with water and shorter cooking time. Whenever possible, cook fruits or vegetables in their skins.
Minimize reheating food.	Prolonged reheating reduces vitamin content.
Do not add fats to vegetables during cooking if you plan to discard the liquid.	Fat-soluble vitamins will be lost in discarded fat. Add fats to vegetables after they are fully cooked and drained.
Do not add baking soda to vegetables to enhance the green color.	Alkalinity destroys much vitamin D, thiamin, and other vitamins.
Store canned foods in a cool place.	Canned foods vary in the amount of nutrients lost, largely because of differences in storage time and temperatures. To get maximal nutritive value from canned goods, serve any liquid packed with the food whenever possible.

The Fat-Soluble Vitamins—A, D, E, and K

Let's look at what we know about the fat-soluble vitamins—vitamins A, D, E, and K.

■ Absorption of Fat-Soluble Vitamins

Vitamins A, D, E, and K are absorbed along with dietary fat. These vitamins then travel with dietary fats through the bloodstream to reach body cells. Special carriers in the bloodstream help distribute some of these vitamins. Fat-soluble vitamins are stored mostly in the liver and fatty tissues.

When fat absorption is efficient, about 40% to 90% of the fat-soluble vitamins are absorbed. Anything that interferes with normal digestion and absorption of fats, however, also interferes with fat-soluble vitamin absorption. For example, people with cystic fibrosis, a disease that often hampers fat absorption, may develop deficiencies of fat-soluble vitamins. Some medications, such as the weight-loss drug orlistat (Xenical), also interfere with fat absorption. (Chapter 10 discusses this drug in detail.) Unabsorbed fat carries these vitamins to the large intestine, where they are excreted in the feces. People with such conditions are especially susceptible to vitamin K deficiency because body stores of vitamin K are lower than those of the other fat-soluble vitamins. Vitamin supplements, taken under a physician's guidance, are part of the treatment for preventing a vitamin deficiency associated with fat malabsorption. Finally, people who use mineral oil as a laxative at mealtimes risk fat-soluble vitamin deficiencies. Because the intestine does not absorb mineral oil, fat-soluble vitamins are eliminated with the mineral oil in the feces.

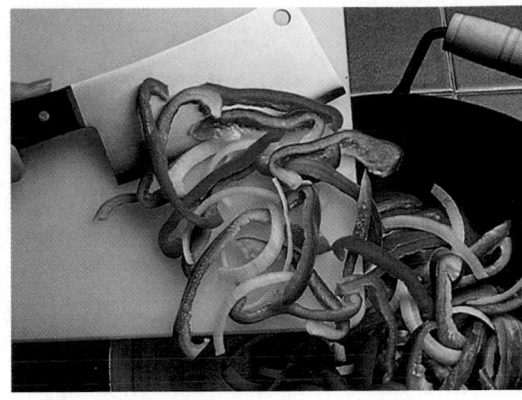

Vegetables are rich sources of provitamin A carotenoids.

Vitamin A

The amount of vitamin A you consume is very important, as both deficiency and toxicity of this vitamin can cause severe problems. In addition, there is a very narrow range of optimal intakes between these two states. Vitamin A is found in foods in a variety of forms. **Retinoids,** or preformed vitamin A, are only found in foods of animal origin, such as fish and organ meats. However, plants contain pigments called **carotenoids,** which can be turned into vitamin A in the body as needed. Since certain carotenoids can be turned into vitamin A, they can be termed **provitamin A.** Currently, only three of the more than 600 carotenoids found in nature are known to serve as provitamin A in humans, but there may be more. Beta-carotene, the orange-yellow pigment in carrots, is the most potent form of provitamin A. Together, preformed vitamin A from animal sources and provitamin A carotenoids make up what is generally called vitamin A.

retinoids Chemical forms of preformed vitamin A; one source is animal foods.

carotenoids Pigment materials in fruits and vegetables that range in color from yellow to orange to red; three of the various carotenoids yield vitamin A. Many are antioxidants.

provitamin A A substance that can be made into a vitamin.

■ Functions of Vitamin A and Carotenoids

Vitamin A plays many important roles in the body. The best known and most clearly understood of its role is in vision. Body changes that occur when vitamin A is lacking provide insight to this and other actions of this fat-soluble nutrient.

Vision

The link between vitamin A and night vision has been known since ancient Egyptian times, when juice extracted from liver was used as a cure for night blindness. Vitamin A performs important functions in light-dark vision, and to a lesser extent, color vision. One form of vitamin A (retinal) allows certain cells in the eye to adjust from bright to dim light (such as after seeing the headlights of an oncoming car). Without

night blindness A vitamin A deficiency condition in which the retina (in the eye) cannot adjust to low amounts of light.

mucus A thick fluid secreted by many cells throughout the body. It contains a compound that has both carbohydrate and protein parts. It acts as a lubricant and means of protection for cells.

xerophthalmia Literally "dry eye." This is a cause of blindness that results from a vitamin A deficiency. The specific cause is linked to a lack of mucus production by the eye, which then leaves it at a greater risk of damage from surface dirt and bacteria.

macular degeneration A painless condition leading to disruption of the central part of the retina (in the eye) and, in turn, blurred vision.

epithelial cells The cells that line the outside of the body and the inside of all external passages within it, such as the GI tract.

Chapter 9 discusses one study that showed that the mineral zinc helps prevent macular degeneration in people who show evidence of the disease, especially when combined with vitamin C and vitamin E.

sufficient dietary vitamin A, the cells in the eye cannot quickly readjust to dim light. This condition is known as **night blindness.**

If vitamin A deficiency progresses, the cells that line the cornea of the eye (the clear window of the eye) also lose their ability to produce **mucus.** The eye then becomes dry. Eventually, when dirt particles scratch the dry surface of the eye, bacteria infect it. The infection soon spreads to the entire surface of the eye and leads to blindness. This disease process is called **xerophthalmia,** which means *dry eye* (review Fig. 8-2).

Vitamin A deficiency is second only to accidents as a worldwide cause of blindness. North Americans are at little risk because of generally good diets. However, people—especially children—in less-developed nations are very susceptible to vitamin A deficiency. Poor vitamin A intakes, low fat intakes that do not allow for sufficient vitamin A absorption, and low stores of vitamin A lessen the ability of the children to meet high needs during rapid childhood growth. Hundreds of thousands of children in developing nations, especially Asia, become blind each year because of vitamin A deficiency and ultimately die from infections. In North America the leading cause of blindness in adults is diabetes; in children, it is accidents. As covered in more detail in Chapter 17, worldwide attempts to reduce this problem have included giving large doses of vitamin A twice yearly and fortifying sugar, margarine, and monosodium glutamate with vitamin A. These food vehicles are used because they are commonly consumed by the populations of less-developed nations. This effort has proven effective in some countries.

Age-related **macular degeneration** is a leading cause of legal blindness among North American adults over the age of 65. The disease is associated with changes in the macular area of the eye, which provides the most detailed vision. Age, smoking, and genetics are risk factors. The macula contains the carotenoids lutein and zeaxanthin in high enough concentrations to impart a yellow color. In one study, the higher the total number of carotenoids (beta-carotene, lutein, and zeaxanthin) consumed in the diet, the lower was the risk for age-related macular degeneration. These carotenoids may also decrease the risk of cataracts in the eyes. Although these are interesting hypotheses, consumption of fruits and vegetables high in carotenoids in general may reduce the risk for these eye disorders rather than the intake of these specific carotenoids. Note that multivitamin and mineral supplements formulated for older adults (e.g., Centrum Silver™) are being marketed as a source of lutein.

Health of Other Cells

Vitamin A maintains the health of cells that line internal and external surfaces of the lungs, intestines, stomach, vagina, urinary tract, and bladder, as well as those of the eyes and skin. These cells (called **epithelial cells**) serve as important barriers to bacterial infection. As just noted for the eye, some epithelial cells secrete mucus, a needed lubricant. Without vitamin A, mucus-forming cells deteriorate and no longer synthesize mucus. Vitamin A deficiency also causes insufficient mucus production in the intestines and lung cells, and poor health of cells in general. Vitamin A deficiency also reduces the activity of certain immune system cells. Together, these effects leave the vitamin A–deficient person at great risk for infections. For many years, vitamin A has been dubbed the "anti-infection" vitamin.

Growth, Development, and Reproduction

Vitamin A participates in the processes of growth, development, and reproduction in several ways. This role has been best illustrated in children experiencing growth retardation as a result of deficiencies of this vitamin, and in whom supplementation with vitamin A has been shown to increase their growth. At the genetic level, vitamin A binds to receptors on DNA to increase synthesis of a variety of proteins. Some of these proteins are required for growth, such as bone growth. In laboratory animals, another consequence of vitamin A deficiency is an inability to reproduce.

Cardiovascular Disease Prevention

Carotenoids may play a role in preventing cardiovascular disease in persons at high risk, possibly linked to carotenoids' antioxidant capability. Until definitive studies are complete, many scientists recommend that we consume a total of at least 5 servings of a combination of fruits and vegetables per day as part of an overall effort to reduce the risk of cardiovascular disease.

Cancer Prevention

Most forms of cancer arise from cells that are influenced by vitamin A. Coupled with its ability to aid immune system activity, vitamin A may be a valuable tool in the fight against cancer. This is especially true for skin, lung, bladder, and breast cancers. Still, because of the potential for toxicity, unsupervised use of megadose vitamin A supplements to reduce cancer risk is not advised.

Carotenoids by themselves also may help prevent cancer, acting again as antioxidants. Population studies show that regular consumption of foods rich in carotenoids decreases the risk of lung and oral cancers. The carotenoid lycopene may decrease skin cancer risk. In contrast, recall from Chapter 1 that recent studies from the United States and Finland failed to show a reduction in lung cancer in male smokers and nonsmokers who were given supplements of the carotenoid beta-carotene for 5 or more years. In fact, beta-carotene use in male smokers increased the number of lung cancer cases compared with the control groups. No comparable studies have been done with women. Although further research continues, most researchers are now convinced that beta-carotene supplementation offers no protection against cancer. The overwhelming advice is to rely on food sources of this or any other carotenoids. Again, the best recommendation is to eat a combination of at least five fruits and vegetables a day (and not smoke).

Cancer of the **prostate gland** is one of the most common cancers among North American men. The dietary carotenoid lycopene (the red pigment found in tomatoes, watermelon, and several other fruits) seems to protect against this type of cancer. The proposed biological role of lycopene again may be that of an antioxidant. Some food companies (e.g., Campbell Soup Company), are even marketing their products as important sources of lycopene.

Vitamin A Analogs for Acne

The acne medication tretinoin (Retin-A) is made of one **analog** form of vitamin A. It is used as a topical treatment (applied to the skin) for acne. It appears to work by altering cell activity in the skin (gene expression role discussed earlier). Another derivative of vitamin A, 13-*cis* retinoic acid (Accutane), is an oral drug used to treat serious acne. Note that taking high doses of vitamin A itself would not be safe. Even Accutane, a less potentially toxic form, can induce toxic symptoms, as well as birth defects in the offspring of women using it during pregnancy. A pregnancy test is required before Accutane is prescribed to women.

■ Vitamin A Sources and Needs

Preformed vitamin A is found in liver, fish, fish oils, fortified milk and yogurt, and eggs. Margarine is also fortified with vitamin A. The provitamin A carotenoids mentioned before are mainly found in dark green and yellow-orange vegetables and some fruits. Carrots, spinach and other greens, winter squash, sweet potatoes, broccoli, mangoes, cantaloupe, peaches, and apricots are examples of such sources. About 65% of the vitamin A in the typical North American diet comes from preformed vitamin A sources, whereas provitamin A dominates in the diet among poor people in other parts of the world (Fig. 8-3).

Among common foods, those especially rich in vitamin A are carrots, spinach and other greens, sweet potatoes, winter squash, romaine lettuce, broccoli, apricots, and

The fundamental role of vitamin A (as retinoic acid) is to bind to DNA to direct protein synthesis (review Fig. 6-1 regarding the role of DNA in protein synthesis). In doing so, vitamin A is said to be affecting **gene expression.**

gene expression Use of DNA information on a gene to produce a protein. This is a major determinant of cell development.

prostate gland A solid, chestnut-shaped organ surrounding the first part of the urinary tract in the male. The prostate gland secretes substances into the semen.

analog A chemical compound that differs slightly from another, usually natural, compound. Analogs generally contain extra or altered chemical groups and may have similar or opposite metabolic effects compared with the native compound. Also spelled *analogue*.

Food Sources of Vitamin A

Food Item and Amount	Vitamin A (micrograms RAE*)
Fried beef liver, 1 ounce	3042
Sweet potato, ½ cup	958
Spinach, ⅔ cup	494
Mango, 1	402
Baby carrots, 5	375
Acorn squash, ⅔ cup	244
Cooked kale, ½ cup	206
Fat-free milk, 1 cup	150
Broccoli, 1 cup	138
Apricot, 3	137
Cheddar cheese, 1 ounce	78
Romaine lettuce, 1 cup	72
Margarine, 1 pat	50
Scallions, 1 tablespoon	32
Peach, 1	26

RDA for adult man, 900 micrograms RAE
RDA for adult woman, 700 micrograms RAE

*Retinol activity equivalents

Figure 8-3 Sources of Vitamin A from MyPyramid. The height of the background color (none, 1/3, 2/3 or completely covered) within each group in the pyramid indicates the average nutrient density for vitamin A in that group. Overall, the vegetables group, fruits group, and certain choices in the meat & beans group provide the richest sources. The grains group contains some foods that are nutrient-dense sources of vitamin A because they are fortified with the vitamin. With regard to physical activity, vitamin A plays no specific role per se in such endeavors.

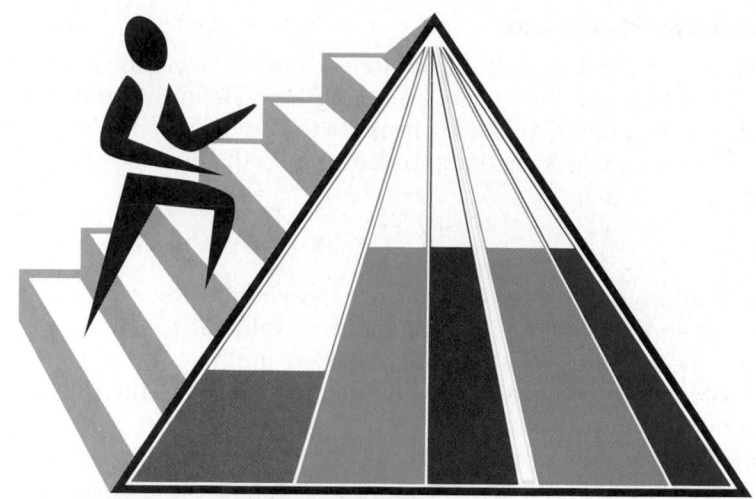

Grains	Vegetables	Fruits	Oils	Milk	Meat & Beans
• Fortified break-fast cereals • Fortified meal replacement bars	• Carrots • Broccoli • Spinach • Squash • Sweet potatoes	• Peaches • Apricots • Cantaloupes • Mangoes • Papayas	• Some forms of palm oil	• Fortified milk • Fortified yogurt • Cheese	• Liver • Eggs

fat-free and low-fat milk. Many of the vegetables listed in Fig. 8-3 are good sources of beta-carotene and the other two provitamin A carotenoids. Note also that marine oils are rich in vitamin A, and that consumption of large amounts of such oils can lead to symptoms of vitamin A toxicity.

Beta-carotene accounts for some of the orange color of carrots. In vegetables such as broccoli, this yellow-orange color is masked by dark-green chlorophyll pigments. Still, green vegetables contain provitamin A. Green, leafy vegetables, such as spinach and kale, have a high concentration of lutein and zeaxanthin. Tomato juice and other tomato products, such as pizza sauce, contain significant amounts of lycopene.

The RDA for vitamin A is 700 to 900 micrograms of retinol activity equivalents (RAEs). These RAE units take into account the activity of both preformed vitamin A and the three carotenoids that also are known to yield vitamin A in humans. The total RAE value for a food is calculated by adding the concentration of preformed vitamin A to the amount of provitamin A carotenoids in the food that will be converted to vitamin A. The Daily Value used on food and supplement labels is 1000 micrograms (5000 IU).

The retinol equivalent (RE) is an older unit for vitamin A. This RE is similar to the RAE but assumed that there was a greater contribution to vitamin A needs from carotenoids than we assume today. Food composition tables and nutrient databases still contain somes values based on this older RE standard, as is the case for Appendix J in this text. It will take some time to update these resources.

Another Bite

Most nutrient amounts in foods, including vitamin A, were formerly expressed in less precise **international units (IUs).** Some food and supplement labels still show the IU value for vitamin A. To compare the older IU standards to current RAE recommendations, assume that for any preformed vitamin A in a food or added to food, 3.3 IU = 1 RAE. The same is true for any beta-carotene added to foods.

There is no easy way to convert IU units to RAE units for foods that naturally contain provitamin A carotenoids, such as carrots, spinach, and apricots. A general rule of thumb is to divide the IU units for foods containing carotenoids by 2, and then divide the result by 3.3 as just discussed.

international unit (IU) A crude measure of vitamin activity, often based on the growth rate of animals in response to the vitamin. Today IUs have largely been replaced by more precise milligram or microgram measures.

Average intakes of vitamin A for North American adult men and women meet the RDA. Most adults in North America have liver reserves of vitamin A that are three to five times greater than needed to provide good health. Thus, the use of vitamin A supplements by most people is unnecessary. At present, there is no separate RDA for beta-carotene or any of the other provitamin A carotenoids.

Deficient vitamin A status in North America may be seen in preschool children who do not eat enough vegetables. The urban poor, older adults, and people with alcoholism or liver disease (which limits vitamin A storage) can also show diminished vitamin A status, especially with respect to stores. Finally, children and adults with severe fat-malabsorption may also experience vitamin A deficiency.

■ Upper Level for Vitamin A

The Upper Level for vitamin A intake is established at 3000 micrograms of preformed vitamin A (3000 RAE or 10,000 IU) per day for adult men and women. This is based on the increases in birth defects and liver toxicity that accompany intakes in excess of 3000 micrograms of vitamin A per day. Above the Upper Level, other possible side effects include an increased risk of hip fracture and poor pregnancy outcomes.

During the early months of pregnancy, a high intake of preformed vitamin A is especially dangerous because it may cause **fetal** malformations and spontaneous abortions. This is because vitamin A binds to DNA and so influences cell development. FDA recommends that women of childbearing age limit their overall intake of preformed vitamin A to a total of about 100% of the Daily Value (1000 micrograms REA or 5000 IU). In addition, it is also important to limit consumption of rich food sources, such as liver. These precautions also apply to women who may possibly become pregnant. Because vitamin A is stored in the body for long periods, women who take large amounts during the months before pregnancy place their fetuses at risk.

The ingestion of large amounts of vitamin A–yielding carotenoids does not cause toxic effects. A high carotenoid concentration in the blood can occur if someone consumes large amounts of carrots or takes pills containing beta-carotene (more than 30 milligrams daily), or if infants eat a great deal of squash. This can turn the skin yellow-orange. The palms of the hand and soles of the feet in particular become colored. This condition does not appear to cause harm and disappears when carotenoid intake decreases. Dietary carotenoids do not produce toxic effects because (1) their rate of conversion into vitamin A is relatively slow and regulated, and (2) the efficiency of carotenoid absorption from the small intestine decreases markedly as oral intake increases.

Vitamin D

Vitamin D is not just a vitamin. It is in fact primarily considered a hormone. Skin cells can convert a cholesterol-like substance to the prohormone vitamin D, using sunlight. Overall, sun exposure provides about 80% to 100% of our vitamin D needs. Liver and kidney cells then convert the prohormone to its active hormone form. The cells that participate in this hormone synthesis are different from those cells that respond mostly to vitamin D, namely bone cells and intestinal cells. This difference between the site of synthesis and action is characteristic of hormones.

The amount of sun exposure needed by individuals to produce vitamin D depends on their skin color, age, time of day, season, and location. Experts recommend that people should expose their hands, face, and arms at least two to three times a week for 25% of the time it takes to turn ones skin pink (e.g., 5 to 10 minutes) to make enough vitamin D. Persons with dark skin would need additional exposure, about 3 to 5 times the amount just recommended (or maybe even more). The large amount of melanin pigment in dark-skin people is a potent natural sunscreen.

Sun exposure is only effective for vitamin D synthesis if sunscreen over SPF 8 is not used during this time, and it is done between about 8:00 A.M. and 4:00 P.M. Still, this

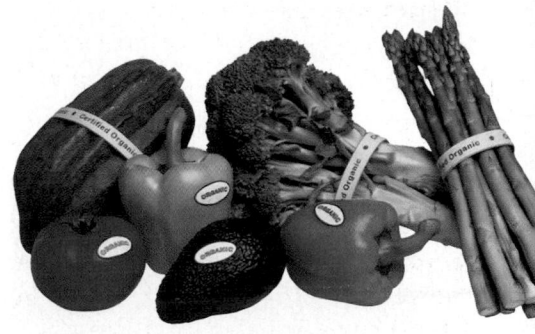

Provitamin A carotenoids are the safest way to meet vitamin A needs.

fetus The developing human life form from 8 weeks after conception until birth.

Vitamin D

↓ **Liver**

25-hydroxyvitamin D

↓ **Kidneys**

1,25-dihydroxyvitamin D (active hormone form)

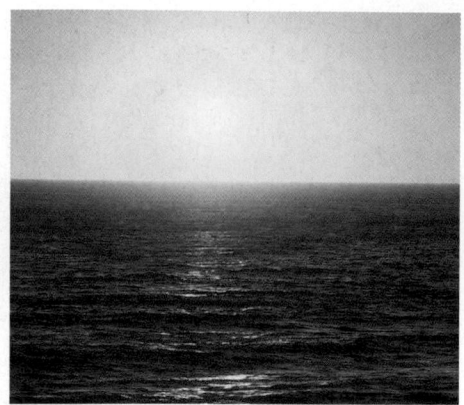

Solar radiation on the skin provides about 80% to 100% of the vitamin D humans use. This is also the most reliable way to maintain vitamin D status. Dietary vitamin D is also effective, but less so.

parathyroid hormone (PTH) A hormone made by the parathyroid glands that increases synthesis of the vitamin D hormone and aids calcium release from bone and calcium conservation by the kidneys, among other functions.

rickets A disease characterized by poor mineralization of newly synthesized bones because of low calcium content. This deficiency disease arises in infants and children from insufficient amounts of the vitamin D hormone in the body.

osteomalacia Adult form of rickets. The weakening of the bones that is seen in this disease is caused by low calcium content. A reduction in the amount of the vitamin D hormone in the body is one cause.

Be careful not to confuse osteomalacia with osteoporosis, another type of bone disorder discussed in Chapter 9.

practice is not effective at all in the winter in northern climates. Some people also may be able to use vitamin D stored from summer months in their adipose cells, but most people in northern climates should find alternate vitamin D sources in the winter months. Overall, anyone who does not receive enough sunshine to synthesize an adequate amount of vitamin D must have a dietary source of the vitamin, but some sun exposure is still important. About 80% of dietary vitamin D is absorbed.

■ Functions of Vitamin D

The main function of the vitamin D hormone (1,25-dihydroxyvitamin D) is to help regulate calcium and bone metabolism. In concert with other hormones, especially **parathyroid hormone (PTH)**, the vitamin D hormone closely regulates blood calcium to supply appropriate amounts of it to all cells. This task entails two main processes: the vitamin D hormone helps regulate absorption of calcium and phosphorus from the intestine and the deposition of calcium in the bones.

Even cells in the brain, pancreas, and pituitary gland appear to be influenced by the vitamin D hormone. More interestingly, the vitamin D hormone is also capable of influencing normal development of some cells, such as skin, colon, prostate, ovary, and breast cells, in turn reducing cancer risk in these sites. The vitamin D hormone also controls the growth of the parathyroid gland, aids in the function of the immune system, and contributes to skin cell development, as well as other functions.

The most obvious result of the vitamin D hormone action is increased calcium and phosphorus deposition in bones. Without adequate calcium and phosphorus deposition during bone synthesis, bones weaken and bow under pressure. A child with these symptoms has the disease **rickets.** Symptoms also include enlarged head, joints, and rib cage and a deformed pelvis (review Fig. 8-2).

Recent studies have shown rickets to be a problem in breastfed infants who receive little sun exposure. For the prevention of rickets, breastfed infants should be provided supplemental vitamin D (under a physician's guidance). Keep in mind, however, that supplements need to be used very carefully to avoid vitamin D toxicity in the infant. Rickets in children is also associated with fat malabsorption, such as that occuring in children with cystic fibrosis.

Osteomalacia, which means *soft bones,* is an adult disease comparable to rickets. It results from inefficient calcium absorption in the intestine or poor conservation of calcium by the kidneys. Both of these calcium-related problems can be caused by vitamin D deficiency. Bones then lose their minerals and become porous and weak and break easily. This leads to fractures in the hip and other bones. One study showed that treatment with 10 to 20 micrograms per day (400 to 800 IU per day) of vitamin D (in conjunction with adequate dietary calcium) greatly decreased fracture risk in older people in nursing homes. Follow-up studies support this role of vitamin D in reducing hip fracture risk. Note that aging decreases production of vitamin D in the skin by about 70% by the time one reaches the age of 70.

Osteomalacia in adults occurs most commonly in people with kidney, stomach, gallbladder, or intestinal disease (especially when most of the intestine has been removed) and in people with cirrhosis of the liver. These diseases affect both vitamin D activation and calcium absorption. Adults with limited sun exposure may also develop the disease as may many African-Americna individuals. Combinations of sun exposure, vitamin D intake, or both can prevent this problem. Older people are advised to get sun exposure during early morning and late afternoon to receive the benefit of vitamin D synthesis without also increasing skin cancer risk.

■ Vitamin D Sources and Needs

Few foods contain appreciable amounts of vitamin D. Rich sources are fatty fish (e.g., sardines and salmon), fortified milk and yogurt, and some ready-to-eat breakfast cereals. In the United States and Canada, milk usually is fortified with 10 micrograms

(400 IU) per quart. Although eggs, butter, liver, and a few brands of margarine contain some vitamin D, large servings must be eaten to obtain an appreciable amount of the vitamin; thus these foods are not considered significant sources.

The Adequate Intake set for vitamin D is 5 micrograms per day (200 IU per day) for people under age 51 and increases two to three times for older adults. (A more accurate RDA could not be set because the amount produced by sunlight exposure is too variable between individuals.) The Daily Value used on food and supplement labels is 10 micrograms (400 IU). As mentioned, young, light-skinned people can synthesize all the vitamin D needed from casual sun exposure. A number of experts suggest older adults, especially those age 70 and over who have limited sun exposure or dark skin, receive about 25 micrograms (1000 IU) from a combination of vitamin D-fortified foods and a multivitamin and mineral supplement, with an individual supplement of vitamin D added if needed.

■ Upper Level for Vitamin D

The Upper Level for vitamin D is 50 micrograms per day (2000 IU per day). Too much vitamin D taken regularly can create problems, especially in some infants and young children. For adults, intakes somewhat above the Upper Level appear to be safe. The Upper Level is based on the risk of overabsorption of calcium and eventual calcium deposits in the kidneys and other organs. The person also suffers the typical symptoms of high blood calcium: weakness, loss of appetite, diarrhea, vomiting, mental confusion, and increased urine output. Calcium deposits in organs cause metabolic disturbances and cell death. However, vitamin D toxicity does not result from tanning in the sun too long because the body regulates the amount made in the skin.

Concept Check

Vitamin A is found in foods as preformed vitamin A and as provitamin A carotenoids. The most fully understood function of vitamin A is its importance in vision. Blindness caused by vitamin A deficiency is a major problem in many parts of the world. Vitamin A is also needed to maintain the health of many types of cells, support the immune system, and promote proper growth and development. Vitamin A and some carotenoids may be important in preventing cancer. However, because taking supplements of preformed vitamin A can be toxic, especially in pregnancy, the best recommendation is to focus primarily on eating plenty of provitamin A–rich foods, such as fruits and vegetables.

Vitamin D is a true vitamin only for people who fail to produce enough from sunlight, such as some older people and those with dark skin. Humans synthesize vitamin D from a cholesterol-like substance by the action of sunlight on their skin. The vitamin D is later acted on by the liver and kidneys to form the hormone 1,25-dihydroxyvitamin D. This hormone increases calcium absorption in the intestine and works with another hormone (PTH) to maintain calcium in bones. Rich food sources of vitamin D are fish oils and fortified milk. Megadose vitamin D intake can be toxic, especially in infancy and early childhood

Vitamin E

North Americans are spending more than $1 billion on vitamin E supplements each year. The following section attempts to sort out fact from fiction in the debate over this high-profile vitamin.

Food Sources of Vitamin D		
Food Item and Amount	Vitamin D (micrograms)	Vitamin D (IU)
Baked herring, 3 ounces	44.4	1775
Smoked eel, 1 ounce	25.5	1020
Baked salmon, 3 ounces	6.0	238
Sardines, 1 ounce	3.4	136
Canned tuna, 3 ounces	3.4	136
1% milk, 1 cup	2.5	99
Fat-free milk, 1 cup	2.5	98
Soft margarine, 1 teaspoon	1.5	60
Italian pork sausage, 3 ounces	1.1	44
Soy milk, 1 cup	1.0	40
Raisin Bran cereal, ¾ cup	1.0	38
Baked bluefish, 3 ounces	0.9	34
Special K cereal, ¾ cup	0.8	30
Cooked egg yolk, 1	0.6	25

Adequate Intake for young adults, 5 micrograms (200 IU)

Figure 8-4 Fat-soluble vitamin E can insert itself into cell membranes, where it helps stop free-radical chain reactions. If not interrupted, these reactions cause extensive oxidative damage to cells and ultimately cell death.

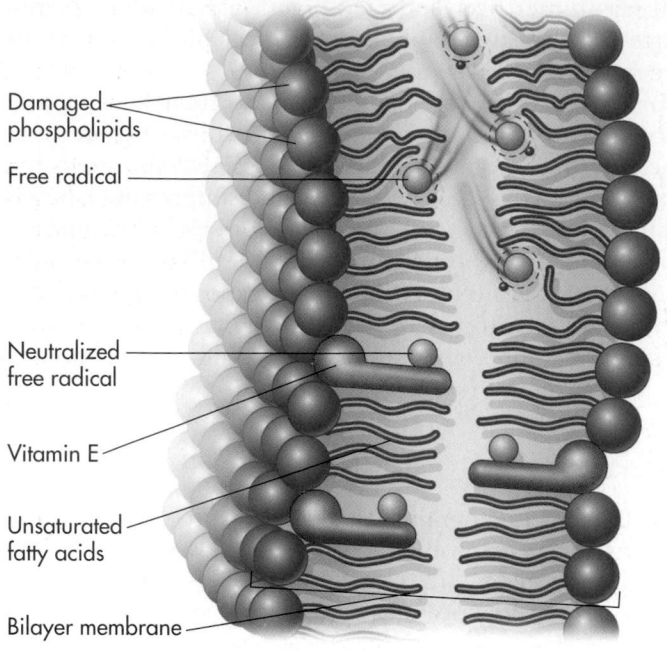

Damaged phospholipids

Free radical

Neutralized free radical

Vitamin E

Unsaturated fatty acids

Bilayer membrane

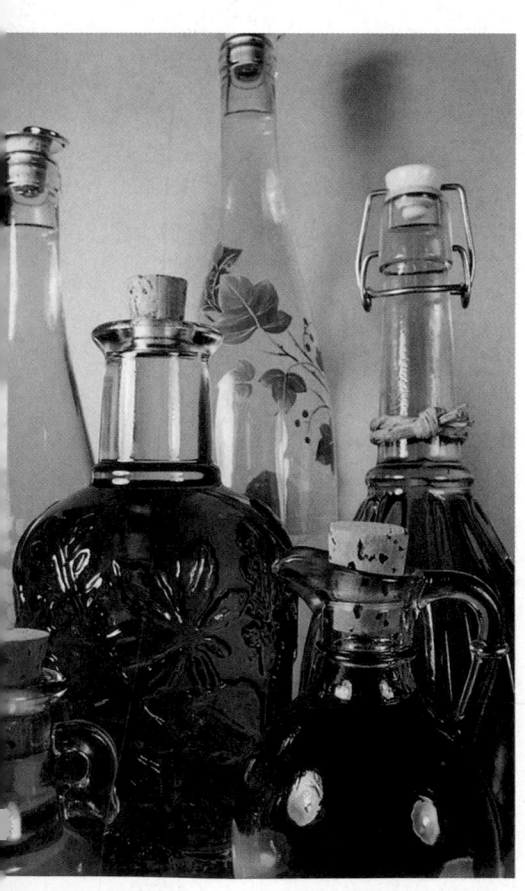

Plant oils are good sources of vitamin E.

■ Functions of Vitamin E

Acting as a fat-soluble antioxidant, vitamin E resides mostly in cell membranes. As discussed in Chapter 5, an antioxidant can form a barrier between a target molecule—an unsaturated fatty acid in a cell membrane, for example—and a compound seeking its electrons (Fig. 8-4). The antioxidant donates electrons or hydrogens to the electron-seeking compound. This protects other molecules or parts of a cell from having electrons stolen.

If vitamin E is not available to do its job, electron-seeking compound(s), known as a free radical(s), can pull electrons from cell membranes, DNA, and other electron-dense cell components. This either alters the cell's DNA, which may increase the risk for cancer, or injures cell membranes, possibly causing the cell to die. Recall from Chapter 7 that free radicals are highly reactive compounds containing an unpaired electron. This free-radical production is a normal result of cell metabolism and immune system function. For example, white blood cells generate free radicals as part of their action to stop infection. Some exposure to free radicals, then, is an important part of life. Overall, however, the body needs antioxidants like vitamin E to carefully regulate this exposure to avoid related undesirable effects.

Cells also do not rely exclusively on vitamin E for protection from free radicals. Many other antioxidant systems exist in cells as well, some of which utilize minerals, such as copper, selenium, and manganese (see Chapter 9 for details). As discussed earlier in this chapter, carotenoids in fruits and vegetables also act as antioxidants. In addition, cells have mechanisms other than antioxidants to repair molecules (such as DNA) that have been damaged by free radicals.

This discussion raises the question of the relative role of vitamin E in oxidant protection in the body. Experts do not know whether megadose vitamin E supplements taken by otherwise healthy people confer any additional protection against cardiovascular disease and cancer than that achieved by improving diet (especially fruit, vegetable, and whole-grain bread and cereal intake), performing regular physical activity, not smoking, and maintaining a healthy body weight. Furthermore, the proven benefits of these lifestyle changes are far greater than the postulated benefits of supplemental antioxidants, including vitamin E, and have the widest scientific support in the battle against these diseases. Thus, as reviewed in Chapter 5, even if antioxidant supplements eventually are clearly determined to be effective in preventing cardio-vascular disease or cancer, they should be used only as an adjunct—not as an alternative—to a healthful lifestyle. In fact, the American Heart Association and a group of leading cardiologists recently stated that it is premature to recommend vitamin E supplements to the general population, based on current knowledge and the failure of major clinical trials to show any benefit (review Chapter 5). This conclusion is in agreement with the latest report on vitamin E by the Food and Nutrition Board of the National Academy of Sciences. In addition, FDA has denied the request of the supplement industry to make a health claim that vitamin E supplements reduce the risk of cardiovascular disease and cancer. Still, some experts recommend vitamin E supplements (100 IU to 400 IU per day), while at the same time noting that evidence supporting this recommendation is sketchy.

Finally, vitamin E can help improve vitamin A absorption if the dietary intake of vitamin A is low. In addition, vitamin E is used to metabolize iron in the cell and help maintain nervous tissue and immune function.

A deficiency of vitamin E causes cell membranes to break down. Unsaturated fatty acids in cell membranes are very sensitive to attack by oxidizing compounds. Because vitamin E neutralizes these agents, it protects cell membranes from damage. When oxidative damage causes the cell membranes of red blood cells to break, it is called **hemolysis.**

■ Vitamin E Sources and Needs

Vitamin E is actually a family of four **tocopherols,** called alpha, beta, gamma, and delta. Alpha-tocopherol is the main form in the human body, whereas gamma-tocopherol is the main form in foods. Major sources of vitamin E include plant oils (e.g., salad dressings and mayonnaise), ready-to-eat breakfast cereals, some fruits and vegetables (e.g., asparagus, tomatoes, and green leafy vegetables), eggs, and margarine. Also, whole grains, nuts (e.g., almonds), and seeds (e.g., sunflower seeds) are good sources of vitamin E. Plant oils are made up of mainly unsaturated fatty acids, and the vitamin E in plant oils protects these unsaturated fats from oxidation. Animal fats and fish oils, on the other hand, have practically no vitamin E (Fig. 8 5). Because vitamin E is very susceptible to destruction by oxygen, metals, light, and especially repeated use in deep-fat frying, the actual vitamin E content of a food depends on how it was harvested, processed, stored, and cooked.

The RDA of vitamin E for adults is 15 milligrams per day of alpha-tocopherol, the most active form of vitamin E. The 15 milligram allotment is equivalent to 22 IU of a natural source and 33 IU of a synthetic source. Typically, North American adults consume about two-thirds of the RDA for vitamin E from food sources. Daily intake of nuts and seeds, ready-to-eat breakfast cereals containing vitamin E, or use of a multivitamin and mineral supplement would close this gap between needs and actual intakes. The Daily Value used on food and supplement labels is 30 IU.

Within the older IU system, 1 IU equals about 0.45 milligrams, based on the synthetic (so called dl **isomer**) form of vitamin E found in most supplements. If vitamin E is from a natural source (so called d isomer), 1 IU equals 0.67 milligrams, because the natural form of vitamin E is more potent than the synthetic form.

The maximum daily dose the body can retain is thought to be 200 milligrams. This would represent 300 IU of the d isomer (200/0.67 = 300) to 450 IU of the dl isomer (200/0.45 = 450).

Cell damage by free radicals occurs over an extended period of time. Therefore, the beneficial effects of vitamin E and other antioxidants in counteracting this damage is most apparent when viewed over the long term. Accordingly, current research cannot rule out a possible benefit of intakes of vitamin E in excess of the RDA for healthy adults. Studies in otherwise healthy men are underway using megadoses of about 600 IU every other day. Results are due by 2007. Recall from Chapter 6 that the resuls from a similar trial in healthy women were generally disappointing.

hemolysis Destruction of red blood cells. The red blood cell membrane breaks down, allowing cell contents to leak into the fluid portion of the blood.

tocopherols The chemical name for some forms of vitamin E. The alpha form is the most potent.

isomers Different chemical structures for compounds that share the same chemical formula.

Food Sources of Vitamin E		
Food Item and Amount	Vitamin E (milligrams)	Vitamin E (IU)
Total Raisin Bran cereal, ¾ cup	22.5	33.5
Sunflower oil, 2 tablespoons	16.3	24.3
Dry-roasted sunflower seeds, 1 ounce	14.3	21.2
Dry-roasted almonds, 1 ounce	7.5	11.1
Safflower oil, 1 tablespoon	5.9	8.7
Canola oil, 2 tablespoons	5.7	8.5
Wheat germ, ¼ cup	5.2	7.7
Almonds, 1 ounce	4.5	6.8
Oil-roasted sunflower seeds, 1 tablespoon	3.4	5.0
Italian dressing, 2 tablespoons	3.1	4.5
Mayonnaise, 1 tablespoon	3.0	4.5
Avocado, 1	2.7	4.0
Chunky peanut butter, 2 tablespoons	2.4	3.6
Mango, 1	2.3	3.5
Peanuts, 1 ounce	2.1	3.1
RDA for adults, 15 milligrams (22 to 33 IU)		

Figure 8-5 Sources of Vitamin E from MyPyramid. The height of the background color (none, 1/3, 2/3 or completely covered) within each group in the pyramid indicates the average nutrient density for vitamin E in that group. Overall, plants oils are the richest source, followed by nuts and seeds in the meat & beans group. With regard to physical activity, vitamin E has no primary role in the related energy metabolism per se, but likely limits some oxidant damage during such endeavors.

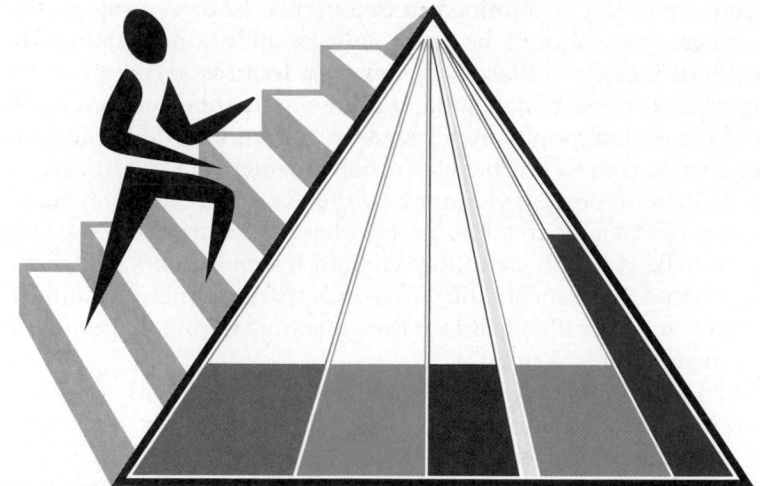

Grains	Vegetables	Fruits	Oils	Milk	Meat & Beans
• Wheat germ (whole grains) • Some fortified breakfast cereals	• Cabbage • Asparagus • Sweet potatoes • Tomatoes	• Apples • Avocados • Mango	• Plant oils • Margarines • Salad dressings	• None	• Nuts • Seeds • Shrimp • Peanut butter

Several populations are especially susceptible to developing marginal vitamin E status. Preterm infants tend to have low vitamin E stores, since this vitamin is transferred from mother to baby during late stages of pregnancy. Hemolysis (described on page 251) is of particular concern for preterm infants, due to red blood cell damage that occurs in the absence of adequate vitamin E. The rapid growth of preterm infants, coupled with the high oxygen needs of their immature lungs, greatly increases the stress on red blood cells. Special formulas and supplements designed for preterm infants can help compensate for lack of vitamin E. Smokers are another group at high risk for vitamin E deficiency, as smoking readily destroys vitamin E in the lungs. Still, one study showed that even using megadoses of vitamin E was ineffective in preventing this damage in smokers. Others at considerable risk of vitamin E deficiency include adults on very low-fat diets or those with fat malabsorption.

◼ Upper Level for Vitamin E

hemorrhage An escape of blood from blood vessels.

The Upper Level for vitamin E is 1000 milligrams per day of supplemental alpha-tocopherol. Excessive amounts of vitamin E can interfere with vitamin K's role in the clotting mechanism, leading to **hemorrhage.** The risk of insufficient blood clotting is especially high if vitamin E is taken in conjunction with anticoagulant medications (e.g., Coumadin or heavy aspirin use). In international units, the Upper Level is 1500 IU for vitamin E isolated from natural sources (so called d isomer; 1000/0.67 = 1500) and 1100 IU for synthetic vitamin E (so called dl isomer; 1000/0.45/2 = 1100). The lower IU value for the synthetic form reflects the greater number of forms present in the synthetic product, only half or less of which contribute to vitamin E activity in cells, but are still absorbed. This Upper Level is set for a healthy population. Again, individuals who are vitamin K deficient or who are taking anticoagulants or heavy doses of aspirin are especially at risk for hemorrhage from megadose vitamin E use.

There is additional concern that taking large amounts of alpha-tocopherol might decrease gamma-tocopherol activity in the body. Gamma-tocopherol is a potentially beneficial form of vitamin E. To compensate, some experts recommend that any vitamin E supplement should contain a mixture of natural tocopherols (i.e., mixed tocopherols). This form is more expensive, however, than natural or synthetic alpha-tocopherol alone.

Vitamin K

A family of compounds known collectively as vitamin K is found in plants, plant oils, fish oils, and meats. One form is also synthesized by bacteria in the human intestine and supplies us with about 10% of the vitamin K we need. The rest comes from diet.

Functions of Vitamin K

Vitamin K is vital for blood clotting, working along with various proteins and calcium. The *K* stands for *koagulation,* as **coagulation** is spelled in Denmark. This spelling is used because a Danish researcher first noted the relationship between vitamin K and blood clotting. Vitamin K contributes to the activation of several blood-clotting factors. Vitamin K also activates proteins present in bone, muscle, and kidneys, thereby imparting calcium-binding potential to these organs. A poor vitamin K intake has been linked to an increase in hip fractures in women because of its effect on various proteins in bone.

At birth a newborn's intestinal tract lacks a sufficient amount of bacteria to produce enough vitamin K to allow for effective blood clotting if the infant is injured or needs surgery. Therefore, vitamin K also is routinely given by injection shortly after birth. In adults, deficiencies of vitamin K have occurred when a person takes antibiotics for a long period (destroying many of the intestinal bacteria that normally produce some of the vitamin K absorbed), and in the presence of severe long-standing fat malabsorption.

Vitamin K Sources and Needs

Major food sources of vitamin K are liver, green leafy vegetables (e.g., kale, turnip greens, dark green lettuce, and spinach), broccoli, peas, and green beans. Other sources are soybean and canola oils, and certain fortified chocolate confections (these also contain extra calcium). Thus, another reason to consume a diet rich in green vegetables is to obtain sufficient vitamin K. Most vitamin K consumed in a day disappears from the body by the next day. Nevertheless, vitamin K is abundant in a balanced diet, and a deficiency is uncommon. Vitamin K is quite resistant to cooking losses.

The Adequate Intake for vitamin K is 90 to 120 micrograms per day for adults. Most North Americans consume at least this much. The Daily Value used on food and supplement labels is 80 micrograms. Older adults may be at risk of a deficiency because of low consumption of green vegetables.

Oral vitamin K generally poses no risk of toxicity, so no Upper Level has been set. The main problem with megadose use is reduced effectiveness of oral medications used to reduce blood clotting (e.g., Coumadin). These medications are used by people with blood-clotting disorders or those who have undergone recent cardiovascular surgery.

Table 8-2 reviews what we have covered so far regarding the fat-soluble vitamins.

Inactive blood-clotting factors

↓ **Action of vitamin K**

Active blood-clotting factors

coagulation Blood clotting; essentially a transition of blood from a liquid cell suspension into a solid, gel-like form.

Food Sources of Vitamin K

Food Item and Amount	Vitamin K (micrograms)
Brussels sprouts, ½ cup	483
Kale, ½ cup	274
Cooked broccoli, ½ cup	211
Turnip greens, 1 cup	138
Spinach, 1 cup	120
Cauliflower, 3 florets	120
Dark green lettuce, 1 cup	118
Raw cabbage, 1 cup	101
Cooked green beans, ½ cup	49
Asparagus spears, 5	38
Boiled egg, 1	31
Sauerkraut, ½ cup	30
Green peas, ½ cup	26
Soybean oil, 1 tablespoon	25
Canola oil, 1 tablespoon	17
Adequate Intake for adults, 90 to 120 micrograms	

Table 8-2 Summary of the Fat-Soluble Vitamins

Vitamin	Major Functions	RDA or Adequate Intake	Dietary Sources	Deficiency Symptoms	Toxicity Symptoms
Vitamin A (preformed vitamin A and provitamin A)	• Promote vision: night and color • Promote growth • Prevent drying of skin and eyes • Promote resistance to bacterial infection and overall immune system function	Females: 700 micrograms RAE Males: 900 micrograms RAE (2300–3000 IU if as preformed vitamin A)	Preformed vitamin A: • Liver • Fortified milk • Fortified breakfast cereals Provitamin A: • Sweet potatoes • Spinach • Greens • Carrots • Cantaloupe • Apricots • Broccoli	• Night blindness • Xerophthalmia • Poor growth • Dry skin	• Fetal malformations • Hair loss • Skin changes • Bone pain • Fractures Upper Level is 3000 micrograms of preformed vitamin A (10,000 IU) based on the risk of birth defects and liver toxicity
Vitamin D	• Increase absorption of calcium and phosphorus • Maintain optimal blood calcium and calcification of bone	5–15 micrograms (200–600 IU)	• Vitamin D fortified milk • Fortified breakfast cereals • Fish oils • Sardines • Salmon	• Rickets in children • Osteomalacia in adults	• Growth retardation • Kidney damage • Calcium deposits in soft tissue Upper Level is 50 micrograms (2000 IU) based on the risk of elevated blood calcium
Vitamin E	• Antioxidant: prevents breakdown of vitamin A and unsaturated fatty acids	15 milligrams alpha-tocopherol (22 IU natural form, 33 IU synthetic form)	• Plant oils • Products made from plant oils • Some greens • Some fruits • Nuts and seeds • Fortified breakfast cereals	• Hemolysis of red blood cells • Nerve degeneration	• Muscle weakness • Headaches • Nausea • Inhibition of vitamin K metabolism Upper Level is 1000 milligrams (1100 IU synthetic form, 1500 IU natural form) based on the risk of hemorrhage
Vitamin K	• Activation of blood-clotting factors • Activation of proteins involved in bone metabolism	90–120 micrograms	• Green vegetables • Liver • Some plant oils • Some calcium supplements	• Hemorrhage • Fractures	No Upper Level has been set

Abbreviations: RAE = retinol activity equivalents; IU = international units

Concept Check

Vitamin E functions primarily as an antioxidant. It can donate electrons to electron-seeking free radical (oxidizing) compounds. By neutralizing these compounds, vitamin E helps prevent cell destruction, especially the destruction of red blood cell membranes. Vitamin E occurs in a wide variety of foods, but its richest sources are plant oils, foods rich in these oils, and nuts. Studies using megadoses of vitamin E are underway. At present, it is not clear if such use provides health benefits.

Vitamin K plays a key role in efficient blood clotting; it contributes to the activation of certain blood-clotting proteins. In addition, vitamin K contributes to the synthesis of the calcium-binding proteins in some organs, such as bones. About 10% of the vitamin K we absorb every day is synthesized by our intestinal bacteria; the rest comes from our diets. The amount in the diet alone generally meets our daily needs. Thus, except for newborns and possibly older adults, a deficiency of vitamin K is unlikely. Green vegetables and certain plant oils are good sources of vitamin K.

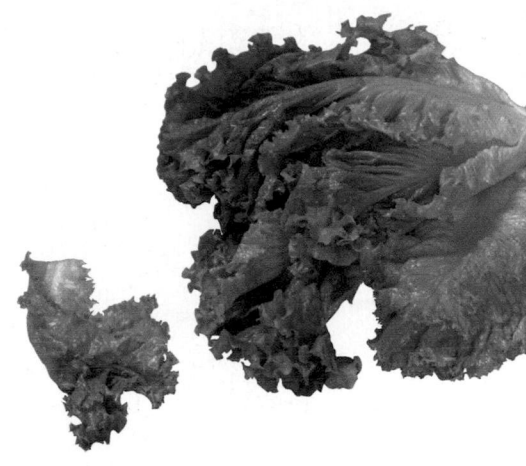

A salad containing dark greens (or other green vegetables) each day provides abundant vitamin K for a diet.

The Water-Soluble Vitamins and Choline

Most water-soluble vitamins are more readily excreted from the body than are fat-soluble vitamins. Since any excess generally ends up in the urine or stool and very little is stored, consuming good sources of the water-soluble vitamins regularly is important. Because they dissolve in water, large amounts of these vitamins can be lost during food processing and preparation. Light cooking methods, such as stir-frying, steaming, and microwaving, best preserve vitamin content (review Table 8-1).

The B vitamins are thiamin, riboflavin, niacin, pantothenic acid, biotin, vitamin B-6, folate, and vitamin B-12. Choline is a related nutrient, but currently is not classified as a vitamin. Vitamin C is also a water-soluble vitamin.

Because the B vitamins often occur in the same foods, a lack of one B vitamin may mean other B vitamins are also low in a diet. The B vitamins function as coenzymes, small molecules that interact with enzymes to enable enzymes to function. In essence, the coenzymes contribute to enzyme activity (review Fig. 8-1).

As coenzymes, the B vitamins play many key roles in metabolism. The metabolic pathways used by carbohydrates, fats, and amino acids all require input from B vitamins. Many B vitamins are interdependent because they participate in the same processes (Fig. 8-6). B vitamin deficiency symptoms typically occur in the brain and nervous system, skin, and GI tract. Cells in these tissues are very metabolically active, and those in the skin and GI tract are also constantly being replaced.

After being ingested, the B vitamins are first broken down from their coenzyme forms into free vitamins in the stomach and small intestine. The vitamins are then absorbed, primarily in the small intestine. Typically, about 50% to 90% of the B vitamins in the diet are absorbed, demonstrating their relatively high **bioavailability**. Once inside cells, the coenzyme forms are resynthesized. Although some vitamins are sold in their coenzyme forms in health-food stores, there is no need to consume the coenzyme forms themselves. These are broken down during digestion and we make them when needed.

Because of their role in energy metabolism, needs for many B vitamins increase somewhat as energy expenditure increases. Still, this is not a major concern since this increase in energy expenditure usually results in a corresponding increase in food intake, which contributes more B vitamins to a diet.

bioavailability The degree to which an ingested nutrient is absorbed and thus is available to the body.

■ B Vitamin Intakes of North Americans

The nutritional health of most North Americans with regard to the B vitamins is generally good. Typical diets contain plentiful and varied natural sources of these vitamins. In addition, many common foods, such as ready-to-eat breakfast cereals, are fortified with one or more of the water-soluble vitamins. In some developing countries, however, deficiencies of the water-soluble vitamins are more common, and the resulting deficiency diseases pose significant public health problems. (A detailed discussion of nutritional deficiencies worldwide is presented in Chapter 17.)

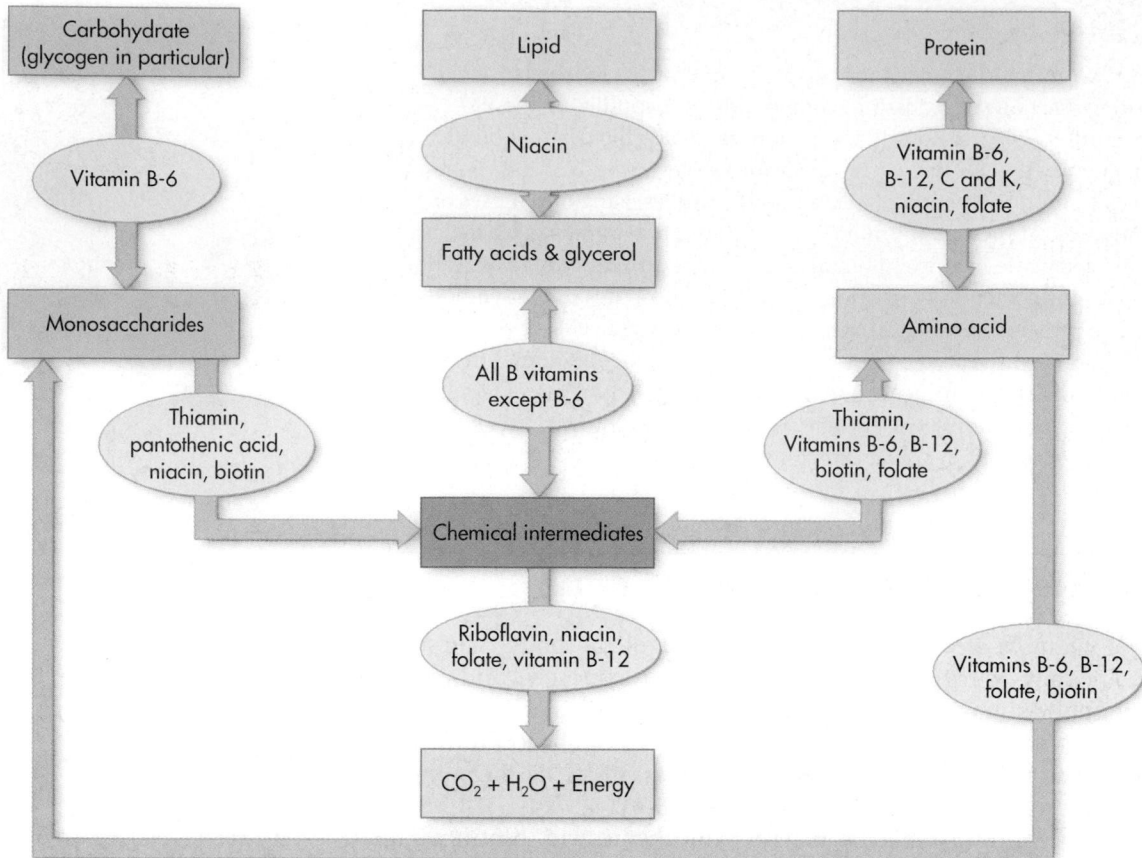

Figure 8-6 Examples of metabolic pathways for which vitamins are essential. The metabolism of energy-yielding nutrients requires vitamin input.

Despite the generally good B vitamin status of North Americans, marginal deficiencies of the water-soluble vitamins may occur in some cases, especially in older people who eat little food, and in people who follow poor dietary patterns. The long-term effects of such marginal deficiencies are as yet unknown, but increased risk of cardiovascular disease, cancer, and cataracts of the eye is suspected. However, in the short run, such a marginal deficiency in most people likely leads only to fatigue or other bothersome and unspecific physical effects. With rare exceptions, healthy adults do not develop the more serious B vitamin deficiency diseases from dietary inadequacies alone. The main exceptions are people with alcoholism. The combination of extremely unbalanced diets and alcohol-induced alterations of vitamin absorption and metabolism creates significant risks for serious nutrient deficiencies among people with alcoholism (review Chapter 7).

The milling of grains leads to losses of vitamins and minerals. In the milling process, seeds are crushed and the germ, bran, and husk layers are discarded, leaving just the starch-containing endosperm in the refined grains. The starch is used to make flour, bread, and cereal products. Unfortunately, many nutrients are lost along with the discarded germ, bran, and husk materials. To counteract these losses, in the United States, bread and cereal products made from milled grains are enriched with four B vitamins (thiamin, riboflavin, niacin, and folic acid) and with the mineral iron. This addition helps protect us from the common deficiency diseases associated with a dietary lack of these nutrients. Unfortunately, these products remain lower in vitamin E, vitamin B-6, potassium, magnesium, fiber, and other nutrients than the whole grains. This is one reason why nutrient experts advocate regular consumption of whole-grain products, such as whole-wheat bread and brown rice, rather than refined grain products.

The Whole-Grain Advantage (whole vs. refined)

Bread:

vitamin E	↑	17%
vitamin B-6	↑	60%
potassium	↑	92%
magnesium	↑	70%
fiber	↑	66%

Rice:

vitamin E	↑	800%
vitamin B-6	↑	93%
potassium	↑	280%
magnesium	↑	450%
fiber	↑	550%

Thiamin

Thiamin (formerly called *vitamin B-1*) is used, among other purposes, to help release energy from carbohydrate. Its coenzyme form participates in reactions in which a carbon dioxide (CO_2) is lost from a larger molecule. This reaction is particularly important in the breakdown of carbohydrates and certain amino acids for energy needs (review Fig. 8-6).

The thiamin deficiency disease is called **beriberi,** a word that means "I can't, I can't" in the Sri Lanka language of Sinhalese. The symptoms include weakness, loss of appetite, irritability, nervous tingling throughout the body, poor arm and leg coordination, and deep muscle pain in the calves. A person with beriberi often develops an enlarged heart and sometimes severe edema.

Beriberi is seen in areas where rice is a staple and polished (white) rice is consumed rather than brown (whole-grain) rice. In most parts of the world, brown rice has had its bran and germ layer removed to make white rice, a poor source of thiamin, unless it is enriched.

Beriberi results when glucose, the primary fuel for brain and nerve cells, cannot be metabolized to release energy. Because the thiamin coenzyme participates in glucose metabolism, problems with body functions associated with brain and nerve action are the first signs of a thiamin deficiency, some after only 10 days on a thiamin-free diet.

▌ Thiamin Sources and Needs

Major sources of thiamin include pork products, whole grains (wheat germ), ready-to-eat breakfast cereals, enriched grains, green beans, milk, orange juice, organ meats, peanuts, dried beans, and seeds (Fig. 8-7).

The adult RDA for thiamin is 1.1 to 1.2 milligrams per day. The Daily Value used on food and supplement labels is 1.5 milligrams. Average daily intakes for men exceed this by 50% or more, and women generally meet the RDA. Some groups, such as low-income

beriberi The thiamin deficiency disorder characterized by muscle weakness, loss of appetite, nerve degeneration, and sometimes edema.

Food Sources of Thiamin

Food Item and Amount	Thiamin (milligrams)
Canned lean ham, 3 ounces	0.9
Pork chops, 4 ounces	0.6
Wheat germ, ¼ cup	0.5
Canadian bacon, 2 ounces	0.5
Acorn squash, 1 cup	0.4
Soy milk, 1 cup	0.4
Flour tortilla, 1	0.4
Ham lunch meat, 2 pieces	0.3
Watermelon, 1 slice	0.2
Fresh orange juice, 1 cup	0.2
Cooked green peas, ½ cup	0.2
Baked beans, ½ cup	0.2
Navy beans, ½ cup	0.2
Corn, ½ cup	0.2

RDA for adults, 1.1 to 1.2 milligrams

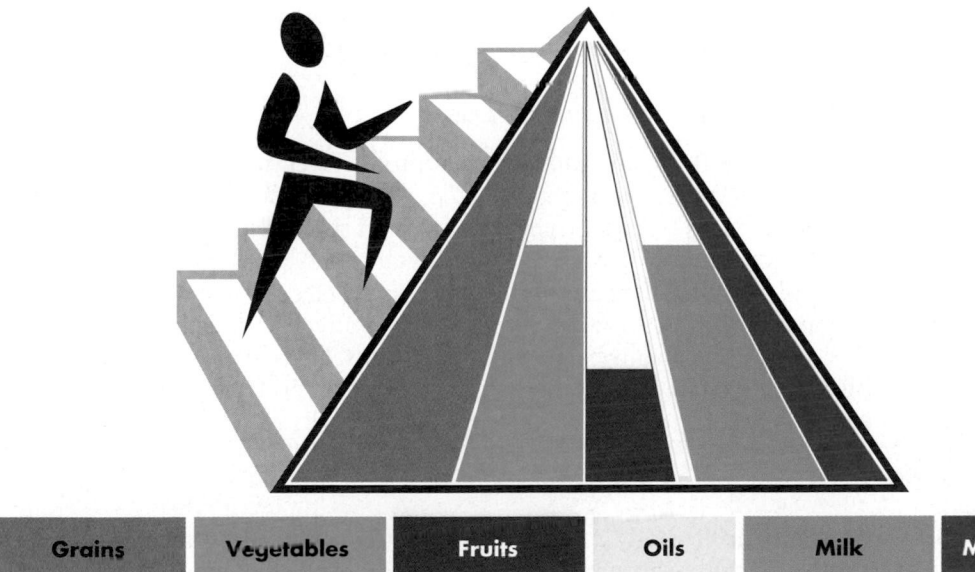

Grains   Vegetables   Fruits   Oils   Milk   Meat & Beans

Figure 8-7 Sources of Thiamin, Riboflaven, and Niacin from MyPyramid. The height of the background color (none, 1/3, 2/3 or completely covered) within each group in the pyramid indicates the average nutrient density for these vitamins in that group. Overall, the meat & beans group and the grains group contain many foods that are nutrient-dense sources of thiamin, riboflavin, and niacin. As well, foods from the milk group are especially rich sources of riboflavin. With regard to physical activity, these vitamins play key roles in the increased energy metabolism that takes place during such endeavors.

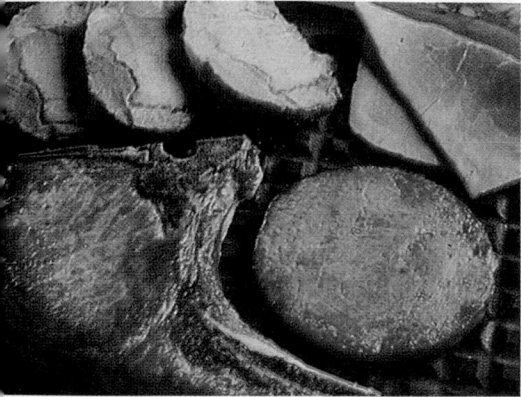

Pork is a good source of thiamin.

Food Sources of Riboflavin	
Food Item and Amount	**Riboflavin (milligrams)**
Multigrain Cheerios, ¾ cup	1.3
Fried beef liver, 1 ounce	1.2
Steamed oysters, 10	1.1
Plain yogurt, 1 cup	0.5
Raw mushrooms, 5	0.5
Braunschweiger sausage, 1	0.4
Cooked spinach, 1 cup	0.4
1% milk, 1 cup	0.4
Buttermilk, 1 cup	0.4
Boiled egg, 1	0.3
Sirloin steak, 3 ounces	0.3
Feta cheese, 1 ounce	0.2
Tortilla, 1	0.2
Lean ham, 3 ounces	0.2
RDA for adults, 1.1 to 1.3 milligrams	

and older people, may barely meet their needs for thiamin. A diet dominated by highly processed and unenriched foods, sugar, fat, and alcohol also creates a potential for thiamin deficiency. Oral thiamin supplements are typically nontoxic since excess thiamin is rapidly lost in the urine. Thus, no Upper Level has been set for thiamin.

Another Bite

People with alcoholism are at the greatest risk for thiamin deficiency because absorption and use of thiamin are profoundly diminished and excretion is increased by consumption of alcohol. Furthermore, the low-quality diet that often accompanies severe alcoholism makes matters worse. Since there is limited thiamin storage in the body, an alcoholic binge lasting 1 to 2 weeks may quickly deplete already diminished amounts of the vitamin and result in deficiency symptoms.

Riboflavin

The name *riboflavin* comes from its yellow color (*flavus* means yellow in Latin). Riboflavin was formerly referred to as *vitamin B-2*.

The coenzyme forms of riboflavin participate in many energy-yielding metabolic pathways. When cells form cellular energy using oxygen-requiring pathways, such as when fatty acids are broken down and burned for energy, the coenzymes of riboflavin are used (review Fig. 8-6). Some vitamin and mineral metabolism also requires riboflavin. In addition, because of its link to the activity of certain enzymes, riboflavin has an antioxidant role in the body, and as well participates in homocysteine metabolism.

The symptoms associated with riboflavin deficiency include inflammation of the mouth and tongue, dermatitis, cracking of tissue around the corners of the mouth (called *cheilosis*), various eye disorders, sensitivity to the sun, and confusion (review Fig. 8-2). Such symptoms develop after approximately 2 months on a riboflavin-poor diet. In addition, riboflavin deficiencies probably do not exist by themselves. Instead, a riboflavin deficiency would occur with deficiencies of niacin, thiamin, and vitamin B-6 because these nutrients often occur in the same foods.

■ Riboflavin Sources and Needs

Major sources of riboflavin are milk and milk products, enriched grains, ready-to-eat breakfast cereals, meat, and eggs (review Fig. 8-7). Vegetables such as asparagus, broccoli, and various greens (e.g., spinach) are also good sources.

The adult RDA of riboflavin is 1.1 to 1.3 milligrams per day. The Daily Value used on food and supplement labels is 1.7 milligrams. On average, daily intakes of riboflavin are slightly above the RDA. As with thiamin, people with alcoholism risk riboflavin deficiency because they generally eat nutrient-poor diets. No specific symptoms indicate that riboflavin taken in megadoses is toxic, so no Upper Level has been set.

Niacin

Niacin functions in the body as one of two related compounds: nicotinic acid and nicotinamide. Niacin was formerly referred to as *vitamin B-3*.

The coenzyme forms of niacin function in many cellular metabolic pathways. In general, when cell energy is being utilized, a niacin coenzyme is used. Synthetic pathways in the cell—those that make new compounds—also often use a niacin coenzyme. This is especially true for fatty acid synthesis (review Fig. 8-6).

Because almost every cellular metabolic pathway uses a niacin coenzyme, a deficiency causes widespread changes in the body. The group of niacin deficiency symptoms is known as *pellagra*, which means rough or painful skin. The symptoms of the disease are **dementia,** diarrhea, and dermatitis (especially on areas of skin exposed to the sun) (review Fig. 8-2). Later, death often results. Early symptoms include poor appetite, weight loss, and weakness.

Pellagra is the only dietary deficiency disease ever to reach epidemic proportions in the United States. It became a major problem in the southeastern United States in the late 1800s and persisted until the late 1930s when standards of living and diets improved. Today, pellagra is rare in Western societies, but can be seen in the developing world.

Another Bite

Niacin in corn is bound by a protein that hampers its absorption. Soaking corn in an alkaline solution, such as lime water (water with calcium hydroxide), releases bound niacin and renders it more usable. Hispanic people in North Americ tradition-ally soak corn in lime water before making tortillas. This treatment is one reason this Hispanic population never experienced much pellagra.

■ Niacin Sources and Needs

Major sources of niacin are poultry, ready-to-eat breakfast cereals, beef, wheat bran, tuna and other fish, asparagus, and peanuts (review Fig. 8-7). Coffee and tea also con-tribute some niacin to the diet. Niacin is very heat stable; little is lost in cooking.

Besides the preformed niacin found in protein foods, we can synthesize niacin from the amino acid tryptophan: 60 milligrams of tryptophan in a diet yield about 1 milligram of niacin. In this manner, we synthesize about 50% of the niacin we need.

The adult RDA of niacin is 14 to 16 milligrams per day. The RDA is expressed as niacin equivalents (NE) to account for niacin received intact from the diet, as well as that made from tryptophan. The Daily Value used on food and supplement labels is 20 milligrams. Intakes of niacin by adults are about double the RDA, without considering the contri-bution from tryptophan. (Note that tables of food composition values also ignore this contribution.) People with alcoholism and those with rare disorders of tryptophan metabolism are generally the only groups to show a niacin deficiency.

■ Upper Level for Niacin

The Upper Level for niacin is 35 milligrams per day of the nicotinic acid form. Effects include headache, itching, and increased blood flow to the skin, causing a general blood vessel dilation or flushing in various parts of the body, especially when intakes are above 100 milligrams per day. In the long run, GI tract and liver damage is possi-ble, so any use of megadoses, including large doses recommended for treatment for cardiovascular disease, requires close physician scrutiny (review Chapter 5).

Concept Check

The B vitamins thiamin, riboflavin, and niacin are all important in the metabolism of carbohydrates, proteins, and fats. Energy metabolism in particular requires adequate amounts of the coenzyme forms of these three vitamins. Deficiency symptoms typically occur in the brain and nervous system, skin, and GI tract. Cells in these tissues are very metabolically active, and those in the skin and GI tract are also constantly being replaced. Enriched grains are adequate sources of all three vitamins, as are ready-to-eat breakfast cereals. Otherwise, pork is an excellent source of thiamin, milk is an excellent source of riboflavin, and protein foods in general—such as chicken—are excellent sources of niacin. Deficiencies of all three vitamins can occur with alcoholism; a thiamin deficiency is the most likely of the three.

dementia A general loss or decrease in mental function.

Food Sources of Niacin	
Food Item and Amount	**Niacin (milligrams)**
Tuna, 3 ounces	11.3
Roasted chicken, 3 ounces	10.1
Peanuts, ½ cup	9.9
Baked salmon, 3 ounces	8.6
Turkey lunch meat, 3 ounces	5.4
Ground beef, 3 ounces	5.0
Raw mushrooms, 5	4.7
Lean steak, 4 ounces	4.5
Chunky peanut butter, 2 tablespoons	4.4
Fried beef liver, 1 ounce	4.1
Raisin Nut Bran cereal, ¾ cup	3.8
Tortilla, 1	2.6
Baked cod, 3 ounces	2.1
Potato, 1	2.1
Broiled halibut, 3 ounces	1.6

RDA for adults, 14 to 16 milligrams

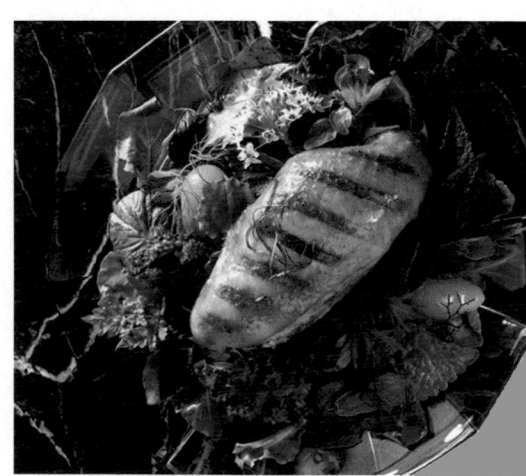

Chicken is a good source of niacin. The tryptophan present can also be metabolized to niacin.

Food Sources of Pantothenic Acid	
Food Item and Amount	**Pantothenic Acid (milligrams)**
Total corn flakes cereal, ¾ cup	11.8
Power bar, 1	10.0
Luna bar, 1	9.9
Sunflower seeds, ¼ cup	2.3
Fried beef liver, 1 ounce	1.7
Raw mushrooms, 5	1.7
Plain yogurt, 1 cup	1.5
Acorn squash, 1 cup	1.2
Peanuts, ½ cup	1.0
1% milk, 1 cup	0.9
Roasted chicken breast, 3 ounces	0.8
Broccoli, 1 cup	0.8
Baked potato, 1	0.7
Legumes, ½ cup	0.7
Cooked egg yolk, 1	0.6
Adequate Intake for adults, 5 milligrams	

Pantothenic Acid

Like the other B vitamins, pantothenic acid helps release energy from carbohydrates, fats, and protein. By forming its coenzyme, pantothenic acid allows many energy-yielding metabolic reactions to occur (review Fig. 8-6). This coenzyme also activates fatty acids so they can yield energy. It is also used in the beginning steps of fatty acid synthesis. Pantothenic acid is so widespread in foods that a nutritional deficiency among healthy people who eat varied diets is unlikely. *Pantothen* actually means "from every side" in Greek.

Pantothenic Acid Sources and Needs

Rich sources of pantothenic acid are sunflower seeds, mushrooms, peanuts, and eggs. Other sources are meat, milk, and many vegetables.

The Adequate Intake set for pantothenic acid is 5 milligrams per day for adults, and we generally consume that amount or more. The Daily Value used on food and supplement labels is 10 milligrams. A deficiency of pantothenic acid might occur in alcoholism along with a very nutrient-deficient diet. However, the symptoms would probably be hidden among deficiencies of thiamin, riboflavin, vitamin B-6, and folate, so the pantothenic acid deficiency might be unrecognizable. No toxicity is known for pantothenic acid, so no Upper Level has been set.

Biotin

In its coenzyme form, biotin aids in fat and carbohydrate metabolism. Biotin assists in the addition of carbon dioxide to other compounds. By doing so, it promotes the synthesis of glucose and fatty acids, while also helping to break down certain amino acids. Symptoms of biotin deficiency include a scaly inflammation of the skin, changes in the tongue and lips, decreased appetite, nausea, vomiting, a form of anemia, depression, muscle pain and weakness, and poor growth.

Biotin Sources and Needs

Food Sources of Biotin	
Food Item and Amount	**Biotin (micrograms)**
Smooth peanut butter, 2 tablespoons	30.1
Cooked lamb liver, 1 ounce	11.6
Boiled egg, 1	9.3
Cooked egg yolk, 1	8.1
Yogurt, 1 cup	7.4
Wheat germ, ¼ cup	7.2
Roasted peanuts, 5	6.5
Wheat bran, ¼ cup	6.4
Fat-free milk, 1 cup	4.9
Salmon, 3 ounces	4.3
Egg noodles, 1 cup	4.0
Swiss cheese, 2 ounces	2.2
Cheddar cheese, 2 ounces	1.7
Raw cauliflower, 1 cup	1.5
American cheese, 2 ounces	1.4
Adequate Intake for adults, 30 micrograms	

Cauliflower, egg yolks, peanuts, and cheese are good sources of biotin. Intestinal bacteria synthesize and supply some biotin, making a biotin deficiency unlikely. However, scientists are not sure how much of the bacteria-synthesized biotin in our intestines is actually absorbed. If intestinal bacterial synthesis is not sufficient, as in people who are missing a large part of the small intestine or who take antibiotics for many months, special attention should be paid to meeting biotin needs. A protein called *avidin* in raw egg whites binds biotin and inhibits its absorption. Consuming many raw egg whites eventually leads to the deficiency disease. Note that cooking denatures avidin in eggs such that it cannot bind biotin.

The Adequate Intake set for biotin is 30 micrograms per day for adults. Our food supply is thought to provide 40 to 60 micrograms per person per day. The Daily Value used on food and supplement labels is 300 micrograms, 10 times our current estimate of needs. Biotin is relatively nontoxic. Large doses have been given over an extended period without harmful side effects to children who exhibit defects in biotin metabolism. Thus, no Upper Level for biotin has been set.

Vitamin B-6

Vitamin B-6 is actually a family of three compounds. All can be changed to the active vitamin B-6 coenzyme. The general vitamin name and form added to foods is called *pyridoxine.*

■ Functions of Vitamin B-6

The coenzymes of vitamin B-6 are needed for the activity of numerous enzymes involved in carbohydrate, protein, and fat metabolism. Because vitamin B-6 is needed in so many areas of metabolism, a deficiency results in widespread symptoms, such as depression, vomiting, skin disorders, irritation of the nerves, and impaired immune response.

A key function of vitamin B-6 concerns protein because metabolizing any amino acid requires the vitamin B-6 coenzyme (review Fig. 8-6). By helping to split the nitrogen group ($-NH_2$) from an amino acid and making it available to another amino acid, the coenzyme participates in reactions that allow a cell to synthesize nonessential (dispensable) amino acids.

Another important role of vitamin B-6 is the synthesis of many neurotransmitters. Recall from Chapter 3 that neurotransmitters allow nerve cells to communicate with each other and with other body cells. In the 1950s, infants fed oversterilized commercial formulas developed vitamin B-6 deficiency symptoms, particularly convulsions. Heat destroyed vitamin B-6 in the formulas. Today, manufacturers are more careful to maintain adequate vitamin B-6 content in formulas.

The vitamin B-6 coenzyme is important for the synthesis of hemoglobin and its function as the oxygen-carrying part of the red blood cell. Vitamin B-6 is also necessary for the synthesis of white blood cells, which perform a major role in the immune system.

Vitamin B-6 participates in various aspects of carbohydrate, fat, and vitamin metabolism. Finally, vitamin B-6 plays a role in homocysteine metabolism.

■ Vitamin B-6 Sources and Needs

Major sources of vitamin B-6 are animal products, ready-to-eat breakfast cereals, potatoes, and milk. Other sources are fruits and vegetables such as bananas, cantaloupes, broccoli, and spinach (Fig. 8-8). Overall, animal sources and fortified products are the

Food Sources of Vitamin B-6

Food Item and Amount	Vitamin B-6 (milligrams)
Baked salmon, 3 ounces	0.8
Baked potato, 1 medium	0.7
Banana, 1	0.7
Avocado, 1	0.6
Roasted chicken breast, 3 ounces	0.5
Acorn squash, 1 cup	0.5
Special K cereal, ¾ cup	0.5
Fried beef liver, 1 ounce	0.4
Roasted turkey lunch meat, 3 ounces	0.4
Sirloin steak, 3 ounces	0.4
Lean ham, 3 ounces	0.4
Watermelon, 1 slice	0.3
Sunflower seeds, ¼ cup	0.3
Cooked spinach, ½ cup	0.2
1% milk, 1 cup	0.1

RDA for adults, 1.3 to 1.7 milligrams

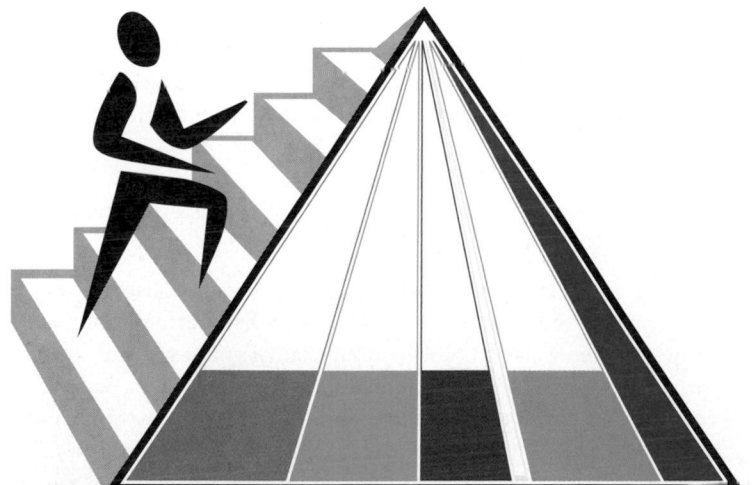

Figure 8-8 Sources of Vitamin B-6 from MyPyramid. The height of the background color (none, 1/3, 2/3 or completely covered) within each group in the pyramid indicates the average nutrient density for vitamin B-6 in that group. Overall, the meat group especially contains many foods that are nutrient-dense sources of vitamin B-6. With regard to physical activity, vitamin B-6 participates in the related energy metabolism during such endeavors.

Grains	Vegetables	Fruits	Oils	Milk	Meat & Beans
• Fortified breakfast cereals • Wheat germ (whole-wheat products)	• Potatoes • Spinach • Cauliflower	• Avocados • Bananas • Dates • Cantaloupe • Watermelon	• None	• Milk • Yogurt • Cottage cheese	• Meat • Poultry • Fish • Beans • Nuts • Seeds

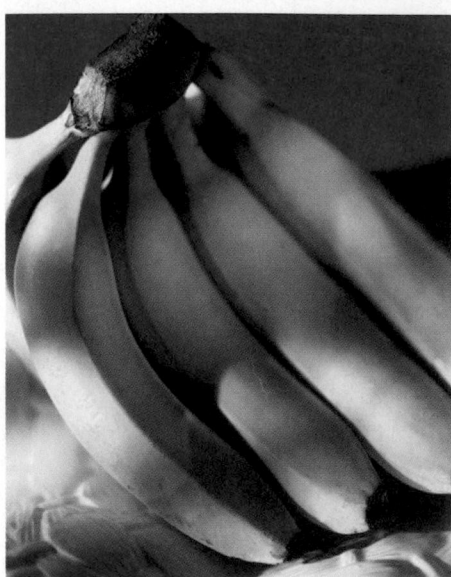

Bananas are a plant source of vitamin B-6.

premenstrual syndrome (PMS) A disorder found in some women a few days before a menstrual period begins. It is characterized by depression, anxiety, headache, bloating, and mood swings. Severe cases are currently termed premenstrual dysphoric disorder (PDD).

Folic acid is more readily absorbed (1.7 times greater) than natural forms of folate. Natural food folate differs from folic acid by containing extra units of the amino acid glutamic acid attached to the structure. These extra units must be removed before absorption, yielding free folic acid.

most reliable because the vitamin B-6 they contain is more absorbable than that in plant foods.

The adult RDA of vitamin B-6 is 1.3 to 1.7 milligrams per day. The Daily Value used on food and supplement labels is 2 milligrams. Average daily consumption of vitamin B-6 for men and women is somewhat above the RDA.

Athletes may need slightly more vitamin B-6 than sedentary adults. The athlete's body processes a great deal of glycogen and ingested protein (in the form of amino acids) for fuel, and the metabolism of these compounds requires vitamin B-6. However, athletes are likely to consume plenty of protein—enough to supply needed amounts of vitamin B-6.

People with alcoholism are susceptible to a vitamin B-6 deficiency because a metabolite formed in alcohol metabolism can displace the coenzyme form from enzymes, increasing its tendency to be destroyed. In addition, alcohol decreases the absorption of vitamin B-6 and decreases the synthesis of its coenzyme form. Cirrhosis and hepatitis (both of which may accompany alcoholism) also disable liver tissue from actively metabolizing vitamin B-6, which in turn decreases synthesis of its coenzyme form.

Carpal tunnel syndrome, a nerve disorder in the wrist, has been treated successfully with large daily doses of vitamin B-6 in some people. However, because of defects in the design of trials, and conflicting data on its effectiveness, vitamin B-6 is currently not routinely recommended for this condition. The inconsistent results of studies of vitamin B-6 and **premenstrual syndrome (PMS)** also make a definitive recommendation for taking vitamin B-6 controversial. Some physicians, however, advise doses of 50 to 100 milligrams per day as a possible part of therapy. Such large doses may also help treat "morning sickness" that develops during pregnancy (see Chapter 13).

■ Upper Level for Vitamin B-6

The Upper Level for vitamin B-6 is 100 milligrams per day, based on the risk of developing nerve damage. Studies have shown that intakes of 2 to 6 grams of vitamin B-6 per day for 2 or more months especially can lead to irreversible nerve damage. Symptoms of vitamin B-6 toxicity include walking difficulties and hand and foot numbness. Some nerve damage in individual sensory neurons is probably reversible, but damage to the ganglia (where many nerve fibers converge) appears to be permanent. With 500 milligram tablets of vitamin B-6 available in health-food stores, taking a toxic dose is quite easy.

Concept Check

Pantothenic acid and biotin both participate in the metabolism of carbohydrate and fat. A deficiency of either vitamin is unlikely; pantothenic acid is found widely in foods, and our need for biotin is partially met by intestinal synthesis from bacteria. Vitamin B-6 is important for protein metabolism, neurotransmitter synthesis, homocysteine metabolism, and other key metabolic functions. Headache, a form of anemia, nausea, and vomiting can result from a vitamin B-6 deficiency. Increased risk of cardiovascular disease is also likely. Animal protein foods, ready-to-eat breakfast cereals, broccoli, spinach, and bananas are some food sources of vitamin B-6. Megadose supplements of vitamin B-6 can lead to nerve damage.

Folate

The term *folate* encompasses a variety of food forms of the vitamin. Folic acid is the chemical form added to foods and present in supplements.

■ Functions of Folate

A key role of the folate coenzymes is to supply or accept single carbon compounds. In this role the coenzymes help form DNA and also metabolize various amino acids and their derivatives, such as homocysteine.

One major result of a folate deficiency is that in the early phases of red blood cell synthesis, the immature cells cannot divide because they cannot form new DNA. The cells grow progressively larger because they can still synthesize enough protein and other cell parts to make new cells. When the time comes for the cells to divide, however, the amount of DNA is insufficient to form two nuclei. The cells then remain in a large immature form, known as a **megaloblast** (review Fig. 8-2).

Because the bone marrow of a folate-deficient person produces mostly immature megaloblast cells, few mature red blood cells (called **erythrocytes**) arrive in the bloodstream. When fewer mature red blood cells are present, the blood's capacity to carry oxygen decreases, causing a form of anemia. In short, a folate deficiency causes megaloblastic anemia (also called **macrocytic anemia**).

The changes in red blood cell formation occur after 7 to 16 weeks on a folate-free diet, depending on the person's folate stores. White blood cell formation is also affected, but to a lesser degree. In addition, cell division throughout the entire body is disrupted. Clinicians focus primarily on red blood cells because they are easy to collect and examine. Other symptoms of folate deficiency are inflammation of the tongue, diarrhea, poor growth, mental confusion, depression, and problems in nerve function.

About 10% of the North American population has a defect in one aspect of folate metabolism. They may need up to twice the RDA to compensate. Currently, testing for this defect is not routine in medical practice, but one day it may be.

Another Bite

Some forms of cancer therapy provide a vivid example of the effects of a folate deficiency on DNA metabolism. A cancer drug, methotrexate, closely resembles a form of folate but cannot act in its place. Because of this resemblance, when methotrexate is taken in high doses, it hampers folate metabolism. In essence, methotrexate crowds out folate in the metabolic pathways. DNA synthesis and, consequently, cell division, then decrease. Because cancer cells are among the most rapidly dividing cells in the body, they are among those first affected. However, other rapidly dividing cells, such as intestinal cells and skin cells, are also affected. Not surprisingly, typical side effects of methotrexate therapy are diarrhea, vomiting, and hair loss. These are also typical symptoms of folate deficiency. Today when patients are given methotrexate, they need to follow a high-folate diet and/or take folic acid supplements because this reduces the toxic side effects of the drug. High supplemental doses generally have little or no influence on methotrexate's effectiveness as a cancer therapy.

A maternal deficiency of folate along with a genetic abnormality related to folate metabolism have been linked to development of **neural tube defects** in the fetus (Fig. 8-9). These defects include spina bifida (spinal cord or spinal fluid bulge through the back) and anencephaly (absence of a brain). About 2000 infants are affected with neural tube defects annually in the United States. Victims of spina bifida exhibit paralysis, incontinence, learning disabilities, and other health problems. Children born with anencephaly die shortly after birth. Adequate folate nutriture is crucial for all women of childbearing age since the neural tube closes within the first 28 days of pregnancy, a time when many women are not even aware that they are pregnant. Hence a recommendation is made that ample folate, specifically 400 micrograms of synthetic folic acid per day, be consumed at least 6 weeks before conception. Note that almost all related research has been done with synthetic folic acid supplementation, and it appears that even women with varied diets may not consume adequate synthetic folic acid to prevent neural tube defects unless specific attention to rich sources is given. Perhaps as many as 70% of these defects could be

megaloblast A large, immature red blood cell that results from the particular cell's inability to divide normally.

erythrocytes Mature red blood cells. These have no nucleus and a life span of about 120 days; they contain hemoglobin, which transports oxygen and carbon dioxide.

macrocytic anemia Anemia characterized by the presence of abnormally large red blood cells.

neural tube defect A defect in the formation of the neural tube occurring during early fetal development. This type of defect results in various nervous system disorders, such as spina bifida. Folate deficiency in the pregnant woman increases the risk that the fetus will develop this disorder.

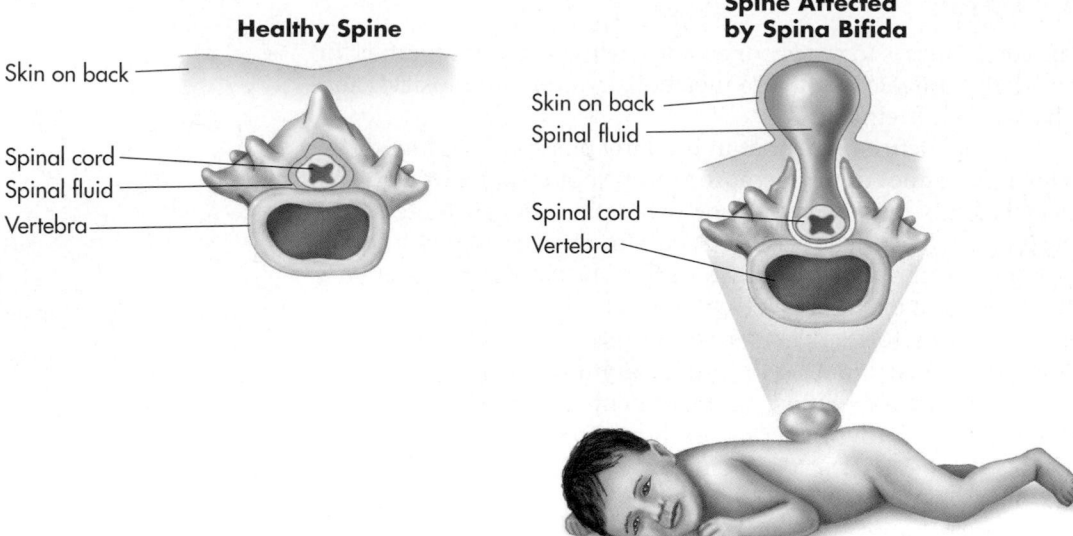

Figure 8-9 Neural tube defects result from a developmental failure affecting the spinal cord or brain in the embryo. Very early in fetal development, a ridge of neural-like tissue forms along the back of the embryo. As the fetus develops, this material develops into both the spinal cord and nerves at the lower end, and into the brain at the upper end. At the same time, the bones that make up the back gradually surround the spinal cord on all sides. If any part of this sequence goes awry, many defects can appear. The worst case is total lack of a brain (anencephaly). Spina bifida, in which the back bones do not form a complete ring to protect the spinal cord, is much more common. Deficient folate status in the mother during the beginning of pregnancy greatly increases the risk of neural tube defects, as does a genetic abnormality in folate metabolism.

avoided by adequate folate status before conception. (Women who have had a child with a neural tube defect are advised to consume 4 milligrams per day of folic acid, beginning at least one month before any future pregnancy. This must be done under strict physician supervision.)

Consuming ready-to-eat breakfast cereals that contain 100% of the Daily Value for folate (this is the same as the RDA) is a good practice for meeting the goal for synthetic folic acid intake. A multivitamin and mineral supplement can also be used to supply adequate synthetic folic acid, but women should be careful to monitor the amount of any accompanying preformed vitamin A content (don't exceed 100% of the Daily Value).

Research is currently underway on the link between folate and cancer protection. Because folate aids in DNA synthesis, it is hypothesized that even mild folate deficiency contributes to abnormal DNA integrity, which in turn affects certain cancer-protecting genes. Meeting the RDA for folate is thought to be one way to reduce cancer risk.

A final function of folate is the formation of neurotransmitters in the brain. Meeting folate needs can improve the depressed state in some cases of mental illness.

■ Folate Sources and Needs

Green, leafy vegetables (*folate* is derived from the Latin word *folium*, which means *foliage* or leaves), organ meats, sprouts, other vegetables, dried beans, and orange juice are the richest sources of folate (Fig. 8-10). The vitamin C in orange juice also reduces folate destruction. Ready-to-eat breakfast cereals, milk, and bread also are important sources of folate for many adults.

Folate is very susceptible to destruction by heat. Food processing and preparation destroy 50% to 90% of the folate in food. This underscores the importance of regularly

Food Sources of Folate

Food Item and Amount	Folate (micrograms)
Asparagus, 1 cup	263
Cooked spinach, 1 cup	262
Cooked lentils, ½ cup	179
Black-eyed peas, ½ cup	179
Romaine lettuce, 1½ cups	114
Great Grains cereal, ¾ cup	114
Tortilla, 1	89
Cooked turnips, ½ cup	85
Cooked broccoli, 1 cup	78
Sunflower seeds, ¼ cup	76
Fresh orange juice, 1 cup	75
Cooked beets, ½ cup	68
Kidney beans, ½ cup	65
Fried beef liver, 1 ounce	62

RDA for adults, 400 micrograms

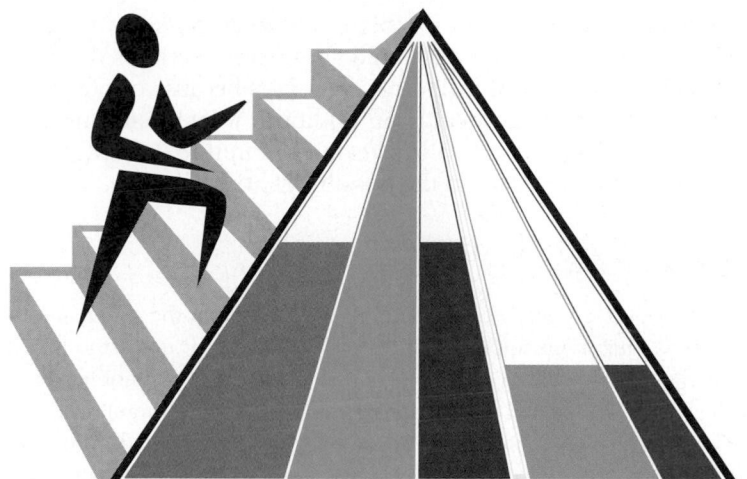

Figure 8-10 Sources of Folate from MyPyramid. The height of the background color (none, 1/3, 2/3 or completely covered) within each group in the pyramid indicates the average nutrient density for folate in that group. Overall, the vegetables group provides the richest sources, but the fruits group and the grains group contain some foods that are nutrient-dense sources of folate. With regard to physical activity, folate plays no specific role in such endeavors.

Grains	Vegetables	Fruits	Oils	Milk	Meat & Beans
• Fortified break-fast cereals • Wheat germ (whole-wheat products) • Enriched grains	• Asparagus • Leafy green vegetables	• Oranges • Strawberries • Cantaloupes and other melons	• None	• Cottage cheese • Yogurt	• Liver • Eggs • Beans • Sunflower seeds

eating fresh fruits and raw or lightly cooked vegetables. As mentioned before, vegetables retain their nutrients best when cooked quickly in minimal water—steaming, stir-frying, or microwaving (review Table 8-1).

The RDA of folate for adults is 400 micrograms per day, as is the Daily Value used on food and supplement labels. Folate recommendations for all but women of child-bearing age are based on dietary folate equivalents (DFE). (As just covered, these women should meet such recommendations with synthetic folic acid.) To compute folate intake in DFE units, one has to determine how much of a day's folate intake comes from food folate and how much comes from synthetic folic acid added to foods. When in doubt, assume all folate in a diet is in the food form, except that coming from ready-to-eat breakfast cereals and refined grain products. Also included in this second category is any folic acid consumed as part of supplements. To calculate the DFE, multiply total synthetic folic acid intake by 1.7, and add that value to the food folate consumed. For example, if a person consumed 300 micrograms as food folate and 200 micrograms from a ready-to-eat breakfast cereal, total folate DFE would be 640 micrograms (300 + 200 × 1.7] = 640). Compared to the RDA of 400 micrograms, this intake would be sufficient.

Prior to 1998, average daily folate intakes in the United States were approximately 320 micrograms for men and 220 micrograms for women. In 1998, the FDA mandated the fortification of grain products with folate with the aim of reducing birth defects of the spine. With this mandate, average intakes have increased by about 200 micrograms per day. Recent studies have shown this practice has decreased rates of neural tube defects in infants as well as decreased blood homocysteine levels in adults in the United States.

Pregnant women need extra folate (a total of 600 micrograms DFE) to accommodate the increased rates of cell division and DNA synthesis in their own bodies and in the developing fetus. A healthy diet easily supplies this much. Still, prenatal care often includes a specially formulated multivitamin and mineral supplement enriched with synthetic folic acid to help compensate for the extra needs associated with pregnancy.

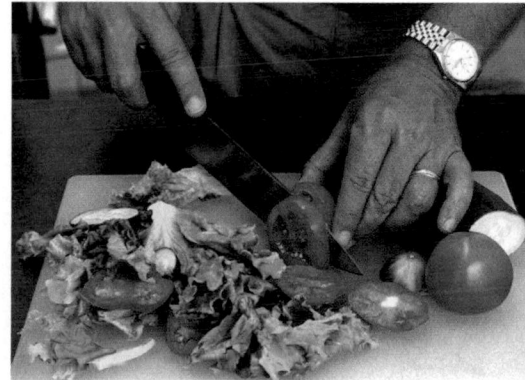

Leafy green vegetables are good sources of folate.

Critical Thinking

Gary has alcoholism and pays no attention to his diet. In addition to the detrimental effects on the liver, excess alcohol consumption can cause deficiencies in certain B vitamins. Explain why this can occur.

Older people are also at risk for folate deficiency, possibly due to a combination of inadequate folate intake and decreased absorption. Perhaps these people fail to consume sufficient amounts of fruits and vegetables because of poverty or physical problems, such as poor dental health. In addition, folate deficiencies often occur with alcoholism, due mostly to poor intake and absorption. Symptoms of a folate-related anemia can alert a physician to the possibility of alcoholism.

Another Bite

The use of dietary folate equivalents (DFEs) instead of the actual amount of folate in a food has some important implications. Typically, many foods will be richer in folate than the Nutrition Facts label suggests since folate content is due primarily to synthetic folic acid added to the foods, such as in enriched grains and ready-to-eat breakfast cereals. This contributes substantially to the DFE calculation. Another implication is that food composition tables (such as the one in the back of this book) and diet analysis software programs (such as that supplied with this book) also underestimate the true folate contribution of a diet compared to folate needs because these have not been updated to DFE units.

■ Upper Level for Folate

The Upper Level for folate is 1 milligram (1000 micrograms), but only refers to the synthetic source. This is because folate naturally present in foods has limited absorption. Large doses of folate can hide the signs of vitamin B-12 deficiency and therefore complicate its diagnosis. Specifically, regular consumption of large amounts of folate can prevent the appearance of an early warning sign of vitamin B-12 deficiency—enlarged red blood cell size. To prevent such masking of vitamin B-12 deficiency, it is the goal of FDA, through its recent enactment of folate fortification of grains, to increase the folate status of women of childbearing age without causing excessive intake (over 1 milligram of synthetic folic acid per day) by other groups. Also, because of risk of masking a vitamin B-12 deficiency, FDA limits supplements for nonpregnant adults and food fortification to 400 microgram amounts.

Vitamin B-12

Vitamin B-12 represents a family of compounds that contain the mineral cobalt. All vitamin B-12 compounds are synthesized by bacteria, fungi, and other lower organisms.

The body's complex means of absorbing vitamin B-12 is unique to this vitamin. Vitamin B-12 in food enters the stomach and is released from other materials by digestion, especially by stomach acid. The free vitamin B-12 in the stomach binds with a substance originally produced by the salivary glands in the mouth, and then later is again freed during digestion. The vitamin B-12 then binds in the small intestine with a compound originally made in the stomach called **intrinsic factor.** The resulting intrinsic factor/vitamin B-12 complex travels to the last portion of the small intestine for absorption. After these digestion steps, approximately 50% of dietary vitamin B-12 is absorbed, depending on the body's need for it. Any failure in this system results in only 1% to 2% absorption of dietary vitamin B-12.

If a defect in the digestion and absorption of vitamin B-12 develops, the person usually takes monthly injections of vitamin B-12, uses vitamin B-12 nasal gels to bypass the need for absorption, or takes megadoses of a supplemental form (300 times the RDA). In this latter case, the vitamin B-12 absorption defect is overcome by providing enough of the vitamin via simple diffusion across the intestinal tract.

About 95% of all cases of vitamin B-12 deficiencies in healthy people result from defective vitamin B-12 absorption, rather than from inadequate intakes. This is especially

intrinsic factor A protein-like compound produced by the stomach that enhances vitamin B-12 absorption.

true for older people. As we age, our stomachs have a decreased ability to synthesize the intrinsic factor needed for vitamin B-12 absorption.

■ Functions of Vitamin B-12

Vitamin B-12 participates in a variety of cellular processes. The most important function is in folate metabolism. Vitamin B-12 is required to convert folate coenzymes to the active forms needed for metabolic reactions, such as DNA synthesis. Without vitamin B-12, reactions that require certain active forms of folate do not take place in the cell. Thus, a vitamin B-12 deficiency can result in symptoms of a folate deficiency. Another vital function of vitamin B-12 is maintaining the myelin sheaths that insulate neurons from each other. People with vitamin B-12 deficiencies have destruction of segments of the myelin sheaths. This destruction eventually causes paralysis and, perhaps, death. Vitamin B-12 also participates in homocysteine metabolism and certain minor metabolic pathways.

In the past, the inability to absorb enough vitamin B-12 eventually led to death, mainly because it destroyed nerves. This phenomenon was called **pernicious anemia** (*pernicious* literally means "leading to death"). Clinically, the anemia looks much like a folate-deficiency anemia, which is characterized by the appearance of many large red blood cells in the bloodstream. However, the true cause of pernicious anemia is poor vitamin B-12 absorption rather than inadequate folate intakes.

Some symptoms of pernicious anemia include weakness, sore tongue, back pain, apathy, and tingling in the extremities. Because we are able to store significant amounts of vitamin B-12, symptoms of nerve destruction generally do not develop until after about 3 years from the onset of the disease. Unfortunately, significant nerve destruction often occurs before the anemia is detected, and this destruction is irreversible. Pernicious anemia and its accompanying nerve destruction generally start after middle age, affecting up to 10% to 20% of older adults. The explanation for this age-associated pernicious anemia is twofold. First, aging is often associated with low production of stomach acid. Thus vitamin B-12 is not properly cleaved from other food components during digestion. Second, aging may be accompanied by reduced output of intrinsic factor, resulting in decreased absorption of the vitamin.

Infants who are breastfed by vegetarian or vegan mothers are at risk for vitamin B-12 deficiency accompanied by anemia and long-term nervous system problems, such as diminished brain growth, degeneration of the spinal cord, and poor intellectual development. The problems may have their origins during pregnancy, when the mother is deficient in vitamin B-12. Because vegan diets supply little vitamin B-12 unless they include vitamin B-12–enriched food or supplements, achieving an adequate vitamin B-12 intake is a key diet planning goal for vegans (review Chapter 6).

■ Vitamin B-12 Sources and Needs

Major sources of vitamin B-12 include meat, milk, ready-to-eat breakfast cereals, poultry, seafood, and eggs. Organ meats (especially liver, kidneys, and heart) are especially rich sources of vitamin B-12. Adults over age 50 are encouraged to seek a synthetic vitamin B-12 source to aid absorption, which can be limited due to reduced intrinsic factor and stomach acid output seen in aging, as just mentioned. Synthetic vitamin B-12 is not food bound, so it doesn't need stomach acid to release it from foods. Thus, it will be more readily absorbed than the food form. Ready-to-eat breakfast cereals and a multivitamin and mineral supplement are two possible synthetic sources.

The RDA of vitamin B-12 for adults is 2.4 micrograms per day. The Daily Value used on food and supplement labels is 6 micrograms. On average, adults consume 2 times the RDA or more. This high intake provides the average meat-eating person with 2 to 3 years' storage of vitamin B-12 in the liver.

It takes a person approximately 20 years of consuming a diet essentially free of vitamin B-12 to exhibit nerve destruction caused by a diet deficiency. (Still, vegans,

pernicious anemia The anemia that results from a lack of vitamin B-12 absorption; it is pernicious because of associated nerve degeneration that can result in eventual paralysis and death.

Food Sources of Vitamin B-12	
Food Item and Amount	**Vitamin B-12 (micrograms)**
Fried beef liver, 1 ounce	31.7
Baked clams, 1 ounce	15.7
Boiled oysters, 2	14.4
Lobster, 3 ounces	2.7
Pot roast, 3 ounces	2.5
Plain yogurt, 1 cup	1.4
Corn Flakes cereal, ¾ cup	1.1
Shrimp, 3 ounces	1.0
1% milk, 1 cup	0.9
Soy milk, 1 cup	0.8
Boiled egg, 1	0.6
Lean ham, 3 ounces	0.6
Beef hot dog, 1	0.5
Ham lunch meat, 2 ounces	0.4

RDA for adults, 2.4 micrograms

People with HIV/AIDS also are at risk of vitamin B-12 deficiency, linked to long-standing malabsorption that they often experience. In a few studies, adequate vitamin B-12 status has been shown to lessen the decline in health experienced by those with HIV/AIDS.

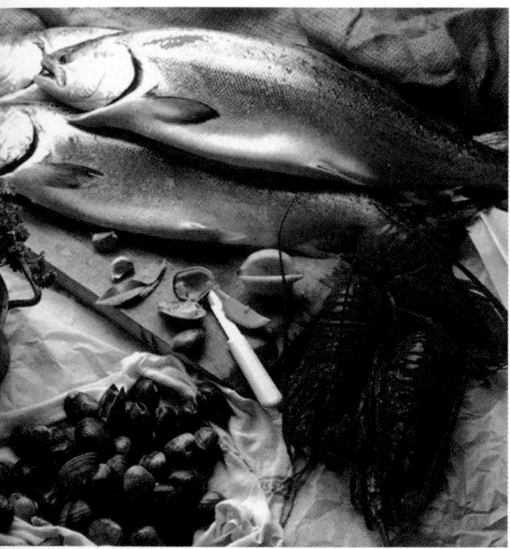

Fish, seafood, and related products are good sources of vitamin B-12.

who eat no animal products, should find a reliable source of vitamin B-12, such as fortified soybean milk, ready-to-eat breakfast cereals, and a form of yeast grown on media rich in vitamin B-12. Use of a multivitamin and mineral supplement containing vitamin B-12 is another option.) As noted earlier, older persons are at significant risk for developing pernicious anemia. This develops after a few years of the loss of vitamin B-12 absorption capacity. The quicker appearance is because of the reduced ability to reabsorb vitamin B-12 that is excreted into the GI tract during digestion, coupled with reduced absorption of dietary sources. Regular physical examinations should test for pernicious anemia in older adults. Vitamin B-12 supplements are essentially nontoxic, so no Upper Level has been set.

Concept Check

Folate is needed for cell division because it influences DNA synthesis. A folate deficiency results in megaloblastic (macrocytic) anemia, as well as elevated blood homocysteine, inflammation of the tongue, diarrhea, and poor growth. Excess folate intake can mask a vitamin B-12 deficiency since these vitamins work together in metabolism. Folate is found in fruits and vegetables, beans, and organ meats. Emphasizing fresh and lightly cooked vegetables in the diet is important because much folate is lost during cooking. Women of childbearing age should meet needs by consuming a source of synthetic folic acid. Folate needs during pregnancy are especially high; a deficiency around time of conception and in the first month of pregnancy may lead to neural tube defects in the fetus.

Vitamin B-12 is necessary for folate metabolism. Without dietary vitamin B-12, folate deficiency symptoms, such as macrocytic anemia, develop. In addition, vitamin B-12 is necessary for maintaining the nervous system. Paralysis can develop from a vitamin B-12 deficiency. Vitamin B-12 also participates in homocysteine metabolism. The absorption of vitamin B-12 requires a number of specific factors. If absorption is inhibited, the resulting deficiency can lead to pernicious anemia and its associated nerve destruction. Concentrated amounts of vitamin B-12 are found only in animal foods; meat-eaters generally have a 2- to 3-year supply stored in the liver. Vegans need to find an alternate source. Vitamin B-12 absorption may decline as we age. Monthly injections, nasal gels, or megadoses can make up for this.

Vitamin C

On long sea voyages, captains often lost half or more of their crews to scurvy, the vitamin C deficiency disease. Its symptoms include weakness, opening of previously healed wounds, slower wound healing, bone pain, fractures, bleeding gums, diarrhea, and pinpoint hemorrhages around hair follicles on the back of the arms and legs. In 1740, the Englishman Dr. James Lind first showed that citrus fruits—two oranges and one lemon a day—could cure scurvy. Fifty years after Lind's discovery, rations for British sailors included limes to prevent scurvy (thus their nickname, limeys).

Vitamin C (ascorbic acid) is a puzzling vitamin. It is found in all living tissues, and most animals synthesize it from the simple sugar glucose. What is strange is that animals who synthesize vitamin C often make quite a lot of it. For instance, a pig produces 8 grams per day (though we do not benefit from it when we eat pork because it is lost in processing). This amount is over 80 times our human RDA of 75 to 90 milligrams. Why some animals make so much vitamin C, whereas other animals, including humans, appear to need so little has fueled much controversy.

Vitamin C is absorbed in the small intestine. About 70% to 90% of vitamin C is absorbed when a person eats between 30 and 180 milligrams of it per day. If someone ingests 1 gram (1000 milligrams) per day, absorption efficiency drops to about 50%.

A common side effect of megadose vitamin C use is diarrhea. The unabsorbed vitamin C stays in the small intestine and attracts water, resulting in diarrhea (see the section on toxicity of vitamin C).

■ Functions of Vitamin C

The best understood function of vitamin C is its role in synthesizing the protein collagen. This protein is highly concentrated in connective tissue, bone, teeth, tendons, and blood vessels. It is very important for wound healing. Vitamin C increases the cross-connections between amino acids in collagen, greatly strengthening the structural tissues it helps form.

A vitamin C deficiency can cause widespread changes in tissue metabolism. Most symptoms of scurvy are linked to a decrease in collagen synthesis, such as in the skin. About 20 to 40 days with no vitamin C intake are required for the first symptoms of scurvy to appear (review Fig. 8-2).

Vitamin C has antioxidants properties. This may allow vitamin C to reduce the formation of cancer-causing nitrosamines in the stomach and also keep the folate coenzymes intact, preventing their destruction. Vitamin C may work as a free radical scavenger. Vitamin C also may aid in reactivating oxidized vitamin E so that it can be reused. The extent to which all this antioxidant activity happens in the body, however, is debatable. It is likely so but not proven as of now. Population studies suggest that vitamin C is effective in helping prevent certain cancers (of the esophagus, mouth, and stomach) and cataracts in the eye, probably because of its antioxidant properties.

Vitamin C enhances iron absorption by keeping iron in its most absorbable form, especially as the mineral travels through the small intestine's alkaline environment. This is seen with a vitamin C intake of 75 milligrams or more at a meal. Increasing intake of vitamin C-rich foods is beneficial for those with poor iron stores. Vitamin C is also necessary for the synthesis of a number of hormones, neurotransmitters, and other compounds, such as bile acids and DNA. It may also contribute to lower blood pressure values.

Finally, vitamin C is vital for the function of the immune system, especially for the activity of certain cells in the immune system. Thus, disease states that increase the need for immune function can increase the need for vitamin C, although we don't know what amount above the RDA is needed (if any). Partly on the basis of this observation, Dr. Linus Pauling gained great notoriety by claiming that vitamin C could combat the common cold. He claimed that 1000 milligrams (1 gram) or more of vitamin C daily could reduce the number of colds for most people by nearly half. As a result of the popularity of his books and the respectability of his scientific credentials, millions of North Americans supplement their diets with vitamin C.

But does vitamin C reliably and effectively work against colds and other infections? Most medical and nutrition scientists disagree with Pauling's views of vitamin C. Numerous well-designed, double-blind studies have not shown megadoses of vitamin C to reliably prevent colds, though it seems to reduce the duration of symptoms by a day or so.

Most vitamin C consumed in large doses in supplements ends up in the feces or the urine. Only a small fraction of such large doses can be used. The kidneys start rapidly excreting this vitamin C beginning at intakes of about 100 milligrams per day. This means that if more than that is ingested, much is quickly excreted. At dosages of 500 milligrams per day, almost all, is excreted.

■ Vitamin C Sources and Needs

Major sources of vitamin C are citrus fruits, green peppers, cauliflower, broccoli, cabbage, strawberries, papayas, and romaine lettuce. Potatoes, ready-to-eat breakfast cereals, and fortified fruit drinks are also good sources of vitamin C (Fig. 8-11). Meeting the servings for fruits and vegetables recommended by MyPyramid can

Food Sources of Vitamin C	
Food Item and Amount	**Vitamin C (milligrams)**
Orange, 1	98
Cooked brussels sprouts, 1 cup	97
Strawberries, 1 cup	94
Grapefruit juice, 1 cup	80
Red peppers, ¼ cup	71
Kiwi fruit, 1	57
Green pepper rings, 5	45
Tomato juice, 1 cup	45
Cooked broccoli, ½ cup	33
Kale, ½ cup	27
Raw cauliflower, ½ cup	23
Sweet potato, 1	17
Baked potato, 1 medium	16
Pineapple chunks, ½ cup	12
Cooked spinach, ½ cup	9
RDA for adults, 75 to 90 milligrams	

Figure 8-11 Sources of Vitamin C from MyPyramid. The height of the background color (none, 1/3, 2/3 or completely covered) within each group in the pyramid indicates the average nutrient density for vitamin C in that group. Overall, the vegetables group and the fruits group contain many foods that are nutrient-dense sources of vitamin C. With regard to physical activity, vitamin C has no primary role in the related energy metabolism per se, but likely limits some oxidant damage during such endeavors.

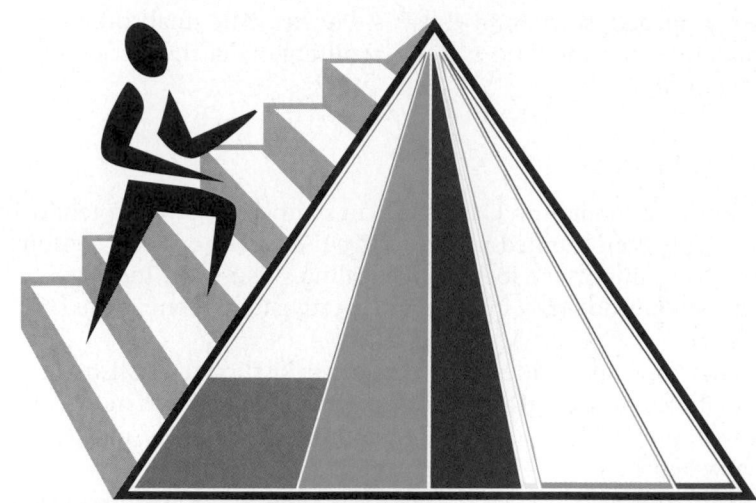

Grains	Vegetables	Fruits	Oils	Milk	Meat & Beans
• Fortified break-fast cereals	• Tomatoes • Potatoes • Cauliflower • Green vegetables	• Citrus fruits • Pineapple • Strawberries	• None	• None	• None

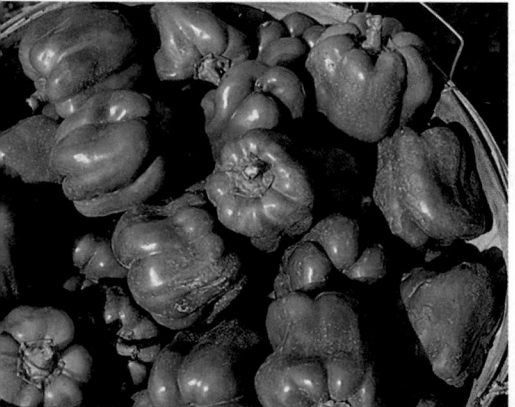

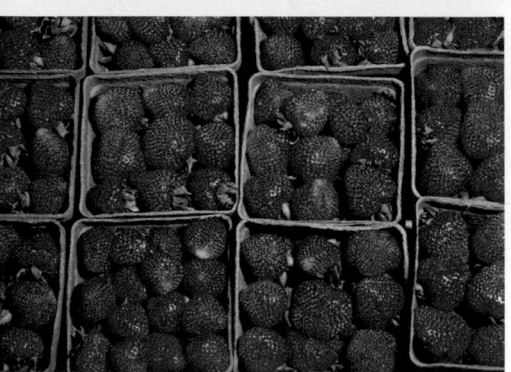

Vegetables such as green peppers are a good source of vitamin C, as are fruits such as strawberries.

easily provide enough vitamin C. Vitamin C is rapidly lost in processing and cooking as it is very unstable in the presence of heat, iron, copper, or oxygen, and is water soluble.

The adult RDA of vitamin C is 75 to 90 milligrams per day. The Daily Value used on food and supplement labels is 60 milligrams. Cigarette smokers need to add an extra 35 milligrams per day to the RDA because of the great stress on their lungs from oxygen and toxic by-products of cigarette smoke. Nearly all North Americans likely meet their daily needs for vitamin C. We consume an average 70 to 100 milligrams per day. Respected nutrition experts who advocate increased use of vitamin C often recommend intakes of about 200 milligrams per day. Still, this amount can be obtained by sufficient fruit and vegetable intake. Today, vitamin C deficiency appears mostly in alcoholic people who eat nutrient-poor diets and in some older persons with inadequate food intakes.

■ Upper Level for Vitamin C

The Upper Level for vitamin C is 2 grams per day. Regularly consuming more than that may cause stomach inflammation and diarrhea. Other purported toxicity symptoms have been discounted.

Figure 8-12 summarizes much of what we have covered about the functions of the vitamins. Note that many vitamins work for a common purpose.

Another Bite

If people want to experiment with large doses of vitamin C, they should alert their physician. High doses of vitamin C can change reactions to medical tests for diabetes (urine) or blood in the feces. Vitamin C can interact with the testing procedures because much of a high dose of vitamin C will not be absorbed, or if absorbed, will be rapidly excreted. Physicians may misdiagnose conditions when large doses of vitamin C are consumed without their knowledge.

Energy Metabolism	Blood Formation (and Clotting*)	Bone Health	Protein Metabolism	Antioxidant Defenses
Thiamin Riboflavin Niacin Pantothenic acid Biotin Vitamin B-12	Vitamin B-6 Vitamin B-12 Folate Vitamin K*	Vitamin A Vitamin D Vitamin K Vitamin C	Thiamin Vitamin B-6 Vitamin C Folate	Vitamin E Vitamin C (likely) Carotenoids Riboflavin (indirect)

Figure 8-12 Vitamins and related nutrients work together to maintain health.

Concept Check

Vitamin C is important in the synthesis of collagen, a major connective tissue protein. A vitamin C deficiency, known as scurvy, causes many changes in the skin and gums, such as small hemorrhages. This is mainly because of poor collagen synthesis. Vitamin C also modestly improves iron absorption, is involved in synthesizing certain hormones and neurotransmitters, and likely acts as a general body antioxidant. Citrus fruits, green peppers, cauliflower, broccoli, strawberries, and ready-to-eat breakfast cereals are good sources of vitamin C. As with folate, eating fresh or lightly cooked foods is important because vitamin C loses a lot of its potency in cooking. High doses of vitamin C can lead to diarrhea and foil various medical tests.

lecithin A group of phospholipid compounds that are major components of cell membranes.

Choline

The dietary component choline is the latest addition to the list of essential nutrients. Choline is part of acetylcholine, a neurotransmitter associated with attention, learning and memory, muscle control, and many other functions. It is also part of phospholipids, such as **lecithin,** the major component of the cell membrane. Finally, choline participates in some aspects of homocysteine metabolism.

There has been only one published study examining the effect of inadequate dietary intake of choline in healthy humans. The study of male volunteers showed decreased choline stores and liver damage when humans were fed choline-deficient total parental (intravenous) nutrition solutions. Based on this one study, plus laboratory animal studies, choline has been deemed essential, but is not yet classified as a vitamin.

Choline Sources and Needs

Choline is widely distributed in foods. Milk, liver, and peanuts are sources. Lecithins often are added to food during processing, so this is yet another source. There is so much choline available in ordinary foods that it is unlikely that a dietary deficiency exists naturally. Choline also can be synthesized from the nonessential (dispensable) amino acid serine.

Food Sources of Choline

Food Item and Amount	Choline (milligrams)
Egg, 1 each	126
Cod, 3 ounces	70
Chicken, 3 ounces	56
Fat-free milk, 1 cup	37
Beef, 3 ounces	36
Yogurt, 1 cup	31
Wheat germ, 2 tablespoons	21
Peanut butter, 2 tablespoons	20
Cottage cheese, ½ cup	20
Orange, 1 each	12
Broccoli, ½ cup	7
Squash, ½ cup	7
Whole-wheat bread, 1 slice	7
Apple, 1 each	7
Romaine lettuce, 4 leaves	6
White bread, 1 slice	3

Adequate Intake for adults; 425 milligrams (women) to 550 milligrams (men)

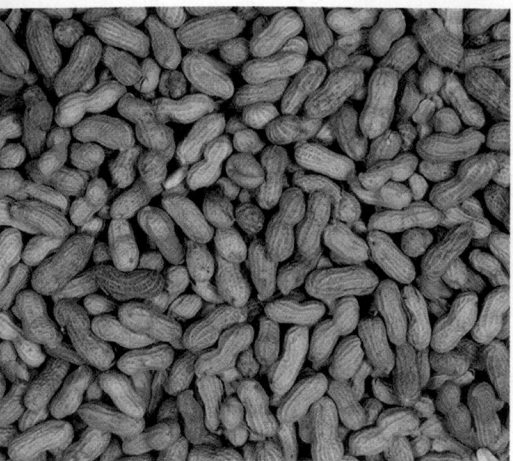

Nuts, such as peanuts, are a good source of choline. Body cells also produce choline.

The Adequate Intake for choline for adults is 425 to 550 milligrams per day. Currently we don't know if a dietary supply is needed at all life stages. Although Adequate Intakes are set for choline, it may be that the choline requirement can be met by body synthesis at some or all stages of life. We consume ample choline from food, at least 700 to 1000 milligrams per day.

∎ Upper Level for Choline

The Upper Level for adults is 3.5 grams per day. This is based on development of a fishy body odor and low blood pressure at excessive intakes.

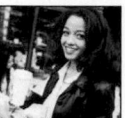

Real Life Scenario Follow-Up

Use of *Nutramega* poses some health risks for Kristen. Taking two to three tablets every 3 hours would mean taking at least 16 tablets per day. This alone would provide an intake of vitamin A, vitamin C, and zinc well in excess of the Upper Levels for these nutrients. Intake of preformed vitamin A would be 1.3 times the Upper Level, intake of vitamin C would be 3.4 times the Upper Level, and intake of zinc would be 3 times the Upper Level. Intake of selenium, however, falls well below the Upper Level set for that nutrient. This is how the math works out.

Vitamin A

33% (0.33) times the Daily Value of 1000 micrograms RAE equals 330 micrograms RAE per tablet. Sixteen tablets would yield 5280 micrograms RAE. The Upper Level is 3000 micrograms RAE for preformed vitamin A. Since 75% of the vitamin A is pre-formed vitamin A, this yields 3960 micrograms RAE of preformed vitamin A (5280 × 0.75 = 3960), or 1.3 times the Upper Level (3960/3000 = 1.3).

Vitamin C

700% (7) times the Daily Value of 60 milligrams equals 420 milligrams per tablet. 16 tablets would yield 6720 milligrams. The Upper Level is 2000 milligrams. This would then yield 3.4 times the Upper Level (6720/2000 = 3.4).

Zinc

50% (0.5) times the Daily Value of 15 milligrams equals 7.5 milligrams per tablet. 16 tablets would yield 120 milligrams. The Upper Level is 40 milligrams. This would then yield 3 times the Upper Level (120/40 = 3).

Selenium

10% (0.1) times the Daily Value of 70 micrograms equals 7 micrograms per tablet. 16 tablets would yield 112 micrograms. This is less than the Upper Level of 400 micrograms.

The maintenance dose of two to three tablets per day poses no risk per se, but *Nutramega* is very expensive compared to the cost of the typical multivitamin and mineral supplement (a 1-month supply would cost about $2 compared to about $15 for *Nutramega*). Overall, Kristen is smart to be concerned about meeting her nutrient needs, but the stress she is under does not increase nutrient needs. A healthy diet as suggested by MyPyramid should be her primary focus. Taking a balanced multivitamin and mineral supplement is also a reasonable practice.

Table 8-3 summarizes much of what we know about the water-soluble vitamins. Now that you have studied the vitamins, review MyPyramid and note how each group can make an important vitamin contribution (Fig. 8-13).

Table 8-3 Summary of the Water-Soluble Vitamins

Vitamin	Major Functions	RDA or Adequate Intake	Dietary Sources*	Deficiency Symptoms	Toxicity Symptoms
Thiamin	• Coenzyme of carbohydrate metabolism • Nerve function	1.1–1.2 milligrams	• Sunflower seeds • Pork • Whole and enriched grains • Dried beans • Peas	*Beriberi* • Nervous tingling • Poor coordination • Edema • Heart changes • Weakness	None
Riboflavin[†]	• Coenzyme of carbohydrate metabolism	1.1–1.3 milligrams	• Milk • Mushrooms • Spinach • Liver • Enriched grains	• Inflammation of the mouth and tongue • Cracks at the corners of the mouth • Eye disorders	None
Niacin	• Coenzyme of energy metabolism • Coenzyme of fat synthesis • Coenzyme of fat breakdown	14–16 milligrams (niacin equivalents)	• Mushrooms • Bran • Tuna • Salmon • Chicken • Beef • Liver • Peanuts • Enriched grains	*Pellagra* • Diarrhea • Dermatitis • Dementia • Death	Upper Level is 35 milligrams from supplements, based on flushing of skin
Pantothenic acid	• Coenzyme of energy metabolism • Coenzyme of fat synthesis • Coenzyme of fat breakdown	5 milligrams	• Mushrooms • Liver • Broccoli • Eggs *Most foods have some.*	• No natural deficiency disease or symptoms	None
Biotin	• Coenzyme of glucose production • Coenzyme of fat synthesis	30 micrograms	• Cheese • Egg yolks • Cauliflower • Peanut butter • Liver	• Dermatitis • Tongue soreness • Anemia • Depression	Unknown
Vitamin B-6[†]	• Coenzyme of protein metabolism • Neurotransmitter synthesis • Hemoglobin synthesis *Many other functions*	1.3–1.7 milligrams	• Animal protein foods • Spinach • Broccoli • Bananas • Salmon • Sunflower seeds	• Headache • Anemia • Convulsions • Nausea • Vomiting • Flaky skin • Sore tongue	Upper Level is 100 milligrams, based on nerve destruction
Folate (folic acid)[†]	• Coenzyme involved in DNA synthesis *Many other functions*	400 micrograms (dietary folate equivalents)	• Green leafy vegetables • Orange juice • Organ meats • Sprouts • Sunflower seeds	• Megaloblastic anemia • Inflammation of tongue • Diarrhea • Poor growth • Depression	None likely Upper Level for adults set at 1000 micrograms for synthetic folic acid (exclusive of food folate), based on masking of B-12 deficiency
Vitamin B-12[†]	• Coenzyme of folate metabolism • Nerve function *Many other functions*	2.4 micrograms *Older adults should use fortified foods or supplements.*	• Animal foods (not natural in plants) • Organ meats • Oysters • Clams • Fortified, ready-to-eat breakfast cereals	• Macrocytic anemia • Poor nerve function	None

(Continued)

Table 8-3 (Continued)

Vitamin	Major Functions	RDA or Adequate Intake	Dietary Sources*	Deficiency Symptoms	Toxicity Symptoms
Vitamin C	• Connective tissue synthesis • Hormone synthesis • Neurotransmitter synthesis • Possible antioxidant activity	75–90 milligrams *Smokers should add 35 milligrams.*	• Citrus fruits • Strawberries • Broccoli • Greens	• Scurvy • Poor wound healing • Pinpoint hemorrhages • Bleeding gums	Upper Level is 2 grams, based on development of diarrhea Can also alter some diagnostic tests
Choline[†]	• Neurotransmitter synthesis • Phospholipid synthesis	425–550 milligrams	Widely distributed in foods and self-synthesized	No natural deficiency	Upper Level is 3.5 grams per day based on development of fishy body odor and reduced blood pressure

*Fortified ready-to-eat breakfast cereals are good sources for most of these vitamins and a common source of B vitamins for many of us.
[†]These nutrients also participate in homocysteine metabolism, which in turn may reduce the risk of developing cardiovascular disease.

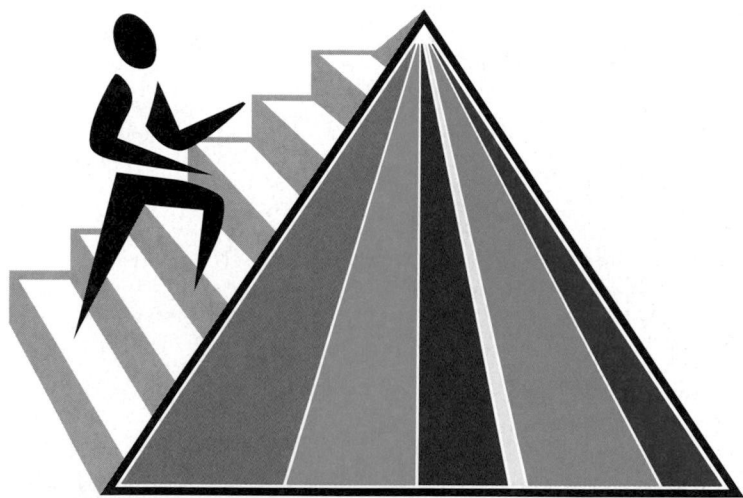

Grains	**Vegetables**	**Fruits**	**Oils**	**Milk**	**Meat & Beans**
• Thiamin • Riboflavin • Niacin • Folic acid	• Vitamin A • Vitamin K • Folate • Vitamin C	• Vitamin A • Vitamin C	• Vitamin E	• Vitamin D • Riboflavin • Vitamin B-12 • Choline	• Thiamin • Riboflavin • Niacin • Biotin • Vitamin B-6 • Vitamin B-12 • Choline

Figure 8-13 Certain groups of MyPyramid are especially rich sources of various vitamins and choline. This is true for those listed. Each may be also found in other groups in the pyramid but in lower amounts. Pantothenic acid is also present in moderate amounts in many groups.

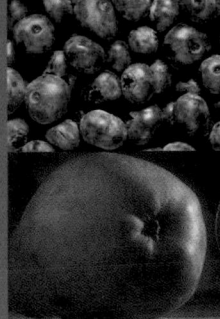

Nutrient Supplements: Who Needs Them and Why?

The term *multivitamin and mineral supplement* has been mentioned many times so far in this textbook. Today, these and other supplements are marketed as cures for anything and everything. This cure-all approach is promoted by the supplement industry and countless health-food stores, pharmacies, and supermarkets.

According to the Dietary Supplement Health and Education Act of 1994 (discussed in Chapter 1), a supplement in the United States is a product intended to supplement the diet that bears or contains one or more of the following dietary ingredients:

- A vitamin
- A mineral
- An herb or another botanical
- An amino acid
- A dietary substance to supplement the diet, which could be an extract or a combination of the first four ingredients in this list

The definition is very broad and covers a wide variety of nutritional substances. The use of dietary supplements is a common practice among North Americans and generates about $17 billion annually for the industry in the United States alone. Recall also from the Looking Further section at the end of Chapter 1 that unless FDA has evidence that a supplement is inherently dangerous or marketed with an illegal claim, it will not regulate such products closely. (The vitamin folate is an exception.) Currently, FDA has limited resources to police supplement manufacturers, and has to act against these manufacturers one at a time. Thus, we cannot rely on FDA to protect us from vitamin and mineral supplement overuse and misuse. We bear that responsibility ourselves, coupled with professional advice from a physician or registered dietitian.

Currently, the supplement makers can make broad claims about their products under the "structure or function" provision of the law, allowing the product onto the market without testing for safety or efficacy. The products, however, cannot claim to prevent, treat, or cure a disease. Since menopause and aging are not diseases per se, products alleging to treat symptoms of these conditions can be marketed without FDA approval. For example, a product that claims to treat hot flashes can be sold without any evidence to prove that the product actually works, but a product that claims to decrease the risk of cardiovascular disease by reducing blood cholesterol must have results from scientific studies that justify the claim.

Why do people take supplements? Reasons that are frequently given include the following:

- To reduce susceptibility to health problems (e.g., colds)
- To prevent heart attacks
- To prevent cancer
- To reduce stress
- To increase "energy"

Should you take a supplement? This is up to you. Currently, opinions vary about the wisdom and safety of supplement use even among knowledgeable scientists. Typically, nutrition scientists have recommended that supplement use is needed only by a few groups. Recently Dr. Alice Lichtenstein and Dr. Robert Russell, as well as the U.S. Preventive Services Task Force, came to the same conclusion, noting there is insufficient evidence to support the recommendation of use of a multivitamin and mineral supplement by the general population. These experts, however, indicate that use by certain groups of people is appropriate (see the next section in this feature for specific examples). On the other hand, over the last few years some reputable nutrition and medical scientists have recommended supplementation of specific nutrients for most (or all) adults.

Because recent research on a variety of nutrient supplements has revealed a lack of product quality, the USP (United States Pharmacopeia) designation is being extended to an increasing number of nutrient supplements. The USP standards designate strength, quality, purity, packaging, labeling, speed of dissolution, and acceptable length of storage of ingredients for drugs. The purpose of applying them to vitamin and mineral supplements is to establish professionally accepted standards for these products. Consumers who buy nutrient supplements should look for a USP label when comparing similar products, such as calcium supplements. If no USP label is present, the next best approach is to purchase nationally advertised brands. Most brand name nutrient supplements aren't labeled USP because the manufacturers prefer to guarantee the products via their brand names.

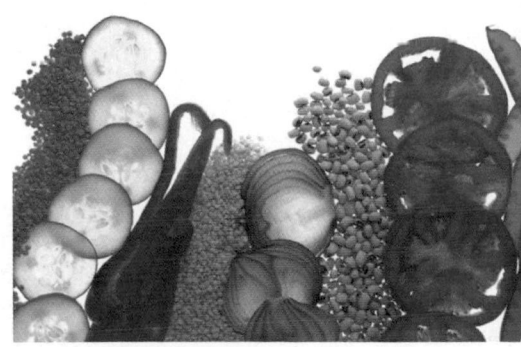

Focus first on foods that meet nutrient needs.

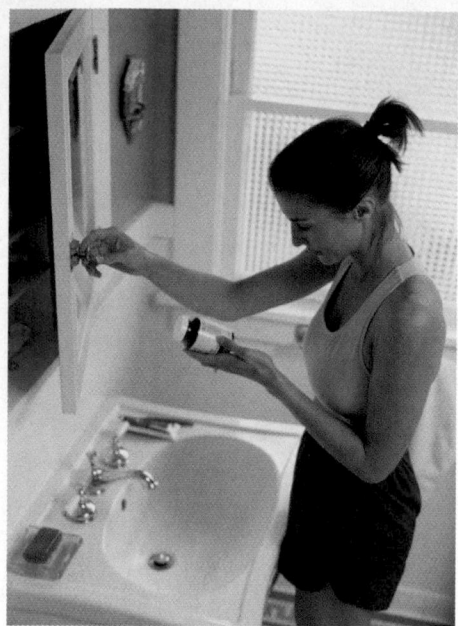

Long-term intake of just three times the Daily Value for some fat-soluble vitamins—particularly preformed vitamin A—can cause toxic effects. Know what you are taking if you use supplements.

As you might guess, generally the people who take supplements in our society are already healthy.

The rationale for widespread use is primarily because many North Americans have been unwilling to change their food habits, such as including ample fruits, vegetables, and whole grains. This gap can leave diets low in the vitamin folate. Adequate folate status when a woman becomes pregnant helps reduce the risk of certain birth defects in her offspring (400 micrograms per day of synthetic folic acid is recommended). Folate also limits homocysteine in the blood, a likely risk factor for cardiovascular disease that can affect all of us. In addition, the committee appointed by the Food and Nutrition Board that set current nutrient standards for vitamin B-12 suggested that adults over age 50 consume vitamin B-12 in a synthetic form, such as that added to ready-to-eat breakfast cereals or present in supplements. Synthetic vitamin B-12 is more easily absorbed than that found in food; this helps compensate for the fall in vitamin B-12 absorption often seen in one's older years.

In his book *Eat, Drink, and Be Healthy* (discussed in Chapter 2), nutrition expert Dr. Walter Willett also recommends that most people take a multivitamin and mineral supplement, citing that this is one inexpensive way to decrease the risk of developing a number of chronic diseases. Recently two articles in the *Journal of the American Medical Association* also supported this recommendation. Still, all these experts, whether they support use of a multivitamin and mineral supplement or not, emphasize that many of the health-promoting effects of foods cannot be found in a bottle. Recall the discussions of phytochemicals in Chapter 2 and the benefits of fiber in Chapter 4. Few or no phytochemicals and no fiber are present in supplements. Multivitamin and mineral supplements also contain little calcium in order to keep the pill size small, and the forms of magnesium, zinc, and copper used in many supplements (oxides) are not as well absorbed as forms found in foods.

Overall, supplement use cannot fix a poor diet in all respects. Uninformed megadose supplement use also can lead to harm—currently, most nutrient toxicity is a result of supplement use. Thus, we are advised to first take a good look at our dietary habits and then improve them, as outlined in Chapter 2 (see also Fig. 8-14). Finally, find out which nutrient gaps remain, and identify food sources that can help. Such a source could be ready-to-eat breakfast cereals to increase vitamin E, folic acid, and vitamin B-6 intake, and as well provide highly absorbable forms of vitamin B-12. One needs to be careful, however, as these products may provide the appropriate amount of nutrients in 1 serving, but the typical consumer may eat more than 1 serving. This can lead to an excessive intake of some nutrients, such as vitamin A, iron, and synthetic folic acid. Calcium-fortified orange juice could be used to increase calcium intake, or milk and yogurt to increase vitamin D and calcium intake.

If supplement use is desired, one should discuss this practice with a physician or registered dietitian, as some supplements can interfere with certain medicines. For example, vitamin B-6 can offset the action of L-dopa (used in treating Parkinson's disease), high intakes of vitamin K or vitamin E alter the action of anticlotting medications, large doses of vitamin C can interfere with certain cancer therapy regimens, excessive zinc intake can inhibit copper absorption, and large amounts of folate can mask signs and symptoms of a vitamin B-12 deficiency (review the section on toxicity of folate in this chapter). Remember, you *can* get too much of a good thing.

People Most Likely to Need Supplements

Various medical and health-related organizations suggest that the following vitamin and mineral supplements can be important for certain groups of healthy people:

- Women of childbearing age may need extra synthetic folic acid if their dietary patterns do not supply the recommended amount (400 micrograms).
- Women with excessive bleeding during menstruation may need extra iron.
- Women who are pregnant or breastfeeding may need extra iron, folate, and calcium.
- People with very low calorie intakes (less than about 1200 kcal per day) may need a range of vitamins and minerals. This is true of some women and many older people.

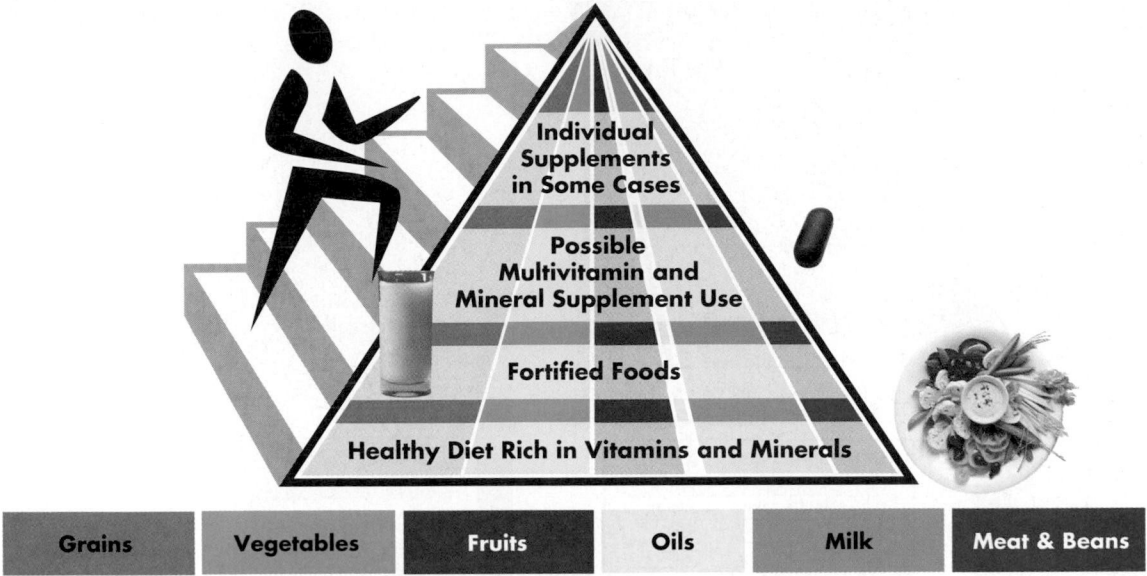

Figure 8-14 Supplement savvy—A MyPyramid approach to the use of nutrient supplementation. Emphasizing the bottom portion of the pyramid is always the first option.

- Strict vegans may need extra calcium, iron, zinc, and vitamin B-12.
- Newborns need a single dose of vitamin K, as directed by a physician.
- Some older infants may need fluoride supplements, as directed by a dentist.
- People with limited milk intake and sunlight exposure may need extra vitamin D. This includes breastfed infants, and many African-American and older people.
- People with lactose maldigestion or lactose intolerance, and those with allergies to dairy products, may need extra calcium.
- Adults over age 50 may need a synthetic source of vitamin B-12.
- People on very low-fat diets or diets low in plant oils and nuts may need some extra vitamin E.

Individuals with certain medical conditions (e.g., vitamin-resistant diseases or long-standing fat malabsorption) and those who use certain medications also may require supplementation with specific vitamins and minerals. Children who are "picky eaters" may require supplementation as well (see Chapter 14). Finally, smokers and alcohol abusers may benefit from supplementation, but cessation of these two activities is far more beneficial than any supplementation.

Which Supplement Should You Choose?

If you decide to take a multivitamin and mineral supplement, which one should you choose? As a start, choose a nationally recognized brand (from a supermarket or pharmacy) that contains about 100% of the Daily Values for the nutrients present. A multivitamin and mineral supplement should also generally be taken with or just after meals to maximize absorption. Make sure also that intake from the total of this supplement, any other supplements used, and highly fortified foods such as ready-to-eat breakfast cereals provide no more than the Upper Level for each vitamin and mineral. (See the inside cover of this textbook for Upper Levels.) This is especially important with regard to preformed vitamin A intake. Two exceptions are (1) both men and older women should make sure any product used is low in iron or iron-free to avoid

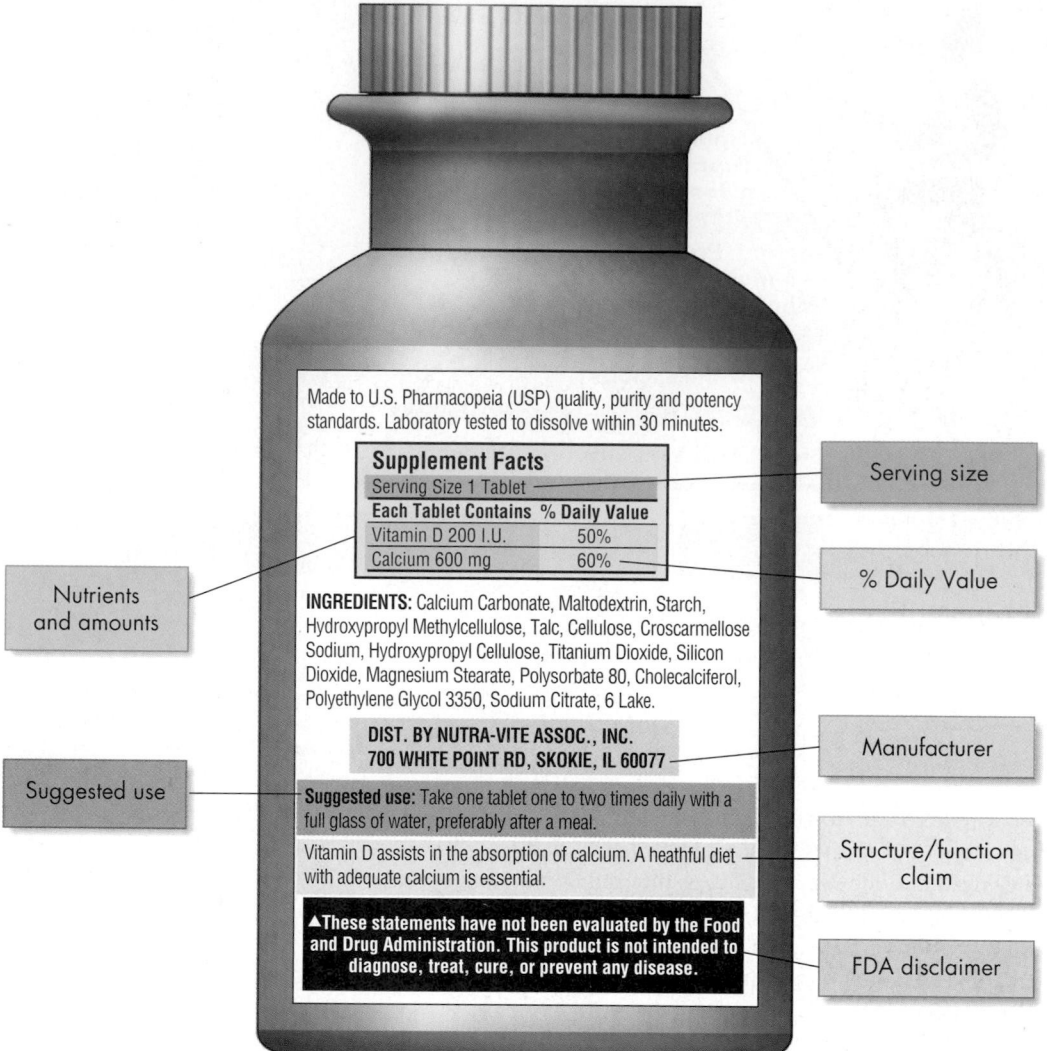

Made to U.S. Pharmacopeia (USP) quality, purity and potency standards. Laboratory tested to dissolve within 30 minutes.

Supplement Facts

Serving Size 1 Tablet

Each Tablet Contains	% Daily Value
Vitamin D 200 I.U.	50%
Calcium 600 mg	60%

INGREDIENTS: Calcium Carbonate, Maltodextrin, Starch, Hydroxypropyl Methylcellulose, Talc, Cellulose, Croscarmellose Sodium, Hydroxypropyl Cellulose, Titanium Dioxide, Silicon Dioxide, Magnesium Stearate, Polysorbate 80, Cholecalciferol, Polyethylene Glycol 3350, Sodium Citrate, 6 Lake.

DIST. BY NUTRA-VITE ASSOC., INC.
700 WHITE POINT RD, SKOKIE, IL 60077

Suggested use: Take one tablet one to two times daily with a full glass of water, preferably after a meal.

Vitamin D assists in the absorption of calcium. A heathful diet with adequate calcium is essential.

▲These statements have not been evaluated by the Food and Drug Administration. This product is not intended to diagnose, treat, cure, or prevent any disease.

Labels: Serving size · % Daily Value · Manufacturer · Structure/function claim · FDA disclaimer · Nutrients and amounts · Suggested use

Figure 8-15 Nutrient supplements display a nutrition label that is different from that of foods. This Supplement Facts label must list the ingredient(s), amount(s) per serving, serving size, suggested use, and % Daily Value if one has been established. Note that this label also includes structure/function claims. Thus, it also must include the FDA warning that these claims have not been evaluated by the agency.

Not exceeding the Upper Level set for sodium and chloride may be hard for many people.

possible iron overload (see Chapter 9 for details), and (2) somewhat exceeding the Upper Level for vitamin D is likely a safe practice for adults. One should read the labels carefully to be sure of what is being taken (Fig. 8-15).

Another consideration in choosing a supplement is avoiding superfluous ingredients, such as para-aminobenzoic acid (PABA), hesperidin complex, inositol, bee pollen, and lecithins. These are not needed in our diets. They are especially common in expensive supplements sold in health-food stores and by mail. In addition, use of l-tryptophan and high doses of beta-carotene or fish oils is discouraged.

Five websites to help you evaluate ongoing claims and evaluate safety of supplements are:

www.acsh.org
www.quackwatch.com
www.ncahf.org
dietary-supplements.info.nih.gov
www.eatright.org

The sites are maintained by groups or individuals committed to providing reasoned and authoritative nutrition and health advice to consumers.

Vitamin-Like Compounds

A variety of vitamin-like compounds are found in the body. These include the following:

- Carnitine, which is needed to transport fatty acids into cell mitochondria
- Inositol, which is part of cell membranes
- Taurine, which is part of bile acids
- Lipoic acid, which participates in carbohydrate metabolism and acts as an antioxidant

All of these vitamin-like compounds can be synthesized by cells using common building blocks, such as amino acids and glucose. Our diets are also a source. In disease states or periods of active growth, synthesis of vitamin-like compounds may not meet needs, so dietary intake can be crucial. The needs for vitamin-like compounds in certain groups of individuals, such as for preterm infants, are being investigated. Although promoted and sold by health-food stores, these vitamin-like compounds need not be included in the diet of the average healthy adult.

Summary

1. Vitamins are carbon-containing compounds we generally need daily in small amounts from foods. They yield no energy directly, but many contribute to energy-yielding chemical reactions in the body and promote growth and development. Many vitamins act as coenzymes, which help enzymes function. Vitamins A, D, E, and K are fat soluble, whereas the B vitamins and vitamin C are water soluble.

2. Vitamin A is a family of compounds that includes several forms of preformed vitamin A. Three forms of carotenoids can also yield vitamin A; some also function as antioxidants. Vitamin A contributes to vision, immune function, and cell development. Vitamin A is found in liver and fish oils; carotenoids are especially plentiful in dark green and orange vegetables. Vitamin A can be quite toxic, even when taken at just 3 times the RDA for preformed vitamin A (the Upper Level). High vitamin A intakes are especially dangerous during pregnancy.

3. Vitamin D is both a hormone and a vitamin. Human skin synthesizes it using sunshine and a cholesterol-like substance. If we don't spend enough time in the sun, such foods as fish and fortified milk can supply the vitamin. The active hormone form of vitamin D helps regulate blood calcium in part by increasing calcium absorption from the intestine. Infants and children who don't get enough vitamin D may develop rickets, and adults develop osteomalacia. Older people, African-Americans, and breastfed infants often need a supplemental source. Vitamin D is potentially a very toxic substance in infancy and early childhood.

4. Vitamin E functions primarily as an antioxidant and is found in plant oils. By donating electrons to electron-seeking, free-radical (oxidizing) compounds, it neutralizes them. This effect shields cell membranes and red blood cells from breakdown. Claims are made about the curative powers of vitamin E, but more information is needed before megadose vitamin E recommendations for healthy adults can be made with certainty. The Upper Level is set at about 50 times adult needs.

5. Vitamin K helps blood clot and increases the calcium-binding potential of some organs. Some vitamin K absorbed each day comes from bacterial synthesis in the intestine, but most comes from foods, primarily green, leafy vegetables. Vitamin K is poorly stored in the body, but our dietary intake alone is usually sufficient. People who can't absorb fat well or who are on antibiotics for long periods may need extra vitamin K. No Upper Level has been set.

6. Thiamin, riboflavin, and niacin play key roles as coenzymes in energy-yielding reactions. They help metabolize carbohydrates, fats, and proteins. Alcoholism and a poor diet can create deficiencies of these three nutrients, which often shows up as symptoms in the brain and nervous system, skin, and GI tract. Enriched grain products are common sources of all three of these vitamins. Only niacin has an Upper Level (2.5 times adult needs).

7. Pantothenic acid, which participates in many aspects of cell metabolism, is widely distributed among foods. Biotin, which participates in glucose production, fatty acid synthesis, and DNA synthesis, can be synthesized by bacteria in the intestine. Biotin comes from foods such as eggs, peanuts, and cheese. No Upper Levels have been set for either vitamin.

8. Vitamin B-6 performs a vital role in protein metabolism, especially in synthesizing nonessential amino acids. It also helps synthesize neurotransmitters and performs other metabolic roles, such as metabolism of homocysteine. Headaches, a form of anemia, nausea, and vomiting result from a B-6 deficiency. Regular consumption of animal protein foods and rich plant sources such as broccoli provide needed vitamin B-6. Taking high doses causes damage to the nervous system. The Upper Level is about 60 times adult needs.

9. Folate plays an important role in DNA synthesis and homocysteine metabolism. Symptoms of a deficiency include generally poor cell division in various areas of the body, megaloblastic anemia, tongue inflammation, diarrhea, and poor growth. Pregnancy puts high demands for folate on the body; deficiency during the first month of pregnancy can result in neural tube defects in offspring. A deficiency can also occur in people with alcoholism. Food sources are leafy vegetables, organ meats, and orange juice. Women of childbearing age need to meet the RDA with synthetic folic acid. Great amounts of folate can be lost in prolonged cooking. Excess folate in the diet can mask a vitamin B-12 deficiency, so an Upper Level has been set at 2½ times adult needs (refers to synthetic folic acid only).

10. Vitamin B-12 is needed to metabolize folate and homocysteine, and maintain the insulation surrounding nerves. A deficiency

results in anemia (because of its relationship to folate) and nerve degeneration. Older people often suffer from inefficient absorption of vitamin B-12, in which case they can benefit from monthly injections or megadoses of the vitamin. Generally a dietary deficiency is unlikely because vitamin B-12 is highly concentrated in animal foods, which constitute a major part of the North American diet. Vitamin B-12 does not occur naturally in plant foods. Vegans need a supplemental source, and adults over age 50 should consume a synthetic source, such as that in ready-to-eat breakfast cereals. No Upper Level has been set.

11. Vitamin C is mainly used to synthesize collagen, a major protein for building connective tissue. A vitamin C deficiency results in scurvy, which is evidenced by poor wound healing, pinpoint hemorrhages in the skin, and bleeding gums. Vitamin C also modestly enhances iron absorption, is likely a general antioxidant, and is needed for synthesizing some hormones and neurotransmitters. Fresh fruits and vegetables, especially citrus fruits, are generally good sources. Because a great amount of vitamin C is lost in cooking, a diet should emphasize fresh or lightly cooked vegetables. Deficiencies can occur in people with alcoholism and those whose diets lack sufficient fruits and vegetables. Smoking makes matters worse for people already at risk. The Upper Level is set at about 20 times adult needs.

12. Choline is a dietary component that is available from a wide variety of foods and is synthesized in the body. It is used to form a neurotransmitter, among other functions, such as homocysteine metabolism. Nutritional needs have recently been set. No natural deficiency of choline has been reported. The Upper Level is set at about 8 times adult needs.

13. The vitamin-like compounds carnitine, inositol, taurine, and lipoic acid, while participating in many important chemical reactions in the body, are not true vitamins because they can be synthesized in the body from readily available building blocks; they are also obtained from the diet.

14. Taking a multivitamin and mineral supplement to help meet nutrient needs is recommended by some experts, while other experts suggest that only some in the population need such supplementation. Taking many nutrient supplements can lead to nutrient-related toxicity, so any such use should be carefully considered. The clearest evidence is for a diet rich in fruits and vegetables and whole-grain breads and cereals, not reliance on supplements.

Study Questions

1. Why is the risk of toxicity greater with the fat-soluble vitamins A and D than with water-soluble vitamins in general?

2. How would you determine which fruits and vegetables displayed in the produce section of your supermarket are likely to provide plenty of carotenoids?

3. What is the primary function of the vitamin D hormone? Which groups of people likely need to supplement their diets with vitamin D, and on what do you base your answer?

4. Describe how vitamin E functions as an antioxidant. Use the term *free radical*.

5. Describe how the RDA, Daily Value, and Upper Level for vitamin B-6 should be used in everyday life. How do the RDA and Daily Value for vitamin B-6 differ?

6. The need for certain vitamins increases as energy expenditure increases. Name two such vitamins and explain why this is the case.

7. Take one of the B vitamins that might be low in the North American diet and explain why the lack might occur.

8. Which vitamins are lost from cereal grains as a result of the "refining" process? Which vitamins must be replaced by law in the subsequent enrichment process?

9. Why does FDA limit the amount of folate that may be included in supplements and fortified foods?

10. Is it necessary for North Americans to consume a great excess of vitamin C to avoid the possibility of a deficiency? Do vitamin C intakes well above the RDA have any negative consequences?

Further Readings

1. ADA Reports: Position of the American Dietetic Association: Fortification and nutritional supplements. *Journal of the American Dietetic Association* 105:1300, 2005.

   The best nutritional strategy for promoting optimal health and reducing the risk of chronic disease is to wisely choose a wide variety of foods. Additional vitamins and minerals from fortified foods and/or supplements can help some people meet their nutritional needs as set by science-based nutrition standards (e.g., the Dietary Reference Intakes).

2. Are you getting enough of this vitamin? *Harvard Health Letter* 30(10):1, 2005

   Those at risk for B-12 deficits include older adults and strict vegans. Although a severe deficiency is fairly unlikely other adults, mild shortfalls may affect balance, memory, and perhaps mood.

3. Aufiero E and others: Pyridoxine hydrochloride treatment of carpal tunnel syndrome: A review. *Nutrition Reviews* 62(3):96, 2004.

   Some, but not all, studies have found megadose vitamin B-6 therapy effective in helping treat carpal tunnel syndrome. This article discusses the latest findings on this topic.

4. Baily LB and others: Folic acid supplements and fortification affect the risk for neural tube defects, vascular disease and cancer: Evolving science. *Journal of Nutrition* 133:1961s, 2003.

   Adequate folic acid status before and during pregnancy reduces the risk of neural tube defects by about 70 percent. The ability of folic acid to reduce the risk of cancer and cardiovascular disease are interesting scientific theories that need more research before clear recommendations can be made.

5. Dawson-Hughes B: Racial/ethnic considerations in making recommendations for vitamin D for adult and elderly men and women. *American Journal of Clinical Nutrition* 80(suppl): 1763S, 2004.

   In the winter months broad-based vitamin D supplementation to 1000 IU/day may be needed to attain adequate vitamin D status in adults. This recommendation would especially benefit African Americans and older adults in general.

6. DeLuca HF: Overview of general physiologic features and functions of Vitamin D. *American Journal of Clinical Nutrition* 80:1689S, 2004.

   Vitamin D is a prohormone produced in skin through ultraviolet irradiation of a form of cholesterol. It is biologically inert and must be metabolized in the liver, then in the kidney, before function. The hormonal form of vitamin D acts through a receptor on the cell nucleus to carry out its many functions, including calcium absorption, phosphate absorption, calcium mobilization in bone, and calcium reabsorption in the kidney. Vitamin D also has several non-calcium-related functions in the body, as described in this overview.

7. Fairfield K, Fletcher R: Vitamins for chronic disease prevention in adults: Scientific review and clinical applications. *Journal of the American Medical Association* 287:3116, 2002 and 287:3127, 2002.

While vitamin deficiency diseases are no longer common in North America, many physicians are suggesting that marginal intakes of many vitamins and minerals consumed by some North Americans may increase the risk of developing some chronic diseases, including cancer and cardiovascular disease. To help ensure optimal intakes of most of the vitamins and minerals, the authors recommend that adult North Americans consume a daily multivitamin and mineral supplement.

8. Fischer LM and others: Ad libitum choline intake in healthy individuals meets or exceeds the proposed Adequate Intake level. *Journal of Nutrition* 135:826, 2005.

Using new and recently published data on the amount of choline in a large number of common foods, the authors report that healthy men and women consumed adequate amounts of choline. The current Adequate Intake level for choline seems to be a good approximation of the actual intake of this nutrient.

9. Food and Nutrition Board, Institute of Medicine: *Dietary Reference Intakes for thiamin, riboflavin, niacin, vitamin B-6, folate, vitamin B-12, pantothenic acid, biotin, and choline.* Washington, DC: National Academy Press, 1998.

Explanation as to how nutrient recommendations were established for the B vitamins and choline, with specific reference to establishing RDA and related standards. The functions of each of the B vitamins and choline are explained.

10. Food and Nutrition Board, Institute of Medicine: *Dietary Reference Intakes for vitamin A, vitamin K, arsenic, boron, chromium, copper, iodine, iron, manganese, molybdenum, nickel, silicon, vanadium, and zinc.* Washington, DC: National Academy Press, 2001.

Recommendations for vitamin A and vitamin K intake are listed. The rationale used to set the RDA or Adequate Intake and Upper Level for these nutrients is discussed in detail.

11. Food and Nutrition Board, Institute of Medicine: *Dietary Reference Intakes for vitamin C, vitamin E, selenium, and carotenoids.* Washington, DC: National Academy Press, 2000.

The functions of antioxidant nutrients, how RDA and related standards were determined, and deficiency and toxicity symptoms are explained. This is the definitive report by the panel of experts on nutrient needs for dietary antioxidants.

12. Food and Nutrition Board, Institute of Medicine: *Dietary Reference Intakes for calcium, phosphorus, magnesium, vitamin D, and fluoride.* Washington, DC: National Academy Press, 1997.

The RDAs and related standards for vitamin D and some minerals are discussed in detail. A major change in setting these new (and all other) estimates of human needs is the use of a specific biolog-ical marker or estimate of current intakes that shows adequacy.

13. Haider A, Shaw JC: Treatment of acne vulgaris. *Journal of the American Medical Association* 292:726, 2004.

Analogs of vitamin A are one potential treatment for acne vulgaris. Since many college students experience this condition, the entire article should be of interest.

14. Holick M: Vitamin D: importance in the prevention of cancers, type 1 diabetes, heart disease, and osteoporosis. *American Journal of Clinical Nutrition* 79:362, 2004.

Adequate sun exposure is very important for maintaining vitamin D status. Anyone who does not obtain adequate sun exposure needs to find it dietary source of vitamin D. Use of a multivitamin and mineral supplement to meet such needs is also appropriate. Besides affecting calcium metabolism, vitamin D might also reduce the risk of certain forms of cancer, such as colon cancer, and as well possibly some autoimmune diseases, such as type 1 diabetes. This article goes into great detail regarding these and other potential benefits of vitamin D.

15. Lichtenstein AH and Russell RM: Essential nutrients: food or supplements? Where should the emphasis be? *Journal of the American Medical Association* 294:351, 2005.

There is insufficient evidence to justify a shift in public health policy from one that emphasizes a food-based diet to fulfill nutrient requirements and promote optimal health to one that emphasizes dietary supplementation. Targeted nutrient supplementation is appropriate in some cases, however, as reviewed by these authors.

16. Maras JE and others: Intake of a-Tocopherol is limited among US adults. *Journal of the American Dietetic Association* 104:567, 2004.

Vitamin E consumption in the US does not generally meet the current RDA. Greater use of nuts, seeds, whole grain breads and cereals, and vitamin E-rich plant oils is advocated to close the gap between intakes and needs.

17. Martinez MA and others: Folate and colorectal neoplasia: relation between plasma and dietary markers of folate and adenoma recurrence. *American Journal of Clinical Nutrition* 79:691, 2004.

Adequate folate nutriture is associated with a lower risk of colon cancer. Intakes of about 600 micrograms per day showed the greatest effect. A healthy diet can easily provide this amount of folate.

18. McNaughton SA and others: Supplement use is associated with health status and health-related behaviors in the 1946 British birth cohort. *Journal of Nutrition* 135: 1782, 2005.

The healthiest people in this large group of people studied were the ones most likely to take supplements. This suggests that the people who actually benefit least from this practice are the ones to do so.

19. Padayatty SJ and others: Vitamin C as an antioxidant: evaluation of its role in disease prevention. *Journal of the American College of Nutrition* 22(1):18, 2003.

Vitamin C has many roles in the body, but its specific action as an antioxidant is still an open question. As little as 10 milligrams per day prevents scurvy; a diet providing 200 milligrams may lead to additional health benefits by saturating blood and tissues in the body. Whether any benefit is because of its potential antioxidant capabilities requires more research.

20. Ribaya-Mercado JD and Blumberg JB: Lutein and zeaxanthin and their potential roles in disease prevention. *Journal of the American College of Nutrition* 23:6:567S, 2004.

Lutein and zeaxanthin are carotenoids found particularly in dark-green leafy vegetables and in egg yolks. They are widely distributed in tissues and are the principal carotenoids in the eye lens and macular region of the retina. Epidemiologic studies indicating an inverse relationship between lutein and zeaxanthin intake and status and both cataract and age-related macular degeneration suggest these compounds can play a protective role in the eye. Some studies show lutein and zeaxanthin may also help reduce the risk of breast cancer, lung cancer, heart disease and stroke.

21. Stover PJ: Physiology of folate and vitamin B-12 in health and disease. *Nutrition Reviews* 62(6):S3, 2004.

This paper reviews the functions of folate and B-12, highlighting the risks of over- and under-consumption.

22. U.S. Preventive Services Task Force: Routine vitamin supplementation to prevent cancer and cardiovascular disease: Recommendations and rationale. *Annals of Internal Medicine* 139:51, 2003.

The health benefits of nutrient supplementation remain uncertain, while there is much evidence to support a diet high in fruit, vegetables, and legumes. Currently the clearest use of supplements is that of folic acid for the prevention of neural tube defects that develop during pregnancy. Other potential benefits of supplementation, such as a lowering of blood homocysteine, need to be established by further studies.

23. Vitamin A: "Magic bullet" that can backfire. *Tufts University Health and Nutrition Letter*, p. 4, February 2005

Vitamin A and its derivatives (e.g., beta-carotene) are micronutrients crucial to growth, immune function, reproductive processes and cell physiology. While it is well-known that very high doses of vitamin A are toxic, it now appears that even moderately high doses can increase chances of birth defects, liver disease, and possibly increase risk for hip fractures in postmenopausal women. In the US, the only people for whom vitamin A supplements are warranted are those who have chronic G.I tract diseases that lead to difficulty in absorbing nutrients.

24. Vitamin excess: Can too much be bad? *Mayo Clinic Health Letter*, p. 4, February 2004.

The potential for vitamin toxicity needs to be considered when considering supplement use. This is especially true for vitamin A and vitamin B-6, and in some cases, vitamin D.

I. *Measuring Your Vitamin Intake Against the RDAs*

 This activity requires you to reexamine the nutritional assessment you did for Chapters 1 and 2. You recorded all the foods and drinks you consumed for 1 day and their quantities. Then you assessed your intake by calculating the total amounts of nutrients you consumed. You were then asked to compare your nutrient intake to the RDAs. Take your completed assessment and look at your intakes of vitamins A, E, C, B-6, B-12, and thiamin, riboflavin, niacin, and folate. Record these numbers in the table. Next, record the RDAs for each of these nutrients from your assessment. Then, record the percentage of the RDA you consumed for each vitamin. Lastly, place a +, −, or = in the space provided, reflecting an intake higher than, lower than, or equal to the RDA.

Vitamin	Intake	RDA	% of RDA	+, −, =
A				
E				
C				
Thiamin				
Riboflavin				
Niacin				
B-6				
Folate				
B-12				

Analysis

1. Which of your vitamin intakes equaled or exceeded the RDA?

   _____

2. Which of your vitamin intakes were below the RDA?

   _____

3. What foods could you eat to improve your dietary intake of vitamins in low amounts in your diet? (Review sources of certain vitamins in this chapter.)

   _____

   _____

II. *Spotting Fraudulent Claims on the Internet*

Search for vitamins and vitamin-like substances that are sold over the Internet. Are the websites found really selling vitamins, or are they actually a cover for selling something else? Compare the price of the vitamins from these sites with the price you would pay at the local supermarket or drug store. Do any of these sites display any disclaimers or warnings about the products? Does the seller make health claims about their products? Based on what you've learned, are the claims reasonable? Can you be sure the supplements contain what they say they do?

Water and Minerals

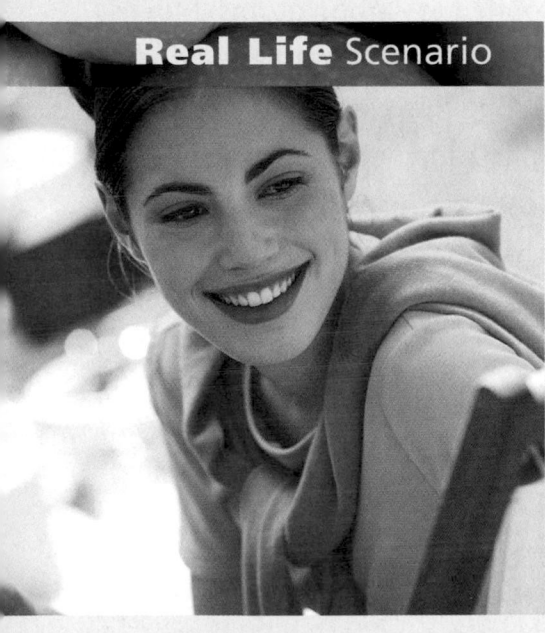

Jana, a sophomore in college, recently gave up drinking milk. She thought this would help her stay slim by avoiding all the calories in milk. Her mother is concerned about her diet change. One of her primary concerns is the future risk of osteoporosis. Jana needs an adequate source of calcium in her diet to allow for continued bone development and maintenance of the bone mass she already has. Jana also recently started smoking, and her only physical activity is practice for the Women's Glee Club.

Jana's diet on a recent day consisted of the following items. For breakfast, she had oatmeal made with water, a banana, and a cup of fruit juice. At midmorning, she bought a snack cake from the vending machine. At lunch, she had vegetable pasta, bread with olive oil, a side salad, 1 ounce of mixed nuts, and a soft drink. For dinner, she had a hamburger sandwich along with mixed vegetables and another soft drink. As an evening snack, she had some cookies and hot tea.

What factors place Jana at risk for osteoporosis in the future? What changes to her current diet could reduce that risk?

Chapter 9 Objectives

Chapter 9 is designed to allow you to:

1. List and briefly explain the functions of water in the body.

2. Classify the minerals as major or trace minerals.

3. List conditions of the body, dietary factors, and other pertinent relationships that influence the absorption, retention, and availability of specific minerals.

4. List key functions of the major and trace minerals.

5. Identify possible deficiency and toxicity symptoms associated with the major and trace minerals.

6. List at least two food sources for each of the major and trace minerals.

7. Describe the processes involving minerals that aid in maintaining bone health as well as those that aid in control of blood pressure.

Check out the **Contemporary Nutrition Online Learning Center**
www.mhhe.com/wardlawcont6 for quizzes, flash cards, other activities, and web links designed to further help you learn about issues surrounding water and minerals.

Chapter 9 Outline

ater—the most versatile medium for a variety of chemical reactions—constitutes the major portion of the human body. Without water, biological processes necessary to life would cease in a matter of days. We must replenish water regularly because the body does not store it per se. We recognize this constant demand for water as thirst. Many nutrients, including minerals, exist in the body dissolved in water. Because the functioning of minerals is related to the characteristics of water, water and its roles in the body are explored first in Chapter 9.

Many minerals, like water, are vital to health. They are considered inorganic because they are typically not bonded to carbon atoms. Minerals are key participants in body metabolism, muscle movement, body growth, water balance, and other wide-ranging processes. Some of the minerals found in our bodies—for example, vanadium and arsenic—may not be necessary to sustain human life. Nevertheless, we know that some mineral deficiencies can cause severe health problems. For this reason, the study of minerals in Chapter 9 also is critical to understanding human nutrition.

Refresh Your Memory

As you begin your study of water and minerals in Chapter 9, you may want to review:

- Cell structure and function, digestion and absorption of nutrients, cardiovascular function, immunity, and endocrine function in Chapter 3
- The functions of vitamin D and vitamin K related to calcium and bone health in Chapter 8
- The role of vitamin C in collagen synthesis in Chapter 8

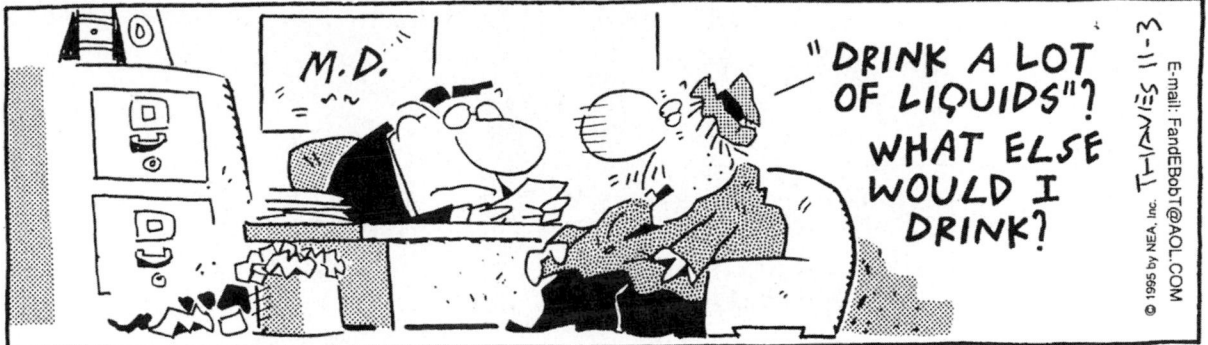

Replacing fluids—water as part of foods, beverages, and water itself—is an important daily task. Why is this so critical for maintaining health? And why are infants, athletes, and older adults particularly at risk for dehydration? In addition, how does water interact with some of the minerals used by the body? Chapter 9 provides some answers.

Water

To appreciate how minerals operate in the body, it helps to understand the nature and general chemical properties of water, as well as its specific nutrient-related functions.

Life as we know it could not exist without water. Acting as a **solvent,** it dissolves many body compounds such as sodium chloride (table salt). Water is the perfect medium for body processes because it enables chemical reactions to occur. Water even participates directly in many of these reactions. It forms the greatest component of the human body, making up 50% to 70% of the body's weight (about 10 gallons or 40 liters). Lean muscle tissue contains about 73% water. Adipose tissue is about 20% water. Thus, as fat content increases (and the percentage of lean tissue decreases) in the body, total body water content drifts toward 50%.

Depending on the amount of fat stores present, an adult can survive for about 8 weeks without eating food but only a few days without drinking water. This occurs not because water is more important than carbohydrate, fat, protein, vitamins, or minerals, but rather because we can not conserve water as well as we can the other components of our diet, nor can we store it per se.

■ Water in the Body—Intracellular and Extracellular Fluid

Water flows in and out of body cells through cell membranes. Water inside cells forms part of the **intracellular fluid**—the fluid within the cells. When water is outside cells or in the bloodstream, it is part of the **extracellular fluid**—that outside cells (Fig. 9-1). Because cell membranes are permeable to water, water shifts freely in and out of cells. For example, if blood volume decreases, water can move from the areas inside and around cells to the bloodstream to increase blood volume. On the other hand, if blood volume increases, water can shift out of the bloodstream into cells and the surrounding areas, leading to edema (review Fig. 6-8 in Chapter 6).

The body controls the amount of water in the intracellular and extracellular compartments mainly by controlling *ion* concentrations. Ions are minerals that have electrical charges, and so are called **electrolytes.** Water is attracted to ions, such as sodium, potassium, chloride, phosphate, magnesium, and calcium. By controlling the movements of ions in and out of the cellular compartments, the body maintains the appropriate amount of water in each compartment using a process called **osmosis.** Overall, where ions go, water follows (Fig. 9-2).

solvent A liquid substance in which other substances dissolve.

intracellular fluid Fluid contained within a cell; it represents about two-thirds of all body fluid.

extracellular fluid Fluid present outside the cells; represents about one-third of all body fluid.

electrolytes Substances that separate into ions in water and, in turn, are able to conduct an electrical current. These include sodium, chloride, and potassium.

osmosis The passage of a solvent such as water through a semipermeable membrane from a less concentrated compartment to a more concentrated compartment.

Figure 9-1 Fluid compartments in the body. Total fluid volume is about 40 liters (about 165 cups).

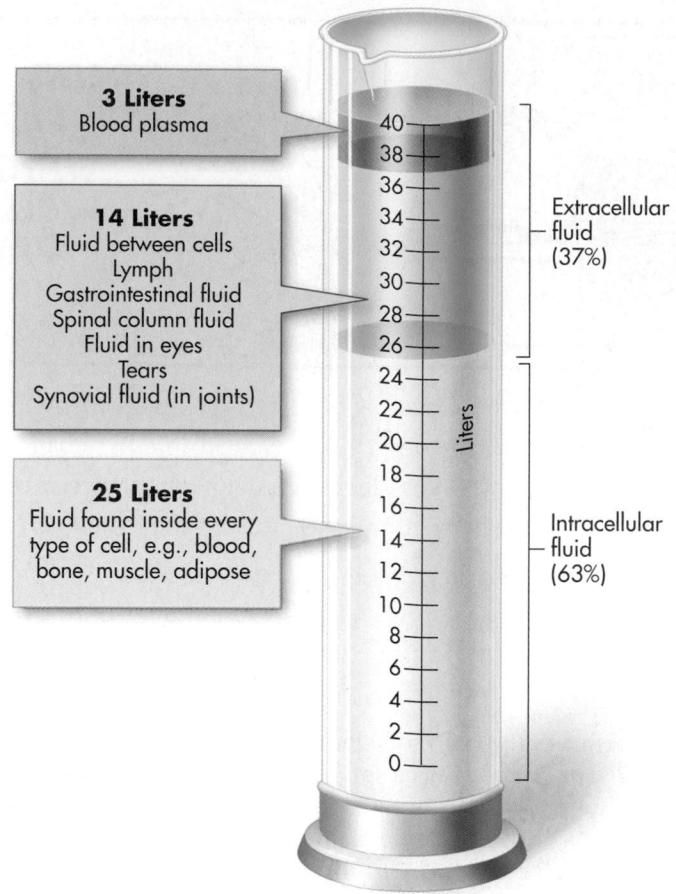

3 Liters
Blood plasma

14 Liters
Fluid between cells
Lymph
Gastrointestinal fluid
Spinal column fluid
Fluid in eyes
Tears
Synovial fluid (in joints)

25 Liters
Fluid found inside every type of cell, e.g., blood, bone, muscle, adipose

Extracellular fluid (37%)

Intracellular fluid (63%)

Liters

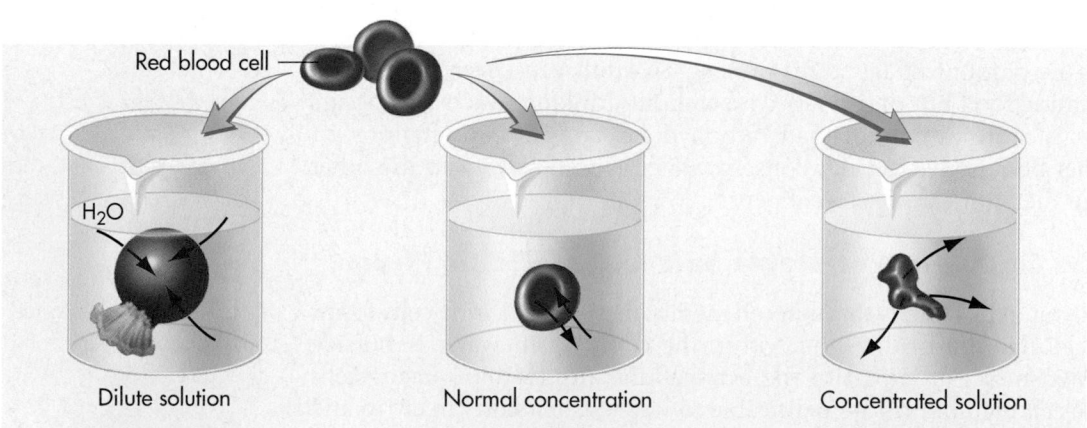

Red blood cell

H_2O

Dilute solution

Normal concentration

Concentrated solution

(a) A dilute solution with a low ion concentration results in swelling (*black arrows*) and subsequent rupture (*puff of red in the lower left part of the cell*) of a red blood cell placed into the solution.

(b) A normal concentration (a concentration of ions outside the cell equal to that inside the cell) results in a typically shaped red blood cell. Water moves into and out of the cell in equilibrium (*black arrows*), but there is no net water movement.

(c) A concentrated solution, with a high ion concentration, causes shrinkage of the red blood cell as water moves out of the cell and into the concentrated solution (*black arrows*).

Figure 9-2 Effects of various ion concentrations in a fluid on red blood cells. This shows the process of osmosis. Fluid is shifting in and out of the red blood cells in response to changing ion concentrations in the flasks.

Positive ions, such as sodium and potassium, end up pairing with negative ions, such as chloride and phosphate. Maintenance of intracellular water volume depends primarily on intracellular potassium and phosphate concentrations. Extracellular water volume depends primarily on the extracellular sodium and chloride concentrations.

■ Water Contributes to Body Temperature Regulation

Water temperature changes slowly because it has a great ability to hold heat. It takes much more energy to heat water than it does to heat fat. Water molecules are attracted to each other, and it takes much energy to separate them. Because water requires so much energy to change states—for example, from a liquid to a gas to evaporate perspiration—it forms an ideal medium for removing heat from the body.

When overheated, the body secretes fluids in the form of perspiration, which evaporates through skin pores. To evaporate water, heat energy is required. So, as perspiration evaporates, heat energy is taken from the skin, cooling it in the process. Each quart (liter) of perspiration evaporated represents approximately 600 kcal of energy lost from the skin and surrounding tissues. For this reason, fever increases one's need for calories.

About 60% of the chemical energy in food is turned directly into body heat; the other 40% is converted to forms of energy cells can use, and almost all of that energy eventually leaves the body in the form of heat. If this heat could not be dissipated, the body temperature would rise enough to prevent enzyme systems from functioning efficiently. Perspiration is the primary way to prevent this rise in body temperature.

Functions of water:

- Chemical processes
- Temperature regulation
- Removal of waste products
- Basis for many body fluids, such as in joints

Another Bite

To cool efficiently, perspiration must be allowed to evaporate. If it simply rolls off the skin or soaks into clothing, perspiration doesn't cool the body as much. Evaporation of perspiration occurs quickly when humidity is low. This is why humans can cool off and therefore tolerate hot, dry climates far better than they do hot, humid climates.

■ Water Helps Remove Waste Products

Water is an important vehicle for transporting waste products from the body. Most unusable substances in the body can dissolve in water and exit the body through the urine.

Urea is a major body waste product. This by-product of protein metabolism contains nitrogen. The more protein we eat in excess of needs, the more nitrogen we excrete—in the form of urea—in the urine. Likewise, the more sodium we consume, the more sodium we excrete in the urine. Overall, the amount of urine a person needs to produce is determined primarily by excess protein and salt intake. By limiting excess protein and salt intakes, it is possible to limit urine output—a useful practice, for example, in space flights. This type of diet is also used to treat some kidney diseases wherein the ability to produce urine is hampered.

urea Nitrogen-containing waste product of protein metabolism; major source of nitrogen in the urine.

A typical urine volume is about 1 liter (1 quart) or more per day, depending mostly on the intake of fluid, protein, and sodium. A somewhat greater urine output than that is fine, but less—especially less than 500 milliliters (2 cups)—forces the kidneys to form very concentrated urine. The simplest way to determine if water intake is adequate is to observe the color of one's urine. Whereas urine should be clear or pale yellow, concentrated urine is very dark yellow in color. The heavy ion concentration in turn increases the risk of kidney stone formation in susceptible people (generally men). Kidney stones are formed from minerals and other substances that have precipitated out of the urine and accumulated in kidney tissues.

Regular intake of water and water-rich fluids are essential to replace daily fluid losses. A recent trend in North America is to carry bottles of water with us.

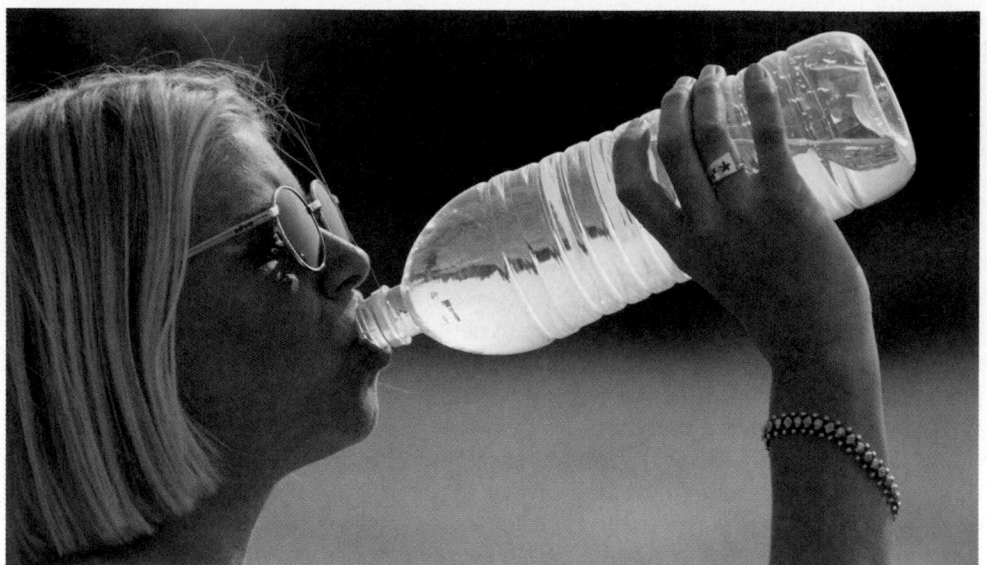

amniotic fluid Fluid contained in a sac within the uterus. This fluid surrounds and protects the fetus during development.

■ Other Functions of Water

Water helps form the lubricants found in knees and other joints of the body. It is the basis for saliva, bile, and **amniotic fluid.** Amniotic fluid acts as a shock absorber surrounding the growing fetus in the mother's womb. Ion concentrations vary in each fluid compartment to accommodate specific needs, such as the ability to transfer nerve impulses.

■ How Much Water Do We Need per Day?

The Adequate Intake for total water intake is 2.7 liters (11 cups) for adult women and 3.7 liters (15 cups) for adult men. This is based primarily on our typical total water intakes from a combination of fluids and foods. For fluid alone this corresponds to about 2.2 liters (9 cups) for women and about 3 liters (13 cups) for men. (Keep in mind also that it does not indicate that water per se must be used to meet fluid needs.) At minimum, adults need 1 to 3 liters of fluid to replace daily water losses.

We consume water in various liquids, such as fruit juice, coffee, tea, soft drinks, and water itself. Note that coffee, tea, and soft drinks often contain caffeine, which increases urine output. However, the fluid consumed from these beverages is not completely lost in urine, so these fluids still help to meet water needs. Foods also supply water; many fruits and vegetables are more than 80% water (Table 9-1). Water as a byproduct of metabolism provides approximately 250 to 350 milliliters (1 to 1½ cups) of additional water.

Much of the water needed is used to produce urine (500 to 1000 milliliters or more). The rest compensates for typical water losses through the lungs (250 to 350 milliliters), feces (100 to 200 milliliters), and skin (450 to 1900 milliliters) (Fig. 9-3). These are just estimates: altitude, caffeine intake, alcohol intake, and humidity can affect these individual losses.

When we consider the large amount of water used to lubricate the gastrointestinal (GI) tract, the loss of only 100 to 200 milliliters of water each day through the feces is remarkable. About 8000 milliliters of water enter the GI tract daily through secretions from the mouth, stomach, intestine, pancreas, and other organs, while the diet supplies an additional 30% to 50% or more. The small intestine reabsorbs most of this water, while the large intestine takes up a lesser—but still important—amount. The kidneys also greatly conserve water. They reabsorb about 97% of the water filtered from waste products.

Table 9-1 Water Content (by Weight) of Various Foods

Food	Water %
Tomato	95
Lettuce	95
Beer	90
Milk	89
Orange	87
Apple	86
Potato	75
Banana	75
Chicken	64
Steak	50
Bread, whole wheat	38
Jam	28
Honey	20
Butter	16
Crackers, saltines	4
Shortening	0

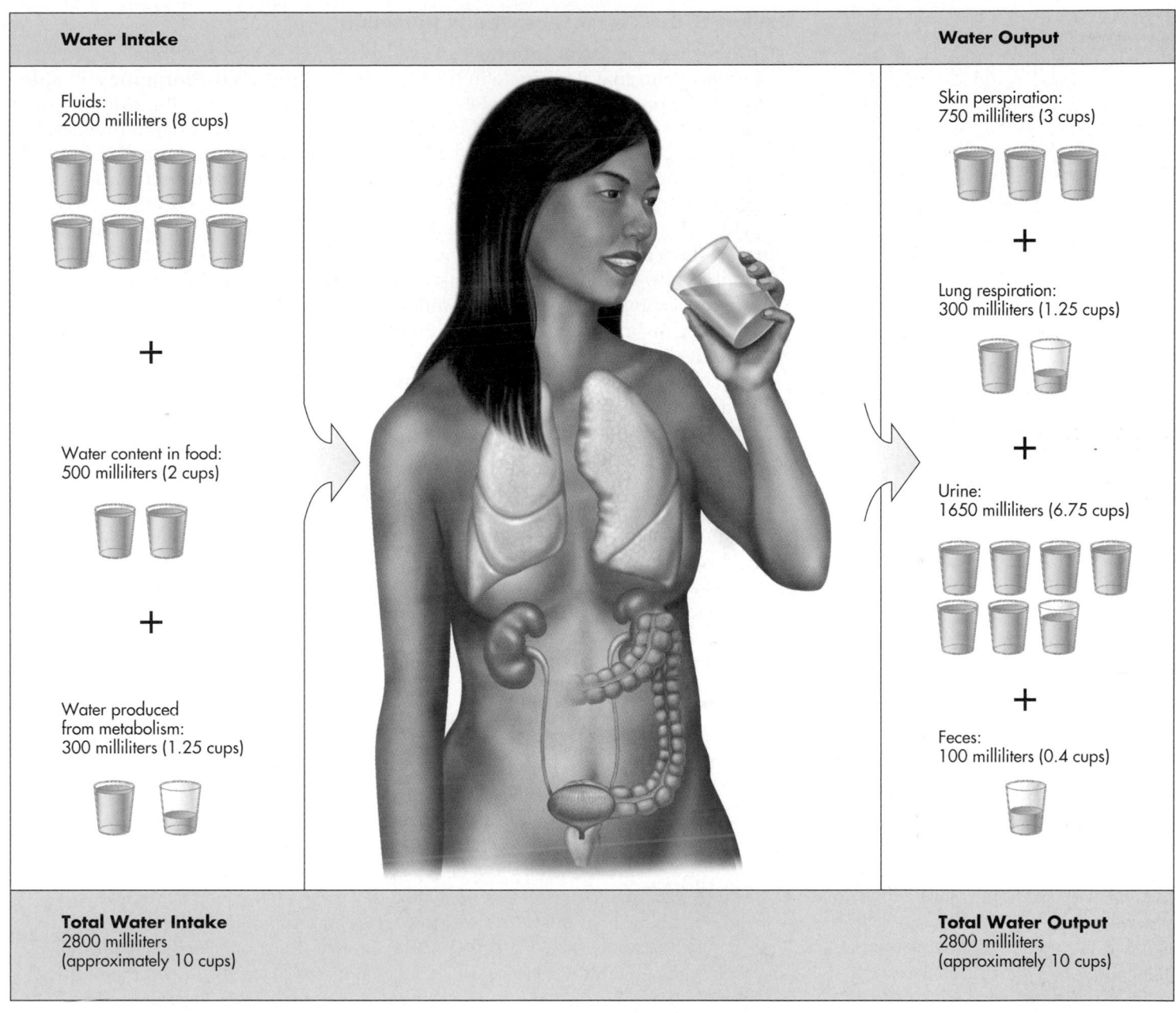

Figure 9-3 Estimate of water balance—intake versus output—in a woman. We primarily maintain body fluids at an optimum amount by adjusting water output to intake. As you can see for this woman, most water comes from the liquids we consume. Some comes from the moisture in more solid foods, and the remainder is manufactured during metabolism. Water output includes that lost via lungs, urine, skin, and feces.

■ Thirst

If you don't drink enough water, your body eventually lets you know by signaling thirst. Your brain is communicating the need to drink. This thirst mechanism can lag behind actual water loss, however, during prolonged exercise and illness, as well as in one's older years. For this reason, athletes especially should monitor fluid status—they should weigh themselves before and after training sessions to determine their rate of water loss and, thus, their water needs. The current goal for athletes is to consume 2½ to 3 cups of fluid for every pound lost (see Chapter 11 for details). Sick children—especially those with fever, vomiting, diarrhea, and increased perspiration—and older persons often need to be reminded to drink plenty of fluids (see Chapters 14 and 15 for details). As Chapter 14 discusses in further detail, infants can easily become dehydrated.

Water can be classified by whether it is hard or soft. Hard water generally comes from underground wells and usually contains calcium, magnesium, and iron. The more minerals the water contains, the harder it is. Soft water has a low content of these minerals and is often produced by replacing other minerals with sodium.

antidiuretic hormone A hormone that is secreted by the pituitary gland and that acts on the kidneys to decrease water excretion.

aldosterone A hormone produced by the adrenal glands that acts on the kidneys to conserve sodium (and therefore water).

Alcohol inhibits the action of antidiuretic hormone. One reason people feel so weak the day after heavy drinking is that they are very dehydrated. Even though they may have consumed a lot of liquid in their drinks, they have lost even more liquid because alcohol has inhibited antidiuretic hormone.

As bottled water becomes more and more popular, the industry now generates more than $3 billion per year. In 1996, FDA instituted definitions for the various types of bottled water on the market; FDA also tests products for microbial and chemical content. For a list of manufacturers that meet federal guidelines, contact the International Bottled Water Association at 1-800-928-3711 or www.nsf.org. Some experts recommend that children not be given bottled water exclusively, as many brands do not contain an adequate fluoride supply to protect against dental caries. For adults, bottled water is typically an unnecessary expense, as it is often very similar to tap water.

cofactor A mineral or other substance that binds to a specific region on a protein, such as an enzyme, and is necessary for the protein's function.

What If the Thirst Message Is Ignored?

Once the body registers a shortage of available water, it increases fluid conservation. Two hormones that participate in this process are **antidiuretic hormone** and **aldosterone.** The pituitary gland releases antidiuretic hormone to force the kidneys to conserve water. The kidneys respond by reducing urine flow. At the same time, as fluid volume decreases in the bloodstream, blood pressure falls. This eventually triggers the release of the hormone aldosterone, which signals the kidneys to retain more sodium and, in turn, more water.

However, despite mechanisms that work to conserve water, fluid continues to be lost via the feces, skin, and lungs. Those losses must be replaced. In addition, there is a limit to how concentrated urine can become. Eventually, if fluid is not consumed, the body becomes dehydrated and suffers ill effects.

By the time a person loses 1% to 2% of body weight in fluids, he or she will be thirsty. Even this small water deficit can cause one to feel tired. At a 4% loss of body weight, muscles lose significant strength and endurance. By the time body weight is reduced by 10% to 12%, heat tolerance is decreased and weakness results. At a 20% reduction, coma and death may soon follow.

■ Is There Such a Thing as Too Much Water?

Too much water—whatever amount the kidneys are unable to excrete—can also lead to ill health, such as low blood electrolyte concentrations, notably sodium. However, an excessive amount would have to approach many quarts (liters) each day. When excessive water overwhelms the kidneys' capacity to excrete, blurred vision is one resulting symptom. Such toxicity risks during athletic events are covered in Chapter 11. Toxicity risks related to bacterial or other contamination of our water supply are covered in Chapter 16.

Concept Check

Because the body can neither readily store nor conserve water, we can survive only a few days without it. Water transports nutrients and waste products, serves as a medium for chemical reactions and as a lubricant, and aids in temperature regulation. Water accounts for 50% to 70% of body weight and distributes itself all over the body—among lean and other tissues (in both intracellular and extracellular fluids) and in urine and other body fluids. The Adequate Intake for total water intake is 2.7 liters (11 cups) for women and 3.7 liters (15 cups) for men. Thirst is the body's first sign of dehydration. If this thirst mechanism is faulty, as it may be during illness or vigorous exercise, hormonal mechanisms also help conserve water by reducing urine output. Excess fluid intake can be hazardous to a person's health.

Minerals—An Overview

The metabolic roles of minerals and the amounts of them in the body vary considerably (Fig. 9-4). Some minerals, such as copper and selenium, work as **cofactors,** enabling various proteins, such as enzymes, to function. Minerals also contribute to many body compounds. For example, iron is a component of red blood cells. Sodium, potassium, and calcium aid in the transfer of nerve impulses throughout the body. Body growth and development also depend on certain minerals, such as calcium and phosphorus. Water balance requires sodium, potassium, calcium, and phosphorus. At all levels—cellular, tissue, organ, and whole body—minerals clearly play important roles in maintaining body functions.

Minerals are categorized based on the amount we need per day. Recall from Chapter 1 that if we require greater than 100 milligrams (1/50 of a teaspoon) of a

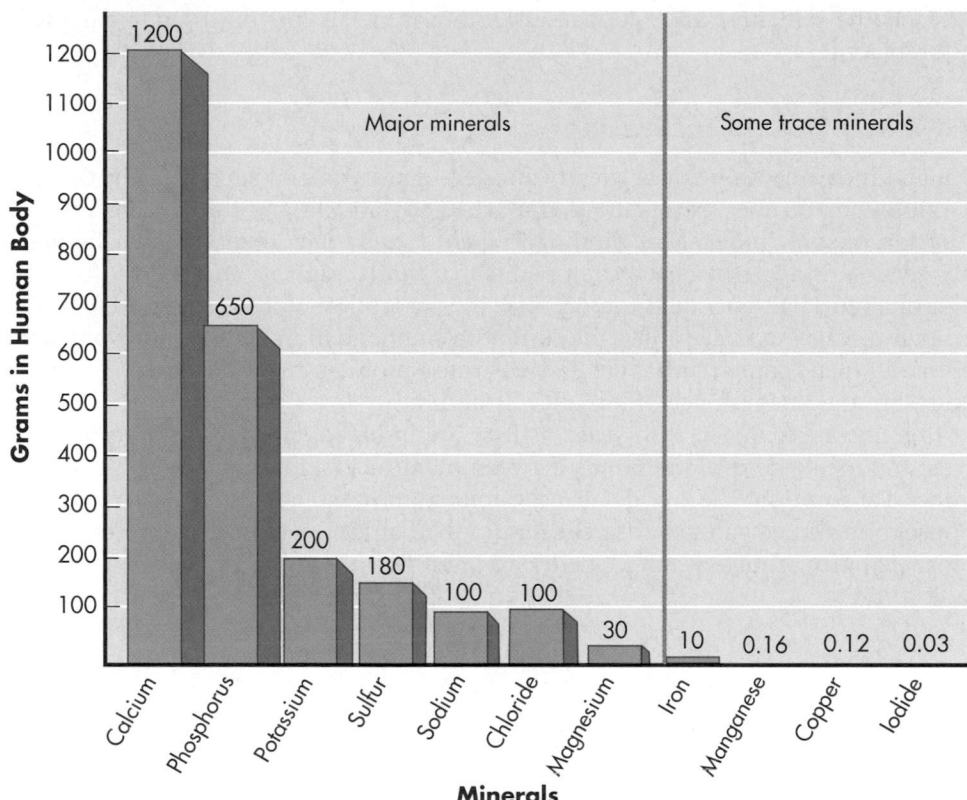

Figure 9-4 Approximate amounts of various minerals present in the average human body. Other trace minerals of nutritional importance not listed include chromium, fluoride, molybdenum, selenium, and zinc.

major mineral A mineral vital to health that is required in the diet in amounts greater than 100 milligrams per day.

trace mineral A mineral vital to health that is required in the diet in amounts less than 100 milligrams per day.

bioavailability The degree to which an ingested nutrient is absorbed and available to the body.

oxalic acid (oxalate) An organic acid found in spinach, rhubarb, and other leafy green vegetables that can depress the absorption of certain minerals present in the food, such as calcium.

mineral per day, it is considered a **major mineral;** otherwise, it is considered a **trace mineral.** Using these criteria, calcium and phosphorus are major minerals and iron and zinc are trace minerals.

The roles and nutritional significance of both the major and the trace minerals are discussed in this chapter. But before examining the properties of the individual minerals, let's consider some topics that apply to all these nutrients.

■ Mineral Bioavailability

Foods offer us a plentiful supply of many minerals, but our bodies vary in their capabilities to absorb and use them. This concept of absorbing variable amounts of a nutrient from food sources is called **bioavailability.** The bioavailability of minerals depends on many factors. The number listed in a food composition table for the amount of a mineral in a food is just a starting point for estimating the actual contribution the food will make to our mineral needs. Spinach, for example, contains plenty of calcium, but only about 5% of it can be absorbed because of the vegetable's high concentration of **oxalic acid (oxalate),** a calcium-binder. Usually, about 25% of dietary calcium is absorbed by adults.

The average North American diet derives minerals from both plant and animal sources. Overall, minerals from animal products are better absorbed than those from plants because binders and fiber (as will soon be discussed) are not present to hinder absorption. The mineral content of plants greatly depends on mineral concentrations of the soil in which they are grown. Vegans must be aware of the potentially poor mineral content of some plant foods and choose some concentrated sources of minerals (review Chapter 6). Soil conditions have less of an influence on the mineral content of animal products since animals may consume a variety of plant products grown from soils of differing mineral contents.

In general, the more refined a plant food—as in the case of white flour—the lower its content of minerals. In the enrichment process, iron is the only mineral added,

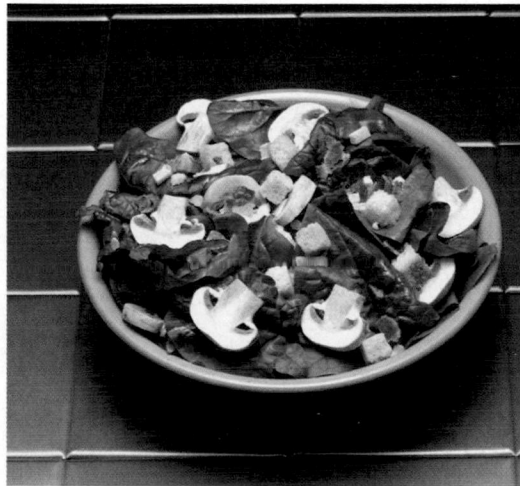

Spinach is often touted as a rich source of calcium, but little of the calcium present is bioavailable—that which is available to the body.

whereas the selenium, zinc, copper, and other minerals lost during refinement are not replaced.

■ Fiber-Mineral Interactions

phytic acid (phytate) A constituent of plant fibers that binds positive ions to its multiple phosphate groups.

Mineral bioavailability can be greatly affected by nonmineral substances in the diet. Components of fiber, especially **phytic acid (phytate)** in grain fiber, can limit absorption of some minerals by binding to them. Oxalic acid, mentioned in the previous section, is another substance in plants that binds minerals and makes them less bioavailable. High-fiber diets can decrease the absorption of iron, zinc, and probably other minerals. An intake above the current recommendation of 25 (adult women) to 38 (adult men) grams of fiber per day may cause problems with mineral status of the body, but the actual degree of this effect is uncertain.

If grains are leavened with yeast, as they are in bread, enzymes produced by the yeast can break some of the bonds between phytic acid and minerals. This increases mineral absorption. The zinc deficiencies found among some Middle Eastern populations are attributed partly to their consumption of unleavened breads, resulting in low bioavailability of dietary zinc. Zinc bioavailability is discussed in greater detail in a later section.

■ Mineral-Mineral Interactions

Many minerals are of similar sizes and electrical charges, such as magnesium, calcium, iron, and copper. Having similar sizes and the same electrical charge causes these minerals to compete with each other for absorption, and therefore they affect each other's bioavailability. Simply stated, an excess of one mineral influences the absorption and metabolism of other minerals. Because of this, people should avoid taking individual mineral supplements unless a dietary deficiency or medical condition specifically warrants it. For example, intake of a large amount of zinc decreases copper absorption. Food sources, however, pose little risk for these mineral interactions, giving us another reason to emphasize foods in meeting nutrient needs.

■ Vitamin-Mineral Interactions

When consumed in conjunction with vitamin C, absorption of certain forms of iron—such as that in plant products—improves. The active vitamin D hormone improves calcium absorption. Many vitamins require specific minerals to act as components in their structure and function. For example, the thiamin coenzyme requires magnesium or manganese to function efficiently.

■ Mineral Toxicities

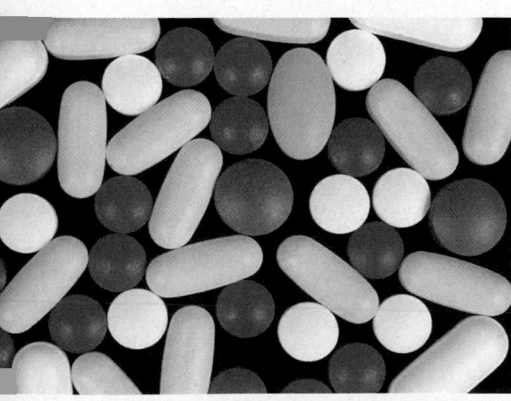

Mineral supplements pose a high risk for toxicity. Generally, mineral intake from a supplement should not exceed 100% of the Daily Value, unless otherwise specified by a physician.

An excessive mineral intake can have toxic results, especially with the trace minerals, such as iron and copper. For many trace minerals, the gap between just enough and too much is quite small. Supplements pose the biggest threat for mineral toxicity, whereas food sources are unlikely culprits. Mineral supplements exceeding current standards for mineral needs—especially those that supply more than 100% of the Daily Values on supplement labels—should be taken only under a physician's supervision. (Note that the Daily Values are for the most part higher than our current standards for mineral needs.) Without close monitoring, doses of minerals should not exceed any Upper Level set on a long-term basis.

The potential for toxicity is not the only reason to carefully consider the use of mineral supplements. Harmful interactions with other nutrients are possible. Also, contamination of mineral supplements—with lead, for example—is a very real possibility. Use of brands approved by United States Pharmacopeia (USP) lessens this risk. In summary, even with the best intentions, people may harm themselves using mineral supplements.

Concept Check

Minerals are vital to the functioning of many body processes. Their bioavailability depends on many factors, including a mineral's interaction with fiber, vitamins, and other minerals. Animal products often yield better mineral absorption than do plants. Still, both animal and plant sources help us meet our mineral needs. Taking megadoses of an individual mineral supplement can greatly diminish the absorption and metabolism of other minerals. In addition, some minerals are potentially toxic in amounts not much in excess of body needs. These are two good reasons to consider carefully any use of mineral supplements, exceeding the Daily Value on the label, and especially so for intakes in excess of any Upper Level set if consumed on a long-term basis.

Major Minerals

Up to now some general characteristics of minerals and how some of them interact with water in the body have been covered. Now let us review the individual properties of the major minerals (also called macrominerals) in the context of the North American diet.

Sodium (Na)

Table salt is our primary dietary source of sodium. This mineral is an essential part of our diets and adds flavor to our foods, but there is concern that an overabundance of sodium in the diet may cause harm.

The human body absorbs almost all sodium that gets eaten. Once absorbed, sodium becomes the major positive ion in extracellular fluid and a key factor for retaining body water. Fluid balance throughout the body depends partly on varied sodium and other ion concentrations among the water-containing compartments in the body. Sodium ions also function in nerve impulse conduction and absorption of some nutrients (e.g., glucose).

A diet low in sodium—coupled with excessive perspiration, persistent vomiting, or diarrhea—has the ability to deplete the body of sodium. This state can lead to muscle cramps, nausea, vomiting, dizziness, and later shock and coma. The likelihood of this happening, however, is low because early kidney responses to low sodium status eventually trigger the body to conserve sodium. This body conservation of sodium demonstrates how important small amounts are to body functions. In addition, a dietary deficiency of sodium is rare.

Only when weight loss from perspiration exceeds 2% to 3% of total body weight (or about 5 to 6 pounds) should sodium losses raise concern. Even then, merely salting foods is sufficient to restore body sodium for most people. Certain endurance athletes, however, may need to consume sports drinks during competition to replace sodium losses from perspiration in order to avoid depletion of sodium (see Chapter 11). Note also that although perspiration tastes salty on the skin, sodium is not highly concentrated in perspiration. Rather, water evaporating from the skin leaves concentrated sodium behind. Perspiration contains about two-thirds the sodium concentration found in blood.

Sodium Sources and Needs

About 80% of the sodium we consume is added during food manufacturing and food preparation at restaurants. Sodium added in cooking provides about 10% of our

For your information, the chemical symbols for the minerals discussed are given next to each mineral heading.

The earliest reference to salt is in The Book of Job written about 300 B.C. At one time, it was the custom to rub salt on newborn babies as a symbol of purity and to ensure their good health. Salt was once so scarce that is was used as money. Caesar's soldiers received part of their pay in common salt. This part of their pay was known as their "salarium", and from this came today's word "salary". The expression "not worth his salt" meant that a man did not earn his wages.

Food Sources of Sodium

Food Item and Amount	Sodium Content (milligrams)
Pepperoni pizza, 2 slices	2045
Ham, sliced, 1 oz	1215
Chicken noodle soup, canned, 1 cup	1106
V8 vegetable juice, 8 oz	620
Macaroni salad, ½ cup	561
Hard pretzels, 1 oz	486
Hamburger with bun, 1 each	474
Green beans, canned, ½ cup	390
Saltine crackers, 6 each	234
Cheddar cheese, 1 oz	176
Peanut butter, 2 tbsp	156
Fat-free milk, 1 cup	127
7 grain bread, 1 slice	126
Animal crackers, 1 oz	112
Grape juice, 1 cup	10

Adequate Intake for young adults, 1500 milligrams

Adequate intake for older adults, 1200 to 1300 milligrams

Table salt is 40% sodium and 60% chloride. Sodium intakes seen in adults of 4 grams or so per day translates to 10 grams or so of salt. A teaspoon of salt contains about 2 grams of sodium (2000 milligrams).

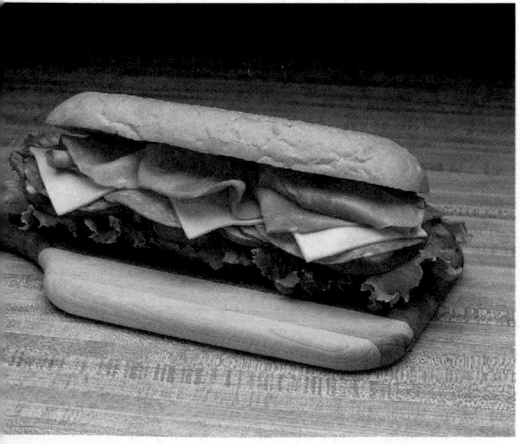

Deli meats, such as ham, are very high in sodium (salt).

intakes, and sodium naturally present in foods provides the rest, again about 10%. Almost all foods naturally contain a little sodium; the higher amount found in milk (about 120 milligrams per cup) is one exception.

The more processed and restaurant food one consumes, generally the higher one's sodium intake. Conversely, the more home cooking one does, the more sodium control that person has. Major contributors of sodium in the adult diet are white bread and rolls, hot dogs and lunch meats, cheese, soups, and foods with tomato sauce, partly because these foods are eaten so often. Other foods that generally are especially high in sodium include salted snack foods, French fries and potato chips, and sauces and gravies.

If we ate only unprocessed foods and added no salt, we would consume about 500 milligrams of sodium per day. In comparison, the Adequate Intake for sodium for adults under age 51 is 1500 milligrams; this is reduced by 100 to 200 milligrams for older adults. (See the inside cover for references to mineral needs for various age groups.) Note that 1500 milligrams is a generous amount; we really need only about 200 milligrams a day to maintain physiological functions. (Additional sodium above needs was added to establish the Adequate Intake in order to allow for a more varied diet where not all foods are low in sodium.)

If we compare 500 milligrams of sodium from unprocessed food with the 2300 to 4700 milligrams or more typically eaten by adults, it is clear that food processing and cooking contribute most of our dietary sodium. As discussed in Chapter 2, nutrition labels list a food's sodium content. When dietary sodium must be severely restricted, attention to food labels is of utmost importance. Under FDA food and supplement labeling rules, the Daily Value for sodium is 2400 milligrams (2.4 grams).

Most humans can adapt somewhat to various dietary salt intakes, though very high intakes can be toxic. For most people, today's sodium intake is simply in tomorrow's urine output. However, approximately 10% to 15% of adults are especially *sodium sensitive*, such as African-Americans and people who have diabetes and/or are overweight. For these people, high sodium intakes can increase blood pressure, whereas lower-sodium diets (about 2000 milligrams daily) often help correct the problem (see the following Looking Further section on minerals and hypertension). Still, keep in mind that other lifestyle factors, such as being overweight and inactive, are more likely to contribute to hypertension.

Scientific groups typically suggest that adults in general reduce sodium intake, mostly to limit the risk of developing hypertension later. It is also a good idea to have your blood pressure checked regularly. If you have hypertension, you should try to reduce your sodium intake as you follow a comprehensive plan to treat this disease. Reducing sodium intake also helps to maintain healthy calcium status, as sodium intake greater than about 2000 milligrams per day can increase urinary calcium loss as the sodium is excreted.

It is actually not that hard to follow a low-sodium diet, but many typical food choices will have to be limited (Table 9-2). At first, foods may also taste quite bland, but eventually you will perceive more flavor as the tongue becomes more sensitive to the salt content of foods. By slowly reducing dietary sodium and substituting lemon juice, herbs, and spices you can eventually become accustomed to a diet that contains minimal sodium daily but does not result in much of a flavor trade-off. Many new cookbooks offer excellent recipes for flavorful low-sodium foods.

■ Upper Level for Sodium

The Upper Level for sodium for adults is 2300 milligrams (2.3 grams). Intakes exceeding this amount typically increase blood pressure. About 95% of North American adults have sodium intakes that exceed the Upper Level.

Table 9-2 Questionnaire for Evaluating Your Sodium Habits with Respect to Typically Rich Sources

HOW OFTEN DO YOU:	Rarely	Occasionally	Often	Regularly (daily)
1. Eat cured or processed meats, such as ham, bacon, sausage, frankfurters, and other luncheon meats?	☐	☐	☐	☐
2. Choose canned or frozen vegetables with sauce?	☐	☐	☐	☐
3. Use commercially prepared meats, main dishes, or canned or dehydrated soups?	☐	☐	☐	☐
4. Eat cheese, especially processed cheese?	☐	☐	☐	☐
5. Eat salted nuts, popcorn, pretzels, corn chips, or potato chips?	☐	☐	☐	☐
6. Add salt to cooking water for vegetables, rice, or pasta?	☐	☐	☐	☐
7. Add salt, seasoning mixes, salad dressings, or condiments—such as soy sauce, steak sauce, catsup, and mustard—to foods during preparation or at the table?	☐	☐	☐	☐
8. Salt your food before tasting it?	☐	☐	☐	☐
9. Ignore labels for sodium content when buying foods?	☐	☐	☐	☐
10. When dining out, choose foods at restaurants with sauces, or foods that are obviously salty?	☐	☐	☐	☐

You can evaluate your sodium habits by completing this questionnaire. The more checks in the "often" or "regularly" columns, the higher your dietary sodium intake. However, not all the habits in the table contribute the same amount of sodium. For example, many natural cheeses such as cheddar are relatively moderate in sodium, whereas processed cheeses and cottage cheese are much higher. To moderate sodium intake, choose lower-sodium foods from each food group more often and balance high-sodium food choices with low-sodium ones.

Concept Check

Sodium is the major positive ion in the extracellular fluid. It is important for maintaining fluid balance and conducting nerve impulses. Sodium depletion is unlikely, since the typical North American's diet has abundant sources of sodium and most of it gets absorbed. Compared to dining out or buying commercially prepared foods, preparation of foods in the home allows greater control over sodium intake. The Adequate Intake for sodium for adults is 1500 milligrams per day. The average adult consumes 2300 to 4700 milligrams or more daily. About 10% to 15% of the population is especially sensitive to sodium, such as overweight individuals and African-Americans. In these people, hypertension can develop as a result of high-sodium diets, but many other lifestyle habits are also important in causing hypertension. Nutrition experts currently suggest that for young adults, sodium intake should be about 1500 milligrams (1.5 grams), and not exceed 2300 milligrams (2.3 grams) on a regular basis. Sodium in the North American diet is provided predominantly through processed and restaurant foods.

Critical Thinking

Mrs. Massa has recently seen and heard a lot about the amount of salt (sodium) in foods. She has been surprised by the number of articles that advise the public to decrease the amount of salt in their food. If sodium is such a bad thing, Mrs. Massa wonders, why do you need to have any at all? How would you respond to her question?

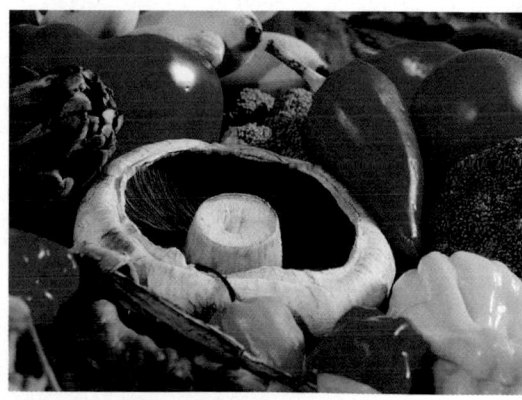

Vegetables in general are a rich source of potassium, as are fruits.

Potassium (K)

Potassium performs many of the same functions as sodium, such as fluid balance and nerve impulse transmission. However, it operates inside, rather than outside cells. Intracellular fluids—those inside cells—contain 95% of the potassium in the body. Also, unlike sodium, potassium is associated with lower rather than higher blood pressure values. We absorb about 90% of the potassium we eat.

Low blood potassium is a life-threatening problem. Symptoms often include a loss of appetite, muscle cramps, confusion, and constipation. Eventually, the heart beats irregularly, decreasing its capacity to pump blood.

Figure 9-5 Sources of Potassium from MyPyramid. The height and background color (none, 1/3, 2/3 or completely covered) within each group in the pyramid indicates the average nutrient density for potassium in that group. Overall, the vegetables group and the fruits group contain many foods that are nutrient-dense sources of potassium, with the milk group and meat & beans group following close behind. With regard to physical activity, potassium is especially needed for the associated cardiovascular functions.

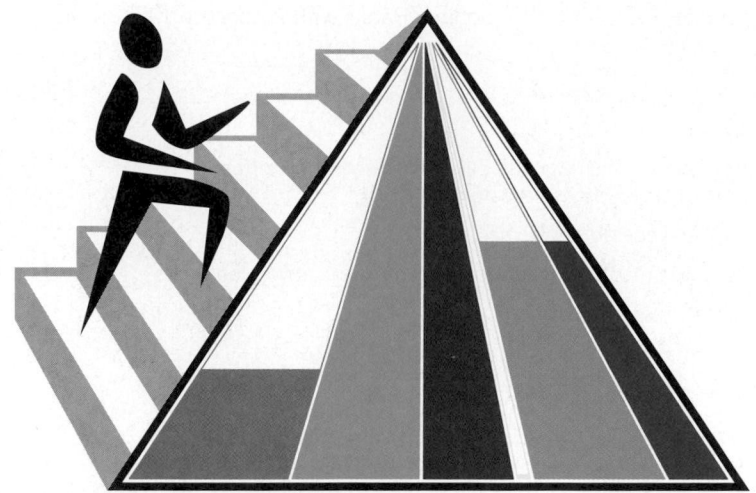

Grains	Vegetables	Fruits	Oils	Milk	Meat & Beans
• Whole-wheat bread • Whole-grain products	• Spinach • Squash • Potatoes • Tomatoes • Lettuce • Lima beans	• Pears • Prunes • Peaches • Avocados • Cantaloupes • Bananas	• None	• Milk • Yogurt • Cottage cheese • Ricotta cheese	• Meat • Chicken • Fish • Shrimp • Beans

Food Sources of Potassium

Food Item and Amount	Potassium (milligrams)
Kidney beans, 1 cup	715
Winter squash, ¾ cup	670
Plain yogurt, 1 cup	570
Orange juice, 1 cup	495
Cantaloupes, 1 cup	495
Lima beans, ½ cup	480
Banana, 1 medium	470
Zucchini, 1 cup	450
Soybeans, ½ cup	440
Artichoke, 1 medium	425
Tomato juice, ¾ cup	400
Pinto beans, ½ cup	400
Baked potato, 1 small	385
Buttermilk, 1 cup	370
Sirloin steak, 3 ounces	345

Adequate Intake for adults, 4700 milligrams

diuretic A substance that increases the flow of urine.

■ Potassium Sources and Needs

Generally, unprocessed foods are rich sources of potassium. This includes fruits, vegetables, milk, whole grains, dried beans, and meats. Major contributors of potassium to the adult diet include milk, potatoes, beef, coffee, tomatoes, and orange juice (Fig. 9-5).

The Adequate Intake for potassium for adults is 4700 milligrams (4.7 grams) per day. The Daily Value used on food and supplement labels is 3500 milligrams. Typically, North Americans consume on average 2000 to 3000 milligrams per day. Thus many of us need to increase our potassium intakes, and preferably by increasing fruit and vegetable intake.

Diets are more likely to be lower in potassium than sodium because we generally do not add potassium to foods. Some **diuretics** used to treat high blood pressure also deplete the body's potassium. Thus, people who take potassium-wasting diuretics need to monitor their potassium intakes carefully. For these people, high-potassium foods are good additions to the diet, as are potassium chloride supplements if prescribed by a physician.

A continually deficient food intake, as may be the case in alcoholism, can result in a severe potassium deficiency that requires medical attention. People with certain eating disorders, whose diets are poor and whose bodies can be depleted of nutrients because of vomiting, are also at risk for severe potassium deficiency (see Chapter 12). Other populations especially at risk for a severe potassium deficiency include people on very low-calorie diets and athletes who exercise heavily. As covered in Chapters 10 and 11, all of these people should compensate for potentially low body potassium by consuming potassium-rich foods.

If the kidneys function normally, typical food intakes will not lead to potassium toxicity. Thus no Upper Level for potassium has been set. When the kidneys function poorly, potassium builds up in the blood. This inhibits heart function, causing slowed heartbeat. If untreated, this can be fatal, as the heart eventually stops beating. Consequently, in cases of reduced kidney function, close control of potassium intake becomes critical.

Chloride (Cl)

In our bodies, chloride—an ion form of chlorine—is an important negative ion for the extracellular fluid. Chlorine, on the other hand, is a very poisonous gas. Chloride ions are a component of the acid produced in the stomach and are also used during immune responses as white blood cells attack foreign cells. In addition, nerve function relies on the presence of chloride. As is the case with sodium, most of the body's chloride is excreted by the kidneys; some is lost in perspiration. It has also been linked to the blood pressure-raising ability of sodium chloride.

A chloride deficiency is unlikely because our dietary sodium chloride (salt) intake is so high. Frequent and lengthy bouts of vomiting—if coupled with a nutrient-poor diet—can contribute to a deficiency because stomach secretions contain much chloride.

∎ Chloride Sources and Needs

A few fruits and some vegetables are naturally good sources of chloride. Chlorinated water is also a source. However, we consume most chloride as salt added to foods. Knowing a food's salt content allows for a close prediction of its chloride content; recall salt is 60% chloride.

The Adequate Intake for chloride for adults is 2300 milligrams per day. This is based on the 40:60 ratio of sodium to chloride in salt (1500 milligrams of sodium in a diet is accompanied by 2300 milligrams of chloride). The Daily Value used on food and supplement labels is 3400 milligrams. If the average adult consumes about 9 grams of salt daily, that yields 5.4 grams (5400 milligrams) of chloride.

∎ Upper Level for Chloride

The Upper Level is 3600 milligrams. Thus the average adult typically consumes an excess amount of this ion.

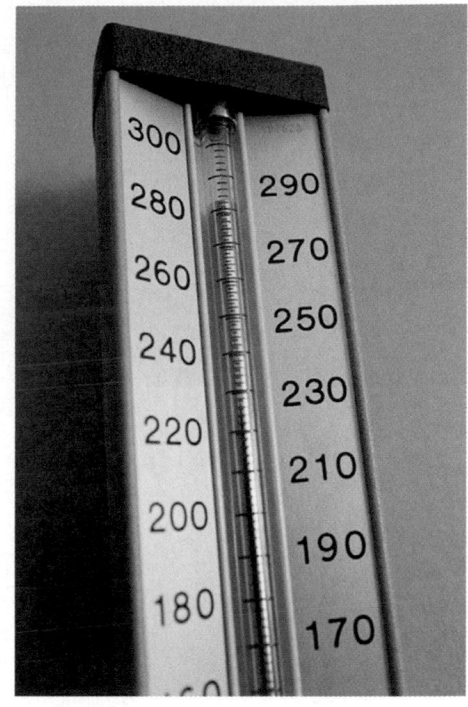

Chloride is likely part of the blood pressure-raising property of sodium chloride (salt).

Concept Check

The functions of potassium closely parallel those of sodium, but whereas sodium is found outside cells, potassium is the main positive ion found inside cells. Potassium is vital to fluid balance and nerve transmission. A potassium deficiency—caused by an inadequate intake of potassium, persistent vomiting, or use of some diuretics—can eventually lead to loss of appetite, muscle cramps, confusion, and heartbeat irregularities. Fruits and vegetables are generally rich sources of potassium. Potassium intake can be toxic if a person's kidneys do not function properly. Chloride is the major negative ion of extracellular fluid. Chloride also functions in digestion as part of stomach acid and in immune and nervous system responses. Deficiencies of chloride are highly unlikely because we eat so much sodium chloride (salt), the major source.

Calcium (Ca)

All cells need calcium, but more than 99% of the calcium in the body is used to strengthen bones and teeth. This calcium represents 40% of all the minerals present in the body and equals about 2.5 pounds (1200 grams). The calcium circulating in the bloodstream supplies the calcium needs of body cells. Growth and bone development require an adequate calcium intake.

Unlike sodium, potassium, and chloride, the amount of calcium in the body depends greatly on its absorption from the diet. Calcium requires an acidic environment in the GI tract to be absorbed efficiently. Absorption occurs primarily in the upper part of the small intestine. This area tends to remain acidic because it receives

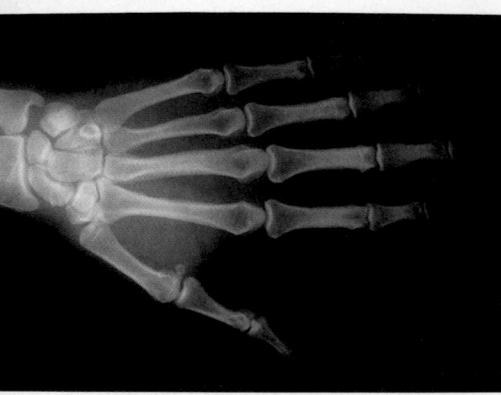

Ninety-nine percent of calcium in the body is in bones.

osteoporosis Decreased bone mass related to the effects of aging, genetic background and poor diet in both genders, and hormonal changes at menopause in women.

tetany A body condition marked by sharp contraction of muscles and failure to relax afterward; usually caused by abnormal calcium metabolism.

the acidic stomach contents. Much calcium absorption in the upper small intestine depends on the active vitamin D hormone.

Adults absorb about 25% of the calcium in the foods eaten, but during times when the body needs extra calcium—such as in infancy and pregnancy—absorption increases to as high as 60%. Young people tend to absorb calcium better than do older people, especially those older than 70.

Many factors enhance calcium absorption, including:

- Blood levels of parathyroid hormone
- The presence of glucose and lactose in the diet
- The flow (motility) of digestive contents through the intestine

On the other hand, several factors limit calcium absorption, such as:

- Large amounts of phytic acid in fiber from grains
- Great excess of phosphorus (and possibly magnesium) in the diet
- Polyphenols (tannins) in tea
- A vitamin D deficiency
- Diarrhea
- Old age

Because we have excellent hormonal systems to control blood calcium, a normal value can be maintained despite an inadequate calcium intake. The bones, however, pay the price. Bones can be seen as a calcium bank. Calcium can be added or withdrawn. Bone loss caused by a net calcium loss from this bank proceeds slowly. Only after many years are clinical symptoms apparent. By not meeting calcium needs, some people—especially women—are most likely setting the stage for future bone fractures.

∎ Functions of Calcium

Forming and maintaining bones are calcium's major roles in the body. This is discussed in detail in the second Looking Further section on minerals and **osteoporosis** found at the end of this chapter. However, calcium is important in many other processes as well. Calcium is essential for blood clotting and for muscle contraction. If blood calcium falls below a critical point, muscles cannot relax after contraction; the body stiffens and shows involuntary twitching, called **tetany.** In nerve transmission, calcium assists in the release of neurotransmitters and permits the flow of ions in and out of nerve cells. Without sufficient calcium, nerve function fails, opening another path to tetany. Finally, calcium helps regulate cellular metabolism by influencing the activities of various enzymes and hormonal responses. It is the hormonal regulation of blood calcium that keeps all of these processes going, even if a person failures to consume enough calcium on a daily basis.

Other Possible Health Benefits of Calcium

Researchers have been examining links between calcium intake and risks for a wide array of diseases. An adequate calcium intake can reduce the risk of colon cancer, especially in people who consume a high-fat diet. A decreased risk of some forms of kidney stones and reduced lead absorption are other possible benefits when calcium is part of a meal. Calcium intakes of 800 to 1200 milligrams per day can also decrease blood pressure, compared with intakes of 400 milligrams per day or less. As covered in Chapter 5, calcium intakes of 1200 milligrams per day in combination with a low-fat, low-cholesterol diet can help people with elevated LDL improve their blood lipid profiles. A link between a low calcium intake and overweight/obesity is also under study. Although the true benefit in this regard is not clear, recent studies suggest that an adequate calcium intake (compared to a very low intake [e.g., 400 milligrams per day]), coupled with a low calorie intake, may promote even more weight loss than the low calorie diet alone. Focusing on dairy sources of calcium is recommended since other components in dairy foods, such as some of the specific dairy proteins present, contribute to this potential weight loss benefit. For women, an adequate calcium intake might also reduce the risk of premenstrual syndrome and high blood pressure that can develop during pregnancy. Overall, the benefits of a diet providing adequate calcium extend beyond bone health.

■ Calcium Sources and Needs

Dairy products, such as milk and cheese, provide about 75% of the calcium in North American diets. The exception is cottage cheese, because most calcium is lost during production. Bread, rolls, crackers, and other foods made with milk products are secondary contributors. Other calcium sources are leafy greens (such as spinach), broccoli, sardines, and canned salmon. However, much of the calcium in some leafy green vegetables, notably spinach, is not absorbed because of the presence of oxalic acid. This effect is not as strong, however, in kale, collard, turnip, and mustard greens. Overall, fat-free milk is the most nutrient-dense (milligrams per kcal) source of calcium because of its high bioavailability and low calorie content, with some of the vegetables just noted following close behind (Fig. 9-6). The new calcium-fortified versions of orange juice and other beverages (e.g., soy milk), as well as calcium-fortified cottage cheese, breakfast cereals, breakfast bars, snacks, and certain chewable chocolate candies, also follow as close competitors. Another source of calcium is soybean curd (tofu) if it is made with calcium carbonate (check the label). Note also that the bones in canned fish, such as salmon and sardines, supply calcium.

Information about calcium is mandatory on food labels. The Daily Value for calcium used for food and supplement labels is 1000 milligrams.

The Adequate Intake for calcium for adults ranges from 1000 to 1200 milligrams per day and is based on the amount of calcium needed each day to offset calcium losses in urine, feces, and other routes. The Adequate Intake for young people includes an additional amount to allow for increases in bone mass during growth and development. In the United States, average calcium intakes are approximately 800 milligrams for women and 1000 milligrams for men. Thus, dietary intakes of calcium by many women,

Food Sources of Calcium

Food Item and Amount	Calcium (milligrams)
Plain yogurt, 1 cup	450
Parmesan cheese, 1 ounce	390
Fortified orange juice, 1 cup	350
Romano cheese, 1 ounce	300
1% milk, 1 cup	300
Buttermilk, 1 cup	285
Swiss cheese, 1 ounce	275
Spinach, 1 cup	250
Salmon (with bones), 3 ounces	210
Cheddar cheese, 1 ounce	200
Total Raisin Bran cereal, ¾ cup	180
Sardines (with bones), 2 ounces	170
Chocolate pudding, ½ cup	160
Tofu, ½ cup	140

Adequate Intake for adults, 1000 milligrams; Adequate Intake for adults over 50, 1200 milligrams

Figure 9-6 Sources of Calcium from MyPyramid. The height and background color (none, 1/3, 2/3 or completely covered) within each group in the pyramid indicates the average nutrient density for calcium in that group. Overall, the milk group especially contains many foods that are nutrient-dense sources, and along with fortified foods, the calcium is quite bioavailable. Additional calcium-fortified foods appear in stores each year and thus will add to the food sources currently listed for various groups. With regard to physical activity, calcium is especially important for related muscle contraction, and as well to maintain a strong skeleton to support the body.

Grains	Vegetables	Fruits	Oils	Milk	Meat & Beans
• Calcium-fortified snack foods • Calcium-fortified flour tortillas • Calcium-fortified breakfast cereals	• Greens • Spinach • Broccoli • Green beans	• Calcium-fortified orange juice	• None	• Milk • Yogurt • Cheese	• Tofu • Almonds • Shrimp • Sardines • Canned salmon

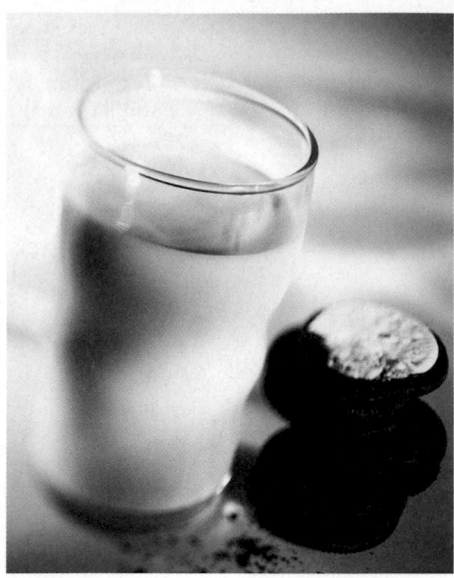

Milk is a rich as well as convenient source of calcium.

especially young women, are below the Adequate Intake, whereas intakes by most men are roughly equivalent to the Adequate Intake. It is also important for vegans to focus on eating good plant sources of calcium as well as on the total amount of calcium ingested.

To estimate your calcium intake, use the rule of 300s. Count 300 milligrams for the calcium provided by foods scattered throughout the diet. Add to that another 300 milligrams for every cup of milk or yogurt or 1.5 ounces of cheese. If you eat a lot of tofu, almonds, or sardines, or drink calcium-fortified beverages, use Table 9-3 or your diet analysis software to get a more accurate calculation of your calcium intake.

Calcium Supplements

Calcium supplements can be used by people who do not like milk or who cannot incorporate enough calcium-containing foods into their diets. Calcium carbonate, the form found in calcium-based antacid tablets, is the most common supplement used. People should take this supplement with or just after meals in doses of about 500 milligrams so that stomach acid produced during digestion can aid with absorption of this mineral. On the other hand, a supplement containing calcium citrate, which is acidic itself, can be taken between or with meals, or at bedtime.

Another Bite

Here is how to determine the calcium content of typical supplements based on the percent of calcium per unit of weight and form of calcium, as listed on the supplement label.

- Calcium carbonate: 40%
- Calcium phosphate (tribasic): 38%
- Calcium citrate: 21%
- Calcium lactate: 13%
- Calcium gluconate: 9%

To calculate the amount of calcium in a supplement, simply multiply the weight of the capsule by the percentage listed above. For example, if 1 tablet of calcium citrate weighs 500 milligrams, it contains 105 milligrams of calcium.

$$500 \text{ milligrams} \times 0.21 = 105 \text{ milligrams}$$

Some calcium supplements are poorly digested because they do not readily dissolve. To test for this, put a supplement in ¾ cup of cider vinegar. Stir every 5 minutes. It should dissolve within 30 minutes.

With calcium supplements, interactions with other minerals are a valid concern. Perhaps most importantly, there is some evidence that calcium supplements may decrease zinc absorption. Therefore, calcium supplements should not be taken with meals rich in zinc. An effect of calcium supplementation on iron absorption is possible; however, this appears to be small over the long term. To be safe, people using a calcium supplement on a regular basis should notify their physician of the practice.

Some calcium supplements also contain lead. Chapter 16 points out that lead produces an array of deleterious effects on the body. Currently, FDA has no standards for lead content in food supplements. However, FDA does plan to regulate the lead content of supplements, including calcium, in the future. Until then, it is important to avoid supplements made from bonemeal, the worst offender when it comes to lead. Tablet or liquid calcium supplements with the USP seal of approval are less likely than others to contain high concentrations of contaminants.

■ Upper Level for Calcium

The Upper Level for calcium intake is 2500 milligrams per day, based on the observation that greater intakes increase the risk for some forms of kidney stones. Excessive calcium intakes by some people also can cause high blood and urinary calcium concentrations, irritability, headache, kidney failure, soft tissue calcification, and decreased absorption of other minerals, as noted above.

Table 9-3 A Tool for Estimating Current Calcium Intake

For all of the following foods, write the number of servings eaten in a day. Total the number of servings in each category and then multiply the total number of servings by the milligrams of calcium for each category. Finally, add the total milligrams to estimate calcium intake for that day.

Food	Serving Size	Number of Servings	Calcium (milligrams)	Total Calcium (milligrams)
Plain low-fat yogurt	1 cup	_____		
Fat-free dry milk powder	½ cup	_____		
	Total servings	_____	× 400	= _____ milligrams
Canned sardines (with bones)	3 ounces	_____		
Fruit-flavored yogurt	1 cup	_____		
Milk: Fat-free, reduced-fat, whole, chocolate, buttermilk	1 cup	_____		
Calcium-fortified soy milk (e.g., Silk)	1 cup	_____		
Parmesan cheese (grated)	¼ cup	_____		
Swiss cheese	1 ounce	_____		
	Total servings	_____	× 300	= _____ milligrams
Cheese (all other hard cheese)	1 ounce	_____		
Pancakes	3	_____		
	Total servings	_____	× 200	= _____ milligrams
Canned pink salmon	3 ounces	_____		
Tofu (processed with calcium)	4 ounces	_____		
	Total servings	_____	× 150	= _____ milligrams
Collards or turnip greens, cooked	½ cup	_____		
Ice cream or ice milk	½ cup	_____		
Almonds	1 ounce	_____		
	Total servings	_____	× 75	= _____ milligrams
Chard, cooked	½ cup	_____		
Cottage cheese	½ cup	_____		
Corn tortilla	1 medium	_____		
Orange	1 medium	_____		
	Total servings	_____	× 50	= _____ milligrams
Kidney, lima, or navy beans, cooked	½ cup	_____		
Broccoli	½ cup	_____		
Carrot, raw	1 medium	_____		
Dates or raisins	¼ cup	_____		
Egg	1 large	_____		
Whole-wheat bread	1 slice	_____		
Peanut butter	2 tablespoons	_____		
	Total servings	_____	× 25	= _____ milligrams
Calcium-fortified orange juice	6 ounces	_____		
Calcium-fortified snack bars	1 each	_____		
Calcium-fortified breakfast bars	½ bar	_____		
	Total servings	_____	× 200	= _____ milligrams
Calcium-fortified chocolate candies	1 each	_____		
Calcium supplements*	1 each	_____	× 500	= _____ milligrams
		Total calcium intake		= _____ milligrams

Other calcium sources to consider include many breakfast cereals (100 to 250 milligrams per cup), and some vitamins/mineral supplements (200 to 500 milligrams or more per tablet).

*Amount varies, so check the label for the amount in a specific product and then adjust the calculation as needed.

Reprinted with permission from *Topics in Clinical Nutrition,* "Putting Calcium into Perspective for Your Clients," G. Wardlaw and N. Weese; 11:1, p. 29. © 1995 Aspen Publishers, Inc.

So, which is better: calcium from food or supplements? Taking 1000 milligrams of calcium carbonate or calcium citrate daily in divided doses (about 500 milligrams per tablet) is probably safe in many instances. However, people often have difficulty adhering to a supplement regimen. If possible, modification of eating habits to include foods that are good sources of calcium is a better plan of action. In addition to this important mineral, foods that contain calcium also supply other vitamins, minerals, phytochemicals, and fats that are needed to support health. Plus, problems associated with excessive consumption of calcium are not likely when foods are one's sources of calcium.

No form of natural calcium, such as coral calcium, is superior to typical supplement forms. People making such claims of superiority have even been prosecuted by the U.S. Federal Trade Commission for false advertising.

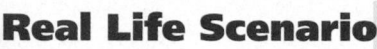

Real Life Scenario Follow-Up

Jana is increasing her chances of developing osteoporosis later in life because of her current high-risk lifestyle. Factors contributing to her potential risk include a poor dietary intake of calcium. Jana needs to find some reliable sources of calcium. These could include calcium-fortified juices, calcium-fortified bread and snack bars, and calcium-fortified chewable chocolate candies. Tofu (made with calcium) is another potential source, as well as calcium-fortified soy milk. Meeting the Adequate Intake of 1000 milligrams per day for her age would not be that hard if she were to make a conscious effort to use these calcium-rich foods and/or incorporate other rich sources. She also should rethink her rationale for avoiding milk. Fat-free milk is very low in calories and provides much calcium. Dairy products such as milk do not lead to weight gain per se. There are even some studies suggesting a regular intake of dairy products rich in calcium may aid in weight loss when on an otherwise calorie-restricted diet.

Concept Check

About 99% of calcium in the body is found in the bones. Aside from its critical role in bone, calcium also functions in blood clotting, muscle contraction, nerve-impulse transmission, and cell metabolism. Calcium requires a slightly acid pH and the vitamin D hormone for efficient absorption. Factors that reduce calcium absorption include a vitamin D deficiency, large amounts of fiber (especially excess wheat bran), and old age in general. Blood calcium is regulated primarily by hormones and does not closely reflect daily intake.

Dairy products are rich food sources of calcium. Other foods, such as calcium-fortified beverages, are rich sources as well. Supplemental forms, such as calcium carbonate, are well-absorbed by most people. However, overzealous supplementation can also result in the development of kidney stones and other health problems.

Phosphorus (P)

Although no disease is currently associated with an inadequate phosphorus intake, a deficiency may contribute to bone loss in older women. The body absorbs phosphorus quite efficiently, about 70% of dietary intake. This high absorption, plus the wide availability of phosphorus in foods, makes this mineral less important than is calcium in diet planning. The active vitamin D hormone enhances phosphorus absorption, as it does for calcium. Blood phosphorus concentration is regulated primarily by kidney excretion. This regulating mechanism differs from that of calcium, wherein changes in the degree of absorption are a more significant factor.

Phosphorus is a component of enzymes, other key metabolic compounds (many of which are involved in energy metabolism), DNA (genetic material), cell membranes, and bone. About 85% of the body's phosphorus is inside bone. The remaining phosphorus circulates freely in the bloodstream and functions inside cells.

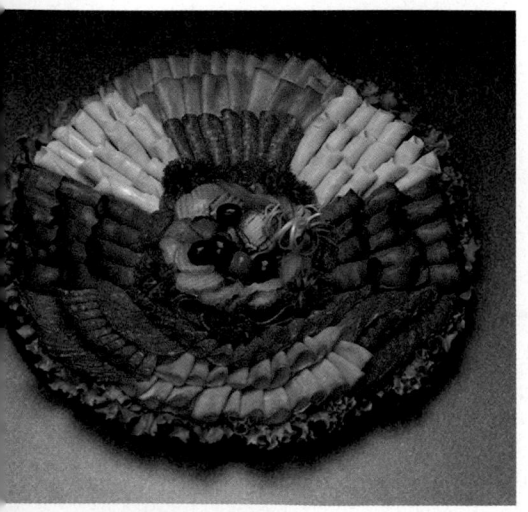

Meats are rich in phosphorus.

■ Phosphorus Sources and Needs

Milk, cheese, meat, and bread provide most of the phosphorus in the adult diet. Breakfast cereals, bran, eggs, nuts, and fish are also good sources. About 20% to 30% of dietary phosphorus comes from food additives, especially in baked goods, cheeses, processed meats, and many soft drinks (about 75 milligrams per 12-ounce—⅓-liter— serving of soft drinks). Next time you have a soft drink, look for a listing of phosphoric acid on the label.

The RDA for phosphorus for adults over age 18 is 700 milligrams daily, based on the amount to maintain normal blood concentrations of phosphorus. The Daily Value used on food and supplement labels is 1000 milligrams. Adults consume from about 1000 to 1600 milligrams of phosphorus per day. Thus, deficiencies of phosphorus are unlikely in healthy adults, especially because it is so efficiently absorbed.

Marginal phosphorus status can be found in preterm infants, vegans, people with alcoholism, older people on nutrient-poor diets, and people with long-term bouts of diarrhea.

■ Upper Level for Phosphorus

The Upper Level for phosphorus intake is 3 to 4 grams per day. Intakes greater than this impair kidney function. High intakes are especially a problem in people with certain kidney diseases. In addition, chronic imbalance in the calcium-to-phosphorus ratio in the diet, resulting from a high phosphorus intake coupled with a low calcium intake, also can contribute to bone loss. This situation most likely arises when the Adequate Intake for calcium is not met, as can occur in adolescents and adults who regularly substitute soft drinks for milk or otherwise underconsume calcium.

Magnesium (Mg)

Magnesium is important for nerve and heart function and aids many enzyme reactions. It is found mostly in the plant pigment chlorophyll, where it functions in respiration. We normally absorb about 40% to 60% of the magnesium in our diets, but absorption efficiency can increase up to about 80% if intakes are low.

Bone contains 60% of the body's magnesium. The rest circulates in the blood and operates inside cells. Over 300 enzymes use magnesium, and many energy-yielding compounds in cells require magnesium to function properly, as does the hormone insulin.

In humans, a magnesium deficiency causes an irregular heartbeat, sometimes accompanied by weakness, muscle pain, disorientation, and seizures. Other possible benefits of magnesium in relation to cardiovascular disease include decreasing blood pressure by dilating arteries and preventing heart rhythm abnormalities. People with cardiovascular disease should closely monitor magnesium intake, especially because they are often on medications such as diuretics that reduce magnesium status. Keep in mind that a magnesium deficiency develops very slowly because our bodies store it readily.

■ Magnesium Sources and Needs

Rich sources for magnesium are plant products, such as whole grains (like wheat bran), broccoli, potatoes, squash, beans, nuts, and seeds. Animal products, such as milk and meats, and even chocolate supply some magnesium, although less than the foods in the magnesium pyramid (Fig. 9-7). Two other sources of magnesium are hard tap water, which contains a high mineral content, and coffee.

The adult RDA for magnesium is about 400 milligrams per day for men and about 310 milligrams per day for women. This is based on the amount needed to offset daily losses. The Daily Value used on food and supplement labels is 400 milligrams. Adult men consume an average of 320 milligrams daily, whereas women consume closer to 220 milligrams daily. This suggests that many of us should improve our intakes of magnesium-rich foods, such as whole-grain breads and cereals. The refined grain products that dominate the diets of many North Americans are poor sources of this

Food Sources of Phosphorus

Food Item and Amount	Phosphorus (milligrams)
Plain yogurt, 1 cup	350
Swiss cheese, 2 ounces	345
Almonds, ½ cup	340
Sunflower seeds, 1 ounce	330
1% milk, 1 cup	235
Cheddar cheese, 1.5 ounces	220
Salmon, 3 ounces	220
Sirloin steak, 3 ounces	210
Raisin Bran cereal, 1 cup	215
Egg, 2 hard-boiled	200
Chicken breast, 3 ounces	180
Roasted turkey, 3 ounces	180
Pot roast, 3 ounces	170
Lean ham, 3 ounces	165
American cheese, 1 slice	155

RDA for adults, 700 milligrams

Food Sources of Magnesium

Food Item and Amount	Magnesium (milligrams)
Spinach, 1 cup	157
Squash, 1 cup	105
Wheat germ, ¼ cup	90
Raisin Bran cereal, 1 cup	90
Navy beans, ½ cup	54
Peanut butter, 2 tablespoons	51
Black-eyed peas, ½ cup	46
Plain yogurt, 1 cup	43
Kidney beans, ½ cup	43
Sunflower seeds, ¼ cup	41
Broccoli, 1 cup	37
Banana, 1 medium	34
1% milk, 1 cup	34
Watermelon, 1 slice	32
Oatmeal, ½ cup	28
Whole-wheat bread, 1 slice	25

RDA for adult men, 400 milligrams
RDA for adult women, 310 milligrams

Figure 9-7 Sources of Magnesium from MyPyramid. The height and background color (none, 1/3, 2/3 or completely covered) within each group in the pyramid indicates the average nutrient density for magnesium in that group. Overall, the vegetables group provides the richest sources. Whole grain choices in the grains group are also rich sources. With regard to physical activity, magnesium is especially needed for the carbohydrate metabolism that takes place in such endeavors.

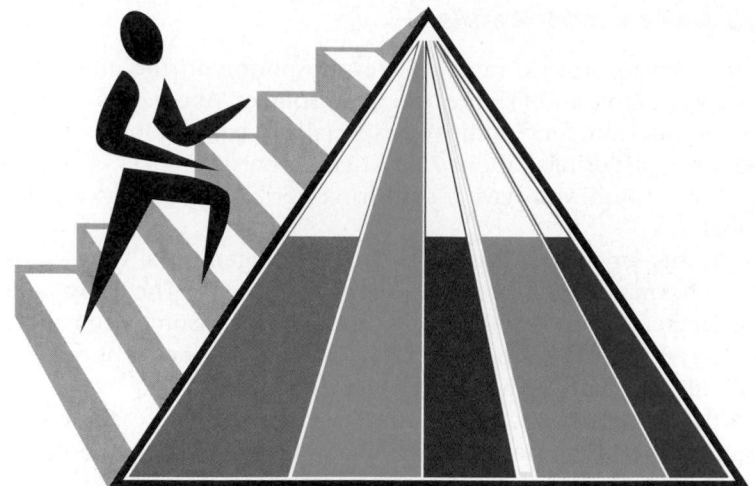

Grains	Vegetables	Fruits	Oils	Milk	Meat & Beans
• Wheat bran • Wheat germ • Whole-grain products	• Spinach • Greens • Broccoli • Lima beans • Potatoes • Squash	• Figs • Peaches • Avocados • Bananas • Berries	• None	• Milk • Yogurt	• Tofu • Nuts • Shrimp • Kidney beans • Sunflower seeds

Diabetes and hypertension have both been linked with low levels of magnesium in the blood. However, the cause for low magnesium in people with these diseases is unclear. Research is currently underway to uncover the potential role of magnesium in treatment and/or prevention of these chronic diseases.

mineral. If dietary means are not enough, a balanced multivitamin and mineral supplement containing approximately 100 milligrams of magnesium can help to close the gap between intake and needs. The typical form used (magnesium oxide) is not as well absorbed as the forms of magnesium found in foods, but still contributes to meeting magnesium needs.

Poor magnesium status is especially found among users of certain diuretics. In addition, heavy perspiration for weeks in hot climates and bouts of long-standing diarrhea or vomiting all cause significant magnesium loss. Alcoholism also increases the risk of a deficiency because dietary intake may be poor and because alcohol increases magnesium excretion in the urine. The disorientation and weakness associated with alcoholism closely resemble the behavior of people with low blood magnesium.

■ Upper Level for Magnesium

The Upper Level for magnesium intake is 350 milligrams per day, based on the risk of developing diarrhea. Note, however, that this guideline refers only to nonfood sources such as antacids, laxatives, or supplements. Magnesium toxicity especially occurs in people who have kidney failure or who overuse over-the-counter medications that contain magnesium, such as certain antacids and laxatives (e.g., milk of magnesia). Older people are at particular risk, as kidney function may be compromised.

▌ Sulfur (S)

Sulfur is found in many important compounds in the body, such as some amino acids (like methionine) and the vitamins biotin and thiamin. Sulfur helps in the balance of acids and bases in the body and is an important part of the liver's drug-detoxifying pathways. Because proteins supply the sulfur we need, it is not an essential nutrient per se. Sulfur is naturally a part of a healthy diet. Sulfur compounds are also used to preserve foods (see Chapter 16).

Table 9-4 summarizes much of what we have covered regarding the major minerals.

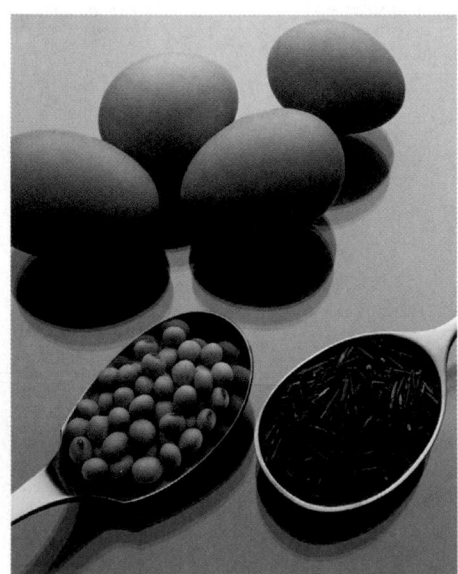

Protein-rich foods supply sulfur in the diet.

Table 9-4 Summary of the Major Minerals

Mineral	Major Functions	RDA, or Adequate Intake	Dietary Sources	Deficiency Symptoms	Toxicity Symptoms
Sodium	• Major positive ion of the extracellular fluid • Aids nerve impulse transmission • Water balance	*Age 19–50 years:* 1500 milligrams *Age 51–70 years:* 1300 milligrams *Age 71 years or more:* 1200 milligrams	• Table salt • Processed foods • Condiments • Sauces • Soups • Chips	• Muscle cramps	• Contributes to hypertension in susceptible individuals • Increases calcium loss in urine • Upper Level is 2300 milligrams
Potassium	• Major positive ion of intracellular fluid • Aids nerve impulse transmission • Water balance	4700 milligrams	• Spinach • Squash • Bananas • Orange juice • Milk • Meat • Legumes • Whole grains	• Irregular heart beat • Loss of appetite • Muscle cramps	• Slowing of the heartbeat, as seen in kidney failure
Chloride	• Major negative ion of extracellular fluid • Participates in acid production in stomach • Aids nerve impulse transmission • Water balance	2300 milligrams	• Table salt • Some vegetables • Processed foods	• Convulsions in infants	• Linked to hypertension in susceptible people when combined with sodium • Upper Level is 3600 milligrams
Calcium	• Bone and tooth structure • Blood clotting • Aids in nerve impulse transmission • Muscle contractions • Other cell functions	*Age greater than 18 years:* 1000–1200 milligrams *Age 9–18 years:* 1300 milligrams	• Dairy products • Canned fish • Leafy vegetables • Tofu • Fortified orange juice (and other fortified foods)	• Increased risk of osteoporosis	• May cause kidney stones and other problems in susceptible people. • Upper Level is 2500 milligrams
Phosphorus	• Major ion of intracellular fluid • Bone and tooth strength • Part of various metabolic compounds • Acid/base balance	*Age greater than 18 years:* 700 milligrams *Age 9–18 years:* 1250 milligrams	• Dairy products • Processed foods • Fish • Soft drinks • Bakery products • Meats	• Possibility of poor bone maintenance	• Impairs bone health in people with kidney failure • Poor bone mineralization if calcium intakes are low • Upper Level is 3 to 4 grams
Magnesium	• Bone formation • Aids enzyme function • Aids nerve and heart function	*Men:* 400–420 milligrams *Women:* 310–320 milligrams	• Wheat bran • Green vegetables • Nuts • Chocolate • Legumes	• Weakness • Muscle pain • Poor heart function	• Causes diarrhea and weakness in people with kidney failure • Upper Level of 350 milligrams, but refers to nonfood sources (e.g., supplements) only
Sulfur	• Part of vitamins and amino acids • Aids in drug detoxification • Acid/base balance	None	• Protein foods	• None observed	• None likely

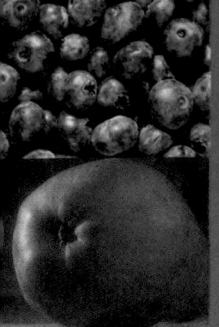

Looking *Further*

Among North Americans, an estimated 1 in 5 adults has hypertension. Over the age of 65, the number rises to 1 in every 2 adults. Only about half of all cases are being treated. Blood pressure is expressed by two numbers. The higher number represents systolic blood pressure, which is the pressure in the arteries when the heart muscle is contracting and pumping blood into the arteries. Optimal systolic blood pressure is 120 millimeters of mercury (mm Hg) or less. The second value is diastolic blood pressure, which is the artery pressure when the heart is relaxed. Optimal diastolic blood pressure is 80 mm Hg or less. Elevations in both systolic and diastolic blood pressure are strong predictors of disease.

Hypertension is defined as sustained systolic pressure exceeding 139 millimeters of mercury (mm Hg) or diastolic blood pressure exceeding 89 mm Hg. Most cases of hypertension (about 95% of cases) have no clear-cut cause. It is described as primary, or essential, in nature (e.g., essential hypertension). Kidney disease, sleep-disordered breathing (sleep apnea), and other causes often lead to the other 5% of cases, known as secondary hypertension. African-Americans are more likely than Caucasians to develop hypertension and to do so earlier in life.

Unless blood pressure is measured periodically, the development of hypertension is easily overlooked. Thus, it's described as a silent disorder, because it usually does not cause symptoms.

Why Control Blood Pressure?

Blood pressure needs to be controlled mainly to prevent cardiovascular disease, kidney disease, strokes and related declines in brain function, poor blood circulation in the legs, problems with vision, and sudden death. All of these conditions are much more likely to be found in individuals with hypertension than in people with normal blood pressure. Smoking and elevated blood lipoproteins make these diseases even more likely. Individuals with hypertension need to be diagnosed and treated as soon as possible, as the condition generally progresses to a more serious stage over time and even resists therapy if it persists for years.

Causes of Hypertension

A family history of hypertension is a risk factor, especially if both parents have (or had) the problem. Blood pressure also usually increases as a person ages. Some increase is caused by atherosclerosis. As plaque builds up in the arteries, the arteries become less flexible and cannot expand. When vessels remain rigid, blood pressure remains high. Eventually, the plaque begins to choke off the blood supply to the kidneys, decreasing their ability to control blood volume and, in turn, blood pressure.

An enzyme secreted by the kidneys and some hormone-like compounds affect blood pressure. Medications are available to reduce their effect.

Overweight people have six times greater risk of having hypertension than lean people. Overall, obesity is considered the number 1 lifestyle factor related to hypertension. This is especially the case in minority populations. Additional blood vessels develop to support excess tissue in overweight and obese individuals, and these extra miles of associated blood vessels increase work by the heart and also blood pressure. Elevated blood insulin concentration associated with insulin-resistant adipose cells is another reason for this link to obesity. Insulin

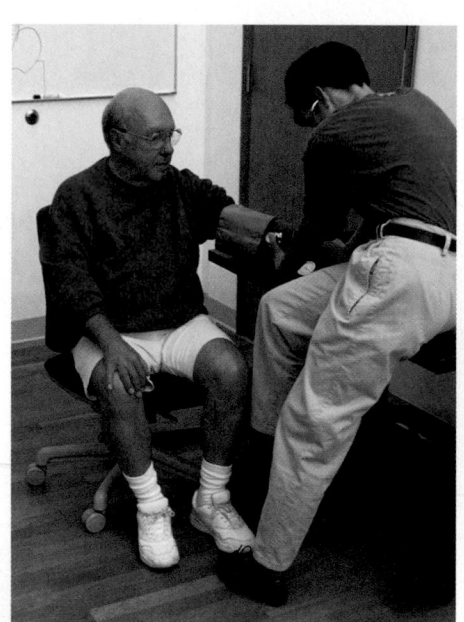

Older adults are particularly at risk of hypertension.

increases sodium retention in the body and accelerates atherosclerosis. A weight loss of as little as 10 to 15 pounds often can help treat hypertension.

Inactivity is considered the number 2 lifestyle factor related to hypertension. If an obese person can engage in regular physical activity (at least 5 days per week for 30 to 60 minutes) and lose weight, blood pressure often returns to normal.

Third, excess alcohol intake is responsible for about 10% of all cases of hypertension, especially in middle-age males and among African-Americans in general. When hypertension is caused by excessive alcohol intake, it is usually reversible. A sensible alcohol intake for people with hypertension is two or fewer drinks per day for men, and one or no drinks per day for women and all older adults. Did you recognize that this is the same recommendation given in the 2005 Dietary Guidelines for Americans? As discussed in Chapter 7, some studies suggest that such a minimal alcohol intake may reduce the risk of ischemic stroke. These data, however, should not be used to encourage alcohol use.

Some people are especially sodium sensitive, particularly African-Americans and older overweight persons. In these people, excess salt leads to fluid retention and a corresponding increase in blood volume, which therefore increases blood pressure. It is not clear whether the sodium ion or the chloride ion is actually most responsible for the effect. Still, as reviewed in this chapter, if one reduces sodium intake, chloride intake naturally falls; the opposite is also true. For the most part, a recommendation to consume less sodium is equivalent to a call for less salt in the diet. Since only some North Americans are very susceptible to increases in blood pressure from salt intake, it is only the number 4 lifestyle factor related to hypertension. It is unfortunate that salt intake receives the major portion of public attention with regard to hypertension. Efforts to prevent hypertension should also focus on obesity, inactivity, and alcohol abuse.

Other Minerals and Blood Pressure

Minerals such as calcium, potassium, and magnesium also deserve attention when it comes to prevention and treatment of hypertension. Recent studies show that a diet rich in these minerals and low in salt can lead to a decrease in blood pressure within days of beginning a specific diet, especially among African-Americans. The response is even similar to that seen with commonly used medications. The diet is called the Dietary Approaches to Stop Hypertension (DASH) diet. The diet takes a standard MyPyramid food plan and adds 1 to 2 extra vegetables and fruits servings and a serving of nuts, seeds, or legumes (beans) 4 to 5 days of the week. All DASH participants also consumed no more than 3 grams of sodium and no more than one to two alcoholic drinks per week. A DASH 2 diet trial tested three daily sodium intakes (3300 milligrams, 2400 milligrams, and 1500 milligrams). People showed a steady decline in blood pressure on the DASH diet as sodium intake declined. Over all, the DASH diet is seen as a total dietary approach to treating hypertension. It is not clear which of the many healthful practices of this diet are responsible for the fall in blood pressure.

Other studies also show a reduction in stroke risk among people who consume a diet rich in fruits, vegetables, and vitamin C (recall that fruits and vegetables are rich vitamin C sources). Overall, a diet low in salt and rich in low-fat and fat-free dairy products, fruits, vegetables, whole grains, and some nuts can substantially reduce hypertension and stroke risk in many people, especially those with hypertension.

Medications to Treat Hypertension

Diuretic medications are one class of drugs used to treat hypertension. These work to reduce blood volume (and therefore blood pressure) by increasing fluid output in the urine. Other medications act by slowing heart rate or by causing relaxation of blood vessels. A combination of two or more medications is commonly required to treat hypertension that does not respond to diet and lifestyle therapy.

Prevention of Hypertension

Many of the risk factors for hypertension and stroke are controllable, and appropriate lifestyle changes can reduce a person's risk (Table 9-5). Experts also recommend that those with hypertension lower blood pressure through diet and lifestyle changes before resorting to blood pressure medications.

Table 9-5 A Nutritional Plan to Minimize Hypertension and Stroke Risk

1. Follow MyPyramid. Also consider going beyond this to include more fruits, vegetables, and some nuts (e.g., DASH diet), especially if one has hypertension.
2. Make sure to meet nutrient recommendations for calcium, potassium, and magnesium.
3. Attain and maintain a healthy body weight.
4. Incorporate regular physical activity (at least five times per week for 30 to 60 minutes per day).
5. Consume alcoholic beverages in moderation, if at all (two drinks per day maximum for men, and one drink per day maximum for women and all older adults).
6. Consume minimal amounts of sodium (salt) and see if this helps.
7. Do not smoke.
8. Maintain blood lipoproteins in the normal range (see Chapter 5).
9. Avoid lead exposure, as this can cause hypertension (see Chapter 16 for strategies).

Concept Check

Phosphorus absorption is quite efficient and is enhanced by the active vitamin D hormone. Urinary excretion mainly controls body content. Phosphorus aids enzyme function and is part of key metabolic compounds and cell membranes. No distinct deficiency symptoms caused by an inadequate phosphorus intake have been reported. Food sources for phosphorus include dairy products, baked goods, and meat. The RDA is met by most North Americans. An excess intake of phosphorus can compromise bone health, if sufficient calcium is not otherwise consumed, and can impair kidney function. Magnesium is required for nerve and heart function; it also aids activity for many enzymes. Food sources of magnesium are whole grains (wheat bran), vegetables, beef, coffee, beans, nuts, and seeds. People using certain diuretics and people with alcoholism are at greatest risk of developing a deficiency. Magnesium toxicity is most likely in people with kidney failure or people using certain forms of laxatives and antacids. Sulfur is a component of certain vitamins and amino acids. The protein we consume supplies sufficient sulfur for the body's needs.

Trace Minerals—An Overview

Information about trace minerals (also called microminerals) is perhaps the most rapidly expanding area of knowledge in nutrition. With the exceptions of iron and iodide, the importance of trace minerals to humans has been recognized only within the last 40 years. Although we need 100 milligrams or less of each trace mineral daily, they are just as essential to good health as are major minerals.

In some cases, discovering the importance of a trace mineral reads like a detective story, and the evidence is still unfolding. In 1961, researchers linked dwarfism in Middle Eastern villagers to a zinc deficiency. Other scientists recognized that a rare form of heart disease in an isolated area of China was linked to a selenium deficiency. In North America, some trace mineral deficiencies were first observed in the late 1960s and early 1970s when the minerals were not added to synthetic formulas used for intravenous feeding.

It is difficult to define precisely our trace mineral needs because we need only minute amounts. Highly sophisticated technology is required to measure such small amounts in both food and body tissues.

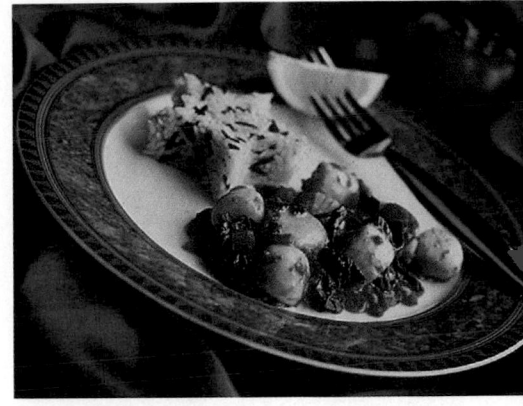

Seafood, like scallops, is a rich source of many trace minerals.

Iron (Fe)

Although the importance of dietary iron has been recognized for centuries, today, iron deficiency is still one of the most common nutrient deficiencies worldwide. Iron is the only nutrient for which young women have a greater RDA than do adult men. Iron is found in every living cell, adding up to about 5 grams (1 teaspoon) for the entire body.

Absorption and Distribution of Iron

The body uses several mechanisms to regulate iron absorption. Controlling absorption is important because our bodies cannot easily eliminate excess iron once it is absorbed. Overall, iron absorption depends on its form in the food, the body's need for it, and a variety of other factors. Iron absorption from foods is about 18% of that present for healthy people, and somewhat higher in people with iron deficiency.

The form of iron in foods especially influences how much is absorbed. About 40% of the total iron in animal flesh is in the form of **hemoglobin** (the same form as in red blood cells) and **myoglobin** (pigment found in muscle cells). This **heme iron** is absorbed about two to three times more efficiently than the simple elemental iron, called **nonheme iron.** Nonheme iron is also present in animal flesh, as well as in eggs, milk, vegetables, grains, and other plant foods.

Consuming heme iron and nonheme iron together increases nonheme iron absorption. A protein factor in meats may also aid nonheme absorption. Overall, eating meat with vegetables and grain products enhances the absorption of all nonheme iron present.

Vitamin C in amounts of about 75 milligrams can increase nonheme iron absorption. So one should consider drinking a glass of orange juice when taking an iron supplement. Consuming more foods rich in vitamin C is particularly desirable if dietary iron is inadequate or if blood iron is low. Iron use in the body is also aided by copper, as explained in the later section on copper.

Several dietary factors interfere with our ability to absorb nonheme iron. Phytic acid and other factors in grain fibers and oxalic acid in vegetables can all bind this iron and reduce its absorption. Polyphenols (tannins) found in tea also reduce nonheme iron absorption. It is a good idea to moderate intake of tannins if one has iron deficiency and keep fiber intake within current recommendations. Zinc supplements, if used, also interfere with nonheme iron by competing with it for absorption.

hemoglobin The iron-containing part of the red blood cell that carries oxygen to the cells and some carbon dioxide away from the cells. The heme iron portion is also responsible for the red color of blood.

myoglobin Iron-containing protein that binds oxygen in muscle tissue.

heme iron Iron provided from animal tissues in the form of hemoglobin and myoglobin. Approximately 40% of the iron in meat is heme iron; it is readily absorbed.

nonheme iron Iron provided from plant sources and animal tissues other than in the forms of hemoglobin and myoglobin. Nonheme iron is less efficiently absorbed than heme iron; absorption is closely dependent on body needs.

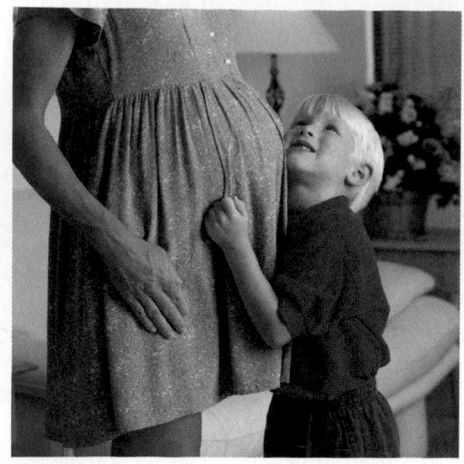

Pregnancy greatly increases iron needs, as does growth in childhood.

Overall, the most important factor influencing nonheme iron absorption is the body's need for it. Iron needs are increased during pregnancy and growth. At high altitudes, the lower oxygen concentration of the air causes an increase in the hemoglobin concentration of blood and thus an increase in iron needs. In a deficiency state, nonheme iron absorption can increase. When iron stores are inadequate, the main blood protein that carries iron readily binds more iron, shifting it from intestinal cells into the bloodstream. If iron stores are adequate and the iron-binding protein in the blood is fully saturated with iron, little will be absorbed from the intestinal cells. It stays bound in the intestinal cells.

By this mechanism, under normal circumstances, iron, especially the nonheme form, is absorbed for the most part as needed. If not needed, when intestinal cells are shed at the end of their 2- to 5-day life cycle, the iron returns to the lumen of the intestinal tract to be excreted. High doses of iron can still be toxic, but absorption is carefully regulated under typical dietary conditions in most people.

Most iron in the body is contained in the hemoglobin molecules of the red blood cells. Some iron is stored in the bone marrow, and a small portion goes to other body cells, such as the liver, for storage. As iron is needed, it can be mobilized from body stores. If dietary intake is chronically inadequate, these iron stores become depleted. Only then do signs of an iron deficiency appear.

■ Functions of Iron

Iron is part of the hemoglobin in red blood cells and myoglobin in muscle cells. Hemoglobin molecules in red blood cells transport oxygen (O_2) from the lungs to cells and assist in the return of some carbon dioxide (CO_2) from cells to the lungs for excretion. In addition, iron is used as part of many enzymes, some proteins, and compounds that cells use in energy production. Iron is also needed for brain and immune function, and contributes to drug detoxification in the liver and to bone health.

If neither the diet nor body stores can supply the iron needed for hemoglobin synthesis, the number of red blood cells decreases in the bloodstream. The blood hemoglobin concentration also falls. Physicians use both the percentage of red blood cells (called the **hematocrit**) and the hemoglobin concentration to assess iron status, along with the amount of iron and iron-containing proteins in the bloodstream. When hematocrit and hemoglobin fall, an iron deficiency is suspected. In severe deficiency, hemoglobin and hematocrit fall so low that the amount of oxygen carried in the bloodstream is decreased. Such a person has anemia, defined as a decreased oxygen-carrying capacity of the blood.

While there are many types of anemia, iron-deficiency anemia is the major type worldwide. About 30% of the world's population is anemic, and about half of those cases are caused by an iron deficiency. Probably about 10% of North Americans in high-risk categories have iron-deficiency **anemia**. This appears most often in infancy, the preschool years, and at puberty for both males and females. Growth, with accompanying expansion of blood volume and muscle mass, increases iron needs, making it difficult to consume enough iron. Women are also very vulnerable during childbearing years from blood loss during menstruation. In addition, anemia is often found in pregnant women, as discussed in Chapter 13. Iron-deficiency anemia in adult men is usually caused by blood loss from ulcers, colon cancer, or hemorrhoids. Finally, athletes can develop this form of anemia, as discussed in Chapter 11.

Clinical symptoms of iron-deficiency anemia primarily include pale skin, fatigue upon exertion, poor temperature regulation, loss of appetite, and apathy. Insufficient iron for the synthesis of red blood cells and key cell compounds may cause the fatigue. Poor iron stores may also decrease learning ability, attention span, work performance, and immune status even before a person is actually anemic.

More North Americans have an iron deficiency without anemia than have iron-deficiency anemia. Their blood hemoglobin values are still normal, but they have no stores to draw from in times of pregnancy or illness, and basic functioning may be at

hematocrit The percentage of blood that is made up of red blood cells.

anemia Generally refers to a decreased oxygen-carrying capacity of the blood. This can be caused by many factors, such as iron deficiency or blood loss.

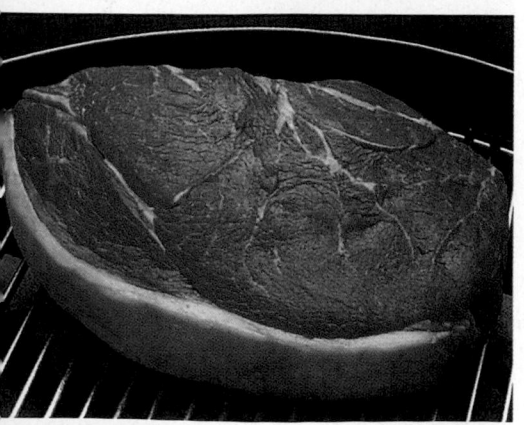

Red meat is a major source of iron in the North American diet. The heme iron present is better absorbed than the nonheme iron found in meats and plants.

decreased levels. That could mean anything from too little energy to perform everyday tasks in an efficient manner to difficulties staying alert in school or on the job.

To speed the cure of iron-deficiency anemia, a person needs to take iron supplements. A physician should also find the cause—an inadequate diet or a bleeding ulcer, for example—so that the anemia does not recur. Changes in diet may prevent iron-deficiency anemia, but supplemental iron is the only reliable cure once it has developed.

■ Iron Sources and Needs

Animal sources contain some heme iron, the most bioavailable form. These then end up our best iron sources. The major iron sources in the adult diet are ready-to-eat breakfast cereals, animal products, and bakery items, such as bread (Fig. 9-8). Most of the iron in these bakery items has been added to refined flour in the enrichment process. Other iron sources are spinach, peas, and legumes, but the iron is less available in these foods than in animal products.

Milk is a very poor source of iron. A common cause of iron-deficiency anemia in children is an overreliance on milk, coupled with an insufficient meat intake. Total vegetarians (vegans) are particularly susceptible to iron-deficiency anemia because of their lack of dietary heme iron.

The daily adult RDA for iron is 8 milligrams for men, as well as for women over 50 years, and 18 milligrams for women ages 19 to 50 years. This is based on the amount needed to counter iron losses. The Daily Value used on food and supplement labels is 18 milligrams.

The higher RDA for young and middle-age women is primarily because of menstrual blood loss. The variation in menstrual blood loss, and hence, loss of iron, makes it difficult to set an RDA for iron for women. Women who menstruate more heavily and longer than average may need even more dietary iron than those who have lighter and shorter flows.

Food Sources of Iron	
Food Item and Amount	**Iron (milligrams)**
Oat bran cereal, 1 cup	15.0
Baked clams, 3 ounces	14.0
Spinach, 1 cup	6.4
Kidney beans, 1 cup	5.3
Pot roast, 4 ounces	3.9
Sirloin steak, 4 ounces	3.8
Parsley, 1 cup	3.7
Fried beef liver, 2 ounces	3.6
Shrimp, 3 ounces	2.7
Braunschweiger sausage, 1 piece	2.7
Flour tortilla, 1	2.4
Garbanzo beans, ½ cup	2.4
Navy beans, ½ cup	2.3
Baked potato, 1	1.7
Artichoke, 1	1.6

RDA for adult men, 8 milligrams
RDA for adult women, 18 milligrams

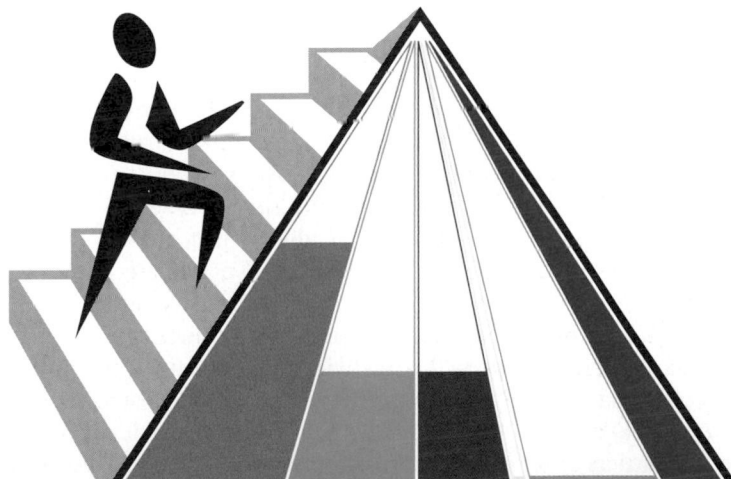

Figure 9-8 Sources of Iron from MyPyramid. The height and background color (none, 1/3, 2/3 or completely covered) within each group in the pyramid indicates the average nutrient density for iron in that group. Overall, the meat & beans group and the grains group contain many foods that are nutrient-dense sources of iron. Still, the iron content of a food containing mostly nonheme iron is only an approximate measure of the amount delivered to body cells, as body need greatly influences the absorption of nonheme iron. With regard to physical activity, iron is especially needed as part of the hemoglobin that carries oxygen in the red blood cell to muscle (and other) cells.

Grains	Vegetables	Fruits	Oils	Milk	Meat & Beans
• Whole grains • Enriched grains • Wheat germ • Oatmeal	• Spinach • Peas • Potatoes • Green beans • Broccoli	• Peaches • Prune juice • Dried apricots	• None	• None	• Beef • Tofu • Beans • Seafood • Organ meats

Most women do not consume 18 milligrams of iron daily. The average daily value is closer to 13 milligrams, while in men it is about 18 milligrams per day. Women can close this gap between average daily intakes and needs by seeking out iron-fortified foods, such as ready-to-eat breakfast cereals that contain at least 50% of the Daily Value. Use of a balanced multivitamin and mineral supplement containing up to 100% of the Daily Value for iron is another option. Consuming more than that much iron is not advised unless a physician suggests otherwise (e.g., compensating for heavy menstrual loss).

Another Bite

The adult human body contains about 21 cups (5 liters) of blood. Blood donations are generally 2 cups (500 milliliters). Thus, a blood donor gives about a tenth of his or her total supply. Healthy people generally can donate blood two to four times a year without harmful consequences. As a precaution, blood banks first screen potential donors' blood for the presence of anemia.

■ Upper Level for Iron

Chapter 8 noted that if men, in general, and older women take a multivitamin and mineral supplement, it should be low in iron or iron-free because of their increased risk for iron toxicity.

The Upper Level for iron is 45 milligrams per day. Higher amounts can lead to stomach irritation. Although iron overload is not as common as iron deficiency, it can be a serious result of misuse because it can easily build up in the body and lead to toxic symptoms. Even a large single dose of 60 milligrams of iron can be life-threatening to a 1-year-old. Children are frequently victims of iron poisoning because iron pills and nutrient supplements containing iron are tempting and available when accessible on kitchen tables and even from cabinets. FDA has recently ruled that all iron supplements must carry a warning about toxicity, and those with 30 milligrams of iron or more per tablet must be individually wrapped.

Smaller doses of iron (but still greater than what is needed) over a long period can also cause problems. A form of iron toxicity, for example, has been observed in an African tribe that brews beer in iron pots. Repeated blood transfusions can also lead to iron toxicity.

hemochromatosis A disorder of iron metabolism characterized by increased iron absorption and deposition in the liver and heart tissue. This eventually poisons the cells in those organs.

In addition, iron toxicity accompanies the genetic disease called hereditary **hemochromatosis.** The disease is associated with a substantial increase in iron absorption. Heme iron poses the greatest risk as body needs do not influence its absorption to a great extent. For people with this disease, iron in the body eventually builds up to dangerous amounts, especially in the blood and liver. Some iron is deposited in the muscles, pancreas, and heart. If not treated, the excess iron deposits contribute to severe organ damage, especially in the liver and heart.

Development of hereditary hemochromatosis requires that a person carry two defective copies of a particular gene. People with one defective gene and one normal gene, called carriers, may also absorb too much dietary iron but not to the same extent as those with two defective genes. About 5% to 10% of North Americans of Northern European descent are carriers of hemochromatosis. Approximately 1 in 250 North Americans has both hemochromatosis genes. These numbers are high considering the fact that many physicians regard hemochromatosis as a rare disease and thus do not routinely test for it.

A reasonable approach is for you to ask to be screened for iron overload at your next visit to a physician (ask for a transferrin saturation test to assess iron stores. A ferritin test may also be added to assess iron stores). Because hemochromatosis can go undetected until a person is in their fifties or sixties, some experts recommend screening for anyone over the age of 20. If the disease goes untreated, many organs will have become irreversibly damaged by one's middle years. If you show evidence of hemochromatosis, it would be wise to undergo therapy. This includes regular blood donations and avoidance of iron-rich foods and iron supplements (see the website www.americanhs.org).

Ideally, consent of a physician should precede any intake of iron from supplements, especially by men. When iron supplements are advised, there should be adequate follow-up so that supplementation does not exceed what is necessary. Probably the only factor keeping many people with hemochromatosis and carriers of one gene from experiencing serious effects of the disease is that they consume only a moderate amount of iron.

Concept Check

Iron is absorbed depending mostly on its form and the body's need for it. Absorption is affected by iron needs but excess iron intake can override the system, leading to toxicity. Nonheme iron absorption increases somewhat in the presence of vitamin C and meat protein and decreases in the presence of large amounts of some components of grain fiber, such as phytic acid. Iron is used in synthesizing hemoglobin and myoglobin, in supporting immune function, and in energy metabolism. An iron deficiency can cause decreased red blood cell synthesis, which can lead to anemia. It is particularly important for women of childbearing age to consume adequate iron, primarily to replace that lost in menstrual blood. Sources include red meat, pork, liver, enriched grains and cereals, and oysters. Iron toxicity usually results from a genetic disorder called hemochromatosis. This disease causes overabsorption and accumulation of iron, which can result in severe liver and heart damage. Because of the risk of toxicity, any use of iron supplements should be supervised by a physician.

Zinc (Zn)

Zinc deficiency was first recognized in humans in the early 1960s in Egypt and Iran. Zinc deficiencies were determined to cause growth retardation and poor sexual development in some groups of people, even though the zinc content of their diets was fairly high. However, the customary diet contained unleavened bread almost exclusively and little animal protein. Unleavened bread is very high in phytic acid and other factors that decrease zinc bioavailability. Parasite infestation and the practice of eating clay and other parts of soil also probably contributed to the severe zinc deficiency.

In North America, zinc deficiencies were first observed in the early 1970s in hospitalized patients who were fed only intravenously via total parenteral nutrition. The protein source in earlier intravenous solutions was based on milk protein or a blood protein, which are both naturally rich in zinc. When the solutions were changed in the early 1970s to include mostly individual amino acids as the protein source, deficiency symptoms quickly developed because amino-acid formulas are low in trace minerals.

Like iron, zinc absorption is influenced by the foods a person ingests. About 40% of dietary zinc is absorbed, especially when animal protein sources are used and when the body needs more zinc. Most people worldwide rely on cereal grains (low in zinc) for their source of protein, calories, and zinc. This makes consuming adequate zinc a problem. In addition, high-dose calcium supplementation with meals decreases zinc absorption. Finally, zinc competes with copper and iron for absorption, and vice versa, when supplemental sources are taken.

■ Functions of Zinc

Up to 200 or so enzymes, such as alcohol dehydrogenase, require zinc as a cofactor for optimal activity. Adequate zinc intake is necessary to support many bodily

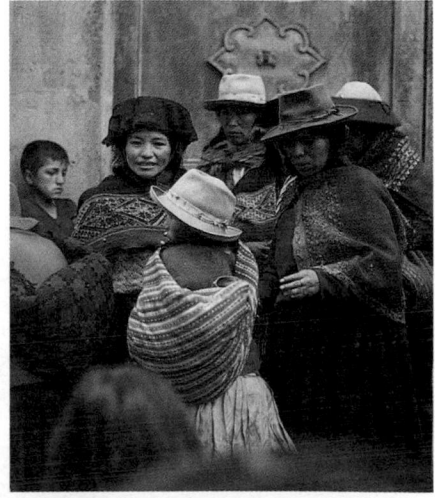

Minimal intakes of protein and zinc limit growth in people worldwide, such as seen in these Bolivian children and adults.

One study has shown that megadose zinc supplements (80 milligrams per day of zinc oxide) reduces the progression of macular degeneration by 25% in people who had a moderate case of the disease. The zinc supplements worked even better when provided in combination with 400 IU of vitamin E, 500 milligrams of vitamin C, and 15 milligrams of beta-carotene. (Copper oxide [2 milligrams] was also included as zinc decreases copper absorption.) Experts suggest that adults who have evidence of moderate macular degeneration talk to their physicians and eyecare specialists about the possibility of following such a protocol.

functions, such as:

- DNA synthesis and function
- Protein metabolism, wound healing, and growth
- Immune function (intakes in excess of the RDA do not provide any extra benefit to immune function)
- Development of sexual organs and bones
- Storage, release, and function of insulin
- Cell membrane structure and function
- Component of two forms of superoxide dismutase, an enzyme that aids in the prevention of oxidative damage to cells. Zinc therefore has an indirect antioxidant function.

Other possible functions of zinc are slowing the progression of macular degeneration of the eye (see the margin for details) and reducing the risk for developing certain forms of cancer.

Symptoms of adult zinc deficiency include an acnelike rash, diarrhea, lack of appetite, reduced sense of taste and smell, and hair loss. In children and adolescents with zinc deficiency, growth, sexual development, and learning ability may also be hampered.

■ Zinc Sources and Needs

In general, protein-rich diets are also rich in zinc. Animal foods supply almost half of an individual's zinc intake. Major sources of zinc are beef, fortified breakfast cereals, milk, poultry, and bread. As with iron, bioavailability is also important to consider for zinc. Animal foods are again our prime sources because zinc from animal sources is not bound by phytic acid. However, good plant sources of zinc—such as whole grains, peanuts, and legumes (beans)—should not be discounted. They can deliver substantial amounts of zinc to body cells (Fig. 9-9). Note also that the form generally used in multivitamin and mineral supplements (zinc oxide) is not as well absorbed as zinc found naturally in foods, but still contributes to meeting zinc needs.

Figure 9-9 Sources of Zinc from MyPyramid. The height and background color (none, 1/3, 2/3 or completely covered) within each group in the pyramid indicates the average nutrient density for zinc in that group. Overall, the meat & beans group and the grains group contain many foods that are nutrient-dense sources of zinc. With regard to physical activity, zinc is especially needed to support muscle growth and muscle healing.

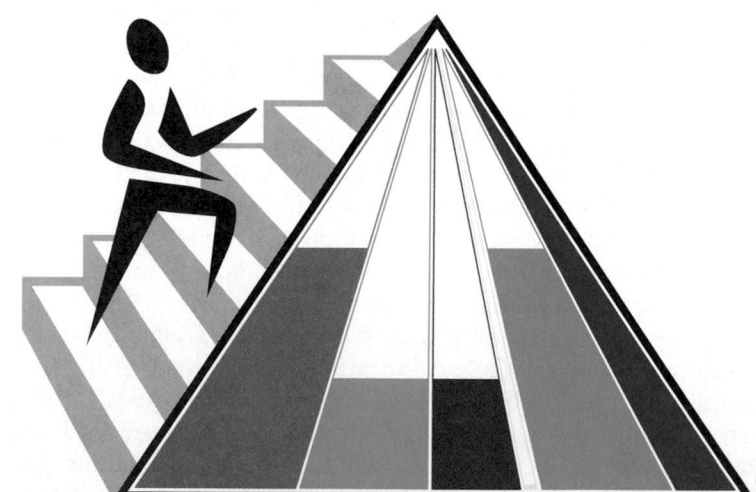

Grains	Vegetables	Fruits	Oils	Milk	Meat & Beans
• Whole-grain breads and cereals • Fortified breakfast cereals	• Spinach • Peas • Asparagus	• Avocados • Dried fruit	• None	• Milk • Yogurt • Cheese	• Beef • Eggs • Beans • Nuts • Shellfish • Poultry

The adult RDA for zinc is 11 milligrams for men and 8 milligrams for women, based on the amount to cover daily losses of zinc. The Daily Value used on food and supplement labels is 15 milligrams. The average North American takes in 10 to 14 milligrams of zinc a day, with men consuming the higher values. There are no indications of moderate or severe zinc deficiencies in an otherwise healthy adult population. It is likely, however, that some North Americans—especially some women, poor children, vegans, older people, and people with alcoholism—have a marginal zinc status. These and other people who show deterioration in taste sensation, recurring infections, poor growth, or depressed wound healing should have zinc status checked.

■ Upper Level for Zinc

The Upper Level for zinc is 40 milligrams per day. Excessive zinc intakes over time can lead to problems by interfering with copper metabolism. The interference with copper metabolism is the basis for setting the Upper Level. An increased risk for prostate cancer is also under study. Overall, if a person uses megadose zinc supplements (e.g., to try to slow macular degeneration), he or she should be under close medical supervision and also take a supplement containing copper (2 milligrams per day). Zinc intakes over 100 milligrams per day also result in diarrhea, cramps, nausea, vomiting, and depressed immune system function, especially if intake exceeds 2 grams per day.

Food Sources of Zinc	
Food Item and Amount	**Zinc (milligrams)**
Steamed oysters, 3	24.9
Sirloin steak, 4 ounces	7.4
Pot roast, 3 ounces	4.6
Special K cereal, 1 cup	3.8
Wheat germ, ¼ cup	3.5
Lamb chops, 3 ounces	2.7
Peanuts, ½ cup	2.4
Black-eyed peas, 1 cup	2.2
Plain yogurt, 1 cup	2.2
Lean ham, 3 ounces	1.9
Swiss cheese, 1.5 ounces	1.7
Ricotta cheese, ½ cup	1.7
Sunflower seeds, 1 ounce	1.5
Cheddar cheese, 1.5 ounces	1.3
Enriched white rice, ½ cup	1.1

RDA for adult male, 11 milligrams
RDA for adult female, 8 milligrams

Another Bite

Many companies are singing the praises of zinc as a cold remedy. Products such as Cold Eeze are lozenges that contain zinc, and their claims are based largely on one study done with 100 participants. The 50 individuals in the experimental group took 13 milligrams of zinc via the lozenges every 2 hours for the duration of their symptoms. Cold symptoms subsided after 4 days in the experimental group and 7 days in the control group. Nausea was a common side effect of the zinc lozenges. Of 10 other follow-up studies, however, only half have shown beneficial results from zinc. This may be due to different bioavailability of various forms of zinc, or simply due to the more bitter flavor of the lozenges used in some studies (may give the impression of potency). Experts also note that we also have no idea of how the zinc would actually treat a cold, if it did. Adults can determine if the benefits outweigh the taste. Zinc expert Dr. Ananda Prasad recommends discontinuing use of zinc lozenges after 3 to 4 days unless they are showing evidence of effectiveness. Any use of such amounts beyond a week or so is potentially dangerous.

▌Selenium (Se)

Selenium exists in many forms that are readily absorbed. Selenium's best understood role is aiding the activity of the enzyme (glutathione peroxidase) that participates in reducing the damage that electron-seeking, free-radical (oxidizing) compounds can do to cell membranes. Thus like zinc, selenium has an indirect antioxidant function. Selenium also contributes to thyroid hormone metabolism and other functions.

In Chapter 8 you saw that vitamin E helps prevent attacks on cell membranes by donating electrons to electron-seeking compounds. Thus, vitamin E and selenium work together toward the same goal. Chapter 8 also discussed how free-radical compounds can cause cancer. Although selenium could prove to have a role in prevention of cancers, such as prostate cancer, it is premature to recommend megadose selenium supplementation for this purpose. Animal studies in this area are conflicting; current studies with humans using supplemental intakes of 200 micrograms per day are under way to help clarify what role, if any, selenium plays in cancer prevention.

Selenium deficiency symptoms in humans include muscle pain and wasting and a certain form of heart damage. In some areas of China, people develop characteristic

Critical Thinking

Tammy read an article about antioxidants and their role in preventing free-radical damage to cells. When Tammy went to the drugstore to take a closer look at such supplements, she saw that selenium was one of the antioxidants in the supplements. Why does selenium deserve consideration as an antioxidant?

Food Sources of Selenium

Food Item and Amount	Selenium (micrograms)
Tuna, 3 ounces	68
Sirloin steak, 5 ounces	47
Lean ham, 3 ounces	42
Clams, 3 ounces	41
Salmon, 3 ounces	40
Egg noodles, 1 cup	35
Chicken breast, 3 ounces	20
Special K cereal, 1 cup	17
Oat bran cereal, 1 cup	14
Whole-wheat bread, 1 slice	10
Cooked oatmeal, ½ cup	10
White bread, 1 slice	9
Raisin Bran cereal, 1 cup	4

RDA for adults, 55 micrograms

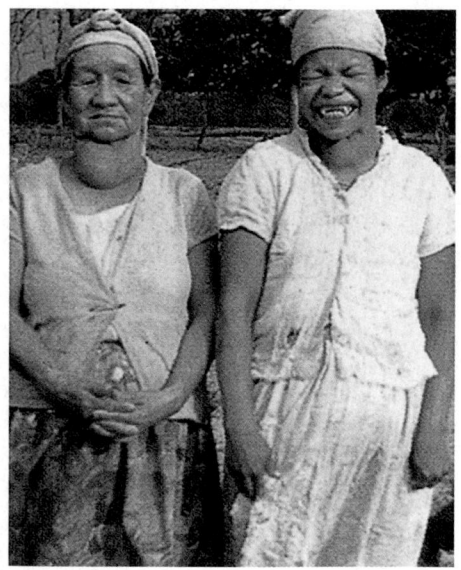

Iodide deficiency leads to a goiter. The mother on the left has a goiter, but is otherwise normal. Her daughter on the right has a goiter and is mentally retarded, deaf, and mute.

goiter An enlargement of the thyroid gland; this is often caused by insufficient iodide in the diet.

muscle and heart disorders associated with inadequate selenium intake. Other factors probably also contribute.

■ Selenium Sources and Needs

Fish, meats (especially organ meats), eggs, and shellfish are good animal sources of selenium. Grains and seeds grown in soils containing selenium are good plant sources. Major selenium contributors to the adult diet are animal and grain products. Because we eat a varied diet of foods supplied from many geographic areas, it is unlikely that low soil selenium in a few locations will mean inadequate selenium in our diets.

The RDA for selenium is 55 micrograms per day for adults. This intake maximizes the activity of selenium-dependant enzymes. The Daily Value used on food and supplement labels is 70 micrograms. In general, adults meet the RDA, consuming on average 105 micrograms of selenium each day.

■ Upper Level for Selenium

The Upper Level for selenium is 400 micrograms per day for adults. This is based on overt signs of selenium toxicity, such as hair loss.

Concept Check

Zinc functions as a cofactor for many enzymes (including those that act as antioxidants) and is important for growth, cell membrane structure and function, immune function, and sense of taste. Beef, seafood, and whole grains are good food sources. As in the case of iron, zinc absorption is regulated according to the body's needs for the mineral. If taken in excess amounts, zinc competes with copper for absorption. Selenium activates an enzyme that helps change electron-seeking, free-radical (oxidizing) compounds into less toxic compounds so these do not attack and break down cell membranes. By helping to dismantle the free-radical compounds, selenium works toward the same goal as vitamin E in providing antioxidant protection to the body. A selenium deficiency results in muscle and heart disorders. Animal products and grains are good selenium sources; however, the selenium content in plants depends on the selenium concentration in the soil. The misuse of both selenium and zinc supplements can readily lead to toxic results.

Iodide (I)

Iodine in foods is actually found in an ion form, called iodide. During World War I, a link was discovered between a deficiency of iodide and the production of a **goiter,** an enlarged thyroid gland. Men drafted from areas such as the Great Lakes Region of the United States had a much higher rate of goiter than did men from some other areas of the country. The soils in these areas have very low iodide contents. In the 1920s, researchers in Ohio found that low doses of iodide given to children over a 4-year period could prevent goiter. That finding led to the addition of iodide to salt beginning in the 1920s.

Today, many nations such as Canada require iodide fortification of salt. In the United States, salt can be purchased either iodized or plain. Check for this on the label of a package of salt next time you are in a grocery store. Some areas of Europe, such as northern Italy, have very low soil levels of iodide, but have yet to adopt an iodide fortification program. People in these areas, especially women, still suffer from goiter, as do people in areas of Latin America, the Indian subcontinent, Southeast Asia, and Africa. About 2 billion people worldwide are at risk of iodide deficiency, and approximately 800 million of these people have suffered the widespread effects of such a deficiency. Eradication of iodide deficiency is a goal of many health-related organizations worldwide.

■ Function of Iodide

The thyroid gland actively accumulates and traps iodide from the bloodstream to support thyroid hormone synthesis. Thyroid hormones are synthesized using iodide and the amino acid tyrosine. These hormones help regulate metabolic rate and promote growth and development throughout the body, including the brain.

If a person's iodide intake is insufficient, the thyroid gland enlarges as it attempts to take up more iodide from the bloodstream. This eventually leads to goiter. Simple goiter is a painless condition, but if uncorrected can lead to pressure on the trachea (windpipe), which may cause difficulty in breathing. Although iodide can prevent goiter formation, it does not significantly shrink a goiter once it has formed. Surgical removal may be required in severe cases.

If a woman has an iodide-deficient diet during the early months of her pregnancy, the fetus suffers iodide deficiency because the mother's body uses up the available iodide. The infant then may be born with short length and develop mental retardation. The stunted growth and mental retardation that results is known as **cretinism**. Cretinism appeared in North America before iodide fortification of table salt began. Today, cretinism still appears in Europe, Africa, Latin America, and Asia.

■ Iodide Sources and Needs

Saltwater fish, seafood, iodized salt, dairy products, and grain products contain various forms of iodide. Sea salt found in health-food stores, however, is not a good source because the iodide is lost during processing.

The RDA for iodide for adults is 150 micrograms in order to support thyroid gland function. This is the same as the Daily Value used on food and supplement labels. A half teaspoon of iodide-fortified salt (about 2 grams) supplies that amount. Most adults consume more iodide than the RDA—an estimated 190 to 300 micrograms daily, not including that from use of iodized salt at the table. This extra amount adds up because dairies and fast food restaurants use it as a sterilizing agent, bakeries use it as a dough conditioner, food producers use it as part of food colorants, and it is added to salt. There is concern, however, that vegans may not consume enough unless iodized salt is used.

■ Upper Level for Iodide

The Upper Level for iodide is 1.1 milligrams per day. When very high amounts of iodide are consumed, thyroid hormone synthesis is inhibited, as in a deficiency. This can appear in people who eat a lot of seaweed, since some seaweeds contain as much as 1% iodide by weight. Total iodide intake then can add up to 60 to 130 times the RDA.

Copper (Cu)

Copper contributes to the metabolism of iron; it operates in processes that form hemoglobin and transport iron. A copper-containing enzyme aids in the release of iron from storage. Copper is needed by enzymes that create cross-links in connective tissue proteins. Copper is also needed by other enzymes, such as those that defend the body against free-radical (oxidizing) compounds (e.g., a form of superoxide dismutase) and those that act in the brain and nervous system. Finally, copper performs in immune system function, blood clotting, and blood lipoprotein metabolism. About 12% to 75% of dietary copper is absorbed, with higher intakes associated with lower absorption. Absorption takes place primarily in the stomach and upper small intestine, with copper excretion via the bile made by the liver and then released by the gallbladder. Phytates, fiber, as well as zinc, and iron supplements, may all interfere with copper absorption. Symptoms of copper deficiency include a form of anemia, low white blood cell count, bone loss, poor growth, and some forms of cardiovascular disease.

Food Sources of Iodide

Food Item and Amount	Iodide (micrograms)
Iodized table salt, ½ teaspoon	195
Plain yogurt, 1 cup	87
Buttermilk, 1 cup	60
1% fat milk, 1 cup	59
Luna bar, 1	38
Soy protein bar, 1	38
Egg, 1 large	35
1% cottage cheese, ½ cup	28
Mozzarella cheese, 1 ounce	10

RDA for adults, 150 micrograms

cretinism The stunting of body growth and poor mental development in the offspring that results from inadequate maternal intake of iodide during pregnancy.

Food Sources of Copper

Food Item and Amount	Copper (micrograms)
Fried beef liver, 3 ounces	3800
Power bar, 1	700
Walnuts, ½ cup	600
Kidney beans, 1 cup	500
Lobster, 3 ounces	400
Molasses, 3 tablespoons	300
Sunflower seeds, 2 tablespoons	300
Shrimp, 3 ounces	300
Raisin Bran cereal, 1 cup	300
Great Grains cereal, 1 cup	300
Black-eyed peas, ½ cup cooked	200
Wheat germ, ¼ cup	200
Milk chocolate, 1 ounce	110
Whole-wheat bread, 1 slice	80

RDA for adults, 900 micrograms

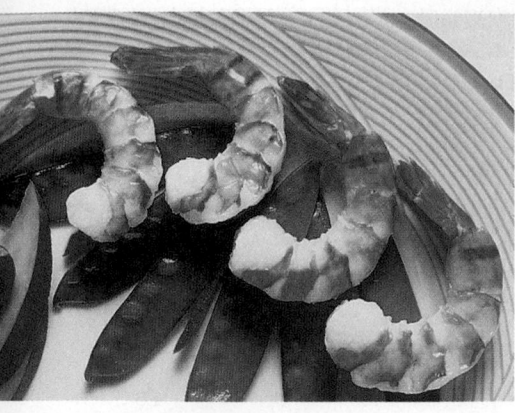

Seafood is one source of copper for a diet.

■ Copper Sources and Needs

Copper is found primarily in liver, seafood, cocoa, legumes, nuts, seeds, and whole-grain breads and cereals.

The RDA for copper is 900 micrograms daily for adults, based on the amount needed for activity of copper-containing proteins and enzymes in the body. The Daily Value used on food and supplement labels is 2 milligrams. The average adult intake is about 1 to 1.6 milligrams per day. Women generally consume the smaller amount. The form of copper typically found in multivitamin and mineral supplements (copper oxide) is not readily absorbed. It is best to rely on food sources to meet copper needs. The copper status of adults appears to be good, though we lack sensitive measures to determine copper status.

The groups most likely to develop copper deficiencies are preterm infants, infants recovering from semistarvation on a milk-dominated diet (which is a poor source of copper), and people recovering from intestinal surgery (during which time copper absorption decreases). Recall that a copper deficiency can also result from overzealous supplementation of zinc, because zinc and copper compete with each other for absorption.

■ Upper Level for Copper

The Upper Limit for copper is 10 milligrams per day. High doses of copper can cause toxicity, including vomiting, at single doses of greater than 10 milligrams. Other forms of toxicity are also possible with megadose uses, such as liver toxicity.

Fluoride (F)

mottling The discoloration or marking of the surface of teeth from fluorosis.

Like chlorine, fluorine (F_2) is a poisonous gas. The fluoride ion (F^-) is the form of this trace mineral essential for human health. This link was found as dentists in the early 1900s noticed a lower rate of dental caries (cavities) in the southwestern United States. These areas contained high amounts of fluoride in the water. The amounts of fluoride were sometimes so high that small spots on the teeth, called **mottling**, appeared. Even though mottled teeth were quite discolored, they contained very few dental caries. After experiments showed that fluoride in the water did indeed decrease the rate of dental caries, controlled fluoridation of water in parts of the United States began in 1945.

Those who grew up drinking fluoridated water generally have 40% to 60% fewer dental caries than people who did not drink fluoridated water as children. Dentists can provide topical fluoride treatments, and schools can provide fluoride tablets, but it is much less expensive and more reliable to simply add fluoride to a community's drinking water. State and private water sources do not always contain enough fluoride, however. When in doubt, contact your local water plant or have the water in your home analyzed for fluoride content. If it is less than 1 part fluoride per million parts of water (e.g., 1 milligram per kilogram or liter of water), talk to your dentist about the best means to obtain the fluoride.

■ Functions of Fluoride

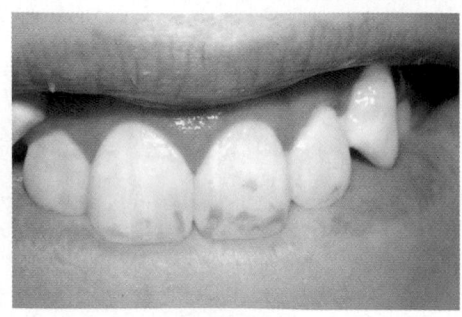

Example of mottling in a tooth caused by overexposure to fluoride.

Dietary fluoride consumed during childhood, when bones and teeth are developing, aids the synthesis of a form of tooth enamel that strongly resists acid. Therefore, teeth become very resistant to dental caries. Fluoride also inhibits metabolism and growth of the bacteria that cause dental caries, and fluoride present in saliva directly inhibits tooth demineralization and enhances tooth remineralization.

Fluoride applied to the surface of the teeth by dentists or from toothpaste or rinses adds additional protection against dental caries. Thus, people of all ages benefit from the topical effects of fluoride, whether or not they consumed fluoridated water or fluoride supplements as children.

■ Fluoride Sources and Needs

Tea, seafood, seaweed, and some natural water sources are the only good food sources of fluoride. Most of our fluoride intake comes from fluoride added to drinking water and toothpaste and from fluoride treatments performed by dentists. Fluoride is not added to bottled water. Therefore, if people such as children consume bottled water, they won't receive fluoride from such water intake.

The Adequate Intake for fluoride for adults is 3.1 to 3.8 milligrams per day. This range of intake provides the benefits of resistance to dental caries without causing ill effects. Typical fluoridated water contains about 1 milligram per liter, which works out to about 0.25 milligrams per cup.

■ Upper Level for Fluoride

The Upper Level for fluoride is set at 1.3 to 2.2 milligrams per day for young children, and 10 milligrams per day for children over 9 years of age and adults, based on skeletal and tooth damage seen with higher doses. Children may swallow large amounts of fluoridated toothpaste as part of daily tooth care, and as a result develop tooth mottling. Not swallowing toothpaste and limiting the amount used to "pea" size are the best ways to prevent this problem. In addition, children under 6 years should have toothbrushing supervised by an adult. Note that fluoride-related mottling only occurs during tooth development, so adults do not develop mottling from their flouride exposure.

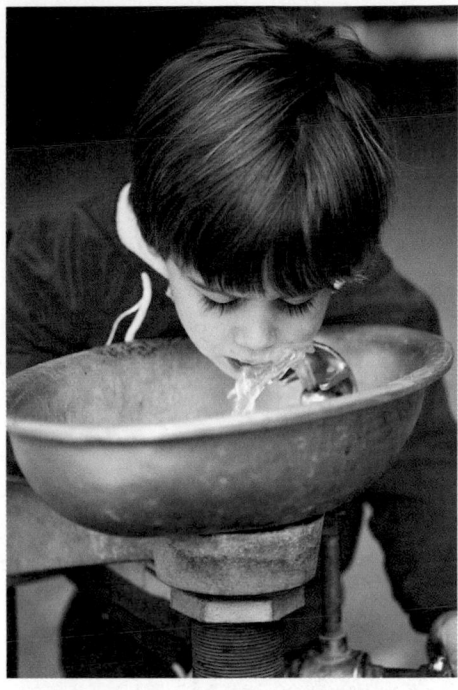

Fluoridated water is responsible for much of the decrease in dental caries throughout North America in recent years.

Concept Check

Iodide is vital for the synthesis of thyroid hormones. A prolonged insufficient intake causes the thyroid gland to enlarge, resulting in a goiter. The use of iodized salt in North America has virtually eliminated this condition. Copper functions mainly in iron and free-radical metabolism, and in the cross-bonding of connective tissue. A deficiency can result in a type of anemia. Good food sources of copper are seafoods, legumes, nuts, dried fruits, and whole grains. Fluoride becomes incorporated into teeth during development and is present in salivary secretions. The presence of this trace mineral makes teeth resistant to acid and bacterial growth, in turn reducing development of dental caries. Fluoride also aids in remineralization of teeth once decay begins. Most of us receive adequate amounts of fluoride from that added to drinking water and toothpaste. An excessive fluoride intake during tooth development can lead to spotted (i.e., mottled) teeth and possibly bone damage.

Chromium (Cr)

The importance of chromium in human diets has been recognized only in the past 40 years. The most-studied function of chromium is the maintenance of glucose uptake into cells. Our current understanding is that chromium enters the cell and acts to enhance the transport of glucose across the cell membrane by aiding insulin function. Marginal to low chromium intakes may contribute to an increased risk for developing type 2 diabetes, but opinions are quite mixed on the true degree of this effect.

A chromium deficiency is characterized by impaired blood glucose control and elevated blood cholesterol and triglycerides. The mechanism by which chromium influences cholesterol metabolism is not known but may involve enzymes that control cholesterol synthesis. Chromium deficiency appears in people maintained on intravenous total parenteral nutrition solutions not supplemented with chromium and in children with malnutrition. Because sensitive measures of chromium status are not available, marginal chromium deficiencies may go undetected.

■ Chromium Sources and Needs

Specific data regarding the chromium content of various foods are scant, and most food composition tables do not include values for this trace mineral. Egg yolks, whole

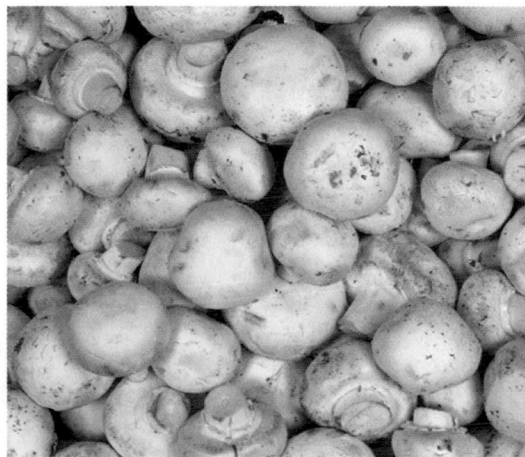

Mushrooms are a good source of chromium.

Chromium supplements have been touted to help with exercise-induced increases in muscle mass and weight loss. Careful research, however, does not support this assertion.

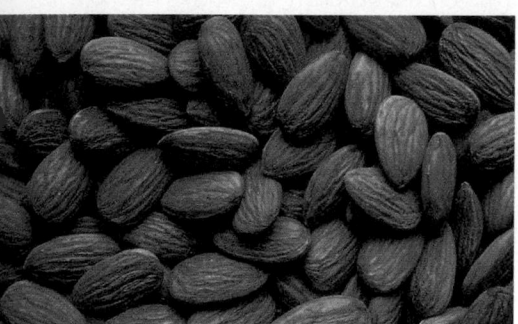

Nuts are rich in manganese.

grains (bran), organ meats, other meats, mushrooms, nuts, and beer are good sources. Yeast is also a source. The amount of chromium in foods is closely tied to the local soil content of chromium. To provide yourself with a good chromium intake, regularly choose whole grains in place of mostly refined grains.

The Adequate Intake for chromium is 25 to 35 micrograms per day, based on the amount present in a balanced diet. The Daily Value used on food and supplement labels is 120 micrograms, about 4 times greater. Average adult intakes in North America are estimated at about 30 micrograms per day, but could be somewhat higher.

No Upper Level for chromium has been set since toxicity for that present in foods has not been observed. Chromium toxicity, however, has been reported in people exposed to industrial waste and in painters who use art supplies with a very high chromium content. Liver damage and lung cancer can result. Because of the risk of toxicity, use of any supplement should normally not exceed the Daily Value set unless supervised by a physician.

Manganese (Mn)

The mineral manganese is easily confused with magnesium. Not only are their names similar, but they also often substitute for each other in metabolic processes. Manganese is needed by some enzymes, such as those used in carbohydrate and free-radical metabolism. The latter is due to a form of superoxide dismutase that contains manganese. Manganese is also important in bone formation.

No human deficiency symptom is associated with a low manganese intake. Animals on manganese-deficient diets suffer alterations in brain function, bone formation, and reproduction. If human diets were low in manganese, these symptoms would probably appear as well. As it happens, our need for manganese is very low, and our diets tend to be adequate in this trace mineral.

Good food sources of manganese are nuts, rice, oats and other whole grains, beans, and leafy vegetables. The Adequate Intake for manganese is 1.8 to 2.3 milligrams to offset daily losses. Average intakes generally fall within this range. The Daily Value used on food and supplement labels is 2 milligrams. Manganese is toxic at high doses.

■ Upper Level for Manganese

The Upper Level is 11 milligrams per day. This is based on the development of nerve damage.

Molybdenum (Mo)

Several human enzymes use molybdenum. No molybdenum deficiency has been noted in people who consume normal diets, though deficiency symptoms have appeared in people maintained on intravenous total parenteral nutrition feedings. These symptoms include increased heart and respiration rates, night blindness, mental confusion, edema, and weakness.

Good food sources of molybdenum include milk and milk products, beans, whole grains, and nuts. The RDA for molybdenum is 45 micrograms to offset daily losses. The Daily Value used on food and supplement labels is 75 micrograms. Our daily intakes average 75 to 110 micrograms.

■ Upper Level for Molybdenum

The Upper Level for molybdenum is 2 milligrams per day. When consumed in high doses, molybdenum causes toxicity in laboratory animals, resulting in weight loss and decreased growth.

Table 9-6 summarizes what we have covered regarding the trace minerals, as does Figure 9-10. Figure 9-11 summarizes the various contributions of groups in MyPyramid to mineral needs.

Table 9-6 A Summary of Key Trace Minerals

Mineral	Major Functions	RDA or Adequate Intake	Dietary Sources	Deficiency Symptoms	Toxicity Symptoms
Iron	• Components of hemoglobin and other key compounds used in respiration • Immune function • Cognitive development	*Men:* 8 milligrams *Women:* 18 milligrams	• Meats • Seafood • Broccoli • Peas • Bran • Enriched breads	• Fatigue • Anemia • Low blood hemoglobin values	• Liver and heart damage (extreme cases) • GI upset • Upper Level is 45 milligrams
Zinc	• Required for nearly 200 enzymes • Growth • Immunity • Alcohol metabolism • Sexual development • Reproduction • Antioxidant protection	*Men:* 11 milligrams *Women:* 8 milligrams	• Seafood • Meats • Greens • Whole grains	• Skin rash • Diarrhea • Decreased appetite and sense of taste • Hair loss • Poor growth and development • Poor wound healing	• Reduced copper absorption • Diarrhea • Cramps • Depressed immune function • Upper Level is 40 milligrams
Selenium	• Part of an antioxidant system	55 micrograms	• Meats • Eggs • Fish • Seafood • Whole grains	• Muscle pain • Weakness • Form of heart disease	• Nausea • Vomiting • Hair loss • Weakness • Liver disease • Upper Level is 400 micrograms
Iodide	• Component of thyroid hormones	150 micrograms	• Iodized salt • White bread • Saltwater fish • Dairy products	• Goiter • Mental retardation • Poor growth in infancy when mother is iodide deficient during pregnancy	• Inhibition of thyroid gland function • Upper Level is 1.1 milligrams
Copper	• Aids in iron metabolism • Works with many antioxidant enzymes • Involved with enzymes of protein metabolism and hormone synthesis	900 micrograms	• Liver • Cocoa • Beans • Nuts • Whole grains • Dried fruits	• Anemia • Low white blood cell count • Poor growth	• Vomiting • Nervous system disorders • Upper Level is 8–10 milligrams
Fluoride	• Increases resistance of tooth enamel to dental caries	*Men:* 3.8 milligrams *Women:* 3.1 milligrams	• Fluoridated water • Toothpaste • Tea • Seaweed (Dental treatments)	• Increased risk of dental caries	• Stomach upset • Mottling (staining) of teeth during development • Bone pain • Upper Level is 10 milligrams for adults
Chromium	• Enhances insulin action	25–35 micrograms	• Egg yolks • Whole grains • Pork • Nuts • Mushrooms • Beer	• High blood glucose after eating	Caused by industrial contamination, not dietary excesses, so no Upper Level has been set
Manganese	• Cofactor of some enzymes, such as those involved in carbohydrate metabolism • Works with some antioxidant systems	1.8–2.3 milligrams	• Nuts • Oats • Beans • Tea	None observed in humans	• Nervous system disorders • Upper Level is 11 milligrams
Molybdenum	• Aids in action of some enzymes	45 micrograms	• Beans • Grains • Nuts	None observed in healthy humans	• Poor growth in laboratory animals • Upper Level is 2 milligrams

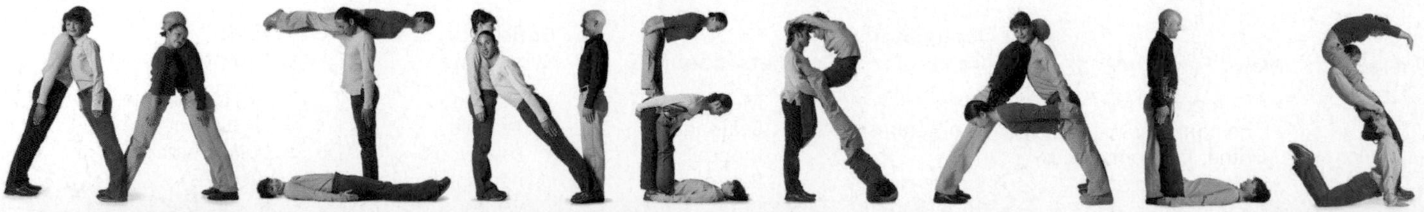

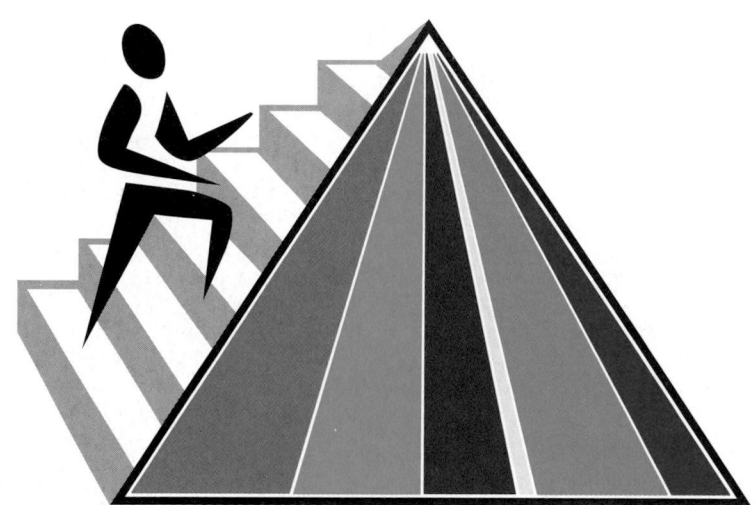

MINERALS

Ion Balance in Cells	Nerve Impulses	Antioxidant Defenses	Blood Formation and Clotting*	Growth and Development	Bone Health	Cell Metabolism
Sodium Potassium Chloride Phosphorus	Sodium Potassium Chloride	Selenium Zinc Copper Manganese	Iron Copper *Calcium	Calcium Phosphorus Zinc Iodide	Calcium Phosphorus Iron Zinc Copper Fluoride Magnesium Manganese	Calcium Phosphorus Magnesium Zinc Chromium Iodide

Figure 9-10 Minerals contribute to many functions in the body. Mineral deficiencies therefore lead to a variety of health problems.

Grains	Vegetables	Fruits	Oils	Milk	Meat & Beans
• Sodium chloride • Calcium— (fortified products) • Phosphorus • Magnesium • Iron • Zinc • Copper • Selenium • Chromium	• Potassium • Magnesium	• Potassium • Boron	• None	• Calcium • Phosphorus • Zinc	• Sodium chloride (processed foods) • Potassium • Phosphorus • Magnesium • Selenium • Iron • Zinc • Copper

Figure 9-11 Certain groups of MyPyramid are especially rich sources of various minerals. This is true for the minerals listed. Each mineal may also be found in other groups, but in lower amounts. Other trace mineals are also present in moderate amounts in many groups. With regard to the grains group, whole-grain varieties are the richest sources of most trace minerals listed.

Concept Check

Chromium contributes to insulin function. The amount of chromium found in food depends on chromium content of the soil on which it was grown. Meats, whole grains, and egg yolks are some good sources. Manganese is a component of bone and is used by many enzymes, including those involved in glucose production. Because our need for manganese is low, deficiencies are rare. Nuts, rice, oats, and beans are good food sources. Molybdenum is another trace mineral required by a few enzymes. Good sources include milk, beans, whole grains, and nuts. Deficiencies have appeared only in people nourished by unsupplemented total parenteral nutrition. The needs for some other trace minerals—such as boron, nickel, arsenic, and vanadium—have not been fully established in humans. If required, these minerals are needed in such small amounts that our current diets are probably adequate sources of them.

Other Trace Minerals

Although a variety of other trace minerals is found in humans, many of them have not yet been shown to be required. The list of minerals in this category includes boron, nickel, vanadium, arsenic, and silicon (Table 9-7). Widespread deficiency symptoms in humans have never been noted, probably because typical diets provide adequate amounts of these minerals and they are needed by very few enzymes and metabolic systems. Their potential for toxicity should make one question any supplementation not supervised by a physician. These trace minerals may achieve more importance as more research is reported.

Table 9-7 A Summary of Trace Minerals for Which Human Needs Have Not Been Established

Mineral	Proposed Function	Estimates of Daily Human Needs	Dietary Sources
Arsenic	• Amino acid and fatty acid metabolism • DNA function	12–25 micrograms	• Fish • Grains • Cereal products
Boron	• Cell membrane function (ion transport) • Hormone metabolism in some cases	1–13 milligrams	• Fruits • Leafy vegetables • Nuts • Beans
Nickel	• Amino acid and fatty acid metabolism	25–35 micrograms	• Chocolate • Nuts • Beans • Whole grains
Silicon	• Bone formation	25–30 milligrams	• Root vegetables • Whole grains
Vanadium	• Mimics action of insulin	10 micrograms*	• Shellfish • Mushrooms • Black pepper

Human needs have not been established in any case; deficiency symptoms have been produced in experimental animals. All of these trace minerals pose a high risk for toxicity. Any supplement use should not exceed the estimates of daily human needs listed above.

*Upper Level is 1.8 milligrams per day (180 times estimated human needs).

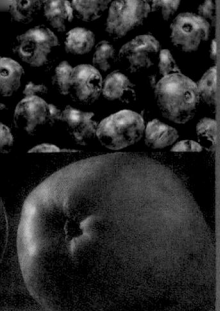

Looking *Further*

Minerals and Osteoporosis

Widespread media attention has made it almost impossible for women to ignore osteoporosis. The crippling effect this disease has on older persons is now recognized as a major medical problem. Osteoporosis leads to approximately 1.5 million bone fractures per year in the United States, usually in the hip, spine, or wrist, leading to about $17 billion per year in health-care costs. Many older women in North America experience osteoporosis-related fractures in their lifetimes.

The slender, inactive woman who smokes is most susceptible to osteoporosis, but any person who lives long enough can suffer from the disease, including men. About 25% of women older than age 50 develop osteoporosis. Among people older than age 80, osteoporosis becomes the rule—not the exception. The spine fractures commonly found in women with osteoporosis cause considerable pain and deformity and decrease physical ability (Fig. 9-12); hip fractures are seen in both men and women with osteoporosis. Not only is this disease debilitating, it also can be fatal. Almost one-quarter of all older persons who suffer hip fractures die within the first year from fracture-related complications.

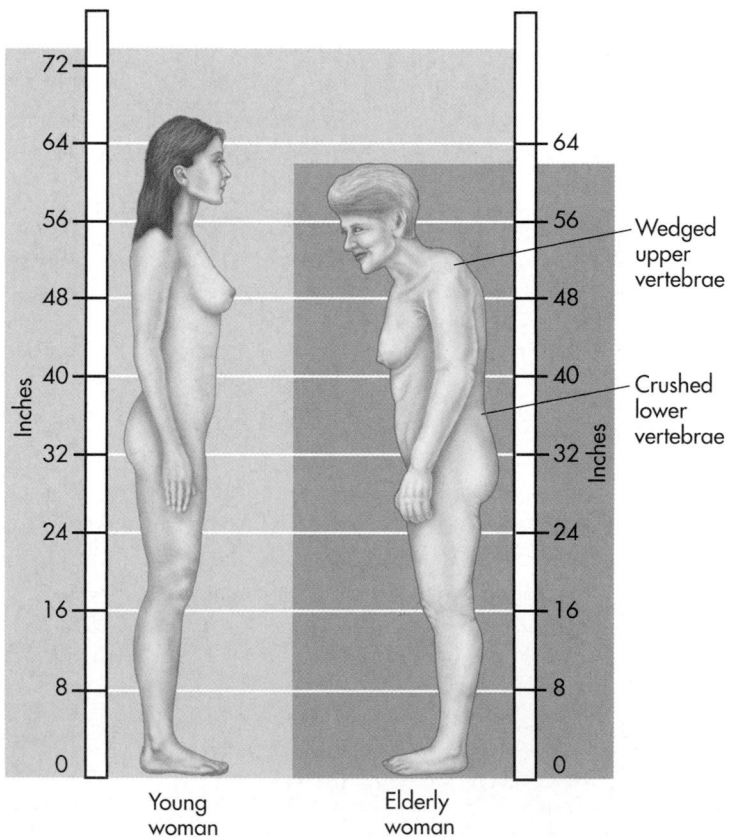

Figure 9-12 Normal and osteoporotic woman. Because osteoporotic bones have less substance, osteoporosis generally leads to loss of height, distorted body shape, fractures, and loss of teeth. Monitoring changes in adult height is one way to detect early evidence of osteoporosis.

A Quick Look at Bone Structure and Strength

To better understand the role calcium plays in bone health and osteoporosis, it is important to understand how bone is constructed. Visual observation of the cross-sections of a bone reveals two primary bone structural types: **cortical bone** and **trabecular bone.** These interact within each bone to form quite an engineering marvel of strength (Fig. 9-13).

The entire outer surface of all bones is composed of cortical bone, which is very dense. The shafts of long bones, such as those of the arm, are almost entirely cortical bone. Trabecular bone is found in the ends of the long bones, inside the spinal vertebrae, and inside the flat bones of the pelvis. Trabecular bone forms an internal scaffolding network for a bone. It supports the outer cortical shell of the bone, especially in heavily stressed areas, such as joints. Another important element is the trabecular bone support network inside a bone. It is especially critical for the horizontal trabeculae to extend continuously—without breaks—between the areas of vertical trabeculae. Any break in the horizontal trabecular beams weakens the support system of a bone and increases the risk for bone fracture. Breaks in the more vertical beams also do the same. And once these beams are broken, there is no way to rebuild them. This is why it is so important to limit bone loss as people age.

cortical bone Dense, compact bone that comprises the outer surface and shafts of bone; also called compact bone.

trabecular bone The spongy, inner matrix of bone, found primarily in the spine, pelvis, and ends of bones; also called spongy or cancellous bone.

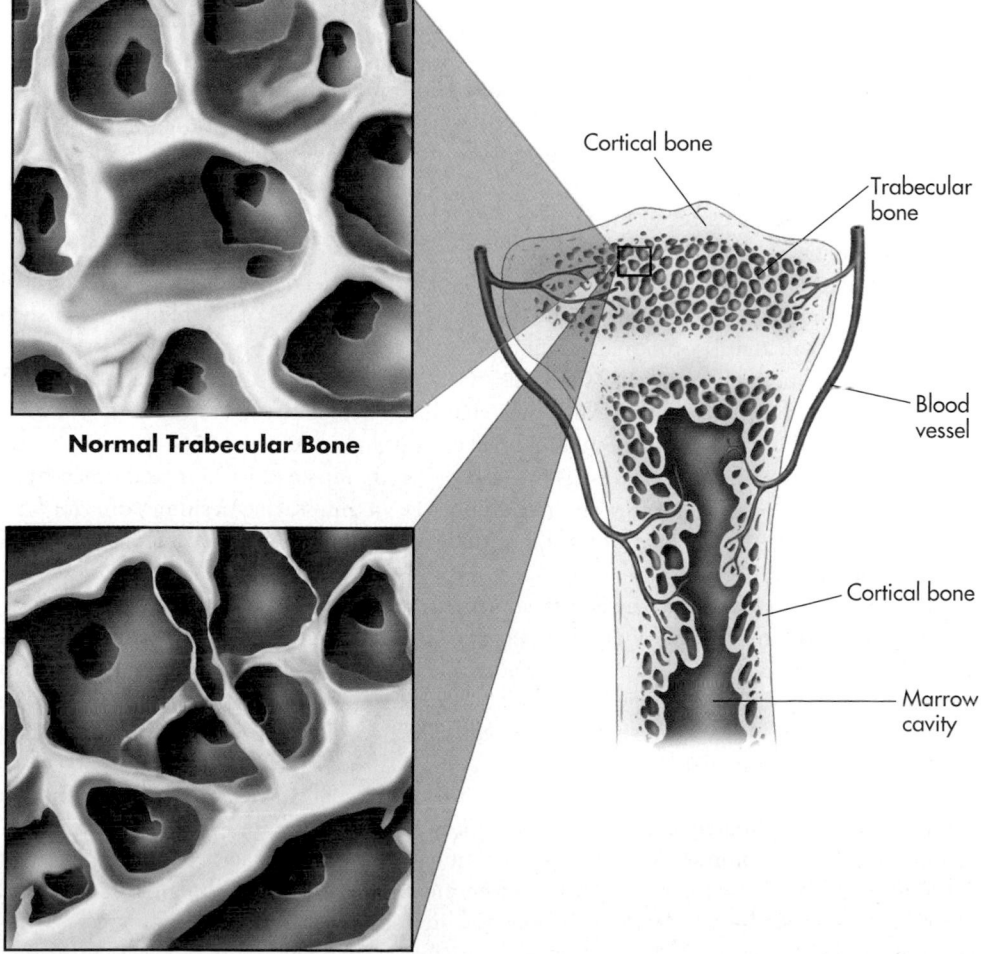

Normal Trabecular Bone

Osteoporotic Trabecular Bone

Cortical bone

Trabecular bone

Blood vessel

Cortical bone

Marrow cavity

Figure 9-13 Cortical and trabecular bone. Cortical bone forms the shafts of bones and their outer mineral covering. Trabecular bone supports the outer shell of cortical bone in various bones of the body, as in the illustration. Note how the osteoporotic bone has much less trabecular bone. This leads to a more fragile bone and is not reversible to any major extent with current therapies.

Table 9-8 Diet and Lifestyle Factors Associated with Bone Status

Positive Diet and Lifestyle Factors	Call to Action
Adequate diet containing a sufficient amount of protein, calcium, phosphorus, magnesium, potassium, vitamin A, vitamin C, vitamin D, vitamin K, iron, zinc, copper, fluoride, and manganese (and boron?)	• Follow MyPyramid with special emphasis on adequate amounts of fruits, vegetables, and low-fat and fat-free dairy products. • Consider use of fortified foods (or supplements) to make up for specific nutrient shortfalls, such as vitamin D and calcium.
Healthy body weight	• Be aware that low body weight (slender figure) increases the risk for low bone mass.
Normal menses	• During childbearing years, seek medical advice if menses cease (such as in cases of anorexia nervosa or extreme athletic training). • Women at menopause and beyond should consider use of current medical therapies to reduce bone loss linked to the fall in estrogen output.
Weight-bearing physical activity	• Perform weight-bearing activity as this contributes to bone maintenance, whereas bed rest and a sedentary lifestyle lead to bone loss. Strength training is especially helpful to bone maintenance.
Negative Diet and Lifestyle Factors	**Call to Action**
Excessive intake of protein, phosphorus, sodium, caffeine, wheat bran, and alcohol	• Moderate intake of these dietary constituents is recommended. Problems primarily arise if adequate calcium is not consumed. • Excessive soft drink consumption is especially discouraged.
Smoking	• Since smoking lowers estrogen output in women, smoking cessation is advised.

Bone Mass Is Related to Age and Gender

Bone strength depends on a person's **bone mass** and **bone mineral density.** The more bone there is, and especially the more densely packed bone crystals are in the bone, the stronger the bone structure. Rapid and continual bone growth and calcification occur throughout the adolescent years, ultimately resulting in what is called *peak bone mass*. In the adolescent growth spurt, bone mass is increasing at the rate of about 8.5% per year. Small increases in bone mass then continue between 20 and 30 years of age.

The ultimate amount of bone built by a person is clearly dependent on gender, race, familial patterns seen in the mother and father, and probably other genetically determined factors, such as the degree of calcium absorption. In addition, men have higher bone mass value than women, and African-Americans have heavier skeletons than Caucasians. As a direct consequence, men and African-Americans in general have a somewhat lower risk of osteoporosis-related fractures than do other populations. Slender, small-framed Caucasian and Asian women show the lowest bone mass values. Peak bone mass is also related to dietary intake of calcium and other nutrients, such as protein, phosphorus, vitamin A, vitamin D, vitamin K, magnesium, iron, zinc, and copper (Table 9-8). Thus, osteoporosis is not just a calcium story—many minerals and other nutrients play a part.

Bone mass varies among young adults; some have much denser bone than others, perhaps because they built more bone when they were young. Some people also may adapt more easily to lower-calcium diets. People who have developed more bone by early adulthood can sustain greater age-related bone loss with less risk of osteoporosis compared with those who have less bone. Thus, osteoporosis is considered to be a "pediatric disease" with geriatric (old age) consequences (Fig. 9-14).

For women, bone loss begins at age 30 and proceeds slowly and continuously to menopause (approximately age 50). It often speeds up at menopause with the decline in estrogen output and continues at a high rate for the next 10 years. By age 65 to 70, the rate of bone loss falls to about the same rate as before menopause. In men, bone loss is slow and steady from around age 30. Overall, this bone loss in both males and females progresses without noticeable symptoms.

bone mass Total mineral substance (such as calcium or phosphorus) in a cross section of bone, generally expressed as grams per centimeter of length.

bone mineral density Total mineral content of bone at a specific bone site divided by the width of the bone at that site, generally expressed as grams per cubic centimeter.

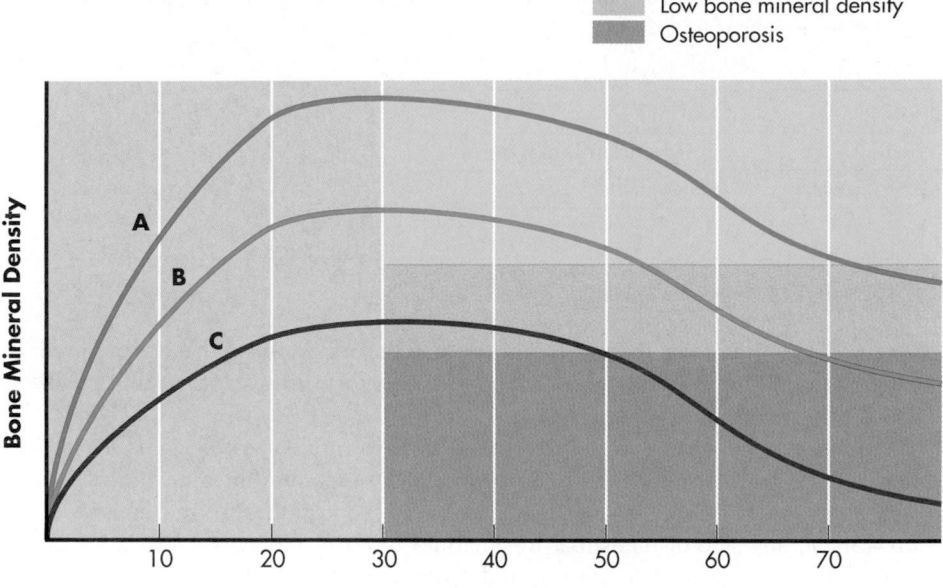

Healthy bone mineral density
Low bone mineral density
Osteoporosis

Figure 9-14 The relationship between peak bone mass and the ultimate risk of developing osteoporosis and related bone fractures. Woman A developed a high peak bone mass by age 30, bone loss was slow and steady between age 30 and age 50, and sped up somewhat after age 50 due to the effects of menopause. Still, by age 75 the woman had a healthy bone mineral density value and did not show evidence of osteoporosis. Woman B developed an average peak bone mass and experienced the same rate of bone loss as woman A. By age 65, woman B had low bone mineral density and evidence of osteoporosis. She was now at risk of related fractures. Woman C achieved a low peak bone mass, and by following the typical pattern for bone loss, at age 50 she already showed evidence of low bone mineral density and osteoporosis. Given the low calcium intakes that are common among young women today, line C is a sobering reality. Ideally by following a diet and lifestyle pattern that contributes to maximal bone mineral density, more women will follow line A, in turn significantly reducing their risk of developing osteoporosis in their lifetimes.

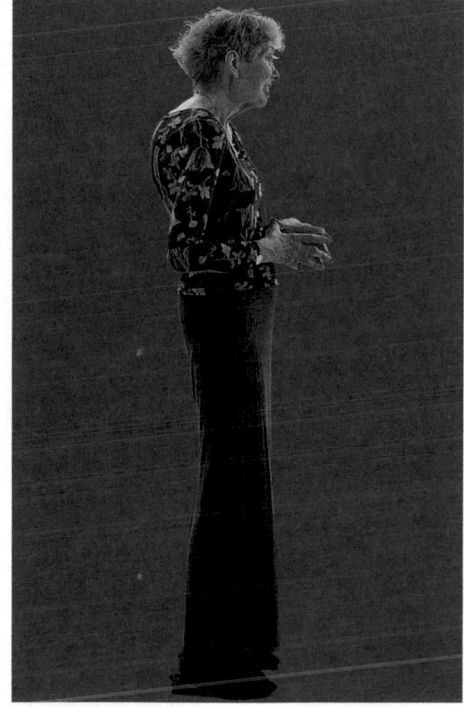

Women with osteoporosis typically develop abnormal curvature of the upper spine. This results from fractures of the weakened vertebrae. This can lead to both physical and emotional pain.

Osteoporosis

Failure to maintain enough bone mass in the body can be caused by the vitamin D deficiency disease osteomalacia, the use of certain medications (such as cortisol and antiseizure drugs), and cancer. If these or similar medical causes are not present, the diagnosis is osteoporosis.

All women age 65 and older should be screened for this disease. The most accurate screening involves a **dual energy X-ray absorptiometry (DEXA) bone scan** of the whole body. (Somewhat less accurate instruments measure bone mineral density at a single site, such as the heel.) Younger women with associated risk factors are advised to do the same at menopause, since the results of the screening would help them decide whether or not medical therapy is an appropriate plan for menopause.

For this DEXA test, a person will lie down on his or her back on a padded table while a movable imaging arm moves over the length of the body. The procedure usually takes about 20 to 30 minutes. The ability of a bone to block the path of radiation is used as a measure of bone mineral density at that bone site. A very low dose of radiation is used for the DEXA—about one-tenth of the exposure from a chest X-ray.

Dual energy X-ray absorptiometry (DEXA) bone scan Method to measure bone density that uses small amounts of X-ray radiation. The ability of a bone to block the path of the radiation is used as a measure of bone density at that bone site.

From the DEXA measurement of bone density, a so called T score is generated, which compares the observed bone density to that of a person at peak bone strength (e.g., age 30). Such a T score is interpreted as follows:

0 to –1	Normal
–1 to –2.4	Low bones mineral density
–2.5 or lower	Osteoporosis

Preventing Osteoporosis

Once osteoporosis is present, there is no way to repair the bone damage that has occurred. This makes prevention important. Strategies for prevention of osteoporosis vary based on age and individual risk factors.

For young women, osteoporosis prevention involves three main elements. First, young women should focus on meeting calcium, vitamin D, protein, and other nutrient needs. Second, since the hormones of regular menstruation contribute to bone maintenance in young women, any sign of menstrual irregularities is reason to see a physician. Note that some non-menstruating female athletes and other women with irregular menstrual cycles (e.g., women with anorexia nervosa) already exhibit low bone mineral density. Third, an active lifestyle that includes weight-bearing physical activity is also important. The increased muscle mass that stems from weight-bearing physical activity is associated with greater bone mineral density, as muscle keeps tension on bone. However, physical activity cannot prevent the bone loss associated with irregular menstruation. Even though female athletes may do plenty of weight-bearing physical activity, they should be closely monitored by a physician if they have irregular menstrual cycles.

Once they have reached menopause, women should discuss approved osteoporosis-related therapies with a physician. The most common medications are **bisphosphonates.** These lessen bone breakdown. Estrogen replacement previously was the most common therapy for bone protection, but since this recently has been shown to increase the risks in some women for cardiovascular disease and strokes, as well as cancers of the breast and ovaries, estrogen replacement is now reserved for short-term use to control menopausal symptoms in most cases.

As age advances, both men and women need to take preventive action. First of all, adults need to accurately track their height. A decrease of more than 1½ inches from young adult height is a sign that significant bone loss is taking place.

Older adults especially need to stay physically active—including some weight-bearing and resistance activities—and they should meet the Adequate Intake for calcium set for their particular age. Regular sun exposure and the consumption of food sources of vitamin D are also very important. If sun exposure and food sources are inadequate, supplements containing up to 25 micrograms (1000 IU) of vitamin D are appropriate (review Chapter 8). The combination of physical activity and meeting calcium and vitamin D needs are most likely to limit bone loss in some areas of the body, such as the hip.

Older adults can also minimize the risk for falls that might lead to fractures by limiting their use of substances that disturb coordination, such as certain medications and alcohol. Likewise, they should take corrective measures if their visual function is impaired. (Hip-protective garments are also available to help reduce hip fracture risk from a fall.)

At any age, smoking and excessive alcohol intake decrease bone mass. Smoking lowers the estrogen concentration in the blood in women, increasing bone loss. Alcohol is toxic to bone cells for both men and women, and alcoholism is probably a major undiagnosed and unrecognized cause of osteoporosis. Excessive intakes of phosphorus, caffeine, and sodium are also discouraged. These are especially problematic when insufficient calcium is consumed.

To find out more about osteoporosis, check out the website of the National Osteoporosis Foundation (www.nof.org) or call (800)464-6700. Another helpful website is that of the National Dairy Council (www.nationaldairycouncil.org).

bisphosphonates Compounds primarily composed of carbon and phosphorus that bind to bone mineral and in turn reduce bone breakdown. Examples are alendronate (Fosamax) and risedronate (Actonel).

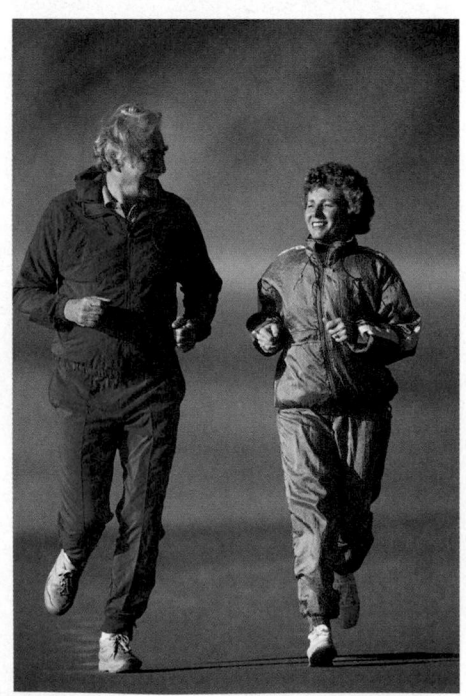

Regular, moderate weight-bearing physical activity contributes to bone health in both men and women. Note that men can also develop osteoporosis as they age.

Summary

1. Water constitutes 50% to 70% of the human body. Its unique chemical properties enable it to dissolve substances as well as serve as a medium for chemical reactions, temperature regulation, and lubrication. Water also helps regulate the acid-base balance in the body. For adults, daily water needs are estimated at 9 cups (women) to 13 cups (men) per day fluid intake in general contributes to meeting this need.

2. Many minerals are vital for sustaining life. For humans, animal products are the most bioavailable sources of most minerals. Supplements of minerals exceeding 100% of the Daily Values listed on the label should be taken only under a physician's supervision. Toxicity and nutrient interactions are especially likely if the Upper Level (when set) is exceeded on a long-term basis.

3. Sodium, the major positive ion found outside cells, is vital in fluid balance and nerve impulse transmission. The North American diet provides abundant sodium through processed foods and table salt. About 10% to 15% of the adult population, such as people who are overweight, is especially sodium-sensitive and at risk for developing hypertension from consuming excessive sodium.

4. Potassium, the major positive ion found inside cells, has a similar function to sodium. Milk, fruits, and vegetables are good sources.

5. Chloride is the major negative ion found outside cells. It is important in digestion as part of stomach acid and in immune and nerve functions. Table salt supplies most of the chloride in our diets.

6. Calcium forms a part of bone structure and plays a role in blood clotting, muscle contraction, nerve transmission, and cell metabolism. Calcium absorption is enhanced by stomach acid and the active vitamin D hormone. Dairy products are important calcium sources. Women are particularly at risk for not meeting calcium needs.

7. Phosphorus aids enzyme function and forms part of key metabolic compounds, cell membranes, and bone. It is efficiently absorbed, and deficiencies are rare, although there is concern about possible poor intake by some older women. Good food sources are dairy products, bakery products, and meats.

8. Magnesium is a mineral found mostly in plant food sources. It is important for nerve and heart function and as an activator for many enzymes. Whole-grain breads and cereals (bran portion), vegetables, nuts, seeds, milk, and meats are good food sources. Sulfur is incorporated into certain vitamins and amino acids.

9. Controlling weight and alcohol intake, exercising regularly, decreasing salt intake, and ensuring adequate potassium, magnesium, and calcium in the diet all can play a part in controlling high blood pressure.

10. Iron absorption depends mainly on the form of iron present and the body's need for it. Heme iron from animal sources is better absorbed than the nonheme iron obtained primarily from plant sources. Consuming vitamin C or meat simultaneously with nonheme iron increases absorption. Iron operates mainly in synthesizing hemoglobin and myoglobin and in the action of the immune system. Women are at great risk for developing iron deficiency, which decreases blood hemoglobin and hematocrit. When this condition is severe, iron-deficiency anemia develops. This decreases the amount of oxygen carried in the blood. Iron toxicity usually results from a genetic disorder called hemochromatosis. This disease causes overabsorption and accumulation of iron, which can result in severe liver and heart damage.

11. Zinc aids in the action of up to 200 enzymes that are important for growth, development, cell membrane structure and function, immune function, antioxidant protection, wound healing, and taste. A zinc deficiency results in poor growth, loss of appetite, reduced sense of taste and smell, hair loss, and a persistent rash. Zinc is best absorbed from animal sources. The richest sources of zinc are oysters, shrimp, crab, and beef. Good plant sources are whole grains, peanuts, and beans.

12. An important role of selenium is decreasing the action of free-radical (oxidizing) compounds. In this way, selenium acts along with vitamin E in providing antioxidant protection. Muscle pain, muscle wasting, and a form of heart damage may result from a selenium deficiency. Meats, eggs, fish, and shellfish are good animal sources of selenium. Good plant sources include grains and seeds.

13. Iodide forms part of the thyroid hormones. A lack of dietary iodide results in the development of an enlarged thyroid gland or goiter. Iodized salt is a major food source.

14. Copper is important for iron metabolism, cross-linking of connective tissue, and other functions, such as enzymes that provide antioxidant protection. A copper deficiency can result in a form of anemia. Copper is found mainly in liver, seafood, cocoa, legumes, and whole grains.

15. Fluoride as part of regular dietary intake or toothpaste use makes teeth resistant to dental caries. Most North Americans receive the bulk of their fluoride from fluoridated water and toothpaste.

16. Chromium aids in the action of the hormone insulin. Egg yolks, meats, and whole grains are good sources of chromium. Manganese and molybdenum are used by various enzymes. One enzyme that uses manganese provides antioxidant protection. Clear deficiencies in otherwise healthy people are rarely seen for any of these three nutrients. Human needs for other trace minerals are so low that deficiencies are uncommon.

17. Women are particularly at risk for developing osteoporosis as they age. Numerous lifestyle and medical options can help reduce this risk, including an adequate intake of calcium and many other minerals.

Study Questions

1. Approximately how much water do you need each day to stay healthy? Identify at least two situations that increase the need for water. Then list three sources of water in the average person's diet.

2. What is the relationship between sodium and water balance, and how is that relationship monitored as well as maintained in the body?

3. Identify four factors that influence the bioavailability of minerals from food.

4. What are two similarities and differences between sodium and potassium? Sodium and chloride?

5. In terms of total amounts in the body, calcium and phosphorus are the first and second most abundant minerals, respectively. What function do these minerals have in common?

6. What are the best food sources for zinc and copper?

7. Describe the symptoms of iron-deficiency anemia and explain possible reasons they occur.

8. Which trace minerals are lost from cereal grains when they are refined? Are any of these nutrients replaced by enrichment?

9. Describe the chief function of fluoride, copper, and chromium in the body.

10. What are the practical consequences of the Daily Values on food and supplement labels exceeding the RDA or Adequate Intake for many trace minerals?

Further Readings

1. ACOG Practice Bulletin: Osteoporosis. *Obstetrics & Gynecology* 103(1):203, 2004.

   Comprehensive look at the diagnosis and treatment of osteoporosis. Many lifestyle factors increase risk, such as a poor diet, inactivity, and smoking. Women especially should work to prevent this disease.

2. ADA Reports: Position of the American Dietetic Association: The impact of fluoride on health. *Journal of the American Dietetic Association* 101:126, 2001.

   The American Dietetic Association reaffirms that fluoride is an important element for all mineralized tissues in the body. Appropriate fluoride intake is beneficial to bone and tooth health.

3. Chobanian AV and others: The seventh report of the joint national committee on the prevention, detection, evaluation, and treatment of high blood pressure. *Journal of the American Medical Association* 289:2560, 2003.

   This article is a comprehensive look at the various lifestyle and medical interventions to prevent and treat hypertension. Key lifestyle factors emphasized are weight reduction, regular physical activity, reduction in salt intake, moderation in alcohol use, and following a healthy diet, such as the DASH diet.

4. Fiske H: Measuring water's benefits & optimal intake recommendations. *Today's Dietitian,* p. 22, January 2003.

   One way to make sure we stay well hydrated is to always have no more than a pale yellow urine. For many of us this is not a challenge as our thirst mechanisms encourage us to drink fluid when needed. All fluids count, even those with caffeine and alcohol (but not quite as much as with water itself).

5. Food and Nutrition Board, Institute of Medicine: *Dietary Reference Intakes for water, potassium, sodium, chloride, and sulfate.* Washington, DC: Standing Committee on the Scientific Evaluation of Dietary Reference Intakes National Academy Press, 2004.

   Dietary standards for water, potassium, sodium, and chloride are discussed. The rationale used to derive the Adequate Intakes, as well as the Upper Levels, are presented along with information on function, intake, and deficiency.

6. Food and Nutrition Board, Institute of Medicine: *Dietary Reference Intakes for calcium, phosphorus, magnesium, vitamin D, and fluoride.* Washington, DC: Standing Committee on the Scientific Evaluation of Dietary Reference Intakes National Academy Press, 1997.

   Dietary standards for many major minerals are discussed. The rationale used to set RDA or Adequate Intakes and Upper Levels for these nutrients is discussed in detail.

7. Food and Nutrition Board, Institute of Medicine: *Dietary Reference Intakes for vitamin A, vitamin K, arsenic, boron, chromium, copper, iodine, iron, manganese, molybdenum, nickel, silicon, vanadium, and zinc.* Washington, DC: Standing Committee on the Scientific Evaluation of Dietary Reference Intakes National Academy Press, 2001.

   Dietary standards for many trace minerals are discussed. The rationale used to set RDA or Adequate Intakes and Upper Levels for these nutrients is discussed in detail.

8. Ford ES, Mokad AH: Dietary magnesium intake in a national sample of U.S. adults. *Journal of Nutrition* 133:2879, 2003.

   Many adults currently do not meet their magnesium needs on a regular basis, particularly women who do not take a multivitamin and mineral supplement on a regular basis, as well as African-Americans in general. Green vegetables, nuts, seeds, dried beans, whole grains, dairy products, and meats are good magnesium sources for a diet.

9. Franchini M and Veneri D: Hereditary hemochromatosis. *Hematology* 10(2):145, 2005.

   Hereditary hemochromatosis is a disorder of iron metabolism characterized by progressive tissue iron overload which leads to irreversible organ damage if not treated in time. Transferrin saturation and serum ferritin are the most reliable tests for the detection of subjects with hereditary hemochromatosis. Therapeutic phlebotomy is the mainstay of treatment. If phlebotomy is started before the onset of irreversible organ damage, the life expectancy of these patients is similar to that of the normal population.

10. Havas S and others: Reducing the public health burden from elevated blood pressure levels in the United States by lowering intake of dietary sodium. *American Journal of Public Health* 94:19, 2004.

    The American public consumes far more sodium than is needed. Most of this sodium is added as salt by food manufacturers and restaurants.

11. Hoolihan L: Beyond calcium. *Nutrition Today* 39(2):69, 2004.

    Meeting one's needs for calcium using dairy products may provide health benefits beyond those attributed to the calcium content alone. This suggests that incorporating dairy products into a diet is a good habit to develop.

12. How to prevent strokes. *Consumer Reports on Health* 16(9):1, 2004.

    Detailed review of the health risks posed by strokes, as well as a look at current treatments. Preventive measures include not smoking, meeting nutrient needs, reducing stress, and controlling diabetes if present.

13. Kuehn BM: Better osteoporosis management a priority: impact predicted to soar with aging population. *Journal of the American Medical Association* 293(20):2453, 2005.

    More than 2 million individuals in the U.S. will experience osteoporosis-related fractures this year, resulting in medical costs estimated to be more than $16.9 billion. By 2025, the number of fractures and the associated costs are expected to rise by 48%. Proper diet and exercise throughout life are now recognized as the most effective measures to maintain bone health.

14. Mitka M: Dash of dissent on salt intake advice. *Journal of the American Medical Association* 291:1686, 2004.

    Low sodium diets especially help some people control blood pressure, but some experts contend that recommending such a diet to all adults does not have strong scientific support. There is no compelling evidence to show low sodium diets harm adults in general. This has led other experts to recommend routine adoption of a low sodium diet.

15. Rosen CJ: Postmenopausal osteoporosis. *New England Journal of Medicine* 353:595, 2005.

    The diagnosis and treatment of osteoporosis, including use of current medications, is reviewed. The author recommends biphosphonates as the most appropriate medication, as well as meeting calcium and vitamin D needs.

16. Schardt D: Potassium: Bones, stones and strokes on the line. *Nutrition Action Health Letter* p. 8, December 2004.

    Potassium is the seventh most plentiful mineral on earth, but it's much too scarce in the American diet. More potassium in our diets would help protect us against high blood pressure, strokes, kidney stones, and bone loss.

17. Stronger bones without the hype. *Consumer Reports on Health* 16(5):1, 2004.

    The article provides detailed answers to typical questions about bone health. A review of the approved osteoporosis medications is also provided.

18. Wright JD and others: Dietary intake of ten key nutrients for public health, United States: 1999–2000. *Advance Data* 334:1, 2003 (April 17).

19. Zimmerman MB: Assessing iodine status and monitoring progress of iodized salt programs. *Journal of Nutrition* 134:1673, 2004.

    Despite remarkable progress in the control of iodide deficiency disorders, they remain a significant global health problem. Assessing the severity of the disorders and monitoring the progress of salt iodization programs are cornerstones of a control strategy. Ensuring sustainability of these programs is one of the great remaining challenges in the global fight to eliminate iodide deficiency.

I. How Does Your Mineral Intake Measure Up?

  To complete this activity, reexamine your nutritional assessment from Chapter 2. Compare your intake of selected minerals with the RDA, AI, or other established standard. Use your completed nutritional assessment to fill out the table. For each mineral, record your intake, the intake recommended, the percentage of that recommendation you consumed, and a +, −, or = to indicate an intake higher, lower, or equal to the recommendations.

Mineral	Intake	RDA/Adequate Intake/ Minimum Needs	% of Needs	+/−/=
Calcium				
Phosphorus				
Sodium				
Potassium				
Iron				
Zinc				

Analysis

1. Which of your mineral intakes equaled or exceeded the RDA (or other standard set)? Do the nutrients for which you exceeded the desired amounts pose a likely risk for toxicity, based on the total amount consumed?

   _____

2. Which of your intakes were below the RDA (or other standard)?

   _____

3. What foods and cooking practices could be emphasized or de-emphasized to modify your weaknesses? Indicate for each food the specific amount of the missing nutrient(s) supplied.

   _____

   _____

   _____

   _____

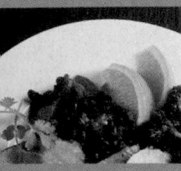

II. Working for Denser Bones

The Looking Further section on osteoporosis in this chapter discussed important information about the disease, which is characterized by thin and brittle bones.

Osteoporosis and related low bone mass affect many adults in North America, especially older women. In fact, one-third of all women experience fractures because of this disease, amounting to about 1.5 million bone fractures per year.

This is a disease you can do something about. Some risk factors can't be changed, but others can. To what degree are you doing the things that can help prevent this debilitating disease? Answer yes or no to the following questions by placing an X in the appropriate blank.

	Yes	No
1. Do you average at least 20 minutes of sun exposure per day to at least your hands and face to get vitamin D, or do you drink vitamin D-fortified milk regularly?	☐	☐
2. Do you engage in weight-bearing physical activity (jogging, brisk walking, etc.) for at least 30 minutes on most or all days of the week?	☐	☐
3. If you are a woman, do you experience regular menstruation?	☐	☐
4. Do you avoid smoking cigarettes?	☐	☐
5. Do you avoid regular consumption of large amounts (greater than one to two drinks per day) of alcohol?	☐	☐
6. Do you consume milk and other dairy products regularly, or substitute other sources to meet at least the Adequate Intake for calcium?	☐	☐
7. Do you moderate intake of phosphorus, sodium, protein, and caffeine?	☐	☐

The more *yes* answers you have, the more you are actively preserving your bone density for the future. Also, remember that this is not just a consideration for women, because if men plan to live well into their eighties and nineties, they are at risk for osteoporosis. In fact, about 14% of all spine fractures and 25% of all hip fractures that are linked to osteoporosis occur in men.

Energy Balance and Weight Control

10

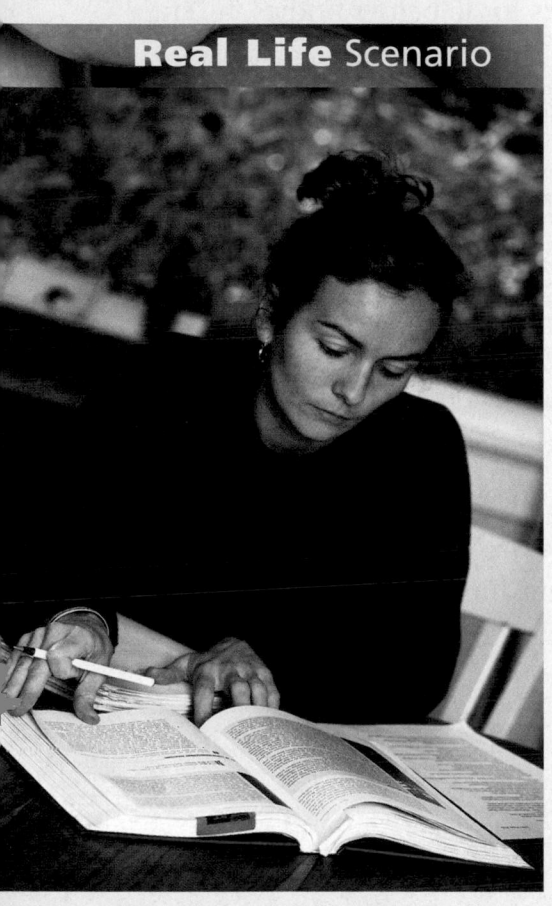

Real Life Scenario

Chris has a hectic schedule. During the day she works full-time at a mail-order warehouse filling orders in the stockroom. At night, three times a week she attends class at the local community college in pursuit of computer certification. On weekends she tries to squeeze in studying and time for her family and friends. Chris has little time to think about what she eats—convenience rules. Unfortunately, over the past few years Chris's weight has been climbing. Watching television a few nights ago, she saw an infomercial for a product that promises she can eat large portions of tasty foods but not gain weight. Famous celebrities support the claim that this product allows one to eat at will and not gain weight. This claim—that by taking this product she can eat whatever she wants and never gain weight—is tempting to Chris. What do you think she should do? What advice can you offer Chris for evaluating weight-loss programs?

Chapter 10 Objectives

Chapter 10 is designed to allow you to:

1. Describe the uses of energy by the body and what constitutes energy balance.

2. Describe various ways to diagnose overweight and obesity.

3. Outline the risks to health posed by overweight and obesity.

4. List and discuss factors affecting energy balance and describe the concept of set point.

5. Describe why and how reduced calorie intake, behavior modification, and increased physical activity fit into a weight-loss plan.

6. Outline the benefits and hazards of various weight-loss methods for severe obesity.

7. Evaluate popular weight-reduction diets and determine which are unsafe, doomed to fail, or both.

Check out the **Contemporary Nutrition Online Learning Center**

www.mhhe.com/wardlawcont6 *for quizzes, flash cards, other activities, and web links designed to further help you learn about energy balance and weight control.*

O f people you see on the street, 29% of the men and 44% of the women are trying to lose weight. Still, despite all their efforts, the ranks of the obese in North America and worldwide are growing. Recall from Chapter 1 that it is estimated that about 1 billion people in the world are overweight. This problem is increasing not only in the United States but also among affluent peoples in Brazil, China, India, Russia, the United Kingdom, and Germany. Excess weight increases the likelihood of many health problems, such as cardiovascular disease, cancer, hypertension, strokes, certain bone and joint disorders, and type 2 diabetes, especially if a person performs minimal physical activity.

Currently, most weight-reduction efforts fizzle before bodies fall into a healthy weight range. Typical popular ("fad") diets are generally monotonous, ineffective, and confusing. They may even endanger some populations, such as children, teenagers, pregnant women, and people with various health disorders. Yet a more logical approach to weight loss is actually very straightforward: (1) Eat less; (2) increase physical activity; and (3) change problematic eating behaviors.

Experts are calling for a national commitment to address the growing weight problem in North America. They suspect that, without a national commitment to weight maintenance and effective new approaches to making our social environment more favorable to maintaining healthy weight, the current trends will not be reversed. Chapter 10 discusses these recommendations to help you understand obesity's, causes, consequences, and potential treatments.

Refresh Your Memory

As you begin your study of weight control in Chapter 10, you may want to review:

- Biological and social dimensions of food intake in Chapter 1
- The concept of energy density and appropriate single serving sizes for foods in Chapter 2
- The causes and consequences of ketosis in Chapter 4
- The fat content of various foods in Chapter 5
- The long-term risks of high-protein diets, especially for some people, in Chapter 6

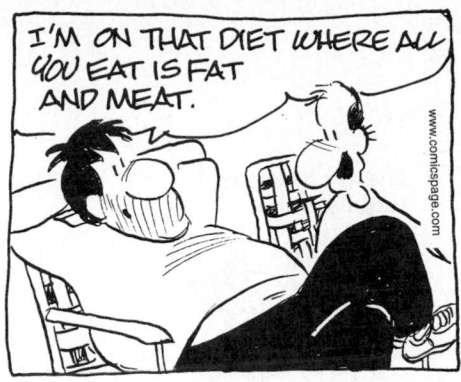 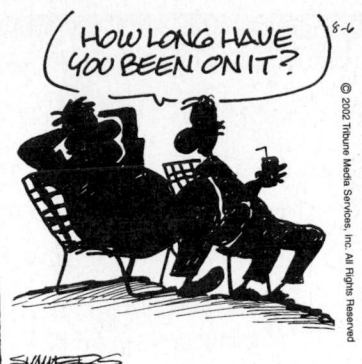 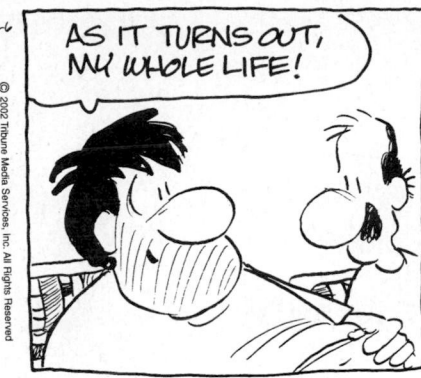

What components make up a successful diet plan? What constitutes a "fad" diet? Why is overweight and obesity a growing problem worldwide? What might be the future consequences of this trend? Chapter 10 provides some answers.

Energy Balance

We begin this chapter with some good news and some bad news. The good news is that if you stay at a healthy body weight, you increase your chances of living a long and healthy life. The bad news is that currently 65% of all North American adults are overweight, significantly more than as recently as the 1980s. Of those, about 45% (30% of the total population) are obese. There is a good chance that any of us could become part of those statistics if we do not pay attention to the prevention of significant weight gain in adulthood. Gaining more than 10 pounds or 2 inches in waist circumference are signals that a re-evaluation of diet and lifestyle is in order.

There is no quick cure for overweight, despite what the advertisements and infomercials claim. Any success comes from hard work and commitment. Currently, a combination of decrease in calorie intake, increase in physical activity, and behavior modification is considered to be the most reliable therapy for the problem of overweight. And without a doubt, the prevention of the problem in the first place is the most successful approach.

The Growing Overweight/Obesity Problem

Adults 20 to 74 who are overweight or obese:

1960–1962	**45%**
1971–1974	**47%**
1976–1980	**47%**
1988–1994	**56%**
1999–today	**64.5%**

■ Positive and Negative Energy Balance

Many of us would benefit from paying more attention to the important concept of **energy balance.** Think of energy balance as an equation:

$$
\begin{array}{ll}
\text{Energy Input} & \text{Energy Output} \\
\text{(calories from food intake)} = & \text{(metabolism; digestion, absorption, and transport} \\
& \text{of nutrients; physical activity)}
\end{array}
$$

The relative size (measured in kcals) of the two sides of this equation can influence energy stores, especially the amount of triglyceride stored in adipose tissue (Fig. 10-1).

When energy input is greater than energy output, the result is **positive energy balance.** The excess calories consumed are stored, which results in weight gain. There are some situations in which positive energy balance is necessary. During pregnancy, a surplus of calories supports the developing fetus. Infants and children require a positive energy balance for growth and development. In adults, however, even a small positive energy balance over time can cause body weight to climb.

On the other hand, if energy input is less than energy output, there is a calorie deficit and **negative energy balance** results. Weight loss occurs as the person is in a

energy balance The state in which energy intake, in the form of food and beverages, matches the energy expended, primarily through basal metabolism and physical activity.

positive energy balance The state in which energy intake is greater than energy expended, generally resulting in weight gain.

negative energy balance The state in which energy intake is less than energy expended, resulting in weight loss.

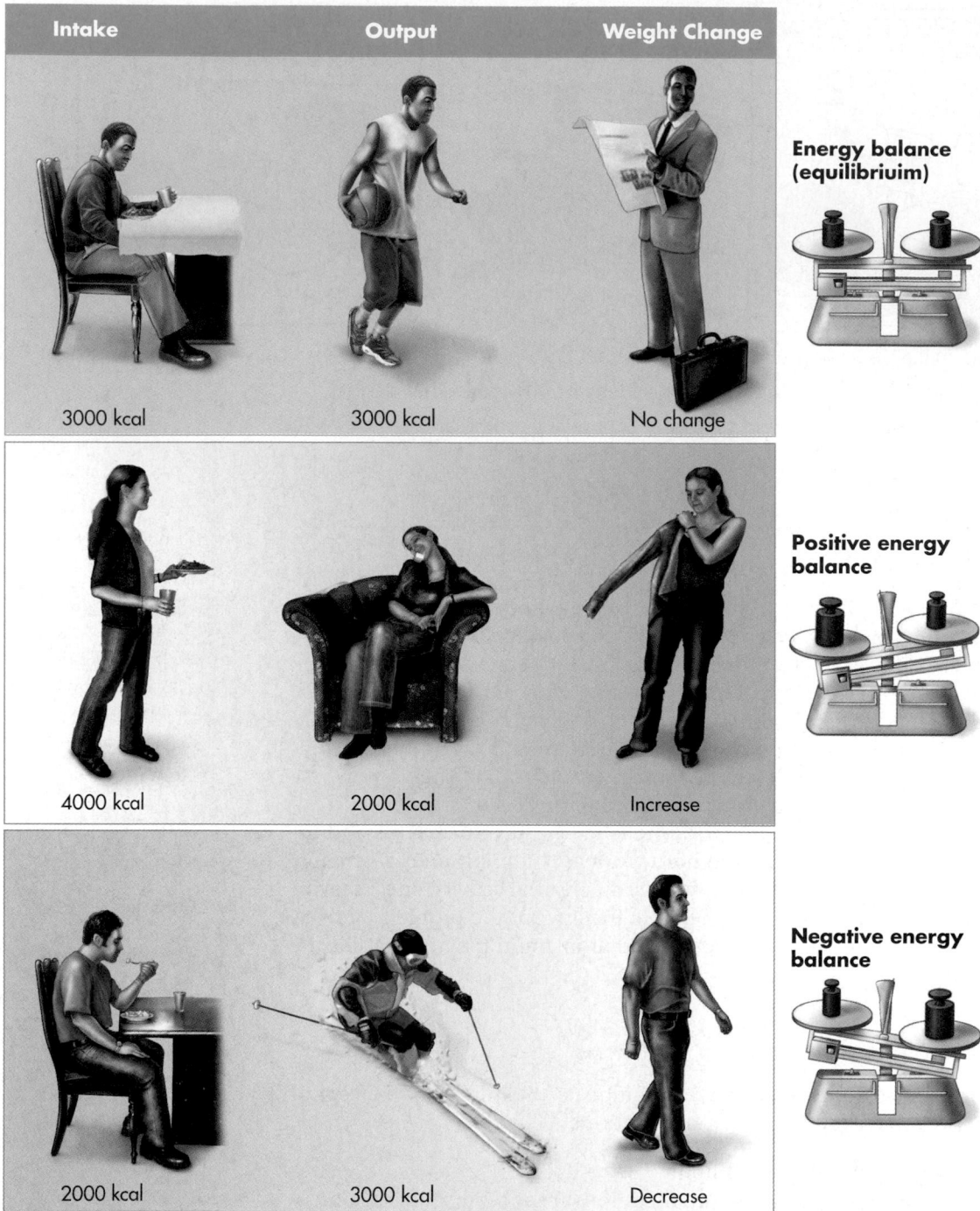

Intake	Output	Weight Change
3000 kcal	3000 kcal	No change
4000 kcal	2000 kcal	Increase
2000 kcal	3000 kcal	Decrease

Energy balance (equilibriuim)

Positive energy balance

Negative energy balance

Figure 10-1 A model for energy balance—input vs. output. This figure depicts energy balance in practical terms.

Critical Thinking

A 26-year-old classmate of yours has been thinking about the process of aging. One of the things she fears most as she gets older is gaining weight. How would you explain energy balance to her?

state of negative energy balance. And even though we think of extra body weight as "fat," this weight loss involves a reduction in both lean and adipose tissue.

As noted in the introduction, the maintenance of energy balance—matching energy intake to energy output over the long term—substantially contributes to health and well-being in adults by minimizing the risk of developing many common health problems. Adulthood is often a time of subtle increases in weight gain, which eventually turns into obesity if left unchecked. The process of aging itself does not cause weight gain; rather the problem stems from a pattern of excess food intake coupled with limited physical activity and slower metabolism. Let's look in detail at the factors that affect the energy balance equation.

■ Energy Intake

Energy needs are met by food intake, represented by the number of calories eaten each day. Determining the appropriate amount and type of food to match energy needs over the long run is a challenge for many of us. Our desire to consume food and ability to use it efficiently are evolutionary survival mechanisms. However, because of modern North American food supplies and accessibility, many of us are now too successful in obtaining food energy. The refrigerator has essentially replaced the need to store body fat—food is always at hand. And given the wide availability of food in vending machines, drive-up windows, social gatherings, and fast-food restaurants—combined with *super-sized* portions—it is no wonder that the average adult is 8 pounds heavier than just 10 years ago. You might say "food hunts man" today. In response to this cultural trend of food being widely available, "defensive eating" (i.e., making careful and conscious food choices, especially in regard to portion size,) on a continual basis is important for many of us.

How much food energy is contained in a meal? A **bomb calorimeter** can be used to determine the amount of energy in a food. The process is described in Figure 10-2. The bomb calorimeter measures the amount of calories that can be derived from carbohydrate, fat, protein, and alcohol. Recall that carbohydrates yield about 4 kcal per gram, proteins yield about 4 kcal per gram, fats yield about 9 kcal per gram, and alcohol yields 7 kcal per gram. These energy figures have been adjusted for (1) digestibility and (2) substances in food, such as fibrous plant parts that burn in the bomb calorimeter but are unusable by the human body for calorie needs. The figures are then rounded to whole numbers. Note, however, that today it is more common to determine the calorie content of a food by simply quantifying its carbohydrate, protein, and fat (and possibly alcohol) content. Then the kcal per gram factors listed above are used to calculate the total kcals. (Recall that Chapter 1 showed how to do this calculation.)

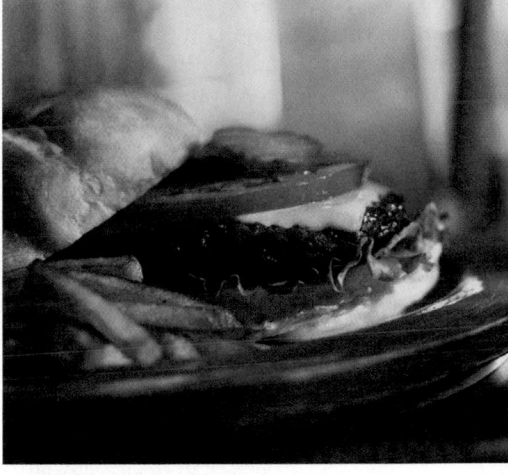

Today we demand food that is immediately available, tastes great, requires little or no preparation, and is served in generous quantities. Of these characteristics, the generous quantities are the most troublesome for many of us. As noted in Chapter 1, a response to the cultural trend of serving large quantities might be to share your meal with another person.

bomb colorimeter An instrument used to determine the calorie content of a food.

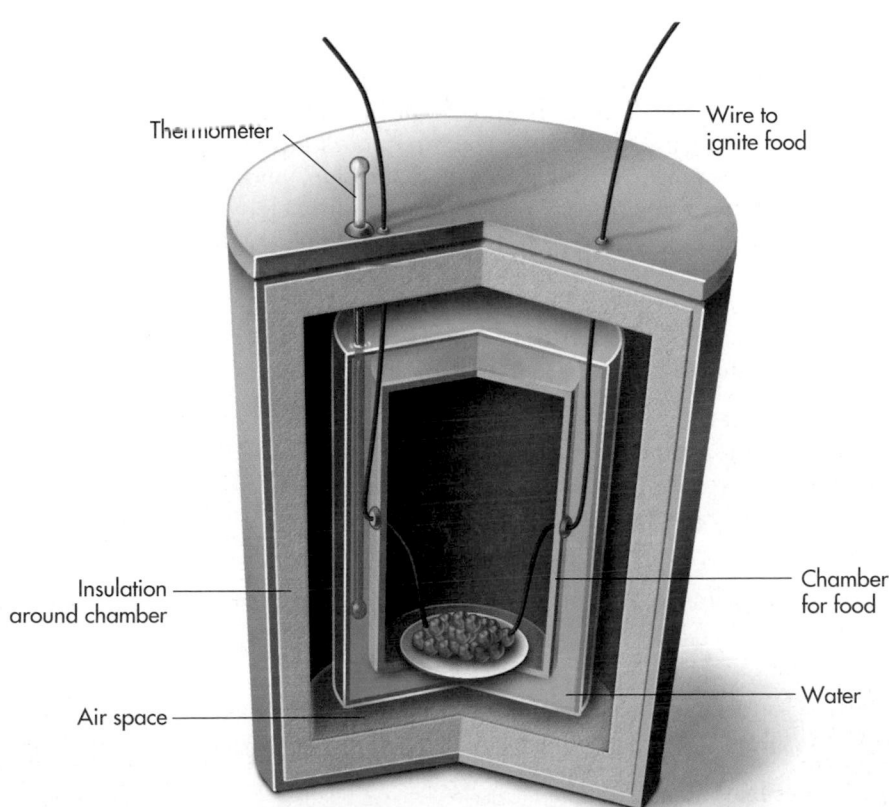

Thermometer

Wire to ignite food

Insulation around chamber

Chamber for food

Air space

Water

Figure 10-2 Cross-section of a bomb calorimeter. A dried portion of food is burned inside a chamber charged with oxygen and surrounded by water to determine energy content. As the food is burned, it gives off heat, which raises the temperature of the water surrounding the chamber. The increase in water temperature indicates the number of kcal contained in the food, because 1 kcal equals the amount of heat needed to raise the temperature of 1 kilogram of water 1 degree Celsius.

Figure 10-3 The components of energy intake and expenditure. This figure incorporates the major variables that influence energy balance. **Remember that alcohol is an additional source of energy for some of us (but is not depicted).** The size of each component shows the relative contribution of that component to energy balance.

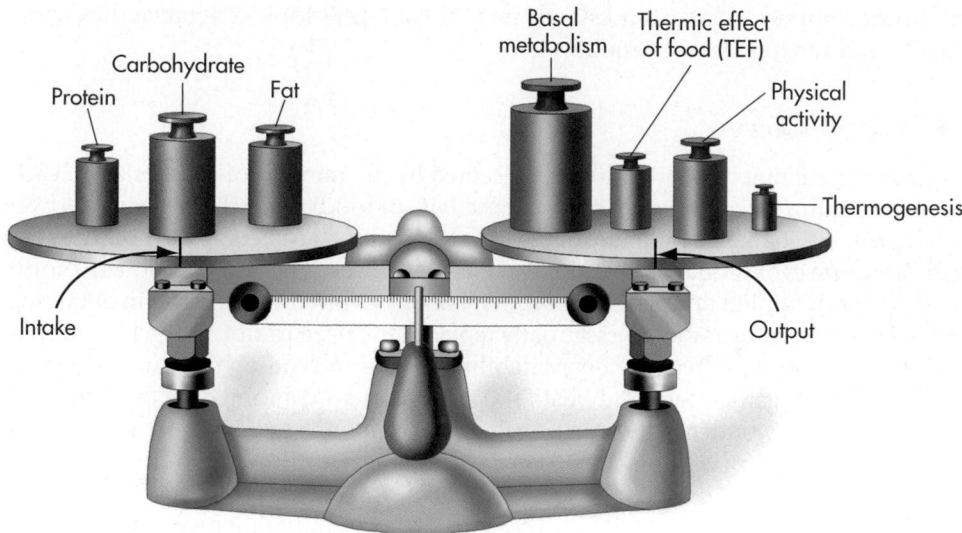

▪ Energy Output

So far, some factors concerning energy intake have been discussed. Now let's look at the other side of the equation—energy output.

The body uses energy for three general purposes: basal metabolism; physical activity; and digestion, absorption, and processing of ingested nutrients. A fourth minor form of energy output, known as thermogenesis, refers to energy expended during fidgeting or shivering in response to cold (Fig. 10-3).

▪ Basal Metabolism

Basal metabolism (expressed as basal metabolic rate [BMR]) represents the minimum amount of calories expended in a fasting state (12 hours or more) to keep a resting, awake body alive in a warm, quiet environment. For a sedentary person, basal metabolism accounts for about 60% to 70% of total energy use by the body. Some of the processes involved include the beating of the heart, respiration by the lungs, and the activity of other organs such as the liver, brain, and kidney. It does not include energy used for physical activity or digestion, absorption, and processing of recently consumed nutrients. If the person is not fasting or completely rested, the term **resting metabolism** is used (expressed as resting metabolic rate [RMR]). An individual's RMR is typically 6% higher than his or her BMR.

To see how basal metabolism contributes to energy needs, consider a 130-pound woman. First, knowing that there are 2.2 pounds for every kilogram, convert her weight into metric units:

$$130 \div 2.2 = 59 \text{ kilograms}$$

Then, using a rough estimate of basal metabolic rate of 0.9 kcal per kilogram per hour for an average female (1.0 kcal per kilogram per hour is used for an average male), calculate her basal metabolic rate:

$$59 \times 0.9 = 53 \text{ kcal per hour}$$

Finally, use this hourly basal metabolic rate to find her basal metabolic rate for an entire day:

$$53 \times 24 = 1272 \text{ kcal}$$

The calculations above give us only an estimate of actual basal metabolism, as it can vary 25% to 30% among individuals. Factors that increase basal metabolism include:

- Greater **lean body mass**
- Larger body surface area

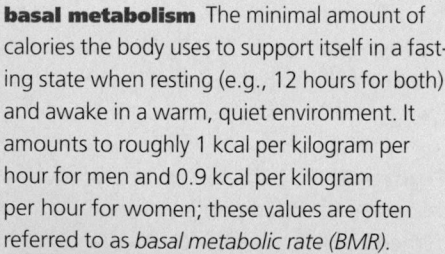

basal metabolism The minimal amount of calories the body uses to support itself in a fasting state when resting (e.g., 12 hours for both) and awake in a warm, quiet environment. It amounts to roughly 1 kcal per kilogram per hour for men and 0.9 kcal per kilogram per hour for women; these values are often referred to as *basal metabolic rate (BMR)*.

resting metabolism The amount of calories the body uses when the person has not eaten in 4 hours and is resting (e.g., 15 to 30 minutes) and awake in a warm, quiet environment. It is roughly 6% higher than basal metabolism due to the less strict criteria for the test; often referred to as *resting metabolic rate (RMR)*.

lean body mass Body weight minus fat storage weight equals lean body mass. This includes organs such as the brain, muscles, and liver, as well as blood and other body fluids.

- Male gender (caused by greater lean body mass)
- Body temperature (fever or cold environmental conditions)
- Thyroid hormones
- Aspects of nervous system activity (release of norepinephrine)
- Pregnancy
- Caffeine and tobacco use. (Still, using the practice of smoking to control body weight is not recommended as too many health risks are increased.)

Of those factors, the amount of lean body mass a person has is the most important one.

In contrast to factors that increase basal metabolism, a low-calorie intake decreases basal metabolism by about 10% to 20% (about 150 to 300 kcal per day) as the body shifts into a conservation mode. This is a barrier to sustained weight loss during dieting that involves an extremely low food intake. In addition, the effects of aging make weight maintenance a challenge. As lean body mass slowly and steadily decreases, basal metabolism declines 1% to 2% for each decade past the age of 30. However, because physical activity aids in maintenance of lean body mass, remaining active as one ages helps to preserve a high basal metabolism and, in turn, aids in weight control.

Energy for Physical Activity

Physical activity increases energy expenditure above and beyond basal energy needs by as much as 25% to 40%. In choosing to be active or inactive, we determine much of our total calorie expenditure for a day. Energy expenditure from physical activity in turn varies widely among people.

Climbing stairs rather than riding the elevator, walking rather than driving to the store, and standing in a bus rather than sitting increase physical activity and, hence, energy use. The alarming rate of and recent increase in obesity in North America are caused in part by our inactivity. Jobs demand less physical activity, and leisure time is often spent slouched before a television or computer.

Thermic Effect of Food (TEF)

In addition to basal metabolism and physical activity, the body uses energy to digest, absorb, and further process the nutrients recently consumed. Energy used for these tasks is referred to as the **thermic effect of food (TEF)**. TEF is analogous to a sales tax—it is like being charged about 5% to 10% for the total amount of calories you eat to cover the cost of processing that food eaten. (We may recognize this increase in metabolism as a warming of the body during and right after a meal.) For every 100 kcal needed for basal metabolism and physical activity, you must eat between 105 and 110 kcal. If your daily calorie intake was 3000 kcal, TEF would account for 150 to 300 kcal. As with other components of energy output, the total amount can vary somewhat among individuals.

Food composition influences TEF. For example, the TEF value for a protein-rich meal (20% to 30% of the calories consumed) is higher than that of a carbohydrate-rich (5% to 10%) or fat-rich (0% to 3%) meal. This is because it takes more energy to metabolize amino acids into fat than to convert glucose into glycogen or transfer absorbed fat into adipose stores. In addition, large meals result in higher TEF values than the same amount of food eaten over many hours.

Thermogenesis

Thermogenesis represents the increase in nonvoluntary physical activity triggered by cold conditions or overeating. Some examples of nonvoluntary activities include shivering when cold, fidgeting, maintenance of muscle tone, and upholding body posture when not lying down. Studies have shown that some people are able to resist weight gain from overfeeding by inducing thermogenesis, while others are not able to do so to a great extent. Thermogenesis goes by other names: thermoregulation, adaptive thermogenesis, and nonexercise activity thermogenesis (NEAT).

While a person is resting, the percentage of total energy use and corresponding energy use by various organs is approximately as follows:

Brain	19%	265 kcal
Skeletal muscle	18%	250 kcal
Liver	27%	380 kcal
Kidney	10%	140 kcal
Heart	7%	100 kcal
Other	19%	265 kcal

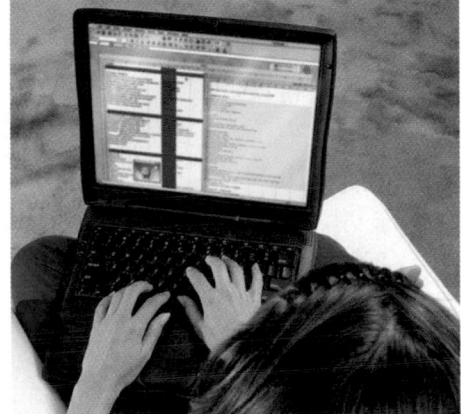

Classwork leads to mental stress but puts little physical stress on the body. Hence, calorie needs are only about 1.5 kcal per minute.

thermic effect of food (TEF) The increase in metabolism that occurs during the digestion, absorption, and metabolism of energy-yielding nutrients. This represents 5% to 10% of calories consumed.

The TEF value for alcohol is 20%.

thermogenesis This term encompasses the ability of humans to regulate body temperature within narrow limits (thermoregulation). Two visible examples of thermogenesis are fidgeting and shivering when cold.

brown adipose tissue A specialized form of adipose tissue that produces large amounts of heat by metabolizing energy-yielding nutrients without synthesizing much useful energy for the body. The unused energy is released as heat.

Another Bite

Brown adipose tissue is a specialized form of adipose tissue that participates in thermogenesis. It is found in small amounts in infants. The brown appearance results from its rich blood flow. Brown adipose tissue contributes to thermogenesis by releasing some of the energy from energy-yielding nutrients into the environment as heat. Adults have very little brown adipose tissue, and its role in adulthood is unknown. It is thought to mostly be important for thermoregulation in infants, in whom brown adipose tissue contributes as much as 5% of body weight. Hibernating animals also make use of brown adipose tissue in the generation of heat to withstand a long winter.

The contribution of thermogenesis to overall calorie needs is fairly small. The combination of basal metabolism and TEF accounts for 70% to 80% of energy used by a sedentary person. The remaining 20% to 30% is used mostly for physical activity, with a small amount used for thermogenesis.

Concept Check

Energy balance involves matching energy intake with energy output. Energy content of food is expressed in kcals and can be determined using a bomb calorimeter. This analysis yields the 4-9-4-7 estimates for the kcals in a gram of carbohydrate, fat, protein, and alcohol, repsectively.

The body uses energy for four main purposes:

1. Basal metabolism (60% to 70% of total energy output) represents the minimal amount of calories needed to maintain the body at rest. Primary determinants of basal metabolic rate include quantity of lean body mass, amount of body surface, and thyroid hormone concentrations in the bloodstream.
2. Physical activity expenditure (20% to 30% of total energy output) represents calorie use for total body cell metabolism above what is needed during rest.
3. Thermic effect of food (5% to 10% of total energy output) represents the calories needed to digest, absorb, and process nutrients recently consumed.
4. Thermogenesis (small, variable percentage of total energy output) includes nonvoluntary, heat-producing activities, such as fidgeting, as well as shivering when cold.

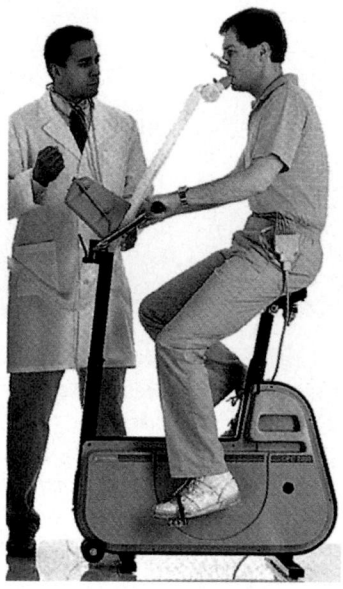

Figure 10-4 Indirect calorimetry. The method of measuring oxygen use and carbon dioxide output can determine calorie use during daily activities.

direct calorimetry A method of determining a body's energy use by measuring heat that is released from the body, usually using an insulated chamber.

indirect calorimetry A method to measure energy use by the body by measuring oxygen uptake. Formulas are then used to convert this gas exchange value into energy use.

Determination of Energy Use by the Body

The amount of energy a body uses can be measured by both direct and indirect calorimetry or can be estimated based on height, weight, degree of physical activity, and age.

Direct and Indirect Calorimetry

Direct calorimetry measures the amount of body heat released by a person. The subject is put into an insulated chamber, often the size of a small bedroom, and body heat released raises the temperature of a layer of water surrounding the chamber. A kcal, as you recall, is related to the amount of heat required to raise the temperature of water. By measuring the water temperature in the direct calorimeter before and after the body releases heat, scientists can determine the energy expended.

Direct calorimetry works because almost all the energy used by the body eventually leaves as heat. However, few studies use direct calorimetry, mostly because of its expense and complexity.

For **indirect calorimetry,** instead of measuring heat output, the most commonly used method measures the amount of oxygen a person consumes (Fig. 10-4). A predictable relationship exists between the body's use of energy and oxygen. For example, when metabolizing a mixed diet of carbohydrate, fat, and protein—a typical blend of energy-yielding nutrients—the human body needs 1 liter of oxygen to yield about 4.85 kcal of energy.

Instruments to measure oxygen consumption for indirect calorimetry are widely used. They can be mounted on carts and rolled up to a hospital bed or carried in backpacks while a person plays tennis or jogs. There are even newly developed handheld instruments (Body Gem). Tables showing energy costs of various forms of exercises rely on information gained from indirect calorimetry studies.

■ Estimates of Energy Needs

As covered in Chapter 2, the Food and Nutrition Board has recently published a number of formulas to estimate energy needs, called Estimated Energy Requirements (EER). Those for adults are shown below (remember to do multiplication and division before addition and subtraction). (Formulas for children, teenagers, pregnant women, and lactating women are listed in Chapters 13 and 14.)

Men 19 years and older

$$EER = 662 - (9.53 \times AGE) + PA \times (15.91 \times WT + 539.6 \times HT)$$

Women 19 years and older

$$EER = 354 - (6.91 \times AGE) + PA \times (9.36 \times WT + 726 \times HT)$$

The variables in the formulas correspond to the following:

EER = Estimated Energy Requirement
AGE = age in years
PA = Physical Activity Estimate (see table below)
WT = weight in kilograms (pounds ÷ 2.2)
HT = height in meters (inches ÷ 39.4)

Physical Activity (PA) Estimates

Activity Level	PA (Men)	PA (Women)
Sedentary (e.g., no exercise)	1.00	1.00
Low activity (e.g., walks the equivalent of 2 miles per day at 3 to 4 mph)	1.11	1.12
Active (e.g., walks the equivalent of 7 miles per day at 3 to 4 mph)	1.25	1.27
Very active (e.g., walks the equivalent of 17 miles per day at 3 to 4 mph)	1.48	1.45

Let's practice using the formula for EER. Consider a man who is 25 years old, 5 feet, 9 inches (1.75 meters), 154 pounds (70 kilograms), and has an active lifestyle. His EER is:

$$EER = 662 - (9.53 \times 25) + 1.25 \times (15.91 \times 70 + 539.6 \times 1.75) = 2997$$

You have determined this man's EER to be about 3000 kcal per day. Remember that this is only an estimate; many other factors, such as genetics and hormones, can affect actual energy needs.

A simple method of tracking your energy expenditure, and thus your energy needs, is to use the forms in Appendix E. Begin by taking an entire 24-hour period and listing all activities performed, including sleep. Record the number of minutes spent in each activity; the total should equal 1440 minutes (24 hours). Next record the energy cost for each activity in kcal per minute following the directions in Appendix E. Multiply the energy cost by the minutes. This gives the energy expended for each activity. Total all the kcal values. This gives your estimated energy expenditure for the day.

Rough guidelines for energy needs (kcals) for adults found in MyPyramid food plan are as follows:

- Sedentary man: 2200–2600
- Sedentary woman: 1800–2000
- Moderately active man: 2400–2800
- Moderately active woman: 2000–2200
- Active man: 2800–3000
- Active woman: 2200–2400

See MyPyramid.gov for a complete listing for ages 2–76+ years. (click on "For Professionals")

Concept Check

Energy use by the body can be measured by direct calorimetry as heat given off and by indirect calorimetry as oxygen used. A person's Estimated Energy Requirement can be estimated based on the following characteristics: gender, height, weight, age, and amount of physical activity.

Women Men

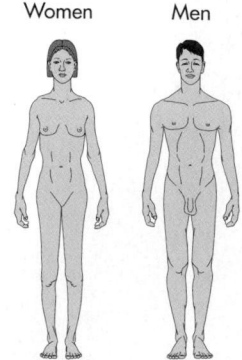

BMI 20

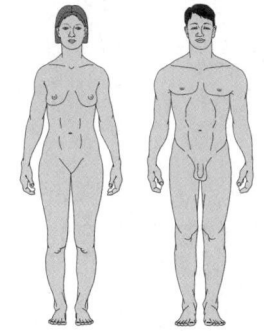

BMI 25

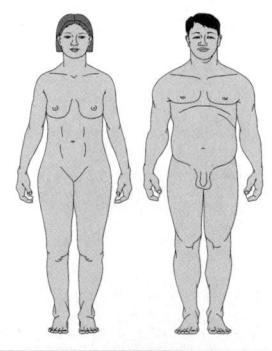

BMI 30

Figure 10-5 Estimates of body shapes at different BMI values.

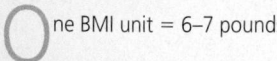

One BMI unit = 6–7 pounds

body mass index (BMI) Weight (in kilograms) divided by height (in meters) squared; a value of 25 and above indicates overweight and a value of 30 and above indicates obesity.

Estimation of a Healthy Weight

Numerous methods are used to establish what body weight should be, typically called *healthy weight*. Several tables exist, generally based on weight-for-height. These tables arise from studies of large population groups. When applied to a population, they provide good estimates of weight associated with health and longevity. However, they do not necessarily indicate the healthiest body weight for each individual. *Athletes with large, lean body mass but low-fat content are a prime example.*

Ideally, family history of weight-related disease and current health conditions should be considered when establishing a healthy weight for an individual, in addition to weight-for-height. Evidence of the following weight-related conditions is important:

- Hypertension
- Elevated LDL-cholesterol
- Family history of obesity, cardiovascular disease, or certain forms of cancer (e.g., uterus, colon)
- Pattern of fat distribution in the body
- Elevated blood glucose

On a more practical note, other questions can be pertinent: What is the least one has weighed as an adult for at least a year? What is the largest size clothing one would be happy with? What weight has one been able to maintain during previous diets without feeling constantly hungry? Overall, the individual, under a physician's guidance, should establish a "personal" healthy weight (or need for weight reduction) based on weight history, fat distribution patterns, family history of weight-related disease, and current health status. This assessment points out how well the person is tolerating any existing excess weight. Thus, current height/weight standards are only a rough guide. Furthermore, a healthy lifestyle may make a more important contribution to a person's health status than the number on the scale. Fit and overweight are not necessarily mutually exclusive (although not often seen together), and neither is thin synonymous with healthy if the person is not also physically active.

■ Using Body Mass Index (BMI) to Set Healthy Weight

For the past 50 years, weight-for-height tables issued by the Metropolitan Life Insurance Company have been the typical way healthy weight was established. These tables considered gender and frame size, predicting the weight range at a specific height that was associated with the greatest longevity. The latest table (issued in 1983) and methods for determining frame size can be found in Appendix G.

Currently **body mass index (BMI)** is the preferred weight-for-height standard (Fig. 10-5). (Still, you may see either standard in medical practice.) Research has shown that body mass index is the weight-for-height standard that is most closely related to body fat content.

Body mass index is calculated as

$$\frac{\text{body weight (in kilograms)}}{\text{height}^2 \text{ (in meters)}}$$

An alternate method for calculating BMI is

$$\frac{\text{weight (pounds)} \times 703}{\text{height}^2 \text{ (inches)}}$$

Table 10-1 lists the BMI for various heights and weights. Health risks from excess weight may begin when the body mass index is 25 or more. A healthy weight-for-height is a BMI 18.5 to 24.9. What is your BMI? How much would your weight need to change to yield a BMI of 25? 30? These are general cut-off values for the presence of overweight and obesity, respectively.

Table 10-1 Body Weight in Pounds According to Height and Body Mass Index (BMI)

Height (Inches)	Healthy BMI						Overweight BMI					Obese BMI		
	19	20	21	22	23	24	25	26	27	28	29	30	35	40
	— Body weight (pounds)													
58	91	96	100	105	110	115	119	124	129	134	138	143	167	191
59	94	99	104	109	114	119	124	128	133	138	143	148	173	198
60	97	102	107	112	118	123	128	133	138	143	148	153	179	204
61	100	106	111	116	122	127	132	137	143	148	153	158	185	211
62	104	109	115	120	126	131	136	142	147	153	158	164	191	218
63	107	113	118	124	130	135	141	146	152	158	163	169	197	225
64	110	116	122	128	134	140	145	151	157	163	169	174	204	232
65	114	120	126	132	138	144	150	156	162	168	174	180	210	240
66	118	124	130	136	142	148	155	161	167	173	179	186	216	247
67	121	127	134	140	146	153	159	166	172	178	185	191	223	255
68	125	131	138	144	151	158	164	171	177	184	190	197	230	262
69	128	135	142	149	155	162	169	176	182	189	196	203	236	270
70	132	139	146	153	160	167	174	181	188	195	202	207	243	278
71	136	143	150	157	165	172	179	186	193	200	208	215	250	286
72	140	147	154	162	169	177	184	191	199	206	213	221	258	294
73	144	151	159	166	174	182	189	197	204	212	219	227	265	302
74	148	155	163	171	179	186	194	202	210	218	225	233	272	311
75	152	160	168	176	184	192	200	208	216	224	232	240	279	319
76	156	164	172	180	189	197	205	213	221	230	238	246	287	328

Each entry gives the body weight in pounds for a person of a given height and BMI (kg/m^2). Pounds have been rounded off. To use the table, find the appropriate height in the far left column. Move across the row to a weight. The number at the top of the column is the BMI for the height and weight.

Another Bite

The concept of body mass index is convenient to use because the values apply to both men and women (i.e., gender neutral). However, any weight-for-height standard is actually a crude measure. Keep in mind, also, that a BMI of 25 to 29.9 is a marker of *overweight* (compared to a standard population) and not necessarily a marker of *overfat*. Many men (especially athletes) have a BMI greater than 25 because of extra muscle tissue. Also, very short adults (under 5 feet tall) may have high BMIs that may not reflect overweight or fatness. For this reason, BMI should be used only as a screening test for overweight or obesity.

Still, overfat and overweight conditions generally appear together. The focus is on BMI in clinical settings mainly because this is easier to measure than total body fat.

Healthy weight is currently the preferred term to use for weight recommendations. Older terms, such as *ideal weight* and *desirable weight*, are no longer used in medical literature.

■ Putting Healthy Weight into Perspective

One current school of thought is to let nature take its course with regard to body weight. According to this proposal, after weight is lost in order to fall within a specific (often unrealistic) height/weight range, people often regain their original weight plus more. In contrast, listening to the body for hunger cues, regularly eating a healthy diet, and remaining physically active (not to be overlooked) eventually helps one maintain an appropriate height/weight value. This concept will be further addressed in the upcoming discussion on treatment for obesity. (It is a cornerstone of the current "size acceptance" movement.) The clearest idea regarding a healthy weight is that it is personal. Weight has to be considered in terms of health, not a mathematical calculation.

Even agreed upon weight standards for BMI are not for everyone. Adult BMIs should not be applied to children, adolescents who are still growing, frail older people, pregnant and lactating women, and highly muscular individuals. Children and pregnant women have unique BMI standards (see Chapters 13 and 14).

In 1994, former U.S. Surgeon General Dr. C. Everett Koop founded the "Shape Up America!" campaign to convince overweight people to lose weight and increase physical activity. According to Dr. Koop, obesity is the number two killer in the United States, just behind smoking. What many North Americans don't understand, he explains, is how serious the problem of excess pounds is.

Energy Imbalance

If calorie intake exceeds output over time, overweight (and often obesity) is a likely result. Often, health problems eventually follow (Table 10-2). In this context, medical experts recommend that an individual's cutoff value for obesity should not be based primarily on body weight but, rather, on the total amount of fat in the body, the location of body fat, and the presence or absence of weight-related medical problems.

Estimating Body Fat Content and Diagnosing Obesity

Body fat can range from 2% to 70% of body weight. Desirable amounts of body fat are about 8% to 24% for men and 21% to 35% for women. In this regard, men with over

Table 10-2 Health Problems Associated with Excess Body Fat

Health Problem	Partially Attributable To
Surgical risk	Increased anesthesia needs, as well as greater risk of wound infections (the latter is linked to a decrease in immune function)
Pulmonary disease and sleep disorders	Excess weight over lungs and pharynx
Type 2 diabetes	Enlarged adipose cells, which poorly bind insulin and poorly respond to the message insulin sends to the cell; less synthesis of factors by enlarged adipose cells that aid insulin action, and greater synthesis of factors by adipose cells that lessen insulin action.
Hypertension	Increased miles of blood vessels found in the adipose tissue, increased blood volume, and increased resistance to blood flow related to hormones made by adipose cells
Cardiovascular disease (e.g., coronary heart disease and stroke)	Increases in LDL-cholesterol and triglyceride values, low HDL-cholesterol, decreased physical activity, and increased synthesis of blood clotting and inflamatory factors by enlarged adipose cells. A greater risk for heart failure is also seen, due in part to altered heart rhythm.
Bone and joint disorders (including gout)	Excess pressure put on knee, ankle, and hip joints
Gallstones	Increased cholesterol content of bile
Skin disorders	Trapping of moisture and microorganisms in tissue folds
Various cancers, such as in the kidney, gallbladder, colon and rectum, and uterus (women) and prostate gland (men)	Estrogen production by adipose cells; animal studies suggest excess calorie intake encourages tumor development
Shorter stature (in some forms of obesity)	Earlier onset of puberty
Pregnancy risks	More difficult delivery, increased number of birth defects, and increased needs for anesthesia
Reduced physical agility and increased risk of accidents and falls	Excess weight that impairs movement
Menstrual irregularities and infertility	Hormones produced by adipose cells, such as estrogen
Vision problems	Cataracts and other eye disorders are more often present
Premature death	A variety of risk factors for disease listed in this Table
Infections	Reduced immune system activity
Liver damage and eventual failure	Excess fat accumulation in the liver
Erectile dysfunction in men	Low grade inflamation caused by excess fat mass and reduced function of the cells lining the blood vessels associated with being overweight

The greater the degree of obesity, the more likely and the more serious these health problems generally become. They are much more likely to appear in people who show an upper-body fat distribution pattern and/or are greater than twice healthy body weight.

24% body fat and women with over about 35% body fat are considered obese. Women need more body fat because some "sex-specific" fat is associated with reproductive functions. This fat is normal and factored into calculations.

To measure body fat content accurately using typical methods, both body weight and body volume of the person must be known. Body weight is easy to measure. Of the typical methods used to estimate body volume, **underwater weighing** is the most accurate. This technique determines body volume using the loss of weight when placed underwater, the relative densities of fat tissue and lean tissue, and a specific mathematical formula. This procedure requires that a subject be totally submerged in a tank of water, and a trained technician needs to direct the procedure (Fig. 10-6). **Air displacement** is another method of determining body volume. Body volume is quantified by measuring the space a person takes up inside a measurement chamber, such as the BodPod (Fig. 10-7). A further method to measure body volume is to simply submerge a person in a tank and observe the level of the water before and after submersion. The volume of the displaced water is then calculated.

Once body volume is known, it can be used along with body weight in the following equation to calculate body density. Then using body density, body fat content finally can be determined.

$$\text{Body density} = \frac{\text{body weight}}{\text{body volume}}$$

$$\% \text{ body fat} = (495 \div \text{body density}) - 450$$

For example, assume that the subject in the underwater weighing tank in Figure 10-6 has a body density of 1.06. The units are grams per centimeter^3. We can use the second formula to calculate that he has 17% body fat ([495 ÷ 1.06] − 450 = 17).

Skinfold thickness is also a common anthropometric method to estimate total body fat content, although there are some limits to its accuracy. Clinicians use calipers to measure the fat layer directly under the skin at multiple sites and then plug these values into a mathematical formula (Fig. 10-8).

The technique of **bioelectrical impedance** is also used to estimate body fat content. The instrument sends a painless, low-energy electrical current to and from the body via wires and electrode patches to estimate body fat. Researchers surmise that

underwater weighing A method of estimating total body fat by weighing the individual on a standard scale and then weighing him or her again submerged in water. The difference between the two weights is used to estimate total body volume.

air displacement A method for estimating body composition that makes use of the volume of space taken up by a body inside a small chamber.

bioelectrical impedance The method to estimate total body fat that uses a low-energy electrical current. The more fat storage a person has, the more impedance (resistance) to electrical flow will be exhibited.

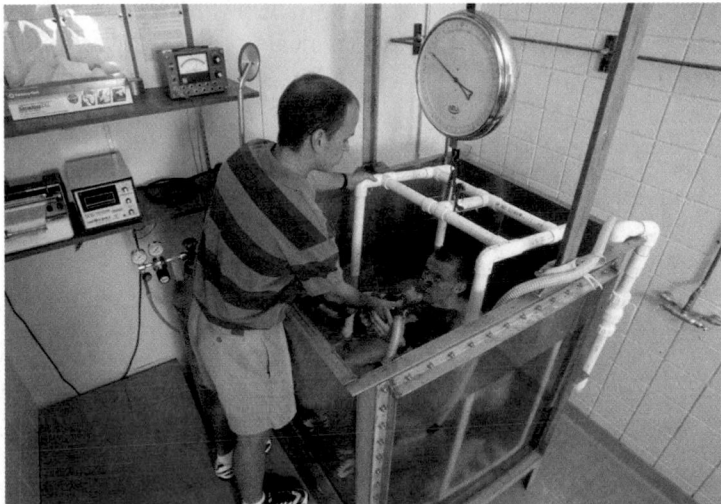

Figure 10-6 Underwater weighing. In this technique the subject exhales as much air as possible and then holds his or her breath and bends over at the waist. Once the subject is totally submerged, the underwater weight is recorded. Using this value, body volume can be calculated.

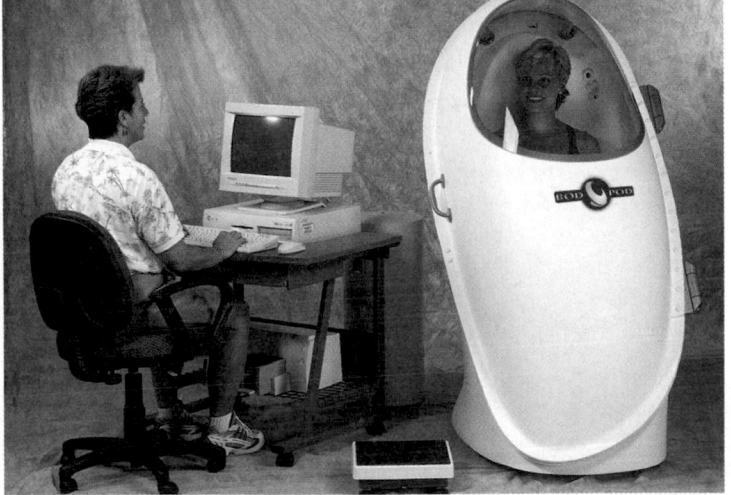

Figure 10-7 BodPod. This device determines body volume based on the volume of displaced air, measured as a person sits in a sealed chamber for a few minutes.

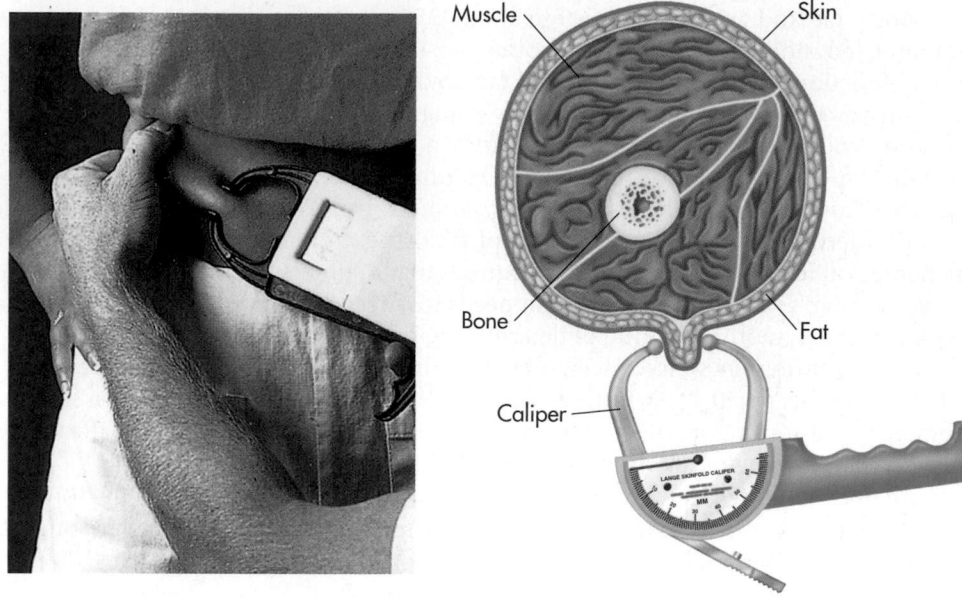

Figure 10-8 Skinfold measurements. Using of proper technique and calibrated equipment, skinfold measurements around the body can be used to predict body fat content in about 10 minutes.

Another method to assess body fat is to measure total-body electrical conductance when placed in an electromagnetic field (TOBEC). Still another method, **near-infrared reactance** exposes the bicep muscle to a beam of near-infrared light. The measuring instrument assesses the interactions of the light beam with fat and lean tissues in the upper arm. After only 2 seconds, this flashlight-size device can give an estimate of body composition. However, experts note that this method, although convenient and inexpensive, is not very accurate.

adipose tissue resists electrical flow more than lean tissue. This is because adipose tissue has a lower electrolyte and water content than lean tissue, and so more adipose tissue proportionately means greater electrical resistance. Within a few minutes, bioelectrical impedance analyzers convert body electrical resistance into an approximate estimate of total body fat, as long as body hydration status is normal (Fig. 10-9).

A further advance in determination of body fat content is use of **dual energy X-ray absorptiometry (DEXA)**. Currently, DEXA is considered the most accurate way to determine body fat, but the equipment is very expensive and not widely available for this use. This X-ray system allows the clinician to separate body weight into three separate components—fat, fat-free soft tissue, and bone mineral. The usual whole-body scan requires about 5 to 20 minutes and the dose of radiation is less than a chest X ray. Obesity, osteoporosis, and other aspects of nutritional health can be investigated using this method (Fig. 10-10).

dual energy X-ray absorptiometry (DEXA) A highly accurate method of measuring body composition and bone mass and density using multiple low-energy X rays.

upper-body obesity The type of obesity in which fat is stored primarily in the abdominal area; defined as a waist circumference more than 40 inches (102 centimeters) in men and more than 35 inches (89 centimeters) in women; closely associated with a high risk for cardiovascular disease, hypertension, and type 2 diabetes.

■ Using Body Mass Index to Define Obesity

BMI offers another way to define obesity (Fig. 10-11).

| 30–39.9 | Obese | Increased health risk |
| 40 or greater | Severely obese | Major health risk. Note that the number of North Americans falling into this category is increasing rapidly. |

■ Using Body Fat Distribution to Further Evaluate Obesity

Where we store fat, as well as how much, can predict health risks, and likely even more than a person's BMI. Some people store fat in upper-body areas. Others hold fat lower on the body. Excess fat in either place generally spells trouble, but each storage space also has its unique risks. Fat deposited in the lower body often resists being shed. However, **upper-body (android) obesity** is more often related to cardiovascular disease, hypertension, and type 2 diabetes. Whereas other adipose cells empty fat directly into general circulation, the fat released from abdominal adipose cells goes straight to

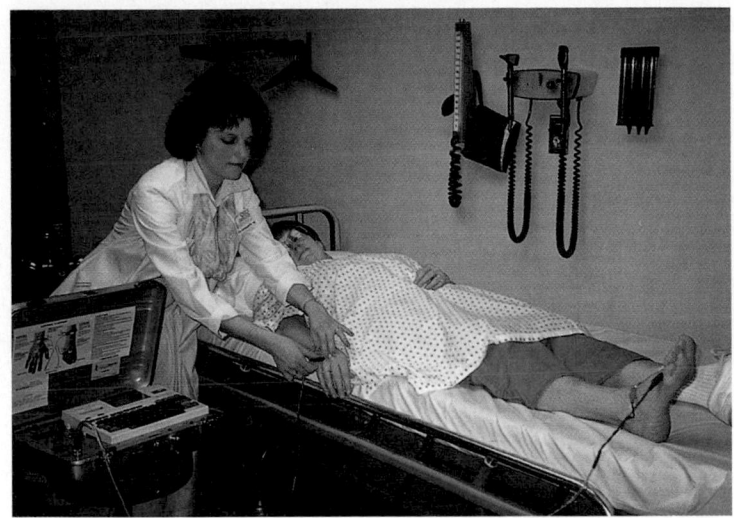

Figure 10-9 Bioelectrical impedance. This method can estimate total body fat in less than 5 minutes and is based on the principle that fat in the body resists the flow of applied low-energy electricity since it is low in water and electrolytes. The degree of resistance to electrical flow is used to estimate body fatness.

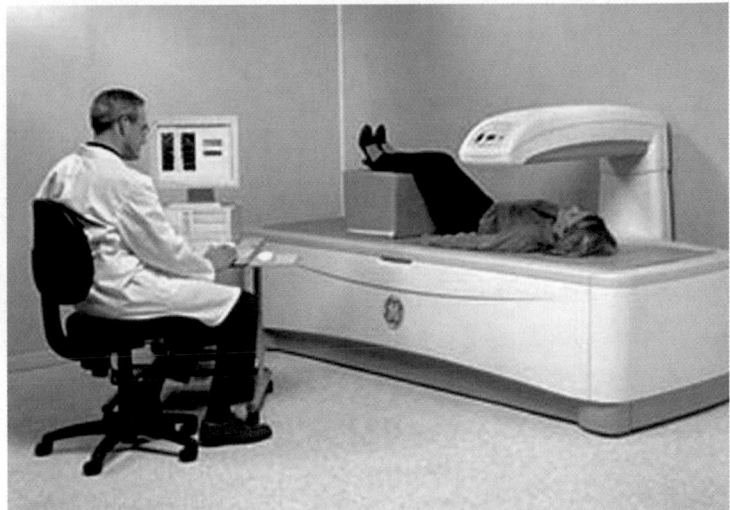

Figure 10-10 Dual energy X-ray absorptiometry (DEXA). This method measures body fat by passing small doses of radiation through the body which a detector then quantifies as fat, lean tissue, or bone. The scanner arm moves from head to toe and in doing so can determine body fat as well as bone density. DEXA is currently considered the most accurate method for determining body fat (as long as the person can fit under the arm of the instrument). The radiation dose is minimal.

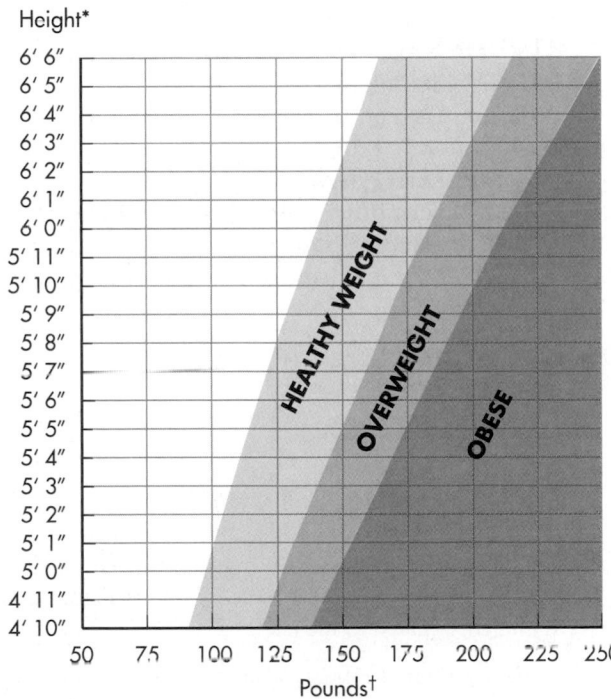

Height*

Figure 10-11 Convenient height/weight table based on BMI; the upper ends of the healthy weight ranges correspond to a body mass index of 25.

* Without shoes.
† Without clothes. The higher weights apply to people with more muscle and bone, such as many men.

the liver, by way of the portal vein found there. This process likely interferes with the liver's ability to clear insulin and alters lipoprotein metabolism by the liver. These adipose cells also make substances that increase inflamation in the body, as well as increase insulin resistance, blood clotting, and blood vessel constriction. All these changes can lead to long-term health problems.

Figure 10-12 Body fat distribution, showing upper-body and lower-body obesity. The upper-body (android) form brings higher risks for ill health associated with obesity. The woman has a waist circumference of 32 inches. The man has a waist circumference of 44 inches. Thus, the man has upper-body obesity, but the woman does not, based on the current cutoff of 40 inches for men and 35 inches for women.

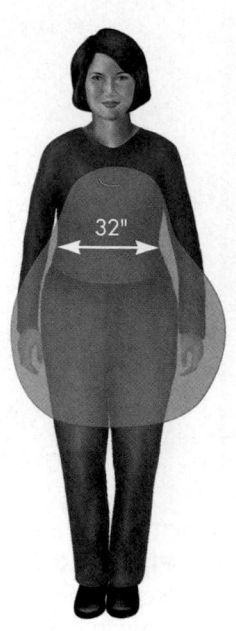
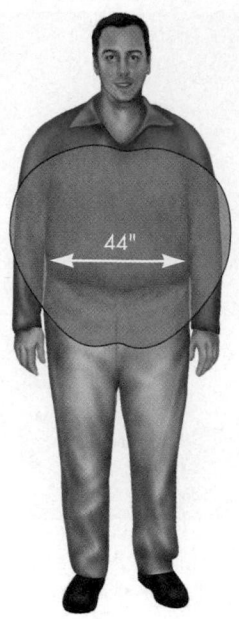

Lower-body obesity   Upper-body obesity

lower-body obesity The type of obesity in which fat storage is primarily located in the buttocks and thigh area.

High blood testosterone (primarily a male hormone) levels apparently encourage upper-body obesity, as does a diet with a high glycemic load, alcohol intake, and smoking. This characteristic male pattern of fat storage appears in the apple shape (large abdomen [pot belly] and small buttocks and thighs). Upper body obesity is assessed by simply measuring the waist at the widest point just above the hips when relaxed. A waist circumference more than 40 inches (102 centimeters) in men and more than 35 inches (88 centimeters) in women indicates such a shape (Fig. 10-12). If BMI is also 25 or more, health risks are significantly increased.

Estrogen and progesterone (primarily female hormones) encourage lower-body fat storage and **lower-body (gynecoid** or **gynoid) obesity**—the typical female pattern. The small abdomen and much larger buttocks and thighs give a pear-like appearance. After menopause, blood estrogen falls, encouraging upper-body fat distribution.

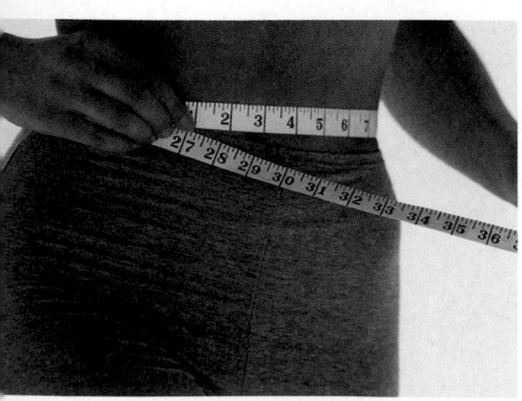

Waist circumference is an important measure of weight-related health risk.

Concept Check

Overweight and obesity typically are associated with excessive body fat storage. The risk of health problems related to being overweight especially increases under the following conditions:

- A man's percentage of body fat exceeds 25%; a woman's exceeds about 35%.
- Excess fat is primarily stored in the upper-body region.
- Body mass index (BMI) is 30 or more (calculated as weight in kilograms divided by height squared in meters).

However, these are merely guidelines. A more individualized approach to assessment is warranted as long as a person is following a healthy lifestyle and has no existing health problems.

Body fat content can be estimated using a variety of methods such as underwater weighing, air displacement, skinfold thickness, bioelectrical impedance, and DEXA. Fat storage distribution further specifies an obese state as either upper body or lower body. Obesity leads to an increased risk for cardiovascular disease, some types of cancer, hypertension, type 2 diabetes, certain bone and joint disorders, and some digestive disorders. The risks for some of these diseases are greater with upper-body fat storage.

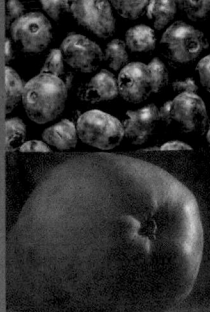
Both genetic and environmental factors can increase the risk for obesity. Experts in the field are at odds over the relative importance of nature versus nurture.

How Does Nature Contribute to Obesity?

Studies in pairs of **identical twins** give us some insight into the contribution of nature to obesity. Even when identical twins are raised apart, they tend to show similar weight gain patterns, both in overall weight and body fat distribution. It appears that nurture—eating habits and nutrition, which varies between twins who are raised apart—has less to do with obesity than nature does. In fact, research suggests that genes account for up to 70% of weight differences between people.

We also inherit specific body types. Tall, thin people appear to have an inherently easier time maintaining healthy body weight. This is probably due to the fact that basal metabolism increases as body surface increases, and therefore taller people use more calories than shorter people, even at rest.

Some rats and mice can have a genetic predisposition to obesity if they inherit a "thrifty metabolism"—one that uses calories frugally. This enables them to store fat more readily than the typical animal. Many of us probably have inherited a thrifty metabolism as well, so that we require fewer calories to get through the day. In earlier times, when food supplies were scarce, a thrifty metabolism would have been a built-in safeguard against starvation. Now, with a general abundance of food, people operating in this low gear require much physical activity and wise

identical twins Two offspring that develop from a single ovum and sperm and, consequently, have the same genetic makeup.

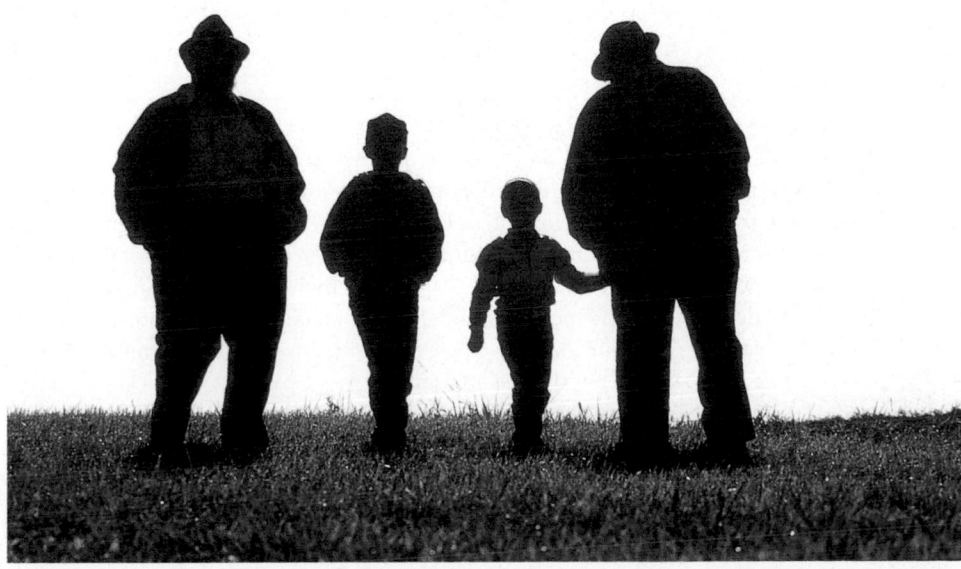

Does the difference in body fat between the grandfathers and the grandsons arise from nature or nurture, or both?

food choices to prevent obesity. If you think you are prone to weight gain, you likely have inherited a thrifty metabolism.

A child with no obese parent has only a 10% chance of becoming obese. When a child has one obese parent (common in our society), that risk advances up to 40%, and with two obese parents, it soars to 80%. Our genes help determine metabolic rate, fuel use, and differences in brain chemistry—all of which affect body weight.

Does the Body Have a Set Point for Weight?

The **set-point** theory of weight maintenance proposes that humans have a genetically predetermined body weight or body fat content, which the body closely regulates. Some research suggests that the hypothalamus monitors the amount of body fat in humans and tries to keep that amount constant over time. Recall from Chapter 1 that the hormone *leptin* forms a communication link between adipose cells and the brain, which allows for some weight regulation.

What evidence supports the set-point theory? In human studies, volunteers who had lost weight through starvation tended to eat in such a way to regain their original weight. In addition, studies in the 1960s using prisoners with no history of obesity found it was hard for some men to gain weight. Also, after an illness is resolved, a person generally regains lost weight.

Physiological measurements also endorse the set-point theory. For example, when calorie intake is reduced, the blood concentration of thyroid hormones falls, which slows basal metabolism. In addition, as weight is lost, the calorie cost of weight-bearing activity decreases, so that an activity that burned 100 kcal before weight loss may only burn 80 kcal after weight loss. Furthermore, with weight loss, the body becomes more efficient at storing fat by increasing the activity of the enzyme *lipoprotein lipase*, which takes fat into cells. All of these changes protect the body from losing weight.

If a person overeats, in the short run, basal metabolism tends to increase. This causes some resistance to weight gain. However, in the long run, resistance to weight gain is much less than resistance to weight loss. When a person gains weight and stays at that weight for a while, the body tends to establish a new set point.

Opponents of the set-point theory argue that weight does not remain constant throughout adulthood—the average person gains weight slowly, at least until old age. Also, if an individual is placed in a different social, emotional, or physical environment, weight can be altered and maintained markedly higher or lower. These arguments suggest that humans, rather than having a set point determined by genetics or the number of adipose cells, actually settle into a particular stable weight based on their circumstances, often regarded as a "settling point."

Overall, the set point is weaker in preventing weight gain than in preventing weight loss. Even with a set point helping us, the odds are in favor of eventual weight gain unless we devote effort to a healthy lifestyle.

Does Nurture Have a Role?

Some would argue that body weight similarities between family members stem more from learned behaviors rather than genetic similarities. Even couples, who have no genetic link, may behave similarly toward food and eventually assume similar degrees of leanness or fatness. Proponents of nurture pose that environmental factors, such as high-fat diets and inactivity, literally shape us. Consider that our gene pool has not changed much in the past 50 years, but the ranks of obese people have grown in what the U.S. Centers for Disease Control and Prevention describe as epidemic proportions over the last 10 years.

Is poverty associated with obesity? Ironically, the answer is often yes. North Americans of lower socioeconomic status, especially females, are more likely to be obese than those in upper socioeconomic groups. Are cultural expectations or socioeconomic stress (e.g., **food insecurity**) the cause of this?

set point Often refers to the close regulation of body weight. It is not known what cells control this set point or how it actually functions in weight regulation. There is evidence, however, that mechanisms exist that help regulate weight.

food insecurity A condition of anxiety regarding running out of either food or money to buy more food.

Adult obesity in women is often rooted in childhood obesity. In addition, relative inactivity, periods of stress or boredom, as well as excess weight gain during pregnancy, contribute to female obesity. (Chapter 13 notes that breastfeeding one's infant contributes to loss of some of the excess fat associated with pregnancy.) These patterns suggest both social and genetic links. Male obesity, however, is not strongly linked to childhood obesity and, instead, tends to appear after age 30. This powerful and prevalent pattern suggests a primary role of nurture in obesity, with less genetic influence.

Nature and Nurture Together

Overall, both nature and nurture influence the tendency toward obesity (Table 10-3). The eventual location of fat storage is strongly influenced by genetics. Consider the possibility that obesity is nurture allowing nature to express itself. Some obese people begin life with a slower basal metabolism, maintain an inactive lifestyle, consume highly-refined, calorie-dense diets. These people in turn are nurtured into gaining weight, promoting their natural tendency toward obesity.

Still, genes do not fully control destiny. With increased physical activity and decreased food consumption, even those with a genetic tendency toward obesity can attain a healthier body weight.

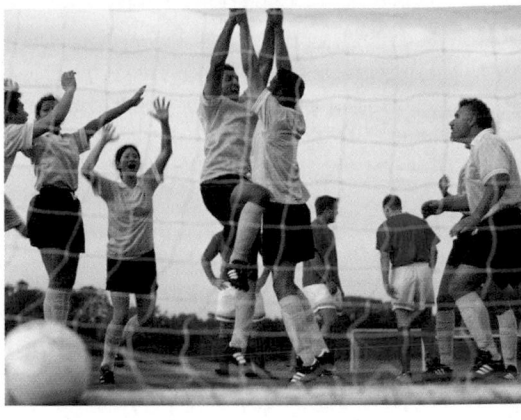

Student life is often full of physical activity. This is not necessarily true for a person's later working life; hence, weight gain is a strong possibility.

Table 10-3 What Encourages Excess Body Fat Stores and Obesity?

Factor	How Fat Storage Is Affected
Age	Excess body fat is more common in adults and middle-age individuals.
Menopause	Increase in abdominal fat deposition is favored.
Gender	Females have more fat.
Positive energy balance	If over a long period, positive energy balance promotes storage of fat.
Composition of diet	Excess calorie intake from a high fat intake, generous alcohol intake, and preference for calorie dense (sugary, fat-rich) foods are likely to contribute to obesity.
Physical activity	Low or decreasing amount of physical activity ("couch potato") affects energy balance and body fat stores.
Basal metabolism	A low value is linked to weight gain.
Thermic effect of food	This is low for some obesity cases.
Increased hunger sensations	Some people especially have trouble resisting the wide food availability typical of modern life, likely linked to the activity of various brain chemicals.
Ratio of fat to lean tissue	A high ratio of fat mass to lean body mass is correlated with weight gain.
Fat uptake by adipose tissue	This is high in some obese individuals and remains high (perhaps even increases) with weight loss.
Variety of social and behavioral factors	Obesity is associated with socioeconomic status; familial conditions; network of friends; busy lifestyles that discourage balanced meals; binge eating; easy availability of inexpensive, "supersized" high-fat food; pattern of leisure activities; television time; smoking cessation; excessive alcohol intake; and number of meals eaten away from home.
Undetermined genetic characteristics	These affect energy balance, particularly via the energy expenditure components, the deposition of the energy surplus as adipose tissue or as lean tissue, and the relative proportion of fat and carbohydrate used by the body.
Race	In some ethnic groups, higher body weight may be more socially acceptable.
Certain medications	Food intake increases.
Childbearing	Women may not lose all weight gained in pregnancy, leading to increased weight gain.
National region	Regional differences, such as high-fat diets and sedentary lifestyles in the Midwest and areas of the South, lead to different rates of obesity in different places.

The total cost attributable to weight-related disease is about $90 billion annually in the United States. Half of this cost is borne by the taxpayers through Medicare and Medicaid.

Treatment of Overweight and Obesity

Treatment of overweight and obesity should be considered similar to that for any chronic disease. This treatment requires long-term lifestyle changes, rather than simply taking medicine for 2 weeks, as for a sore throat, or following a quick fix promoted by a popular (also called fad) diet book. We often, however, view a "diet" as something one goes on temporarily, only to resume prior (typically poor) habits once satisfactory results have been achieved. It is mostly for this reason that so many people regain lost weight. In place of this, healthy, active living with dietary modifications one can live with should be the emphasis for both overweight and obese, as well as lean, people. Let's explore why obesity must be regarded as such and in response treated appropriately.

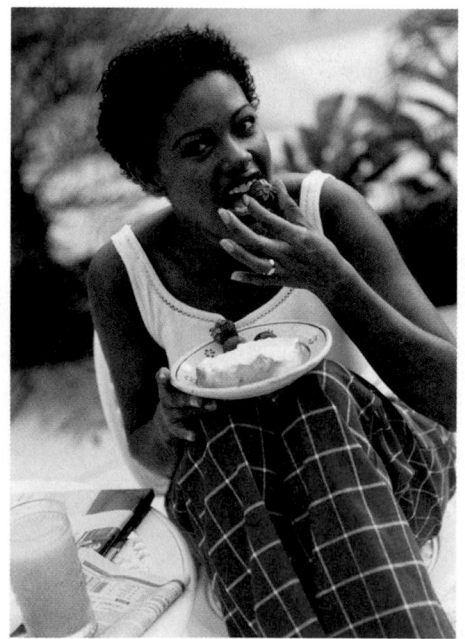

Making a commitment to a healthier diet and lifestyle can be a daunting challenge for many individuals. However, a sound weight-loss plan does not require you to completely avoid certain favorite foods. A more practical strategy may include substituting lower-calorie choices, choosing high-calorie treats less often, and limiting portion sizes.

Rate of Loss

- [ ] Slow and steady weight loss, rather than rapid weight loss, is encouraged.
- [ ] Goal is 1 pound or so of loss of fat storage per week.
- [ ] A period of weight maintenance for a few months following a loss of 10% of body weight.
- [ ] Evaluation of need for further dieting before more weight loss begins.

Flexibility

- [ ] Ability to participate in normal activities (e.g., parties, restaurants).
- [ ] Adaptations to individual habits and tastes.

Intake

- [ ] Nutritional needs are met (except for calories).
- [ ] Common foods are included, with no certain foods being promoted as magical.
- [ ] Use of a fortified ready-to-eat breakfast cereal or balanced multivitamin/mineral supplement is recommended, especially when consuming less than 1600 kcal per day.
- [ ] Use MyPyramid as a pattern for food choices.

Behavior Modification

- [ ] Maintenance of healthy lifestyle (and weight) is a key concern; there is a lifetime focus.
- [ ] Changes are reasonable and can be maintained.
- [ ] Social support is encouraged.
- [ ] Plans for relapse so one does not quit after a setback.

Overall Health

- [ ] Screening by a physician is required for persons with existing health problems, those over 40 (men) to 50 (women) years of age who plan to substantially increase physical activity, and those who plan to lose weight rapidly.
- [ ] Regular physical activity, proper rest, stress reduction, and other healthy changes in lifestyle are encouraged.
- [ ] Underlying psychological weight issues are addressed, such as depression or marital stress.

Figure 10-13 Characteristics of a sound weight-loss diet. How many ☑ does the diet plan that you may be considering have?

■ What to Look for in a Sound Weight-Loss Plan

A dieter can try to devise a plan of action by seeking advice from a health professional, such as a registered dietitian, or by consulting current literature. Either way, a sound weight-loss program (Fig. 10-13) should especially include these components:

1. Control of calorie intake. One recommendation is to decrease calorie intake by 100 kcal per day (and increase physical activity by 100 kcal per day). This should allow for slow and steady weight loss.
2. Increased physical activity.
3. Acknowledgment that maintenance of a healthy weight requires lifelong changes in habits, not simply a short-term weight-loss period.

A one-sided approach that focuses only on restricting calories is a difficult plan of action. Instead, adding physical activity and an appropriate psychological component will contribute to success in weight loss and eventual weight maintenance (Fig. 10-14).

Another Bite

Rapid weight loss cannot consist primarily of fat loss because a high calorie deficit is needed to lose a large amount of adipose tissue. Adipose tissue, which is mostly fat, contains about 3500 kcal per pound. Weight loss as fat includes adipose tissue plus supporting lean tissues, and represents approximately 3300 kcal per pound (about 7.2 kcal per gram). Therefore, to lose 1 pound of adipose tissue per week, calorie intake must be decreased by approximately 500 kcal per day, or physical activity must be increased by 500 kcal per day. Alternately, a combination of both strategies can be used. Diets that promise 10 to 15 pounds of weight loss per week cannot ensure that the weight loss is from adipose tissue stores alone. Subtracting enough calories from one's daily intake to lose that amount of adipose tissue simply is not possible. Lean tissue and water, rather than adipose tissue, account for the major part of the weight lost during these dramatic weight-loss programs.

■ Weight Loss in Perspective

All of these principles point to the importance of preventing obesity. This concept has wide support because conquering the disorder is so difficult. Public health strategies to address the current obesity problem must speak to all age groups. There is a particular need to focus on children and adolescents because patterns of excess weight and sedentary lifestyle developed during youth may form the basis for a lifetime of weight-related illness and increased mortality. In the adult population, attention should be directed toward weight maintenance and increased physical activity.

Concept Check

Obesity is a chronic disease that necessitates lifelong treatment. Emphasis should be placed especially on preventing obesity, since overcoming this disorder is very difficult. Appropriate weight-loss programs have the following characteristics in common: (1) They meet nutritional needs; (2) they can adjust to accommodate habits and tastes; (3) they emphasize readily obtainable foods; (4) they promote changing habits that discourage overeating; (5) they encourage regular physical activity; and (6) they help change obesity-promoting beliefs and rally healthy social support.

Weight-Control Objectives from *Healthy People 2010*

Increase by 40% the proportion of adults who are at a healthy weight (body mass index between 18.5 and 25).

Reduce by 50% the proportion of adults who are obese (body mass index of 30 or more).

Reduce by 50% the proportion of children and adolescents who are overweight or obese.

As you read brochures, articles, or research reports about specific diet plans, look beyond the weight loss promoted by the diet's advocate to see if the reported weight loss was maintained. If the weight maintenance aspect was missing, then the program was not successful.

For more information on weight control, obesity, and nutrition, visit the Weight-Control Information Network (WIN) at www.niddk.nih.gov/health/nutrit/win.htm or call 800-WIN-8098. Complete guidelines for weight management are available at www.nhlbi.nih.gov/guidelines/index.htm. Other websites include www.caloriecontrol.org, www.weight.com, www.obesity.org, and www.cyberdiet.com.

Figure 10-14 Weight-loss tripod. Successful weight loss (and maintenance) is analogous to a camera on a tripod. The three legs are controlling calorie intake, performing regular physical activity, and correcting "problem" behaviors. If one leg is missing, the tripod will tip over. Similarly, without one of these three principles, weight loss and later maintenance become unlikely.

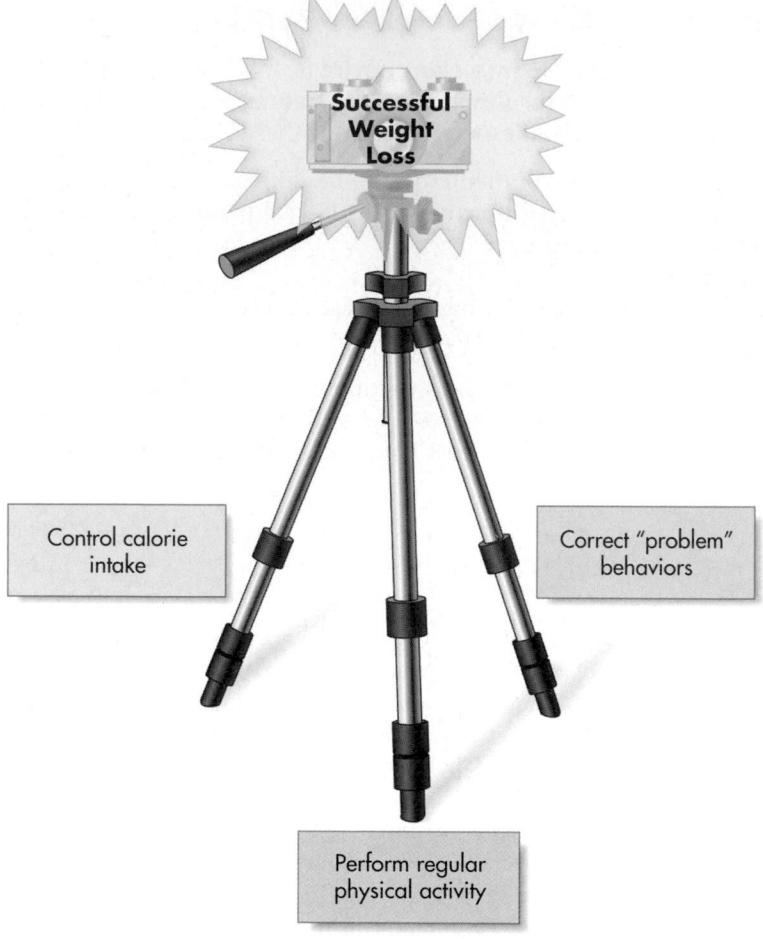

Successful Weight Loss

Control calorie intake

Correct "problem" behaviors

Perform regular physical activity

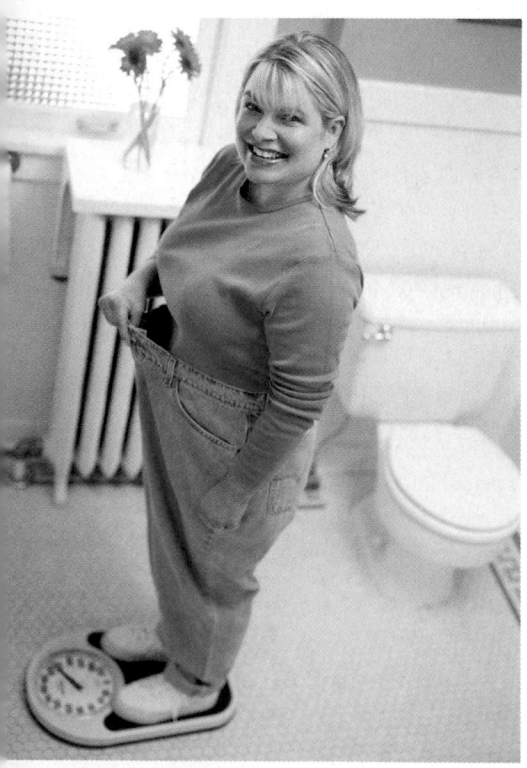

Slow, steady weight loss is one of the characteristics of a sound weight-loss program.

Control of Calorie Intake—The Main Key to Weight Loss and Weight Maintenance

A goal of losing 1 pound or so of stored fat per week may require limiting calorie intake to 1200 kcal per day for women and 1500 kcal for men. The calorie allowance could also be higher for very active people. Keep in mind that, in our very sedentary society, decreasing calorie intake is vital because it is difficult to burn much energy without ample physical activity. With regard to consuming fewer calories, some experts suggest consuming less fat (especially saturated fat and *trans* fat), while others suggest consuming less carbohydrate, especially refined (high glycemic load) carbohydrate sources. Protein intakes somewhat in excess of what is typically needed by adults are also receiving attention. Using all these approaches simultaneously is also fine. At this time the low-fat, high-fiber approaches have been the most successful in long-term studies. There is no long-term evidence of the effectiveness of the other approaches. Finding what works for an individual is a process of trial and error. In addition, the notion that any type of diet has a "metabolic advantage" (i.e. promotes greater calorie use by the body) is nonsense, despite the marketing claims for low carbohydrate diets.

One way for a dieter to monitor calorie intake at the start of a weight-loss program is by reading labels. Label reading is important, because many foods are more energy dense than people suppose (Fig. 10-15). Another method is to write down food intake for 24 hours and then calculate calorie intake from the food table in Appendix E or by using your diet analysis software, adjusting future food choices as needed. Because people often underestimate portion size when recording food intake, measuring cups and a food weighing scale can help.

Table 10-4 shows how to start reducing calorie intake. As you should realize by now, it is best to consider eating healthy a lifestyle change, rather than simply a

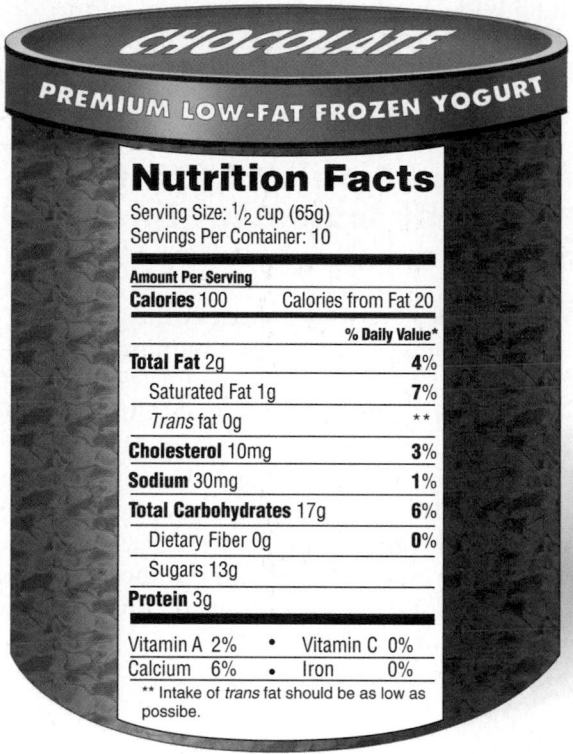

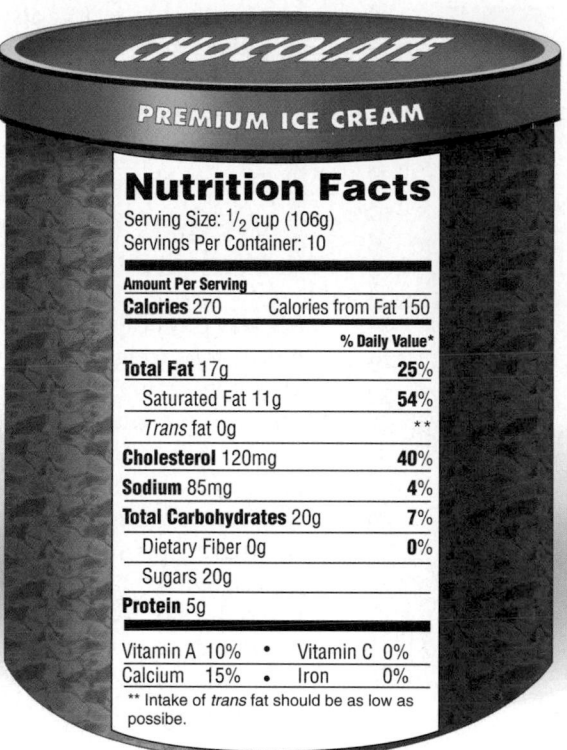

Figure 10-15 Reading labels helps you choose foods with fewer calories. Which of these frozen desserts is the best choice, per ½ cup serving, for a person on a weight-loss diet? The % Daily Values are based on a 2000 kcal diet.

Table 10-4 Saving Kcal: Ideas to Help Get Started

Instead of	Try	Number of Kcal Saved
3 oz well-marbled meat (prime rib)	3 oz lean meat (eye of round)	140
½ chicken breast, batter-fried	½ chicken breast, broiled with lemon	175
½ cup beef stroganoff	3 oz lean roast beef (or use a fat-reduced recipe)	210
½ cup home-fried potatoes	1 medium baked potato	65
½ cup green bean-mushroom casserole	½ cup cooked green beans	50
½ cup potato salad	1 cup raw vegetable salad	140
½ cup pineapple chunks in heavy syrup	½ cup pineapple chunks canned in juice	25
2 tbsp bottled French dressing	2 tbsp low-calorie French dressing	150
⅛ 9-inch apple pie	1 baked apple, unsweetened	308
3 oatmeal-raisin cookies	1 oatmeal raisin cookie	125
½ cup ice cream	½ cup ice milk	45
1 danish pastry	½ English muffin	150
1 cup sugar-coated corn flakes	1 cup plain corn flakes	60
1 cup whole milk	1 cup 1% low-fat milk	45
7-fluid-oz gin and tonic	6-fluid-oz wine cooler made with sparkling water	150
1-oz bag potato chips	1 cup plain popcorn	120
1/12 8-inch white layer cake with chocolate frosting	1/12 angel food cake, 10-inch tube	185
12 fluid ounce regular beer	12 fluid ounce light beer	40

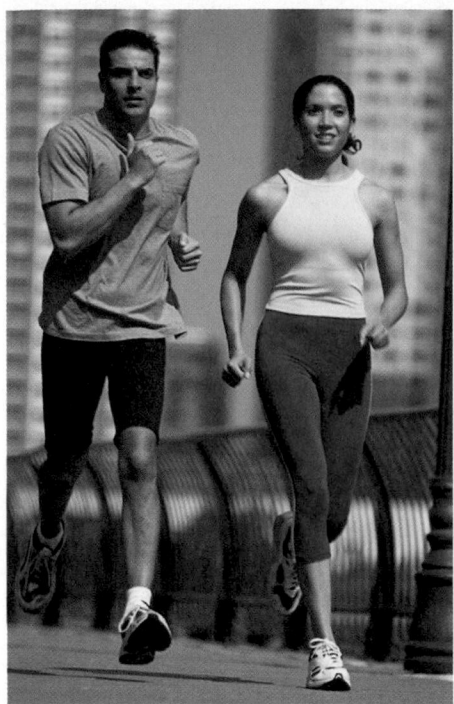

Physical activity complements any diet plan. Making exercise part of your daily routine can benefit nearly everyone, especially those who are trying to lose weight or maintain weight loss.

The motivation to lose weight and keep it off generally comes with a proverbial "flip of the switch," in which the desire to lose weight finally becomes more important than the desire to overeat.

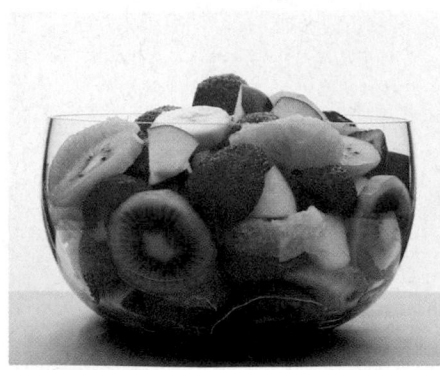

Fruit is a great low-cal snack—high nutrient density and low in calories.

weight-loss plan. Note also that liquids deserve attention, since liquid calories do not stimulate satiety mechanisms to the same extent as solid foods. The corresponding advice from experts is to use beverages that have few or no calories and limit sugar-sweetened beverages.

Regular Physical Activity—A Second Key to Weight Loss and Especially Important for Later Weight Maintenance

Regular physical activity is very important for everyone, especially those who are trying to lose weight or maintain a lower body weight. Calorie burning is enhanced. Therefore, it greatly complements a reduction in calorie intake for weight loss (but does not substitute for it). Many of us rarely do more than sit, stand, and sleep. Obviously, more calories are used during physical activity than at rest. In addition, expending only 100 to 300 extra kcal per day above and beyond normal daily activity, while controlling calorie intake, can lead to a steady weight loss. Furthermore, physical activity has so many other benefits, including a boost for overall self-esteem. The latest advice for adults on physical activity and body weight from the 2005 Dietary Guidelines is: to maintain body weight and prevent weight gain: 60 minutes per day; maintenance of weight loss: 60 to 90 minutes per day.

Another Bite

Spot-reducing by using diet and physical activity is not possible. "Problem" local fat deposits can be reduced in size, however, using suction lipectomy. Lipectomy means surgical removal of fat. A pencil-thin tube is inserted into an incision in the skin, and the fat tissue, such as that in the buttocks and thigh area, is suctioned. This procedure carries some risks, such as infection; lasting depressions in the skin; and blood clots, which can lead to kidney failure and sometimes death. The procedure is designed to help a person lose about 4 to 8 pounds per treatment. Cost is about $1600 per site; total costs range as high as $2600 to $9000.

Adding any of the activities in Table 10-5 to one's lifestyle can increase calorie use. Duration and regular performance, rather than intensity, are the keys to success with this approach to weight loss. One should search for activities that can be continued over time. In this regard, walking vigorously 3 miles per day can be as helpful as aerobic dancing or jogging, if it is maintained. Moreover, activities of lighter intensity are less likely to lead to injuries. Some resistance exercises (weight training) also should be added to increase lean body mass and, in turn, fat use (see Chapter 11). And as lean muscle mass increases, so will one's overall metabolic rate. An added benefit of including exercise in a weight reduction program is maintenance of bone health.

Unfortunately, opportunities to expend calories in our daily lives are diminishing as technology systematically eliminates almost every reason to move our muscles. The easiest way to increase physical activity is to make it an enjoyable part of a daily routine. To start, one might pack a pair of sneakers and walk around the parking lot before coming home after school or work every day. Other ideas are avoiding elevators in favor of stairs, parking the car farther away from the shopping mall, or getting up to change the channels on the television.

Behavior Modification—A Third Strategy for Weight Loss

Controlling calorie intake, so important to weight loss, also means modifying *problem* behaviors. Only the dieter can decide what behaviors keep him or her from reaching for the wrong foods at the wrong times for the wrong reasons.

Table 10-5 Approximate Calorie Costs of Various Activities, and Specific Calorie Costs Projected for a 150-Pound (68 kilogram) Person

Activity	Kcal per kilogram per Hour	Total kcal per Hour	Activity	Kcal per kilogram per Hour	Total kcal per Hour
Aerobics—heavy	8.0	544	Horseback riding	5.1	346
Aerobics—medium	5.0	340	Jogging—medium	9.0	612
Aerobics—light	3.0	204	Ice skating (10 MPH)	5.8	394
Backpacking	9.0	612	Jogging—slow	7.0	476
Basketball—vigorous	10.0	680	Lying—at ease	1.3	89
Cycling (5.5 MPH)	3.0	204	Racquetball—social	8.0	544
Bowling	3.9	265	Roller skating	5.1	346
Calisthenics—heavy	8.0	544	Running or jogging (10 MPH)	13.2	897
Calisthenics—light	4.0	272	Downhill skiing (10 MPH)	8.8	598
Canoeing (2.5 MPH)	3.3	224	Sleeping	1.2	80
Cleaning (female)	3.7	253	Swimming (.25 MPH)	4.4	299
Cleaning (male)	3.5	236	Tennis	6.1	414
Cooking	2.8	190	Volleyball	5.1	346
Cycling (13 MPH)	9.7	659	Walking (2.5 MPH)	3.0	204
Dressing/showering	1.6	106	Walking (3.75 MPH)	4.4	299
Driving	1.7	117	Water skiing	7.0	476
Eating (sitting)	1.4	93	Weight lifting—heavy	9.0	612
Food shopping	3.6	245	Weight lifting—light	4.0	272
Football—touch	7.0	476	Window cleaning	3.5	240
Golf	3.6	244	Writing (sitting)	1.7	118

The values in Table 10-5 refer to total energy expenditure, including that needed to perform the physical activity, plus that needed for basal metabolism, the thermic effect of food, and thermogenesis. Use your diet analysis software for your personal estimate.

A pedometer is a device that monitors activity as steps. Cost is minimal. An often-stated goal for activity is to take at least 10,000 steps per day—typically we take half that many or less. A pedometer tracks this activity.

What events start (or stop) eating? What factors influence food choices? Psychologists often use terms such as *chain-breaking, stimulus control, cognitive restructuring, contingency management,* and *self-monitoring* when discussing behavior modification (Table 10-6). These factors help place the problem in perspective and organize the intervention strategy into manageable steps.

Chain-breaking separates behaviors that tend to occur together—for example, snacking on chips while watching television. Although these activities do not have to occur together, they often do. Dieters may need to break the chain reaction (see Rate Your Plate at the end of this Chapter for more details).

Stimulus control puts us in charge of temptations. Options include pushing tempting food to the back of the refrigerator, removing fat-laden snacks from the kitchen counter, and avoiding the path by the vending machines. Provide a positive stimulus by keeping low-fat snacks available to satisfy hunger/appetite. Note that alcohol and foods offer quick, easy stress relief. We need to plan healthful alternatives.

Cognitive restructuring changes our frame of mind. For example, after a hard day, respond with a walk or satisfying talk with a friend instead of a binge. Replace eating reactions to stress with healthful, relaxing alternatives.

Labeling some foods as "off limits" sets up an internal struggle to resist the urge to eat that food. This hopeless battle can keep us feeling deprived. We lose the fight. Managing food choices with the principle of moderation is best. If a favorite food

chain-breaking Breaking the link between two or more behaviors that encourage overeating, such as snacking while watching television.

stimulus control Altering the environment to minimize the stimuli for eating—for example, removing foods from sight and storing them in kitchen cabinets.

cognitive restructuring Changing one's frame of mind regarding eating—for example, instead of using a difficult day as an excuse to overeat, substituting other pleasures for rewards, such as a relaxing walk with a friend.

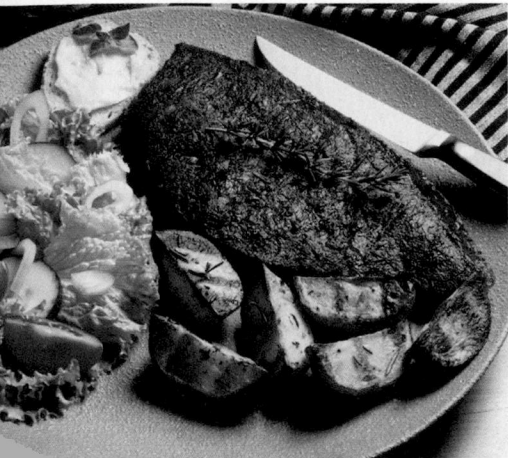

We are faced with many opportunities to overeat, in this case meat. It takes much perseverance to eat sensibly.

Table 10-6 Behavior Modification Principles for Weight Loss

Shopping
1. Shop for food after eating—buy nutritious foods.
2. Shop from a list; limit purchases of irresistible "problem" foods. Shopping for fresh foods around the perimeter of the store first helps.
3. Avoid ready-to-eat foods.
4. Put off food shopping until absolutely necessary.

Plans
1. Plan to limit food intake as needed.
2. Substitute periods of physical activity for snacking.
3. Eat meals and snacks at scheduled times; don't skip meals.

Activities
1. Store food out of sight, preferably in the freezer, to discourage impulsive eating.
2. Eat all food in a "dining" area.
3. Keep serving dishes off the table, especially dishes of sauces and gravies.
4. Use smaller dishes and utensils.

Holidays and Parties
1. Drink fewer alcoholic beverages.
2. Plan eating behavior before parties.
3. Eat a low-calorie snack before parties.
4. Practice polite ways to decline food.
5. Don't get discouraged by an occasional setback.

Eating Behavior
1. Put fork down between mouthfuls.
2. Chew thoroughly before taking the next bite.
3. Leave some food on the plate.
4. Pause in the middle of the meal.
5. Do nothing else while eating (for example, reading, watching television).

Reward
1. Plan specific rewards for specific behavior (behavioral contracts).
2. Solicit help from family and friends and suggest how they can help you. Encourage family and friends to provide this help in the form of praise and material rewards.
3. Use self-monitoring records as basis for rewards.

Self-Monitoring
1. Note the time and place of eating.
2. List the type and amount of food eaten.
3. Record who is present and how you feel.
4. Use the diet diary to identify problem areas.

Cognitive Restructuring
1. Avoid setting unreasonable goals.
2. Think about progress, not shortcomings.
3. Avoid imperatives such as *always* and *never*.
4. Counter negative thoughts with positive restatements.

Portion Control
1. Make substitutions, such as a regular hamburger instead of a "quarter pounder" or cucumbers instead of croutons in salads.
2. Think small. Order the entrée and share it with another person. Order a cup of soup instead of a bowl or an appetizer in place of an entrée.
3. Use a doggie bag. Ask your server to put half the entrée in a doggie bag before bringing it to the table.

As we said at the start of this Chapter, many of us need to become "defensive eaters." Know when to refuse food after satiety registers, and reduce portion sizes.

Successful weight losers and maintainers from the National Weight Control Registry:

• Eat a low-fat, high-carbohydrate diet (on average 25% of calorie intake as fat).
• Eat breakfast almost every day.
• Self-monitor by regularly weighing oneself and keeping a food journal.
• Exercise for about 1 hour per day.
• Eat at restaurants only once or twice per week.

Other recent studies support this approach, especially the last four characteristics.

becomes troublesome, place it off limits only temporarily, until it can be enjoyed in moderation.

Contingency management prepares us for potential pitfalls and high-risk situations. We might rehearse in advance some appropriate responses to pressures—such as food being passed at a party.

Did you keep a record of what you ate and what catalysts urged you to pick up the fork or put it down as suggested in Rate Your Plate in Chapter 1? If so, you already know one key tool in modifying behavior—**self-monitoring.** A self-monitoring record can reveal patterns—such as unconscious overeating—that may explain problem eating habits. This record can encourage new habits to counteract unwanted behaviors. Obesity experts note that this is the key behavioral tool to use in any weight-loss program.

Overall, it's important to *address specific* problems, such as snacking, compulsive eating, and mealtime overeating. Behavior modification principles end up as critical components of weight reduction and maintenance. Without behavior modification, it is difficult to make lifelong lifestyle changes needed to meet weight-control goals.

■ Relapse Prevention Is Important

Preventing relapse is actually thought to be the hardest part of weight control—even harder than losing weight. A dieter can tolerate an occasional lapse but needs to plan for lapses. The key is not to overreact, but take charge immediately. Change responses such as "I ate that cookie; I'm a failure" to "I ate that cookie, but I did well to stop after only one!" An occasional cookie is fine; a pound of cookies in an afternoon deserves reconsideration. When dieters lapse from their diet plan, newly learned food habits should steer them back toward the plan. This should enable dieters to avoid the lapse-relapse-collapse trap. Without a strong behavioral program for **relapse prevention** in place, a lapse frequently turns into a relapse. Once a pattern of poor food choices begins, dieters may feel that they have failed and stray further from the plan. As the relapse lengthens, the diet plan collapses, and dieters fall short of their weight-loss goal. Even with a good behavioral plan, one may fail at a diet. Losing weight is difficult. Overall, maintenance of weight loss is fostered by the "3 *Ms*": motivation, movement, and monitoring.

■ Social Support Aids Behavioral Change

Healthy social support is helpful in weight control. Helping others understand how they can be supportive can make weight control easier. Family and friends can provide praise and encouragement. A registered dietitian or other weight-control professional can keep dieters accountable and help them learn from difficult situations. Long-term contact with a professional can be quite helpful for later weight maintenance. Groups of individuals attempting to lose weight or maintain losses can provide empathetic support.

> **Concept Check**
>
> Increasing physical activity in daily life should be part of any weight-loss plan. Daily activity, such as walking and stair climbing, is recommended. Behavior modification can improve conditions for losing weight. One key step is to break behavior chains that encourage overeating, such as snacking while watching television. Another tactic is to modify the environment to reduce temptation; for example, put foods into cupboards to keep them out of sight. In addition, rethinking attitudes about eating—for example, substituting pleasures other than food as a reward for coping with a stressful day—can be important for altering undesirable behavior. Advanced planning to prevent and deal with lapses is vital, as is rallying healthy social support. Finally, careful observation and recording of eating habits can reveal subtle cues that lead to overeating. Overall, weight loss and maintenance are fostered by controlling calorie intake, performing regular physical activity, and modifying "problem" behaviors.

contingency management Forming a plan of action to respond to a situation in which overeating is likely, such as when snacks are within arm's reach at a party.

self-monitoring Tracking foods eaten and conditions affecting eating; actions are usually recorded in a diary, along with location, time, and state of mind. This is a tool to help people understand more about their eating habits.

relapse prevention A series of strategies used to help prevent and cope with weight-control lapses, such as recognizing high-risk situations and deciding beforehand on appropriate responses.

Critical Thinking

With regard to readiness to lose weight, what would you say to a young woman who has just had a baby, needs to find a new job, and recently has gone back to school part-time?

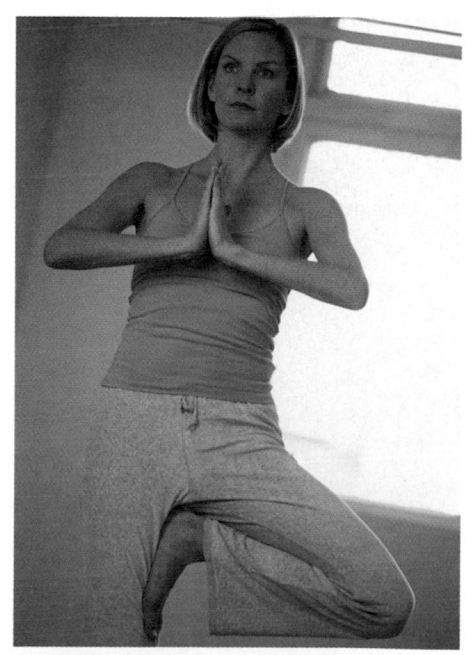

Individuals who successfully maintain their weight loss employ a variety of strategies to cope with the stresses and challenges of changing problem behaviors.

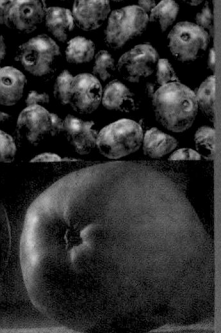

Looking *Further*

Popular Diets—Why All the Commotion?

A well-known example of the effectiveness of monotony contributing to weight loss is the experience of Jared Fogle. He ate primarily Subway sandwiches for 11 months and lost 245 pounds. He notes however that this is not a miracle diet—it takes a lot of hard work to lead to the success he experienced. There are also many other examples where diet monotony has led to weight loss.

Meals replacement formulas to replace a meal or snack are appropriate to use 1 to 2 times per day, if one desires. These are not a "magic bullet" for weight loss, but have been shown to help some people lose weight.

Many overweight people try to help themselves by using the latest popular (also called fad) diet book. But, as you will see, most of these diets do not help, and some can actually harm those who follow them (Table 10-7).

Recently, weight-loss experts came together at the request of the USDA to evaluate weight-loss diets. They came to this conclusion: Forget these fads when it comes to dieting. Most of the popular diets are nutritionally inadequate and include certain foods that people would not normally choose to consume in large amounts. The experts stated that eating less of one's favorite foods and becoming more physically active can be much more effective when trying to implement a weight-loss diet. People need a plan that they can live with in the long run so that weight control becomes permanent. The goal should be weight control over a lifetime, not immediate weight loss. Every popular diet leads to some immediate weight loss simply because daily intake is monitored and monotonous food choices are typically part of the plan. Overall, a traditional moderate diet coupled with regular physical activity is adequate for weight loss.

How to Recognize a Dubious Popular Diet

The criteria for evaluating weight-loss programs with regard to their safety and effectiveness were discussed previously. In contrast, dubious popular diets typically share some common characteristics:

1. They promote quick weight loss. This is the primary temptation that the dieter falls for. As mentioned before, this initial weight loss primarily results from water loss and lean muscle mass depletion.
2. They limit food selections and dictate specific rituals, such as eating only fruit for breakfast or cabbage soup every day.
3. They use testimonials from famous people and tie the diet to well-known cities, such as Beverly Hills and New York.
4. They bill themselves as cure-alls. These diets claim to work for everyone, whatever the type of obesity or the person's specific strengths and weaknesses.
5. They often recommend expensive supplements.
6. No attempts are made to change eating habits permanently. Dieters follow the diet until the desired weight is reached and then revert to old eating habits—they are told, for example, to eat rice for a month, lose weight, and then return to old habits.
7. They are generally critical of and skeptical about the scientific community. The fact that the medical and dietetic professions cannot provide a quick fix for overweight has led to some of the public to seek advice from those who appear to have the answer.

Probably the cruelest characteristic of these diets is that they essentially guarantee failure for the dieter. The diets are not designed for permanent weight loss. Habits are not changed, and the food selection is so limited that the person cannot follow the diet in the long run. Although dieters assume they have lost fat, they have actually lost mostly muscle and other lean tissue mass. As soon as they begin eating normally again, much of the lost tissue is replaced. In a matter of weeks, most of the lost weight is back. The dieter appears to have failed, when actually the diet has failed. The gain and loss cycle is called weight cycling or yo-yo dieting. This whole scenario can add more blame and guilt, challenging the self-worth of the dieter. It can also come with some health costs, such as increased upper-body fat deposition. If someone needs help losing weight, professional help is advised. It is unfortunate that current trends suggest that people are spending more time and money on "quick fixes" rather than on such professional help.

Table 10-7 Summary of Popular Diet Approaches to Weight Control

Approach	Examples	Characteristics	Outcomes
Moderate calorie restriction	The Set-Point Diet Slim Chance in a Fat World Weight Watcher's Diet Mary Ellen's Help Yourself Diet Plan The Beyond Diet Staying Thin The Callaway Diet	Generally 1200 to 1800 kcal per day, with moderate fat intake Reasonable balance of macronutrients Encourage exercise May use behavioral approach	Acceptable if a multivitamin and mineral supplement is used and permission of family physician is granted
Living Without Dieting Volumetrics Lose the Last 10 Pounds Dieting with the Duchess Dieting for Dummies The Wedding Dress Diet Dr. Shapiro's Picture Perfect Diet			
Restricted carbohydrate	Dr. Atkins' New Diet Revolution Calories Don't Count Miracle Diet for Fast Weight Loss Woman Doctor's Diet for Women The Doctor's Quick Weight Loss Diet The Complete Scarsdale Medical Diet Four Day Wonder Diet	Generally less than 100 grams of carbohydrate per day	Ketosis; reduced exercise capacity due to poor glycogen stores in the muscles; excessive animal fat intake; constipation, headaches, halitosis (bad breath), and muscle cramps
Endocrine Control Diet Enter the Zone Protein Power The Five-Day Miracle Diet Healthy for Life Carbohydrate Addicts Diet Sugar Busters South Beach Diet (especially initial phases)			
Low fat	The Rice Diet Report The Macrobiotic Diet (some versions) The Pritikin Diet Eat More, Weigh Less The 35+ Diet 20/30 Fat and Fiber Fat to Muscle Diet T-Factor Diet Fit or Fat Two-Day Diet Complete Hip and Thigh Diet	Generally less than 20% of calories from fat Limited (or elimination of) animal protein sources; also limited fats, nuts, seeds	Flatulence; possibly poor mineral absorption from excess fiber; limited food choices sometimes leads to deprivation Not necessarily to be avoided, but certain aspects of many of the plans possibly unacceptable
The Maximum Metabolism Diet The Pasta Diet The McDougall Plan Ultrafit Diet Stop the Insanity G-Index Diet Outsmarting the Female Fat Cell Foods That Cause You to Lose Weight Lean Bodies Turn Off the Fat Genes			
Novelty diets	Dr. Abravenel's Body Type and Lifetime Nutrition Plan (or his other books) Dr. Berger's Immune Power Diet Fit for Life The New Hilton Head Metabolism Diet The Beverly Hills Diet Dr. Debetz Champagne Diet Sun Sign Diet F-Plan Diet Fat Attack Plan Autohypnosis Diet The Princeton Diet The Diet Bible Eat to Succeed	Promotes certain nutrients, foods, or combinations of foods as having unique, magical, or previously undiscovered qualities	Malnutrition; no change in habits which leads to relapse; unrealistic food choices lead to possible bingeing
The Underburner's Diet Eat to Win Paris Diet Cabbage-Soup Diet Eat Great, Lose Weight Eat Smart Think Smart Promotes certain nutrients, Scentsational Weight Loss Eat Right 4 Your Type The Greenwich Diet 3 Season Diet Metabolize God's Diet The Weigh Down Diet			

People on diets often fall within a non-overweight BMI of 18.5 to 25. Rather than worrying about weight loss, these individuals should be focusing on a healthy lifestyle that allows for weight maintenance. Incorporating necessary lifestyle changes and learning to accept one's particular body characteristics should be the overriding goals.

The dieting mania can be viewed as mostly a social problem, stemming from unrealistic weight expectations (especially for women) and lack of appreciation for the natural variety in body shape and weight. Not every woman can look like a fashion model, nor can every man look like a Greek god, but all of us can strive for good health and, if physically possible, an active lifestyle.

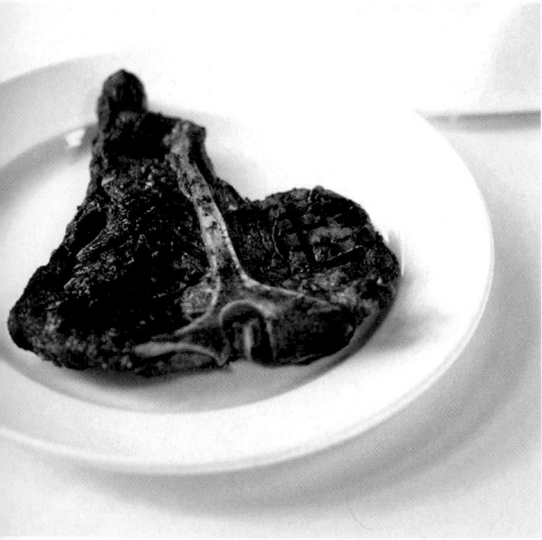

In time, the very-low-carbohydrate, high-protein diets typically leave a person wanting more variety in meals, and so the diets are abandoned. Dropout rates are very high on these diets.

Types of Popular Diets

Low- or Restricted-Carbohydrate Approaches

This is currently the most common form of popular diets. The low-carbohydrate intake leads to less glycogen synthesis, and therefore less water in the body (about 3 grams of water are stored per gram of glycogen). As discussed in Chapter 4, a very-low-carbohydrate intake also forces the liver to produce needed glucose. The source of carbons for this glucose is mostly tissue proteins. Thus, a low-carbohydrate diet results in protein tissue loss (which is about 72% water), as well as urinary loss of essential ions, such as potassium. Since protein tissue is mostly water, the dieter loses weight very rapidly. When a normal diet is resumed, the protein tissue is rebuilt and the weight is regained.

Low-carbohydrate diets primarily work in the short run because they limit total food intake. And in long-term studies these diets have not shown a distinct advantage compared to diets that simply limit calorie intake in general.

Diet plans that use a low-carbohydrate approach are the Dr. Atkins' New Diet Revolution, the Scarsdale Diet, and the Four-Day Wonder Diet. More moderate approaches are found in the various Zone diets (40% of calorie intake as carbohydrate), Sugar Busters diet, and the South Beach diet (especially initial phases).

Low-Fat Approaches

The very-low-fat diet turns out to be a very-high-carbohydrate diet. These diets contain approximately 5% to 10% of calories as fat. The most notable are the Pritikin Diet and the Dr. Dean Ornish "Eat More, Weigh Less" diet plans. This approach is not harmful for healthy adults, but it is difficult to follow. People get bored with this type of diet very quickly because they cannot eat many of their favorite foods. These dieters eat primarily grains, fruits, and vegetables, which most people cannot do for very long. Eventually, the person wants some foods higher in fat or protein. These diets are just too different from the typical North American diet for many adults to follow consistently, but may be acceptable for some people.

Novelty Diets

A variety of diets are built on gimmicks. Some novelty diets emphasize one food or food group and exclude almost all others. A rice diet was designed in the 1940s to lower blood pressure; now it has resurfaced as a weight-loss diet. The first phase consists of eating only rice and fruit. On the Beverly Hills Diet, you eat mostly fruit.

The rationale behind these diets is that you can eat only rice or fruit for just so long before becoming bored and, in theory, reducing your calorie intake. However, chances are that you will abandon the diet entirely before losing much weight.

The most questionable of the novelty diets propose that "food gets stuck in your body." Fit for Life, the Beverly Hills Diet, and Eat Great, Lose Weight are examples. The supposition is that food gets stuck in the intestine, putrefies, and creates toxins, which invade the blood and cause disease. In response, recommendations are to not consume meat with potatoes, or consume fruits only after noon. These recommendations make no physiological sense.

Quackery Is Characteristic of Many Popular Diets

Many popular diets fall under the category of quackery—people taking advantage of others. They usually involve a product or service that costs a considerable amount of money. Often, those offering the product or service don't realize that they are promoting quackery, because they were victims themselves. For example, they tried the product and by pure coincidence it worked for them, so they wish to sell it to all their friends and relatives.

Numerous other gimmicks for weight loss have come and gone and are likely to resurface. If in the future an important aid for weight loss is discovered, you can feel confident that major journals, such as the *Journal of the American Dietetic Association,* the *Journal of the American Medical Association,* or *The New England Journal of Medicine,* will report it. You don't need to rely on paperback books, infomericals, billboards, or newspaper advertisements for information about weight loss.

Real Life Scenario Follow-Up

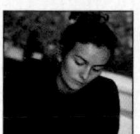

As you have probably surmised, Chris will just be wasting his money if he buys the product seen in the infomercial. Unfortunately, regulation of the supplement industry currently is woefully lacking. In the future, if there is a meaningful breakthrough in weight loss and weight control, authorities such as the Surgeon General's Office or the National Institutes of Health will make North Americans aware of that fact. At this time, Chris would be better off simply paying more attention to what he is eating and trying to find time for daily physical activity.

Professional Help for Weight Loss

The first professional to see for advice about a weight-loss program is one's family physician. Doctors are best equipped to assess overall health and the appropriateness of weight loss. The physician may then recommend a registered dietitian for a specific weight-loss plan and answers to diet-related questions. Registered dietitians are uniquely qualified to help design a weight-loss plan because they understand both food composition and the psychological importance of food. Exercise physiologists can provide advice about programs to increase physical activity. The expense for such professional interventions is tax deductible in the United States in some cases (see a tax advisor) and often covered by health insurance plans if prescribed by a physician.

Many communities have a variety of weight-loss organizations. These include self-help groups, such as Take Off Pounds Sensibly and Weight Watchers. Other programs, such as Jenny Craig and Physicians' Weight Loss Center, are less desirable for the average dieter. Often, the employees are not registered dietitians or other appropriately trained health professionals. These programs also tend to be expensive because of their requirements for intense counseling or mandatory diet foods and supplements. In addition, the Federal Trade Commission has charged these and other commercial diet-program companies with misleading consumers through unsubstantiated weight-loss claims and deceptive testimonials.

■ Medications for Weight Loss

People who are candidates for medications for obesity include those with a BMI of 30 or more, or a BMI of 27 to 29.9 with weight-related conditions, such as type 2 diabetes, cardiovascular disease, hypertension, or excess waist circumference; those with no contraindications to use of the medication; and those ready to undertake lifestyle change. Success with medications has been shown only in those who also modify their behavior, decrease calorie intake, and increase physical activity. Drug therapy alone has not been found to be successful. In addition, if a person has not lost at least 4.4 pounds (2 kilograms) after 4 weeks, it is not likely that the person will benefit from further use of the medication.

Currently three main classes of medications are used. An **amphetamine**-like medication (phenteramine [Fastin or Ionamin]) prolongs the activity of epinephrine and norepinephrine in the brain. This therapy is effective for some people in the short run but has not yet been proven effective in the long run. Most state medical boards currently limit use to 12 weeks unless the person is participating in a medical study using the product. The medication should not be used in pregnant or nursing women or those under 18 years of age.

Sibutramine (Meridia) is a second class of medication that has been approved by FDA for weight loss. It enhances both norepinephrine and serotonin activity in the

North Americans are willing to try almost anything to shed unwanted pounds. Operation Waistline is a program designed by the U.S. Federal Trade Commission to terminate fraudulent claims being made by weight-loss charlatans with regard to diet products. The program hopes to put an end to the $6 billion spent annually in the United States on counterfeit products. Recently the Enforma Natural Products Corporation had to pay $10 million in response to false claims for its "Fat Trapper" product.

amphetamine A group of medications that induce stimulation of the central nervous system, and have other effects in the body. Abuse is linked to physical and psychological dependence.

Recently a woman developed liver failure after using a so-called weight-loss aid called usnic acid. Her purchase was via the Internet. Today more than ever, let the buyer beware concerning any purported weight-loss aid not prescribed by a physician.

brain by reducing reuptake of these neurotransmitters by nerve cells. The neurotransmitters then remain active in the brain for a longer period of time, and so prolong a sense of reduced hunger. The most common side effects are constipation, dry mouth, insomnia, and a mild increase in blood pressure in some people. Thus, sibutramine should be used with caution in people with a history of hypertension (or cardiovascular disease). Studies have shown that it is effective in helping some people who already eat healthy diets, but just eat too much. The main effect is to moderately reduce appetite so that people eat less. Sibutramine is safe and effective only when combined with a comprehensive weight-control program and when supervised by a physician.

The third class of medication approved by FDA for weight loss is orlistat (Xenical). This medication inhibits lipase enzyme action in the small intestine, reducing fat digestion by about 30%. This cuts absorption of dietary fat by one-third for about 2 hours when taken along with a meal containing fat. This malabsorbed fat simply is deposited in the feces. *Fat intake has to be controlled*, however, because large amounts of fat in the feces cause numerous side effects, such as gas, bloating, and oily discharge. Interestingly, orlistat use can actually remind the person to follow a fat-controlled diet, as the symptoms resulting from consuming a high-fat meal are unpleasant and quickly develop. Orlistat is taken with each meal containing fat.

Since the malabsorbed fat also carries fat-soluble vitamins into the feces, the person taking orlistat must take a multivitamin and mineral supplement at bedtime. In this way, any micronutrients not absorbed during the day can be replaced; fat malabsorption from the dinner meal will not greatly influence micronutrient absorption in the late evening.

Overall, in skilled hands, prescription medications can aid weight loss in some instances. However, they do not replace the need for reducing calorie intake, modifying "problem" behaviors, and increasing physical activity, both during and after therapy. And, more often than not, any weight loss during drug treatment can be attributed mostly to the individual's hard work at balancing calorie intake with output.

The only two weight-loss medications approved by FDA for long-term use are sibutramine (Meridia) and orlistat (Xenical). Drug companies are working on many other types of medications, and have high hopes some of these will prove to be safe and effective for weight loss.

■ Treatment of Severe Obesity

Severe (morbid) obesity—weighing at least 100 pounds over healthy body weight (or twice one's healthy body weight)—requires professional treatment. Because of the serious health implications of severe obesity, drastic measures may be necessary. Such treatments are recommended only when traditional diets fail. Drastic weight-loss procedures are not without side effects, both physical and psychological, making careful monitoring by a physician a necessity.

Very-Low-Calorie Diets

very-low-calorie diet (VLCD) Known also as *protein-sparing modified fast (PSMF)*, this diet allows a person 400 to 800 kcal per day, often in liquid form. Of this, 120 to 480 kcal is carbohydrate, and the rest is mostly high-quality protein.

If more traditional diet changes have failed, treating severe obesity with a **very-low-calorie diet (VLCD)** is possible, especially if the person has obesity-related diseases that are not well controlled (e.g., hypertension, type 2 diabetes). Some researchers believe that people with body weight greater than 30% above their healthy weight are appropriate candidates. Optifast is one such commercial program. In general, the diet allows a person to consume 400 to 800 kcal per day, often in liquid form. (These diets were previously known as protein-sparing modified fasts.) Of this amount, about 30 to 120 grams (120 to 480 kcal) is carbohydrate. The rest is high-quality protein, in the amount of about 70 to 100 grams per day (280 to 400 kcal). This low carbohydrate intake often causes ketosis, which may decrease hunger. However, the main reasons for weight loss are the minimal energy consumption and the absence of food choice. About 3 to 4 pounds can be lost per week; men tend to lose at a faster rate than women. When physical activity and resistance training augment this diet, a greater loss of adipose tissue occurs. Careful monitoring by a physician is crucial throughout this very restrictive form of weight loss. Major health risks include heart problems and gallstones.

Weight regain remains a nagging problem, especially without a behavioral and physical activity component. If behavioral therapy and physical activity supplement a long-term support program, maintenance of the weight loss is more likely but still difficult. Any program under consideration should include a maintenance plan. Today, antiobesity medications also may be included in this phase of the program.

Gastroplasty

Gastroplasty (gastric bypass surgery, also called stomach stapling) is the primary surgical procedure used today for treating severe obesity. The most common and effective approach (the Roux-en-Y gastric bypass procedure) works by reducing the stomach capacity to about 30 milliliters (the volume of one egg or shot glass) and bypassing a short segment of the upper small intestine (Fig. 10-16). Weight loss is promoted mainly because overeating of solid foods is now less likely due to rapid satiety and discomfort or vomiting with overeating. About 75% of people with severe obesity eventually lose 50% or more of excess body weight with this method. In addition, the surgery's success at long-term maintenance often leads to dramatic health improvements, such as reduced blood pressure and elimination of type 2 diabetes. Risk of death from the surgery itself is about 2%, especially if the surgeon has performed less than 20 of the procedures, because it is a very demanding surgery. Risks of the surgery include bleeding, blood clots, hernias, and severe infections. In the long run nutrient deficiencies can develop if the person is not adequately treated in the years following the surgery. Anemia and bone loss might then be the result.

Current patient selection criteria for gastroplasty include:

- BMI should be greater than 40.
- BMI between 35 and 40 is considered when there are serious obesity-related health concerns.
- Obesity must be present for a minimum of 5 years, with several nonsurgical attempts to lose weight.
- There should be no history of alcoholism or major psychiatric disorders.

The person also must consider that the surgery is costly ($20,000 to $40,000 or more) and may not be covered by medical insurance. In addition, follow-up surgery is often needed after weight loss to correct stretched skin, which was previously filled

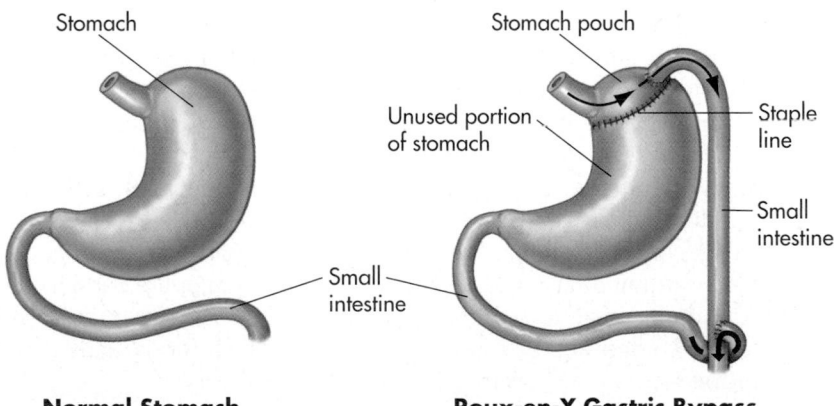

Normal Stomach   **Roux-en-Y Gastric Bypass**

Figure 10-16 The Roux-en-Y procedure is the most common and most effective form of gastric bypass surgery for treatment of severe obesity. In this technically demanding procedure, the upper portion of the stomach is separated from the lower portion by stapling to create a small pouch, and a lower segment of the small intestine is attached to the pouch. The stomach pouch is about the size of an egg or shot glass, but may stretch to about 2 to 3 times that size over time. (Compare that to the original stomach capacity of 4 cups [32 ounces]). Food travels through the stomach pouch into the relocated portion of the small intestine, and eventually into the main flow of the small intestine.

Another common surgical is the lap-band procedure, where a band is placed around the upper portion of the stomach, creating a small stomach pouch. A salt solution can be injected into the band through a port attached to the abdominal wall in order to adjust the size of the pouch over time. Much less common is biliopancreatic diversion (often called a "duodenal switch" procedure), where stomach volume is reduced surgically by 75% and much of the intestinal tract is bypassed using surgical rearrangement. This combination leads to less food consumption and significant nutrient malabsorption. Because of the latter, it has yet to gain much acceptance by surgeons.

with fat. Furthermore, the surgery necessitates major lifestyle changes, such as the need to plan frequent, small meals. Therefore, the dieter who has chosen this drastic approach to weight loss faces months of difficult adjustments.

> ## Concept Check
>
> Severely obese people who have failed to lose weight with conservative weight-loss strategies may consider other options. Their doctors may recommend undergoing surgery such as reducing the volume of the stomach to approximately 30 milliliters or following a very-low-calorie diet plan containing 400 to 800 kcal per day. Careful monitoring by a physician is crucial in both cases.

Treatment of Underweight

underweight A body mass index below 18.5. The cutoff is less precise than for obesity because this condition has been less studied.

Underweight can be caused by a variety of factors, such as cancer, infectious disease (e.g., tuberculosis), digestive tract disorders (e.g., chronic inflammatory bowel disease), and excessive physical activity. Genetic background may also lead to a higher resting metabolic rate, a slight body frame, or both. Significant underweight is also associated with increased death rates, especially when combined with cigarette smoking. Health problems associated with underweight include the loss of menstrual function, low bone mass, complications with pregnancy and surgery, and slow recovery after illness. We frequently hear about the risks of obesity, but seldom of underweight. In our culture, being underweight is much more socially acceptable than being obese.

Sometimes being underweight requires medical intervention. A physician should be consulted first to rule out hormonal imbalances, depression, cancer, infectious disease, digestive tract disorders, excessive physical activity, and other hidden disease, such as a serious eating disorder (see Chapter 12 for a detailed discussion of eating disorders).

The causes of underweight are not altogether different from the causes of obesity. Internal and external satiety-signal irregularities, the rate of metabolism, hereditary tendencies, and psychological traits can all contribute to underweight.

In growing children, the demand for calories to support physical activity and growth can cause underweight. During growth spurts in adolescence, active children may not take the time to consume enough calories to support their needs. Moreover, gaining weight can be a formidable task for an underweight person. An extra 500 kcal per day may be required to gain weight, even at a slow pace, in part because of the increased expenditure of energy in thermogenesis. In contrast to the weight loser, the weight gainer may need to increase portion sizes.

When underweight requires a specific intervention, one approach for treating adults is to gradually increase their consumption of calorie-dense foods, especially those high in vegetable fat. Italian cheeses, nuts, and granola can be good calorie sources with low saturated-fat content. Dried fruit and bananas are good fruit choices. If eaten at the end of a meal, they don't cause early satiety. The same advice applies to salads and soups. Underweight people should replace such foods as diet soft drinks with good calorie sources, such as fruit juices and smoothies.

Encouraging a regular meal and snack schedule also aids in weight gain and maintenance. Sometimes people who are underweight have experienced stress at work or have been too busy to eat. Making regular meals a priority may not only help them attain an appropriate weight but also help with digestive disorders, such as constipation, which are sometimes associated with irregular eating times.

Excessively physically active people can reduce activity. If their weight remains low, they can add muscle mass through a resistance training (weight-lifting) program, but they must increase their calorie intake to support that physical activity. Otherwise, weight gain will be hindered.

If these efforts fail to achieve a healthy weight, they should at least prevent the health problems associated with being underweight. After achieving that, they may have to accept their lean frames.

Summary

1. Energy balance considers energy intake and energy output. Negative energy balance occurs when energy output surpasses energy intake, resulting in weight loss. Positive energy balance occurs when calorie intake is greater than output, resulting in weight gain.

2. Basal metabolism, the thermic effect of food, physical activity, and thermogenesis account for total energy use by the body. Basal metabolism, which represents the minimum amount of calories required to keep the resting, awake body alive, is primarily affected by lean body mass, surface area, and thyroid hormone concentrations. Physical activity is energy use above that which is expended at rest. The thermic effect of food describes the increase in metabolism that facilitates digestion, absorption, and processing of the nutrients recently consumed. Thermogenesis is heat production caused by shivering when cold, fidgeting, and other stimuli. In a sedentary person, about 70% to 80% of energy use is accounted for by basal metabolism and the thermic effect of food.

3. A person of healthy weight shows good health and performs daily activities without weight-related problems. A body mass index (weight in kilograms ÷ height^2 in meters) of 18.5 to 25 is one measure of healthy weight, although weight in excess of this value may not lead to ill health. A healthy weight is best determined in conjunction with a thorough health evaluation by a physician.

4. A body mass index of 25 to 29.9 represents overweight. Obesity is defined as a total body fat percentage over 25% (men) or 35% (women), or a body mass index of 30 or more.

5. Fat distribution greatly determines health risks from obesity. Upper-body fat storage, as measured by a waist circumference greater than 40 inches (102 centimeters)(men) or 35 inches (88 centimeters) (women) suggests higher risks of hypertension, cardiovascular disease, and type 2 diabetes than does lower-body fat storage.

6. A sound weight-loss program meets the dieter's nutritional needs by emphasizing a wide variety of low-calorie bulky foods; adapts to the dieter's habits; consists of readily obtainable foods; strives to change poor eating habits; stresses regular physical activity; and stipulates the participation of a physician if weight is to be lost rapidly or if the person is over the age of 40 (men) or 50 (women) and plans to perform substantially greater physical activity than usual.

7. A pound of adipose tissue contains about 3500 kcal. Loss or gain of a pound of adipose tissue—the fat itself plus lean support tissue—represents approximately 3300 kcal. Thus, if energy output exceeds calorie intake by about 500 kcal per day, a pound of adipose tissue can be lost per week.

8. Physical activity as part of a weight-loss program should be focused on duration rather than intensity. Ideally, vigorous activity for 60 minutes should be part of each day to prevent adult weight gain.

9. Behavior modification is a vital part of a weight-loss program because the dieter may have many habits that discourage weight maintenance. Specific behavior modification techniques, such as stimulus control and self-monitoring, can be used to help change problem behavior.

10. Medications to blunt appetite, such as phenteramine (Fastin) and sibutramine (Meridia), can aid weight-reduction strategies. Orlistat (Xenical) reduces fat absorption from a meal when taken with the meal. Weight-loss drugs are reserved for those who are obese or have weight-related problems, and they must be administered under close physician supervision.

11. The treatment of severe obesity may include surgery to reduce stomach volume to approximately 30 milliliters (1 ounce) or very-low-calorie diets containing 400 to 800 kcal per day. Both of these measures should be reserved for people who have failed at more conservative approaches to weight loss. They also require close medical supervision.

12. Underweight can be caused by a variety of factors, such as excessive physical activity and genetic background. Sometimes being underweight requires medical attention. A physician should be consulted first to rule out underlying disease. The underweight person may need to increase portion sizes and learn to like calorie-dense foods. In addition, encouraging a regular meal and snack schedule aids in weight gain, as well as weight maintenance.

Study Questions

1. After re-examining the nature and nurture aspects of weight control, propose two hypotheses for the development of obesity.

2. Propose two hypotheses for the development of obesity, based on the four contributors to energy expenditure.

3. Define a healthy weight in a way that makes the most sense to you.

4. Describe a practical method to define obesity in a clinical setting.

5. What are the two most convincing pieces of evidence that both genetic and environmental factors play significant roles in the development of obesity?

6. List three health problems that obese people typically face. Describe a possible reason that each problem arises.

7. When searching for a sound weight-loss program, what three key characteristics would you look for?

8. Why is the claim for quick, effortless weight loss by any method always misleading?

9. Define the term *behavior modification*. Relate it to the terms *stimulus control*, *self-monitoring*, *chain-breaking*, *relapse prevention*, and *cognitive restructuring*. Give examples of each.

10. Why should the treatment of obesity be viewed as a lifelong commitment rather than just a short episode of weight loss?

Further Readings (See also the May 2005 Supplement on Obesity in the *Journal of the American Dietetic Association*)

1. Blackburn GL: Solutions in weight control: lessons from gastric surgery. *American Journal of Clinical Nutrition* 82:248S, 2005.

   Surgery is currently the only proven way to achieve significant long-term weight loss, improve obesity-related health problems, reduce the risk of premature death, and improve quality of life in a large proportion of obese individuals. Roux-en-Y gastric bypass, the most widely performed procedure in the United States, achieves permanent, significant weight loss in more than 90% of cases of severe obesity.

2. Booth KM and others: Obesity and the built Environment. *Journal of the American Dietetic Association* 105:S110, 2005.

   Obesity is linked with many features of the "built environment": residence, neighborhood, resources, television, walkability, land use, and sprawl. Lower socioeconomic status neighborhoods are a primary concern, as residents in these areas may have less access to recreational facilities or food stores with healthful, affordable options. In the future, neighborhoods should be designed in ways that promote physical activity

3. Dansinger ML and others: Comparison of the Atkins, Ornish, Weight Watchers, and Zone diets for weight loss and heart disease risk reduction: a randomized trial. *Journal of the American Medical Association* 293:43, 2005.

   All four popular diets (Atkins, Ornish, Weight Watchers, Zone) are equally effective for helping adults lose weight. Because success in this study directly correlated with adherence to the diet, it makes sense to help patients choose the diet that is easiest for them to follow, rather than preferentially encouraging one diet over any other.

4. Davison KK, Birch LL: Lean and weight stable: Behavioral predictors and psychological correlates. *Obesity Research* 12:1085, 2004.

   Being at a healthy weight and avoiding large weight fluctuations during adulthood are linked with patterns of healthy eating and regular physical activity, lower dietary restraint, and less reliance on dieting attempts. These lifestyle behavioral patterns may emerge during childhood; intervention efforts should focus on this age period.

5. Ello-Martin JA and others: The influence of food portion size and energy density on energy intake: implications for weight management. *American Journal of Clinical Nutrition* 82:236S, 2005.

   Providing larger food portions can lead to significant increases in calorie intake. One strategy to address this effect of portion size is decreasing the energy density of foods. Eating satisfying portions of low-energy-dense foods maintains satiety while reducing calorie intake.

6. Foster GD and others: Behavioral treatment of obesity. *American Journal of Clinical Nutrition* 82:230S, 2005.

   The behavior change process is facilitated through the use of self-monitoring, goal-setting, and problem solving. Behavior therapy can help individuals develop a set of skills (such as eating a low-calorie, low-fat diet) to achieve a healthier weight.

7. Hill JO and others: Obesity and the environment: Where do we go from here? *Science* 299:853, 2003.

   The obesity epidemic shows no signs of abating. There is an urgent need to push back against the environmental forces that are producing gradual weight gain in the population. A moderate decrease in calorie intake (100 kcal) and greater physical activity (100 kcal) are advocated by the authors.

8. Hu FB: Protein, body weight, and cardiovascular health *American Journal of Clinical Nutrition* 82:242S, 2005.

   It may be beneficial to partially replace refined carbohydrates with protein sources low in saturated fat. Plant sources of protein and fat, such as nuts, legumes, soy, and vegetable oils, may provide even greater health benefits in place of refined carbohydrates and animal products.

9. Hu FB and others: Adiposity as compared with physical activity in predicting mortality among women. *The New England Journal of Medicine* 351:2694, 2004.

   Both BMI and level of physical activity are important and independent predictors of mortality; a higher level of physical activity does not however appear to negate the risk associated with significant adiposity. Women who are both lean and physically active had the lowest mortality in this study.

10. Jakicic JM and Otto AD: Physical activity considerations for the treatment and prevention of obesity. *American Journal of Clinical Nutrition* 82:226S, 2005.

    Physical activity is an important component of long-term weight control, and therefore adequate levels of activity should be prescribed to combat the obesity epidemic. Although there is evidence that 30 minutes of moderate-intensity physical activity may improve health outcomes, a growing body of scientific literature suggests that at least 60 minutes of moderate-intensity physical activity may be necessary to maximize weight loss and prevent significant weight regain.

11. Klein S and others: Clinical implications of obesity with specific focus on cardiovascular disease. *Circulation* 110:2952, 2004.

    Obesity adversely affects cardiac function, increases the risk factors for coronary heart disease, and is an independent risk factor for cardiovascular disease. The risk of developing coronary heart disease is directly related to obesity-related risk factors. In contrast, modest weight loss can affect the entire cluster of coronary heart disease factors simultaneously.

12. Li Z and others: Meta-analysis: Pharmacologic treatment of obesity. *Annals of Internal Medicine* 142(7):532, 2005.

    Sibutramine, orlistat, and phentermine promote weight loss for at least 6 months when given along with recommendations for diet (and other behavioral and exercise interventions). The amount of extra weight loss attributable to these medications is modest, but still may be clinically significant. Use of each of these medications is reviewed in detail.

13. Lofgren I and others: Waist circumference is a better predictor than body mass index of coronary heart disease risk in overweight premenopausal women. *Journal of Nutrition* 134:1071, 2004.

    Although neither BMI nor waist circumference provides a complete picture of overall risk, the waist circumference classification of the subjects from the present study revealed stronger associations with multiple risk factors for chronic disease. This finding suggests that waist circumference should be used to screen the general population.

14. Nielsen SJ, Popkin BM: Patterns and trends in food portion sizes, 1977–1998. *Journal of the American Medical Association* 289:450, 2003.

    Portion sizes and calorie intake for specific food types have increased markedly, with the greatest increases for food consumed in fast-food establishments and in the home. In response, adults should

strive for reduced portion sizes such that smaller amounts of food will be eaten at each meal. In addition, the public needs better education about control of portion size; simply educating the public about which foods to eat is not enough.

15. Ornish D: Was Dr Atkins Right? *Journal of the American Dietetic Association* 104: 537, 2004.

    The safest way to lose weight in the long run is to focus on reducing fat and refined carbohydrate intake. Whole foods and complex carbohydrates should instead be emphasized.

16. Periera MA and others: The fast-food track to obesity and insulin resistance. *Lancet* 365: 36, 2005.

    Participants in this study who reported more than 2 fast-food visits each week gained significantly more weight and had a twofold increase in insulin resistance, compared with participants who reported fewer than 1 weekly fast-food visit. Thus, the growing use of fast food restaurants needs to be reexamined by many if us.

17. Pittler MH, Ernst E: Dietary supplements for body-weight reduction: a systematic review. *American Journal of Clinical Nutrition* 79:529, 2004.

    Evidence for most dietary supplements as aids in reducing body weight is not convincing. None of the reviewed dietary supplements in the article, such as chromium and chitosan, can be recommended for over-the-counter use.

18. Schulz M and others: Identification of a food pattern characterized by high-fiber and low-fat food choices associated with low prospective weight change in the EPIC-Potsdam cohort. *Journal of Nutrition* 135:1183, 2005.

    Low-fat, high-fiber, high-carbohydrate food choices, such as whole-grain bread, fruits, grains and cereals, may help adults maintain body weight or to prevent excess weight gain over time. Although the predictive value of this dietary pattern was confined to nonobese subjects, this study lends support to the current recommendations regarding macronutrient composition of the diet.

19. Wing RR, Phelan S: Long-term weight loss maintenance. *American Journal of Clinical Nutrition* 82:222S, 2005.

    National Weight Control Registry members provide evidence that long-term weight loss maintenance is possible and help identify the specific approaches associated with long-term success. The article reviews the habits of these participants, such as regularly eating breakfast, self-monitoring weight, and meeting the goal of 60 minutes of physical activity.

20. Weighing in on the South Beach Diet. *Tufts University Health & Nutrition Letter* 22:1 2004 (May).

    The South Beach Diet has not been proven to be effective and contains both scientific inconsistencies and inaccurate statements. This low-carbohydrate plan amounts to just another low-calorie plan because of the foods it limits. It has no unique aspect that contributes to weight loss.

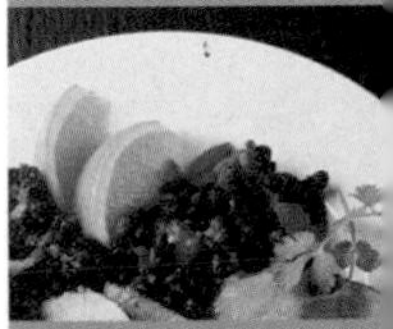

I. A Close Look at Your Weight Status

Determine the following two indices of your body status: body mass index and waist circumference.

Body Mass Index (BMI)

Record your weight in pounds: _____ lb
Divide your weight in pounds by 2.2 to determine your weight in kilograms: _____ kilograms
Record your height in inches: _____ in
Divide your height in inches by 39.3 to determine your height in meters: _____ meters
Calculate your BMI using the following formula:
BMI = weight (kilograms)/height^2 (meters)
BMI = _____ kg/ _____ m^2 = _____

Waist Circumference

Use a tape measure to measure the circumference of your waist (at the umbilicus with stomach muscles relaxed).
Circumference of waist (umbilicus) = _____ in

Interpretation

1. When BMI is greater than 25, health risks from obesity often begin. It is especially advisable to consider weight loss if your BMI exceeds 30. Does yours exceed 25 (or 30)?
   Yes _____   No _____

2. When a person has a BMI greater than 25 and a waist circumference of more than 40 inches (102 centimeters) in men or 35 inches (88 centimeters) in women, there is an increased risk of cardiovascular disease, hypertension, and type 2 diabetes. Does your circumference exceed the standard for your gender?
   Yes _____   No _____

3. Do you feel you need to pursue a program of weight loss?
   Yes _____   No _____

Application

From what you've learned in Chapter 10, what habits can you change in patterns of eating and physical activity to lose weight and help ensure maintenance of any loss?

_____

_____

_____

II. An Action Plan to Change or Maintain Weight Status

Now that you have assessed your current weight status, do you feel that you would like to make some changes? Following is a step-by-step guide to behavioral change. This process can be useful even for those who are satisfied with their current weight, as it can be applied to changing exercise habits, self-esteem, and a variety of other behaviors (Fig. 10-17).

Becoming Aware of the Problem

By calculating your current weight status, you have already become aware of the problem, if one exists. From here, it is important to find out more information about the cause of the problem and whether it is worth working toward a change.

1. What are the factors that most influence your eating habits? Do you eat due to stress, boredom, or depression? Is volume of food your problem, or do you eat mainly the wrong foods for you? Take some time to assess the root causes of your eating habits.

Figure 10-17 A model for behavior change. It starts with awareness of the problem and ends with the incorporation of new behaviors intended to address the problem.

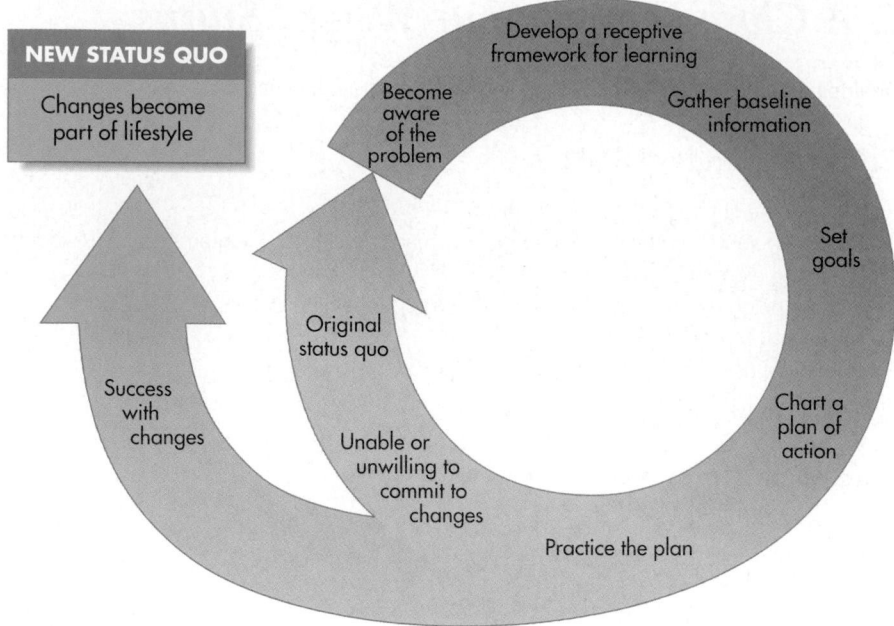

NEW STATUS QUO

Changes become part of lifestyle

Develop a receptive framework for learning

Become aware of the problem

Gather baseline information

Set goals

Original status quo

Success with changes

Chart a plan of action

Unable or unwilling to commit to changes

Practice the plan

2. Once you have more information about your specific eating practices, you must decide if it is worth changing these practices. A benefits and costs analysis can be a useful tool in evaluating whether or not it is worth your effort to make life changes. Use the following example as a guide for listing benefits and costs pertinent to your own situation (Fig. 10-18).

Setting Goals

What can we accomplish, and how long will it take? Setting a realistic, achievable goal and allowing a reasonable amount of time to pursue it increase the likelihood of success.

1. Begin by determining the final outcome you would like to achieve. If you are trying to change your eating behaviors to be more healthy, list your reasons for doing so (e.g., overall health, weight loss, self-esteem).

Overall goal:

_____

_____

Reasons to pursue goal:

_____

_____

_____

2. Now list several steps that will be necessary to achieve your goal. Keep in mind, however, that it is generally best to change only a few specific behaviors at first—walking briskly for 60 minutes each day, reducing fat intake, using more whole-grain products, and not eating after 7 P.M. Attempting small and perhaps easier dietary changes first reduces the scope of the problem and increases the likelihood of success.

Steps toward achieving goal:

1. _____

2. _____

3. _____

Note that, if you are having trouble deciphering the steps needed to achieve your goal, health professionals are an excellent resource for aid in planning.

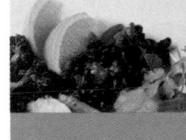

Benefits and Costs Analysis

1 Benefits of changing eating habits?

What do you expect to get, now or later, that you want?
What may you avoid that would be unpleasant?

feel better physically and psychologically
look better

2 Benefits of not changing eating habits?

What do you get to do that you enjoy doing?
What do you avoid having to do?

no need for planning
can eat without feeling guilty

3 Costs involved in changing eating habits?

What do you have to do that you don't want to do?
What do you have to stop doing that you would rather continue doing?

take time to plan meals and shop
must give up some food volume

4 Costs of not changing eating habits?

What unpleasant or undesirable effects are you likely to experience now or in the future?
What are you likely to lose?

creeping weight gain
low self-esteem and poor health

Figure 10-18 Benefits and costs analysis applied to increasing physical activity. This process helps put behavior change into the context of total lifestyle.

Measuring Commitment

Now that you have collected information and know what is required to reach your goal, you must ask yourself, "Can I do this?" Commitment is an essential component in the success of behavioral change. Be honest with yourself. Permanent change is not quick or easy. Once you have decided that you have the commitment required to see this through, continue on to the following sections.

Making It Official with a Contract

Drawing up a behavioral contract often adds incentive to follow through with a plan. The contract could list goal behaviors and objectives, milestones for measuring progress, and regular rewards for meeting the terms of the contract. After finishing a contract, you should sign it in the presence of some friends. This encourages commitment.

Initially, plans should reward positive behaviors, and then they should focus on positive results. Positive behaviors, such as regular physical activity, eventually lead to positive outcomes, such as increased stamina.

Figure 10-19 is a sample contract for increasing physical activity. Keep in mind that this sample contract is only a suggestion; you can add your own ideas as well.

Psyching Yourself Up

Once your contract is in place, you need to psych yourself up. Discouragement from peers and your own temptations to stray from your plan need to be anticipated. Psyching yourself up can enable you to progress toward your goals in spite of others' attitudes and opinions.

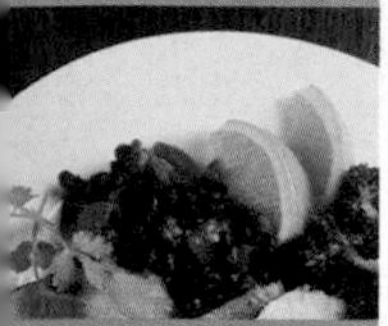

Name _Alan Young_

Goal

I agree to _ride my exercise bike_
(specify behavior)

under the following circumstances _for 30 minutes, 4 times per week in the evening_
(specify where, when, how much, etc.)

Substitute behavior and/or reinforcement schedule _I will reinforce myself if I've achieved my goal after a month with a weekend off campus with my roommate._

Environmental planning

In order to help me do this, I am going to (1) arrange my physical and social environment by _buying a new portable CD player_

and (2) control my internal environment (thoughts, images) by _coordinating riding the bike with the first T.V. watching I do in the evening_

Reinforcements

Reinforcements provided by me daily or weekly (if contract is kept):
I will buy myself a new piece of clothing for off campus trip

Reinforcements provided by others daily or weekly (if contract is kept):
at the end of a month if I've completed my goal my parents will buy me a fitness club membership for winter.

Social support

Behavior change is more likely to take place when other people support you. During the quarter/semester please meet with the other person at least three times to discuss your progress.

The name of my "significant helper" is: _Mr. and Mrs. Young_

This contract should include:

1. Baseline data (one week)
2. Well-defined goal
3. Simple method for charting progress (diary, counter, charts, etc.)
4. Reinforcements (immediate and long-term)
5. Evaluation method (summary of experiences, success, and/or new learnings about self).

Figure 10-19 Alan's behavior contract. Completing such a contract can help generate commitment to behavior change. What would your contract look like?

Almost everyone benefits from some assertiveness training when it comes to changing behaviors. The following are a few suggestions. Can you think of any others?

- No one's feelings should be hurt if you say, "No, thank you," firmly and repeatedly when others try to dissuade you from a plan. Tell them you have new diet behavior and your needs are important.

- You don't have to eat a lot to accommodate anyone—your mother, business clients, or the chef. For example, at a party with friends, you may feel you have to eat a lot to participate, but you don't. Another trap is ordering a lot just because someone else is paying for the meal.

- Learn ways to handle put-downs—inadvertent or conscious. An effective response can be to communicate feelings honestly, without hostility. Tell criticizers that they have annoyed or offended you, that you are working to change your habits and would really like understanding and support from them.

Practicing the Plan

Once you've set up a plan, the next step is to implement it. Start with a trial of at least 6 to 8 weeks. Thinking of a lifetime commitment can be overwhelming. Aim for a total duration of 6 months of new activities before giving up. We may have to persuade ourselves more than once of the value of continuing the program. The following are some suggestions to help keep a plan on track:

- *Focus on reducing, but not necessarily extinguishing, undesirable behaviors.* For example, it's usually unrealistic to say, "I'll never eat a certain food again." It's better to say, "I won't eat that *problem* food as often as before."

- *Monitor progress.* Note your progress in a diary and reward yourself according to your contract. While conquering some habits and seeing improvement, you may find yourself quite encouraged, even enthusiastic, about your plan of action. That can give you the impetus to move ahead with the program.

- *Control environments.* In the early phases of behavioral change, try to avoid problem situations, such as parties, coffee breaks, and favorite restaurants. Once new habits are firmly established, you can probably more successfully resist the temptations of these environments.

Re-evaluating and Preventing Relapse

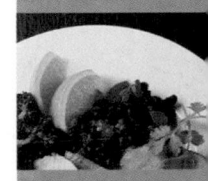

After practicing a program for several weeks to months, it is important to reassess the original plan. In addition, you may now be able to pinpoint other problem areas for which you need to plan appropriately.

1. Begin by taking a close and critical look at your original plan. Does it actually lead to the goals you set? Are there any new steps toward your goal that you feel capable of adding to your contract? Do you need new reinforcements? It may even be necessary to make a new contract. For permanent change, it is worth this time of reassessment.

2. In practicing your plan over the past weeks or months, you have likely experienced relapses. What triggered these relapses? To prevent a total retreat to your old habits, it is important to set up a plan for such relapses. You can do this by identifying high-risk situations, rehearsing a response, and remembering your goals.

You may have noticed a behavior chain in some of your relapses. That is, the relapse may stem from a series of interconnected habitual activities. The way to break the chain is to first identify the activities, pinpoint the weak links, break those links, and substitute other behaviors. Figure 10-20 illustrates a sample behavior chain and a substitute activities list. Consider compiling your own list based on your behavior chains.

Epilogue

If you have used the activities in this section, you are well on your way to permanent behavioral change. Recall that this exercise can be used for a variety of desired changes, including quitting smoking, increasing physical activity, and improving study habits. It is by no means an easy process, but the results can be well worth the effort. Overall, the keys to success are motivation (keeping the problem in the forefront of your mind), having a plan of action, securing the resources and skills needed for success, and looking for help from family, friends, or a group.

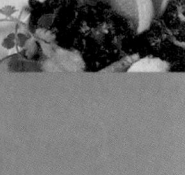

ALTERNATIVE ACTIVITY SHEET

SUBSTITUTE ACTIVITIES

Pleasant activities
1. *Singing / washing hair*
2. *Reading comics / biking*
3. *Sewing / calling a friend*

Necessary activities
1. *Ironing*
2. *Vacuuming*
3. *Straightening apartment*

Situations when used
1. *Wanted ice cream — delayed with bath*
2. *Wanted wheat thins — cleaned up apt.*
3. *Wanted snack — went for walk*
4. *Wanted cookies — did dishes first*
5. *Saw leftovers — went for bike ride*
6. *Tempted by cookies — set timer*
7. *Wanted snack — read comics*

BEHAVIOR CHAIN

Identify the links in your eating response chain on the following diagram. Draw a line through the chain where it was interrupted. Add the link you substituted and the new chain of behavior this substitution started.

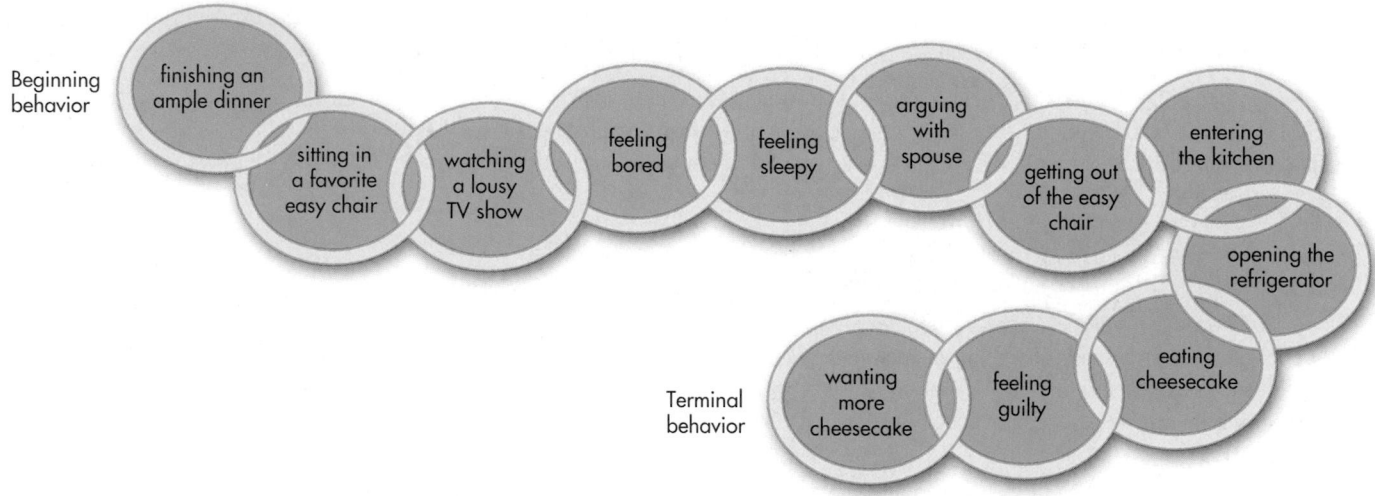

Figure 10-20 Identifying behavior chains. This is a good tool for understanding more about your habits and pinpointing ways to change unwanted habits. The earlier in the chain you substitute a nonfood link, the easier it is to intervene. Four types of behaviors can be substituted in an ongoing behavior chain.

1. Fun activities (taking a walk, reading a book)
2. Necessary activities (cleaning a room, balancing your checkbook)
3. Incompatible activities (taking a shower)
4. Urge-delaying activities (setting a kitchen timer for 20 minutes before allowing yourself to eat)

Using activities to interrupt behavior patterns that lead to inappropriate eating (or inactivity) can be a powerful means of changing habits.

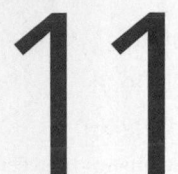

Nutrition:

Fitness and Sports

11

Real Life Scenario

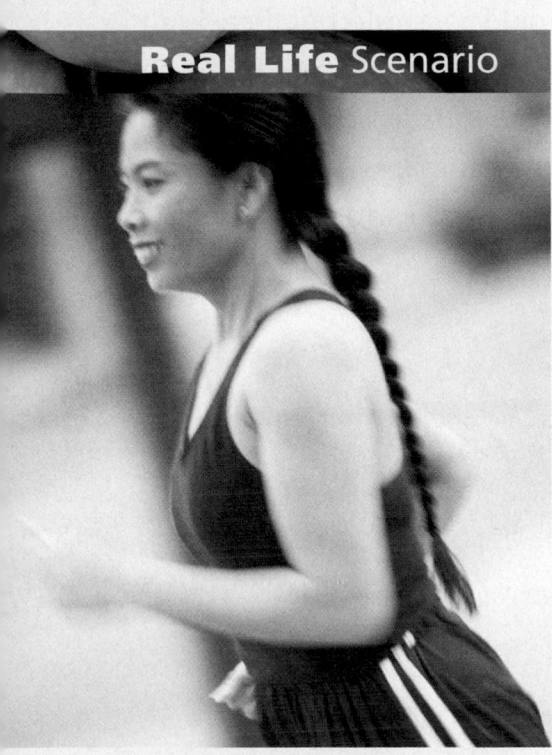

Marcella is training for a 10K run coming up in 3 weeks. She has read a lot about sports nutrition, and especially about the importance of eating a high-carbohydrate diet while in training. She also has been struggling to keep her weight in a range that she feels contributes to better speed and endurance. Consequently, she is also trying to eat as little fat as possible. Unfortunately, over the past week her workouts in the afternoon have not met her expectations. Her run times are slower, and she shows signs of fatigue after just 20 minutes into her training program.

Her breakfast yesterday was a large bagel, a small amount of cream cheese, and orange juice. For lunch, she had a small salad with fat-free dressing, a large plate of pasta with tomato marinara sauce and broccoli, and a diet soft drink. For dinner, she had a small broiled chicken breast, a cup of rice, some carrots, and iced tea. Later, she snacked on fat-free pretzels.

What advice would you provide Marcella regarding her training diet? Note current strengths and weaknesses. Is her diet likely contributing to her recent fatigue during workouts?

Chapter 11 Objectives

Chapter 11 is designed to allow you to:

1. List five positive health-related outcomes of a physically active lifestyle.

2. Design a fitness regimen.

3. Describe when and how glycogen, blood glucose, fat, and protein are used to meet energy needs during different types of physical activity.

4. Differentiate between anaerobic and aerobic use of glucose and identify advantages and disadvantages of each.

5. Show how muscles and related organs adapt to an increase in physical activity.

6. Outline how to estimate an athlete's calorie needs and discuss the general principles for meeting overall nutrient requirements in the training diet.

7. Examine the problems associated with rapid weight loss by dehydration and outline the importance of water and/or sports drinks during exercise.

8. Understand the importance of maintaining a healthy status of various vitamins and minerals during training.

9. List several ergogenic aids and describe their effects, if any, on an athlete's performance.

A thletes invest a lot of time and effort in training. Because they often seek ways to enhance their diets to improve performance, athletes make easy targets for purveyors of nutrition misinformation. Still, most athletes don't want to miss out on any advantage, whether real or perceived, that might give them the winning edge.

Although good eating habits can't substitute for physical training and genetic endowment, proper diet choices are crucial for top-notch performance, contributing to endurance and helping to speed the repair of injured tissues.

Looking at our population in general, experts might disagree on how much carbohydrate, protein, and fat we should consume, but there is no argument over the health benefits of regular physical activity. It is even beneficial for overweight people who remain at that excess weight.

In Chapter 11, you will discover how physical fitness benefits the entire body, and how nutrition relates to fitness and sports performance.

Refresh Your Memory

As you begin your study of nutrition for fitness and sports in Chapter 11, you may want to review:

- The current trend of consuming "energy bars" in Chapter 1
- The components of the cell in Chapter 3
- The concept of glycemic load in Chapter 4
- The various food sources of carbohydrates, proteins, and lipids in Chapters 4–7
- Food sources of calcium and iron in Chapter 9

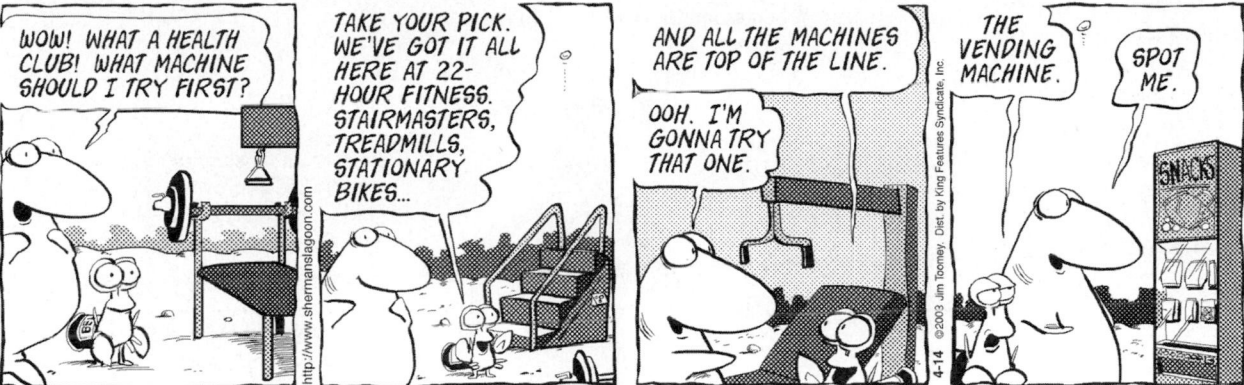

Why is regular physical activity—including some strength-building activities—generally advocated for all of us? What benefits accrue from this practice? How do strength-training and endurance athletes need to tailor their diets to support their vigorous physical activities? Chapter 11 provides some answers.

The Close Relationship between Nutrition and Fitness

The ability to engage routinely in vigorous physical activity requires good health. The ability to perform also depends on a nutritious diet that supplies all the needed nutrients.

Once muscles have nutrients available to them, what determines the type of fuel they will use? Athletes have a say in that decision, depending on how physically fit the athletes are and how hard each one performs. This physical fitness—defined as the ability to perform moderate to vigorous activity without undue fatigue—especially affects fat use by the body. As one's level of physical fitness improves, so does one's ability to mobilize fat stores for energy needs—especially during activities that last for 20 minutes or more.

Beyond affecting fuel use, the benefits of regular physical activity include enhancement of several aspects of heart function, less injury, better sleep habits, and improvement in body composition (less body fat, more muscle mass). Physical activity also can reduce stress and positively affect blood pressure, blood cholesterol, blood glucose regulation, and immune function. In addition, it aids in weight control, both by raising resting energy expenditure for a short period of time after exercise and by increasing overall energy expenditure. See Figure 11-1 for a further look at the benefits of a physically active lifestyle.

Unfortunately, as noted in Chapter 10, many North American adults lead sedentary lives. Most adults do not practice moderate to vigorous physical activity on a regular basis, and about half of all adults quit an exercise program within 3 months of onset. Does this discussion motivate you to assess your activity patterns and improve them as needed? The first Looking Further section in this chapter will help you plan your exercise program.

Healthy People 2010 has set a number of specific objectives for U.S. adults related to physical activity:

- Reduce by 50% the proportion of adults engaging in no leisure-time physical activity (currently 27% of adults).
- Double the proportion of adults engaging regularly, preferably daily, in moderate physical activity for at least 30 minutes per day (currently 45% of adults). (Note

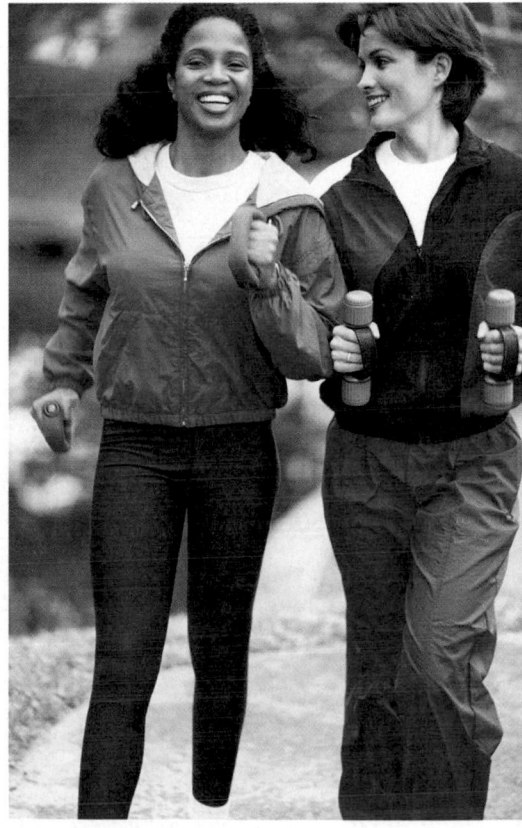

What is the best exercise? One you enjoy.

Figure 11-1 Exercise is medicine—the benefits of regular, moderate physical activity. There is also evidence that regular physical activity slows the aging process.

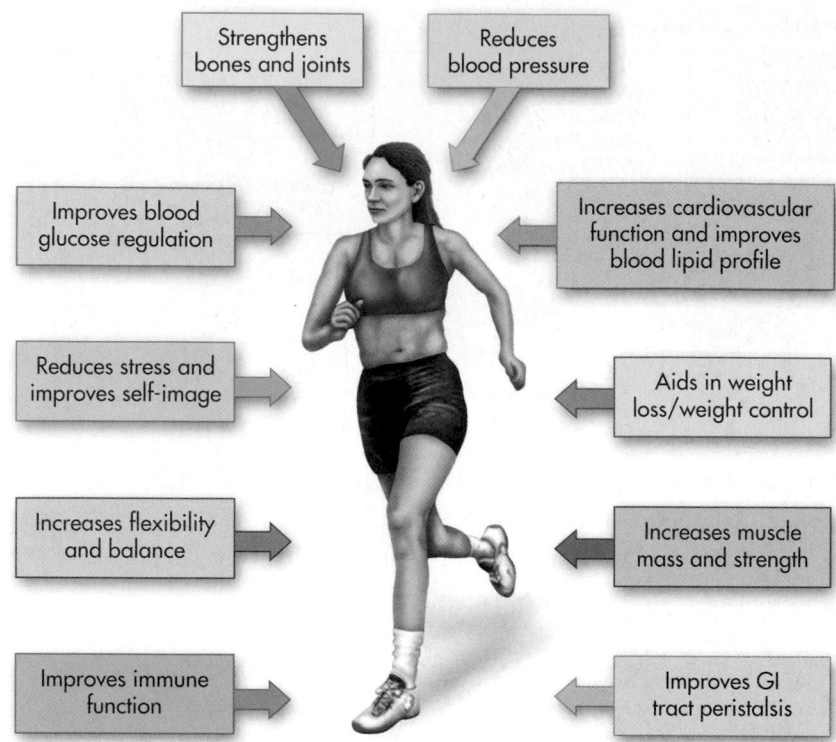

Strengthens bones and joints

Reduces blood pressure

Improves blood glucose regulation

Increases cardiovascular function and improves blood lipid profile

Reduces stress and improves self-image

Aids in weight loss/weight control

Increases flexibility and balance

Increases muscle mass and strength

Improves immune function

Improves GI tract peristalsis

that the Food and Nutrition Board recommends 60 minutes per day, especially if weight loss/weight control is an issue.)

- Increase by 50% the proportion of adults who perform physical activities that enhance and maintain muscular strength and endurance (currently 19% of adults).

To help yourself stay with an exercise program, experts recommend the following:

- Start slowly.
- Vary your activities; make it fun.
- Include friends and others.
- Set specific attainable goals and monitor progress.
- Set aside a specific time each day for exercise; build it into your routine, but make it convenient.
- Reward yourself for being successful in keeping up with your goals.
- Don't worry about occasional setbacks; focus on the long-term benefits to your health.

Another Bite

Consider applying the dietary principles of variety, balance, and moderation to your exercise plan:

- Variety: Enjoy many different activities to exercise different muscles.
- Balance: Different activities have different benefits, so balance your exercise pattern. For overall fitness, you need exercises that build cardiovascular endurance, muscular strength, and flexibility.
- Moderation: Exercise to keep fit without overdoing it. You don't need a heavy workout every day to achieve fitness.

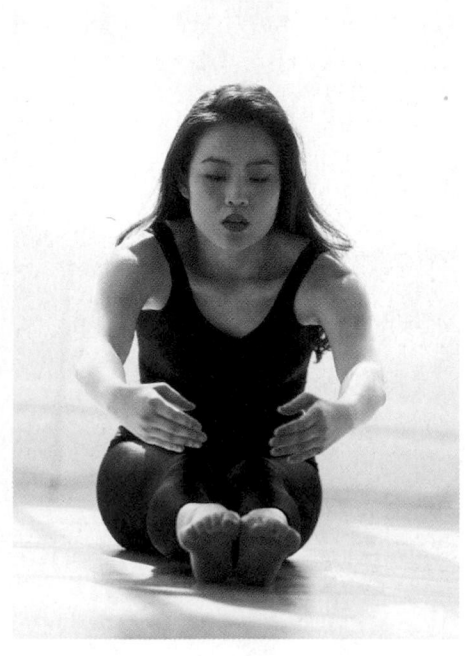

Stretching should be part of an overall fitness plan.

Energy Sources for Exercising Muscles

To allow for the many benefits of locomotion, muscle cells need a specific form of energy for contraction. Muscle (and other) cells cannot directly use the energy released from breaking down glucose or triglycerides. Rather, body cells must first convert food energy (i.e., calories) to **adenosine triphosphate (ATP)**.

The chemical bonds between phosphates in ATP and related molecules are high-energy bonds. Using the energy obtained from foodstuffs, cells make ATP from its breakdown product **adenosine diphosphate (ADP)** and a phosphate group (abbreviated Pi). Conversely, to release energy from ATP, cells partially break the compound down into ADP and Pi. The released energy is used for many cell functions.

$$ADP + Energy\ from\ food + Pi \rightarrow ATP$$

$$ATP \rightarrow Energy\ to\ do\ work + ADP + Pi$$

Essentially, ATP is the immediate source of energy for body functions (Table 11-1). The primary goal in the use of any fuel, whether carbohydrate, fat, or protein, is to make ATP. A resting muscle cell contains only a small amount of ATP that can be used immediately. If no resupply of ATP were possible, this amount of ATP could keep the muscle working maximally for only about 2 to 4 seconds. Fortunately, another type of high-energy compound—**phosphocreatine (PCr)**—is present in muscle cells and can

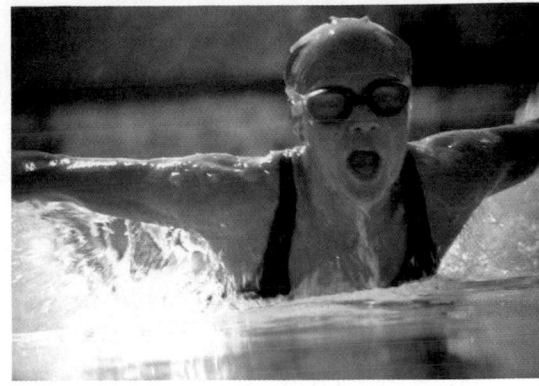

Bursts of muscle activity use a variety of energy sources, including PCr and ATP.

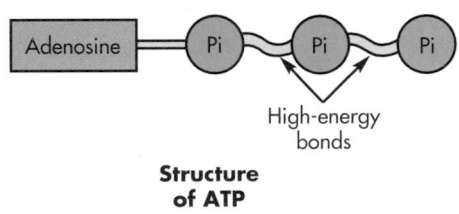

High-energy bonds

Structure of ATP

adenosine triphosphate (ATP) The main energy currency for cells. ATP energy is used to promote ion pumping, enzyme activity, and muscular contraction.

adenosine diphosphate (ADP) A breakdown product of ATP. ADP is synthesized into ATP using energy from foodstuffs and a phosphate group (abbreviated Pi).

phosphocreatine (PCr) A high-energy compound that can be used to re-form ATP. It is used primarily during bursts of activity, such as lifting and jumping.

Table 11-1 Energy Sources Used by Resting and Working Muscle Cells

Source/System*	When in Use	Examples of an Exercise
ATP	At all times	All types
Phosphocreatine (PCr)	All exercise initially; short bursts of exercise thereafter	Shotput, high jump
Carbohydrate (anaerobic)	High-intensity exercise, especially lasting 30 seconds to 2 minutes	200-yard (about 200 meters) sprint
Carbohydrate (aerobic)	Exercise lasting 2 minutes to 3 hours or more; the higher the intensity (for example, running a 6-minute mile), the greater the use	Basketball, swimming, jogging
Fat (aerobic)	Exercise lasting more than a few minutes; greater amounts are used at lower exercise intensities.	Long-distance running, long-distance cycling; much of the fuel used in a 30-minute brisk walk is fat.
Protein (aerobic)	Low amount during all exercise; slightly more in endurance exercise, especially when carbohydrate fuel is lacking	Long-distance running

*Note that at any given time, more than one system is operating.

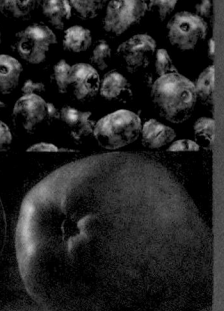

Looking Further

For healthy people, a gradual increase to a goal of regular physical activity is recommended. Men 40 years of age or older and women 50 years of age or older who have been inactive for many years, or who have an existing health problem, should discuss their fitness goals with their physician before increasing activity. Health problems that require medical evaluation before beginning an exercise program are obesity, cardiovascular disease (or family history of it), hypertension, diabetes (or family history), shortness of breath after mild exertion, and arthritis.

Phase 1: Getting Started Means Getting Going

During the first phase of a fitness program to promote health, you should begin to incorporate short periods of physical activity into the daily routine. This includes walking, taking the stairs instead of the elevator, house cleaning, gardening, and other activities that cause you to "huff and puff" a bit. The goal is a total of 30 minutes of this moderate type of physical activity on most (and preferably all) days. If necessary, this can be broken up into increments lasting at least 10 minutes. Experts suggest starting with short intervals, building up to a total of 30 minutes of activity incorporated into each day's tasks. If there is not much time for activity, you can even go for more intensity in the activities over shorter periods to get the same benefits.

The easiest way to increase physical activity is to make it part of a daily routine, similar to other regular activities, such as eating. You do not need to join a gym or attend aerobic classes. Daily activities can meet the Phase 1 goal. Many people find that the best time to exercise is when they need an energy pick-me-up or a break from work. Rather than abandoning an exercise program entirely when obstacles impede you, strive to use any small periods of available time, such as breaks between classes or "coffee breaks" at work. Once you reap the benefits of exercise, you will tend to spend more time at it.

Clearly, many of the activities recommended for Phase 1 are not very vigorous. Although Phase 1 is recommended for those starting an exercise program, fitness experts have not given up on the value of more vigorous physical activity. They're just making concessions to human nature. Still, most of the possible benefits from physical activity are seen if this Phase 1 goal is met.

Phase 2: Guidelines for Achieving and Maintaining Even Greater Physical Fitness

Once you can perform physical activity for 30 minutes per day, turn your attention to more specific activities, such as increasing muscle mass and strength, to reap even more benefits.

Warm-up

Stretch the whole torso for 5 to 10 minutes. Start with smaller muscle groups (arms) and work toward larger muscle groups (legs and abdomen).

Do 5 to 10 more minutes of low-intensity exercises, such as walking, slow jogging, or any slow version of anticipated activity. This warms up your muscles so that muscle filaments slide more easily over one another to increase range of motion and decrease the risk of injury.

■ Aerobic Workout

Daily aerobic activity is recommended. To start, an aerobic workout prescription considers mode, duration, frequency, intensity, and progression.

Mode: The mode of exercise is the type of exercise prescribed. It must be one that uses large muscle groups in a rhythmic fashion, such as brisk walking, running, and cycling.

Duration: Duration is the amount of time spent in an exercise session. It should generally last at least 20 to 30 minutes, depending on intensity, not counting time for warm-up and cooldown. Ideally, this should be continuous (without stopping) exercise, but multiple 10-minute bouts with rest periods in between are also acceptable.

Frequency: The frequency of the exercise describes the number of times that the activity is performed. The frequency of exercise should be at least five times per week. Daily exercising will lead to even further benefits related to physical fitness.

Intensity: Intensity is defined as the level of exertion that indicates the degree of energy expenditure required to sustain the activity. In other words, intensity is used to describe how hard you are working and to what extent you can maintain that intensity over time. Health benefits beyond phase 1 are especially seen when you can achieve a moderate level of intensity of exercise.

There are a few ways to determine the intensity of exercise. A popular and simple method is to use a percentage of your age-predicted maximum heart rate. To find maximum heart rate, subtract your age from 220. Multiplying maximum heart rate by 0.60 and 0.90 will result in a range of heart rates, sometimes called the *target zone*. For a 20-year-old person beginning an exercise program, maximum heart rate equals 200 beats per minute ($220 - 20 = 200$). Then, (200×0.6) and (200×0.9) yields a target zone of 120 to 180 beats per minute. Measuring heart rate (pulse) is easy: Stop and count your pulse for 10 seconds and then multiply that number by 6 to determine your heart rate for one minute. There are also watches available that contain heart rate monitors.

At the initiation of an exercise program, aim for the lower end of the target zone. As you progress and become more physically fit, you can work up to a higher heart rate. As with many of the prediction formulas, calculation of maximum heart rate is just an estimate. Medications, such as those for hypertension and other health conditions, may impact heart rate. If you have health concerns, a physician can help to personalize the target zone.

Another way of determining the intensity of exercise is the Rating of Perceived Exertion scale (RPE). One version includes a range of 1 to 10, with each number corresponding to a subjective feeling of exertion. For example, the number 0 is "nothing at all" (sitting at a table) and the number 10 is considered close to maximal effort or "very, very strong" (all-out sprint) (Figure 11-2).

When using the RPE scale, the goal is to aim for the number 4, which corresponds to the beginning of "somewhat strong." This is the point at which you begin to see significant fitness results. You should be working hard, but still be able to talk to an exercise partner (sometimes called the "talk test").

Progression: Progression, the final component, describes how the frequency, intensity, and duration of exercise have increased over a period of time. The first 3 to 6 weeks of your new exercise program are the initiation, or "getting started," phase. This phase corresponds to the time it takes for your body to adapt to the exercise program. The next 5 or 6 months

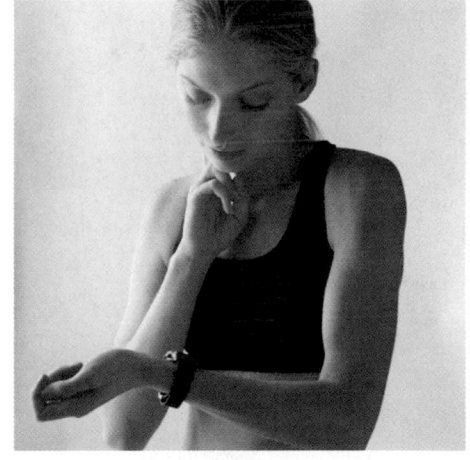

Taking one's pulse determines if exercise output is in the target zone.

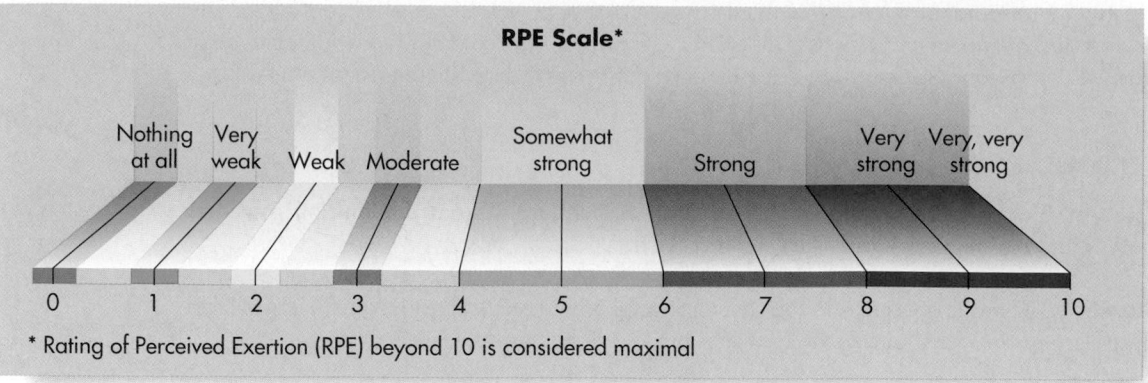

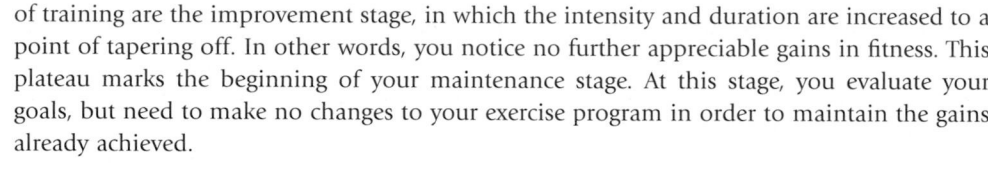

* Rating of Perceived Exertion (RPE) beyond 10 is considered maximal

Figure 11-2 Rating of Perceived Exertion Scale. When exercising, a rating of 4 or above is advocated for building/maintaining physical fitness.

of training are the improvement stage, in which the intensity and duration are increased to a point of tapering off. In other words, you notice no further appreciable gains in fitness. This plateau marks the beginning of your maintenance stage. At this stage, you evaluate your goals, but need to make no changes to your exercise program in order to maintain the gains already achieved.

∎ Strength Training Workout

Strength training should be done at least 2, and preferably 3, days per week. To start, it is recommended that a group of 8 to 10 exercises be performed in a circuit (all in one exercise session) to condition major muscle groups of the upper body and lower body. When selecting the proper weight to use, make sure that the weight allows you to perform one (or more) set(s) of at least 8 repetitions, but no more than 12. (However, 10 to 15 repetitions is fine for older adults using lighter weights.) Proper form during these exercises is also important. Generally, if more than 12 repetitions can be performed with relative ease, the weight can then be increased in moderate increments.

∎ Cool-down

During cool-down follow a reverse pattern of warm-up: 5 to 10 minutes of low-intensity activity and 5 to 10 minutes of stretching. The same exercises performed during warm-up are appropriate. The cool-down is essential to the prevention of injury and soreness.

∎ Further Considerations

Including several types of enjoyable physical activities in a fitness program may also be helpful. For example, jogging one day might be followed by swimming the next day. Adding variety to a program not only keeps you mentally fresh but also strengthens different muscle groups and reduces risk of injury. This also keeps the program interesting. An exercise partner may offer additional motivation.

Vigorous programs for overweight people should be non-weight-bearing activities, such as swimming, water aerobics, and bicycling. Note also that even if weight loss is not possible, overweight people still benefit from regular physical activity.

Whatever physical activities you choose to include in your fitness program, they should be enjoyable. This way they can become routine. Consider convenience, cost, and options for bad weather so that when motivation wanes, you are not adding further obstacles. Overall, do what you enjoy, but start out small, committing to keeping on track and maintaining reasonable expectations. Positive results may take a month or so to be noticeable.

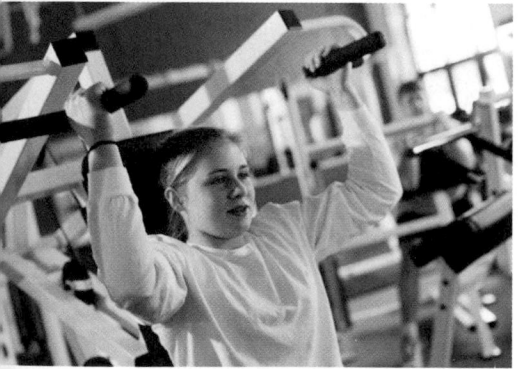

Resistance activities help round out a total fitness plan.

be quickly broken down to release enough energy to make more ATP. This helps resupply ATP until use of carbohydrate and fat fuels begins in earnest. Overall, cells must constantly and repeatedly use and then re-form ATP, using a variety of energy sources.

Phosphocreatine Is the First Line of Defense for Resupplying ATP in Muscles

As soon as ATP stored in muscle cells begins to be used, another source of energy just mentioned, PCr, is used to produce ATP. An enzyme in the muscle cell is activated to split PCr into phosphate and **creatine.** This releases energy that can be used to re-form ATP from its breakdown products. If no other source of energy for ATP resupply were available, PCr could probably maintain maximal muscle contractions for about 10 seconds. Because other ATP resupply sources kick in, however, PCr ends up as a source of energy for events lasting about 1 minute or less.

$$PCr + ADP \rightarrow ATP + Cr$$

The main advantage of PCr is that it can be activated instantly and can replenish ATP at rates fast enough to meet the energy demands of the fastest and most powerful actions, including jumping, lifting, throwing, and sprinting. The disadvantage of PCr is that not much of it is made and stored in the muscles.

Carbohydrate Fuel for Muscles

Carbohydrates are an important fuel for muscles. The most useful form of carbohydrate fuel is the simple sugar glucose, available to all cells from the bloodstream. As you will recall from Chapter 4, glucose is stored as glycogen in the liver and muscle cells. Blood glucose is maintained by the breakdown of liver glycogen. Breakdown of glycogen stored in a specific muscle also helps meet the carbohydrate demand of that muscle, but the actual amount of glycogen stored in muscle is limited (about 350 grams, which would yield about 1400 kcal).

Depending on whether or not oxygen is available to exercising muscles, use of glucose to make ATP can be either anaerobic or aerobic.

Anaerobic Glucose Breakdown Yields Energy Fast

When oxygen supply in the muscle is limited (anaerobic conditions), glucose is broken down into a three-carbon compound called **pyruvic acid.** The pyruvic acid accumulates in the muscle and is then converted to **lactic acid.** Only about 5% of the total amount of ATP that could be formed from complete breakdown of glucose, is released through this anaerobic process (glucose → → lactic acid).

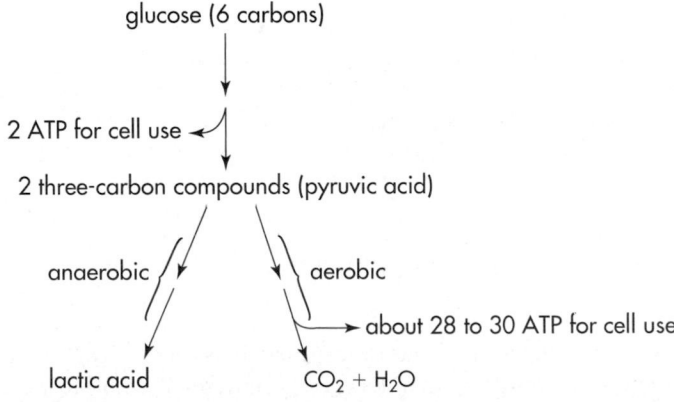

ATP yield from aerobic versus anaerobic glucose utilization.

The advantage of anaerobic glucose breakdown is that it is the fastest way to resupply ATP, other than PCr breakdown. It therefore provides most of the energy needed

creatine An organic (i.e. carbon-containing) molecule in muscle cells that serves as a part of a high-energy compound (termed creatine phosphate or phosphocreatine) capable of synthesizing ATP from ADP.

Strength-training athletes have begun to use creatine supplements (see the second Looking Further section at the end of this Chapter for details).

pyruvic acid A three-carbon compound formed during glucose metabolism; also called *pyruvate*.

lactic acid A three-carbon acid formed during anaerobic cell metabolism; a partial breakdown product of glucose; also called *lactate*.

for events that require a quick burst of energy, ranging from about 30 seconds to 2 minutes. Examples of activities that primarily rely on anaerobic glucose breakdown include sprinting 400 meters or swimming 100 meters.

The two major disadvantages of the anaerobic process are that (1) the high rate of ATP production cannot be sustained for long periods of time, and (2) the rapid accumulation of lactic acid greatly increases the acidity of the muscle. Acidity inhibits the activities of key enzymes in the muscle cells, slowing anaerobic ATP production and causing short-term fatigue. We learn by trial-and-error a pace that will control muscle lactate concentrations during these anaerobic events.

For the most part, lactic acid builds up in active muscle cells until it is released into the bloodstream. The liver (and the kidneys, to some extent) takes up the lactic acid and resynthesizes it into glucose. Glucose can then reenter the bloodstream, where it is available for cell uptake and breakdown. The heart can also use the lactic acid directly for its energy needs, as can less active muscle cells situated near active ones.

Aerobic Glucose Breakdown Is a Sustained Energy Source

If plenty of oxygen is available in the muscle (aerobic conditions), such as when the exercise is of low to moderate intensity, the bulk of the three-carbon pyruvic acid is shuttled to the mitochondria of the cell, where it is further and fully metabolized into carbon dioxide (CO_2) and water (H_2O) (Fig. 11-3). This aerobic breakdown of glucose yields approximately 95% of the ATP made from complete glucose metabolism (glucose $\rightarrow \rightarrow CO_2 + H_2O$).

Aerobic glucose breakdown supplies more ATP than does the anaerobic process, but it releases the energy more slowly. This slower rate of aerobic energy supply can be sustained for hours. One reason is that the end products are carbon dioxide and water, not lactic acid. Aerobic glucose breakdown makes a major energy contribution to activities that last anywhere from 2 minutes to 3 hours or more. Examples of such activities include jogging or distance swimming (review Table 11-1).

Critical Thinking

Marty started going to the gym about 8 weeks ago. At first, he noticed that he began "huffing and puffing" about 7 minutes into his aerobic workout. Now, however, he can work out for about 25 minutes without tiring. What is a possible explanation for this ability to work out longer?

Another Bite

As people start exercising regularly four or five times per week, they experience a "training effect." Initially, these individuals might be able to exercise for 20 minutes before tiring. Months later, exercise can be extended to an hour before they feel tired. During the months of training, muscle cells have produced more mitochondria and thus can burn more fat. Training also increases the number of capillaries in muscles, which increases oxygen supply to the muscles. As a result, lactic acid production from anaerobic glucose metabolism decreases. Because it contributes to short-term muscle fatigue, the less lactic acid produced, the longer the exercise can be sustained. Other contributors to the training effect include increased aerobic efficiency of the heart and muscles, and elevations in muscle triglyceride content, with an enhanced ability of muscles to use triglycerides for energy needs.

Many researchers have studied the ability of various types of carbohydrate feedings to maximize glucose supply to muscles during prolonged exercise. Overall, the techniques have succeeded. Carbohydrate feedings of about 30 to 60 grams per hour during strenuous endurance exercise that lasts 1 hour or more, such as cycling, can aid in maintaining adequate blood glucose, resulting in a delay of fatigue by 30 to 60 minutes. This attention to carbohydrate intake also helps one tolerate vigorous training on a daily basis.

As blood glucose declines during exercise, so does mental function. Cyclists refer to this diminished mental ability as "bonking." Note that the fall in blood glucose is related to depletion of liver glycogen, not muscle glycogen, since liver glycogen is used

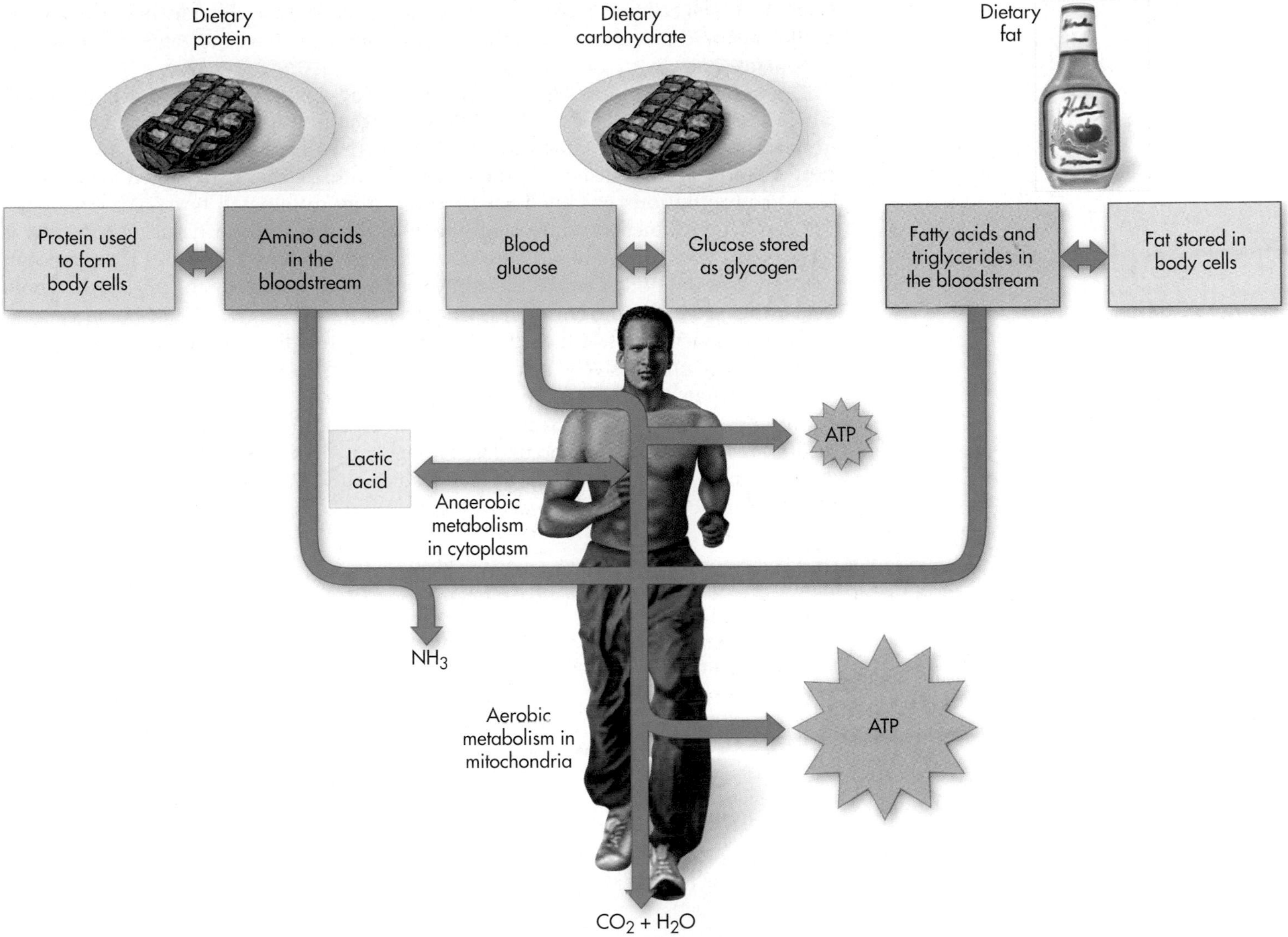

Dietary
protein

Dietary
carbohydrate

Dietary
fat

| Protein used to form body cells | ⟷ | Amino acids in the bloodstream | | Blood glucose | ⟷ | Glucose stored as glycogen | | Fatty acids and triglycerides in the bloodstream | ⟷ | Fat stored in body cells |

Lactic
acid

ATP

Anaerobic
metabolism
in cytoplasm

NH_3

Aerobic
metabolism in
mitochondria

ATP

$CO_2 + H_2O$

Figure 11-3 Simplified view of ATP formation from carbohydrate, fat, and protein. Along with phosphocreatine (PCr) all three nutrients may be used for ATP synthesis, but glucose and fatty acids are primary sources. Glucose may be broken down anaerobically, or may undergo complete aerobic metabolism. The products of fatty acid breakdown are channeled into aerobic metabolism. Although limited, products of amino acid breakdown are channeled into the aerobic pathway as well. Recall also from Chapters 8 and 9 that many vitamins and minerals participate in these metabolic pathways.

to maintain blood glucose. A later section, "Sports Drinks," discusses this topic of carbohydrate replacement during exercise in more detail (see Figure 11-5 on page 396).

Carbohydrate intake during exercise is not as important in shorter events (e.g., one-half hour or so) since the muscles do not take up much blood glucose during short-term exercise, relying instead primarily on their glycogen stores for fuel. This is because the action of the hormone insulin to increase glucose uptake by muscles is blunted by other hormones, such as epinephrine and glucagon, that increase initially during exercise.

■ Fat: The Main Fuel for Prolonged Low-Intensity Activity

When fat stores in body tissues begin to be broken down for energy, each triglyceride first yields three fatty acids and a glycerol. The majority of the stored energy is found in the fatty acids. During physical activity, the fatty acids are released from various adipose tissue depots into the bloodstream and travel to the muscles, where they are

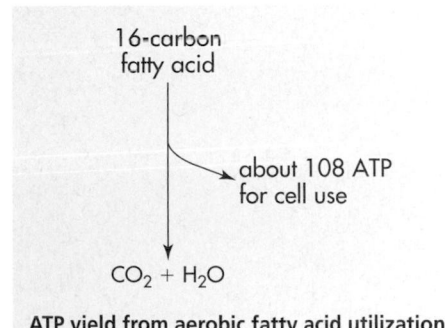

16-carbon
fatty acid

about 108 ATP
for cell use

$CO_2 + H_2O$

ATP yield from aerobic fatty acid utilization.

taken into each cell and broken down aerobically to carbon dioxide and water. Some of the fat stored in muscles also is used, especially as activity increases from a low to a moderate pace.

The rate at which muscles use fatty acids partly depends on the concentration of fatty acids in the bloodstream. In other words, the more fatty acids that are released from adipose tissue stores into the bloodstream, the more fat will be used by the muscles. Recently, some cyclists and other endurance athletes have attempted to raise their blood concentrations of fatty acids by consuming caffeinated beverages. This practice can actually increase fatty acid release from the adipose tissue depots and is therefore helpful to certain athletes, but it is illegal under NCAA rules if the amount of caffeine in the body exceeds the equivalent of 6 to 8 cups of coffee (see the Looking Further section at the end of this Chapter).

Fat, as a general muscle fuel, is not a very useful fuel for intense, brief exercise, but it becomes a progressively more important energy source as duration increases, especially when exercise remains at a low or moderate (aerobic) rate for more than 20 minutes (Fig. 11-4). The reason for this is that some of the steps involved in fat breakdown simply cannot occur fast enough to meet the ATP demands of short-duration, high-intensity exercise. If fat were the only available fuel, we would be unable to exercise beyond a fast walk or jog.

Figure 11-4 Rough estimates of fuel use during various forms of physical activity. With regard to the weightlifting session, carbohydrate use could be somewhat greater and fat use somewhat less if the session is intense and fast-paced (e.g., circuit training). Fat use generally is higher since much of the time spent weight lifting is for rest periods and equipment-related.

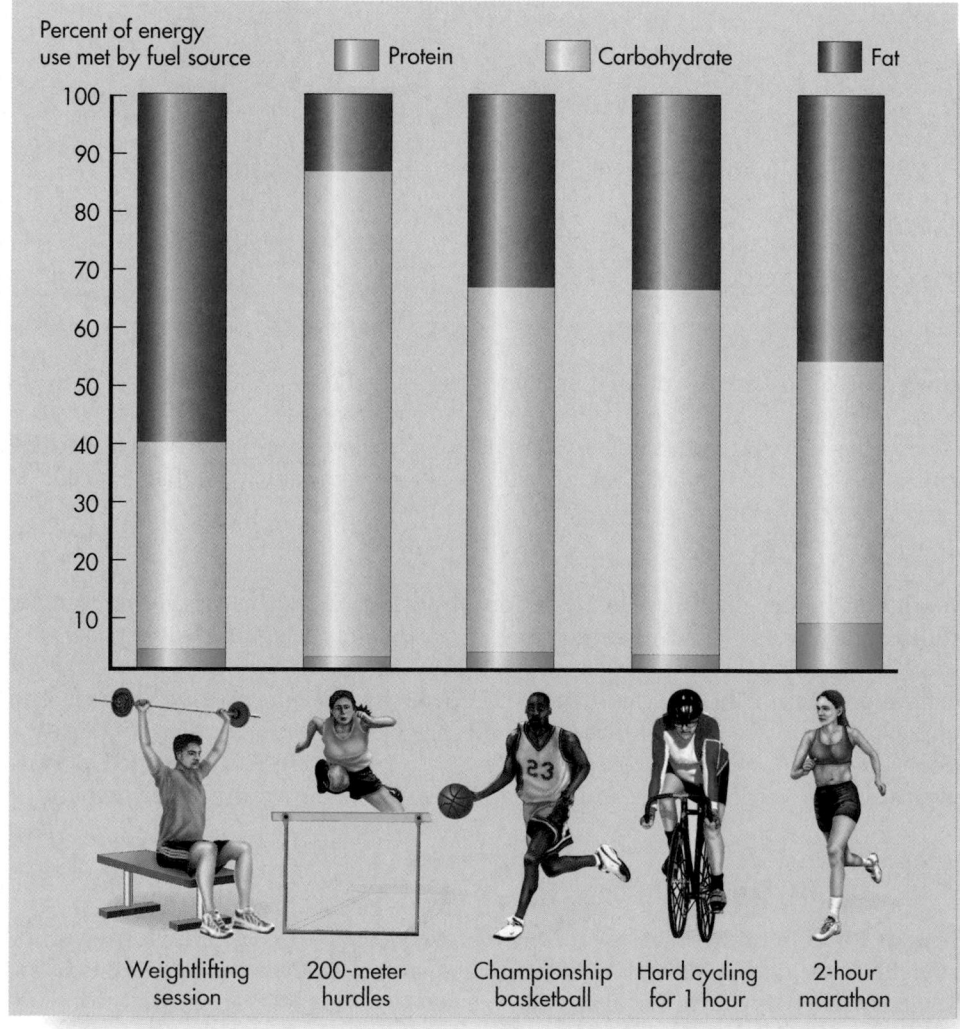

The advantage of fat fuel is that it provides stores of energy in a relatively concentrated form, and we generally have a lot of it stored. For a given weight of fuel, fat supplies more than twice as much energy as carbohydrate does. For very lengthy activities at a moderate pace (for example, hiking) or even sitting at a desk for 8 hours a day, fat supplies about 70% to 90% of the energy required. Carbohydrate use is much less. As intensity increases, such as in a 3-hour marathon run at a competitive pace, muscles use about a 50:50 ratio of fat to carbohydrate. In comparison, for short events, such as a 100-meter sprint or even a 1500-meter race, the contribution of fat used to resupply ATP is minimal. To summarize, remember that the only fast-paced (anaerobic) fuel we eat is carbohydrate; slow and steady (aerobic) activity uses much fat in addition to carbohydrate.

■ Protein: A Minor Fuel Source, Primarily for Endurance Exercise

Although amino acids derived from protein can be used to fuel muscles, their contribution is relatively small, compared with that of carbohydrate and fat. As a rough guide, only about 5% of the body's general energy needs, as well as the typical energy needs of exercising muscles, is supplied by the metabolism of amino acids.

During endurance exercise, proteins can contribute importantly to energy needs, perhaps as much as 10% to 15%, especially as glycogen stores in the muscle are exhausted. Most of the energy supplied from protein comes from metabolism of the branched-chain amino acids—leucine, isoleucine, and valine. Because a normal diet provides enough protein to supply this amount of fuel, protein or amino acid supplements are not needed. Contrary to what many athletes believe, protein is used for fuel less in resistance types of exercise (e.g., weightlifting) than in endurance exercise (e.g., running) (review Fig. 11-4). The primary muscle fuels for weightlifting are phosphocreatine (PCr) and carbohydrate for the brief bursts of activity, with fat providing energy during the resting stages, and little use of protein overall. Despite this fact, high-protein products such as Pro-Complex, Amino Fuel 2000, High Voltage Protein Drink, and Instant Egg Protein are marketed specifically to weightlifters and bodybuilders in nearly every health-food and fitness store. Note also that consuming high-carbohydrate, moderate-protein foods immediately after a weight-training workout enhances the muscle-building effect of the activity, most likely by increasing the concentrations of insulin and growth hormone released into the blood and contributing to protein synthesis. Still, it is impossible to increase muscle mass simply by eating protein. Putting physical strain on muscle through strength training or other physical activity is needed.

Concept Check

Adenosine triphosphate (ATP) is the main form of energy used by cells. Cells use food energy to form ATP. Phosphocreatine (PCr) can rapidly re-form ATP from its breakdown product adenosine diphosphate (ADP), but PCr supplies are limited. Carbohydrate metabolism to form ATP begins as glucose becomes available from the absorption of carbohydrates from the diet or glycogen breakdown. In a muscle cell, each glucose molecule is broken down through a series of steps to yield either lactic acid or carbon dioxide (CO_2) plus water (H_2O). The process that occurs when glucose is broken down into carbon dioxide and water is called *aerobic* because oxygen is used. The conversion of glucose to lactic acid is called *anaerobic* because no oxygen is used. The anaerobic process allows the cell to quickly re-form ATP and supports the demand for energy during intense exercise. Fat is a key aerobic fuel for muscle cells, especially at low exercise outputs. At rest and during light activity, muscles burn primarily fat for energy needs. In comparison, little protein generally is used to fuel muscles. At most, protein supplies 10% to 15% of energy needs during endurance activities, especially when glycogen stores are depleted.

Fatty acids can come from all over the body, not necessarily from depots near the active muscles. **This is why spot reducing does not work.** Exercise can tone the muscles that are near adipose tissue but does not preferentially use those stores. If this was not the case, we would all have lean cheeks and necks, because muscles in that vicinity are regularly used.

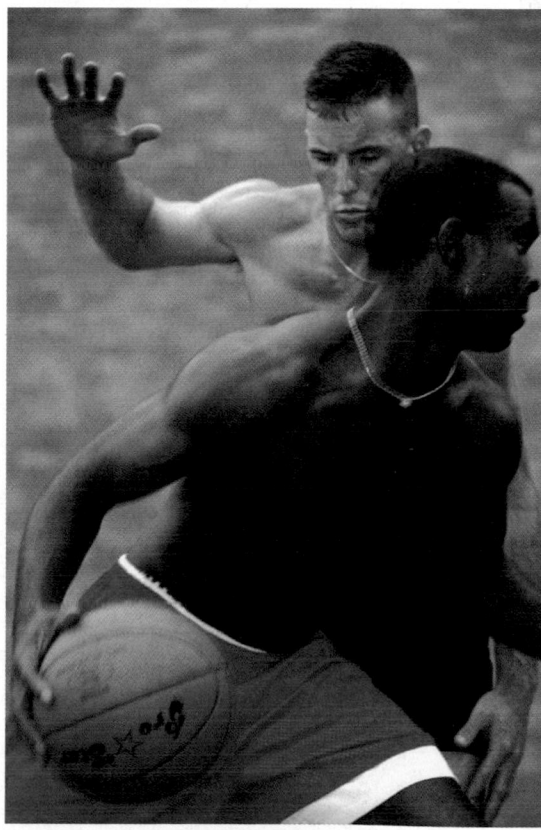

The calories needed to perform come from carbohydrate, fat, and protein. The relative mix depends on the pace.

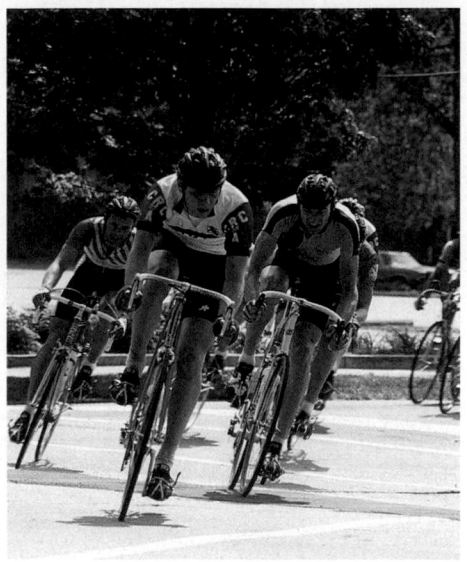

Athletes often expend much energy. In such cases, their increased food intake should easily provide ample protein and other nutrients to support activity.

Power Food: Dietary Advice for Athletes

Athletic training and genetic makeup are two very important determinants of athletic performance. A good diet won't substitute for either factor, but diet can help to enhance and maximize an athlete's potential. On the other hand, a poor diet can seriously harm performance.

■ Calorie Needs

Athletes need varying amounts of calories, depending on each athlete's body size, body composition, and on the type of training or competition being considered. A small person may need only 1700 kcal daily to sustain normal daily activities without losing body weight; a large, muscular man may need 4000 kcal. These rough estimates can be viewed as starting points that need to be individualized by trial and error for each athlete.

An estimate of the calories required to sustain moderate activity is 5 to 8 kcal per minute. The calories required for sports training or competition then have to be added to those used just to carry on normal activities. For example, an hour of bowling requires few calories in addition to that required to sustain normal daily living. At the other extreme, a 12-hour endurance bicycle race over mountains can require an additional 4000 kcal per day. Therefore, some athletes may need as much as 7000 kcal or more daily just to maintain body weight while training, whereas others may need 1700 kcal or less. If an athlete experiences daily fatigue, the first consideration should be whether he or she is consuming enough food. Up to six meals per day may be needed, including one before each workout.

How can we know if an athlete is getting enough calories? Estimating daily intake from a food diary kept by the athlete is one way. Another step is to estimate the athlete's body fat percentage via skinfold measurements, bioelectrical impedance, or underwater weighing (review Chapter 10). Body fat should be the typical amount found for athletes in the specific sport practiced. This corresponds to 5% to 18% for most male athletes and 17% to 28% for most female athletes. The next step is to monitor body weight changes on a daily or weekly basis. If body weight starts to fall, calories should be increased; if weight rises and it is because of increases in body fat, the athlete should eat less.

Another Bite

Wrestlers, boxers, judoists, jockeys, and oarsmen often try to lose weight before a competition, so that they can be certified to compete in a lower weight class. This helps them gain a mechanical advantage over an opponent of smaller stature. They usually lose this weight before stepping on the scale for weight certification. Athletes can lose up to 22 pounds (10 kilograms) of body weight as water in 1 day by sitting in a sauna, exercising in a plastic sweat suit, or taking diuretic drugs, which speed water loss from the kidneys. Losing as little as 2% of body weight by dehydration, however, can adversely affect endurance performance, especially in hot weather. A pattern of repeated weight loss or gain of more than 5% of body weight by dehydration carries risk of kidney malfunction and heat-related illness. Death is also a possibility.

To prevent future deaths from such weight loss in athletes, the National Collegiate Athletic Association and many states have authorized physicians or athletic trainers to set safe weight and body fat content minimums (e.g., 7% or more of total body weight) for their athletes in weight-class sports. Under new guidelines, athletes are assigned to weight classes at the beginning of the season and are not allowed to "cut weight" to gain a competitive advantage. If athletes, such as wrestlers, wish to compete in a lower-body-weight class and have enough extra fat stores, they should begin a gradual, sustained reduction in calorie intake long before the competitive season starts.

If the body composition test shows that an athlete has too much body fat, the athlete should lower food intake by about 200 to 500 kcal per day, while maintaining a regular exercise program, until the desirable fat percentage is achieved. Reducing fat intake is the best nutrient-related approach. On the other hand, if an athlete needs to gain weight, increasing food intake by 500 to 700 kcal per day will eventually lead to the needed weight gain. A mix of carbohydrate, fat, and protein is advised, coupled with exercise to make sure this gain is mostly in the form of lean tissue, and not fat stores.

■ Carbohydrate Needs

Anyone who exercises vigorously, especially for more than 1 hour per day on a regular basis, needs to consume a diet that includes moderate to high amounts of carbohydrates. The diet should include a variety of foods, such as those recommended by MyPyramid. Numerous servings of grains, starchy vegetables, and fruits provide enough carbohydrate to maintain adequate liver and muscle glycogen stores, especially for replacing glycogen losses from workouts on the previous day. Relatively low-carbohydrate/high-protein diets, such as *The Zone Diet*, are not recommended. Recall that Chapter 10 discussed the Zone Diet. The carbohydrate content of this diet is only 40% of calories, rather than the 60% or more that is typically recommended for athletes.

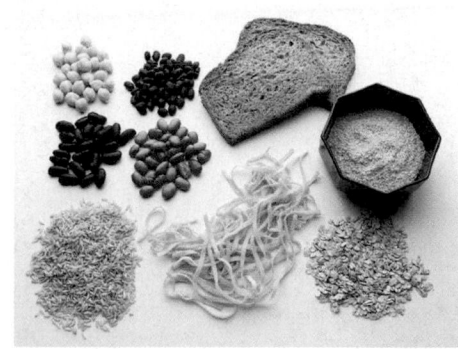

High carbohydrate foods should form the basis of the diet for athletes.

Carbohydrate intake should be at least 5 grams per kilogram body weight. People engaged in aerobic training and endurance activities (duration 60 minutes or more per day) may need as much as 7 grams per kilogram body weight. When exercise duration approaches several hours per day, the carbohydrate recommendation increases to up to 10 grams per kilogram of body weight. In other words, triathletes and marathoners should consider eating close to 500 to 600 grams of carbohydrates daily, and even more if necessary, to (1) prevent chronic fatigue and (2) load the muscles and liver with glycogen. Attention to carbohydrate intake is especially important when performing multiple training bouts in a day, such as swim practices, or heavy training on successive days, as in cross-country running. Depletion of carbohydrate ranks just behind depletion of fluid and electrolytes as a major cause of fatigue. Table 11-2 shows sample menus, based on MyPyramid, for diets providing food energy ranging from 1500 to 5000 kcal per day. In addition, the Exchange System described in Appendix C is a very useful tool for planning all types of diets, including high-carbohydrate diets for athletes.

As noted above, athletes should obtain at least 60% of their total energy needs from carbohydrate (rather than the 50% typical of most North American diets), especially if exercise duration is expected to exceed 2 hours and total caloric intake is about 3000 kcal per day or less. Diets containing 4000 to 5000 kcal per day can be as low as 50% carbohydrate, as these will still provide sufficient carbohydrate (e.g., 500 to 600 grams or so per day).

Note that one does not have to give up any specific food when planning a high-carbohydrate diet. The focus is to include more high-carbohydrate foods while moderating concentrated fat sources. Sports nutritionists emphasize the difference between a high-carbohydrate meal and a high-carbohydrate/high-fat meal. Before endurance events, such as marathons or triathlons, some athletes seek to increase their carbohydrate reserves by eating foods such as potato chips, French fries, banana cream pie, and pastries. Although such foods contain carbohydrate, they also contain a lot of fat. Better high-carbohydrate food choices include pasta, rice, potatoes, bread, fruit and fruit juices, and many breakfast cereals (check the label for carbohydrate content) (Table 11-3). Sports drinks appropriate for carbohydrate loading, such as GatorLode and UltraFuel, can also help. Consuming a moderate rather than a high amount of fiber during the final day of training is a good precaution to reduce the chances of bloating and intestinal gas during the next day's event.

For athletes who compete in continuous, intense aerobic events lasting more than 60 to 90 minutes (or in shorter events taking place more than once within a 24-hour period), a **carbohydrate-loading** regimen can help to maximize the amount of energy

Critical Thinking

Joe is a wrestler who qualified for the 125-pound weight classification in the annual state high school competition. After a few matches, Joe began to feel dizzy and faint. He was disqualified because he was unable to continue the match. Later, the coach found out that Joe had spent 2 hours in the sauna before weighing in, which had made him dehydrated. What are the consequences of dehydration? What can you suggest as a safer alternative for weight loss?

carbohydrate loading A process in which a very high carbohydrate intake is consumed for 6 days before an athletic event while tapering exercise duration in an attempt to increase muscle glycogen stores.

Table 11-2 Sample Daily Menus Based on MyPyramid That Provide Various Total Calorie Intakes

1500 kcal Diet	2000 kcal Diet	3000 kcal Diet	4000 kcal Diet	5000 kcal Diet
Breakfast	**Breakfast**	**Breakfast**	**Breakfast**	**Breakfast**
Fat-free milk, 1 cup	Fat-free milk, 1 cup	Fat-free milk, 1 cup	Orange, 1	Cheerios, 2 cups
Cheerios, ½ cup	Cheerios, 1 cup	Cheerios, 2 cups	Cheerios, 2 cups	Bran muffins, 2
Bagel, ½	Bagel, ½	Bagel, 1	Fat-free milk, 1 cup	Orange, 1
Cherry jam, 2 tsp	Cherry jam, 1 tbsp	Cherry jam, 2 tsp	Bran muffins, 2	Fat-reduced milk, 1 cup
Margarine, 1 tsp	Margarine, 1 tsp	Margarine, 1 tsp		
		Oat bran muffins, 2	**Snack**	**Snack**
Lunch	**Lunch**		Chopped dates, ¾ cup	Low-fat yogurt, 1 cup
Chicken breast (roasted), 2 oz	Chicken breast (roasted), 2 oz	**Lunch**		Chopped dates, 1 cup
Figs, 1	Wheat bread, 2 slices	Chicken breast (roasted), 2 oz	**Lunch**	
Fat-free milk, ½ cup	Mayonnaise, 1 tsp	Wheat bread, 2 slices	Romaine lettuce, 1 cup	**Lunch**
Banana, 1	Raisins, ¼ cup	Provolone cheese, 1 oz	Garbanzo beans, 1 cup	Apple juice, 1 cup
	Cranberry juice, 1½ cups	Mayonnaise, 1 tsp	Grated carrots, ½ cup	Chicken enchilada, 1
Snack	Banana, 1	Raisins, ⅓ cup	French dressing, 2 tbsp	Romaine lettuce, 1 cup
Oatmeal-raisin cookie, 1		Cranberry juice, 1½ cups	Macaroni and cheese, 3 cups	Garbanzo beans, 1 cup
Low-fat fruit yogurt, 1 cup	**Snack**	Low-fat fruit yogurt, 1 cup	Apple juice, 1 cup	Shredded carrots, ¾ cup
	Oatmeal-raisin cookies, 3			Chopped celery, ½ cup
	Low-fat fruit yogurt, 1 cup	**Snack**	**Snack**	Seasoned croutons, 1 oz
Dinner		Banana, 1	Wheat bread, 2 slices	French dressing, 2 tbsp
Spaghetti w/meatballs, 1 cup	**Dinner**	Oatmeal-raisin cookies, 3	Margarine, 1 tsp	Wheat bread, 2 slices
Romaine lettuce, 1 cup	Broiled beef sirloin, 3 oz		Jam, 2 tbsp	Margarine, 1 tbsp
Italian dressing, 2 tsp	Romaine lettuce, 1 cup	**Dinner**		
Green beans, ½ cup	Italian dressing, 2 tsp	Broiled beef sirloin, 3 oz	**Dinner**	**Snack**
Cranberry juice, 1½ cups	Green beans, 1 cup	Romaine lettuce, 1 cup	Skinless turkey breast, 2 oz	Banana, 1
	Fat-free milk, ½ cup	Garbanzo beans, 1 cup	Mashed potatoes, 2 cups	Bagel, 1
		Italian dressing, 2 tsp	Peas and onions, 1 cup	Cream cheese, 1 tbsp
18% protein (68 grams)	17% protein (85 grams)	Spinach pasta noodles, 1½ cups	Banana, 1	
64% carbohydrate (240 grams)	63% carbohydrate (315 grams)	Margarine, 1 tsp	Fat-free milk, 1 cup	**Dinner**
19% fat (32 grams)	20% fat (44 grams)	Green beans, 1 cup		Fat-reduced milk, 1 cup
		Fat-free milk, ½ cup	**Snack**	Beef sirloin, 5 oz
			Pasta, 1 cup cooked	Mashed potatoes, 2 cups
		17% protein (128 grams)	Margarine, 2 tsp	Spinach pasta noodles, 1½ cups
		62% carbohydrate (465 grams)	Parmesan cheese, 2 tbsp	Grated parmesan cheese, 2 tbsp
		21% fat (70 grams)	Cranberry juice, 1 cup	Green beans, 1 cup
				Oatmeal-raisin cookies, 3
			14% protein (140 grams)	
			61% carbohydrate (610 grams)	**Snack**
			26% fat (116 grams)	Cranberry juice, 2 cups
				Air-popped popcorn, 4 cups
				Raisins, ⅓ cup
				14% protein (175 grams)
				63% carbohydrate (813 grams)
				24% fat (136 grams)

stored in the form of muscle glycogen for the event. (Note, however, that this amount of activity applies to few athletes.) In one possible regimen, during the week prior to the event, the athlete gradually reduces the intensity and duration of exercise ("tapering") while simultaneously increasing the percentage of total calories supplied by carbohydrate.

For example, consider the carbohydrate-loading schedule of a 25-year-old man preparing for a marathon. His typical calorie needs are about 3500 kcal per day. Six days before competition, he completes a final hard workout of 60 minutes. On that day, carbohydrates contribute 45% to 50% of his total calorie intake. As he goes through the rest of the week, the duration of his workouts decreases to 40 minutes, and then to about 20 minutes by the end of the week. Meanwhile, he increases the amount of carbohydrate in his diet to reach 70% to 80% of total calorie intake as

Table 11-3 Grams of Carbohydrate Based on Serving Size of Typical Carbohydrate-Rich Foods

Starches—15 grams Carbohydrate per Serving (80 kcal)

One Serving

½–¾ cup dry breakfast cereal*	¼ large baked potato
½ cup cooked breakfast cereal	¼ bagel (4 ounces)
½ cup cooked grits	½ English muffin
⅓ cup cooked rice	1 slice bread
⅓ cup cooked pasta	¾ oz pretzels
⅓ cup baked beans	6 saltine crackers
½ cup cooked corn	1 pancake, 4 inches in diameter
½ cup cooked/dry beans	2 taco shells (add 45 kcal)

Vegetables—5 grams Carbohydrate per Serving (25 kcal)

One Serving

½ cup cooked vegetables
1 cup raw vegetables
½ cup vegetable juice
Examples: carrots, green beans, broccoli, cauliflower, onions, spinach, tomatoes, vegetable juice

Fruits—15 grams Carbohydrate per Serving (60 kcal)

One Serving

½ cup canned fruit or berries	17 grapes (small)
½ cup fruit juice	½ grapefruit 1½ figs (dried)
1 small apple or orange	3 dates
8 apricots (dried)	1 peach
1 small banana	1¼ cups watermelon cubes

Milk—12 grams Carbohydrate per Serving

One Serving

1 cup milk	1 cup soymilk
⅔ cup plain low-fat yogurt	

Sweets—15 grams Carbohydrate per Serving (variable calories)

One Serving

2-inch square typical slice of cake	½ cup ice cream
2 small cookies	½ cup sherbet

Modified from *Exchange Lists for Meal Planning* by the American Diabetes Association and American Dietetic Association, 2003, Chicago, American Dietetic Association.

*Note that the carbohydrate content of dry cereal varies widely. Check the labels of the ones you choose and adjust serving size accordingly.

the week continues. Total calorie intake should decrease as exercise time decreases throughout the week. On the final day before competition, he rests while maintaining the high-carbohydrate intake.

Carbohydrate Loading Regimen

Days Before Competition	6	5	4	3	2	1
Exercise time (minutes)	60	40	40	20	20	Rest
Carbohydrate (grams)	450	450	450	600	600	600

This carbohydrate-loading technique usually increases muscle glycogen stores by 50% to 85% over typical conditions (that is, when dietary carbohydrate constitutes only about 50% of total calorie intake).

A potential disadvantage of carbohydrate loading is that additional water (about 3 grams) is incorporated into the muscles along with each gram of glycogen. Although it aids in maintaining hydration, for some individuals this additional water weight and related muscle stiffness detract from their sports performance, making carbohydrate loading inappropriate. Athletes considering a carbohydrate-loading regimen

Appropriate Activities for Carbohydrate Loading

Marathons
Long-distance swimming
Cross-country skiing
30-kilometer runs
Triathlons
Tournament-play basketball
Soccer
Cycling time trials
Long-distance canoe racing

Inappropriate Activities for Carbohydrate Loading

American football games
10-kilometer or shorter runs
Walking and hiking
Most swimming events
Single basketball games
Weightlifting
Most track and field events

Consuming excessive amounts of protein has drawbacks. As noted in Chapter 6, it increases calcium loss somewhat in the urine. It also leads to increased urine production, possibly compromising body hydration. It also may lead to kidney stones in people with a history of this or other kidney problems. Finally, enough carbohydrate fuel may not be consumed on such a diet, leading to fatigue.

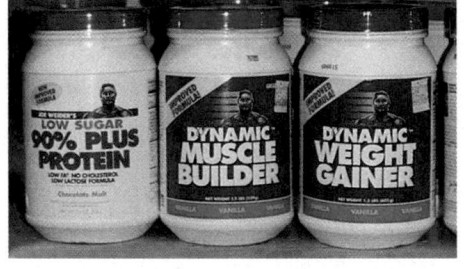

High-protein products, which are often marketed to athletes, are unnecessary. The same holds true for high-protein bars, a current trend in marketing products to athletes.

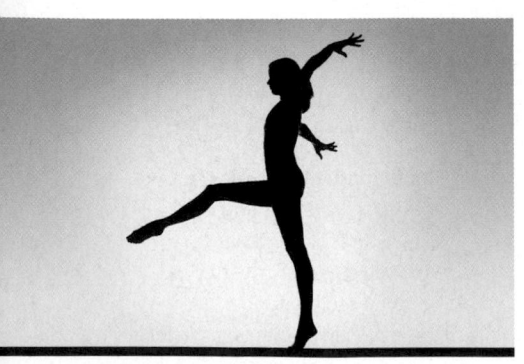

Weight-restricted athletes especially should make sure they are consuming enough protein as well as other essential nutrients.

should try it during training (and well before an important competition) to experience its effects on performance. They can then determine whether it is worth the effort. Note also that carbohydrate feeding during a competition provides about the same advantage as carbohydrate loading prior to the event. In fact, expert advice is currently shifting away from carbohydrate loading and more toward this second method, coupled with a daily diet high in carbohydrate. In addition, remember the importance of the "training effect" discussed in "Another Bite" on page 384.

■ Fat Needs

A diet containing up to 35% of calories from fat is generally recommended for athletes. Rich sources of monounsaturated fat, such as canola oil, should be emphasized, and saturated fat and *trans* fat intake should be limited.

■ Protein Needs

Typical recommendations for protein intake in the sports nutrition literature for most athletes range from 1.0 to 1.6 grams of protein per kilogram of body weight. This is considerably higher than the RDA of 0.8 grams per kilogram body weight for nonathletes recommended by the Food and Nutrition Board for all adults, including athletes (Table 11-4).

For athletes beginning a strength-training program, some experts recommend up to 1.7 grams of protein per kilogram of body weight. That is more than twice the RDA for protein. To date, the value of such an excessive protein intake during the initial phases of strength training has not been supported by sufficient research. In addition, protein intakes above this amount simply result in an increased use of amino acids for energy needs; no further increase in muscle protein synthesis is seen. Note also that calorie needs for strength training itself are not the reason for the high protein recommendation, as the fuel used in this activity is primarily phosphocreatine and carbohydrate. The extra protein, theoretically, is required for the synthesis of new muscle tissue brought on by the loading effect of strength training. Once the desired muscle mass is achieved, protein intake need not exceed 1.2 grams per kilogram of body weight.

Table 11-4 summarizes recommended ranges of protein intakes for various types of activity. Any athlete not specifically on a low-calorie regimen can easily meet these protein recommendations simply by eating a variety of foods (review Table 11-2). To illustrate, a 123-pound (53-kilogram) woman who is performing endurance activity can consume 64 grams of protein (53 × 1.2) during a single day by including 3 ounces of chicken (one chicken breast), 3 ounces of beef (a small, lean hamburger), and two glasses of milk in her diet. Similarly, a 180-pound (77-kilogram) man who aims to gain muscle mass through strength training needs to consume only 6 ounces of chicken (a large chicken breast), ½ cup of cooked beans, a 6-ounce can of tuna, and three glasses

Table 11-4 Current Recommendations for Protein Intake Based on kilograms Body Weight*

Activity Group	grams/kilograms	Amount for a 70-kilogram Person (grams)
Sedentary	0.8	56
Strength trained, maintenance	1.0–1.2	70–84
Strength trained, gain muscle mass	1.5–1.7	105–119
Moderate intensity endurance activities	1.2	84
High-intensity endurance training	1.6	112

*Calculate kilograms by dividing pounds by 2.2.

Source: Burke L, Deakin V: Clinical Sports Nutrition, McGraw-Hill, Roseville NSW2069, Australia, 2000.

of milk to achieve an intake of 130 grams of protein (77 × 1.7) in a day. And, for both athletes, these calculations do not even include the protein present in grains or vegetables they will also eat. As you can see, simply by meeting their calorie needs, many athletes consume much more protein than is required. Despite marketing claims, protein supplements are an expensive and unnecessary part of a fitness plan.

Athletes who either feel they must significantly limit their calorie intake or are vegetarians should specifically determine how much protein they eat. They should make sure to follow a diet that provides at least 1.2 grams of protein per kilogram of body weight per day, the upper recommendation for most athletes.

■ Vitamin and Mineral Needs

Vitamin and mineral needs are the same or slightly higher for athletes, compared with those of sedentary adults. Still, because athletes usually have such high calorie intakes, they tend to consume plenty of vitamins and minerals. An exception is athletes consuming low-calorie diets (about 1200 kcal or less), such as seen with some female athletes participating in events in which maintaining a low body weight is crucial. These diets may not meet B-vitamin and other micronutrient needs. Vegetarian athletes are also a concern. In these cases, consuming fortified foods, such as ready-to-eat breakfast cereals, or a balanced multivitamin and mineral supplement is recommended.

Athletes' needs for vitamin E and vitamin C may be somewhat greater because of the potential antioxidant protection these nutrients provide; this effect could be especially important in the face of high oxygen use by muscles. Still, the use of large doses of vitamin E and vitamin C requires more study and is not currently an accepted part of the dietary guidance for athletes. Experts such as Dr. Priscilla Clarkson suggest simply following a diet containing foods rich in antioxidants, such as fruits, vegetables, whole-grain breads and cereals, and vegetable oils. In addition, there is evidence that antioxidant systems in the body increase in activity as exercise training progresses. There is also speculation that the "oxidant stress" produced during exercise might have benefits, such as for muscle adaptation to exercise, and so trying to block this process may not be wise.

Iron Deficiency Impairs Performance

Since iron is involved in red blood cell production, oxygen transport, and energy production, a deficiency of this mineral can noticeably detract from optimal athletic performance. The potential causes for iron deficiency in athletes vary. As in the general population, female athletes are most susceptible to low iron status due to monthly menstrual losses. Special diets followed by athletes, such as low-calorie and vegetarian (especially vegan) diets are likely to be low in iron. Distance runners should pay special attention to iron intake, because their intense workouts may lead to gastrointestinal bleeding. Another concern is *sports anemia*—which occurs because exercise causes blood plasma volume to expand, particularly at the start of a training regimen before the synthesis of red blood cells increases. This results in dilution of the blood. In this case, even if iron stores are adequate, blood iron tests may appear low.

Sports anemia is not detrimental to performance, but it is hard to differentiate between sports anemia and true anemia. If iron status is low and not replenished, iron-deficiency anemia and markedly impaired endurance performance can eventually result. Although true anemia (noted as a depressed blood hemoglobin level) is not that common among athletes, it is a good idea, especially for adult women athletes, to have their iron status checked at the beginning of a training season and at least once during midseason, and to monitor dietary iron intake.

Any blood test indicating low iron status—sports anemia or not—is cause for follow-up. For some, the use of iron supplements may be advisable. However, indiscriminate use of iron supplements is not advised because toxic effects are possible.

Recall from Chapter 8 that any supplement use especially should not exceed any Upper Levels set over the long term. As well, men should be cautious about any use of supplements containing iron.

At one time in his career, long-distance runner Alberto Salazar experienced problems sleeping and performed poorly because of low iron intake and related iron-deficiency anemia.

It is important that physicians investigate the cause of the deficiency since iron deficiency can be caused by blood loss. If caught early, some serious medical conditions such as this can be treated or prevented.

Some studies have suggested that iron deficiency without anemia may also have a negative effect on physical activity and performance. Also, once depleted, iron stores can take months to replenish. For this reason, athletes must be especially careful to meet iron needs.

Calcium Intake Deserves Attention, Especially in Women

Athletes, especially women trying to lose weight by restricting their intake of dairy products, can have marginal or low dietary intakes of calcium. This practice compromises optimal bone health. Of still greater concern are women athletes who have stopped menstruating because their arduous exercise training and low body fat content interferes with the normal secretion of the reproductive hormones. Disturbing reports show that female athletes who do not menstruate regularly have far less dense spinal bones than both nonathletes and female athletes who menstruate regularly. This places them at increased risk for bone fractures during training and competition, and osteoporosis in later life. This combination of risks outweighs the benefits of weight-bearing exercise on bone density. This topic is discussed further in Chapter 12, with respect to the female athlete triad, and in Chapter 9, where osteoporosis was reviewed in detail.

Research has clearly documented the importance of regular menstruation to maintain bone mineral density. Current studies show that a woman runner who does not menstruate regularly may also have a higher risk for the development of a **stress fracture.** Thus, female athletes whose menstrual cycles become irregular should consult a physician to ascertain the cause. Decreasing the amount of training or increasing energy intake and body weight often restores regular menstrual cycles. If irregular menstrual cycles persist, severe bone loss (much of which is not reversible) and osteoporosis can result. Extra calcium in the diet does not necessarily compensate for the effects of menstrual irregularities, but inadequate dietary calcium can make matters worse.

A Focus on Fluid Needs

Water (fluid) needs for an average adult are about 9 cups per day for women and 13 cups per day for men. Athletes need this and generally even more water to maintain the body's ability to regulate internal temperature and to keep cool. Most energy released during metabolism appears immediately as heat. Furthermore, heat production in contracting muscles can rise 15 to 20 times above that of resting muscles. Unless this heat is quickly dissipated, heat exhaustion, heat cramps, and deadly heatstroke may ensue. In fact, typically three to five athletes die each year of heatstroke. In 2001, both college football players and a professional football player died this way.

Heat exhaustion occurs when heat stress causes loss of body fluid and then depletion of blood volume. Maintaining adequate body fluid is important. As environmental temperature rises above 95°F (35°C), virtually all body heat is lost through the evaporation of sweat from the skin. Sweat rates during prolonged exercise range from 3 to 8 cups (750 to 2000 milliliters) per hour. However, as the humidity rises, especially when it rises above 75%, evaporation slows and sweating becomes an inefficient way to cool the body. The result is rapid fatigue, increased work for the heart, and difficulty with prolonged exertion. Clearly, the combination of high heat and humidity (e.g., 95°F and 90% humidity) can be as dangerous as extreme cold.

Increased body temperature associated with dehydration is evident when the amount of water loss only exceeds 2% of body weight, especially in hot weather. This dehydration then leads to a decline in endurance, strength, and overall performance. Wearing football equipment in hot weather can lead to a loss of 2% of body weight in

stress fracture A fracture that occurs from repeated jarring of a bone. Common sites include bones of the foot.

heat exhaustion The first stage of heat-related illness that occurs because of depletion of blood volume from fluid loss by the body. This increases body temperature and can lead to headache, dizziness, muscle weakness, and visual disturbances, among other effects.

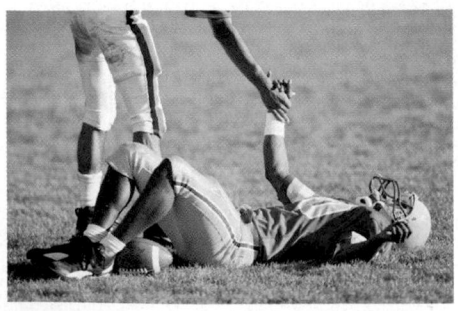

Dehydration, which can lead to illness and death, is a problem that must be avoided during physical activity.

30 minutes. Marathon runners have been shown to lose 6% to 10% of body weight during a race.

Common symptoms of heat exhaustion include profuse sweating, headache, dizziness, nausea, vomiting, muscle weakness, visual disturbances, and flushing of the skin. A person with heat exhaustion should be taken to a cool environment immediately, and excess clothing should be removed. The body should be sponged with tap water. Fluid replacement, as tolerated, then should suffice to correct the condition.

Heat cramps are a frequent complication of heat exhaustion, but they may appear without other symptoms of dehydration. Cramps usually occur in individuals who have exercised for several hours in a hot climate, experienced significant sweating, and who have consumed a large volume of water without replacing sodium losses. It is important not to confuse heat cramps with other forms of muscle cramps, such as those caused by GI tract upset. Heat cramps occur in skeletal muscles, including those of the abdomen and extremities. They consist of a contraction lasting 1 to 3 minutes at a time. The cramp moves down the muscle and is associated with excruciating pain. The best way to prevent heat cramps is to exercise moderately at first and to have adequate salt intake before engaging in long, strenuous activity in the heat, and not become dehydrated.

Heatstroke can occur when the internal body temperature reaches 104 °F or more. Related symptoms include nausea, confusion, irritability, poor coordination, seizures, and coma (in severe cases). Exertional heatstroke results from high blood flow to exercising muscles, which overloads the body's cooling capacity. Sweating generally ceases, and the body temperature may become dangerously high. If left untreated, circulatory collapse, nervous system damage, and death are likely. The death rate from heat stroke is high, approximately 10%.

Many individuals faint during heatstroke, and their skin becomes hot and dry. Cooling the skin with ice packs or cold water is the usual recommended immediate treatment until medical help can be summoned. To decrease the risk of developing heatstroke, athletes should watch for rapid body-weight changes (2% or more of body weight), replace lost fluids, and avoid exercising under extremely hot, humid conditions.

Athletes must avoid becoming dehydrated since dehydration during exercise sets the stage for heat exhaustion, heat cramps, and potentially fatal heatstroke. Fluid intake during exercise, when possible, should be adequate to minimize body-weight loss; following this practice is a good idea even when sweating can go unnoticed, such as when swimming or during the winter.

The recommended fluid status goal is a loss of no more than 2% of body weight during exercise. Athletes should first calculate 2% of their body weight and then by trial and error determine how much fluid they must take in to avoid losing more than this amount of weight during exercise. This determination will be most accurate if an athlete is weighed before and after a typical workout. For every 1 pound (½ kilogram) lost, 2½ to 3 cups (about 0.75 liters) of water should be consumed during exercise or immediately afterward. Experts now recommend a total of 2½ to 3 cups of water per pound lost, rather than the previous recommendation of 2 cups per pound, as some of the fluid replacement will quickly be lost via increased sweating after exercise and increased urine output. Much of this fluid replacement will have to take place after exercise since it is difficult to consume enough fluid during exercise to prevent weight loss. If weight change can't be monitored, urine color is another measure of hydration status. Urine color should be no more yellow than that of lemonade.

Thirst is a late sign of dehydration and so is not a reliable indicator of an athlete's need to replace fluid during exercise. An athlete who drinks only when thirsty is likely to take 48 hours to replenish fluid loss. After several days of training, an athlete relying on thirst as an indicator can build up a fluid debt that will impair performance. The following fluid replacement approach can meet athletes' fluid needs in most cases:

- Freely drink beverages (e.g., water, diluted fruit juice, sports drinks) during the 24-hour period before an event, even if not particularly thirsty.
- Drink 1½ to 2½ cups of fluid (400 to 600 milliliters) 2 to 3 hours before exercise.

heat cramps A frequent complication of heat exhaustion. They usually occur in people who have experienced large sweat losses from exercising for several hours in a hot climate and have consumed a large volume of water. The cramps occur in skeletal muscles and consist of contractions for 1 to 3 minutes at a time.

heatstroke Heatstroke can occur when internal body temperature reaches 104°F. Sweating generally ceases if left untreated, and blood circulation is greatly reduced. Nervous system damage may ensue, and death is likely. Often the skin of individuals who suffer heatstroke is hot and dry.

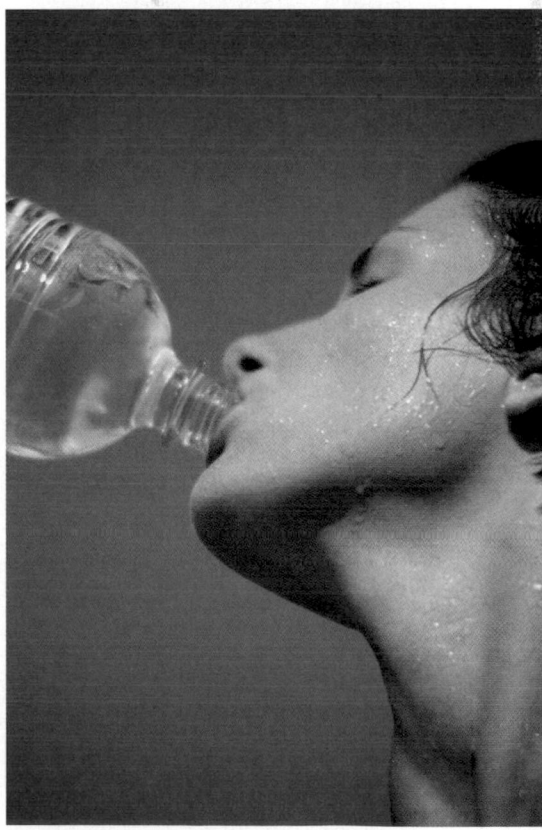

Fluid intake during physical activity is important.

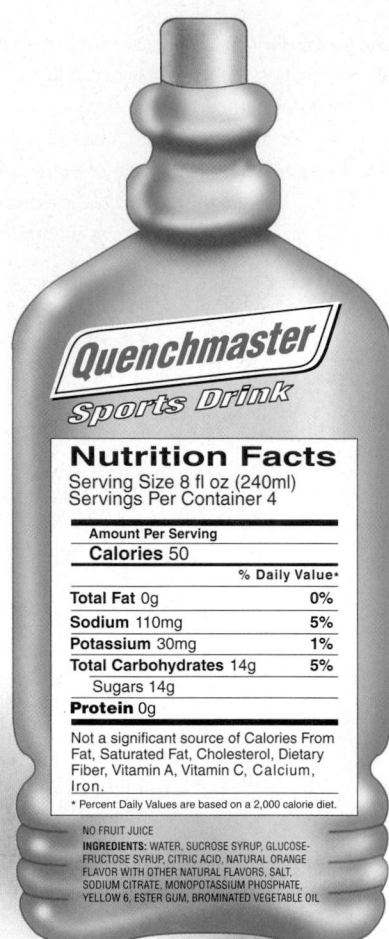

Figure 11-5 Sports drinks for fluid and electrolyte replacement typically contain a form of simple carbohydrate plus sodium and potassium. The various sugars in this product total 14 grams per 1 cup (240 milliliters) serving. In percentage terms based on weight, the sugar content is about 6% ([14 grams sugar per serving ÷ 240 grams per serving] × 100 = 5.8%). Sports drinks typically contain about 6% to 8% sugar. This provides ample glucose and other monosaccharides to aid in fueling working muscles, and it is well tolerated. Drinks with a sugar content above 10%, such as soft drinks or fruit juices, may cause stomach distress, and so are not recommended.

This allows time for both adequate hydration and excretion of excess fluid.

- During events lasting more than 30 minutes, consume about ½ to 1½ cups (150 to 350 milliliters) of fluid every 15 to 20 minutes beginning at the start of the exercise. Consuming more than 1 quart (1 liter) per hour can cause discomfort. On hot days, cold drinks are preferable to help cool the body. Again, the athlete should not wait until he or she feels thirsty. In many cases, athletes, especially children and teenagers, need to be reminded to do this.
- Within 4 to 6 hours after exercise, about 2½ to 3 cups of fluid should be consumed for every pound lost, as just mentioned. It is also important that weight be restored before the next exercise period. Skipping fluids before or during events will almost certainly cause problems. Note also that since caffeine has a dehydrating effect on the body, fluids containing it should not be part of any hydration plan before, during, or after exercise. Alcoholic beverages also have a diuretic effect.

Sports Drinks

A question that often arises is whether to drink water or a sports-type carbohydrate-electrolyte drink (e.g., All Sport, Exceed Energy Drink, Gatorade, PowerAde, and Amino Force) during competition (Fig. 11-5). For sports that require less than 60 minutes of exertion or when total weight loss is less than 5 to 6 pounds, the primary concern is replacing the water lost in sweat, because losses of carbohydrate stores and electrolytes (sodium, chloride, potassium, and other minerals) are not usually very great. Although electrolytes are lost in sweat, the quantities lost in exercise of brief to moderate duration can be easily replaced later by consuming normal foods, such as orange juice, potatoes, and tomato juice. Keep in mind that sweat is about 99% water and only 1% electrolytes and other substances.

When exercise extends beyond 60 minutes, electrolyte (especially sodium) and carbohydrate replacement becomes increasingly important. Use of sports drinks during these longer bouts of exercise—even more so in hot weather—now offers several distinct advantages over water alone.

Water by itself, as you have learned, increases blood volume to allow for efficient cooling and transport of potential cellular fuels and waste products. The addition of carbohydrate to a sports drink supplies glucose to muscles as they become depleted of glycogen, and thus can enhance performance when administered during endurance activities (see the later section on carbohydrate replacement). Carbohydrate also adds flavor, which encourages athletes to drink. Finally, the electrolytes in sports drinks help to maintain blood volume, enhance the absorption of water and carbohydrate from the intestine, and stimulate thirst. For these reasons, some experts prefer sports drinks over water for all athletes.

Overall, the decision to use a sports drink hinges primarily on the duration of the activity. As the projected duration of continuous activity approaches 60 minutes or longer, the advantages of the use of a sports drink over plain water clearly emerge. However, athletes should first experiment with sports drinks during practice, instead of trying them for the first time during competition.

It is also possible for some athletes to drink too much water. Endurance athletes (especially poorly trained individuals) may compete at relatively low exercise intensities for prolonged periods of time and therefore may not sweat as much as one might predict. Thus, water losses are not very high. In addition, some of these athletes have used one-half strength Coca-Cola as their fluid-replacement beverage, which is relatively low in sodium, and they drink this at every rest stop. This combination leads to an eventual fall in blood sodium, which is not desirable. Drinking less fluid, choosing a sports drink containing sodium (usually in the form of sodium chloride), and not gaining weight during the activity can help prevent this problem.

Specialized Dietary Advice for Before, During, and After Endurance Exercise

A light meal supplying up to 1000 kcal should be eaten about 2 to 4 hours before an endurance event to top off muscle and liver glycogen stores, prevent hunger during the event, and provide extra fluid. The longer the period before an event, the larger the meal can be, as there will be more time available for digestion. A pre-event meal should consist primarily of carbohydrate (about 200 grams), have little fat or fiber, and include a moderate amount of protein (Table 11-5). A meal eaten 1 hour or so before an event should be blended or liquid to promote rapid stomach emptying. Examples are low-fat smoothies, juices, and sports drinks.

Table 11-5 Convenient Pre-event Meals

Breakfast

Cheerios, ¾ cup	450 kcal
Reduced-fat milk, 1 cup	82% carbohydrate
Blueberry muffin, 1	(92 grams)
Orange juice, 4 oz	
or	
Low-fat fruit yogurt, 1 cup	482 kcal
Plain bagel, ½	68% carbohydrate
Apple juice, 4 oz	(84 grams)
Peanut butter (for bagel), 1 tbsp	
or	
Whole-wheat toast, 1 slice	507 kcal
Jam, 1 tsp	73% carbohydrate
Apple, 1 large	(98 grams)
Reduced-fat milk, 1 cup	
Oatmeal, ½ cup	
(with Reduced-fat milk, ½ cup)	

Lunch or Dinner

Chili; with beans, 8 oz	900 kcal
Baked potato with sour cream and chives	65% carbohydrate
Chocolate Frosty	(150 grams)
or	
Spaghetti noodles, 2 cups	761 kcal
Spaghetti sauce, 1 cup	66% carbohydrate
Reduced-fat milk, 1½ cups	(129 grams)
Green beans, 1 cup	
or	
Orange, 1 large	829 kcal
Reduced-fat milk, 1½ cups	70% carbohydrate
Chicken noodle soup, 1 cup	(160 grams)
Saltine crackers, 12	
Buttered beans, 1 cup	
Corn, 1 cup	
Angel food cake, 1 slice	

With regard to the timing of preactivity meals, the rule of thumb is to allow 4 hours for a big meal (about 1200 kcal), 3 hours for a moderate meal (about 800 to 900 kcal), 2 hours for a light meal (about 400 to 600 kcal), and an hour or less for a snack (about 300 kcal).

Rule of Thumb for Approximate Pre-event Carbohydrate Intake		
Hours Before	Grams per kilogram Body Weight	For a 70-kilogram Person
1	1	70
2	2	140
3	3	210
4	4	280

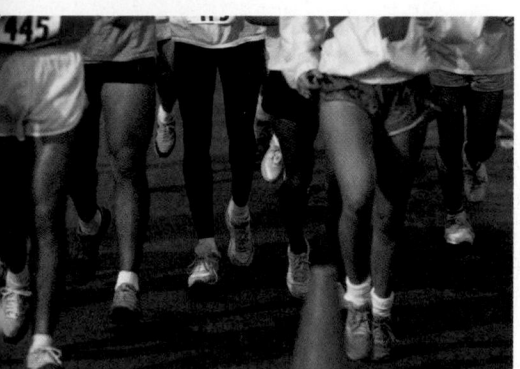

Carbohydrate intake during endurance exercise helps maintain this source of energy for the body.

Good food choices for a pre-event meal include spaghetti, muffins, bagels, pancakes with fresh fruit topping, oatmeal with fruit, baked potato topped with yogurt or a small amount of sour cream, toasted bread with jam, bananas, apples, oranges, pears, plums, nuts, and low-sugar breakfast cereals with reduced-fat or fat-free milk. Liquid meal-replacement formulas, such as Carnation Instant Breakfast, also can be used. Foods especially rich in fiber should be eaten the previous day to help empty the colon before an event, but they should not be eaten the night before or in the morning before the event. Foods to avoid are those that are fatty or fried, such as sausage, bacon, sauces, and gravies.

■ Replenishing Fuel during Endurance Exercise

We've already established the importance of consuming adequate fluids during endurance exercise. For sporting events that are longer than 60 minutes, consumption of carbohydrate during activity can also improve athletic performance. This is because prolonged exercise depletes muscle glycogen stores and low levels of blood glucose lead to fatigue, both physically and mentally. When the supply of carbohydrate calories runs low, athletes often complain of "hitting the wall," the point at which maintaining a competitive pace seems impossible. One way to overcome this obstacle is to maintain normal blood glucose concentrations by carbohydrate feedings. As mentioned before, a general guideline for endurance events is to consume 30 to 60 grams of carbohydrate per hour; however, an athlete should experiment during training sessions to establish the level that leads to optimal performance.

In the previous section on fluid needs, you learned that sports drinks are a good source of carbohydrate calories during endurance events. They supply the necessary fluid, electrolytes, and carbohydrate to keep an athlete performing at his or her best. As an alternative to sports drinks, some athletes have begun to use carbohydrate gels (e.g., PowerGel and Clif Shot) and energy bars (e.g., PowerBar). Check the label on these products to gauge the amount of gel or bar that provides 30 to 60 grams of carbohydrate per hour. Gels contain about 25 grams of carbohydrate per serving, and depending on the type, popular energy bars range from 2 to 45 grams of carbohydrate per serving (Table 11-6). Sports drinks, by comparison, contain about 14 grams of carbohydrate per 8-oz serving.

The wide range of carbohydrate content in energy bars is due to a variety of marketing trends in the sports supplement industry. Some advertise a high-carbohydrate content (about 40 grams), including most varieties of PowerBars, as well as Clif and Boulder bars. Bars based on the "Zone Diet," which is not very effective for supporting endurance activity, the Balance and Prozone bars provide about 20 grams of carbohydrate. High-protein varieties, such as Met-Rx and Twinlab Protein Fuel, are marketed more toward strength-trained rather than endurance-trained athletes. (As discussed earlier, these are rarely needed.) Based on your knowledge of fuels to support aerobic activity, you can see that the high-carbohydrate varieties make the most sense for endurance events. Overall, choosing a bar with about 40 grams of carbohydrate and no more than 10 grams of protein, 4 grams of fat, and 5 grams of fiber is recommended. The bars are also typically fortified with vitamins and minerals, often to 100 percent of the Daily Values. As such, these bars can be seen as

Another Bite

Why hasn't fat been mentioned as a way to improve athletic performance during an endurance event? While it is true that fat is used along with carbohydrate as fuel during prolonged aerobic activity, the processes of digestion, absorption, and metabolism of fat are relatively slow. Therefore, consumption of fat during activity is not likely to translate into better athletic performance.

Table 11-6 Calorie and Macronutrient Contents of Popular Energy Bars and Gels

Product	Calories (kcal)	Carbohydrates (grams)	Protein (grams)	Fat (grams)
PowerBar Performance (chocolate)	230	45	10	2
PowerBar ProteinPlus (cookies & cream)	230	38	24	5
PowerBar PowerGel (lemon lime)	110	28	0	0
Luna Bar (cherry-covered chocolate)	180	28	10	4
Clif Bar (chocolate chip)	250	45	10	5
Clif Shot (viva vanilla)	100	24	0	0
Balance Bar (chocolate)	200	22	14	6
Balance Satisfaction (chocolate crisp)	280	47	12	6
Boulder Bar (chocolate)	210	42	10	4

Overall, choosing energy bars is preferable to choosing candy bars and packaged cakes. When used in sports situations, energy bars can be handy. Better yet, however, is to eat a variety of wholesome foods; these offer more health-protective compounds. This is also a less expensive choice, especially for day-to-day snacking. An additional concern is that micronutrient toxicity might occur if numerous bars are eaten in a day, as many are highly fortified. Vitamin A and iron are two nutrients of special concern in this regard.

a convenient, although somewhat expensive, source of nutrients. The highly fortified nature of these bars may also lead to nutrient toxicities if overused, such as with vitamin A.

If solid sources of carbohydrate are one's preference, it is interesting to note that fig cookies, Gummy Bears, and jellybeans can also yield a quick source of glucose, and with a much lower cost. However, any carbohydrate-containing food, including energy bars and gels, must be accompanied by fluid to also achieve adequate hydration.

■ Carbohydrate Intake during Recovery from Prolonged Exercise

Carbohydrate-rich foods providing 1 to 2 grams of carbohydrate per kilogram body weight should be consumed within 2 hours after extended (endurance) exercise, and the sooner the better. Immediately after exercise is when glycogen synthesis is greatest, as the muscles are very insulin-sensitive at this point. This process should then be repeated over the next 2-hour interval. Athletes who are training hard can consume a simple sugar candy, sugared soft drink, fruit or fruit juice, or a sports-type carbohydrate supplement right after training as they attempt to reload their muscles with glycogen. Later, bread, mashed potatoes, and rice can contribute to additional carbohydrate consumption. All of these high-glycemic-load carbohydrates especially contribute to glycogen synthesis. Adding some rich protein sources is also recommended, with carbohydrate to protein in a 3:1 ratio. For a 154-pound (70-kilogram) athlete, this corresponds to about 70 grams of carbohydrate and 25 grams of protein in each 2-hour interval (Table 11-7 contains sample meals of this composition). In summary,

It cannot be emphasized enough that any nutrition strategies should be tested during practice and trial runs before being used in a meet or key event. An athlete should never try a new food or beverage on the day of competition. Some food items and beverages may not be well tolerated, and the day of competition is not the time to find this out.

For more information on sports nutrition, visit the Gatorade Sport Science Institute web page (www.gssiweb.com). For more information on sports medicine, visit www.physsportsmed.com. This home page of *The Physician and Sportsmedicine* journal details current issues in sports medicine, including injury prevention, nutrition, and exercise. Also helpful are the web pages of the American College of Sports Medicine (www.acsm.org), Centers for Disease Control and Prevention (www.cdc.gov/nccdphp/dnpa), and the American Council on Exercise (www.acefitness.org).

Table 11-7 Sample Postexercise Meals for Rapid Muscle Glycogen Replacement

Option 1
1 regular bagel
2 tbsp peanut butter, smooth
8 fl oz fat-free milk
1 medium banana
562 kcal, 77 grams carbohydrate, 23 grams protein, 18 grams fat

Option 2
1 packet Carnation Instant Breakfast
8 oz fat-free milk
1 medium banana
1 tbsp peanut butter
Blend until smooth
438 kcal, 70 grams carbohydrate, 17 grams protein, 10 grams fat

Option 3
1.5 cans GatorPro (11 fl oz per can)
559 kcal, 89 grams carbohydrate, 26 grams protein, 11 grams fat

the following are key factors for achieving the most rapid replenishment of muscle glycogen after exercise: (1) availability of adequate carbohydrate, (2) ingestion of carbohydrate as soon as possible after completion of exercise, (3) selection of high-glycemic-load carbohydrates, (4) combination of carbohydrate and protein foods, rather than either carbohydrate or protein alone.

Fluid and electrolyte (i.e., sodium and potassium) intake is also an essential component of an athlete's recovery diet. This helps replenish body fluids as quickly as possible. This is especially important if two workouts a day are performed or if the environment is hot and humid. If food and fluid intake is sufficient to restore weight loss, it generally will also supply enough electrolytes to meet needs during recovery from endurance activities.

Concept Check

All athletes would do well to plan a diet following MyPyramid. High-carbohydrate foods should be emphasized, and these should dominate in pre-event meals. Protein intake above twice the RDA is not supported by scientific evidence. Most athletes easily consume enough protein from typical food choices. If nutrient supplements are used, dosages generally should not exceed the Upper Level set for each nutrient. Fluid should be consumed as liberally as possible before, during, and after an event. Carbohydrate and electrolytes in the fluid are especially helpful to help delay fatigue and maintain electrolyte balance when exercise duration is expected to exceed 60 minutes.

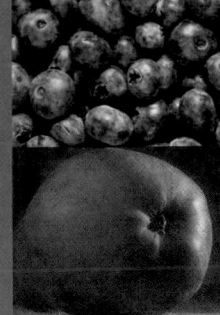

Evaluating Ergogenic Aids to Enhance Athletic Performance

Diet manipulation to improve athletic performance is not a recent innovation. As long as 30 years ago, American football players were encouraged on hot practice days to "toughen up" for competition by liberally consuming salt tablets before and during practice and by not drinking water. Now it is widely recognized that this practice can be fatal. Today's athletes are as likely as their predecessors to experiment with artichoke hearts, bee pollen, dried adrenal glands from cattle, seaweed, freeze-dried liver flakes, gelatin, and ginseng. These are just some of the ineffective substances used by athletes in hopes of gaining an **ergogenic** (work-producing) edge.

Based on what is known at this time, today's athletes can benefit from recent scientific evidence documenting the ergogenic properties of a few dietary substances. These ergogenic aids include sufficient water and electrolytes, lots of carbohydrates, and a balanced and varied diet consistent with MyPyramid. Protein and amino acid supplements are not among those aids because athletes can easily meet protein needs from foods, as Table 11-2 demonstrated. The use of nutrient supplements should be designed to meet a specific dietary shortcoming, such as an inadequate iron intake. These and other aids, which often have dubious benefits and may pose health risks, must be given close scrutiny before use. The risk-benefit ratio of any ergogenic aid merits careful evaluation.

As summarized in Table 11-8, no scientific evidence supports the effectiveness of many substances touted as performance-enhancing aids. Many are useless; some are dangerous. Athletes should be skeptical of any substance until its ergogenic effect is scientifically verified. FDA has a limited ability to regulate these dietary supplements (review Chapter 1), and the manufacturing processes for dietary supplements are not as tightly regulated by FDA as they are for prescription drugs. Some supplements may contain substances that will cause athletes to "test positive" for various banned substances. This was demonstrated in the 2002 Winter Olympics. Recent studies also have called into question the quality control associated with the manufacturing of dietary supplements. Many do not contain the substance and/or the amount listed on the label.

These results add yet another worry for the athlete. Not only must he or she determine whether there is evidence that a dietary supplement is safe and effective (FDA does not closely regulate dietary supplements), but must also question if the dietary supplement contains what it is supposed to contain.

ergogenic Work-producing. An ergogenic aid is a mechanical, nutritional, psychological, pharmacological, or physiological substance or treatment that is intended to directly improve exercise performance.

Note that the stimulant ephedra was taken off the market by FDA in April, 2004.

Another Bite

The NCAA's Committee on Competitive Safeguards and Medical Aspects of Sports has developed lists of supplements that are permissible and nonpermissible for athletic departments to dispense. Following are key examples:

Permissible	Nonpermissible
Vitamins and minerals	Amino acids
"Energy" bars (if no more than 30% protein)	Creatine
Sports drinks	Glycerol
Meal replacement drinks such as Ensure Plus or Boost	HMB
	L-carnitine
	Protein powders

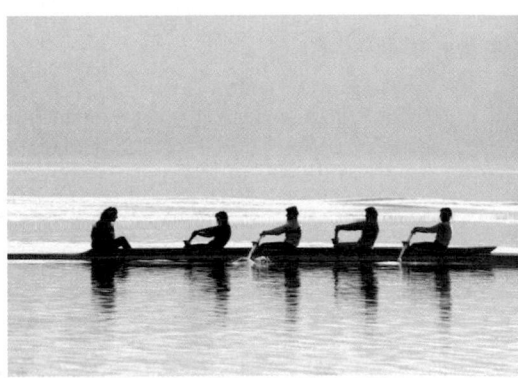

Attention to carbohydrate and fluid needs—along with meeting overall nutrient needs—is the most important ergogenic aid.

Even substances whose ergogenic effects have been supported by systematic scientific studies should be used with caution, as the testing conditions may not match those of the intended use. Finally, rather than waiting for a magic bullet to enhance performance, athletes are advised to concentrate their efforts on improving their training routines and sport techniques, while consuming well-balanced diets as described in this chapter.

Table 11-8 An Evaluation of Ergogenic Aids Currently in the Limelight

Substance/Practice	Rationale	Reality
Useful in Some Circumstances		
Creatine	Increase phosphocreatine (PCr) in muscles to keep ATP concentration high	Use of 20 grams per day for 5 to 6 days and then a maintenance dose of 2 grams per day may improve performance in those who undertake repeated bursts of activity, such as in sprinting and weightlifting. Some of the muscle weight gain noted with use results from water contained in muscles. Endurance athletes do not benefit from use. Little is known about the safety of long-term creatine use. Continual use of high doses has led to kidney damage in a few cases. Cost: $25 to $65 per month.
Sodium Bicarbonate (baking soda)	Counter lactic acid buildup	Partially effective in some circumstances, such as wrestling, but induces nausea and diarrhea. The dose used is 300 milligrams/kilogram, given 1 to 3 hours before exercise. Cost: nil.
Caffeine	Increase use of fatty acids to fuel muscles, promote psychological effects	Drinking two to three 5-ounce cups of coffee (equivalent to 3 to 9 milligrams of caffeine per kilogram of body weight) about 1 hour before events lasting about 5 minutes or longer is useful for some athletes; benefits are less apparent in those who have ample stores of glycogen, are highly trained, or habitually consume caffeine; intake of more than about 600 milligrams (six to eight cups of coffee) elicits a urine concentration illegal under NCAA rules (greater than 15 micrograms per milliliter). A possible side effect is reduced body hydration and shakiness. Cost: $0.08 per 300 milligrams.
Possibly Useful, Still Under Study		
Beta-hydroxy-beta methylbutyric acid (HMB)	Decrease protein catabolism, causing a net growth-promoting effect	Research in livestock and humans suggests that supplementation with this substance may increase muscle mass. Still, safety and effectiveness of long-term HMB use in humans is unknown. Cost: $100 per month.
Glutamine (an amino acid)	Enhance immune function, preserve lean body mass	Some preliminary studies show decreased occurrence of upper respiratory tract infections in athletes with use. It also may promote muscle growth, but long-term studies are lacking. Protein foods are a rich source of glutamine. Cost: $10 to $20 per month for 1 to 2 grams per day.
Branched-chain amino acids (BCAA) (leucine, isoleucine, valine)	Important energy source, especially when carbohydrate stores are depleted	Supplementation of BCAA (7 to 20 grams per day) during exercise can increase BCAA in the blood when it has been lowered due to exercise, but there is no consistent evidence of improved performance. Carbohydrate feeding, by delaying use of BCAA as fuel, may negate the need for BCAA supplementation. Preliminary studies show that BCAA use increases muscle mass more than does carbohydrate supplementation alone in swimmers, but there are no studies regarding resistance training. Protein-rich foods are also rich in BCAA. Cost: $20 per month.
Chondroitin and glucosamine	Aid in repair of joint damage	Most of the positive evidence is for repair of knee damage in older people. May be of use to athletes experiencing knee damage, but reliable evidence is lacking. Cost: $30 per month.
Dangerous or Illegal Substances/Practices		
Anabolic steroids (and related substances, such as androstenedione)	Increase muscle mass and strength	Although effective for increasing protein synthesis, anabolic steroids are illegal in the United States unless prescribed by a physician. They have numerous potential side effects, such as premature closure of growth plates in bones (thus possibly limiting the adult height of a teenage athlete), bloody cysts in the liver, increased risk of cardiovascular disease, increased blood pressure, and reproductive dysfunction. Possible psychological consequences include increased aggressiveness, drug dependence (addiction), withdrawal symptoms (such as depression), sleep disturbances, and mood swings (known as "roid rage"). Use of needles for injectable forms adds further health risk. Banned by the International Olympic Committee.

Table 11-8 (continued)

Substance/Practice	Rationale	Reality
Growth hormone	Increase muscle mass	At critical ages may increase height; may also cause uncontrolled growth of the heart and other internal organs and even death; potentially dangerous; requires careful monitoring by a physician. Use of needles for injections adds further health risk. Banned by the International Olympic Committee.
Blood doping	To enhance aerobic capacity by injecting red blood cells harvested previously from the athlete, or alternately the athlete may use the hormone erythropoietin (Epogen) to increase red blood cell number	May offer aerobic benefit; very serious health consequences are possible, including thickening of the blood, which puts extra strain on the heart; is an illegal practice under Olympic guidelines.
Gamma hydroxybutyric acid (GHB)	Promoted as a steroid alternative for bodybuilding	FDA has never approved it for sale as a medical product; is illegal to produce or sell GHB in the United States. GHB-related symptoms include vomiting, dizziness, tremors, and seizures. Many victims have required hospitalization, and some have died. Clandestine laboratories produced virtually all of the chemical accounting for GHB abuse. FDA is working with the U.S. Attorney's office to arrest, indict, and convict individuals responsible for the illegal operations.

Substances that are promoted to athletes but have yet to show any clear ergogenic effects include pyruvic acid (pyruvate), glycerol, ribose, medium chain triglycerides, L-carnitine, conjugated linoleic acid (CLA), bovine colostrum, insulin, and amino acids not already mentioned in this section. Any use of these products is not recommended at this time. Note that these substances are defined in the glossary.

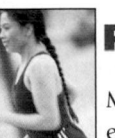

Real Life Scenario Follow-Up

Marcella is correct in following a high-carbohydrate diet. However, in her effort to minimize her fat intake, she is probably not consuming enough calories, protein, iron, and calcium to support her training routine. She has fallen into the bagel, pasta, and pretzel routine that sports nutritionists warn is not conducive to peak performance. Marcella's performance would improve if she also had a high-protein source at each meal. She could include milk with breakfast and possibly some low-fat yogurt or low-fat cheese at lunch. She should have a carbohydrate/protein snack before her workout, such as half a sandwich with fruit and some water. The sandwich and fruit will help provide her with fuel to support her vigorous training. During her workouts, she could consume a sports drink to meet fluid needs and supply some carbohydrate, or she could consume water, along with a few fig cookies or other high-carbohydrate food. In the evenings, she could substitute oil and vinegar dressing for the fat free dressing on her salad and cheese and crackers for the pretzels to improve protein intake. Overall, it is important for Marcella to fuel her body before, during, and after workouts.

Summary

1. A gradual increase in regular physical activity is recommended for all healthy persons. A minimum plan includes 30 minutes of physical activity on most (or all) days; 60 minutes per day provides even more benefit, especially if weight control is an issue. An intense program lasting about 60 minutes should begin with warm-up exercises to increase blood flow and warm the muscles, and end with cooldown exercises. Regular resistance activities and stretching add further benefits.

2. Human metabolic pathways extract chemical energy from food and transform it into ATP, the compound that provides energy for body functions.

3. In carbohydrate fuel use, glucose is broken down into the three-carbon compound pyruvic acid, yielding some ATP. This is metabolized further via the aerobic pathway to form carbon dioxide (CO_2) and water (H_2O) or via the anaerobic pathway to form lactic acid.

4. At rest, muscle cells mainly use fat for fuel. For intense exercise of short duration, muscles mostly use phosphocreatine (PCr) for energy. During more sustained intense activity, muscle glycogen breaks down to lactic acid, providing a small amount of ATP. For endurance exercise, both fat and carbohydrate are used as fuels; carbohydrate is used increasingly as activity intensifies. Little protein is used to fuel muscles.

5. Anyone who exercises regularly should consume a diet that meets calorie needs and is moderate to high in carbohydrates and fluid, and adequate in other nutrients such as iron and calcium.

6. Athletes should consume enough fluid to both minimize loss of body weight and ultimately restore preexercise weight. Sports drinks help replace fluid, electrolyte, and carbohydrate replacement. Their use especially should be considered when continuous activity lasts beyond 60 minutes.

7. Plenty of carbohydrates should be in the pre-event meal, especially for endurance athletes. High-glycemic-load carbohydrates should be consumed by an athlete within 2 hours after a workout to begin restoration of muscle glycogen stores. Some protein in the meal is also helpful.

Study Questions

1. How does greater physical fitness contribute to greater overall health? Explain the process.

2. The store of ATP in muscle is rapidly depleted once muscle contraction begins. For physical activity to continue, ATP must be resupplied immediately. Describe how this occurs after initiation of exercise and at various times thereafter.

3. What is the difference between anaerobic and aerobic exercise? Explain why aerobic metabolism is increased by a regular exercise routine.

4. What is glycogen? How is it used during exercise?

5. Is fat from adipose tissue used as an energy source during exercise? If so, when?

6. What are some typical measures used to assess whether an athlete's calorie intake is adequate?

7. List five specific nutrients that athletes need and the appropriate food sources from which these nutrients can be obtained.

8. What conditions might contribute to the inability to get all required nutrients from food, thus requiring use of a multivitamin and mineral supplement?

9. What advice would you give your neighbor, who is planning to run a 5-kilometer (km) race, concerning fluid intake before and during the event?

10. One of your friends, a competitive athlete, asks your opinion about an amino acid supplement sold in a local sporting-goods store. She has read that such supplements can help improve athletic performance. What would you tell her about the general effectiveness of such products?

Further Readings

1. Almond, CSD and others: Hyponatremia among runners in the Boston Marathon. *The New England Journal of Medicine* 352:1550, 2005.

   Low blood sodium (technically called hyponatremia) is a potential problem if runners drink too much water during a prolonged race. This is especially seen in poorly trained runners in comparison to elite athletes. Any fluid replacement needs to be carefully monitored to avoid weight gain during prolonged physical activity.

2. American College of Sports Medicine and others: Nutrition and athletic performance, *Medicine & Science in Sports & Exercise* 32:2130, 2000.

   The athlete who wants to optimize exercise performance needs to follow good nutrition and hydration practices, use supplements and ergogenic aids carefully, minimize severe weight-loss practices, and eat a variety of foods in adequate amounts. The various recommendations for carbohydrate, protein, fat, vitamins, minerals, and fluids in Chapter 11 were taken from this article.

3. Blair SN, Church TS: The fitness, obesity, and health equation. *Journal of the American Medical Association* 292:1232, 2004.

   Most of the health benefits from physical activity come with only 30 minutes at a moderate pace performed at least 5 days per week. This is true for both lean and overweight individuals. Brisk walking, swimming, bicycling, or daily activities such as gardening and house work, contribute to meeting this goal.

4. Coyle EF: Fluid and fuel intake during exercise. *Journal of Sports Science* 22: 39, 2004.

   Regular fluid and carbohydrate intake are crucial to maintain performance during prolonged physical activity. In the post recovery period, fluid, carbohydrate, and protein intake deserve the most attention in diet planning. The article provides the scientific support for such advice.

5. Dunford, M: Supplements for athletes. Safe? Effective? *Today's Dietitian* p.24, March 2005.

The supplements that have the most support in the sports nutrition literature are creatine for weight lifters and caffeine for some aerobic sports. A number of other supplements reviewed in this article have little or no support for use, including chromium and ribose. The author recommends visiting the web site www.ais.org.au/nutrition/supp-program.asp to learn more about the various supplements marketed to athletes.

6. Glazer, J.L.: Management of heat stroke and heat exhaustion *American Family Physician* 71:2133, 2005.

Heat exhaustion and heat stroke are common and preventable conditions that affect athletes (and other individuals such as older adults). Treatment of heat exhaustion involves putting the person in a cool shady environment and ensuring adequate hydration. Treating heat stroke is much more complicated, as outlined in the article.

7. Harber, VJ: Energy balance and reproductive function in active women. *Canadian Journal of Applied Physiology* 29:48, 2004.

It is very important for female athletes engaged in rigorous training programs to meet their calorie needs. If not, the resulting negative calorie balance will likely lead to a variety of menstrual cycle disturbances that can lead to other health problems. The article discusses this problem in detail and provides treatment strategies for problems that may develop.

8. Laaksonen, DE and others: Physical activity in the prevention of Type 2 diabetes: the Finnish Diabetes Prevention Study. *Diabetes* 54: 158, 2005.

Regular physical activity can substantially reduce the risk of developing type 2 diabetes in high risk individuals. People who increased their activity from moderate to vigorous amounts reduce their risk of developing type 2 diabetes by 65% compared to people who remained inactive. Even typical low intensity activities, such as walking, confered similar benefits in this study.

9. Lukaski, HC: Vitamin and mineral status: affects on physical performance. *Nutrition* 20:632, 2004.

Physically-active people generally consume sufficient vitamins and minerals to support such activity. The clearest indication for use of vitamin and mineral supplements by athletes is to treat existing nutrition deficiencies, or bridge gaps in nutrient intake versus nutrient needs. Use of vitamin and mineral supplements does not improve measures of performance in people consuming adequate diets.

10. Make the most of your exercise minutes. *Consumer Reports on Health*, p. 1, November 2003.

Key considerations when designing an exercise program are to include alternating bouts of vigorous and easier exercise to give muscles a chance to recover; alternating among exercises to work different muscles; and finding ways to make one's whole day more physically active. The article goes on to provide much guidance surrounding exercise protocols.

11. Nieman, DC and others: Vitamin E and immunity after the Kona Triathlon World Championship. *Medicine and Science in Sports and Exercise* 36:1328, 2004.

Athletes in this study who were provided 800 IU of vitamin E per day for two months before their triathlon event showed a greater degree of whole body oxidant damage compared to athletes who did not consume the supplement. The authors caution that megadose use of vitamin E supplements by athletes promotes lipid oxidation and inflammation during exercise, and so should not be recommended.

12. Powers, SK and others: Dietary antioxidants and exercise. *Journal of Sports Sciences* 22:81, 2004.

After careful review of the scientific literature, the authors could find little evidence for the effectiveness of antioxidant supplements in preventing exercise-related muscle damage. Therefore, they recommend that antioxidant supplements cannot be recommended at this time.

13. Rankin, JW and others: Effect of post-exercise supplement consumption on adaptations to resistance training. *Journal of the American College of Nutrition* 23:322, 2004.

Consuming either a combination of carbohydrate and protein or carbohydrate alone after weightlifting leads to adaptations to such resistance training. There was some indication that the combination of protein and carbohydrate together was more beneficial than consuming carbohydrate alone.

14. Ross, R and others: Exercise induced reduction in obesity and insulin resistance in women: a randomized control trial. *Obesity Research* 12:789, 2004.

Following a regular exercise program for 14 weeks resulted in a reduction in total and abdominal obesity in this study. Adding caloric restriction to the exercise program was associated with even more substantial decrease in those parameters, as well as a decrease in insulin resistance.

15. Sinclair, LM, Hinton, PS: Prevalence of iron deficiency with and without anemia in recreationally active men and women. *Journal of the American Dietetic Association* 105:975, 2005

Both males and female athletes are at risk of exhibiting poor iron stores and even iron deficiency anemia, with females being at much higher risk. The authors recommend that athletes be screened for iron deficiency anemia, and as well have their current state of iron storage tested. Poor iron status can lead to poor work performance, and therefore should be avoided.

16. Thompson PD and others: Exercise and physical activity in the prevention and treatment of atherosclerotic cardiovascular disease. *Circulation* 107:3109, 2003.

The American Heart Association supports the recommendation from the Centers for Disease Control and Prevention (CDC) and the American College of Sports Medicine (ACSM) that individuals should engage in 30 minutes or more of moderate-intensity physical activity (such as brisk walking) on most (preferably all) days of the week. Such activity is beneficial in both the prevention and treatment of cardiovascular disease.

17. Tipton KD, Wolfe RR: Protein and amino acids for athletes. *Journal of Sports Science* 22: 65, 2004.

A well-balanced diet can easily meet the protein needs of athletes. There is no need to consume more than 2 grams of protein per kilogram of body weight, even for strength-training athletes. In fact, an intake of more than 1.7 grams of protein per kilogram of body weight just results in the extra protein being used to meet calorie needs.

18. Williams MH: *Nutrition for health, fitness & sport.* 7th ed. Boston: McGraw-Hill, 2005.

Excellent textbook for reviewing nutrient needs of athletes, as well as learning more about ergogenic aids; also provides a detailed look at metabolism in exercise.

19. Why everyone needs strength training. *UC Berkeley Wellness Letter*, p. 4, May 2004.

Strength-training is an important part of an overall active lifestyle. One to three sets of 8 to 15 repetitions is sufficient for a specific exercise.

20. Zanker, CL, Cooke, CB: Energy balance, bone turnover and skeletal health in physically active individuals. *Medicine and Science in Sports and Exercise* 36:1372, 2004.

A physically-active life style contributes to maintenance of bone health; however, skeletal problems can result in underweight women who no longer have menstrual periods. The authors stress the importance for women meeting calorie needs during exercise in order to avoid this problem. There is even some evidence that the same problem can happen in men who do not meet calorie needs, but is not specifically linked to a sex hormone deficiency as it is in women. Thus the key factor in the disturbance of skeletal health is a calorie deficit.

I. Is Your Diet Measuring Up to the Numbers?

In Chapter 11, several key nutrients were discussed in relation to exercise performance. The following guidelines were mentioned, not only for athletes but for everyone maintaining generally good fitness.

- Eat a moderate to high amount of carbohydrates (generally 60% or more of total calorie intake).

- Athletes generally should eat a minimum of 1.2 grams of protein per kilogram of body weight.

- Consume the recommended amounts of vitamins and minerals, making sure iron and calcium intakes are adequate (especially for women).

- Consume enough fluid, to maintain weight during prolonged exercise or in hot conditions.

Review the results of the dietary assessment you completed in Chapter 2. Remember that you analyzed a 1-day food intake. Now answer the following questions, whether or not you consider yourself an athlete.

1. What percentage of your calorie intake came from carbohydrate? Was your carbohydrate intake 60% or more of your total calorie intake?

   _____

2. Did you eat at least 0.8 grams of protein per kilogram of body weight? If you are an athlete, did you consume at least 1.2 grams per kilogram of body weight? Did intake exceed 2 grams per kilogram of body weight or 35% of total calorie intake?

   _____

   _____

3. Did you consume your estimated needs of all vitamins and minerals, especially iron and calcium? Which ones were below the current nutrient standards?

   _____

   _____

4. For nutrients low in your diet, list one rich food source for each nutrient (see Chapters 8 through 9).

   _____

   _____

5. Did you consume sufficient fluid—about 9 cups (women) to 13 cups (men) is a good starting point?

   _____

   _____

6. What can you do to improve your dietary intake to aid general fitness and, if you are an athlete, to promote maximal performance in your chosen event(s)?

   _____

   _____

   _____

   _____

   _____

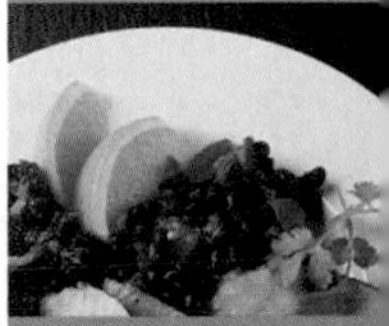

II. *Evaluating Protein Intake—A Case Study*

Mark is a college student who has been lifting weights at the student recreation center. The trainer at the center recommended a protein drink to help Mark build muscle mass. Answer the questions below about Mark's current food intake and determine whether a protein drink is needed to supplement Mark's diet.

1. The following is a tally of yesterday's intake.

Breakfast	Frosted Mini-Wheats cereal, 2 oz 1% milk, 1½ cups Orange juice, chilled, 6 oz Glazed yeast doughnut, 1 Brewed coffee, 1 cup
Lunch	Double hamburger with condiments, 1 French fries, 30 Cola, 12 oz Medium apple, 1
Dinner	Frozen lasagna w/meat, 2 pieces 1% milk, 1 cup Looseleaf lettuce, chopped, 1 cup Creamy Italian salad dressing, 2 tsp Medium tomato, ½ Whole carrot, raw, 1
Evening snack	Vanilla ice milk, 1 cup Hot fudge chocolate topping, 2 tsp Soft chocolate chip cookies, 2

Evaluate Mark's diet using Appendix J or NutritionCalc Plus—is he meeting the minimum recommendations of MyPyramid?

_____

2. Mark's weight has been stable at 70 kilograms (154 pounds). Determine his protein needs based on the RDA (0.8 grams per kilogram).

a. Mark's estimated protein RDA: _____

b. What are the maximum recommendations for protein intake for strength-training athletes?_____

c. Calculate the maximum protein recommendation for Mark. _____

_____

3. An analysis of the total calorie and protein content of Mark's current diet is 3470 kcal, 125 grams of protein (14% of total calories supplied by protein). This diet is representative of the food choices and amounts of food that Mark chooses on a regular basis.

a. What is the difference between Mark's estimated protein needs as an athlete (from number 2) and the amount of protein that his current diet provides? _____

b. Is his current protein intake inadequate, adequate, or excessive? _____ _____

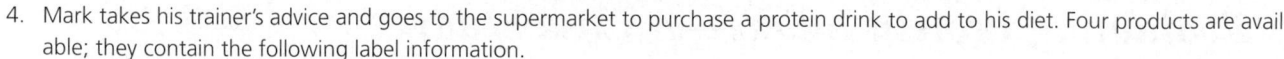
4. Mark takes his trainer's advice and goes to the supermarket to purchase a protein drink to add to his diet. Four products are available; they contain the following label information.

	Amino Fuel	Joe Weider's Sugar-Free 90% Plus Protein	Joe Weider's Dynamic Muscle Builder	Victory Super Mega Mass 2000
Serving size	3 tbsp	3 tbsp	3 tbsp	¼ scoop
Kcal	104	110	103	104
Protein (grams)	15	24	10	5

The trainer recommends adding the supplement to Mark's diet two times a day. Mark chooses the Muscle Builder protein drink.

a. How much protein would be added to Mark's diet daily from two servings of the supplement alone (prior to mixing it with a beverage)?

b. Mark mixes the powder with the milk he already consumes at breakfast and dinner. How much protein total would Mark now consume in 1 day? (Add the protein amount from the nutrition analysis to the value from question 4a.)

c. What is the difference between Mark's estimated protein needs as an athlete and this total value?

5. What is your conclusion—does Mark need the protein supplement?

Answers to Calculations

2a. Mark's estimated protein RDA: 70 kilograms × 0.8 grams per kilogram = 56 grams.
2b. Maximum recommendation for protein intake for athletes = 1.8 grams per kilogram.
2c. Applied to Mark: 1.8 × 70 = 126 grams.
3a. Difference between Mark's estimated maximum protein needs if an athlete and the amount of protein provided by his current diet: 126 − 125 = 1 gram protein.
3b. Mark's current diet is adequate.
4a. Two servings of protein supplement alone = 20 grams of protein.
4b. Mark's total protein consumption: 125 grams + 20 grams = 145 grams protein.
4c. Difference between Mark's estimated maximum protein needs as an athlete and total value (from above): 145 grams − 126 grams = 19 grams protein.

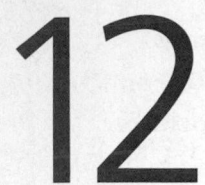

Eating Disorders:
Anorexia Nervosa, Bulimia Nervosa, and Other Conditions

12

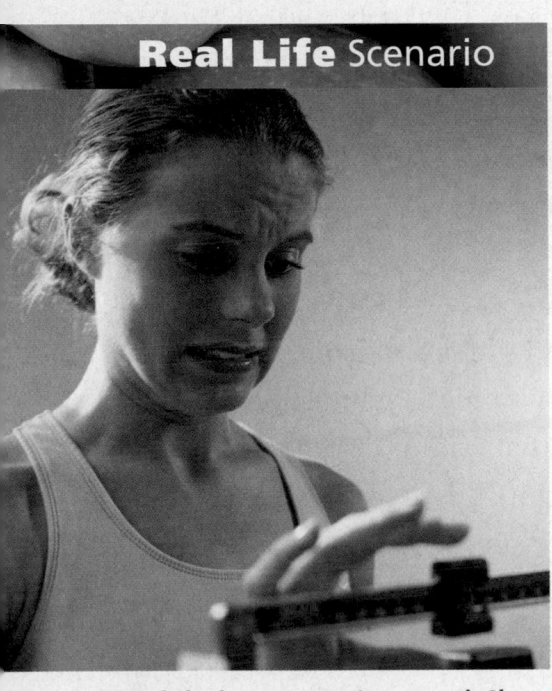

Real Life Scenario

At age 16, Sarah suddenly became self-conscious about her body when her peers criticized her about being overweight. She began exercising to an aerobics video for an hour each day and found that she had success in losing weight; this was the beginning of her obsession to be thin. Next, Sarah turned to eating less food to lose even more weight and began eliminating certain foods from her diet, such as candy and meat. She increased her water and vegetable intake and chewed sugarless gum to curb her appetite. Once she began dieting, it was impossible for her to stop. She really enjoyed having a high degree of self-control over her body. Still, she was literally obsessed with food, even staring at others while they were eating a meal. She occasionally cooked large meals and then refused to eat all but a few bites. By the time Sarah was 19 years old and 5 feet 6 inches tall, her weight had dropped from 150 pounds to 85 pounds in 20 months. Her family was concerned about her weight status, demanding that she go to a physician for an evaluation. Sarah was not happy about this idea but believed that her family would stop pestering her if she just did this. Sarah did not think she had a problem; she truly thought she was still grotesquely overweight. She did notice, however, that she was intolerant of cold temperatures and was concerned that she had not menstruated in a year.

Does Sarah have an eating disorder? What types of therapy do you think the physician will suggest for Sarah? Where could she go for such therapy? What is the likelihood that she will fully recover from her condition?

> Check out the **Contemporary Nutrition Online Learning Center**
> www.mhhe.com/wardlawcont6 for quizzes, flash cards, other activities, and web links designed
> to further help you learn about eating disorders.

Chapter 12 Objectives

Chapter 12 is designed to allow you to:

1. Contrast healthy attitudes toward uses of food with behavior patterns that could lead to unhealthy uses of food.

2. Outline the causes of, effects of, typical persons affected by, and treatment for anorexia nervosa.

3. Outline the causes of, effects of, typical persons affected by, and treatment for bulimia nervosa.

4. Describe still other forms of eating disorders: binge-eating disorder and the female athlete triad.

5. Relate the presence of eating disorders to current social trends.

6. Describe methods to reduce the development of eating disorders, including the use of warning signs to identify early cases.

Chapter 12 Outline

Many of us occasionally eat until we're stuffed and uncomfortable, such as at Thanksgiving dinner. Faced with savory and tempting foods, we find that we can't easily stop eating. Usually we forgive ourselves, vowing not to overeat the next time. Nevertheless, many of us have problems controlling our food intake and body weight. Although progressive weight gain can eventually lead to medical problems, it is usually associated with simple overeating, coupled with too little physical activity.

Actually, obesity is the most common eating disorder in our society; however, the eating disorders explored in Chapter 12 involve much more severe distortions of the eating process. The eating disorders discussed here are just as if not more serious than obesity, and can develop into life-threatening conditions if left untreated. What's most alarming about these disorders—anorexia nervosa, bulimia nervosa, binge-eating disorder, and the female athlete triad—is the increasing number of cases reported each year.

Some people are more susceptible to these eating disorders than other people are—for genetic, psychological, and physical reasons. Successful treatment of eating disorders, therefore, is complex and must go beyond nutritional therapy. And keep in mind that eating disorders are not restricted to any socioeconomic class or ethnicity. They can also strike at any age in both females and males. Let's examine the causes and treatments of these conditions in detail, because these eating disorders touch many of our lives.

Refresh Your Memory

As you begin your study of eating disorders, such as anorexia nervosa and bulimia nervosa, in Chapter 12, you may want to review:

- The effects of neurotransmitters on food intake in Chapter 1
- The role of genetic risk in disease susceptibility in Chapter 3
- The effects and treatment of osteoporosis in Chapter 9
- The effects and treatment of iron-deficiency anemia in Chapter 9
- Calculation of BMI in Chapter 10

FOR BETTER OR FOR WORSE

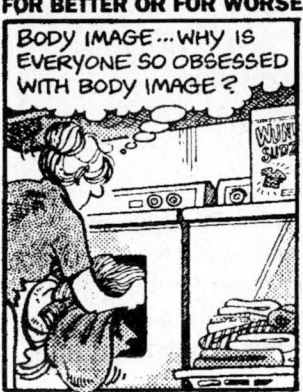 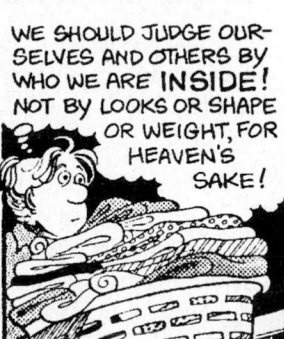 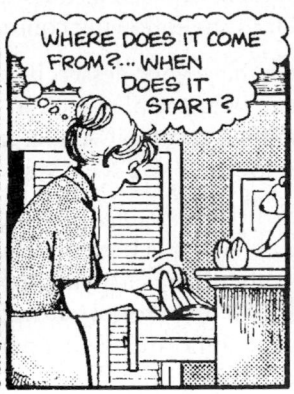 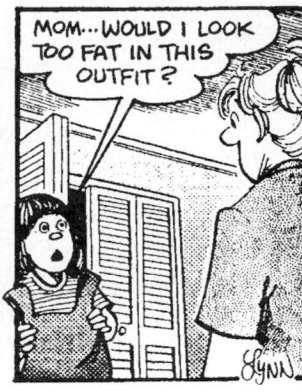

Concern with body image often starts early in life. Why do you think this is so? What recent societal trends have fostered this concern? Are some people more vulnerable, based on genetics and environment? Chapter 12 provides some answers.

From Ordered to Disordered Eating Habits

Eating—a completely instinctive behavior for animals—serves an extraordinary number of psychological, social, and cultural purposes for humans. Eating practices may take on religious meanings; signify bonds within families and ethnic groups; and provide a means to express hostility, affection, prestige, or class values. Within the family, supplying, preparing, and distributing food may be a means of expressing love, hatred, or even power.

We are bombarded daily with images of our society's portrayal of the "ideal" body. Dieting is promoted to achieve this ideal body—eternally young and admired. Television programs, billboard advertisements, magazine pictures, movies, and newspapers suggest that an ultraslim body will bring happiness, love, and ultimately, success. This fantasy notion is contradictory to the fact that much of society is becoming fatter, even obese. In response to this social pressure, some of us take an extreme approach—the pathological pursuit of weight control or weight loss.

It is difficult to resist comparing ourselves to the "ideal" body. Not everyone can look like a fashion model. People who are overly impressed by these messages, especially those with genetic, psychological, and physical influences, may be more likely than others to develop eating disorders in an effort to close the gap between reality and the perceived ideal.

Given the multiple functions associated with normal eating and the media bombardment with the ideal body image, it is not surprising that some people progress from typical responses to hunger and satiety cues to obsessive weight-loss behaviors, and then to a full-blown eating disorder.

Food: More than Just a Source of Nutrients

From birth, we link food with personal and emotional experiences. As infants, we associate milk with security and warmth, so the breast or bottle becomes a source of comfort as well as food. As noted in Chapter 1, even when older, most people continue to derive comfort and great pleasure from food. This is both a biological and a psychological phenomenon. Food can be a symbol of comfort, but eating can also stimulate the release of certain neurotransmitters (e.g., serotonin) and *natural opioids* (including **endorphins**), which produce a sense of calm and euphoria in the human body. Thus, in times of great stress some people turn to food for a druglike, calming effect.

Early in life, we develop images of "acceptable" and "unacceptable" body types. Of all the attributes that constitute attractiveness, many people view body weight as the most important, partly because we can control our weight somewhat. Fatness is the most dreaded deviation from our cultural ideals of body image, the one most derided and shunned, even among schoolchildren.

Progression from Ordered to Disordered Eating

Attention to hunger and satiety signals; limitation of calorie intake to restore weight to a healthful level

↓

Some disordered eating habits begin as weight loss is attempted, such as very restricted eating

↓

Clinically evident eating disorder recognized

endorphins Natural body tranquilizers that may be involved in the feeding response and function in pain reduction.

disordered eating Mild and short-term changes in eating patterns that occur in relation to a stressful event, an illness, or a desire to modify one's diet for a variety of health and personal appearance reasons.

eating disorder Severe alterations in eating patterns linked to physiological changes. The alterations are associated with food restriction, binge eating, purging, and fluctuations in weight. They also involve a number of emotional and cognitive changes that affect the way a person perceives and experiences his or her body.

anorexia nervosa An eating disorder involving a psychological loss or denial of appetite, followed by self-starvation; related in part to a distorted body image and to various social pressures commonly associated with puberty.

bulimia nervosa An eating disorder in which large quantities of food are eaten at one time (binge eating) and then purged from the body by vomiting, or misuse of laxatives, diuretics, or enemas. Alternate means to counteract the caloric excess use are fasting and excessive exercise.

binge-eating disorder An eating disorder characterized by recurrent binge eating and feelings of loss of control over eating that has lasted at least 6 months. Binge episodes can be triggered by frustration, anger, depression, anxiety, permission to eat forbidden foods, and excessive hunger.

Food is also used as a reward or a bribe. Haven't you heard or spoken something similar to the following comments?

You can have your dessert if you eat five more bites of your vegetables.
You can't play until you clean your plate.
I'll eat the broccoli if you let me watch TV.
If you love me, you'll eat your dinner.

On the surface, using food as a reward or bribe seems harmless enough. Eventually, however, this practice encourages both caregivers and children to use food to achieve goals other than satisfying hunger and nutrient needs. Food may then become much more than a source of nutrients. Regularly using food as a bargaining chip can contribute to abnormal eating patterns. Carried to the extreme, these patterns can lead to **disordered eating.**

Disordered eating can be defined as mild and short-term changes in eating patterns that occur in response to a stressful event, an illness, or even a desire to modify the diet for a variety of health and personal appearance reasons. The problem may be no more than a bad habit, a style of eating adapted from friends or family members, or an aspect of preparing for athletic competition. While disordered eating can lead to weight loss or weight gain, as well as certain nutritional problems, it rarely requires in-depth professional attention. If, however, disordered eating becomes sustained, distressing, or starts to interfere with everyday activities linked to physiological changes, it may require professional intervention.

■ Overview of Anorexia Nervosa and Bulimia Nervosa

Given the common practice of dieting in North America, it can sometimes be difficult to tell where disordered eating stops and an **eating disorder** begins. Indeed, many eating disorders start with a simple diet. Eating disorders then go on to involve physiological changes associated with food restriction, binge eating, purging, and fluctuations in weight. They also involve a number of emotional and cognitive changes that affect the way a person perceives and experiences his or her body, such as feelings of distress or extreme concern about body shape or weight. Eating disorders are not due to a failure of will or behavior; rather, they are real, treatable medical illnesses in which certain maladaptive patterns of eating take on a life of their own.

The main types of eating disorders are **anorexia nervosa** and **bulimia nervosa.** A third type, **binge-eating disorder,** has been suggested but has not yet been approved as a formal psychiatric diagnosis. More than 5 million people in North America have one of these disorders; females outnumber males 5 to 1. Eating disorders frequently (85% of the time) develop during adolescence or early adulthood but some reports indicate their onset can occur during childhood or later in adulthood. Eating disorders frequently co-occur with other psychological disorders such as depression, substance abuse, and anxiety disorders. *People who suffer from eating disorders, especially anorexia nervosa and bulimia nervosa, can experience a wide range of physical health complications, including serious heart conditions and kidney failure, which may even lead to death.* Recognition of eating disorders as important and treatable diseases, therefore, is critical.

Currently, up to 5% of women in North America develop some form of anorexia nervosa or bulimia nervosa in their lifetimes. This section provides a brief description of the characteristics and diagnoses of the two primary eating disorders that primarily afflict those of college age and younger. A detailed discussion of these and related disorders, including treatment, then follow.

Anorexia nervosa is characterized by extreme weight loss, a distorted body image, and an irrational, almost morbid, fear of obesity and weight gain. Anorexic patients irrationally believe they are fat, even though others constantly comment on their thin physique. Some anorexics realize they are thin but continue to be haunted by certain areas of their bodies that they believe to be fat (such as thighs, buttocks, and stomach).

Common to both eating disorders, *nervosa* refers to an attitude of disgust with one's body. The term *anorexia* implies a loss of appetite; however, a denial of one's appetite more accurately describes the behavior of people with anorexia nervosa. By rough estimate, approximately 1 in 200 (0.5%) adolescent girls in North America eventually develops anorexia nervosa. This high number may be due to the tendency for females to blame themselves for weight gain typical of their age group. Men only account for approximately 10% of the cases of anorexia nervosa, partly because the ideal image conveyed for men is big and muscular. Among men, athletes are most prone to develop this (and other) eating disorders, especially those who participate in sports that require weight classes, such as boxers, wrestlers, and jockeys. Other activities that may foster eating disorders in men include swimming, dancing, and modeling.

Bulimia nervosa (*bulimia* means "great [ox] hunger") is characterized by episodes of binge eating followed by attempts to purge the calories consumed by vomiting or misusing laxatives, diuretics, or enemas. People with this disorder may be difficult to identify because they keep their binge-purge behaviors secret, and their symptoms are not obvious. Four percent or more of adolescent and college-age women suffer from bulimia nervosa. And, as with anorexia nervosa, about 10% of the cases occur in men.

Specific criteria are used by clinicians to diagnose eating disorders (e.g., *Diagnostic and Statistical Manual of Mental Disorders* of the American Psychiatric Association). Some characteristics are listed in Table 12-1. It is possible that people exhibit some symptoms of eating disorders, but not enough to enable a medical worker to diagnose one of the two diseases. Also, as suggested in the diagnostic criteria, some people show characteristics of both anorexia nervosa and bulimia nervosa because the diseases overlap considerably. About half of the women diagnosed as having anorexia nervosa eventually develop bulimic symptoms. As shown in Table 12-1, bulimic characteristics also can be seen in anorexia nervosa, which blurs the distinction. Still, appreciating

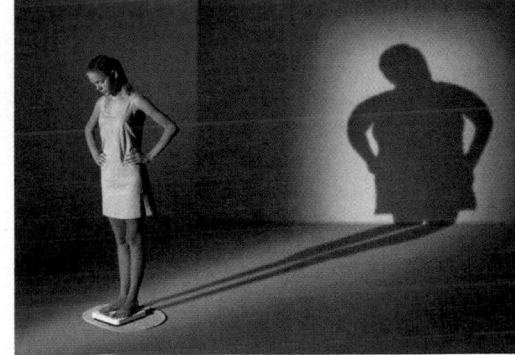

Self-image is an important part of adolescence. For people with eating disorders, the difference between the real and desired body images may be too difficult to accept. See the website www.4women.gov/bodyimage/index.htm

Table 12-1 Typical Characteristics of Anorexic and Bulimic Persons

Anorexia Nervosa	Bulimia Nervosa
• Rigid dieting causing dramatic weight loss, generally to less than 85% of what would be expected for one's age (or BMI of 17.5 or less) • False body perception—thinking "I'm too fat," even when extremely underweight; relentless pursuit of control • Rituals involving food, excessive exercise, and other aspects of life • Maintenance of rigid control in lifestyle; security found in control and order • Feeling of panic after a small weight gain; intense fear of gaining weight • Feelings of purity, power, and superiority through maintenance of strict discipline and self-denial • Preoccupation with food, its preparation, and observing another person eat • Helplessness in the presence of food • Lack of menstrual periods (after what should be the age of puberty) for at least 3 months • Possible presence of bingeing and purging practices	• Secretive binge eating; generally not overeating in front of others • Eating when depressed or under stress • Bingeing on a large amount of food, followed by fasting, laxative or diuretic abuse, self-induced vomiting, or excessive exercise (at least twice a week for 3 months) • Shame, embarrassment, deceit, and depression; low self-esteem and guilt (especially after a binge) • Fluctuating weight (±10 pounds or 5 kilograms) resulting from alternate bingeing and fasting • Loss of control; fear of not being able to stop eating • Perfectionism, "people pleaser"; food as the only comfort/escape in an otherwise carefully controlled and regulated life • Erosion of teeth, swollen glands • Purchase of syrup of ipecac, a compound sold in pharmacies that induces vomiting

Those who exhibit only one or a few of these characteristics may be at risk but probably do not have either disorder. They should, however, reflect on their eating habits and related concerns and take appropriate action, such as seeking a careful evaluation by a physician.

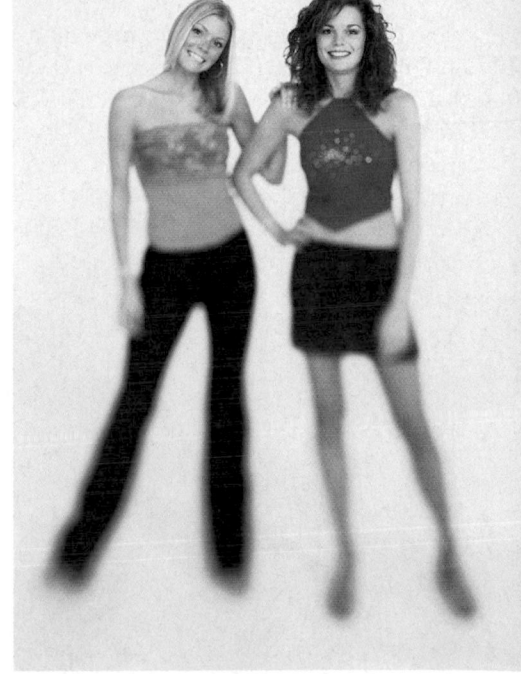

Maintaining an anorexic body type is an all too common goal in today's culture.

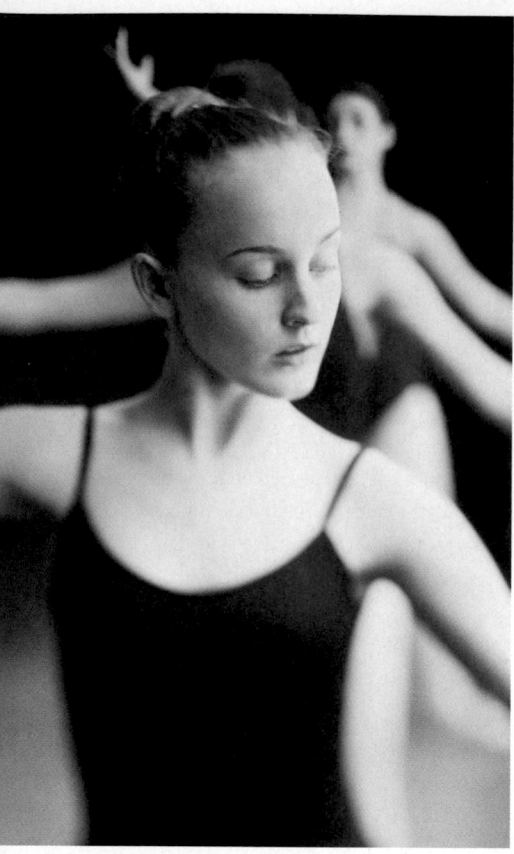

Eating disorders are commonly seen in people who must maintain low body weight, such as ballet dancers.

Our passion for thinness may have its roots in the Victorian era of the nineteenth century, which specialized in denying "unpleasant" physical realities, such as appetite and sexual desire. Flappers of the 1920s cemented the twentieth century trend for thinness. Since 1922, the BMI values of Miss America winners has steadily decreased; during the last three decades, most winners had a BMI in the "underweight" range (less than 18.5).

A person with anorexia nervosa may use the disorder to gain attention from the family, sometimes in hopes of holding the family together.

the differences between the disorders helps us to understand the various approaches to prevention and treatment.

Until recently, most researchers have reported that eating disorders primarily affect middle- and upper-class Caucasian women. Now, studies show greater similarities in the rates of body dissatisfaction and disordered eating behaviors across ethnic and cultural groups. Perhaps minorities with eating disorders have been less likely to seek help in the past due to fear of shame or stigma, lack of resources, or language barriers. It seems more likely, however, that health care workers are less likely to diagnose non-Caucasians as having eating disorders. Previously, it seemed that non-Caucasian cultures were more accepting of larger body shapes, but mainstream pressures for thinness now seem to cut across racial differences. In fact, our overall cultural change itself may be associated with increased vulnerability to eating disorders.

Do you know someone who is at risk of these eating disorders? If so, suggest that the person seek a professional evaluation because, the sooner treatment begins, the better the chances for recovery. However, do not try to diagnose eating disorders in your friends or family members. Only a professional can exclude other possible diseases and correctly evaluate the diagnostic criteria required to make a diagnosis of anorexia nervosa or bulimia nervosa. Once an eating disorder is diagnosed, immediate treatment is advisable. As a friend, the best you can do is to encourage an affected person to seek professional help. Note that such help is commonly available at student health centers and student guidance/counseling facilities on college campuses.

There are no simple causes of eating disorders, and there are no simple treatments. Stress may have an especially strong role in the development of eating disorders. An underlying commonality seems to be the lack of appropriate coping mechanisms as individuals begin to reach adolescence and young adulthood, coupled with dysfunctional family relationships.

A few research studies have investigated the possible link between genetic factors and the development of eating disorders. These studies have involved a comparison of identical twins with fraternal twins and the incidence of eating disorders. In general, these studies have shown that identical twins have a higher likelihood of sharing eating disorders than do fraternal twins. This indicates that genetics may play a strong role in development of such disorders, since identical twins share the same DNA. Identifying genes that cause eating disorders eventually could help in tailoring prevention efforts to those who are at risk, but affected individuals would still need the same counseling that is part of therapy today.

A Closer Look at Anorexia Nervosa

Anorexia nervosa evolves from a dangerous mental state to an often life-threatening physical condition. As first described in the early medical literature in 1689, people suffering from this disorder think they are fat and intensely fear obesity and weight gain. They lose much more weight than is healthful. Although food is entwined in this disease, it stems more from psychological conflict.

About 10% of people with anorexia nervosa eventually die from the disease—from suicide, heart ailments, and infections. About one quarter of those with anorexia nervosa recover within 6 years, whereas the rest simply exist with the disease or go on to develop another form of eating disorder. The longer someone suffers from this eating disorder, the poorer the chances for complete recovery. A young patient with a brief episode and a cooperative family has a better outlook than those without these factors. Overall, prompt and vigorous treatment with close follow-up improves the chances for success.

Anorexia nervosa may begin as a simple attempt to lose weight. A comment from a well-meaning friend, relative, or coach suggesting that the person seems to be gaining weight or is too fat may be all that is needed. The stress of having to maintain a certain weight to look attractive or competent on a job can also lead to disordered eating. Physical changes associated with puberty, the stress of leaving childhood, or the loss of a friend may serve as another trigger for extreme dieting. Leaving home for boarding school or college or starting a job can reinforce the desire to appear more "socially acceptable." Still, looking "good" does not necessarily help people deal with anger, depression, low self-esteem, or past experiences with sexual abuse. If these issues are behind the disorder and are not resolved as weight is lost, the individual may intensify efforts to lose weight "to look even better," rather than work through unresolved psychological concerns.

During adolescence, a period of turbulent sexual and social tensions, teenagers seek—and are often expected—to establish separate and independent lives. While declaring independence, they seek acceptance and support from peers and parents and react intensely to how they think others perceive them. At the same time, their bodies are changing, and much of the change is beyond their control. In response to the adolescent's or teenager's lack of control and coping mechanisms, dieting may start and then lead to a failure to gain appropriate weight-for-height. This may not be readily identified as a problem because the child has not actually lost any weight. Stunting (failure to grow in height) may also occur if inadequate calories are ingested during a period of growth. If anorexia develops before puberty, sexual maturation and menstruation also may be delayed.

Teens with chronic illnesses, such as type 1 diabetes or asthma, are at even greater risk for disordered eating. Any evidence of poor weight gain/maintenance or excessive exercise among these individuals needs to be investigated as a possible sign of disordered eating.

Extreme dieting is the most important predictor of an eating disorder. (Adolescents expressing concern about their weight should be advised to focus on exercise, which does not appear to impart a risk for subsequent problems.) Once dieting begins, a person developing anorexia nervosa does not stop. The result is a long period of rigidly self-enforced semistarvation, practiced almost with a vengeance, in a relentless pursuit of control. Anorexia nervosa may eventually lead to bingeing on large amounts of food in a short time, then purging. Purging occurs primarily through vomiting, but laxatives, diuretics, and enemas are also used. Thus, a person with anorexia nervosa may exist in a state of semistarvation or may alternate periods of starvation with periods of bingeing and purging.

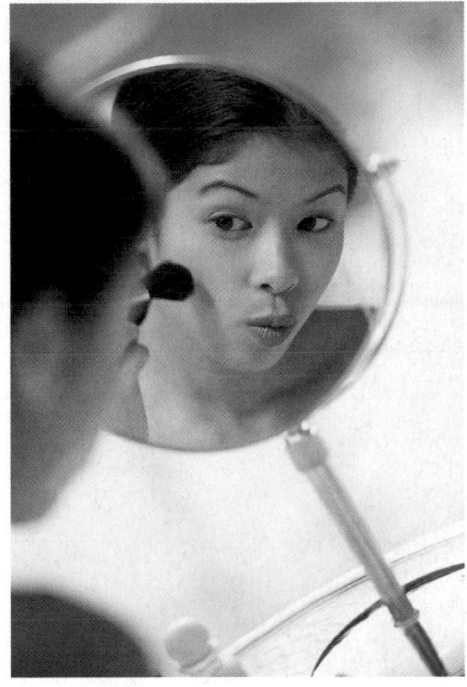

Concern over appearance begins early in life; a focus on a healthful outlook with regard to body weight should also begin at this time.

Another Bite

Recently, a 19-year-old woman with a body weight of 60 pounds was admitted on an emergency basis to the Ohio State University Hospitals. She had lost 55 pounds in the previous 6 months and was at great risk of impending death. Upon interview, she said she started dieting and could not stop. She was transferred out-of-state to a clinic specializing in eating disorders.

▪ Profile of the Typical Person with Anorexia Nervosa

A person with anorexia nervosa refuses to eat enough food to maintain an acceptable weight. This refusal is a hallmark of the disease, whether or not other practices, such as binge-purge cycles, appear. The most typical anorexic person is a Caucasian female from the middle or upper socioeconomic class. Perhaps her mother also has distorted views of desirable body shape and acceptable food habits. The girl is often described by parents and teachers as responsible, meticulous, and obedient.

She is competitive and often obsessive. Her parents set high standards for her. At home, she may not allow clutter in her bedroom. Physicians note that, after a physical examination, she may fold her examination gown very carefully and clean up the examination room before leaving. Even though such behavior may seem odd, only a skilled professional can tell the difference between anorexia nervosa and other adolescent complaints, such as delayed puberty, fatigue, and depression.

By severely limiting calorie intake for long periods, adolescent girls and young adult women greatly compromise their nutritional status, impair their reproductive systems, and restrict growth. The harm produced by milder, shorter periods of diet restriction is not clear. Evidence, however, suggests that even moderate diet restriction, if continued, contributes to the risks for various forms of anemia, future pregnancy complications and delivery of low-birth-weight infants, and permanently reduced bone mass.

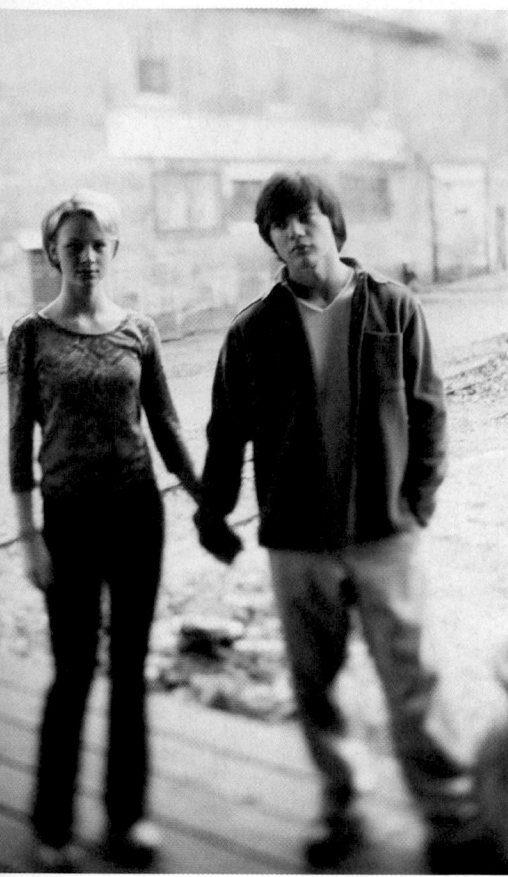

Anorexia nervosa occurs much more frequently in young women than in young men.

Parents may not consider a teenager mature enough to make decisions. If the teen disagrees and the situation is very tense, she may turn to purging or starving as a way to show her power: "You may try to control my life, but I can do anything I want with my body."

In the words of one young woman, "I couldn't get angry, because it would be like destroying someone else, like my mother. It felt like she would hate me forever. I got angry through anorexia nervosa. It was my last hope. It's my own body and this was my last-ditch effort."

A common thread underlying many—but not all—cases of anorexia nervosa is conflict within the family structure, typically with an overbearing mother and an emotionally absent father. When family expectations are always too high—including those regarding body weight—frustration results, and leads to fighting. Overinvolvement, rigidity, overprotection, and denial are typical daily transactions of such families.

Issues of control are central to the development of anorexia nervosa. Often, the eating disorder allows an anorexic person to exercise control over an otherwise powerless existence. Losing weight may be the first independent success the person has had. People with anorexia evaluate their self-worth almost entirely in terms of self-control. Some sexually abused children develop anorexia nervosa, believing that if they control their appetite for food, sexual relations, and human contact, they will feel in control and competent and will eliminate shameful feelings. Moreover, food restriction, which arrests development and shuts down sexual impulses, may be a strategy to prevent future victimization and guilt feelings. Often anorexic persons feel hopeless about human relationships and socially isolated because of their dysfunctional families. They focus on food, eating, and weight instead of human relationships.

■ Early Warning Signs

A person developing anorexia nervosa exhibits important warning signs. At first, dieting becomes the life focus. The person may think, "The only thing I am good at is dieting. I can't do anything else." This innocent beginning often leads to very abnormal self-perceptions and eating habits, such as cutting a pea in half before eating it. Other habits include hiding and storing food and or spreading food around a plate to make it look as if much has been eaten. An anorexic person may cook a large meal and watch others eat it while refusing to eat anything. Anorexic persons may also exercise compulsively to the point that it is obsessive and driven. Exercise can interfere with life activities or occur at unusual times or settings—for example, doing squats while brushing teeth.

As the disorder progresses, the range of foods may narrow and be rigidly divided into safe and unsafe ones, with the list of safe foods becoming progressively shorter. For people developing anorexia nervosa, these practices say "I am in control." These people may be hungry, but they deny it, driven by the belief that good things will happen by just becoming thin enough. It becomes a question of willpower.

People with anorexia become irritable and hostile and begin to withdraw from family and friends. School performance generally crumbles. They refuse to eat out with family and friends, thinking, "I won't be able to have the foods I want to eat," or "I won't be able to throw up afterward."

Anorexic persons see themselves as rational and others as irrational. They also tend to be excessively critical of themselves and others. Nothing is good enough. Because it cannot be perfect, life appears meaningless and hopeless. A sense of joylessness colors everything.

As stress increases in the person's life, sleep disturbances and depression are common. Many of the psychological and physical problems associated with anorexia nervosa arise from insufficient calorie intake, as well as deficiencies of nutrients, such as thiamin and vitamin B-6. For the latter reason, a multivitamin and mineral supplement is typically prescribed in therapy. For a female, the combination of problems—coupled with lower and lower body weight and fat stores—causes menstrual periods to cease. This may be the first sign of the disease that a parent notices, and represents an additional hallmark of the disease.

Ultimately, an anorexic person eats very little food; 300 to 600 kcal daily is not unusual. In place of food, the person may consume up to 20 cans of diet soft drinks and chew many pieces of sugarless gum each day.

■ Physical Effects of Anorexia Nervosa

Rooted in the emotional state of the victim, anorexia nervosa produces profound physical effects. The anorexic person often appears to be skin and bones. Body weight less than 85% of that expected is one clinical indicator of anorexia nervosa. This percentage can be calculated using the Metropolitan Life Insurance Company tables (see Appendix G), but it is important to note that the body build and weight history should also be used when estimating an appropriate weight. BMI is a more reliable indicator of the degree of malnourishment; generally, a BMI of 17.5 or less indicates a severe case (review Chapter 10 for more on BMI). For children under age 18, growth charts should be used to assess weight status (see Chapter 14).

The state of semistarvation disturbs many body systems as it forces the body to conserve energy stores as much as possible (Fig. 12-1). This attempt to conserve energy stores is the cause of most of the physical effects. Thus, many complications can be reversed by returning to a healthy weight, provided the duration of the insult has not been too long. The following are predictable effects caused by hormonal responses to and deficient nutrient intakes from semistarvation:

- Lowered body temperature and cold intolerance from loss of insulating fat layer
- Slowed metabolic rate from decreased synthesis of thyroid hormones
- Decreased heart rate as metabolism slows, leading to premature fatigue, fainting, and an overwhelming need for sleep. Other changes in heart function may occur as well, including loss of heart tissue and irregular heart rhythm.
- Iron-deficiency anemia, which leads to further weakness
- Rough, dry, scaly, and cold skin, which may show multiple bruises because of the loss of the protective fat layer normally present under the skin

Critical Thinking

Jennifer is an attractive 13-year-old. However, she's very compulsive. Everything has to be perfect—her hair, her clothes, even her room. Since her body is beginning to mature, she's quite obsessed with having perfect physical features as well. Her parents are worried about her behavior. The school counselor told them to look for certain signs that could indicate an eating disorder. What might those signs be?

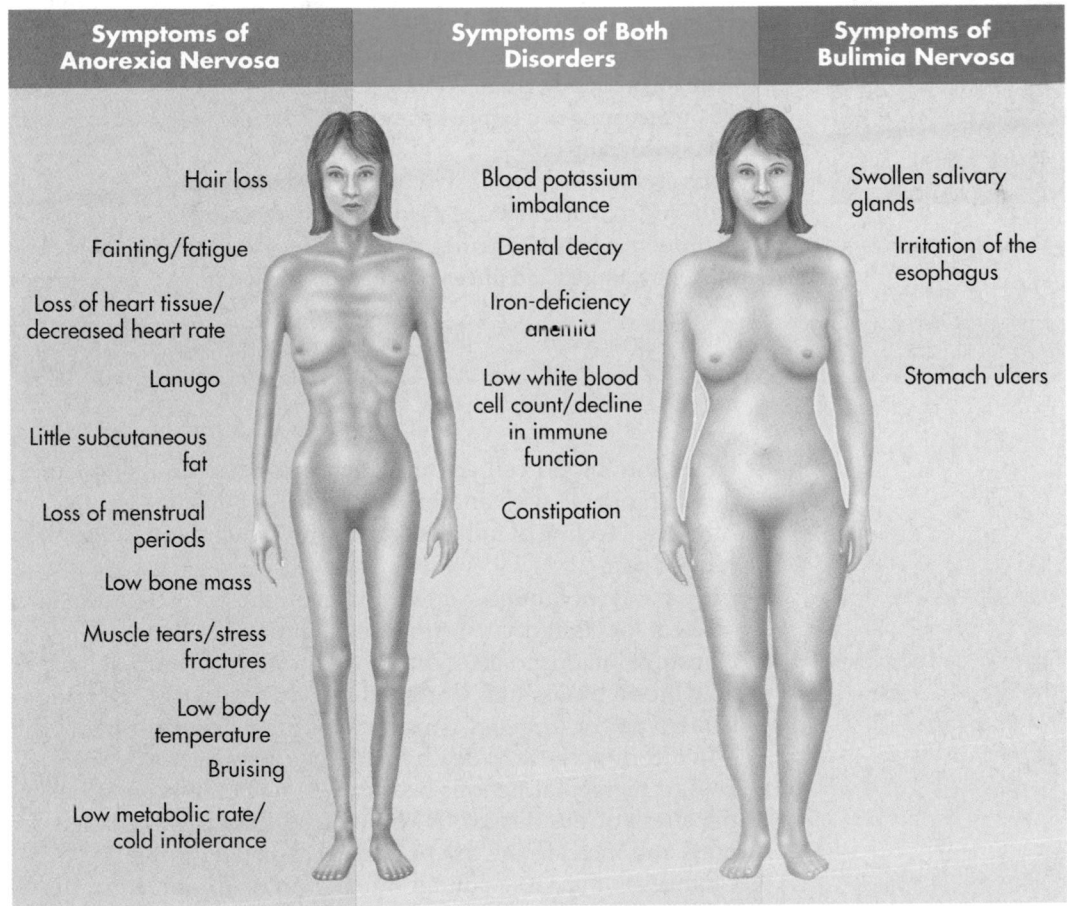

Figure 12-1 Signs and symptoms of eating disorders. A vast array of physical effects are associated with anorexia nervosa and bulimia nervosa. This figure contains many, but is not an exhaustive list of all potential consequences. These physical effects can also serve as warning signs that a problem exists. Professional evaluation is then indicated.

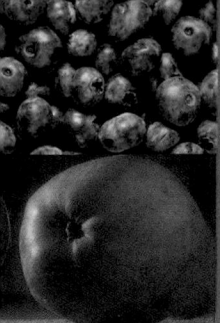

Looking *Further*

Thoughts of an Anorexic Woman

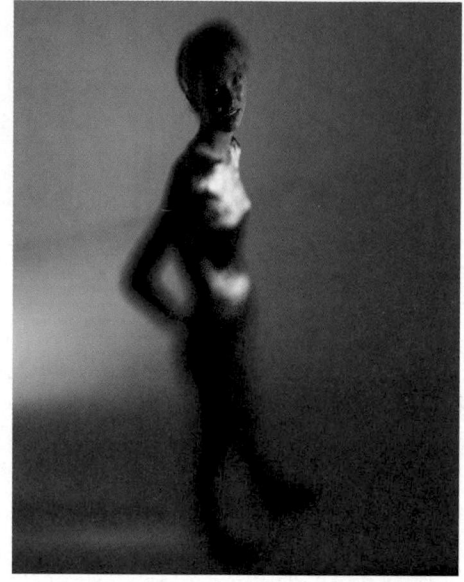

A history of anorexia nervosa can harm physical as well as mental health.

It was the spring of my freshman year of high school, and I had just turned 15. I wanted to get a leading role in the upcoming high school musical *West Side Story.* I thought I should lose some weight to look more attractive to the student director Shawn, so I decided to give up "junk" food. The next day my friend Sandra looked at my lunch, spread out neatly on a napkin before me, and squawked, "Dill pickles?! Who brings dill pickles for lunch in a zip-lock baggie?" The other girls at the table fell into a fit of hysterics. "Casting for *West Side Story* is coming up," I said, "and I gave up 'junk' food to try to lose a few pounds." One of my friends thought it would be funny to give me an M&M—just to smell. Ha, ha. I put it in a little Tupperware container and kept it for days in my backpack as a reminder.

Every once in a while, I did smell it.

For the next few weeks there were times when I would find myself cracking open the refrigerator door and just staring down what I knew to be a deliciously crunchy, crisp, and cold Kit Kat bar in the dairy bin. I didn't eat it though. At the mall with my friends (since at 15, that's about all my parents allowed me to do), Bridgette and Nora wanted to stop and get a Cinna-Bun. They chided me, but I didn't budge. The Cinna-Buns smelled so good. But as I sat opposite them in the food court and watched them overdramatize its ooey-gooey goodness, I felt a sense of pride that I could make a decision and stick with it. I could see that they were jealous of my willpower.

When Easter came around, I took a look at the contents of the Easter basket my mom insisted on preparing and turned up my nose at it. I had proven to myself that I could resist temptation . . . why stop now?

I was eventually offered only a minor part in the musical, but I wasn't that disappointed. I was looking so much better as the pounds kept coming off. Every morning, just after going to the bathroom and before getting any breakfast, I would pop onto the scale in my mom's bathroom. One hundred and fifteen pounds and still going. At 5 feet 7 inches, that wasn't too bad.

lanugo Downlike hair that appears after a person has lost much body fat through semi-starvation. The hair stands erect and traps air, acting as insulation for the body to compensate for the relative lack of body fat, which usually functions as insulation.

- Low white blood cell count, which increases the risk of infection—one cause of death in people with anorexia nervosa
- Abnormal feeling of fullness or bloating, which can last for several hours after eating
- Loss of hair
- Appearance of **lanugo**—downy hairs on the body that trap air to partially counteract heat loss that occurs with loss of fat tissue
- Constipation due to deterioration of the gastrointestinal tract and abuse of laxatives
- Low blood potassium, worsened by potassium losses during vomiting and use of some types of diuretics. This increases the risk of heart rhythm disturbances, another leading cause of death in anorexic people.
- Loss of menstrual periods because of low body weight, low body fat content, and the stress of the disease. Accompanying hormonal changes cause a loss of bone mass and increase the risk of osteoporosis later in life.
- Changes in neurotransmitter function in the brain, which leads to depression
- Eventual loss of teeth caused by acid erosion of tooth enamel if frequent vomiting occurs. Until vomiting ceases, one way to reduce this effect on teeth is to rinse the mouth with water right away and brush the teeth as soon as possible. Loss of teeth (along with low bone mass) can be lasting signs of the disease, even if the other physical and mental problems are resolved.

Also at this time, I started running, and my friend Laura became my running partner. She was getting in shape for the next season of field hockey. After school, we met in the locker room, changed out of our school clothes, and out we went. I had never been much of an athlete—I thought that being part of a team, whether in sports or academics, diluted the excellence I could achieve on my own. Running, however, could just be me and the road—no mediocrity there.

Cheese and butter had made it to the "no" list by the time I was 16 and down to 105 pounds. Fat-free was my mantra. In fact, for my 16th birthday, my friends threw a little surprise party for me. Nora, knowing I would put up a fight, made me a cake. "It's your birthday! You can have a piece of cake!" I politely said no, that I would cut it for everyone else, but I really didn't want any. They pestered me and Nora started to feel offended, so finally I took a few bites so she wouldn't burst into tears. It had been so long since I'd had so much sugar. I felt bloated and sick. I ate nothing for the rest of the day, and only 6 saltines, 1 apple, and 2 stalks of celery the next day. Those foods were on the "yes" list. Salads also were okay, but only lettuce with salt and vinegar. I told my parents that the dissections in biology class had given me a distaste for meat, but really, I just didn't want all those calories. For a while, I craved food day and night, but I was getting better and better at holding my ground.

By my senior year, I was skipping lunches altogether, opting instead to hang out in the library and read over my AP Bio text. "Where were you at lunch today?" Bridgette would ask later. "Oh, I had some reading to do. The AP exam is going to be tough." At 100 pounds, I was getting closer to finding out what "tough" really meant.

Even though Laura moved out of state, I didn't give up on exercising. Now, the stair stepper in the gym was my favorite. I'd take my microbiology notes, prop them up in front of me, and step-step-step until I had burned 400 kcal. I felt so efficient being that I could multi-task. Sometimes I'd go twice a day. As senior year wore on, though, it got harder and harder to get up in the morning and put on my tennis shoes. And then one morning, in the shower, I just collapsed under the stream of hot water.

I ended up in this hospital bed with an IV tube in my arm. At 92 pounds, my body was starving. As it turns out, if you don't give your body any fuel, you start to cannibalize yourself, in a sense. My body had been so hungry, my muscles had been wasting away, and the episode in the shower was due to a problem with my heart. It's a problem I have created . . . not my parents or my distant group of friends . . . just me. My mom was there, next to me, caressing the arm with the IV tube, putting her whole life on hold because of me. Isn't this what I'd wanted—to be in control of my own destiny?

Where do I go from here?

- Muscle tears and stress fractures in athletes because of decreased bone and muscle mass

A person with this disorder is psychologically and physically ill and needs help.

■ Treatment of Anorexia Nervosa

People with anorexia often sink into shells of isolation and fear. They deny that a problem exists. Frequently, their friends and family members meet with them to confront the problem in a loving way. This is called an *intervention*. They present evidence

Concept Check

Anorexia nervosa is an eating disorder characterized by semistarvation. It is found primarily—but not exclusively—in adolescent girls, starting at or around puberty. People with anorexia dwindle essentially to skin and bones yet still believe they are fat. Semistarvation produces hormonal changes and nutrient deficiencies, which lower body temperature, slow the heart rate, decrease immune response, stop menstrual periods, and contribute to hair, muscle, and bone loss. It is a very serious disease, which often produces lifelong consequences and may be fatal.

Erika Goodman, former dancer with the Joffrey Ballet, is now in her fifties and is crippled from osteoporosis resulting from years of restricting food intake in order to maintain a low body weight. Her food restriction led to irregular or absent menstrual periods for many years.

of the problem and encourage immediate treatment. Treatment then requires a multidisciplinary team of experienced physicians, registered dietitians, psychologists, and other health professionals working together. An ideal setting is an eating disorders clinic in a medical center. Outpatient therapy generally begins first. This may be extended to 3 to 5 days per week. Day hospitalization (6 to 12 hours) is another option, as is total hospitalization. Hospitalization is necessary once a person falls below 75% of expected weight, experiences acute medical problems, and/or exhibits severe psychological problems or suicidal risk. Still, even in the most skilled hands at the finest facilities, efforts may fail. This tells us that the prevention of anorexia nervosa is of utmost importance.

Once a medical team has gained the cooperation and trust of an anorexic person, the team attempts to work together to restore a sense of balance, purpose, and future possibilities. As previously stated, anorexia nervosa is usually rooted in psychological conflict. However, the anorexic person who has been barely existing in a state of semi-starvation cannot focus on much besides food. Dreams and even morbid thoughts about food will interfere with therapy until sufficient weight is regained.

Nutrition Therapy

The first goal of nutrition therapy is to gain the person's cooperation and trust, with the ultimate objective of increasing oral food intake. Ideally, weight gain must be enough to raise the metabolic rate to normal and reverse as many physical signs of the disease as possible. Food intake is designed first to minimize or stop any further weight loss. Then, the focus shifts to restoring appropriate food habits. After this, the expectation can be switched to slowly gaining weight. A gain of 2 to 3 pounds per week is appropriate. Tube and/or intravenous (IV) feeding is used only if immediate renourishment is required, as this can frighten the person and cause him or her to distrust medical staff.

Persons with anorexia nervosa need considerable reassurance during the refeeding process because of uncomfortable and unfamiliar effects—such as bloating, increase in body heat, and increase in body fat. This is a frightening process because these changes can symbolize a loss of control. Rapid changes in electrolytes and minerals in the blood associated with refeeding, especially potassium, phosphorus, and magnesium, can be dangerous. Therefore, monitoring blood levels of these minerals is of critical importance during the process of incorporating more food into the diet.

In addition to helping persons with anorexia nervosa reach and maintain adequate nutritional status, the registered dietitian on the medical team provides accurate nutrition information throughout the treatment, promotes a healthy attitude toward food, and helps the person learn to eat in response to natural hunger and satiety cues. The focus then turns to identify healthy and adequate food choices that promote weight gain to achieve and maintain a clinically estimated goal weight (e.g., BMI of 20 or more).

Because excessive physical activity prevents weight gain, professionals must help anorexic persons moderate their activity. At many treatment centers, moderate bed rest is used in the early stages of treatment to help promote weight gain.

Experienced professional help is the key. An anorexic person may be on the verge of suicide and starvation. In addition, anorexic people are often very clever and resistant to therapy. They may try to hide weight loss by wearing many layers of clothes, putting coins in their pockets or underwear, and drinking numerous glasses of water.

Psychological and Related Therapy

Once the physical problems of anorexia nervosa are addressed, the treatment focus shifts to the underlying emotional problems that led to excessive dieting and other symptoms of the disorder. To heal, these anorexic persons must reject the sense of accomplishment they have associated with an emaciated body and begin to accept themselves at a healthy body weight. If therapists can discover reasons for the disorder,

A young woman in a self-help group for those with anorexia nervosa explained her feelings to the other group members: "I have lost a specialness that I thought it gave me. I was different from everyone else. Now I know that I'm somebody who's overcome it, which not everybody does."

A disturbing trend is the attempt to promote eating disorders as a way of life. Some anorexic individuals have personified their illness into a role model named "Ana," who tells them what to eat and mocks them when they don't lose weight. Ana web sites reject the serious health risks of anorexia behaviors and instead dispense unsafe "thinspiration" to vulnerable individuals.

they can develop strategies for restoring normal weight and eating habits that involve resolving psychological conflicts. Education about the medical consequences of semi-starvation is also helpful. A key aspect of psychological treatment is showing affected individuals how to regain control of other facets of their lives and cope with difficult situations. As eating evolves into a normal routine, they can turn to previously neglected activities.

Therapists may use **cognitive behavior therapy,** which involves helping the person confront and change irrational beliefs about body image, eating, relationships, and weight. Underlying issues that may be the cause for the disease, such as sexual abuse, also must be identified and addressed by the therapist.

Family therapy often is important in treating anorexia nervosa, especially for younger persons who still live with their families. It focuses on the role of the illness among family members, the reactions of individual family members, and ways in which their subconscious behavior might contribute to the abnormal eating patterns. Frequently, a therapist finds family struggles at the heart of the problem. As the disorder resolves, patients must relate to family members in new ways to gain the attention that was needed and previously tied to the disease. For example, the family may need to help the young person ease into adulthood and accept its responsibilities as well as its advantages.

Self-help groups for anorexic (and bulimic) people, as well as their families and friends, represent nonthreatening first steps into treatment. Others can also attend to get a sense of whether they really do have an eating disorder.

Food is the drug of choice in the treatment of anorexic patients. Generally, medications are not effective in management of the primary symptoms of anorexia nervosa. Fluoxetine (Prozac®) and related medications may stabilize recovery once 85% of expected body weight has been attained. These medications work by prolonging serotonin activity in the brain, which in turn regulates mood and feelings of satiety. A variety of other pharmacologic agents may have some role in treating mood changes, anxiety, or psychotic symptoms associated with anorexia nervosa, but they have limited value unless weight gain is also achieved.

With professional help, many people with anorexia nervosa can lead normal lives. Although they may not be totally cured, anorexic individuals do not have to depend on unusual eating habits to cope with daily problems. They recover a sense of normality in their lives. No universal approach exists, because each case is unique. Establishing a strong relationship with either a therapist or another supportive person is an especially important key to recovery. Once anorexic persons feel understood and accepted by another person, they can begin to build a sense of self and exercise some autonomy. As they learn alternative coping mechanisms, they can relinquish their dysfunctional relationships with food, and instead develop healthy personal relationships.

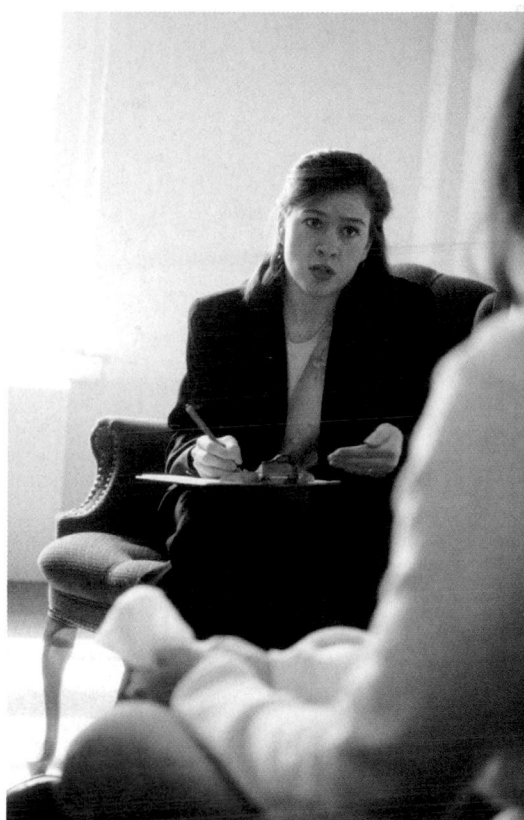

Early treatment for an eating disorder, such as anorexia nervosa, improves chances of success.

cognitive behavior therapy Psychological therapy in which the person's assumptions about dieting, body weight, and related issues are confronted. New ways of thinking are explored and then practiced by the person. In this way, an individual can learn new ways to control disordered eating behaviors and related life stress.

Real Life Scenario Follow-Up

Sarah does have the characteristics to be diagnosed with anorexia nervosa because she refuses to maintain a healthy weight-for-height, is at a weight below 85% of that expected, has a distorted view of her appearance, and has had no menstrual periods for over 3 consecutive months.

Sarah would need to be hospitalized initially, due to her low BMI of 13.8. While in the hospital, her treatment would most likely consist of moderate bed rest to promote weight gain and an intake of 1000 to 1600 kcal initially, which is then increased by increments of about 100 to 200 kcal every few days until an acceptable rate of weight gain is achieved. The goal is to achieve a body weight that is at least 90% of an expected weight for her age, such as a BMI of at least 19. This weight goal should also allow for resumption of menstrual periods. The physician would likely

Singer Karen Carpenter's death from complications of anorexia nervosa in 1983 increased awareness of the serious nature of this disease. Currently, the average time for recovery from anorexia nervosa is 7 years; many insurance companies cover only a fraction of the estimated $150,000 cost of treatment.

prescribe a multivitamin and mineral supplement, along with supplements of calcium as needed to make sure intake is in the range of 1200 to 1500 milligrams. This overall practice will correct vitamin and mineral deficiencies that exist, and the calcium in particular will contribute to bone maintenance. A team of health professionals, most likely consisting of a physician, registered dietitian, and psychologist, would provide therapy. Sarah's cooperation would be the most important element for therapy to be successful. She needs to realize she has a problem and that she needs help, and she must be willing to accept the assistance these professionals are willing to offer. The team, especially the psychologist, may use cognitive behavior therapy to help Sarah improve her self-image.

Sarah's outlook for recovery is not good unless she realizes she has a problem. Even if she is willing to accept the therapy and counseling, a relapse is likely to occur. Only about 50% of anorexia nervosa patients have been found to recover fully from the disease. Since Sarah's disordered eating habits have been in place for about 6 years, her problem is deep-rooted. The chances of recovery are greater if a vigorus treatment program is reinforced with close follow-up.

Concept Check

To relieve the semistarved condition of most anorexic persons, the initial treatment focuses on moderately increased food intake and slow weight gain. Once this is accomplished, psychotherapy can begin to uncover the causes of the disease and help the individual develop the skills needed to return to a healthy life. Family therapy can be an important tool in treatment, whereas medications have a limited role.

A Closer Look at Bulimia Nervosa

Bingeing and purging (via vomiting) was evident in pre-Christian Roman times, but was practiced in a group setting. The eating disorder bulimia nervosa is generally practiced in private. It was first described in the medical literature in 1979.

Bulimia nervosa involves episodes of binge eating followed by various means to purge the food. It is most common among young adults of college age, although some high school students are also at risk. Susceptible people often have genetic factors and lifestyle patterns that predispose them to becoming overweight, and many try frequent weight-reduction diets as teenagers. Like people with anorexia nervosa, those with bulimia nervosa are usually female and successful. Unlike anorexic individuals, however, they are usually at or slightly above a normal weight. Females with bulimia nervosa are also more likely to be sexually active than those with anorexia nervosa.

The person with bulimia nervosa may think of food constantly. But unlike the anorexic person, who turns away from food when faced with problems, the bulimic person turns toward food in critical situations. Also, unlike those with anorexia nervosa, people with bulimia nervosa recognize their behavior as abnormal. These people often have very low self-esteem and are depressed. Approximately half of the people with bulimia nervosa have major depression. Lingering effects of child abuse may be one reason for these feelings. Many bulimic persons report that they have been sexually abused. They appear competent to outsiders, while they actually feel out of control, ashamed, and frustrated.

Bulimic people tend to be impulsive, which may be expressed in behaviors such as stealing, increased sexual activity, drug and alcohol abuse, self-mutilation, or attempted suicide. Some experts have suggested that part of the problem may actually arise from an inability to control responses to impulse and desire. Some studies have demonstrated that bulimic people tend to come from disengaged families—ones that are loosely organized. In these families, roles for family members are not clearly defined, rules are disregarded, and a great deal of conflict exists. (In comparison, anorexic people tend to have families so actively engaged that roles may be too well defined.)

■ Typical Behavior in Bulimia Nervosa

It is likely that many people with bulimic behavior are never diagnosed; the diagnostic criteria specify that a person must binge and purge at least twice a week for 3 months. People with bulimia nervosa lead secret lives, hiding their abnormal eating habits. Moreover, it is impossible to recognize the disorder simply by appearance. Because most diagnoses of bulimia nervosa rely on self-reports, current estimates of the number of cases are probably low. The disorder, especially in its milder forms, may be much more widespread than commonly thought.

For intake to qualify as a binge, an atypically large amount of food must be consumed in a short time, and the person must exhibit a lack of control over his or her behavior. Among sufferers of bulimia nervosa, bingeing often alternates with attempts to rigidly restrict food intake. Elaborate food rules are common, such as avoiding all sweets. Thus, eating just one cookie or donut may cause individuals with this disorder to feel as though they have broken a rule. At that point, in the mind of a bulimic person, the objectionable food must be eliminated. Usually this leads to further overeating, partly because it is easier to regurgitate a large amount of food than a small amount.

Binge-purge cycles may be practiced daily, weekly, or across longer intervals. A specific time often is set aside. Most binge eating occurs at night, when other people are less likely to interrupt, and usually lasts from ½ to 2 hours. A binge can be triggered by a combination of stress, boredom, loneliness, and depression. It often follows a period of strict dieting and thus can be linked to intense hunger. The binge is not at all like normal eating; once begun, it seems to propel itself. The person not only loses control, but generally doesn't even taste or enjoy food during a binge. This separates the practice from simple overeating.

Most commonly, bulimic people consume cakes, cookies, ice cream, and other high-carbohydrate convenience foods during binges because these foods can be purged relatively easily and comfortably by vomiting. In a single binge, foods supplying 3000 kcal or more may be eaten. Purging follows in hopes that no weight will be gained. However, even when vomiting follows the binge, 33% to 75% of the calories taken in is still absorbed, inevitably causing some weight gain. When laxatives or enemas are used, about 90% of the calories are absorbed, as laxatives act in the large intestine, which is beyond the point of most nutrient absorption. Clearly, the belief that purging soon after bingeing will prevent excessive calorie absorption and weight gain is a misconception.

At the onset of bulimia nervosa, sufferers often induce vomiting by placing their fingers deep into the mouth. They may bite down on these fingers inadvertently, resulting in bite marks and scars around the knuckles that are a characteristic sign of this disorder. Once the disease is established, however, a person may be able to vomit simply by contracting the abdominal muscles. Vomiting may also occur spontaneously.

Another way bulimic persons attempt to compensate for a binge and control their weight is by engaging in excessive exercise to expend a large amount of calories. In this practice, referred to as "debting," bulimic individuals try to estimate the amount of calories eaten during a binge, and then exercise to counteract the excess.

People with bulimia nervosa are not proud of their behavior. After a binge, they usually feel guilty and depressed. Over time, they experience low self-esteem, feel hopeless about their situation, and are caught in a vicious cycle of obsession (Fig. 12-2). Compulsive lying, shoplifting to obtain food, and drug abuse can further intensify these feelings. Bulimic people discovered in the act of bingeing by a friend or family member may order the intruder to "get out" and "go away." Sufferers gradually distance themselves from others, spending more and more time preoccupied by and engaging in bingeing and purging.

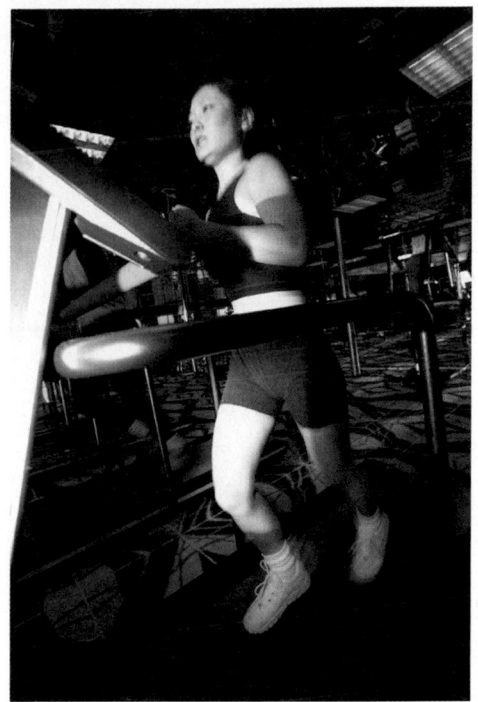

Excessive exercising can be one component of bulimia if it is used as a way to offset the calorie intake from a binge. Exercise is considered excessive when it is done at inappropriate times or settings, or when a person does it despite injury or other medical complications.

Figure 12-2 Bulimia nervosa's vicious cycle of obsession.

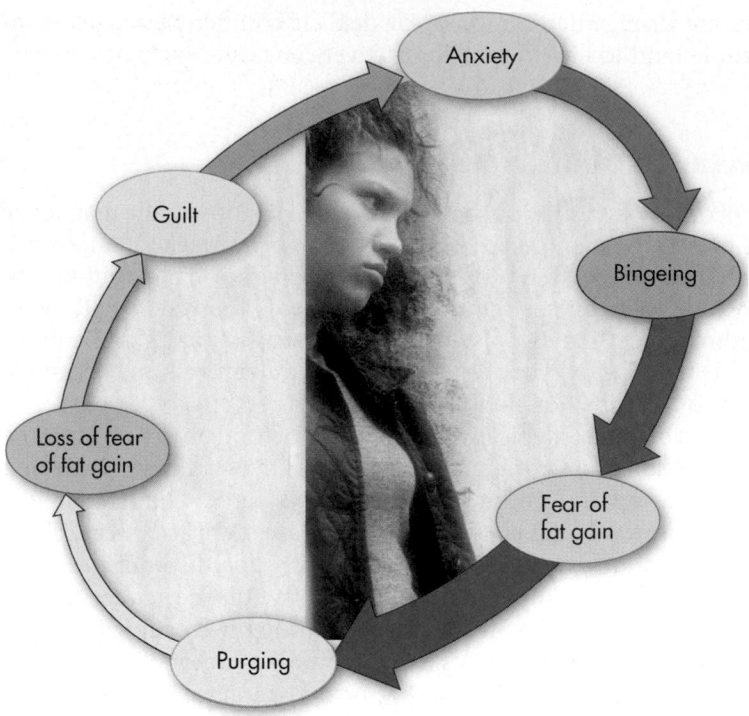

∎ Health Problems Stemming from Bulimia Nervosa

The vomiting that many bulimic sufferers induce is a physically destructive method of purging. Indeed, the majority of health problems associated with bulimia nervosa, as noted below, arise from vomiting:

- Repeated exposure of teeth to the acid in vomit causes demineralization, making the teeth painful and sensitive to heat, cold, and acids. Eventually, the teeth may decay severely, erode away from fillings, and finally fall out (Fig. 12-3). Dental professionals are sometimes the first health professionals to notice signs of bulimia nervosa. As noted earlier it is important to rinse the mouth with water after any vomiting episode, especially before brushing the teeth.
- Blood potassium can drop significantly with regular vomiting or the use of certain diuretics. This can disturb the heart's rhythm and even produce sudden death.
- Salivary glands may swell as a result of infection and irritation from persistent vomiting.
- Stomach ulcers and bleeding and tears in the esophagus develop in some cases.
- Constipation may result from frequent laxative use.
- Ipecac syrup, sometimes used to induce vomiting, is toxic to the heart, liver, and kidneys. It has caused accidental poisoning when taken repeatedly.

Overall, bulimia nervosa is a potentially debilitating disorder that can lead to death, usually from suicide, low blood potassium, or overwhelming infections.

∎ Treatment of Bulimia Nervosa

Therapy for bulimia nervosa, as for anorexia nervosa, requires a team of experienced clinicians. Bulimic individuals are less likely than those with anorexia to enter treatment in a state of semistarvation. However, if a bulimic person has lost significant weight, this must be treated before psychological treatment begins. Although clinicians

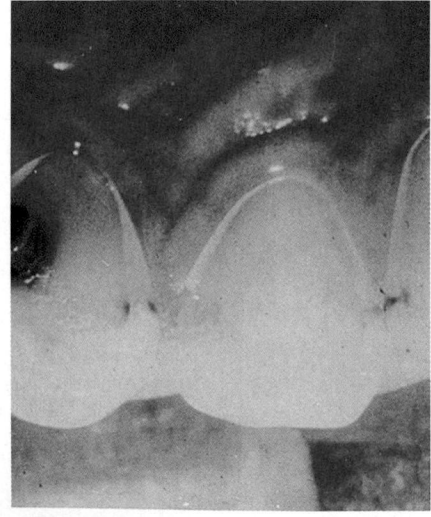

Figure 12-3 Excessive tooth decay is common in bulimic patients.

have yet to agree on the best therapy for bulimia nervosa, they generally agree that treatment should last at least 16 weeks. Hospitalization may be indicated in cases of extreme laxative abuse, regular vomiting, substance abuse, and depression, especially if physical harm is evident.

The first goal of treatment for bulimia nervosa is to decrease the amount of food consumed in a binge session in order to decrease the risk of esophageal tears from related purging by vomiting. A decrease in the frequency of this type of purging will also decrease damage to the teeth.

The primary aim of psychotherapy is to improve a persons' self-acceptance and help one to be less concerned about body weight. Cognitive behavior therapy is generally used. Psychotherapy helps correct the all-or-none thinking typical of bulimic persons: "If I eat one cookie, I'm a failure and might as well binge." The premise of this therapy is that, if abnormal attitudes and beliefs can be altered, normal eating will follow. In addition, the therapist guides the person in establishing food habits that will minimize bingeing: avoiding fasting, eating regular meals, and using alternative methods—other than eating—to cope with stressful situations. Group therapy is often useful to foster strong social support. One goal of therapy is to help bulimic persons accept some depression and self-doubt as normal.

Although pharmacological agents should not be used as the sole treatment for bulimia nervosa, studies indicate that some medications may be beneficial in conjunction with other therapies. Fluoxetine (Prozac®) is the only antidepressant that has been approved by FDA for use in the treatment of bulimia nervosa, but physicians also may prescribe other similar forms of antidepressants, other classes of psychiatric medications, or certain antiseizure medications.

Nutritional counseling has two main goals: correcting misconceptions about food and re-establishing regular eating habits. Bulimic persons are given information about bulimia nervosa and its consequences. Avoiding binge foods and not constantly stepping on a scale may be recommended early in treatment. The primary goal, however, is to develop a normal eating pattern. To achieve this goal, some specialists encourage these individuals to develop daily meal plans and keep a food diary in which they record food intake, internal sensations of hunger, environmental factors that precipitate binges, and thoughts and feelings that accompany binge-purge cycles. Keeping a food diary not only is an accurate way to monitor food intake but also may help identify situations that seem to trigger binge episodes. With the help of a therapist, bulimic persons can develop alternative coping strategies.

In general, the focus is not on stopping bingeing and purging per se but on developing regular eating habits. Once this is achieved, the binge-purge cycle should start to break down. Individuals are discouraged from following strict rules about healthy food choices, because this simply mimics the typical obsessive attitudes associated with bulimia nervosa. Rather, encouraging a mature perspective on nutrient intake— that is, regular consumption of moderate amounts of a variety of foods balanced among the food groups—helps one overcome this disorder.

Setting time limits for the completion of meals and snacks is important for people with eating disorders. Many bulimic persons eat very quickly, reflecting their difficulties with satiety. Suggesting that the person put his or her utensil down after each bite is a behavioral technique that a therapist might try during recovery for bulimia. (In comparison, many anorexic persons eat in an excessively slow manner—for example, taking 1 hour to eat a muffin cut into tiny, bite-size pieces.)

People with bulimia nervosa must recognize that they have a serious disorder that can have grave medical complications if not treated. Because relapse is likely, therapy should be long term. Note that those with bulimia nervosa need professional help because they can be very depressed and are at a high risk for suicide. About 50% of people with bulimia nervosa recover completely from the disorder. Others continue to struggle with it to varying degrees for the rest of their lives. This fact underscores the need for prevention because treatment is difficult.

The binge-purge cycle can create an initial state of euphoria in the person. Giving up this euphoria has been equated to giving up an addiction. Still, it is important to do so.

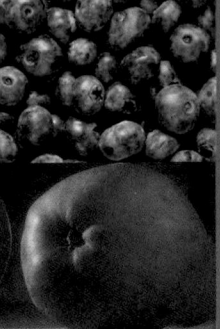

Looking *Further*

Thoughts of a Bulimic Woman

I am wide awake and immediately out of bed. I think back to the night before, when I made a new list of what I wanted to get done and how I wanted to be. My husband is not far behind me on his way into the bathroom to get ready for work. Maybe I can sneak onto the scale to see what I weigh this morning before he notices me. I am already in my private world. I feel overjoyed when the scale says that I stayed the same weight as I was the night before, and I can feel that slightly hungry feeling. Maybe it will stop today; maybe today everything will change. What were the projects I was going to get done?

We eat the same breakfast, except that I take no butter on my toast, no cream in my coffee, and never take seconds (until Doug gets out the door). Today I am going to be really good, and that means eating certain predetermined portions of food and not taking one more bite than I think I am allowed. I am very careful to see that I don't take more than Doug. I judge myself by his body. I can feel the tension building. I wish Doug would hurry up and leave so I can get going!

As soon as he shuts the door, I try to get involved with one of the myriad responsibilities on my list. I hate them all! I just want to crawl into a hole. I don't want to do anything. I'd rather eat. I am alone; I am nervous; I am no good; I always do everything wrong anyway; I am not in control; I can't make it through the day, I know it. It has been the same for so long. I remember the starchy cereal I ate for breakfast. I am into the bathroom and onto the scale. It measures the same, but I don't want to stay the same! I want to be thinner! I look into the mirror. I think my thighs are ugly and deformed looking. I see a lumpy, clumsy, pear-shaped wimp. There is always something wrong with what I see. I feel frustrated, trapped in this body, and I don't know what to do about it.

I float to the refrigerator knowing exactly what is there. I begin with last night's brownies. I always begin with the sweets. At first I try to make it look like nothing is missing, but my appetite is huge and I resolve to make another batch of brownies. I know there is half of a bag of cookies in the bathroom, thrown out the night before, and I polish them off immediately. I take some milk so my vomiting will be smoother. I like the full feeling I get after downing a big glass. I get out six pieces of bread and toast one side of each in the broiler, turn them over and load them with pats of butter, and put them under the broiler again until they are bubbling. I take all six pieces on a plate to the television and go back for a bowl of cereal and a banana to have along with them. Before the last piece of toast is finished, I am already preparing the next batch of six more pieces. Maybe another brownie or five, and a couple of large bowls full of ice cream, yogurt, or cottage cheese.

My stomach is stretched into a huge ball below my rib cage. I know I'll have to go into the bathroom soon, but I want to postpone it. I am in never-never land. I am waiting, feeling the pressure, pacing the floor in and out of the rooms. Time is passing. Time is passing. It is getting to be time. I wander aimlessly through each of the rooms again, tidying, making the whole house neat and put back together. I finally make the turn into the bathroom. I brace my feet, pull my hair back and stick my finger down my throat, stroking twice, and get up a huge pile of food. Three times, four times, and another pile of food. I can see everything come back. I am so glad to see those brownies because they are so fattening. The rhythm of the emptying is broken and my head is beginning to hurt. I stand up feeling dizzy, empty, and weak. The whole episode has taken about an hour.

From Hall L, Cohn L: *Bulimia—A Guide to Recovery.* Gurze Books: Carlsbad, CA, 1992.

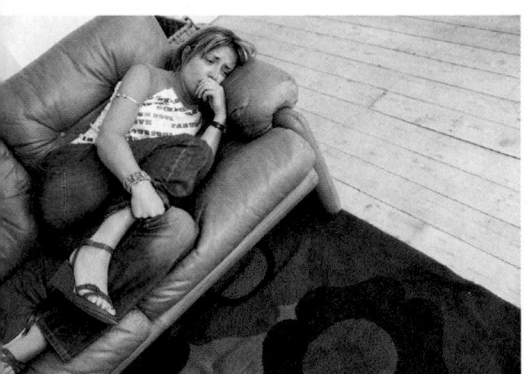

Bulimic episodes add to the despair felt in this disorder.

Concept Check

Bulimia nervosa is characterized by episodes of binge eating followed by purging, usually by vomiting. Vomiting is very destructive to the body, often causing severe dental decay, stomach ulcers, irritation of the esophagus, and blood potassium imbalances. Treatment using nutrition counseling and psychotherapy attempts to restore normal eating habits, to help the person correct distorted beliefs about diet and lifestyle, and to find tools to cope with the stresses of life. Medications, such as fluoxetine (Prozac®), can aid recovery when added to this regimen.

Other Examples of Disordered Eating: Binge-Eating Disorder and the Female Athlete Triad

In recent years, two other conditions—binge-eating disorder (mentioned in the introduction) and the **female athlete triad**—have been recognized as requiring professional treatment. Although these disordered eating patterns share some characteristics of anorexia nervosa and bulimia nervosa, each has distinctive qualities.

female athlete triad A condition characterized by disordered eating, lack of menstrual periods (amenorrhea), and osteoporosis.

▪ Binge-Eating Disorder

The typical characteristics for binge-eating disorder are listed in Table 12-2. Generally, it can be defined as binge-eating episodes not accompanied by purging (as typifies bulimia nervosa) at least two times per week for at least 6 months. First officially described in 1994, today health care professionals recognize binge-eating disorder as a growing, complex, and potentially serious problem.

Approximately 30% of subjects in organized weight-control programs have binge-eating disorder, whereas among the general U.S. population about 4 million have this disorder. However, many more people in the general population are likely to have

Table 12-2 Some Characteristics of Binge-Eating Disorder

A. Recurrent episodes of binge eating, an episode being characterized by both of the following:
   (1) Eating, in a discrete period of time (e.g., within any 2-hour period), an amount of food that is definitely larger than most people would eat during a similar period of time in similar circumstances
   (2) A sense of lack of control during the episodes (e.g., a feeling that one can't stop eating or control what or how much one is eating)

B. During most binge episodes, at least three of the following occur:
   (1) Eating much more rapidly than usual
   (2) Eating until feeling uncomfortably full
   (3) Eating large amounts of food when not feeling physically hungry
   (4) Eating alone because of being embarrassed by how much one is eating
   (5) Feeling disgusted with oneself, depressed, or very guilty after overeating

C. Marked distress regarding binge eating

D. The binge eating occurs, on average, at least 2 days a week for 6 months.

E. The behavior does not occur only during the course of bulimia nervosa or anorexia nervosa.

Based on information from the *Diagnostic and Statistical Manual of Mental Disorders*, Fourth Edition (DSM-IV-TR). Washington DC: American Psychiatric Association, 2000.

Another eating disorder under study is night eating syndrome. In this disorder people feel they need to eat food in order to fall asleep again once awakened in the night. It may also take place during sleep walking. This night eating can contribute to weight gain, so affected persons are urged to seek treatment. For more information see the August 2004 edition of *Today's Dietitian*,

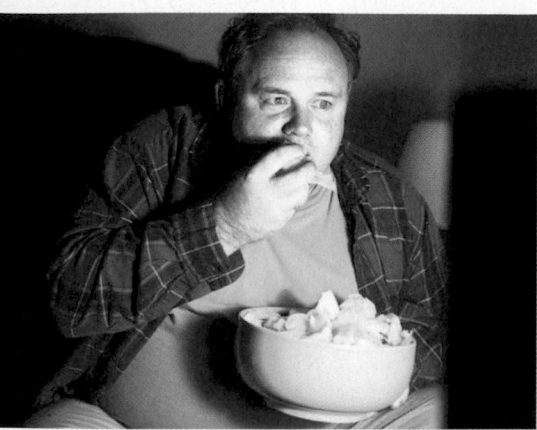

Binge-eating disorder is seen in both men and women.

As noted in Chapter 2, spreading one's dietary intake into numerous, small meals (grazing) over a day actually provides some health advantages if overall calorie intake remains appropriate.

People with binge-eating disorder may come from families with alcoholism or may have suffered sexual abuse. Members of such dysfunctional families often do not know how to deal effectively with emotions. They cope by turning to substances. Family members learn to cover up dysfunctional patterns for the alcoholic person and to nurture him or her at the expense of each other and their own needs.

less severe forms of the disorder that do not meet all the criteria that describe the problem. The number of cases of binge-eating disorder is far greater than that of either anorexia nervosa or bulimia nervosa. This disorder is also more common among the severely obese and those with a long history of frequent restrictive dieting, although obesity is not a criterion for having binge-eating disorder.

Development and Characteristics of Binge-Eating Disorder

Individuals with binge-eating disorder (about 40% of whom are males) often perceive themselves as hungry more often than normal. They usually started dieting at a young age, began bingeing during adolescence or in their early twenties, and did not succeed in commercial weight-control programs. Almost half of those with severe binge-eating disorder exhibit clinical depression. Some people also may have a genetic predisposition for this disorder.

Typical binge eaters isolate themselves and eat large quantities of a favorite food. Stressful events and feelings of depression or anxiety can trigger this behavior. Giving themselves permission to eat a forbidden food can also precipitate a binge. Other triggers include loneliness, anxiety, self-pity, depression, anger, rage, alienation, and frustration. They sometimes binge on whatever is easy to eat in large amounts—noodles, rice, bread, leftovers. Characteristically, however, binge eaters consume foods that carry the social stigma of "junk" or "bad" foods—ice cream, cookies, sweets, potato chips, and similar snack foods.

In general, people engage in binge eating to induce a sense of well-being and perhaps even numbness, usually in an attempt to avoid feeling and dealing with emotional pain and anxiety. They eat without regard to biological need and often in a recurrent, ritualized fashion. Some people with this disorder eat food continually over an extended period, called *grazing;* others cycle episodes of bingeing with normal eating. For example, someone with a stressful or frustrating job might come home every night and graze until bedtime. Another person might eat normally most of the time but find comfort in consuming large quantities of food when an emotional setback occurs.

Although people with anorexia nervosa and bulimia nervosa exhibit persistent preoccupation with body shape, weight, and thinness, binge eaters do not necessarily share these concerns. Thus, neither purging nor prolonged food restriction is characteristic of binge-eating disorder. Some physicians classify binge-eating disorder as an addiction to food, involving psychological dependence. The person becomes attached to the behavior itself and has a drive to continue it, senses only limited control over it, and needs to persist at it despite negative consequences. Food is used to reduce stress, produce feelings of power and well-being, avoid feelings of intimacy with others, and avoid life problems. Note that obesity and binge eating are not necessarily linked. Not all obese people are binge eaters, and, although obesity may result from trying to numb emotional pain with food, it is not necessarily an outcome of binge eating.

Binge-eating disorder is most likely to develop in people who never learned to express and deal appropriately with their feelings. Rather than face their problems, they turn to food. They continue to do the things that perpetuate the experiences of frustration, anger, and pain. The frustration will continue because they never confront the basic problem. Binge eating makes them feel they cannot control the behavior pattern and therefore cannot control their lives. Worse, the binge eating usually increases feelings of guilt, embarrassment, and shame.

Often, people who practice binge eating have been shaped by families who do not address and express feelings in healthful ways. The parents nurture and comfort their children with food rather than engage in healthy exchanges of self-disclosure of feelings and potential solutions. Members of such families learn to eat in response to emotional needs and pain instead of hunger. Those who regularly practice binge eating may grow up nurturing others instead of themselves, avoiding their own feelings and taking little time for themselves. Not knowing how to satisfy their personal and emotional needs in more healthful ways, people in these families turn to food.

For some people, frequent dieting beginning in childhood or adolescence is a precursor to binge-eating disorder. During periods when little food is eaten, they get very hungry and obsessive about food. When allowed to eat more food, they feel driven to eat in a compulsive, uncontrolled way. The pattern of strict dieting alternating with binge eating may continue over time.

Help for the Person with Binge-Eating Disorder

Those with binge-eating disorder must learn to eat in response to hunger—a biological signal—rather than in response to emotional needs or external factors (such as the time of day or the simple presence of food). Counselors often direct binge eaters to record their perceptions of physical hunger throughout the day and at the beginning and end of every meal. These people must learn to respond to a prescribed amount of fullness at each meal. They should initially avoid weight-loss diets because feelings of food deprivation can lead to more disruptive emotions and a greater sense of unmet needs. Diets are likely to encourage more intense problems, such as extreme hunger. Many people with binge-eating disorder may experience difficulty in identifying personal emotional needs and expressing emotions. Because this problem is a common predisposing factor in binge eating, communication issues should be addressed during treatment. Binge eaters often must be helped to recognize their own buried emotions in anxiety-producing situations, and then encouraged to share them with their therapist or therapy group. Learning simple but appropriate phrases to say to oneself can help stop bingeing when the desire is strong.

Self-help groups, such as Overeaters Anonymous, aim to help recovery from binge-eating disorder. Their treatment philosophy, which parallels that of Alcoholics Anonymous, attempts to create an environment of encouragement and accountability to overcome this eating disorder. Dietary advice typically ranges from avoiding restraint in eating in general to limiting binge foods. Some experts feel that learning to eat all foods—but in moderation—is an effective goal for binge eaters. This practice can prevent the feelings of desperation and deprivation that come from limiting particular foods. Antidepressants, such as fluoxetine (Prozac®), and other types of medications also have been found to help reduce binge eating in these individuals by decreasing depression. Overall, people who have this disorder are usually unsuccessful in controlling it on their own. Professional help is advised.

■ Female Athlete Triad

Women participating in appearance-based and endurance sports are at risk of developing an eating disorder. One study of college-age female athletes found that 15% of swimmers, 62% of gymnasts, and 32% of all varsity athletes exhibited disordered eating patterns. Estimates of eating disorders for college women not involved in competitive sports are much lower.

In addition to disordered eating, college women athletes tend to experience irregular menstruation more frequently than other college women. Disordered eating, particularly food restriction and stress, can precipitate this, causing women to have less dense and weaker bones than normal because of lower estrogen concentrations in the blood. Some of these young women have bone mass values equivalent to those of 50- to 60-year-olds, increasing their risk for bone and stress fractures during sports as well as general activities. Much of the bone loss is irreversible.

The American College of Sports Medicine (ACSM) has named this syndrome "female athlete triad" because it consists of three parts: disordered eating, lack of menstrual

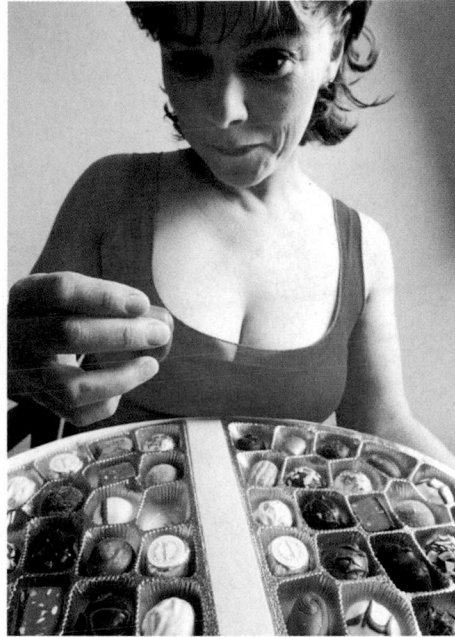

Professional help is advised for people with a binge-eating disorder.

A female high school athlete recently admitted her 3-year struggle with anorexia nervosa and bulimia nervosa. Even after her athletic performance declined and she suffered a sports-related injury, which sidelined her for a year and required surgery, she continued to think that controlling both her weight and eating behaviors would make her the best—academically and physically. This example demonstrates several important points about eating disorders: certain groups of people are at greater risk for developing eating disorders; these people are often high achievers and are very careful about concealing their eating disorder; and eating disorders such as the female athlete triad, bulimia nervosa, and anorexia nervosa frequently overlap.

Figure 12-4 The female athlete triad occurs when the athlete has disordered eating, lack of menstrual periods, and osteoporosis. Stress fractures and recurrent fatigue also occur. This triad often is seen in appearance-related sports, such as gymnastics. Long-term health is at risk; thus, early treatment is most beneficial.

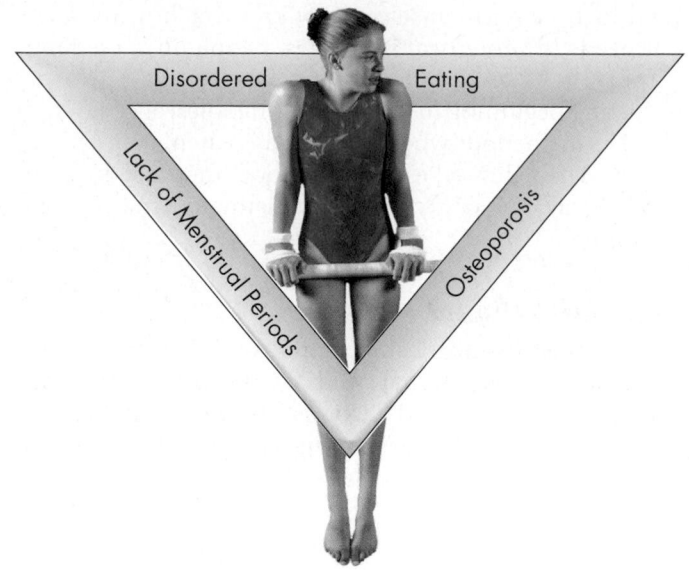

It is often difficult to get female athletes to accept necessary treatment plans. They frequently have a single-minded approach to their sport, while ignoring future health consequences.

periods, and osteoporosis (Fig. 12-4). The ACSM has issued a plea to teachers, coaches, health professionals, and parents to educate female athletes about the triad and its health consequences.

Many coaches/trainers and even some health professionals wrongly believe that loss of menstrual periods is a normal consequence of a high level of physical activity. However, loss of menstrual periods in female athletes stems from a dramatic decrease in female reproductive hormones, particularly estrogen. Loss of estrogen has other negative consequences on the body, such as fragile bones, as just mentioned. Correcting the hormonal imbalance and menstrual irregularities by increasing caloric intake should increase bone mass. During therapy, a physician may prescribe a multivitamin and mineral supplement as well as calcium supplements as needed to maintain an intake of 1200 to 1500 milligrams (review the Real Life Scenario Follow-Up for recommended treatment of anorexia nervosa).

Those exhibiting symptoms of the female athlete triad should seek treatment from a multidisciplinary team of health professionals. Involving the coach or trainer in therapy is usually a key factor in the success of the treatment plan. Suggestions for treatment are as follows:

- Reduce preoccupation with food, weight, and body fat.
- Gradually increase meals and snacks to an appropriate amount.
- Achieve an appropriate weight-for-height.
- Establish regular menstrual periods.
- Decrease training time and/or intensity by 10% to 20%.

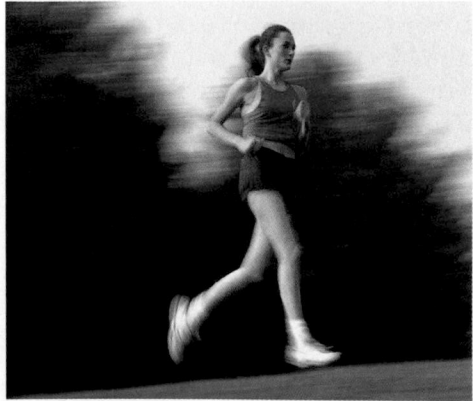

Low body weight coupled with excessive exercise can lead to cessation of menstrual periods, and ultimately female athlete triad.

Another Bite

The tragic case of Christy Henrich illustrates why anyone at risk for the female athlete triad should seek professional help. As a young teenager, Christy weighed 95 pounds and was 4 feet 11 inches tall. She showed promise as a gymnast but was told that she was too fat to excel in gymnastics. Christy continued her training but often starved herself, some days consuming just an apple and frequently purging by vomiting. Her success in gymnastics continued, but at age 22 her weight had fallen to 52 pounds, and she died from the effects of long-term semistarvation.

Prevention of Eating Disorders

A key to developing and maintaining healthful eating behavior is to realize that some concern about diet, health, and weight is normal. It is also normal to experience variation in what we eat, how we feel, and even how much we weigh. For example, it is normal to experience some minimal weight change (up to 2 to 3 pounds) throughout the day and even more over the course of a week. A large weight fluctuation or ongoing weight gain or weight loss is more likely to indicate that a problem is present. If you notice a large change in your diet, how you feel, or your body weight, it is a good idea to consult your personal physician. Treating physical and emotional problems early helps lead you to peace of mind and good health.

With a view on society as a whole, many people begin to form opinions about food, nutrition, health, weight, and body image prior to or during puberty. Parents, friends, and professionals working with young adults should consider the following advice for preventing eating disorders:

- Discourage restrictive dieting and meal skipping. Fasting is also discouraged (except for religious occasions).
- Provide information about normal changes that occur during puberty.
- Correct misconceptions about nutrition, healthy body weight, and approaches to weight loss.
- Carefully phrase weight-related recommendations and comments and use them with caution.
- Don't overemphasize numbers on a scale. Instead, primarily promote healthful eating.
- Encourage normal expression of disruptive emotions.
- Encourage children to eat only when they're hungry.
- Teach the basics of proper nutrition and regular physical activity in school and at home.
- Provide adolescents with an appropriate, but not unlimited, degree of independence, choice, responsibility, and self-accountability for their actions.
- Increase self-acceptance and appreciation of the power and pleasure emerging from one's body.
- Enhance tolerance for diversity in body weight and shape, and personal food choices.
- Build respectful environments, supportive relationships.
- Encourage coaches to be sensitive to weight and body-image issues among athletes.
- Emphasize that thinness is not necessarily associated with better athletic performance.

Our society as a whole can benefit from a fresh focus on healthful food practices and a healthful outlook toward food and body weight.

Overall, the challenge facing many North Americans is achieving a healthy body weight without excessive dieting. This means adopting and maintaining sensible eating habits, a physically active lifestyle, and realistic and positive attitudes and emotions while practicing creative ways to handle stress. Because eating disorders develop in part from certain cultural values, changing these values might reduce the pressures predisposing some people to various types of disordered eating behavior. Some feminists, for example, assert that true liberation means being free to find one's natural weight. Women who combine careers and motherhood are saying that they have more important things to worry about; some fashion leaders are tolerating more curves; exercise programs are encouraging regular brisk walking, rather than mostly jogging and working out. Finally, writers, therapists, and registered dietitians are working to help women accept their bodies, as noted in the "size acceptance" approach discussed in Chapter 10.

Critical Thinking

Tom, a high school teacher, is concerned about eating disorders. He wants to try to prevent young adults from falling into the discouraging traps of anorexia nervosa and bulimia nervosa. What are some of the topics and issues he should discuss with students in his health classes?

Not only is treatment of eating disorders far more difficult than prevention, these disorders also have devastating effects on the entire family. For this reason, caregivers and health care professionals alike must emphasize the importance of an overall healthful diet that focuses on moderation, as opposed to restriction and perfection. Restricted diets are especially detrimental to children because they do not supply enough calories to sustain growth. In response, nutritional counseling can assure caregivers that including some sweets and fast-food in a child's diet is appropriate (see Chapter 14 for more details).

Another Bite

For further information on eating disorders, contact:

Academy for Eating Disorders, 6728 McClean Village Dr., McLean, VA 22101; 703-556-9222; www.acadeatdis.org

American Anorexia Bulimia Association, 165 West 46th St., #1108, New York, NY 10036; 212-575-6200; www.aabainc.org/home.html

The National Eating Disorders Organization, 603 Stewart St., Suite 803, Seattle, WA 98101; 206-382-3587 or 800-931-EDAP; www.nationaleatingdisorders.org

Harvard Eating Disorders Centers, 356 Boylston St., Boston, MA 02116; 617-236-7766; www.hedc.org

The National Institute of Mental Health has recently published a concise review of eating disorders (www.nimh.nih.gov/publicat/eatingdisordersmenu.cfm).

Concept Check

Food bingeing (without purging) and grazing are two characteristic behaviors of binge-eating disorder. Treatment addresses the deeper emotional issues that undermine healthy eating practices, while shifting the person's focus away from food deprivation and restrictive diets and toward more normal eating behaviors. The female athlete triad consists of disordered eating, amenorrhea, and osteoporosis, and most commonly affects those in appearance-related and endurance sports. Parents, coaches, teachers, and health professionals need to initiate efforts to prevent and treat this problem.

Summary

1. Anorexia nervosa is most common among high-achieving, perfectionist girls from families marked by conflict, high expectations, rigidity, and denial. The disorder usually starts with dieting in early puberty and proceeds to the near-total refusal to eat. Early warning signs include intense concern about weight gain and dieting, as well as abnormal food habits, such as cooking food that they won't allow themselves to eat.

2. Anorexic persons become irritable, hostile, overly critical, and joyless; they tend to withdraw from family and friends. Eventually, anorexia nervosa can lead to numerous physical effects, including a profound decrease in body weight and body fat, a fall in body temperature and heart rate, iron-deficiency anemia, a low white blood cell count, hair loss, constipation, low blood potassium, and the loss of menstrual periods. Those with anorexia nervosa are in a state of physical illness.

3. Treatment of anorexia nervosa includes increasing food intake to support gradual weight gain. Psychological counseling attempts to help establish regular food habits and to find means of coping with the life stresses that led to the disorder. Hospitalization may be necessary, as well as use of certain medications.

4. Bulimia nervosa is characterized by secretive bingeing on large amounts of food within a short time span, and then purging by vomiting or misusing laxatives, diuretics, or enemas. Alternately, fasting and excessive exercise may be used. Both men and women are at risk. Vomiting as a means of purging is especially destructive to the body; it can cause severe tooth decay, stomach ulcers,
irritation of the esophagus, low blood potassium, and other problems. Bulimia nervosa poses a serious health problem and is associated with significant risk of suicide.

5. Treatment of bulimia nervosa includes psychological as well as nutritional counseling. During treatment, bulimic persons learn to accept themselves and to cope with problems in ways that do not involve food. Regular eating patterns are developed as these bulimic persons begin to plan meals in an informed, healthful manner. Certain medications can be a helpful addition to the regimen.

6. Binge-eating disorder, which is more widespread than either anorexia nervosa or bulimia nervosa, is most common among people with a history of frequent, unsuccessful dieting. Binge eaters typically either practice bingeing without purging or grazing (i.e., eating continually over extended periods). Emotional disturbances are often at the root of this disordered form of eating. Treatment addresses deeper emotional issues, discourages food deprivation and restrictive diets, and helps restore normal eating behaviors. Certain medications may be a useful addition to this therapy.

7. The female athlete triad consists of disordered eating, loss of menstrual periods, and osteoporosis. It is particularly common in appearance-related and endurance sports. If not corrected, this disorder eventually leads to decreased athletic performance and general health problems.

Study Questions

1. What are the typical characteristics of a person with anorexia nervosa? What may influence a person to begin rigid, self-imposed dietary patterns?
2. List the detrimental physical and psychological side effects of bulimia nervosa. Describe important goals of the psychological and nutrition therapy used to treat bulimic patients.
3. What is the current thinking concerning medication use for anorexia nervosa and bulimia nervosa?
4. Explain the role of excessive exercise in eating disorders.
5. How might parents significantly contribute to the development of an eating disorder? Suggest an attitude that a parent or an adult friend of yours displayed that may not have been conducive to developing a normal relationship to food.
6. Based on your knowledge of good nutrition and sound dietary habits, answer the following questions:
   a. How can repeated bingeing and purging lead to significant nutrient deficiencies?
   b. How can significant nutrient deficiencies contribute to major health problems in later life?
   c. A friend asks you, the nutrition expert, if it is okay to "cleanse" the body by eating only grapefruit for a week. What is your response?
7. How, in your opinion, has society contributed to the development of various forms of disordered eating? Provide an example.
8. List the three symptoms that constitute the female athlete triad. What is the major health risk associated with loss of menstrual periods in the female athlete?
9. How does binge-eating disorder differ from bulimia nervosa? Describe the factors that contribute to the development and treatment of binge-eating disorder.
10. Provide two recommendations to reduce the problem of eating disorders in our society.

Further Readings

1. ADA Reports: Position of the American Dietetic Association: Nutrition intervention in the treatment of anorexia nervosa, bulimia nervosa, and eating disorders not otherwise specified (EDNOS). *Journal of the American Dietetic Association* 101:810, 2001.

   Eating disorders are complex and serious illnesses, as described in detail in this article. To be effective in treating individuals who suffer from these illnesses, the expert interaction between professionals in many disciplines is required.

2. American Academy of Pediatrics: Identifying and treating eating disorders. *Pediatrics* 111:204, 2003.

   Eating disorders are becoming more common in our society. This article reviews the current diagnostic and treatment options for such disorders.

3. American Psychiatric Association: Practice guidelines for the treatment of patients with eating disorders (revision). *American Journal of Psychiatry* 157(suppl):4, 2000.

   People with eating disorders display a broad range of symptoms that occur along a continuum between those of anorexia nervosa and those of bulimia nervosa. The care of these people requires a comprehensive array of approaches to provide the best chance of treatment success.

4. Jackson K: Eating disorders revealed. *Today's Dietitian* p. 37, March 2004.

   Eating disorders are often hard to recognize as individuals may hide the various practices. This article discusses the many characteristics of eating disorders that can be used in the diagnosis.

5. Jackson K Exercise abuse: Too much of a good thing. *Today's Dietitian* p. 51, March 2005.

   Regularly performing an excessive amount of exercise has deleterious effects on the body, including the skeleton. This author discusses the problem of exercise abuse and reviews treatment options.

6. Kouba S and others: pregnancy and neonatal outcomes in women with eating disorders. *Obstetrics and Gynecology* 105: 255, 2005.

   Pregnant women with past or ongoing eating disorders such as anorexia nervosa and bulimia nervosa have a greater risk for delivering infants with low birth weight. The authors suggest that these women receive careful medical follow up during pregnancy.

7. Lamberg L: Advances in eating disorders: Offer food for thought. *Journal of the American Medical Association* 290:1437, 2003.

   The latest research shows that genetic background provides a major risk factor for the development of eating disorders, and is possibly implicated in 50% to 80% of cases. The current thinking is that today's societal emphasis on thinness brings out the genetic propensity in certain individuals to develop an eating disorder.

8. Mehler PS: Bulimia nervosa. *The New England Journal of Medicine* 349:875, 2003.

   The combination of cognitive behavior therapy and antidepressant medications provides the best hope for treatment of bulimia nervosa. Nutritional counseling also has a role, such as addressing concerns about specific "forbidden" foods.

9. Miller KK and others: Medical findings in outpatients with anorexia nervosa. *Archives of Internal Medicine* 165: 561, 2005.

   Medical problems are typically seen in people with anorexia nervosa. Examples are lowered immune system status and bone loss with related history of bone fractures.

10. Pritts SD, Susman J: Diagnosis of eating disorders in primary care. *American Family Physician* 67:297, 2003.

    Eating disorders can lead to devastating medical and psychological consequences. Treatment, as outlined in this article, needs to be instituted as soon as possible to improve chances of a successful outcome.

11. Shanta-Retelny V: Binge eating into obesity. *Today's Dietitian* p. 34, May 2004.

    Binge-eating disorder is a common problem in people seeking therapy for obesity. The combination of cognitive behavior therapy and certain psychiatric and antiseizure medications currently provides the greatest likelihood for successful therapy. Not skipping meals is a key part of the nutrition therapy.

12. Yager J, Andersen AA: Anorexia nervosa. *The New England Journal of Medicine* 353:1481, 2005.

    Excellent review of eating disorders by noted experts. Both diagnosis and treatment are highlighted.

I. Assessing Risk of Developing an Eating Disorder

British investigators have developed a five-question screening tool called the SCOFF Questionnaire for recognizing eating disorders:[†]

1. Do you make yourself *S*ick because you feel full?

2. Do you lose *C*ontrol over how much you eat?

3. Have you lost more than *O*ne stone (about 13 pounds) recently?

4. Do you believe yourself to be *F*at when others say you are thin?

5. Does *F*ood dominate your life?

Two or more positive responses suggest an eating disorder.

1. After completing this questionnaire, do you feel that you might have an eating disorder or the potential to develop one?

   _____

   _____

2. Do you think any of your friends might have an eating disorder?

   _____

   _____

3. What counseling and education resources exist in your area or on your campus to help with a potential eating disorder?

   _____

   _____

4. If a friend has an eating disorder, what do you think is the best way to assist him or her in getting help?

   _____

   _____

[†]Morgan JF and others: The SCOFF Questionnaire, *British Medical Journal* 319:1467, 1999.

II. Helping Prevent Eating Disorders

You have been asked to speak to a junior high school class about eating disorders. What are four major points that you would make to help prevent disordered eating in this population?

1. _____

2. _____

3. _____

4. _____

Here are points you may consider:

1. Extreme thinness is oversold in the media. Extremely low weight (i.e., BMI of less than 17.5) is generally not healthy.

2. Self-induced vomiting is dangerous. Damage to the teeth, stomach, and esophagus often results.

3. Loss of menstrual periods is a sign of illness. It is important to see a physician about this. Bone deterioration is a common result.

4. The treatment of eating disorders in early phases aids success. These diseases are difficult to treat once firmly established.

Pregnancy and Breastfeeding

13

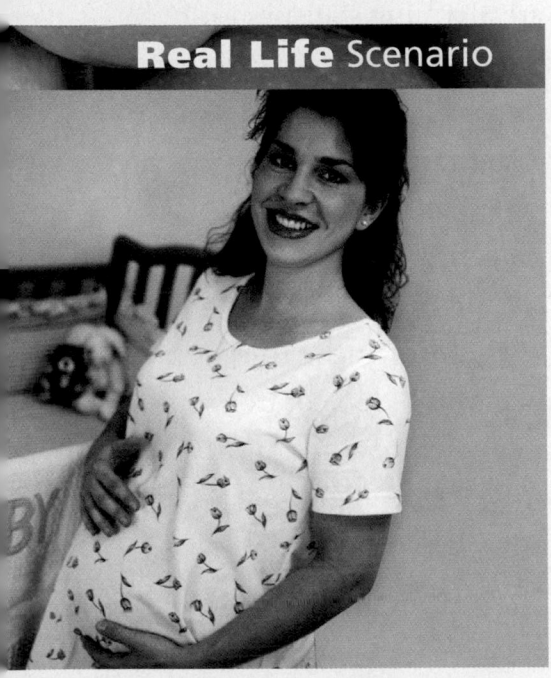

Tracey and her husband of 4 years have decided that they are ready to prepare for Tracey's first pregnancy. Tracey has been reading everything she can find on pregnancy because she knows that her prepregnancy health is important to the success of her pregnancy.

She just turned 25 and is in the recommended childbearing age of 20 to 35 years. She knows she should avoid alcohol, especially because alcohol is particularly toxic to the growing fetus in the first weeks of pregnancy, and she could become pregnant and not know about it right away. Tracey is not a smoker, does not take any medications, and limits her coffee intake to 4 cups a day and soft drink intake to 3 colas per day.

Based on her reading, she has decided to breastfeed her infant and has already inquired about childbirth classes. She has modified her diet to include some extra protein, along with more fruits and vegetables. Recently, she started a running program 5 days a week, and she plans to continue running throughout her pregnancy. She has also started taking an over-the-counter vitamin and mineral supplement.

Tracey and her husband think that they have covered all the key areas of prepregnancy care. List a few positive attributes of her current practices you support. Can you identify some potential problems and what information they may have missed?

Chapter 13 Objectives

Chapter 13 is designed to allow you to:

1. List major physiological changes that occur in the body during pregnancy and how nutrient needs are altered.

2. List factors that predict a successful pregnancy outcome, and some that do not.

3. Specify the optimal weight gain during pregnancy for the normal adult woman.

4. Plan an adequate, balanced meal plan for a pregnant or lactating woman using MyPyramid as a basis.

5. Identify the nutrients that may need to be supplemented during pregnancy and explain the reason for each.

6. Explain the typical discomforts of pregnancy that can be minimized by dietary changes.

7. Describe the physiological processes involved in breastfeeding, as well as some advantages of breastfeeding for both the infant and mother.

Check out the **Contemporary Nutrition Online Learning Center**
www.mhhe.com/wardlawcont6 *for quizzes, flash cards, activities, and web links designed to further help you learn about nutrition for pregnant and breastfeeding women.*

Pregnancy can be a very special time. Along with the responsibility of shaping a child's health and personality comes the prospective exhilaration of watching a child develop and grow. Those involved often feel an overriding desire to produce a healthy baby, which can arouse new interest in nutrition and health information. They usually want to do everything possible to maximize their chances of having a robust, lively newborn.

Despite these intentions, the infant mortality rate in North America is higher than that seen in many other industrialized nations. In Canada, about 6.1 of every 1000 infants per year die before their first birthday, while in the United States it is 6.9. These are alarming statistics for two countries that have such a high per capita expenditure for health care compared to many other countries in the world. And compare that to Sweden at roughly 3 of every 1000 infants. In addition, in the United States, about 20% of pregnant women receive inadequate prenatal care in the early months of pregnancy. Expectant teenagers are at the highest risk for this.

Producing a healthy baby is not just a matter of luck. True, some aspects of fetal and newborn health are beyond our control. Still, conscious decisions about social, health, and nutritional factors during pregnancy significantly affect the baby's future. Choosing to breastfeed the infant adds further benefits. Let's examine how eating well during pregnancy and breastfeeding can help a baby to have a healthy start in life.

Refresh Your Memory

As you begin your study of nutrition in pregnancy and breastfeeding in Chapter 13, you may want to review:

- Typical fortification in meal replacement bars in Chapter 1 and ready-to-eat breakfast cereals in Chapter 2
- Causes and effects of ketosis in Chapter 4
- Components of the macronutrient classes—carbohydrates, proteins, and lipids—in Chapters 4 to 6, especially omega-3 fatty aids
- Alcohol content of various beverages in Chapter 7
- Food sources of folate in Chapter 8 and calcium, iron, and zinc in Chapter 9
- Calculation of body mass index in Chapter 10

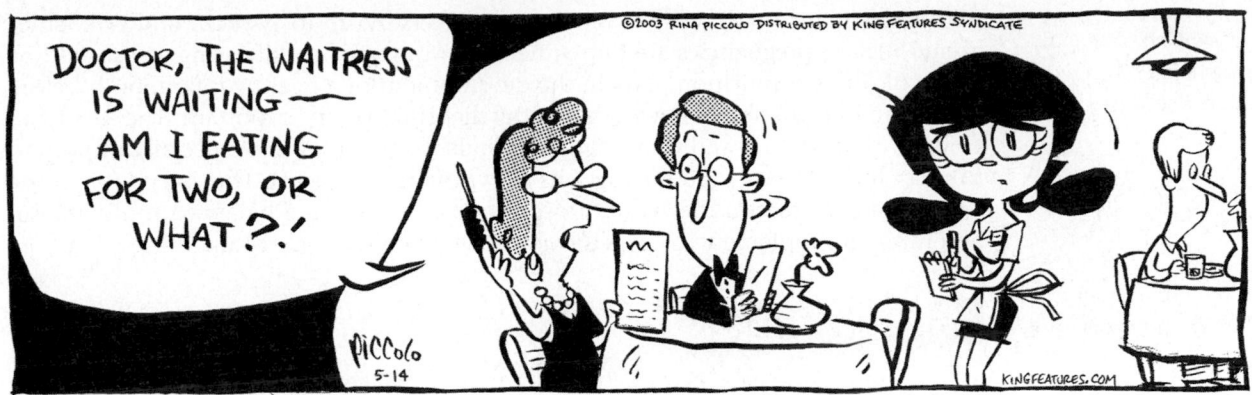

Which diet and lifestyle habits contribute to a successful pregnancy? Which are likely to be harmful? Why should a woman begin to prepare for pregnancy months before conception of her new baby? When pregnant, does the mother need to "eat for two"? Chapter 13 provides some answers.

© Rina Piccolo. Reprinted with special permission of King Features Syndicate.

Planning for Pregnancy

Because many practices or conditions of the mother can harm the developing fetus, planning for pregnancy is very important. The following are some potentially harmful habits that can be modified when planning to have a baby:

- Lack of enough synthetic folic acid in the diet (at least 3 months before becoming pregnant)
- Any amount of alcohol consumption
- Use of certain medicines, such as aspirin and related NSAIDs (e.g., ibuprofen [Advil]), as well as typical medicines used to treat the common cold
- Use of illegal drugs, such as marijuana and cocaine
- Job-related hazards and stresses
- Smoking
- Inadequate intake of other nutrients, such as too little iron, magnesium, and zinc
- Excess vitamin A intake and megadose use of other nutrient supplements
- Heavy caffeine use
- Lack of medical treatment with HIV-positive status or AIDS
- Poor control of ongoing diabetes or hypertension
- X-ray exposure, including dental X rays

Women need to pay attention to these risks in the months before conception. This precaution is necessary because women often do not suspect they are pregnant during the first few weeks after conception and may not seek medical attention until after the first 2 to 3 months of pregnancy.

Still, even without fanfare, the child-to-be grows and develops daily. For that reason, the health and nutrition habits of a woman who is trying to become pregnant—or has the potential to become pregnant—are particularly important. Although some aspects of fetal and newborn health are beyond control, a woman's conscious decisions about social, health, and nutritional factors affect her infant's health and future. Much research suggests that an adequate vitamin and mineral intake at least 8 weeks before conception and then during pregnancy can help prevent birth defects such as neural tube defects (review Figure 8-9 in Chapter 8). Neural tube defects especially have been linked to a folate deficiency. Recall from Chapter 8 that neural tube defects develop within 28 days after conception, and that adequate folate status before and during this

Healthy People 2010 includes a goal of increasing to 80% the number of pregnancies that begin with optimal folate status from the current estimate of 21%, in an effort to reduce the occurrence of neural tube defects.

Any use of herbal therapies should be approved by a physician as well.

embryo In humans, the developing offspring in utero from about the beginning of the third week to the end of the eighth week after conception.

ovum The egg cell from which a fetus eventually develops if the egg is fertilized by a sperm cell.

fetus The developing life form from about the beginning of the ninth week after conception until birth.

placenta An organ that forms in the uterus in pregnant women. Through this organ, oxygen and nutrients from the mother's blood are transferred to the fetus, and fetal wastes are removed. The placenta also releases hormones that maintain the state of pregnancy.

zygote The fertilized ovum; the cell resulting from the union of an egg cell (ovum) and sperm until it divides.

part of pregnancy reduces the risk of such defects by up to 70%. In addition, since about 50% of pregnancies are unplanned, all women of childbearing age should be aware of the role nutrition plays in the development of a healthy infant, both before and during pregnancy. Following a healthy diet is then very important. The American College of Obstetrics and Gynecology reminds women that it is especially important to meet folate needs (400 micrograms of synthetic folic acid). This is possible if the woman makes careful dietary choices. Alternately, adding a balanced multivitamin and mineral supplement to one's diet is also appropriate for meeting this goal.

Another Bite

Women who have previously given birth to an infant with a neural tube defect such as spina bifida should consult their physician about the need for folate supplementation; an intake of 4 milligrams of synthetic folic acid per day at least one month prior to conception is recommended, but must be taken under a physician's supervision.

Prenatal Growth and Development

For 8 weeks after conception, a human **embryo** develops from a fertilized **ovum** into a **fetus.** For about another 32 weeks, the fetus continues to develop. When its body finally matures, the infant is born. Until birth, the mother nourishes it via a **placenta,** an organ that forms in her uterus to accommodate the growth and development of the fetus (Fig. 13-1). The role of the placenta is to exchange nutrients, oxygen and other gases, and waste products between the mother and the fetus.

Early Growth—The First Trimester Is a Very Critical Time

In the formation of the human organism, egg and sperm first unite, producing the **zygote** (Fig. 13-2). From this point, the reproductive process occurs very rapidly:

- Within 30 hours—zygote divides in half to form 2 cells.
- Within 4 days—cell number climbs to 128 cells.

Figure 13-1 The fetus in relationship to the placenta. The placenta is the organ through which nourishment flows to the fetus.

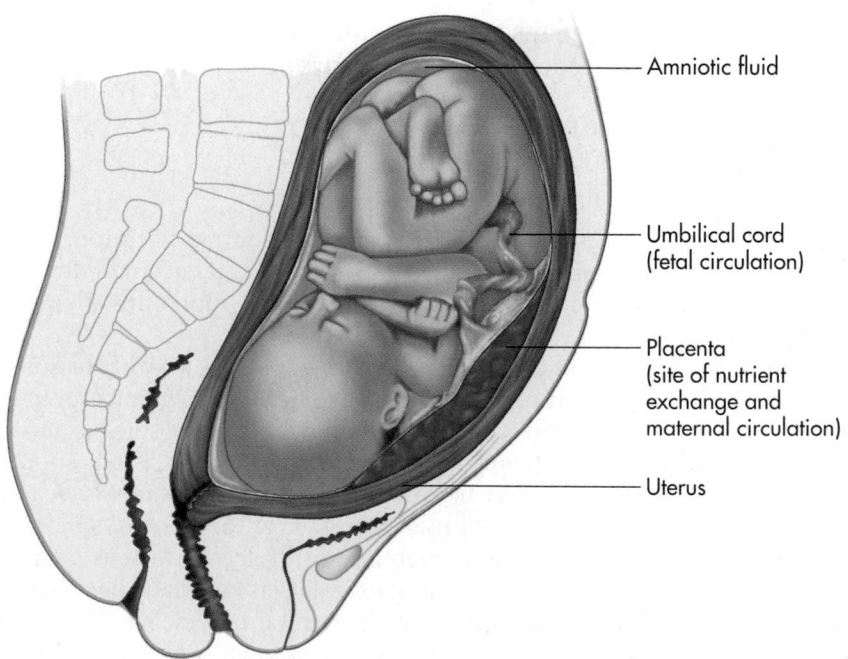

Amniotic fluid

Umbilical cord
(fetal circulation)

Placenta
(site of nutrient
exchange and
maternal circulation)

Uterus

- At 14 days—the group of cells is called an embryo.
- Within 35 days—heart is beating, embryo is ¹/₃₀ of an inch (8 millimeters) long, eyes and limb buds are clearly visible.
- At 8 weeks—the embryo is known as a fetus.
- At 13 weeks (end of first trimester)—most organs are formed, and the fetus can move.

For purposes of discussion, the duration of pregnancy—normally, 38 to 42 weeks—is commonly divided into three periods, called **trimesters.** Growth begins in the first trimester with a rapid increase in cell number. This type of growth dominates embryonic and later fetal development. The newly formed cells then begin to grow larger. Further growth is then a mix of increases in cell number and cell size. By the end of 13 weeks—the first trimester—most organs are formed and the fetus can move (see Fig. 13-2).

As the embryo or fetus develops, nutritional deficiencies and other insults have the potential to impose damage or risk to organ systems. For example, adverse reactions to medications, high intakes of vitamin A, exposure to radiation, or trauma can alter or arrest the current phase of fetal development, and the effects may last a lifetime

trimesters Three 13- to 14-week periods into which the normal pregnancy of 38 to 42 weeks is divided somewhat arbitrarily for purposes of discussion and analysis. Development of the offspring, however, is continuous throughout pregnancy, with no specific physiological markers demarcating the transition from one trimester to the next.

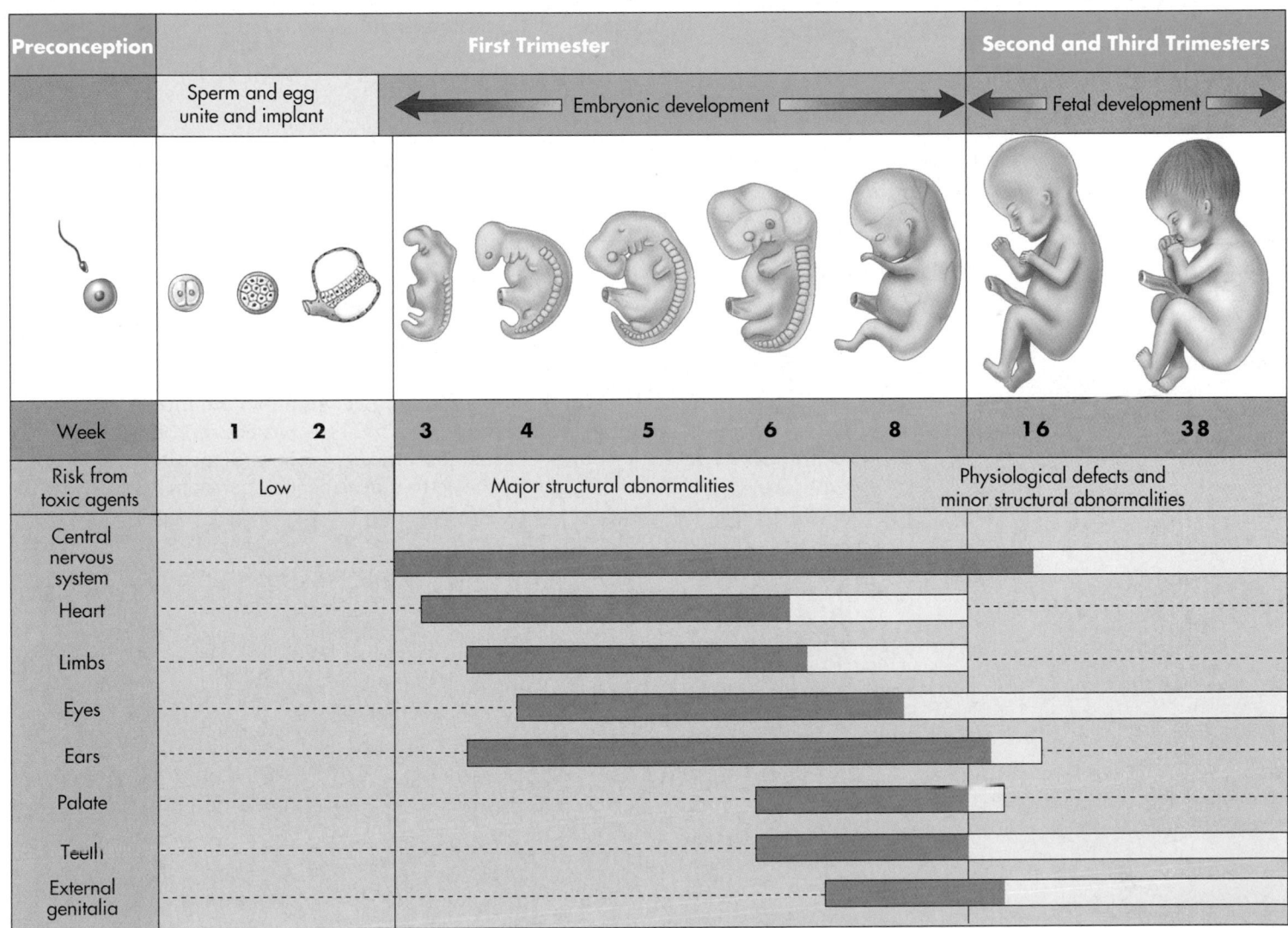

Figure 13-2 Harmful effects of toxic agents during pregnancy. Vulnerable periods of fetal development are indicated with orange bars. The orange shading indicates the time of greatest risk to the organ. The most serious damage to the fetus from exposure to toxins is likely to occur during the first 8 weeks after conception, two-thirds of the way through the first trimester. As the white bars in the chart shows, however, damage to vital parts of the body—including the eyes, brain, and genitals—can also occur during the last months of pregnancy.

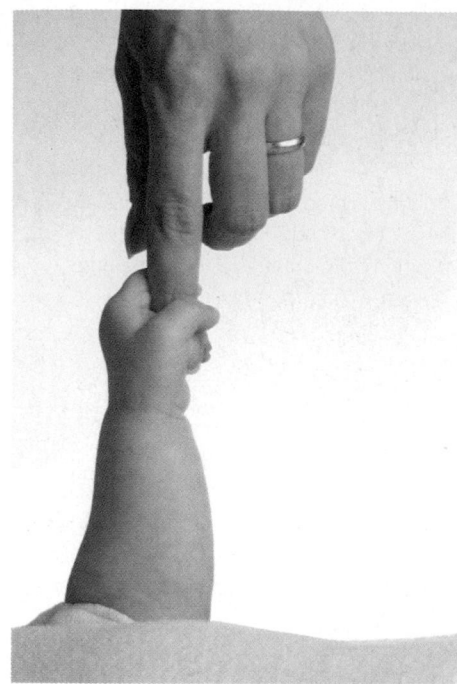

The time to begin thinking about prenatal nutrition is before becoming pregnant. This includes making sure folic acid intake is adequate (400 micrograms of synthetic folic acid per day) and that any supplemental intake of preformed vitamin A does not exceed 100% of the Daily Value (1000 micrograms RAE or 5000 IU).

spontaneous abortion Cessation of pregnancy and expulsion of the embryo or nonviable fetus prior to 20 weeks gestation. This is the result of natural causes, such as a genetic defect or developmental problem; also called *miscarriage*.

(review Fig. 13-2). The most critical time for these potential problems is during the first trimester. Most **spontaneous abortions**—premature terminations of pregnancy that occur naturally—happen at this time. Currently, about one-half or more of all pregnancies end in this way, often so early that a woman does not even realize she was pregnant. (An additional 15% to 20% are lost before normal delivery.) Early spontaneous abortions usually result from a genetic defect or fatal error in fetal development. Smoking, alcohol abuse, use of aspirin and NSAIDs, and illicit drug use raise the risk for spontaneous abortion.

A woman should avoid substances that may harm the developing fetus, especially during the first trimester. This holds true, as well, for the time when a woman is trying to become pregnant. As previously mentioned, she is unlikely to be aware of her pregnancy for at least a few weeks. In addition, the fetus develops so rapidly during the first trimester that, if an essential nutrient is not available, the fetus may be affected even before evidence of the nutrient deficiency appears in the mother.

For this reason, the quality—rather than the quantity—of one's nutritional intake is most important during the first trimester. In other words, women should consume the same amount of calories, but the foods chosen should be more nutrient dense. Although some women lose their appetite and feel nauseated during the first trimester, they should be careful to meet nutrient needs as much as possible.

Another Bite

Although a mother's decisions, practices, and precautions during pregnancy contribute to the health of her fetus, she cannot guarantee her fetus good health because some genetic and environmental factors are beyond her control. She and others involved in the pregnancy should not hold an unrealistic illusion of control.

■ Second Trimester

By the beginning of the second trimester, a fetus weighs about 1 ounce. Arms, hands, fingers, legs, feet, and toes are fully formed. The fetus has ears and begins to form tooth sockets in its jawbone. Organs continue to grow and mature, and, with a stethoscope, physicians can detect the fetus's heartbeat. Most bones are distinctly

A healthy 1-week-old baby. At birth, a baby usually weighs about 7.5 pounds and is 20 inches long.

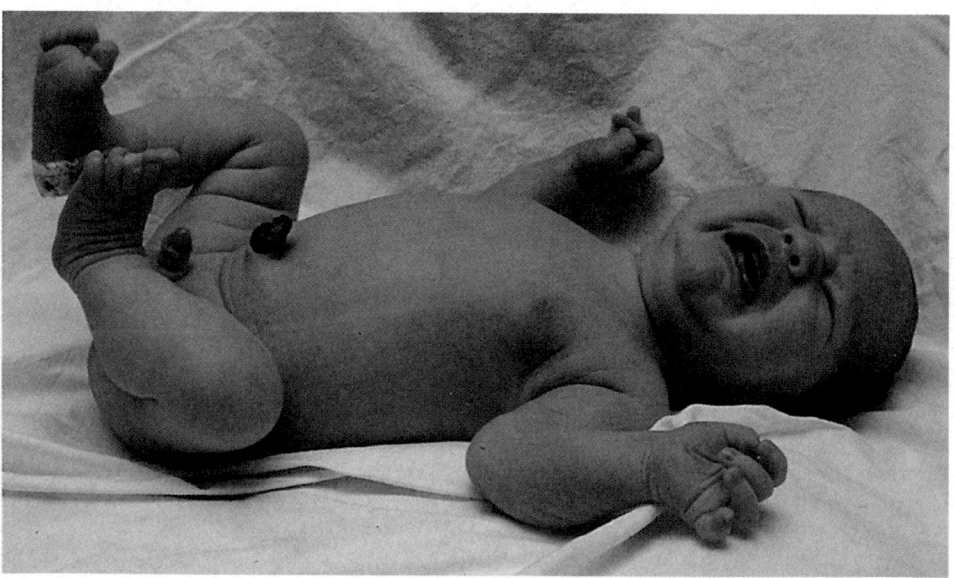

evident through the body. Eventually, the fetus begins to look more like an infant. It may suck its thumb and kick strongly enough to be felt by the mother. As was shown in Figure 13-2, the fetus can still be affected by exposure to toxins, but not to the degree seen in the first trimester.

During the second trimester, the mother's breast weight increases by approximately 30% due to the development of milk-producing cells and the deposition of 2 to 4 pounds of fat for **lactation.** This stored fat serves as a reservoir for the extra calories needed to produce breast milk.

■ Third Trimester

By the beginning of the third trimester, a fetus weighs about 2 to 3 pounds. The third trimester is a crucial time for fetal growth. The fetus will double in length and will multiply its weight by three to four times. An infant who is born after about 26 weeks of **gestation** has a good chance of survival if cared for in a nursery for high-risk newborns. However, the infant will not contain the stores of minerals (mainly iron and calcium) and fat that are normally accumulated during the last month of gestation. This and other medical problems, such as a poor ability to suck and swallow, complicate nutritional care for preterm infants. Note also that the fetus takes higher priority than the mother with regard to iron, and will deplete the stores of the mother. If the mother is not meeting her iron needs, she can be severely depleted after delivery.

At 9 months, the fetus usually weighs about 7 to 9 pounds (3 to 4 kilograms) and is about 20 inches (50 centimeters) long. A soft spot on the top of the head indicates where the skull bones (fontanels) are growing together. The bones finally close by the time the baby is about 12 to 18 months of age.

▌ Definition of a Successful Pregnancy

One common criterion of a successful pregnancy is the protection of the mother's physical and emotional health, so that she can return to her prepregnancy health status. As for the infant, two widely accepted criteria are (1) a gestation period longer than 37 weeks and (2) a birth weight greater than 5.5 pounds (2.5 kilograms). Sufficient lung development, which is likely to have occurred by 37 weeks' gestation, is critical to the survival of a newborn. The longer the gestation, the greater the ultimate birth weight and maturation state, leading to fewer medical problems.

Low-birth-weight (LBW) infants are those weighing less than 5.5 pounds (2.5 kilograms) at birth. Most commonly, LBW is associated with **preterm** birth. Note that hospital-related costs of caring for low-birth-weight newborns total more than $2 billion per year in the United States, ranging from $20,000 to $200,000 per infant. Compare this with an average hospital-related cost of $4300 for a normal delivery and an average of $800 for preventive prenatal care. Full-term and preterm infants who weigh less than the expected weight for their duration of gestation, the result of insufficient growth, are described as **small for gestational age (SGA).** Thus, a full-term infant weighing less than 5.5 pounds at birth is SGA but not preterm, whereas a preterm infant born at 30 weeks' gestation is probably low birth weight without being SGA. Infants who are SGA are more likely than normal-weight infants to have medical complications, including problems with blood glucose control, temperature regulation, growth, and development in the early weeks after birth.

The newborn's quality of life must also be considered in rating the success of a pregnancy. Overall, the goal of prepregnancy and prenatal care is aimed to ensure that the baby is born healthy, on time, and with the mental, physical, and physiological capabilities to take advantage of whatever life offers, while also protecting the mother's health.

lactation The period of milk secretion following pregnancy; typically called *breastfeeding.*

gestation The period of intrauterine development of offspring, from conception to birth; in humans, gestation lasts for about 40 weeks after the woman's previous menstrual period.

low birth weight (LBW) Referring to any infant weighing less than 2.5 kilograms (5.5 pounds) at birth; most commonly results from preterm birth.

preterm An infant born before 37 weeks of gestation; also referred to as *premature.*

small for gestational age (SGA) Referring to infants who weigh less than the expected weight for their length of gestation. This corresponds to less than 2.5 kilograms (5.5 pounds) in a full-term newborn. A preterm infant who is also SGA will most likely develop some medical complications.

A goal of *Healthy People 2010* is to reduce low birth weight and preterm births by one-third.

Studies from Britain suggest infants who are small for gestational age are likely to develop obesity, diabetes, hypertension, and other health problems during later adult years. Reduced growth of the liver, the pancreas, the kidneys, and other organs during gestation is one possible reason. This increase in health risk is likely to be more pronounced if the infants also fail to gain enough weight in the first year of life.

To help ensure the optimal health of both the mother and her offspring, adequate nutrition, especially meeting folate needs from a synthetic source starting at least 3 months before pregnancy begins, is vital both before and during pregnancy. Organs and body parts in the offspring begin to develop very soon after conception. The first trimester is a critical period when inadequate nutrient intake or alcohol and drug use can result in birth defects.

Infants born after 37 weeks of gestation who weigh more than 5.5 pounds (2.5 kilograms) have the fewest medical problems at birth. To reduce infant and maternal medical problems or death, the expectant mother, family, and medical care providers should take the steps necessary to allow the mother to carry the baby in her uterus for the entire 9 months which in turn contributes to adequate growth. Good nutrition and health practices aid in this goal.

Pregnancy leads to increased nutrient needs for the mother. Meeting these nutrient needs is an important step toward a successful pregnancy.

Effect of Nutritional Status on Pregnancy Success

Is attention to good nutrition worth the effort? Yes; evidence shows that the effort is justified. Extra nutrients and calories are used for fetal growth, as well as for the changes the mother's body undergoes to accommodate the fetus. Her uterus and breasts grow, the placenta develops, her total blood volume increases, the heart and kidneys work harder, and stores of body fat increase.

Although it is difficult to predict what degree of poor nutrition will affect each pregnancy, a daily diet containing only 1000 kcal has been shown to greatly restrict fetal growth and development. Increased maternal and infant death rates seen in famine-stricken areas of Africa supply further evidence.

Genetic background can explain very little of the observed differences in birth weight between developed and developing countries. Both environmental factors and nutritional factors are more important. The worse the nutritional condition of the mother at the beginning of pregnancy, the more valuable a healthy prenatal diet and/or use of prenatal supplements are in improving the course and outcome of her pregnancy.

Increased Nutrient Needs to Support Pregnancy

It is important to realize that pregnancy is a time of increased nutrient needs. It is equally important to recognize the need for individual assessment and counseling of mothers-to-be, as the nutritional and health status of each woman is different. Still, there are some general principles that are true of most women with regard to increased nutrient needs.

Increased Calorie Needs

To support the growth and development of the fetus, pregnant women need to increase their calorie intake. Calorie needs during the first trimester are essentially the same as for the nonpregnant woman. However, during the second and third trimesters, it is necessary for a pregnant woman to consume approximately 350 to 450 kcal more per day than her prepregnancy needs (the upper end of the range is needed in the third trimester).

Rather than seeing this as an opportunity to fill up on sugary desserts or fat-filled snacks, these extra calories should be in the form of nutrient-dense foods. For example, throughout the day, about six whole-wheat crackers, 1 ounce of cheese, and ½ cup of fat-free milk would supply the extra calories (and also some calcium). Although she "eats for two," the pregnant woman must not double her normal calorie intake. The "eating for two" concept refers more appropriately to increased needs for several vitamins and minerals. Micronutrient needs are increased by up to 50% during pregnancy, whereas calorie needs during the second and third trimesters represent only about a 20% increase.

If a woman is active during her pregnancy, she may need to increase her calorie intake by even more than the estimated 350 to 450 kcal per day. Her greater body weight requires more calories for activity. While pregnancy is not the time to begin an intense fitness regimen, women can generally take part in most low- or moderate-intensity activities during pregnancy. Walking, cycling, swimming, or light aerobics for 30 minutes or more on most days of the week is generally advised, and may actually promote an easier delivery. A few types of activities can potentially harm the fetus and should be avoided, especially those with inherent risk of falls and abdominal trauma. Examples of exercises to avoid, especially during the second and third trimesters, include downhill skiing, weightlifting, soccer, basketball, horseback riding, certain calisthenics (e.g., deep knee bends), any contact sports (e.g., hockey), and scuba diving. Because many women find that they are inactive during the later months, partly because of their increased size, an extra 350 to 450 kcal in their daily diets is usually enough.

Women with high-risk pregnancies, such as those experiencing premature labor contractions, may need to restrict their physical activity. To ensure optimal health for both herself and her infant, a pregnant woman should first consult her physician about physical activity and possible limitations.

■ Adequate Weight Gain

Adequate weight gain for a mother is one of the best predictors of pregnancy outcome. Her diet should allow for approximately 2 to 4 pounds (0.9 to 1.8 kilograms) of weight gain during the first trimester and then a subsequent weight gain of 0.75 to 1 pound (0.3 to 0.5 kilogram) weekly during the second and third trimesters. A healthy goal for total weight gain for a woman of normal weight (based on BMI; Table 13-1) averages about 25 to 35 pounds (11.5 to 16 kilograms). Adolescents and African-American women, who often have smaller babies, are strongly advised to aim for the greater amount. Women carrying twins should gain 35 to 45 pounds, and those carrying triplets should gain 50 pounds (23 kilograms).

For women with a low BMI, the goal increases to 28 to 40 pounds (12.5 to 18 kilograms). The goal decreases to 15 to 25 pounds (7 to 11.5 kilograms) for women at a high BMI, and 15 pounds (7 kilograms) or more for an obese woman. Figure 13-3 shows why the typical recommendation begins at 25 pounds.

A weight gain of between 25 and 35 pounds for a woman starting at normal weight has repeatedly been shown to yield optimal health for both mother and fetus if gestation lasts at least 38 weeks. The weight gain should yield a birth weight of 7.5 pounds (3.5 kilograms). Although some extra weight gain during pregnancy is usually not harmful

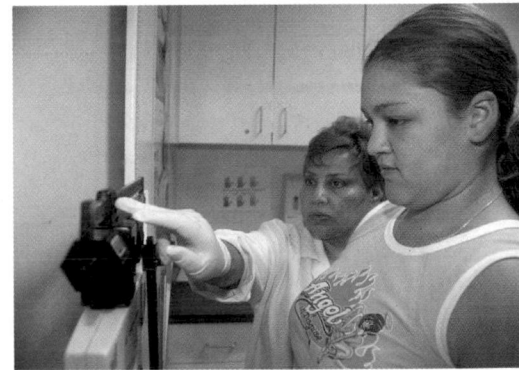

Weight gain should be carefully monitored during pregnancy.

During pregnancy, women in North America are more likely to gain excess weight and make poor food choices than to eat too little.

Table 13-1 Recommended Weight Gain in Pregnancy Based on Prepregnancy Body Mass Index (BMI)

	Total Weight Gain*	
Prepregnancy BMI Category	**(pounds)**	**(kilograms)**
Low (BMI less than 19.8)	28 to 40	12.5 to 18
Normal (BMI 19.8 to 25.9)	25 to 35	11.5 to 16
High (BMI 26 to 29)	15 to 25	7 to 11.5
Obese (BMI greater than 29)	15 (or more)	7 (or more)

Reprinted with permission from *Nutrition During Pregnancy and Lactation,* Copyright 1992 by the National Academy of Sciences. Courtesy of the National Academy Press, Washington, DC.

*The listed values are for pregnancies with one fetus. Short women (less than 62 inches) should strive for gains at the lower end of the ranges. For women of normal BMI who are carrying twins, the range is 35 to 45 pounds (16 to 20 kilograms). Adolescents within 2 years of beginning menses and African-American women should strive for gains at the upper end of the ranges.

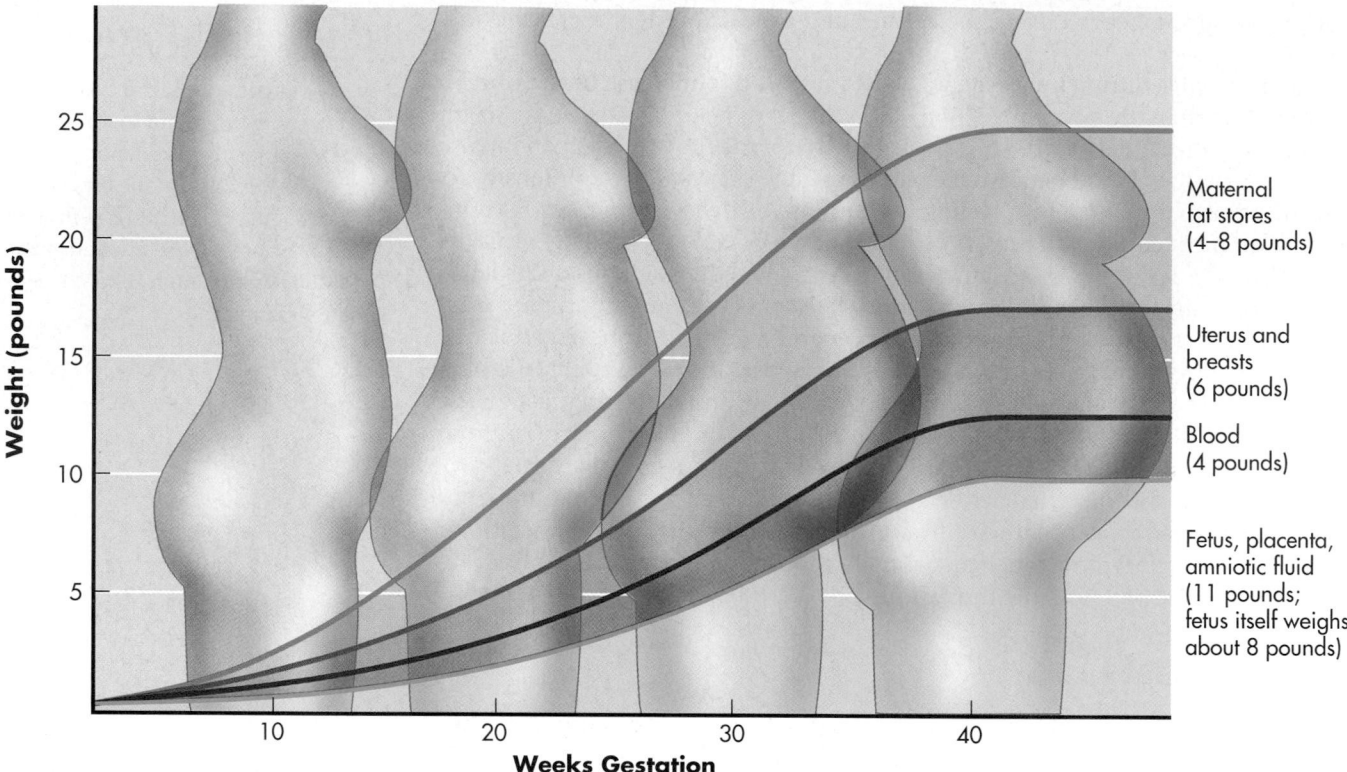

Figure 13-3 The components of weight gain in pregnancy. A weight gain of 25 to 35 pounds is recommended for most women. Note that the various components total about 25 pounds.

(about 5 to 10 pounds), it can set the stage for a pattern of weight gain during the child-bearing years if the mother does not return to her approximate prepregnancy weight.

Weight gain during pregnancy, especially in the teenage years, should generally follow the pattern in Figure 13-3. Monitoring weekly records of a pregnant woman's weight gain helps assess how much to adjust her food intake. Weight gain is a key issue in prenatal care and a concern of many mothers-to-be. Remember that inadequate weight gain can cause many problems.

If a woman deviates from the desirable pattern, she should make the appropriate adjustment. For example, if a woman begins to gain too much weight during her pregnancy, she should not lose weight to get back on track. Even if a woman gains 35 pounds in the first 7 months of pregnancy, she must still gain more during the last 2 months. She should simply slow the increase in weight to parallel the rise on the prenatal weight gain chart. In other words, the sources of the unnecessary calories should be found and minimized. Alternately, if a woman has not gained the desired weight by a given point in pregnancy, she shouldn't gain the needed weight rapidly. Instead, she should slowly gain a little more weight than the typical pattern to meet the goal by the end of the pregnancy. A registered dietitian can help make any needed adjustments.

■ Increased Protein and Carbohydrate Needs

The RDA for protein increases by an additional 25 grams per day during pregnancy. A cup of milk alone contains 8 grams. Many nonpregnant women already consume protein in excess of their needs and therefore do not need to increase protein intake any further. However, all women should check to make sure they are actually eating enough protein (and as well enough calories so this protein is not used for energy needs).

The RDA for carbohydrate increases to 175 grams daily. This amount prevents ketosis, which can harm the fetus (see the Looking Further section on the effects of nutrition and other factors on pregnancy outcome). Most women already consume this amount and more.

■ Increased Vitamin Needs

Vitamin needs generally increase from prepregnancy RDAs/Adequate Intakes by up to 30% for most of the B vitamins, and even greater for vitamin B-6 (45%) and folate (50%). It is important to note that vitamin A needs only increase by 10%, so a specific focus on this vitamin is not needed. And remember, excess amounts of vitamin A are very harmful to the developing fetus.

The extra amount of vitamin B-6 and other B vitamins (except folate) needed in the diet is easily met via wise food choices, such as a serving of a typical ready-to-eat breakfast cereal and some animal protein sources. Folate needs, however, often merit specific diet planning and possible vitamin supplementation. Because the synthesis of DNA, and therefore cell division, requires folate, this nutrient is especially crucial during pregnancy. Ultimately, both fetal and maternal growth depend on an ample supply of folate. Red blood cell formation, which requires folate, increases during pregnancy. Serious folate-related anemia therefore can result if folate intake is inadequate. The RDA for folate increases during pregnancy to 600 micrograms DFE per day. This is a critical goal in the nutritional care of a pregnant woman. Increasing folate intakes to meet 600 micrograms DFE per day for a pregnant woman can be achieved through either dietary sources or a supplemental source of folic acid, or a combination of both. Choosing a diet rich in synthetic folic acid, such as from ready-to-eat breakfast cereals or meal replacement bars (look for approximately 50% to 100% of the Daily Value), is especially helpful in meeting folate needs. Recall from Chapter 8 that synthetic folic acid is much more easily absorbed than the various forms of folate found naturally in foods.

■ Increased Mineral Needs

Mineral needs generally increase during pregnancy, especially the requirements for iodide and iron. Zinc needs also increase. (Calcium needs do not increase, but still may deserve special attention since many women have deficient intakes.)

Pregnant women need the extra iodide (total of 220 micrograms per day) for prevention of goiter. Typical iodide intakes are enough if the woman uses iodized salt. Animal proteins or a fortified ready-to-eat breakfast cereal in the diet can easily provide enough extra zinc. The extra iron (total of 27 milligrams per day) is needed to synthesize the greater amount of hemoglobin needed during pregnancy and to provide iron stores for the fetus. Women often need a supplemental source of iron, especially if they do not consume iron-fortified foods, such as highly fortified breakfast cereals containing close to 100% of the Daily Value for iron (18 milligrams). Because iron supplements decrease appetite and can cause nausea and constipation, if used these should be taken between meals or just before going to bed. Milk, coffee, or tea should not be consumed with an iron supplement because these beverages have substances that interfere with iron absorption. Eating foods rich in vitamin C along with nonheme iron–containing foods and iron supplements helps increase iron absorption from those sources. Pregnant women who are not anemic may wait until the second trimester, when pregnancy-related nausea generally lessens, to start iron supplementation if needed.

The consequences of iron-deficiency anemia—especially during the first trimester—can be severe. Negative outcomes include preterm delivery, low-birth-weight infants, and increased risk for fetal death in the first weeks after birth.

■ Food Plan for Pregnant Women

One approach to a diet that supports a successful pregnancy is based on MyPyramid. For an active 24-year-old woman, about 2200 kcal are recommended (the same as recommended for such a woman when not pregnant). The plan should include:

- 3 cups of calcium-rich foods from the milk group or use of calcium-fortified foods to make up for any gap between calcium intake and need
- 6 ounce-equivalents from the meat & beans group

pica The practice of eating nonfood items, such as dirt, laundry starch, or clay.

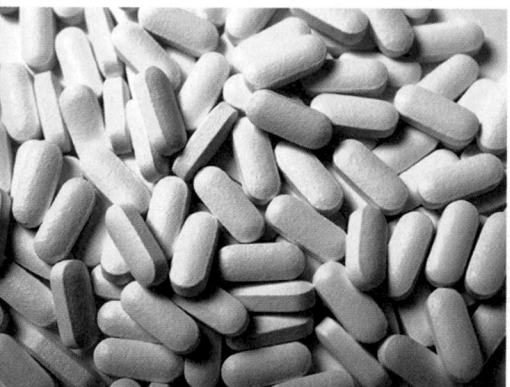

Pregnancy, in particular, is not a time to self-prescribe vitamin and mineral supplements. For example, although vitamin A is a routine component of prenatal vitamins, it is important to note that intakes over three times the RDA for vitamin A has been shown to have toxic effects on the fetus.

Mercury can harm the nervous system of the fetus. Thus recently FDA warned pregnant women to avoid swordfish, shark, king mackerel, and tile fish because of possible high mercury contamination. Largemouth bass are also implicated. In general, intake of other fish and shellfish should not exceed 12 ounces per week. Note also that since canned albacore tuna is a potential mercury source, it should not be consumed in amounts exceeding 6 ounces per week.

- 3 cups from the vegetable group
- 2 cups from the fruit group
- 7 ounce-equivalents from the grain group
- 6 teaspoons of oil

Specifically, choices from the milk group should include low-fat or fat-free versions of milk, yogurt, and cheese. These foods supply extra protein, calcium, and carbohydrate, as well as other nutrients. Choices from the meat & beans group should include both animal and vegetable sources. Besides protein, these foods help provide the extra iron and zinc needed. The vegetable and fruit group choices provide a variety of vitamins and minerals. One cup from this combination should be a good vitamin C source, and 1 cup should be a green vegetable or other rich source of folate. Choices from the grain group should focus on whole-grain and enriched foods. One ounce of a whole-grain, ready-to-eat breakfast cereal significantly contributes to meeting many vitamin and mineral needs. Finally, inclusion of plant oils in the diet contributes essential fatty acids. Discretionary calories (up to about 300 kcal) can then be added to allow for weight maintenance.

In the second and third trimesters, about 2600 kcal are recommended for this woman. The plan should now include:

- 3 cups of calcium-rich foods from the milk group or use of calcium-fortified foods
- 6 ½ ounces-equivalents from the meat & beans group
- 3 ½ cups from the vegetable group
- 2 cups from the fruit group
- 8 ounce-equivalents from the grain group
- 7 teaspoons of oil

Discretionary calories (up to about 400 kcal) can then be added to allow for gradual weight gain. Table 13-2 illustrates one daily menu based on the 2600 kcal plan for pregnancy for women in the second or third trimesters. This menu meets the extra nutrient needs associated with pregnancy. Women who need to consume more than this—and some do for various reasons—should incorporate additional fruits, vegetables, and whole-grain breads and cereals, not poor nutrient sources such as desserts and sugared soft drinks.

■ Use of Prenatal Vitamin and Mineral Supplements

Special supplements formulated for pregnancy are prescribed routinely for pregnant women by most physicians. Some are sold over the counter, while others are dispensed by prescription because of their high synthetic folic acid content (1000 micrograms), which could pose problems for others, such as older people (review Chapter 8). These supplements are very high in iron (27 milligrams per pill). There is no evidence that use of such supplements causes significant health problems in pregnancy, aside perhaps from the combined amounts of supplementary and dietary vitamin A. During pregnancy, supplemental preformed vitamin A should not exceed 3000 micrograms RAE per day (15,000 IU per day). Toxicity of vitamin A is linked with birth defects (review

Table 13-2 Sample 2600 kcal Daily Menu That Meets the Nutritional Needs of Most Pregnant and Breastfeeding Women

	Vitamin B-6	Folate	Iron	Zinc	Calcium
Breakfast					
1 cup Kellogg's Smart Start cereal	✓	✓	✓	✓	✓
1 cup orange juice		✓			
1 cup fat-free milk	✓				✓
Snack					
2 tbsp peanut butter	✓	✓	✓	✓	
2 stalks of celery		✓			
1 slice whole-wheat toast		✓	✓	✓	
1 cup plain low-fat yogurt	✓				✓
½ cup strawberries					
Lunch					
2 cups spinach salad with 2 tbsp oil and vinegar dressing		✓			✓
½ tomato					
1 slice whole-wheat toast		✓	✓	✓	
1 ½ ounce provolone cheese	✓				✓
Snack					
5 whole-wheat crackers		✓	✓	✓	
1 cup grape juice					
Dinner					
3 ounces lean hamburger, broiled (with condiments)	✓		✓	✓	
½ cup baked beans	✓	✓	✓	✓	
1 hamburger bun		✓	✓		
½ sliced tomato					
1 cup cooked broccoli		✓			✓
1 tsp soft margarine					
Iced tea					
Snack					
Granola bar (2 ounces)		✓	✓	✓	
½ banana	✓				
Discretionary calories of up to 400 kcal*					

This diet meets nutrient needs for pregnancy and lactation. Lack of a check (✓) indicates a poor source of the nutrient. The vitamin- and mineral-fortified breakfast cereal used in this example makes an important contribution to meeting nutrient needs. Fluids can be added as desired. Total intake of fluids, such as water, should be 10 cups or so per day.

*Amount of discretionary calories will vary based on the actual food choices made within each MyPyramid group.

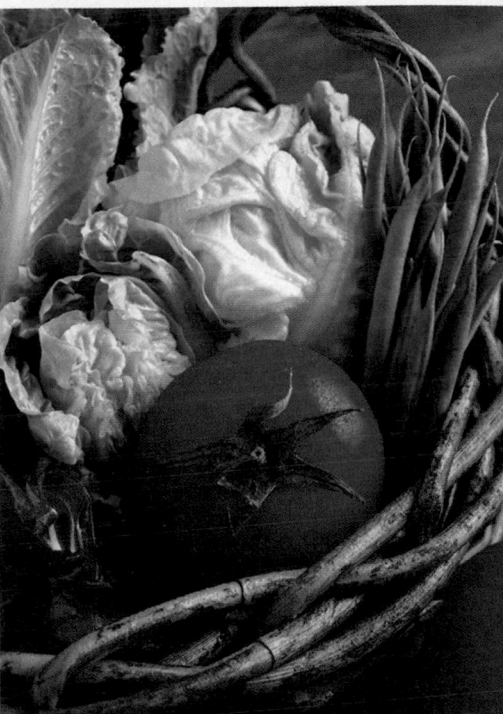

A salad each day provides many nutrients for the prenatal diet.

Chapter 8). This occurs mainly during the first trimester. The primary instances when prenatal supplements especially may contribute to a successful pregnancy are with poor women, teenagers, those with a generally deficient diet, women carrying multiple fetuses, those that smoke or use alcohol or illegal drugs, and vegans.

■ Pregnant Vegetarians

Women who are either lactoovovegetarian(s) or lactovegetarian(s) generally do not face special difficulties in meeting their nutritional needs during pregnancy. Like nonvegetarian women, they should be concerned primarily with meeting vitamin B-6, iron, folate, and zinc needs.

On the other hand, for a vegan, careful diet planning during preconception and pregnancy is crucial to insure sufficient protein, vitamin D (or sufficient sun exposure), vitamin B-6, iron, calcium, zinc, and especially a supplemental source of vitamin B-12. The basic vegan diet listed in Chapter 6 should be modified to include more grains, beans, nuts, and seeds to supply the necessary extra amounts of some of these nutrients. And as just mentioned, use of a prenatal multivitamin and mineral supplement also is generally advocated to help fill micronutrient gaps. Note, however, that although these are high in iron, this is not true for calcium (200 milligrams per pill). If iron and calcium supplements are used, they should not be taken together, to avoid possible competition for absorption.

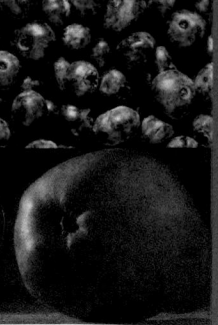

Looking *Further*

Effects of Nutritional and Other Factors on Pregnancy Outcome

In North America, maternal death as a result of childbirth is uncommon—only about 11 deaths in every 100,000 live births. The infant mortality rate, however, is much higher: for each 100,000 live births, about 600 to 700 infants die within the first year. The infant death rate among African-Americans is more than double the rates among Whites and Hispanics in the United States. Such grim and discomforting statistics can be attributed largely to the current number of teenage pregnancies and to inadequate prenatal care, as well as marginal nutritional health among poor pregnant women. Also, many factors other than nutrition affect the health of mother and fetus.

Low Socioeconomic Status

Several characteristics that are typical of low socioeconomic status, such as poverty, inadequate health care, poor health practices, lack of education, and unmarried status are associated with problems in pregnancy. Currently, in the United States about 31% of all births are to unwed mothers, many of whom are poor.

Closely Spaced and Multiple Births

Siblings born in succession to a mother with less than a year between birth and subsequent conception are more likely to be born with low birth weights than are those farther apart in age. The risks of low birth weight, preterm birth, or small size for gestational age are 30% to 40% higher for infants conceived less than 6 months following a birth compared to those conceived 18 to 23 months following a birth. These poor outcomes are probably linked to a lack of enough time to rebuild nutrient stores that were depleted by the pregnancy.

Similarly, multiple births (i.e., twins) increase the risk for preterm birth.

Teenage Pregnancy

About half a million teenagers give birth in the United States each year, accounting for about 13% of all births. In Canada, the comparable statistics are about half that amount. Teenage pregnancy poses special health problems for both the mother and child. Young women continue maturing into physical adulthood for 5 years after the onset of menstruation (**menarche**). Because the average age for menarche is 13 years in the United States, a woman younger than 18 years is not as physically ready to be pregnant as she will be later. However, by age 16, birth outcomes begin to improve.

Pregnant teens frequently exhibit a variety of other risk factors that can complicate pregnancy and pose a risk to the fetus. For instance, teenagers are more likely than adult women to be underweight at the beginning of pregnancy and to gain too little weight during pregnancy. In addition, their bodies generally lack the maturity needed to carry a fetus safely. Sixteen percent of low-birth-weight infants are born to teenage mothers. This is true even if the mothers receive adequate prenatal care.

Advanced Maternal Age

The risks of low birth weight and preterm delivery increase modestly, but progressively, with maternal age beyond 35 years. Given close monitoring, however, a woman older than 35 has an

menarche The onset of menstruation. Menarche usually occurs around age 13, 2 or 3 years after the first signs of puberty start to appear.

excellent chance of producing a healthy infant. Most women in this age group exhibit typical pregnancy-related problems, which usually are manageable if under close medical supervision.

Inadequate Prenatal Care

If prenatal care is inadequate, delayed, or absent, untreated maternal nutritional deficiencies can deprive a developing fetus of needed nutrients. In addition, untreated chronic diseases, such as hypertension or diabetes, increase the risk of fetal damage. Without prenatal care, a woman is three times more likely to deliver a low-birth-weight baby—one who will be 40 times more likely to die during the first 4 weeks of life than a normal-birth-weight infant. Although the ideal time to start prenatal care is before conception, about 20% of women in the United States receive no prenatal care throughout the first trimester—a critical time to positively influence the outcome of pregnancy.

Lifestyle Factors

Smoking, use of some medications, alcohol consumption, and illicit drug use during pregnancy all lead to harmful effects. (Use of a sauna or hot tub also can cause problems.) Smoking is linked to preterm birth and low birth weight and appears to increase the risk of birth defects, sudden infant death, and childhood cancer. Problem drugs include aspirin (especially when used heavily), hormone ointments, nose drops and related "cold" medications, rectal suppositories, weight-control pills, and medications prescribed for previous illnesses.

Marijuana is the most common illegal drug used during the reproductive years. For pregnant women, marijuana use is very risky and potentially can result in reduced blood flow and oxygen to the uterus and placenta and poor fetal growth. Low birth weight and higher risk of premature delivery often are seen in infants whose mothers used marijuana during pregnancy. Cocaine use also has devastating consequences for the developing fetus.

Conclusive evidence shows that repeated consumption of four or more alcoholic drinks at one sitting harm(s) the fetus. Such binge drinking is especially perilous during the first 12 weeks of pregnancy, as this is when critical early developmental events take place in utero. Although scientists don't know whether pregnant women must totally eliminate alcohol use to avoid risk of damage to the fetus, women are advised not to drink any alcohol during pregnancy or when there is a chance pregnancy might occur—until a safe level can be established. The embryo (and, at later stages, the fetus), has no means of detoxifying alcohol.

Women with chronic alcoholism produce children with a recognizable pattern of malformations called **fetal alcohol syndrome (FAS)**. A diagnosis of FAS is based mainly on poor fetal and infant growth, physical deformities (especially of facial features), and mental retardation (Fig. 13-4). The infant is frequently irritable and may develop hyperactivity and a short attention span. Limited hand-eye coordination is common. Defects in vision, hearing, and mental processing often develop over time.

Exactly how alcohol causes these defects is not known. One line of research suggests that alcohol, or products produced by the metabolism of alcohol (acetaldehyde), cause faulty movement of cells in the brain during early stages of nerve cell development or block the action of certain brain neurotransmitters. In addition, inadequate nutrient intake, reduced nutrient and oxygen transfer across the placenta, cigarette smoking commonly associated with alcohol intake, drug use, and possibly other factors contribute to the overall result.

Body Weight and Weight Gain

Obesity leads to an increased rate of hypertension and diabetes during pregnancy. The need for surgery and other complications during delivery likewise increase with obesity. These pregnancies require intense monitoring and are linked to an increase in risk of birth defects in the infant, primarily because the fetus can grow very large.

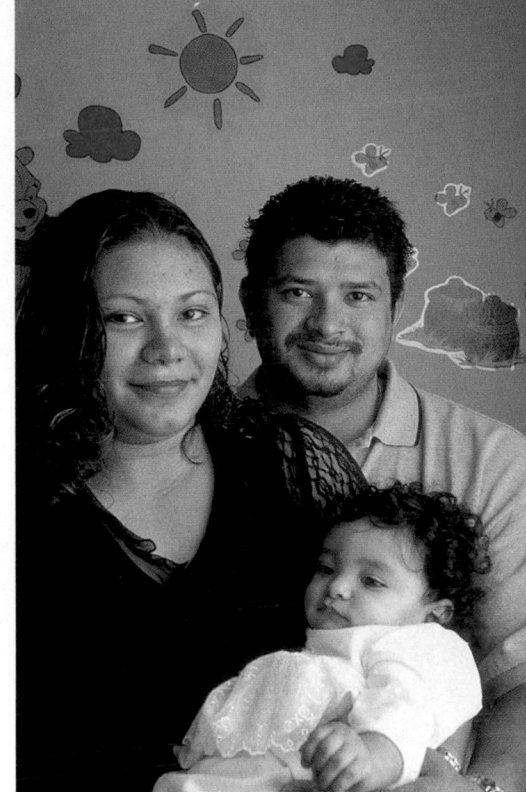

Delivering a healthy baby is more than just luck. Many nutrition- and health-related practices need to be considered.

fetal alcohol syndrome (FAS) A group of irreversible physical and mental abnormalities in the infant that result from the mother's consuming alcohol during pregnancy.

Pregnant women should recognize that many cough syrups contain alcohol. Cases have been reported of infants with FAS born to mothers who consumed generous amounts of such cough syrups but no other alcoholic beverages.

Figure 13-4 Fetal alcohol syndrome. The facial features shown are typical of affected children. Additional abnormalities in the brain and other internal organs accompany fetal alcohol syndrome but are not immediately apparent from simply looking at the child. Milder forms of alcohol-induced changes from a lower alcohol exposure to the fetus are known as **fetal alcohol effects.** In this case behavior problems without physical effects, such as altered facial features, are seen.

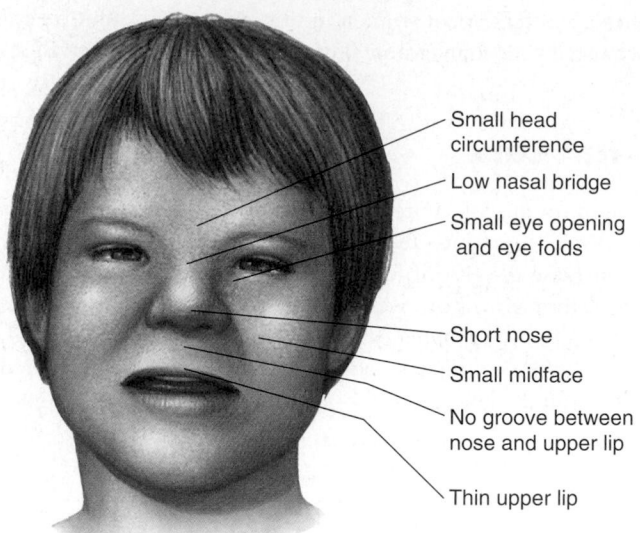

Small head circumference

Low nasal bridge

Small eye opening and eye folds

Short nose

Small midface

No groove between nose and upper lip

Thin upper lip

fetal alcohol effect (FAE) Hyperactivity, attention deficit disorder, poor judgment, sleep disorders, and delayed learning as a result of prenatal exposure to alcohol.

On the other hand, inadequate weight gain, especially among underweight women, increases the risk of preterm birth and infants of low birth weight. Underweight women also often have borderline vitamin and mineral intakes and need to build up body stores. They should try to reach healthy weight by the end of the first trimester and meet the weight-gain goals listed in earlier in the Chapter.

Prenatal Ketosis

Ketosis can result from fasting and is not desirable for the growing fetus. Ketone bodies are thought to be poorly used by the fetal brain, implying possible slowing of fetal brain development. Since a pregnant woman can develop significant ketosis after only 20 hours of fasting, experts oppose crash diets or fasting for more than 12 hours during pregnancy. Eating at least 175 grams of carbohydrate every day prevents such ketosis. Even nonpregnant women usually eat this amount and more.

Caffeine Consumption

Caffeine decreases the mother's absorption of iron and may reduce blood flow through the placenta. In addition, the fetus is unable to detoxify caffeine. Animal experiments have shown that the risk of spontaneous abortion increases in the first trimester and early in the second trimester with heavy caffeine consumption (greater than 500 milligrams, or the equivalent of about 5 cups of coffee per day). In addition, as caffeine intake increases, so does the risk of delivering a low-birth-weight infant. Heavy caffeine use during pregnancy may also lead to caffeine withdrawal symptoms in the newborn. Drinking no more than three cups of coffee and no more than four cups of caffeinated soft drinks per day during pregnancy, or when pregnancy is possible, is advocated. Paying attention to caffeine intake from tea, over-the-counter medicines containing caffeine, and chocolate is also important.

Aspartame Use

Phenylalanine, a component of aspartame (NutraSweet® and Equal®), causes concern for some pregnant women. High amounts of phenylalanine in maternal blood disrupt fetal brain development if the mother has a disease known as *phenylketonuria* (review Chapter 4). If the mother does not have this condition, however, it is unlikely that the baby will be affected by moderate aspartame use.

Listeria and Toxoplasmosis Infections

Infection by the bacterium *Listeria monocytogenes* causes mild flulike symptoms, such as fever, headache, and vomiting, about 7 to 30 days after exposure. However, pregnant women, newborn infants, and people with depressed immune function may suffer more severe symptoms, including spontaneous abortion and serious blood infections. In these high-risk people, 25% of infections may be fatal. Because unpasteurized milk, soft cheeses made from raw milk (brie, Camembert, feta, and blue cheeses), and raw cabbage can be sources of *Listeria* organisms, it is especially important that pregnant women (and other people at high risk for infection) avoid these products. Experts advise consuming only pasteurized milk products and cooking meat, poultry, and seafood thoroughly to kill this and other foodborne organisms. It is unsafe in pregnancy to eat any raw meats or other raw animal products, uncooked hot dogs, or any undercooked poultry.

Toxoplasmosis is another infection that causes birth defects, leading to about 3000 such cases per year in the United States. Pregnant women should limit exposure to the organism that causes toxoplasmosis by avoiding contact with cat feces (have someone else clean the cat's litter box or wear gloves), avoiding contact with kittens, bird feces, and garden soil (by wearing garden gloves), and by not eating raw or undercooked meat. Chapter 16 covers foodborne illness, such as *Listeria* and toxoplasmosis infections, in more detail.

Many of the risk factors described in this Looking Further section are avoidable. The goal of a reduction in maternal and infant deaths requires that more attention be paid to these problems.

USDA warns pregnant women to thoroughly cook (e.g., microwave) all ready-to-eat meats, including hot dogs and cold cuts, until they are steaming to reduce risk of listeria infections.

Concept Check

Calorie needs increase by an average of about 350 to 450 kcal per day during the second and third trimesters of pregnancy, respectively. Weight gain should be slow and steady up to a total of 25 to 35 pounds for a woman of normal weight (i.e., prepregnancy BMI of 19.8 to 25.9). Protein and certain vitamin and mineral needs increase during pregnancy. Most important to consider are vitamin B-6, folate, iron, iodide, and zinc. A pregnant woman's diet should be varied and generally follow a MyPyramid pattern. A prenatal multivitamin and mineral supplement is commonly prescribed but may not be necessary, depending on one's diet and current health status. Taking too many supplements—especially vitamin A—can be hazardous to the fetus.

■ Prenatal Care and Counseling

The chances of producing a healthy baby are maximized with education, an adequate diet, and early and consistent prenatal medical care. Also, avoiding the controllable risks discussed in this Chapter—especially smoking, over-supplementation with vitamin A, and use of certain medications, illegal drugs, and alcohol—will promote a healthier outcome of pregnancy for both the mother and the baby. If anemia, AIDS, diabetes, or hypertension are present or developing, these conditions must be carefully addressed to minimize complications during pregnancy. Treating ongoing infections is also important, as is avoiding x-ray exposure.

Ideally, women should receive examinations and counseling before becoming pregnant and continue during pregnancy. Many potential problems that develop during pregnancy can be diagnosed and quickly treated medically.

Food habits cannot be predicted from income, education, or lifestyle. Although some women already have good dietary habits, most can benefit from nutritional advice. All should be reminded of habits that may harm the growing fetus, such as severe dieting or

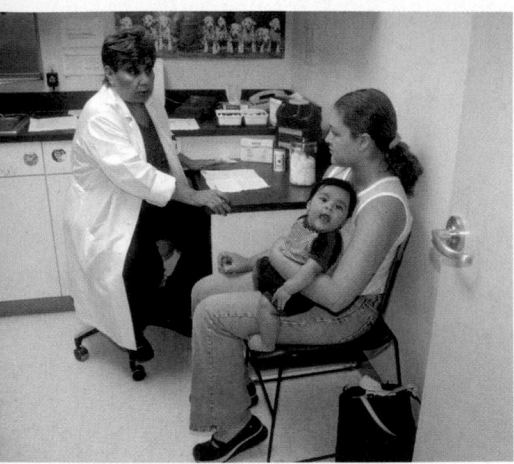

In the United States, low-income pregnant women and their infants (and children) benefit from the nutritional and medical attention provided by the WIC program.

fasting. By focusing on appropriate prenatal care, nutrient intake, and health habits, parents give their fetus—and, later, their infant—the very best chance of thriving.

Several U.S. government programs provide high-quality health care and foods to reduce infant mortality. These are designed to alleviate the effects of poverty and insufficient education and nutrient intake. An example of such a program is the Special Supplemental Nutrition Program for Women, Infants, and Children (WIC). This program offers health assessments and vouchers for foods that supply high-quality protein, calcium, iron, and vitamins A and C to pregnant women, infants, and children (up to age 5 years) from low-income populations. The WIC program is available in all areas of the United States and has a staff trained to help women have healthy babies. More than 7 million women, infants, and young children are currently benefiting from this program, but many eligible pregnant women are not participating in this program.

Real Life Scenario Follow-Up

From a dietary standpoint, Tracey is smart to take a close look at her protein intake because needs will increase somewhat during pregnancy. More fruits and vegetables will provide some fiber to help prevent constipation, which is common in the later stages of pregnancy. These foods also supply folate, and her use of an over-the-counter vitamin and mineral supplement provides an ample amount of synthetic folic acid. Still, she should discuss this supplement use with her physician and would probably eventually benefit more from a prenatal supplement, as this will have more iron than over-the-counter multivitamin and mineral supplements. Her diet may not have enough calcium, so she should pay as much attention to consuming some extra calcium as she does for protein. Avoiding alcohol is a smart move.

Many experts would say that she is consuming too much caffeine and would be wise to cut down coffee and caffeine-containing soft drinks to a total of three servings or less per day. Her exercise routine is probably too vigorous if she hasn't already been practicing regular running. Tracey should not begin a new exercise routine upon becoming pregnant unless it is at a moderate pace, such as brisk walking or stationary biking (spinning).

A goal of *Healthy People 2010* is 100% abstinence from alcohol, cigarettes, and illicit drugs by pregnant women.

Concept Check

Infants born after 37 weeks of gestation and weighing more than 5.5 pounds (2.5 kilograms) have the fewest medical problems at birth. Limiting the factors that increase the risk of having a preterm or small-for-gestational-age infant is a worthwhile goal for individuals and for society as a whole. Such contributing high-risk factors, besides an inadequate diet in general, include low socioeconomic status; closely spaced births; inadequate or absent prenatal care; cigarette smoking; alcohol consumption; aspirin and NSAID use; illegal drug use, such as cocaine and marijuana; teenage pregnancy; obesity; inadequate prenatal weight gain; heavy caffeine use; *Listeria* and toxoplasmosis infections; and prenatal ketosis. Adequate nutrition can reduce the risk of many medical problems in pregnancy.

Physiological Changes of Concern during Pregnancy

During pregnancy, the fetus's needs for oxygen, nutrients, and excretion increase the burden on the mother's lungs, heart, and kidneys. Although a mother's digestive and metabolic systems work very efficiently, some discomfort accompanies the changes her body undergoes to accommodate the fetus.

■ Heartburn, Constipation, and Hemorrhoids

Hormones (such as progesterone) produced by the placenta relax muscles in both the uterus and the gastrointestinal tract. This often causes heartburn as stomach acid refluxes into the esophagus (review Chapter 3). When this occurs, the woman should avoid lying down after eating, eat less fat so that foods pass more quickly from the stomach into the small intestine, and avoid spicy foods she cannot tolerate. She should also consume most liquids between meals to decrease the volume of food in the stomach after meals, and thus relieve some of the pressure that encourages reflux. Women with more severe cases may need antacids or related medications.

Constipation often results as the intestinal muscles relax during pregnancy. It is especially likely to develop late in pregnancy, as the fetus competes with the GI tract for space in the abdominal cavity. To offset these discomforts, a woman should perform regular exercise and consume more fluid, fiber, and dried fruits, such as prunes (dried plums). The Adequate Intake for fiber in pregnancy is 28 grams, slightly more than for the nonpregnant woman. Fluid needs are 10 cups per day. These practices can help prevent constipation and a problem that frequently accompanies it, hemorrhoids. Straining during elimination can lead to hemorrhoids, which are already more likely to occur during pregnancy because of other body changes. A reevaluation of the need and dose of iron supplementation also should be considered, as high iron intakes are linked to constipation.

■ Edema

Placental hormones cause various body tissues to retain fluid during pregnancy. Blood volume also greatly expands during pregnancy. The extra fluid normally causes some swelling (edema). There is no reason to restrict salt severely or use diuretics to limit mild edema. However, the edema may limit physical activity late in pregnancy and occasionally requires a woman to elevate her feet to control the symptoms. Overall, edema generally spells trouble only if hypertension and the appearance of extra protein in the urine accompany it (see a following section, "Pregnancy-Induced Hypertension").

■ Morning Sickness

About 70% to 85% of pregnant women experience nausea during the early stages of pregnancy. This nausea may be related to the increased sense of smell induced by pregnancy-related hormones circulating in the bloodstream. Although commonly called "morning sickness," pregnancy-related nausea may occur at any time and persist all day. It is often the first signal to a woman that she is pregnant. To help control mild nausea, pregnant women can try the following: avoiding nauseating foods, such as fried or greasy foods; cooking with good ventilation to dissipate nauseating smells; eating saltine crackers or dry cereal before getting out of bed; avoiding large fluid intakes early in the morning; and eating smaller, more frequent meals. Because the iron in prenatal supplements triggers nausea in some women, changing the type of supplement used or postponing use until the second trimester may provide relief in some cases. If a woman thinks her prenatal supplement is related to morning sickness, she should discuss switching to another supplement with her physician.

Overall, if a food sounds good to a pregnant woman with morning sickness, whether it is broccoli, soda crackers, or lemonade, she should eat it and eat when she can, while also striving to follow her prenatal diet. The American College of Obstetricians and Gynecologists recommends the following for the prevention and treatment of nausea and vomiting of pregnancy:

- History of use of a balanced multivitamin and mineral supplement at the time of conception
- Use of megadoses of vitamin B-6 (10–25 milligrams taken 3 to 4 times a day), especially coupled with the antihistamine doxylamine (10 milligrams) with each dose
- Ginger may also be helpful (350 milligrams taken 3 times per day).

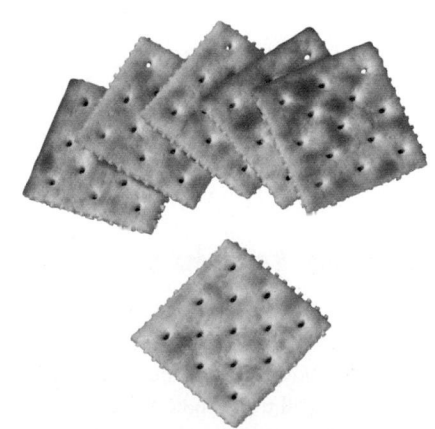

A few saltine crackers upon waking or between meals can help lessen the nausea that often accompanies morning sickness.

Usually, nausea stops after the first trimester; however, in about 10% to 20% of cases, it can continue throughout the entire pregnancy. In cases of serious nausea, the preceding practices offer little relief. Excessive vomiting can cause dangerous dehydration and must be avoided. When vomiting persists (about 0.5% to 2% of all pregnancies), medical attention is needed.

■ Anemia

To supply fetal needs, the mother's blood volume expands to approximately 150% of normal. The number of red blood cells, however, increases by only 20% to 30%, and this occurs more gradually. As a result, a pregnant woman has a lower ratio of red blood cells to total blood volume in her system. This hemodilution is known as **physiological anemia.** It is a normal response to pregnancy, rather than the result of inadequate nutrient intake. If during pregnancy, however, iron stores and/or dietary iron intake are not sufficient to meet needs, any resulting iron-deficiency anemia requires medical attention.

■ Gestational Diabetes

Hormones synthesized by the placenta decrease the efficiency of insulin. This leads to a mild increase in blood glucose, which helps supply calories to the fetus. If the rise in blood glucose becomes excessive, this leads to **gestational diabetes,** often beginning in weeks 20 to 28, particularly in women who have a family history of diabetes or who are obese. Other risk factors include maternal age over 25 and gestational diabetes in a prior pregnancy. In North America, gestational diabetes develops in about 4% of pregnancies; however, it increases to 7% in the Caucasian population. Today, pregnant women often are screened for diabetes at 24 to 28 weeks by checking for elevated blood glucose concentration 1 to 2 hours after consuming 50 to 100 grams of glucose. If gestational diabetes is detected, a special diet that distributes low glycemic load carbohydrates throughout the day needs to be implemented. Sometimes insulin injections are also needed. Regular physical activity also helps control blood glucose.

The primary risk of uncontrolled diabetes during pregnancy is that the fetus can grow quite large. This is a result of the oversupply of glucose from maternal circulation coupled with an increased production of insulin by the fetus, which allows fetal tissues to take up building materials for growth. The mother may require a Cesarean section if the size of the fetus is not compatible with a vaginal delivery. Another threat is that the infant may have low blood glucose at birth, because of the tendency to produce extra insulin that began during gestation. Other concerns are the potential for early delivery and increased risk of birth trauma and malformations. Although gestational diabetes often disappears after the infant's birth, it increases the mother's risk of developing diabetes later in life, especially if she fails to maintain a healthy body weight. Recent studies show that infants of mothers with gestational diabetes may also have higher risks of developing obesity and type 2 diabetes as they grow to adulthood. For all these reasons, proper control of gestational diabetes (and any diabetes present in the mother before pregnancy) is extremely important.

■ Pregnancy-Induced Hypertension

Pregnancy-induced hypertension is a high-risk disorder and occurs in about 3% to 5% of pregnancies. In its mild forms, it is also known as *preeclampsia* and, in severe forms, as *eclampsia*. Early symptoms include a rise in blood pressure, excess protein in the urine, edema, changes in blood clotting, and nervous system disorders. Very severe effects, including convulsions, can occur in the second and third trimesters. If not controlled, eclampsia eventually damages the liver and kidneys, and mother and fetus both may die. The populations most at risk for this disorder are women under age 17 or over age 35, and those who have had multiple-birth pregnancies. A family history

---

physiological anemia The normal increase in blood volume in pregnancy that dilutes the concentration of red blood cells, resulting in anemia; also called *hemodilution*.

gestational diabetes A high blood glucose concentration that develops during pregnancy and returns to normal after birth; one cause is the placental production of hormones that antagonize the regulation of blood glucose by insulin.

pregnancy-induced hypertension A serious disorder that can include high blood pressure, kidney failure, convulsions, and even death of the mother and fetus. Although its exact cause is not known, an adequate diet (especially adequate calcium intake) and prenatal care may prevent this disorder or limit its severity. Mild cases are known as *preeclampsia;* more severe cases are called *eclampsia* (formerly called *toxemia*).

Critical Thinking

Sandy, who is 4 months pregnant, has been having heartburn after meals, constipation, and difficult bowel movements. As a student of nutrition, you understand the digestive system and the role of nutrition in health. What remedies might you suggest to Sandy to relieve her problems?

of pregnancy-induced hypertension in the mother's or father's side of the family, diabetes, African-American race, and a woman's first pregnancy also raise risk. A diet inadequate in vitamin E, vitamin C, calcium, zinc, and other nutrients may also be part of the cause (conflicting research results at this time).

Pregnancy-induced hypertension resolves once the pregnancy ends, making delivery the most reliable treatment for the mother. However, since the problem often begins before the fetus is ready to be born, physicians in many cases must use treatments to prevent the worsening of the disorder. Bed rest and magnesium sulfate are currently the most effective treatment methods, although their effectiveness varies. Magnesium likely acts to relax blood vessels, and so leads to a fall in blood pressure. Several other treatments, such as various antiseizure and antihypertensive medications, are under study.

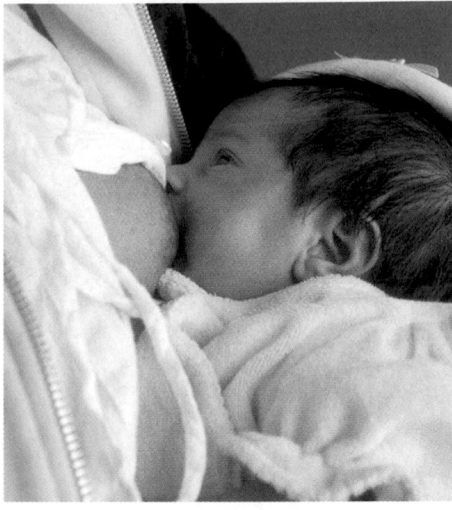

Breastfeeding is the preferred way to feed a young infant.

Concept Check

Heartburn, constipation, hemorrhoids, nausea and vomiting, edema, anemia, and gestational diabetes are possible discomforts and complications of pregnancy. Changes in food habits can often ease these problems. Pregnancy-induced hypertension, with high blood pressure and kidney failure, can lead to severe complications or even death of both the mother and fetus if not treated.

Breastfeeding

Breastfeeding the new infant further fosters his or her health, and so complements the attention given to diet during pregnancy. The American Dietetic Association and the American Academy of Pediatrics recommend breastfeeding exclusively for the first 6 months, with the continued combination of breastfeeding and infant foods until 1 year. The World Health Organization goes beyond that to recommend breastfeeding (with appropriate solid food introduction; see Chapter 14) for at least 2 years. Still, surveys show that only about 70% of North American mothers now begin to breastfeed their infants in the hospital, and at 4 and 6 months only 33% and 20%, respectively, are still breastfeeding their infants. The number falls to 18% at 1 year of age. These statistics refer to Caucasian women; minority women are even less likely to be breastfeeding at these time intervals.

Women who choose to breastfeed usually find it an enjoyable, special time in their lives and their relationship with their new infant. Still, bottle feeding with an infant formula is also safe for infants, as discussed in Chapter 14, but does not equal the benefits derived from human milk in all aspects. If a woman doesn't breastfeed her child, breast weight returns to normal very soon after birth.

Many of the benefits of breastfeeding can be found in Table 13-3 and at www.4woman.gov./Breastfeeding/index.htm, sponsored by the U.S. Surgeon General.

■ Ability to Breastfeed

Almost all women are physically capable of breastfeeding their children (see later section "Medical Conditions Precluding Breastfeeding" for exceptions). In most cases, problems encountered in breastfeeding are due to a lack of appropriate information. Anatomical problems in breasts, such as inverted nipples, can be corrected during pregnancy. Breast size generally increases during pregnancy and is no indication of success in breastfeeding. Most women notice a dramatic increase in the size and weight of their breasts by the third or fourth day of breastfeeding. If these changes do not occur, a woman needs to speak with her physician or a lactation consultant.

Breastfed infants must be followed closely over the first days of life to ensure that feeding and weight gain are proceeding normally. Monitoring is especially important with a mother's first child, because the mother will be inexperienced with the technique of breastfeeding. Currently, mothers and healthy infants are commonly

Healthy People 2010 has set a goal of 75% of women breastfeeding their infants at time of hospital discharge, 50% breastfeeding for 6 months, and 25% still breastfeeding at 1 year.

discharged from the hospital 1 to 2 days after delivery, whereas 20 years ago they stayed in the hospital for 3 or 4 days or longer. One result of such rapid discharge is a decreased period of infant monitoring by health care professionals. Incidents have been reported of infants developing dehydration and in turn blood clots soon after hospital discharge when breastfeeding did not proceed smoothly. Careful monitoring in this first week by a physician or lactation consultant is advised.

First-time mothers who plan to breastfeed should learn as much as they can about the process early in their pregnancy. Interested women should learn the proper technique, what problems to expect, and how to respond to them. Overall, breastfeeding is a learned skill, and mothers need knowledge to breastfeed safely, especially with the first child.

■ Production of Human Milk

lobules Saclike structures in the breast that store milk.

prolactin A hormone secreted by the mother that stimulates the synthesis of milk.

During pregnancy, cells in the breast form milk-producing cells called **lobules** (Fig. 13-5). Hormones from the placenta stimulate these changes in the breast. After birth, the mother produces more **prolactin** hormone to maintain the changes in the breast and therefore the ability to produce milk. During pregnancy, breast weight increases by about 1 to 2 pounds.

The hormone prolactin also stimulates the synthesis of milk. Infant suckling stimulates prolactin release from the pituitary gland. Milk synthesis then occurs as an infant nurses. The more the infant suckles, the more milk is produced. Because of this, even twins (and triplets) can be breastfed adequately.

Most protein found in human milk is synthesized by breast tissue. Some proteins also enter the milk directly from the mother's bloodstream. These proteins include immune factors (e.g., antibodies) and enzymes. Fats in human milk come from both

Figure 13-5 The anatomy of the breast. Many types of cells form a coordinated network to produce and secrete human milk.

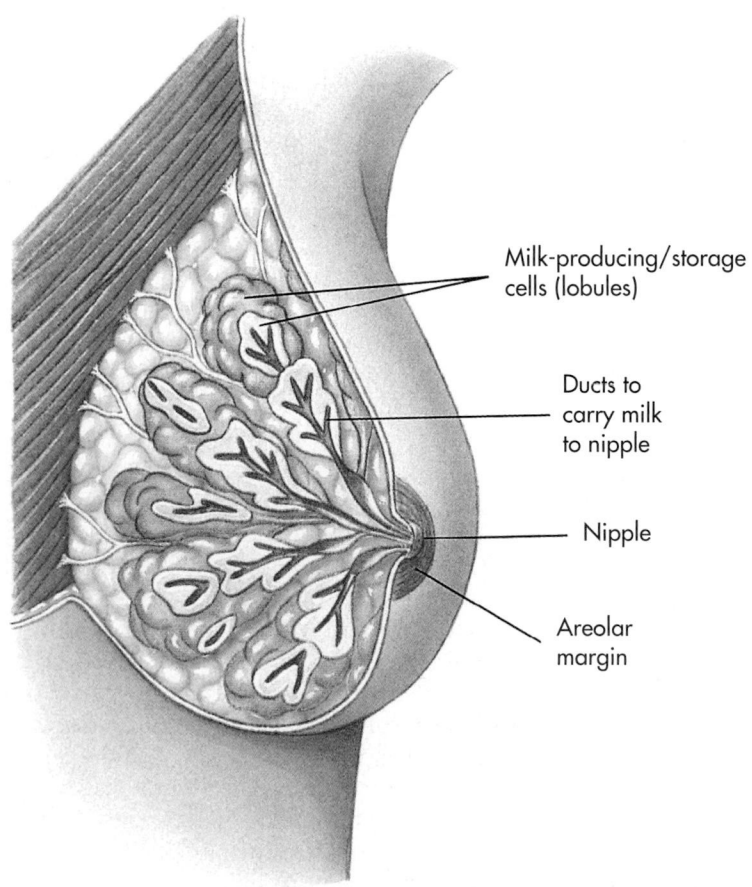

Milk-producing/storage cells (lobules)

Ducts to carry milk to nipple

Nipple

Areolar margin

the mother's diet and those synthesized by breast tissue. The sugar galactose is synthesized in the breast, whereas glucose enters from the mother's bloodstream. Together, these sugars form lactose, the main carbohydrate in human milk.

■ Let-Down Reflex

An important brain-breast connection—commonly called the **let-down reflex**—is necessary for breastfeeding. The brain releases the hormone **oxytocin** to allow the breast tissues to let down (release) the milk from storage sites (Fig. 13-6). It then travels to the nipple area. A tingling sensation signals the let-down reflex shortly before milk flow begins. If the let-down reflex doesn't operate, little milk is available to the infant. The infant then gets frustrated, and this can frustrate the mother.

The let-down reflex is easily inhibited by nervous tension, a lack of confidence, and fatigue. Mothers should be especially aware of the link between tension and a weak let-down reflex. They need to find a relaxed environment where they can breastfeed.

After a few weeks, the let-down reflex becomes automatic. The mother's response can be triggered just by thinking about her infant or seeing or hearing another one cry. At first, however, the process can be a bit bewildering. Because she cannot measure the amount of milk the infant takes in, a mother may fear that she is not adequately nourishing the infant.

As a general rule, a well-nourished breastfed infant should (1) have six or more wet diapers per day after the second day of life, (2) show a normal weight gain, and (3) pass at least one or two stools per day that look like lumpy mustard. In addition, softening of the breast during the feeding helps indicate that enough milk is being consumed. Parents who sense their infant is not consuming enough milk should consult a physician immediately because dehydration can develop rapidly.

It generally takes 2 to 3 weeks to fully establish the feeding routine: Infant and mother both feel comfortable, the milk supply meets infant demand, and initial

let-down reflex A reflex stimulated by infant suckling that causes the release (ejection) of milk from milk ducts in the mother's breasts; also called *milk ejection reflex.*

oxytocin A hormone secreted by the pituitary gland. It causes contraction of the musclelike cells surrounding the ducts of the breasts and the smooth muscle of the uterus.

Disposable diapers can absorb so much urine that it is difficult to judge when they are wet. A strip of paper towel laid inside a disposable diaper makes a good wetness indicator. Alternatively, cloth diapers may be used for a day or two to assess whether nursing is supplying sufficient milk.

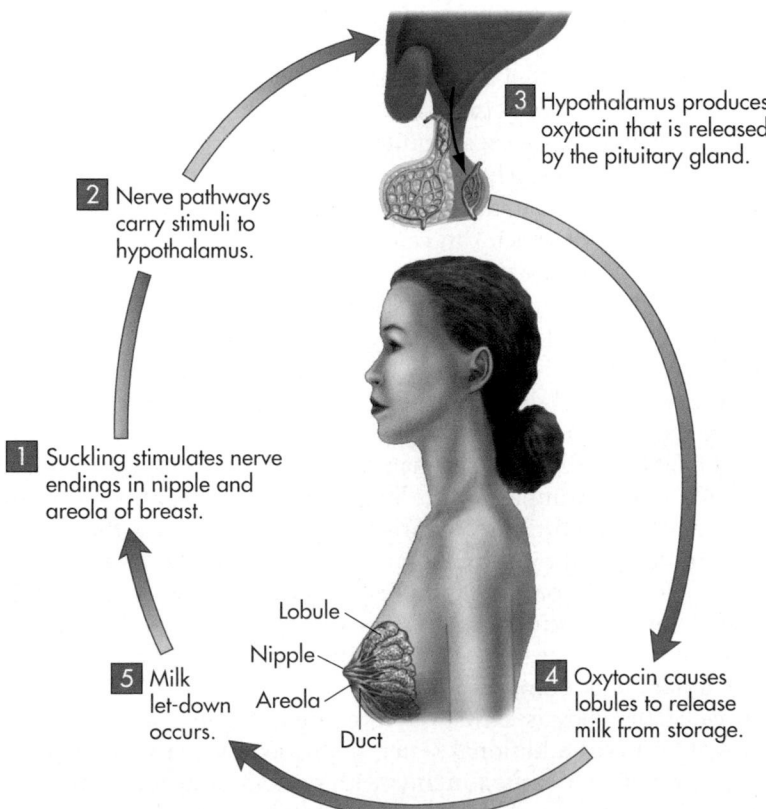

3 Hypothalamus produces oxytocin that is released by the pituitary gland.

2 Nerve pathways carry stimuli to hypothalamus.

1 Suckling stimulates nerve endings in nipple and areola of breast.

Lobule

Nipple

5 Milk let-down occurs.

Areola

Duct

4 Oxytocin causes lobules to release milk from storage.

Figure 13-6 Let-down reflex. Suckling sets into motion the sequence of events that lead to milk let-down, the flow of milk into ducts of the breast.

nipple soreness disappears. Establishing the breastfeeding routine requires patience, but the rewards are great. The adjustments are easier if supplemental formula feedings are not introduced until breastfeeding is well established, after at least 3 to 4 weeks. Then it is fine if a supplemental bottle or two of infant formula per day is needed.

▪ Nutritional Qualities of Human Milk

Human milk is very different in composition from cow's milk. Unless altered, cow's milk should never be used in infant feeding until the infant is at least 12 months old. Cow's milk is too high in minerals and protein and does not contain enough carbohydrate to meet infant needs. In addition, the major protein in cow's milk is harder for an infant to digest than the major proteins in human milk. The proteins in cow's milk also may spur allergies in the infant. Finally, certain compounds in human milk presently under study show other possible benefits for the infant.

Colostrum

colostrum The first fluid secreted by the breast during late pregnancy and the first few days after birth. This thick fluid is rich in immune factors and protein.

Lactobacillus bifidus **factor** A protective factor secreted in the colostrum that encourages growth of beneficial bacteria in the newborn's intestines.

At the end of pregnancy the first fluid made by the human breast is **colostrum.** This thick, yellowish fluid may leak from the breast during late pregnancy and is produced in earnest for a few days to a week after birth. Colostrum contains antibodies and immune system cells, some of which pass unaltered through the infant's immature GI tract into the bloodstream. The first few months of life are the only time when we can readily absorb whole proteins across the GI tract. These immune factors and cells protect the infant from some GI tract diseases and other infectious disorders, compensating for the infant's own immature immune system during the first few months of life.

One component of colostrum, the *Lactobacillus bifidus* factor, encourages the growth of *Lactobacillus bifidus* bacteria. These bacteria limit the growth of potentially toxic bacteria in the intestine. Overall, breastfeeding promotes the intestinal health of the breastfed infant in this way.

Mature Milk

Human milk composition gradually changes until it achieves the normal composition of mature milk several days after delivery. Human milk looks very different from cow's milk. (Table 14-1 in Chapter 14 provides a direct comparison.) Human milk is thin and almost watery in appearance and often has a slightly bluish tinge. Its nutritional qualities, however, are quite impressive.

Human milk's proteins form a soft, light curd in the infant's stomach and are easy to digest. Some human milk proteins bind iron, reducing the growth of iron-requiring bacteria, some of which can cause diarrhea. Still other proteins offer the important immune protection already noted.

The lipids in human breast milk are high in linoleic acid and cholesterol, which are needed for brain development. Breast milk also contains long-chain omega-3 fatty acids, such as docosahexaenoic acid (DHA). This polyunsaturated fatty acid is used for the synthesis of tissues in the brain and the rest of the central nervous system, and in the retina of the eye.

The fat composition of human milk changes during each feeding. The consistency of milk released initially (fore milk) first resembles that of skim milk. It later has a greater fat proportion, similar to whole milk. Finally, the milk released after 10 to 20 minutes (hind milk) is essentially like cream. Babies need to nurse long enough (e.g., a total of 20 or more minutes) to get the calories in the rich hind milk to be satisfied between feedings and to grow well. The overall calorie content of human milk is about the same as that of infant formulas (67 kcal per 100 milliliters).

Human milk composition also allows for adequate fluid status of the infant, provided the baby is exclusively breastfed. A question commonly asked is whether the infant needs additional water, if stressed by hot weather, diarrhea, vomiting, or fever. Providing breastfed infants with up to 4 ounces of water a day from a bottle is fine. Note, however, that greater amounts of supplemental water can lead to brain disorders, low blood sodium, and other problems. Thus, extra water should be given only with a physician's guidance.

■ Food Plan for Women Who Breastfeed

Nutrient needs for a breastfeeding mother change to some extent from those of the pregnant woman in the second and third trimester (see the inside cover of this book). There is a decrease in folate and iron needs and an increase in the needs for calories, vitamins A, E, and C, riboflavin, copper, chromium, iodide, manganese, selenium, and zinc. Still, these increased needs of the breastfeeding mother will be met by the general diet plan proposed for a woman in the latter stages of pregnancy. Recall that each day this diet plan includes at least:

- 3 cups of calcium-rich foods such as from the milk group or use of calcium-fortified foods to make up for any gap between calcium intake and need
- 6 ½ ounce-equivalents from the meat & beans group
- 3 ½ cups from the vegetable group
- 2 cups from the fruit group
- 8 ounce-equivalents from the grain group
- 7 teaspoons of oil

Discretionary calories (up to about 400 kcal) can then be added to allow for weight maintenance or gradual weight loss, whichever is needed.

Table 13-2 provided a menu for such a plan. Substituting a soyburger (veggie burger) for the hamburger in that menu would make this a practical guide for a lactovegetarian woman as well.

As in pregnancy, a serving of a highly fortified ready-to-eat breakfast cereal (or use of a balanced multivitamin and mineral supplement) is advised to help meet extra nutrient needs. And, as mentioned for pregnant women, breastfeeding mothers should consume fish at least twice a week (or 1 gram per day of omega-3 fatty acids from a fish oil supplement) because the omega-3 fatty acids present in fish are secreted into breast milk and are likely to be important for development of the infant's nervous system.

Milk production requires approximately 800 kcal every day. The Estimated Energy Requirement during lactation is an extra 400 to 500 kcal daily above prepregnancy recommendations. The difference between that needed for milk production and the recommended intake—about 300 kcal—should allow a gradual loss of the extra body fat accumulated during pregnancy, especially if breastfeeding is continued for 6 months or more and the woman performs some physical activity. This shows just one of the natural benefits of following pregnancy with at least several months of breastfeeding.

After giving birth, women are often eager to shed the excess "baby fat." Breastfeeding, however, is no time for crash diets. A gradual weight loss of 1 to 4 pounds per month in the nursing mother is appropriate. At significantly greater rates of weight loss—when calories are restricted to less than about 1500 kcal per day—milk output decreases. A reasonable approach for a breastfeeding mother is to eat a balanced diet that supplies at least 1800 kcal per day, has moderate fat content, and includes a variety of dairy products, fruits, vegetables, and whole grains.

To promote the best possible feeding experience for the infant, there are several other dietary factors to consider. Hydration is especially important during breastfeeding; the woman should drink fluids every time her infant nurses. Drinking about 13 cups of fluids per day encourages ample milk production. Poor health habits, such as smoking cigarettes or drinking more than two alcoholic drinks a day, can decrease milk output. To avoid exposure to harmful levels of mercury, precautions concerning fish that are likely to contain mercury should extend past pregnancy for the breastfeeding mother. Breastfeeding women also may want to avoid eating peanuts or peanut butter, as several studies have shown that peanut allergens pass into breast milk, potentially increasing the infant's risk for peanut allergy.

Most substances that the mother ingests are secreted into her milk. For this reason, she should limit intake of or avoid all alcohol and caffeine and check all medications with a pediatrician. Some mothers believe that some foods, such as garlic and chocolate, flavor the breast milk and upset the infant. If a woman notices a connection between a food she eats and the infant's later fussiness, she could consider avoiding that food. However, she might experiment again with it later, as infants become fussy for other reasons. Some researchers, on the other hand, feel that the passage of flavors from the mother's diet into her milk affords an opportunity for the infant to learn about the flavor of the foods of its family long before solids are introduced. These researchers suspect that bottle-fed infants are missing significant sensory experiences that, until recent times in human history, were common to all infants.

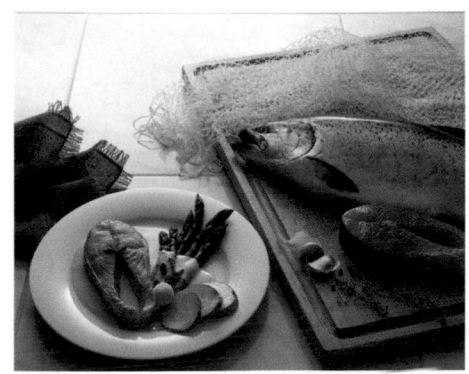

Eating fish at least twice a week will help breastfeeding women ensure that their infants receive important omega-3 fatty acids. It is important however to avoid those fish that are likely contaminated with mercury (listed on page 446).

Concept Check

Recognition of the importance of breastfeeding has contributed to its greater popularity in recent years. Almost all women have the ability to breastfeed. The hormone prolactin stimulates breast tissue to synthesize milk. Some components of human milk come directly from the mother's bloodstream. Infant suckling triggers a let-down reflex, which releases the milk. The more an infant nurses, the more milk is synthesized. The nutrient composition of human milk is very different from that of cow's milk and changes as the infant matures. The first fluid produced, colostrum, is rich in immune factors. The diet for breastfeeding is generally similar to that for pregnancy, except for necessary additional fluids. For teenage mothers in general, four servings from the milk, yogurt, and cheese group and/or calcium-fortified foods are recommended.

■ Breastfeeding Today

As noted already, the vast majority of women are capable of breastfeeding and their infants benefit from it. The many benefits are listed in Table 13-3. Nonetheless, a woman's decision to breastfeed depends on a variety of factors, some of which may make breastfeeding impractical or undesirable for a woman. Mothers who don't want to breastfeed their infants should not feel compelled to do so. Breastfeeding provides distinct advantages, but none so great that a woman who decides to bottle feed should feel she is significantly compromising her infant.

Advantages of Breastfeeding

Just as the milk of all mammals is the perfect nutrition source for the young of that species, human milk is tailored to meet infant nutrient needs for the first 4 to 6 months of life. The possible exceptions are the relative lack of fluoride, iron, and vitamin D. Infant supplements, used under the guidance of a pediatrician, can supply these and are often recommended, especially vitamin D. The American Academy of Pediatrics recommends all breastfed infants be given 200 IU of vitamin D per day

Table 13-3 Advantages of Breastfeeding

Infant
• Bacteriologically safe
• Always fresh and ready to go
• Provides antibodies while infant's immune system is still immature, as well as substances that contribute to maturation of the immune system
• Contributes to maturation of gastrointestinal tract via *Lactobacillus bifidus* factor; decreases incidence of diarrhea and respiratory disease
• Reduces risk of food allergies and intolerances, as well as some other allergies
• Establishes habit of eating in moderation, thus decreasing possibility of obesity later in life by about 20%
• Contributes to proper development of jaws and teeth for better speech development
• Decreases ear infections
• May enhance nervous system development (by providing the fatty acid DHA) and eventual learning ability
• May reduce the risk of later developing hypertension and other chronic diseases, such as diabetes

Mother
• Contributes to earlier recovery from pregnancy due to the action of hormones that promote a quicker return of the uterus to its prepregnancy state
• Decreases the risk of ovarian and premenopausal breast cancer
• Potential for quicker return to prepregnancy weight
• Potential for delayed ovulation and therefore reducing chances of pregnancy (short term however)

until they are consuming that much from food, such as, at least 2 cups (0.5 liters) of infant formula per day. Some sun exposure also helps in meeting vitamin D needs. Fluoride may be found in the household water supply. If it is not present in adequate amounts or the infant is not receiving tap water, a fluoride supplement should be considered and a dentist consulted. Vitamin B-12 supplements are recommended for the breastfed infant whose mother is a complete vegetarian (vegan).

Fewer Infections Breastfeeding reduces the infant's overall risk of developing infections. This is partially because an infant can use the antibodies in human milk. Breastfed infants also have fewer ear infections (otitis media) because they do not sleep with a bottle in their mouths. Experts strongly discourage allowing any infants to sleep with a bottle in their mouths, because when that happens, milk can pool in the mouth, back up through the throat, and eventually settle in the ears, creating a growth medium for bacteria. Infant ear infections are a common problem. By avoiding these problems, parents can decrease discomfort for the infant, avoid related trips to the doctor, and prevent possible hearing loss. Tooth decay from nighttime bottles is another likely consequence of sleeping with a bottle in the mouth (see Chapter 14).

Fewer Allergies and Intolerances Breastfeeding also reduces the chances of some allergies, especially in allergy-prone infants (see Chapter 14). The key time to attain this benefit from breastfeeding is during the first 4 to 6 months of an infant's life. A longer commitment than 4 to 6 months is best, but the first few months are most critical. Breastfeeding for even just the first few weeks is beneficial. Another benefit of breastfeeding is that infants are better able to tolerate human milk than formulas. Formulas sometimes must be switched several times until caregivers find the best one for the infant.

Convenience and Cost Breastfeeding frees the mother from the time and expense involved in buying and preparing formula and washing bottles. Human milk is ready to go and sterile. This allows the mother to spend more time with her baby.

Possible Barriers to Breastfeeding

Widespread misinformation, the mother's need to return to a job, and social reticence all serve as barriers to breastfeeding.

Misinformation Probably the major barriers to breastfeeding are misinformation, such as the idea that one's breasts are too small, and the lack of role models. One positive note has been the widespread increase in the availability of lactation consultants over the past several years. These consultants are a valuable resource for new mothers in the adjustment to breastfeeding. If a woman is interested in breastfeeding, she should find support by talking to women who have experienced it successfully because they can be an invaluable help to the first-time mother. The first-time mother should find a friend she can call on for advice. In almost every community, a group called La Leche League offers classes in breastfeeding and advises women who have problems with it (800-LALECHE or www.lalecheleague.org). Other resources are www.breastfeeding.com, www.breastfeeding.org, and www.nal.usda.gov/wicworks.

Return to an Outside Job Working outside the home can complicate plans to breastfeed. One possibility after a month or two of breastfeeding is for the mother to express and save her own milk. She can use a breast pump or manually express milk into a sterile plastic bottle or nursing bag (used in a disposable bottle system). Saving human milk requires careful sanitation and rapid chilling. It can be stored in the refrigerator for 3 days or be frozen for 3 months. There is a knack to learning how to express milk, but the freedom can be worth it, because it allows others to feed the infant the mother's milk. A schedule of expressing milk and using supplemental formula feedings is most successful if begun after 1 to 2 months of exclusive breastfeeding. After 1 month or so, the baby is well adapted to breastfeeding and probably feels enough emotional security and other benefits from nursing to drink both ways.

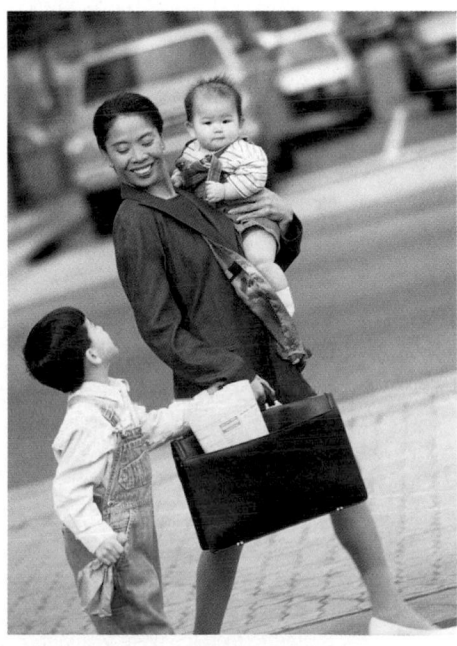

Breastfeeding a baby once returning to work is possible, but requires planning.

Frozen human milk should not be thawed in a microwave. The heat can destroy immune factors in the milk and create hot spots, which may scald the infant's tongue.

Some women can juggle both a job and breastfeeding, but others find it too cumbersome and decide to formula-feed. A compromise—balancing some breastfeedings, perhaps early morning and night, with infant formula feedings during the day—is possible. However, too many supplemental infant formula feedings decrease milk production.

Social Concerns   Another barrier for some women is embarrassment about nursing a child in public. Historically our society has stressed modesty and has discouraged public displays of breasts—even for as good a cause as nourishing babies. In the United States, no state or territory has a law prohibiting breastfeeding. However, indecent exposure (including the exposure of women's breasts) has long been a common law or statutory offense. During the 1990s, some individual states, such as Florida and North Carolina, began to clarify the right to breastfeed and to decriminalize public breastfeeding. Since then, several other states have passed similar laws. Women who feel reluctant should be reassured that they do have social support and that breastfeeding can be done very discreetly with little breast exposure.

Medical Conditions Precluding Breastfeeding   Breastfeeding may be ruled out by certain medical conditions in either the infant or mother. For example, breastfeeding may be detrimental to infants with phenylketonuria; the high concentration of phenylalanine in breast milk may overwhelm the impaired ability of these infants to metabolize this amino acid, leading to production of toxic products.

Certain medications, which pass into the milk and adversely affect the nursing infant, are best avoided while breastfeeding. In addition, a woman in North America or other developed regions of the world who has a serious chronic disease (such as tuberculosis, AIDS, or HIV-positive status) or who is being treated with chemotherapy medications should not breastfeed. A final group can include immature mothers and those with psychiatric problems.

Breastfeeding mothers should get their physician's permission before embarking on a vigorous exercise program. Breastfeeding women must also take care to drink plenty of fluids before and after workouts and should avoid exercising when fatigued.

Environmental Contaminants in Human Milk

There is some legitimate concern over the levels of various environmental contaminants in human milk. However, the benefits from human milk are very well established and the risks from environmental contaminants are still largely theoretical. Thus, it is probably best to continue with what has been shown to work until sufficiently strong research data contradict it. A few measures a woman could take to counteract some known contaminants are to (1) avoid freshwater fish from polluted waters, (2) carefully wash and peel fruits and vegetables, and (3) remove the fatty edges of meat, as pesticides concentrate in fat. In addition, a woman should not try to lose weight rapidly while nursing (more than ¾ to 1 pound per week) because contaminants stored in her fat tissue might then enter her bloodstream and affect her milk. If a woman questions whether her milk is safe, especially if she has lived in an area known to have a high concentration of toxic wastes or environmental pollutants, she should consult her local health department.

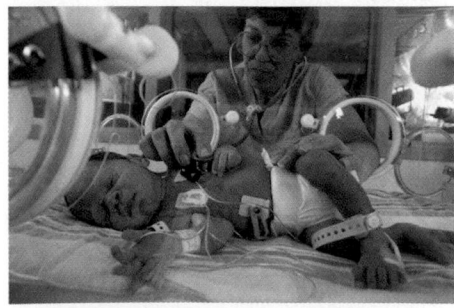

If human milk is used to feed the preterm infant, fortification of the milk with certain nutrients is often needed.

Another Bite

There is no universal answer to whether a woman can breastfeed a preterm infant. In some cases, human milk is the most desirable form of nourishment, depending on infant weight and length of gestation. If so, it must usually be expressed from the breast and fed through a tube until the infant's sucking and swallowing reflex develops. This type of feeding demands great maternal dedication. Fortification of the milk with such nutrients as calcium, phosphorus, sodium, and protein is often necessary to match the preterm infant's rapid growth. In other cases, special feeding problems may prevent the use of human milk or necessitate supplementing it with formula. Sometimes total parenteral nutrition (intravenous feeding) is the only option. Working as a team, the pediatrician, neonatal nurses, and registered dietitian must guide the parents in this decision.

Concept Check

Human milk supplies most of an infant's nutritional needs for the first 6 months, although supplementation with vitamin D, iron, and fluoride may be needed. Breastfeeding is often more convenient than formula feeding. Compared with formula-fed infants, breastfed infants have fewer intestinal, respiratory, and ear infections and are less susceptible to some allergies and food intolerances. Despite the advantages of breastfeeding, misinformation, job responsibilities, and social reticence may dissuade a mother from breastfeeding. A combination of breastfeeding and formula feeding is possible when a mother is regularly away from the infant and is not able to express and store her milk for later use. Breastfeeding is not desirable if a mother has certain diseases or must take medication potentially harmful to the infant. The preterm infant, depending on its condition, may benefit from consuming human milk.

Summary

1. Adequate nutrition is vital during pregnancy to ensure the well-being of both the infant and mother. Poor maternal nutrition and use of some medications, especially during the first trimester, can cause birth defects. Growth restriction and altered development can also occur if these insults happen later in pregnancy.

2. Infants born preterm (before 37 weeks gestation) usually have more medical problems at and following birth than normal infants.

3. A woman typically needs an additional 350 to 450 kcal per day during the second and third trimesters of pregnancy to meet her calorie needs. A better measure of meeting energy needs is adequate weight gain. This should occur slowly, reaching a total of 25 to 35 pounds in a woman of healthy weight.

4. Protein, carbohydrate, fiber, vitamin, and mineral needs increase during pregnancy. Following a plan based on MyPyramid is recommended. A supplemental source of iron, in particular, may be needed. Folate nutriture especially should be adequate at the time of conception. Any nutrient supplement use needs to be guided by a physician, as an excess intake of vitamin A and other nutrients during pregnancy can have harmful effects on the fetus.

5. The factors that contribute to poor pregnancy outcome include inadequate health care in general and prenatal care in particular, teenage pregnancy, closely spaced births, smoking, alcohol consumption, illicit drug use (such as cocaine), insufficient carbohydrate intake (less than 175 grams per day), heavy caffeine use, and various infections, such as *Listeria*.

6. Pregnancy-induced hypertension, gestational diabetes, heartburn, constipation, nausea, vomiting, edema, and anemia are all possible discomforts and complications of pregnancy. Nutrition therapy can help minimize some of these problems.

7. Almost all women are able to breastfeed their infants. The nutrient composition of human milk is very different from that of unaltered cow's milk and is much more desirable. Colostrum, the first fluid produced by the human breast, is very rich in immune factors. Mature milk is rich in protein and in lactose. The diet plan recommended for the second and third trimesters of pregnancy is also appropriate for meeting the nutrient needs of the lactating woman, except more fluids in general should be consumed.

8. For the infant, the advantages of breastfeeding over formula feeding are numerous, including fewer intestinal, respiratory, and ear infections and fewer allergies and food intolerances. Moreover, breastfeeding is also less expensive and possibly more convenient for the mother than formula feeding. However, an infant can be adequately nourished with formula if the mother chooses not to breastfeed. Breastfeeding is not desirable if the mother has certain diseases or must take medication potentially harmful to the infant. Likewise, breastfeeding is not advised for infants with certain medical conditions, including some preterm infants.

Study Questions

1. Provide three key pieces of advice for parents seeking to maximize their chances of having a healthy infant. Why did you identify those specific factors?

2. Outline current weight-gain recommendations for pregnancy. What is the basis for these recommendations?

3. Identify four key nutrients for which intake should be significantly increased during pregnancy.

4. How is the MyPyramid diet for an average woman adapted to meet the increased nutrient needs of pregnancy?

5. Why does teenage pregnancy receive so much attention these days? At what age do you think pregnancy is ideal? Why?

6. Give three reasons a woman should give serious consideration to breastfeeding her infant.

7. Describe the physiological mechanisms that stimulate milk production and release. How can knowing about these help mothers breastfeed successfully?

8. What guidelines can a woman use to determine whether her breastfed infant is receiving sufficient nourishment?

9. How should the basic food plan suitable for pregnancy be modified during breastfeeding?

10. Where can first-time mothers go for help in establishing successful breastfeeding?

Further Readings

1. ADA Reports: Position of the American Dietetic Association: Nutrition and lifestyle for a healthy pregnancy outcome. *Journal of the American Dietetic Association* 102:1479, 2002.

   The key components of a healthy lifestyle during pregnancy include appropriate weight gain; consumption of a variety of foods; appropriate and timely vitamin and mineral intake; avoidance of alcohol, tobacco, and other harmful substances; and safe food handling. Vitamin and mineral supplementation is appropriate for some nutrients, particularly in certain situations, such as for vegans.

2. ADA Reports: Position of the American Dietetic Association: Promoting and supporting breastfeeding. *Journal of the American Dietetic Association* 105: 810, 2005.

   The American Dietetics Association strongly supports the breastfeeding of infants. This article discusses the benefits from breastfeeding that accrue to the mother and infant, as well as dietary considerations that need to addressed, such as avoiding consumption of species of fish known to contain high amounts of mercury.

3. Allen LH: Multiple micronutrients in pregnancy and lactation: An overview. *American Journal of Clinical Nutrition* 81:1206S, 2005.

   Numerous nutrients contribute to a healthy outcome of pregnancy, including many B vitamins and iron. The author notes in many cases diet changes allow women to meet these needs, but in some cases supplementation is needed, such as for poor women. With respect to diet changes, these should begin before pregnancy so a woman has a healthy status in the fist weeks while she is pregnant but still does not know this is the case.

4. Crowther CA and others: Effect of treatment of gestational diabetes mellitus on pregnancy outcomes. *The New England Journal of Medicine* 352: 2477, 2005.

   This study found that treating gestational diabetes when it develops is important in order to improve the health of the mother, fetus, and ultimately the infant. Diet changes and regular blood glucose monitoring are important parts of the therapy; in some cases insulin injections are also need to control blood glucose.

5. Field CJ: The immunological components of human milk and their effect on immune development in infants. *Journal of Nutrition* 135:1, 2005.

   Human milk contains many factors that improve immune function in the infant. This article reviews a number of these quite complex factors.

6. Green NS: Folic acid supplementation and prevention of birth defects. *Journal of Nutrition* 132:2356S, 2002.

   If all women began pregnancy with adequate folate status, neural tube birth defects could be decreased by up to 70%. The current recommendation is for all women of childbearing age to consume 400 micrograms of synthetic folic acid daily. Women who have given birth to a child with a neural tube defect should consume 4000 micrograms (4 milligrams) of synthetic folic acid per day in anticipation of a possible pregnancy.

7. Hulsey TC and others: Maternal prepregnant body mass index and weight gain related to low birth weight in South Carolina. *Southern Medical Journal* 98:411, 2005.

   A healthy weight at conception and adequate weight gain during pregnancy contributed to a substantial reduction in low birth weight infants in this study. For example, women with inadequate weight gains had about a 1.5 to 2 times greater risk of delivering a low birth weight infant.

8. Kabiru KW, Raynor BD: Obstetric outcomes associated with increase in BMI category during pregnancy. *American Journal of Obstetrics and Gynecology* 191: 928, 2004.

   Obesity in pregnant women leads to a high risk for complications in the pregnancy, and so requires careful monitoring by the physician. Such potential complications in this study included gestational diabetes and the need for cesarean deliveries.

9. Kelly, AKW: Practical exercise advice during pregnancy. The *Physician and SportsMedicine* 33(6):24, 2005.

   It is safe for pregnant women to exercise if they are experiencing uncomplicated pregnancies. The author notes that in fact many positive effects of exercise during pregnancy are possible. Most non-weight bearing exercises, (e.g., swimming) and walking are safe for pregnant women. These should begin with 15 minutes of exercise three times a week and progressing as tolerated. The author discusses how to monitor women as they increase their physical activity.

10. King JC: The risk of maternal nutritional depletion and poor outcomes increases in early or closely spaced pregnancies. *Journal of Nutrition* 133:1732S, 2003.

    An adequate supply of nutrients is probably the single most important environmental factor affecting pregnancy outcome. A short interval between pregnancies or an early pregnancy within 2 years of the onset of menstrual periods increases the risk for preterm birth and growth-retarded infants. Maternal nutrient depletion arising from closely spaced pregnancies is one cause of these poor pregnancy outcomes. Supplementation with food and micronutrients during the interpregnancy period may improve pregnancy outcomes and maternal health among women with early or closely spaced pregnancies.

11. Koebnick C and others: Long-term ovo-lacto vegetarian diet impairs vitamin B-12 status in pregnant women. *Journal of Nutrition* 134: 3319, 2004.

    Pregnant women consuming a long term predominantly vegetarian diet had an increased risk of developing a vitamin B-12 deficiency in this study. Attention to vitamin B-12 intake is thus merited in women who are vegetarians, and this needs to done before they become pregnant.

12. Kramer MS and others: Infant growth and health outcomes associated with 3 compared with 6 months of exclusive breastfeeding. *American Journal of Clinical Nutrition* 78:291, 2003.

    Exclusive breastfeeding for 6 months in this study was associated with a lower risk of infant GI tract infections. In addition, there were no demonstrable adverse health effects of this practice in the infant's first year of life.

13. Moore, VM, Davies, MJ: Diet during pregnancy, neonatal outcomes and later health. Reproduction, Fertility, and Delivery 17:341, 2005.

    Altering the maternal diet before and during pregnancy can induce permanent changes in the offspring birth size and adult health/life span. Consequences of inadequate maternal nutrition for the offspring depend on the specific time in gestation that they occur. The authors emphasize the importance of improving diet before a woman becomes pregnant in order to protect her health and the health of her offspring.

14. Pawley, N., Bishop, NJ: Prenatal and infant predictors of bone health: The influence of vitamin D. *American Journal of Clinical Nutrition* 80:1748S, 2004.

    Women who are vitamin D-deficient during pregnancy deliver infants with disturbed skeletal development, and in some cases even with evidence of rickets and fractures. Populations at risk for vitamin D deficiency are those for which, for environmental, cultural, or medical reasons, exposure to sunlight is poor and the dietary intake of vitamin D is low. Especially in these cases, attention to meeting vitamin D needs is very important.

15. Prather, CM: Pregnancy-related constipation. *Current Gastroenterology Reports* 6:402, 2004.

    Constipation is a common complaint in pregnancy. In most cases, dietary measures such as increased fiber are sufficient to treat the disorder. As pointed out in this article, any laxative use needs to be reviewed by a physician as some are not appropriate for use during pregnancy.

16. Rosenburg, TJ and others: Maternal obesity and diabetes as risk factors for adverse pregnancy outcomes: Differences among 4 racial/ethnic groups. *American Journal of Public Health* 95:1545, 2005.

    In this large population-based study obesity and diabetes were clearly associated with adverse pregnancy outcomes. This highlights the need for women to control these conditions as best as possible during their child-bearing years in order to protect the health of their future infant.

17. Wagner, LK: Diagnosis and managements of preeclampsia. *American Family Physician* 70:2317, 2004.

    Preeclampsia is a multisystem disorder of unknown cause. It effects about 5-7% of pregnancies and is a significant cause of both illness and death in the mother and fetus. Management requires careful monitoring of the mother and fetus once the disorder develops. Currently, magnesium sulfate is the major therapy used, but medications to control related hypertension may also be employed. This article reviews preeclampsia in detail.

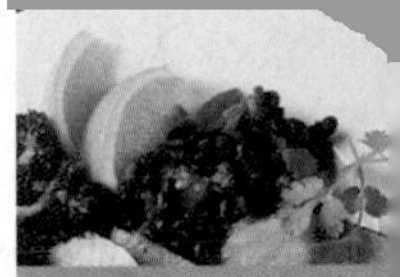

I. Targeting Nutrients Necessary for Pregnant Women

This chapter mentioned that pregnant women may have difficulty meeting their increased needs for folate, vitamin B-6, iron, and zinc. List six foods rich in each of these nutrients next to the appropriate heading below. Refer to Chapters 8 and 9 if necessary.

Nutrient	Foods	Nutrient	Foods
Folate	_____	Iron	_____
	_____		_____
	_____		_____
	_____		_____
	_____		_____
Vitamin B-6	_____	Zinc	_____
	_____		_____
	_____		_____
	_____		_____
	_____		_____

1. Foods rich in more than one of these nutrients would be especially valuable for pregnant women. Write on the line below any foods you listed that are good sources of more than one of these critical nutrients.

   _____

2. The needs for folate, vitamin B-6, iron, and zinc increase during pregnancy. For which of these nutrients can pregnant women usually obtain adequate intakes from dietary sources?

   _____

3. Which of these nutrients are commonly taken in supplement form during pregnancy?

   _____

   _____

4. Why might it be hard for pregnant women to meet their increased needs for these nutrients from food alone?

   _____

   _____

II. *Putting Your Knowledge About Nutrition and Pregnancy to Work*

 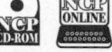 A college friend, Angie, tells you that she is newly pregnant. You are aware that she usually likes to eat the following foods for her meals:

Breakfast

Skips this meal, or eats a granola bar
Coffee

Lunch

Sweetened yogurt, 1 cup
Small bagel with cream cheese
Occasional piece of fruit
Regular caffeinated soda, 12 ounces

Snack

Chocolate candy bar

Dinner

2 slices of pizza, macaroni and cheese, or 2 eggs with 2 slices of toast
Seldom eats a salad or vegetable
Regular caffeinated soda, 12 ounces

Snacks

Pretzels or chips, 1 ounce
Regular caffeinated soda, 12 ounces

1. Using NutritionCalc Plus, or Appendix J, evaluate Angie's diet for protein, carbohydrate, iron, vitamin B-6, folate, and zinc. How does her intake compare with the recommended amounts for pregnancy?

   _____

   _____

   _____

2. Now redesign her diet and make sure that her intake meets pregnancy needs for carbohydrates, protein, folate, vitamin B-6, and zinc. (Hint: Fortified foods, such as breakfast cereal, are generally nutrient-rich foods, which can more easily help meet one's needs.) Increase the iron content as well, but it still may be below the RDA for pregnancy.

   _____

   _____

   _____

Nutrition from Infancy through Adolescence

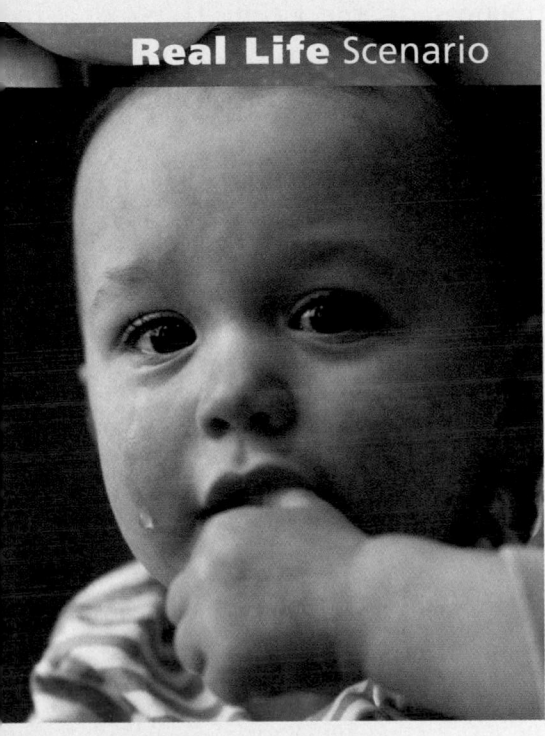

Real Life Scenario

Damon is a 7-month-old boy who has been taken into a clinic for a routine checkup. On examination, he was found to be moderately underweight relative to his age and body length. His physician scheduled a follow-up appointment in 3 months. At the 10-month-visit, Damon appeared sluggish and was now even more underweight for his age and length.

A registered dietitian interviewed Damon's 16-year-old mother to collect information on Damon's dietary intake. His intake over the previous 24 hours consisted of two bottles of infant formula, three 8 ounce bottles of Kool-Aid, and a hot dog. However, the mother was still in school, and at night she often left Damon with the neighbor, so that she could go out with friends for a few hours. Thus, she was not aware of all that he ate.

What problems do you think are present in Damon's diet? What potential dangers await Damon if his growth continues to lag behind?

Chapter 14 Objectives

Chapter 14 is designed to allow you to:

1. Describe the extent to which nutrition affects infant growth and physiological development.

2. Identify diet guidelines to meet the basic nutritional needs for normal growth and development for an infant and discuss some do's and don'ts associated with infant feeding.

3. List several challenges parents might face in dealing with childhood eating habits.

4. List the nutrients often found to be lacking in the diets of infants, toddlers, preschoolers, and teenagers and make recommendations to remedy the problems.

Check out the **Contemporary Nutrition Online Learning Center**
www.mhhe.com/wardlawcont6 for quizzes, flash cards, other activities, and web links designed to further help you learn about issues surrounding nutrition from infancy through adolescence.

As humans grow through early years into young adulthood, our needs for calories and nutrients change. Infants need more calories, protein, vitamins, and minerals per pound of body weight than young and older adults to support their rapid pace of growth and development. The growth rate of children is slower than that of infants, therefore children's needs and intake are proportionately less. The erratic eating behaviors of young children pose major challenges for parents and other caregivers. In turn, childhood becomes an important time to establish healthful habits, including those related to food choice and physical activity.

Family behaviors wield important influences on the child. Thus, education designed to change children's eating behaviors must be directed simultaneously at the main caregivers. Parents and other caregivers usually determine what foods are purchased and how they are prepared. To help children adopt a lifelong healthy dietary intake, a variety of foods should be introduced at home, fast-food and sugared soft drinks should be limited to a few times per week or less, and new foods should be introduced regularly. Maintaining a healthful eating (and physical activity) pattern should continue as children grow into teenagers. In exploring all these stages of life, Chapter 14 looks at the key role nutrients play and how food choices should be tailored to meet changing needs.

Refresh Your Memory

As you begin your study of nutrition from infancy through adolescence in Chapter 14, you may want to review:

- MyPyramid and the 2005 Dietary Guidelines in Chapter 2
- Diagnosis and treatment of type 2 diabetes in Chapter 4
- The immune system in Chapter 3
- Common sources of saturated fat, cholesterol, and *trans* fat in Chapter 5
- Vegetarianism in "Looking Further: Vegetarian Diets" in Chapter 6
- Rich sources of calcium, iron, and zinc in Chapter 9
- The concept of body mass index (BMI) and the treatment of obesity, including typical medications prescribed in Chapter 10
- The benefits of regular physical activity in Chapter 11
- Anorexia nervosa and other eating disorders in Chapter 12

MARVIN

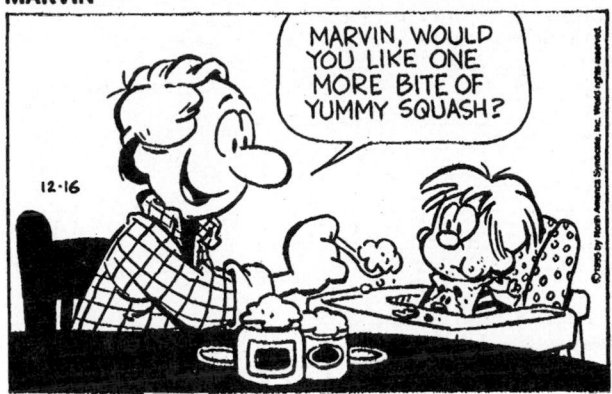
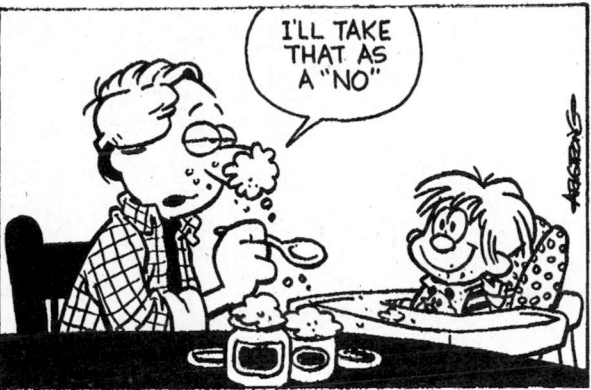

At what age should an infant be fed solid foods? Which foods are most appropriate for those early stages of solid food introduction? Which foods should not be fed to infants? Why? Chapter 14 provides some answers.

MARVIN © Reprinted with special permission of King Features Syndicate, Inc.

Nutrition and Child Health—An Introduction

Current statistics describing the nutrition and overall health among children and adolescents in North America have shown both positive and negative trends. On a positive note, more children are receiving vaccinations than ever before, fewer teenagers are giving birth, and the poverty rate for children has fallen considerably. In contrast to this good news, the number of children and teenagers with obesity and type 2 diabetes is rising, and physical activity in general is on the decline as more time is spent sitting in front of computer screens and television sets. Low calcium intakes are also receiving much attention, as soft drinks have replaced much of the milk that children and teenagers previously consumed on a daily basis. Fruits, vegetables and whole grains are also often in short supply in their diets. In this chapter, we will look at these trends and their effects on nutrition and overall health of this age group.

Infant Growth and Nutrition Needs

During infancy, attitudes toward foods and the whole eating process begin to take shape. If parents and other caregivers practice good nutrition and are flexible, they can lead an infant into lifelong healthful food habits. An infant that starts life in such an environment has a good chance of starting life with the nutrients needed to support brain and body growth spurts, and as well developing a willingness to try new foods. However, these physical and psychological advantages alone don't guarantee that a child will thrive.

Children also need specific attention focused on them; they need to grow in a stimulating environment, and they need a sense of security. For example, children hospitalized for growth failure gain weight more quickly when more caring stimulation, such as holding and rocking the infant, accompanies needed nutrients.

The Growing Infant

All babies seem to do is eat and sleep. There's a good reason for this. An infant's birth weight doubles in the first 4 to 6 months and triples within the first year. Never again

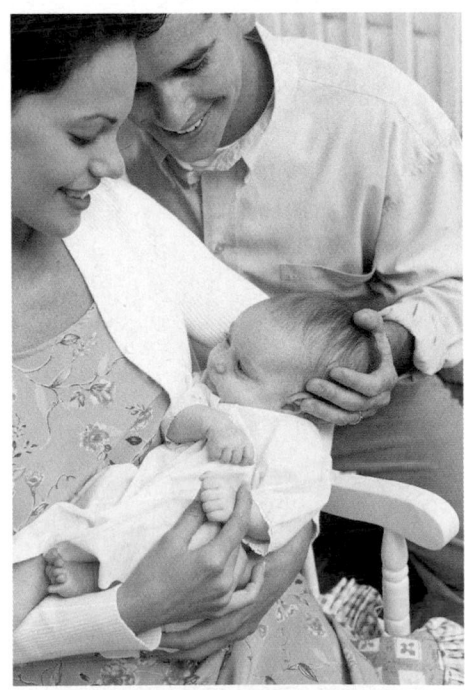

Children benefit from the love and attention of adults.

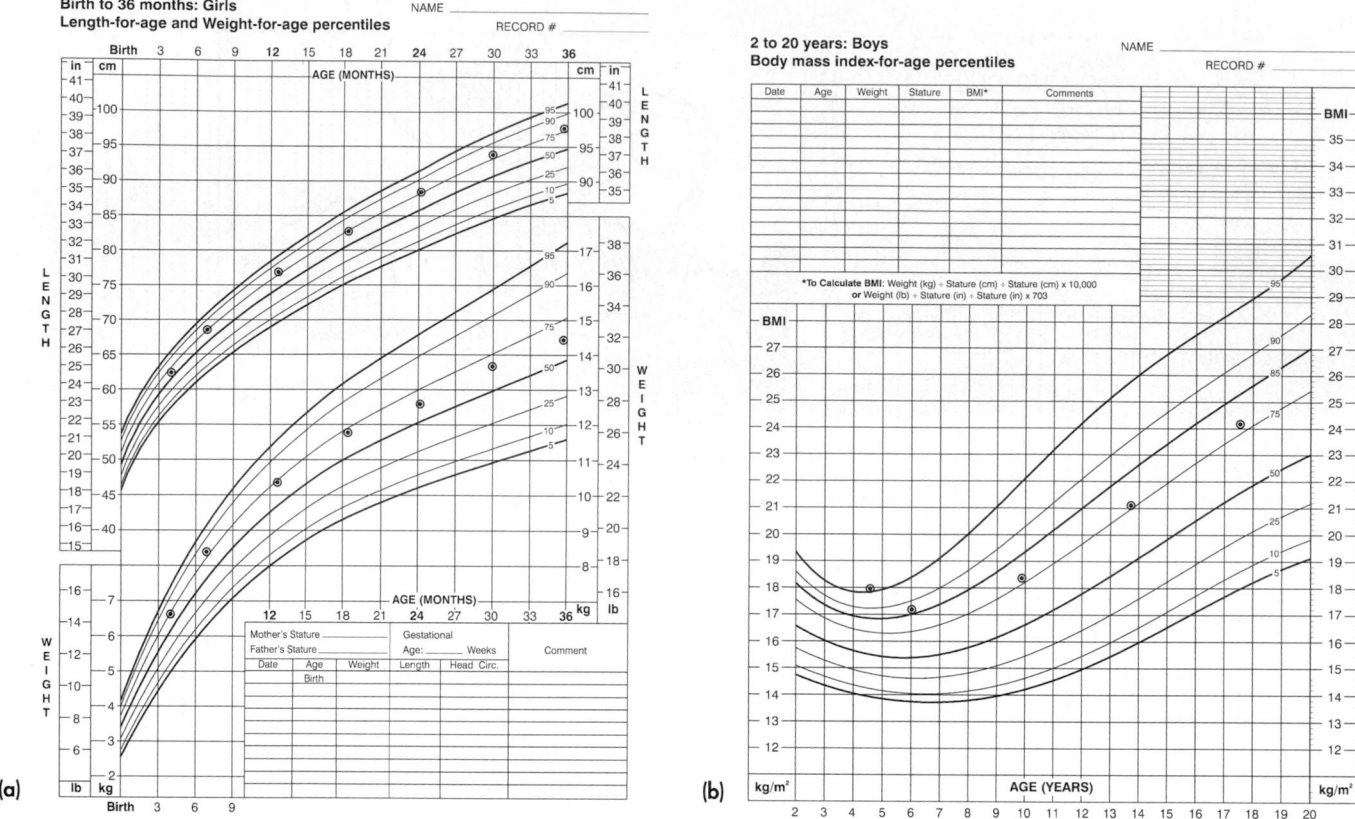

Figure 14-1 Growth charts for assessment of children in the growing years. The growth of a youngster is plotted to show how the charts are used in health care settings. (a) Growth charts used to assess length (height) and weight in young girls. A certain weight and length (height) correspond to a percentile value, which is a ranking of the person among 100 peers. This chart shows that at 36 months of age the girl was at the 75th percentile for length and the 62nd percentile for height. (b) Growth charts used to assess weight-for-height relationships in boys ages 2 to 20 years. Today, these charts for older children and adolescents typically utilize BMI for the evaluation. At 6 years of age the boy was at the 85th percentile for BMI.

Source: Developed by the National Center for Health Statistics in collaboration with the National Center for Chronic Disease Prevention and Health Promotion (2000). www.cdc.gov/growthcharts. Revised November 21, 2000.

is growth so rapid. Such rapid growth requires a lot of nourishment and sleep. After the first year, growth is slower; it takes 5 more years to double the weight seen at 1 year. An infant also increases in length in the first year by 50% and then continues to gain height through the teen years. These gains are not necessarily continuous—spurts of growth alternate with plateaus. Height is essentially maximized by age 19, although increases of several inches may occur in the early twenties, especially for boys (Fig. 14-1). Head size in proportion to total height shrinks from one-fourth to one-eighth during the climb from infancy to adulthood.

The human body needs a lot more food to support growth and development than it does to merely maintain its size once growth ceases. When nutrients are missing at critical phases of this process, growth and development may slow or even stop. In countries of the developing world today, about one-third of the children under 5 years of age are short and underweight for their ages. Poor nutrition—called **undernutrition**—is at the heart of the problem. This occurs to a lesser extent in North America. The undernourished children are simply smaller versions of nutritionally fit children. In poorer countries, when breastfeeding ceases, children are often fed a high-carbohydrate, low-protein diet. This diet supports some growth but does not allow children to attain their full genetic potential. To grow, children must consume adequate amounts of calories, protein, calcium, iron, zinc, and other nutrients.

undernutrition Failing health that results from a long-standing dietary intake that is not enough to meet nutritional needs.

■ Effect of Undernutrition on Growth

As with the fetus in utero, the long-term effects of nutritional problems in infancy and childhood depend on the severity, timing, and duration of the nutritional insult to cell processes.

The single best indicator of a child's nutritional status is growth, particularly weight gain in the short run and length (height) in the long run. Mild zinc deficiencies in North American children have been linked to poor growth. Improving the diets of these children then leads to improved growth. Overall, eating a poor diet as an infant or a child hampers the cell division that occurs at that critical stage. Consuming an adequate diet later usually won't compensate for lost growth, however, as the hormonal and other conditions needed for growth will not likely be present. In addition, growth ceases in girls and boys when the skeleton reaches its final size. This happens as growth plates at the ends of the bones fuse, which begins around 14 years of age in girls and 15 years of age in boys. The final stages of this process end at about 19 years of age in girls and 20 years of age in boys. Furthermore, muscles can increase in diameter later in life but their linear growth is limited by the length of the shorter bone.

For these reasons, a 15-year-old Central American girl who is 4 feet 8 inches tall cannot attain the adult height of a typical North American girl simply by eating better. Girls experience their peak rate of growth right before the onset of the menses. Once the time for growth ceases (in women, this is about 5 years after they start menstruating), a sufficient nutrient intake helps maintain health and weight but cannot make up for lost growth.

■ Assessment of Infant Growth and Development

Health professionals assess a child's increases in height and weight by comparing them with typical growth patterns recorded on charts (review Fig. 14-1). The charts contain **percentile** divisions, which represent the typical measurements for 90% to 96% of children. A percentile represents the rank of the person among 100 peers matched for age and gender. If a young boy, for example, is at the 90th percentile of height-for-age, he is shorter than 10% (of children) and taller than 89% (of children). A child at the 50th percentile is considered average. Fifty children will be taller than this child; 49 will be shorter.

Individual growth charts are available for both males and females. For ages ranging from birth to 36 months, options for growth charts include weight-for-age, length-for-age, weight-for-length, and head circumference-for-age. For males and females who are 2 to 20 years old, growth charts are available to determine weight-for-age and height-for-age; however, the preferred growth chart for children and adolescents is body mass index (BMI)-for-age. For adults, BMI has fixed cutoff points (for example, a BMI of 25 for an adult is considered overweight). As Figure 14-1 shows, this is not true for children, as BMI is both gender- and age-specific.

Infants and children should have their growth assessed during regular health checkups. It takes 1 to 3 years for the genetic potential (in terms of percentile ranking on growth charts) of infant growth to be established. By 3 years of age, a child's measurements, such as length (height)-for-age, should generally track along the established percentile. If the child's growth doesn't keep up with its length-for-age percentile, the physician needs to investigate whether a medical or nutritional problem is impeding the predicted growth. Inappropriate weight gain—too little or too much—should also be investigated.

Infants born preterm may catch up in growth in 2 to 3 years. This requires that the child move up in the percentiles. If this occurs—especially in length-for-age—it is usually no cause for alarm. On the other hand, moving up in the percentiles for weight-for-height can be disturbing if the child approaches the 80th to 90th percentiles. A child at the 85th percentile or above for BMI is considered at risk for overweight. At or above the 95th percentile, the child is considered overweight. At the 95th percentile,

percentile Classification of a measurement of a unit into divisions of 100 units.

Children under 2 to 3 years of age are measured lying on their backs with knees unflexed, so the term *length* is used rather than *height*.

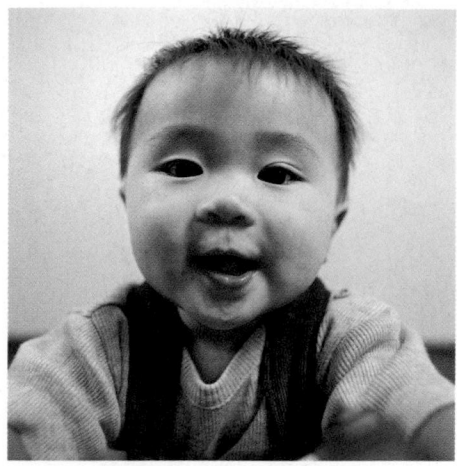

Brain growth is faster in infancy than in any other stage of life. Therefore an infant's head needs to be larger in comparison to the body in order to allow for such growth.

the diagnosis of obesity can also be established if the physical exam of the child indicates he or she is truly overfat. This is generally the case at this percentile.

Another Bite

The brain grows faster in infancy than at any other time of life. To accommodate the growth, an infant's head circumference must be very large in proportion to the rest of the body. The rapid growth stops at about 18 months of age. The rest of the body eventually grows to reach a typical proportion to head size. In early physical checkups, a health professional usually measures the head circumference as another means of assessing growth, especially brain growth. How nutritional status affects brain development and intelligence quotient (IQ) is difficult to measure because scientists have not determined how to separate the effects of nature from those of nurture. However, several studies have determined that breastfed babies have higher IQs than do babies who were fed with infant formula. At the same time, studies from Central America suggest that IQ after age 5 years relates more closely to the amount of schooling a child receives than to nutritional intake during childhood.

■ Adipose Tissue Growth

Since 1970, researchers have speculated that overfeeding during infancy may increase the numbers of adipose tissue cells. Today, we know that the number of adipose cells can also increase as adulthood obesity develops. Still, if calorie intake is limited during infancy to keep down the number of adipose cells, the growth of other organ systems may also be severely restricted. Special concern revolves around body growth and development, especially brain and nervous system development. In addition, most overweight infants become normal-weight preschoolers without excessive diet restrictions. For these reasons, it's unwise to greatly restrict diet, and especially fat intake in infants. After the first 12 months, fat intake can range from 30% to 40% of calorie intake for ages 1 to 3 years, and 25% to 35% for older children (and teenagers).

■ Failure to Thrive

Occasionally, an infant doesn't grow much in the first few months. Physical problems that may contribute to restricted growth range from poor oral cavity development, infections, and heart irregularities to constant diarrhea associated with intestinal problems. However, more than half the infants who fail to thrive have no apparent disease. Sometimes the cause is poor infant-parent interaction. This stems from misinformation, lack of a parent role model, or too little concern about the child's welfare. In general, the problems arise from the parents' inexperience, rather than intentional negligence. When health professionals encounter an infant who is failing to thrive, the true causes need to be identified and then treated.

Children older than 2 years are less likely to experience failure to thrive because they can often get food for themselves. Younger children, for the most part, are limited to what caregivers provide.

Concept Check

Growth occurs rapidly during infancy: Birth weight doubles in about 4 to 6 months and triples within the first year. Undernutrition in childhood can irreversibly inhibit growth and maturation, so that an individual never attains his or her full genetic potential for height. Infant and child growth is assessed by tracking body weight, length (height), and head circumference over time. Body mass index (BMI) is generally used to assess weight-for-height after 2 years of age. It is not desirable for infants to become overweight, although no evidence strongly indicates that overweight infants become overweight adults. However, severe calorie restriction is not recommended for infants because it may slow the growth of organ systems. When infants do not grow properly, their failure to thrive may stem from physical disorders or inadequate care, including inappropriate feeding practices.

■ Infant Nutritional Needs

Infants' nutritional needs vary as they grow, and these differ from adult needs in both amount and proportion. Initially, human milk or infant formula (generally using heat-treated cow's milk as a base) supplies needed nutrients. Solid foods are not needed until around 6 months. Even after solid foods are added, the basis of an infant's diet for the first year is still human milk or infant formula. Because of the critical importance of adequate nutrition in infancy and the difficulties encountered in feeding some infants, there is more discussion in this chapter on this developmental period than on the later periods of childhood.

Calories

Calorie needs (based on Estimated Energy Requirements) in infancy are **(89 kcal × weight of infant [kilogram]) + 75** from 0 to 3 months. From 4 to 6 months, such needs are **(89 kcal × weight of infant [kilogram]) + 44;** from 7 to 12 months it is **(89 kcal × weight of infant [kilogram]) − 78.** Based on body weight comparisons, at 6 months of age this amounts to about 700 kcal daily, and is two to four times more calories per kilogram of body weight than adults need. Infants need an easy way to get this amount of calories. Either human milk or infant formula is ideal for the first few months. Both are high in fat and supply about 640 kcal per quart of fluid (about 670 kcal per liter; Table 14-1). Later, human milk or infant formula, supplemented by solid foods, can provide even more calories and variety as well for the maturing infant.

The infant's high calorie needs are primarily driven by rapid growth and high metabolic rate. The high metabolic rate is caused in part by the ratio of the infant's body surface to its weight. More body surface allows more heat loss from the skin; the body must use extra calories to replace that heat.

Carbohydrate

Carbohydrate needs in infancy are 60 grams per day at 0 to 6 months, and 95 grams per day at 7 to 12 months. These needs are based on the typical intakes of human milk

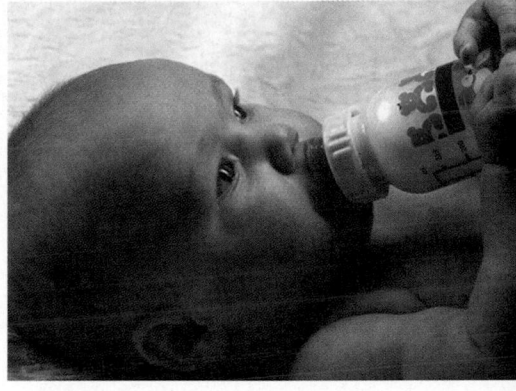

Infants who are formula-fed should remain on formula until 1 year of age.

Table 14-1 Composition of Human and Cow's Milk and Infant Formulas per liter. At 3 Months of Age Infants Typically Consume 0.75 to 1 liter of Human Milk or Formula per Day.

	Energy (kcal)	Protein (grams)	Fat (grams)	Carbohydrate (grams)	Minerals* (grams)
Milk					
Human milk	670**	11	45	70	2
Cow's milk, whole†	670	36	36	49	7
Cow's milk, fat-free†	360	36	1	51	7
Casein/Whey-Based Formulas					
Similac	680	14	36	71	3
Enfamil	670	15	37	69	3
Good Start	670	16	34	73	3
Soybean Protein-Based Formulas					
ProSobee	670	20	35	67	4
Isomil	680	16	36	68	4
Transition Formulas/Beverages‡					
Similac Toddler's Best	670	25	33	75	3
Enfamil Next Step	670	17	33	74	3
Carnation Follow-Up	670	17	27	88	3

*Calcium, phosphorus, and other minerals.

**Rough estimate; ranges from 650–700 kcal per liter.

†Not appropriate for infant feeding, based primarily on high protein and mineral content.

‡For use after 6 months of age or later (see label).

by breastfed infants and their eventual use of solid foods. Both carbohydrate goals are satisfied by usual intakes of infants on a proper diet.

Protein

Daily protein needs in infancy are about 9 grams per day for younger infants and about 14 grams per day for older infants. These needs also are based on the typical intakes of human milk by breastfed infants for 0 to 6 months, and then on the needs for growth for older infants. About half of total protein intake should come from essential (indispensable) amino acids. As with carbohydrate, protein needs are easily satisfied by either human milk or infant formula. Protein intake should not greatly exceed this standard. Excess nitrogen and minerals supplied by high-protein diets would exceed the ability of an infant's kidneys to excrete the waste products of protein metabolism, thus putting much stress on overall kidney function.

In North America, infant protein deficiency is unlikely, except in cases of mistakes in formula preparation, such as when an infant's formula is excessively diluted with water. Protein deficiency may also be induced by elimination diets used to detect food **allergies** (hypersensitivities). As foods are eliminated from the diet, infants may not be offered enough protein to compensate for the high-protein sources no longer present (see the Looking Further section later in this chapter).

Fat

Infants need about 30 grams of fat per day. Essential fatty acids should make up about 15% of total fat intake (about 5 grams per day). Both recommendations are again based on the typical intakes of human milk by breastfed infants, and the eventual intake from of solid foods. Fats are an important part of the infant's diet because they are vital to the development of the nervous system. As a concentrated source of calories, fat also helps resolve the potential problem of the infant's high calorie needs and small stomach capacity. Again, this is not an age to greatly restrict fat intake (Fig. 14-2).

Arachidonic acid (AA) and docosahexaenoic acid (DHA) are two long-chain fatty acids that have very important roles in infant development. The nervous system, especially the brain and eyes, depend on these fatty acids for proper development. During the last trimester, DHA and AA provided by the mother accumulate in the brain and retinas of the eyes in the fetus. Infants who are breastfed are able to continue to acquire these fatty acids from human milk, especially if their mothers are regularly eating fish. Until recently, no infant formulas sold in the United States included AA or DHA, but certain brands are now available with both AA and DHA. These are particularly useful for feeding preterm infants.

Vitamins of Special Interest

As noted in Chapter 8, vitamin K is routinely given by injection to all infants at birth. Formula-fed infants receive the rest of the vitamins they need from the formula. Breastfed infants should be given a vitamin D supplement (200 IU per day) until they are weaned to infant formula and are consuming at least 500 milliliters of it. Breastfed infants whose mothers are total vegetarians (vegans) should also receive vitamin B-12 in supplement form.

Minerals of Special Interest

Infants are born with some internal stores of iron. However, by the time birth weight doubles (4 to 6 months of age), iron stores are generally depleted if not otherwise part of the diet. If the mother was iron deficient during the pregnancy, these iron stores will be exhausted even sooner. As you will recall from Chapter 9, iron-deficiency anemia can lead to poor mental development in infants. To maintain a desirable iron status, the American Academy of Pediatrics recommends that formula-fed infants should be given an iron-fortified formula from birth. Low-iron infant formulas are sometimes prescribed to treat infants with various GI tract problems but their use is discouraged. In contrast, breastfed infants at about 6 months of age need solid foods to supply extra

allergy A hypersensitive immune response that occurs when immune bodies produced by us react with a protein we sense as foreign (an antigen).

Looking at Table 14-1 it is easy to see why fat-free milk products are not recommended for infants—these do not supply adequate fat and calories to meet needs. Fat-free (and reduced fat and whole milk as well) also would provide too much protein and minerals if it were used to meet calorie needs.

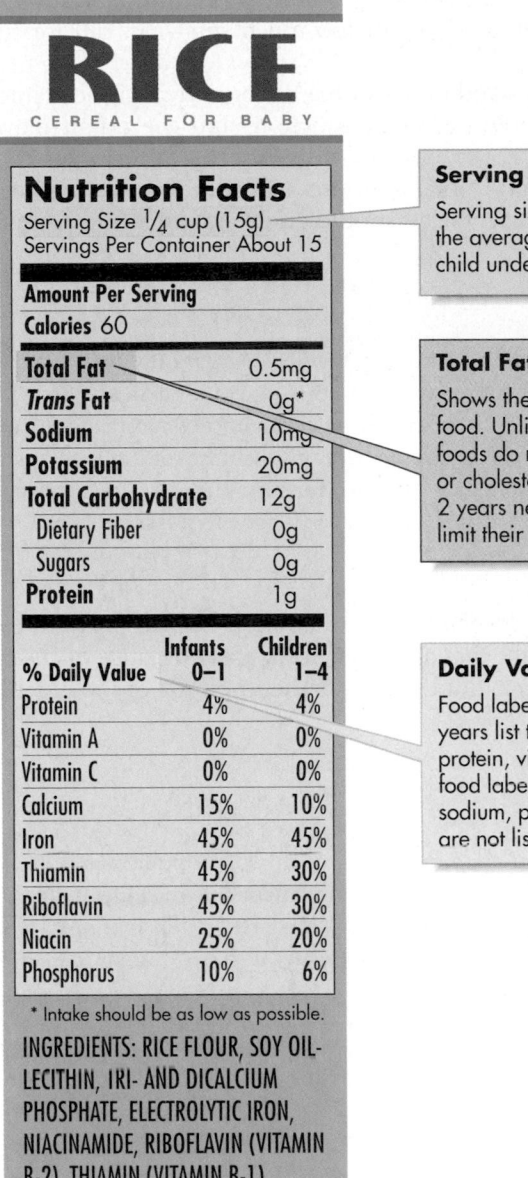

Nutrition Facts

Serving Size 1/4 cup (15g)
Servings Per Container About 15

Amount Per Serving	
Calories 60	
Total Fat	0.5mg
Trans Fat	0g*
Sodium	10mg
Potassium	20mg
Total Carbohydrate	12g
Dietary Fiber	0g
Sugars	0g
Protein	1g

% Daily Value	Infants 0–1	Children 1–4
Protein	4%	4%
Vitamin A	0%	0%
Vitamin C	0%	0%
Calcium	15%	10%
Iron	45%	45%
Thiamin	45%	30%
Riboflavin	45%	30%
Niacin	25%	20%
Phosphorus	10%	6%

* Intake should be as low as possible.

INGREDIENTS: RICE FLOUR, SOY OIL-LECITHIN, IRI- AND DICALCIUM PHOSPHATE, ELECTROLYTIC IRON, NIACINAMIDE, RIBOFLAVIN (VITAMIN B-2), THIAMIN (VITAMIN B-1).

Serving Size

Serving sizes for infant foods are based on the average amount eaten at one time by a child under 2 years.

Total Fat

Shows the amount of total fat in a serving of the food. Unlike adult food labels, labels on infant foods do not list calories from fat, saturated fat, or cholesterol, since infants and toddlers under 2 years need fat. Parents should not attempt to limit their infant's fat intake.

Daily Values

Food labels for infants and children under 4 years list the Daily Value percentages for protein, vitamins, and minerals. Unlike adult food labels, Daily Values for fat, cholesterol, sodium, potassium, carbohydrate, and fiber are not listed.

Figure 14-2 The labels on infant foods, like those on adult foods, contain a Nutrition Facts panel. However, the information provided on infant food labels differs from that on adult food labels, especially with respect to total fat, saturated fat, and cholesterol content (see Fig. 2-10 for a comparison). Note also that some cereal brands are fortified with various other micronutrients.

iron. In fact, this need for iron is a major consideration in the decision to introduce solid foods. Some physicians recommend liquid iron supplements from birth or by 1 month of age for breastfed infants, especially if the infant shows evidence of iron deficiency.

To aid in tooth development, fluoride supplements are recommended for breastfed infants after 6 months of age. The same holds true for formula-fed infants if the water supply used in home formula preparation—either tap or bottled water—does not contain fluoride. Note that formula manufacturers use fluoride-free water in formula preparation. Parents should consult their dentist for advice on meeting their infant's fluoride needs.

Infants also need adequate amounts of zinc and iodide to support growth. However, when human milk and infant formula are provided in quantities to meet calorie needs, sufficient zinc and iodide are generally supplied.

Water

An infant needs about 3 cups (700 to 800 milliliters) of water per day. Infants typically consume enough human milk or formula to supply this amount. In hot climates,

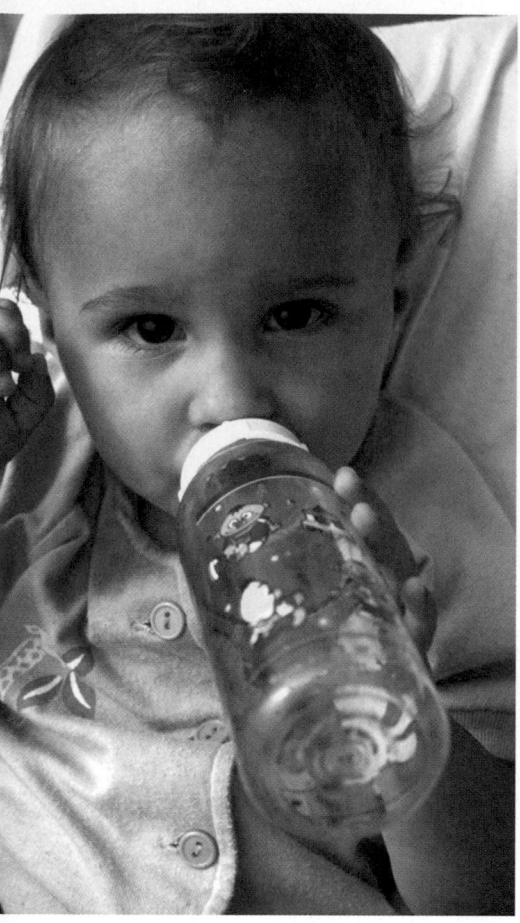

Supplemental fluids should be limited to 4 ounces per day unless the infant's physician prescribes a larger amount.

Parents should consult a physician when choosing an appropriate infant formula. Not all formula-like products are designed for infant use. A 5-month-old girl was admitted to a hospital in Arkansas with symptoms of heart failure, rickets, inflamed blood vessels, and possible nerve damage after being fed Soy Moo (a soy beverage sold in health stores) since 3 days of age. The symptoms suggest severe vitamin deficiencies.

however, supplemental water may be necessary. Furthermore, any conditions that lead to water loss—diarrhea, vomiting, fever, or too much sun—can call for supplemental water.

Infants are easily dehydrated, a condition that has serious effects if not remedied. Dehydration can result in rapid loss of kidney function, and the infant may then require hospitalization for rehydration. Special fluid-replacement formulas containing electrolytes such as sodium and potassium are available in supermarkets and pharmacies to treat dehydration. A physician should guide any use of these products.

Another Bite

Note that, in some stores, bottled water products marketed specifically for infants may be placed alongside infant formulas and electrolyte-replacement solutions. This placement may give parents and caregivers the mistaken impression that bottled water products are an appropriate feeding supplement or substitute for fluid replacement for infants; they are not and should not be used for such purposes. It is important to remember that excessive fluid can also be harmful, especially to the brain.

Overall, it is best to limit supplemental fluids to about 4 ounces (120 milliliters) per day, unless the physician thinks that a greater need exists because of disease or other conditions. In sum, extremes in fluid intake—either too little or too much—can lead to health problems.

Concept Check

Most nutrient needs in the first 6 months are met by human milk or infant formula. Breastfed infants need a vitamin D supplement and possibly an iron supplement; formula-fed infants and breastfed infants may need fluoride supplements after 6 months of age. Infants usually receive enough water from the human milk or infant formula they drink.

■ Formula Feeding for Infants

Breastfeeding was covered in detail in Chapter 13. Let's now focus on formula feeding. You'll recall that a major advantage of breastfeeding is the provision of immune protection to the infant. Overall, in areas of the world where high standards for water purity and cleanliness are common, formula feeding is a safe alternative for infants (but generally is not as beneficial as breastfeeding).

Formula Composition

Infants cannot tolerate cow's milk as such because of its high protein and mineral content. Cow's milk is perfect for the greater growth needs of calves, but not for human infants. Thus, cow's milk must be altered by formula manufacturers to be safe for infant feeding. Altered forms of cow's milk, known as infant formulas, must conform to strict federal guidelines for nutrient composition and quality. Formulas generally contain lactose and/or sucrose for carbohydrate, heat-treated proteins from cow's milk, and vegetable oils for fat (review Table 14-1). Soy protein–based formulas are available for infants who can't tolerate lactose or the types of proteins found in cow's milk. If the soybean-based formula is not tolerated, the next step is to try a predigested formula in which the proteins have been broken down into small polypeptides and amino acids. A variety of other specialized formulas also are available for specific medical conditions. In any case, it is important to use an iron-fortified formula unless a physician recommends otherwise.

Some transition formulas/beverages have been introduced for older infants and toddlers (review Table 14-1). Some of these products are intended for use after 6 months of age if the infant is consuming solid foods, whereas others are intended for use only by toddlers. These transition products are lower in fat than human milk or standard infant formulas; their iron content is higher than that of cow's milk, and their overall mineral content is generally more like that of human milk than cow's milk. According to the manufacturers, the advantages of these transition formulas/beverages over standard formulas for older infants and toddlers include reduced cost and better flavor. Parents should consult their physician with regard to the use of these products.

Formula Preparation

Some infant formulas come in ready-to-feed form. These are poured into a clean bottle and fed immediately. Room-temperature formula is acceptable for many infants. Otherwise, to warm a bottle of formula, a caregiver can run hot water over it or place it briefly in a pan of simmering water. Note that infant formulas should not be heated in a microwave oven because hot spots may develop, which can burn the infant's mouth and esophagus.

Powdered and concentrated fluid formula preparations are also commonly used. All utensils used in preparing formula from these preparations should be washed and thoroughly rinsed. Powdered or concentrated formulas are poured into a bottle, to which clean, cold water is added (following label directions) and then mixed. The formula is then warmed, if desired, and fed immediately to the infant. Hot water from the faucet should not be used to make formula, since it poses a risk for high lead content (see Chapter 16). Cold water poses much less risk.

Refrigerating prepared formula for 1 day is safe. However, formula left over from a feeding should be discarded because it will be contaminated by bacteria and enzymes from the infant's saliva. If well water is used, it should be boiled before making formula for at least the infant's first 3 months of life, and it should be analyzed for excessive concentration of naturally occurring nitrates, which can lead to a severe form of anemia. Note that, if nitrates are high in municipal water systems, consumers will be warned (such as in a local newspaper) not to use the water for making infant formula until the concentration falls to a safe amount. Alternatively, if water contaminants are of concern, formula can be mixed with bottled nursery water, which is available alongside infant formula in most supermarkets.

Feeding Technique

Because infants swallow a lot of air as they ingest either formula or human milk, it's important to burp an infant after either 10 minutes of feeding or 1 to 2 ounces (30 to 60 milliliters) has been consumed from a bottle and again at the end of feeding. Spitting up a bit of milk is normal at this time.

When the infant begins acting full, bottle feeding should be stopped, even if some milk is left in the bottle. Common cues that signal that an infant has had enough include turning the head away, being inattentive, falling asleep, and becoming playful. Generally, the infant's appetite is a better guide than standardized recommendations concerning feeding amounts. Breastfeeding infants usually have had enough to eat after about 20 minutes. Although it's difficult to tell how much milk breastfed infants are getting, they also give signs when full. By carefully observing bottle-feeding or breastfeeding infants and responding to their cues appropriately, caregivers not only can be assured that the infants' calorie needs are being met but also can foster a climate of trust and responsiveness.

Once fed, an infant should not be placed on its stomach. Placing the infant on its back is recommended by the American Academy of Pediatrics. The reason that an infant should not be placed on its stomach is because this sleeping position has been linked to sudden infant death syndrome (SIDS). The Back to Sleep campaign, started in 1994 in the United States, has reduced SIDS by 40%.

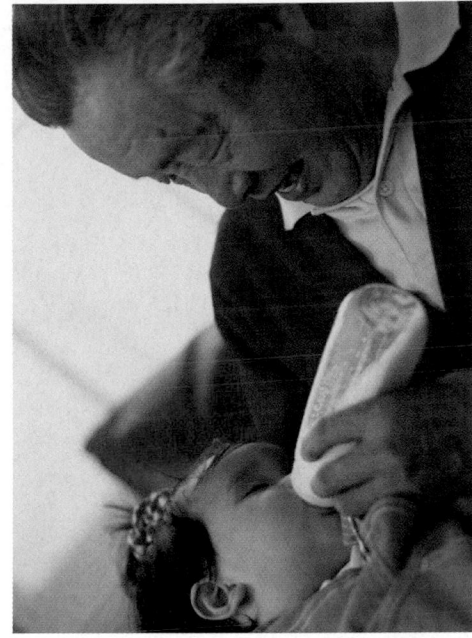

Careful attention during feeding allows the caregiver to notice the infant's signal as to when the feeding should cease.

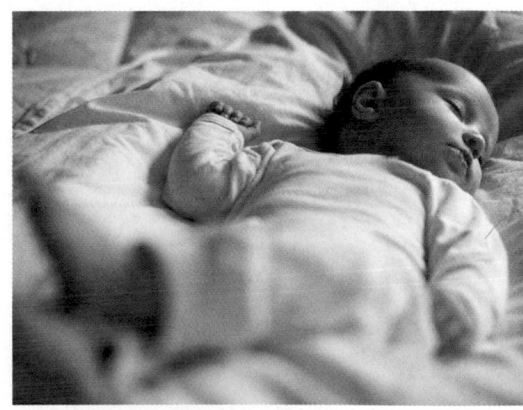

The Back to Sleep campaign advises that infants be placed on their backs for sleeping.

Table 14-2 Sample Daily Menu for a 1-Year-Old Child*

Breakfast	Snack
1 to 2 tbsp applesauce	½ ounce cheddar cheese
¼ cup Cheerios	4 wheat crackers
½ cup whole milk	½ cup whole milk
Snack	**Dinner**
½ hard-cooked egg	1 ounce hamburger (crumbled)
½ slice wheat toast with ½ tsp margarine	1 to 2 tbsp mashed potatoes with ½ tsp margarine
½ cup orange juice	1 to 2 tbsp cooked carrots (cut in strips, not coins)
	½ cup whole milk
Lunch	**Snack**
1 ounce roasted chicken, minced	½ banana
1 to 2 tbsp rice with ½ tsp margarine	2 oatmeal cookies (no raisins)
1 to 2 tbsp cooked peas	½ cup whole milk
½ cup whole milk	

Nutritional Analysis	
Total energy (kcal)	1100
% energy from	
Carbohydrate	40%
Protein	19%
Fat	41%

*This diet is just a start. A 1-year-old may need more or less food. In those cases, serving sizes should be adjusted. The milk can be fed by cup; some can be put into a bottle if the child has not been fully weaned from the bottle. The juice should be fed in a cup.

The Back to Sleep campaign, however, has led to a problem known as flattened head syndrome (clinically known as positional plagiocephaly). Infant skulls are soft and therefore can change in shape. Flattened head syndrome can occur if an excessive amount of an infant's day is spent on his or her back, or against a highchair/car seat. In response to this concern the American Academy of Pediatrics has recommended periodic repositioning of an infant's head while asleep and allowing for time on his or her stomach while awake. In addition, some infants may need to wear specially fitted helmets to correct the shape of their head.

▪ Expanding the Infant's Mealtime Choices

By about 6 months of age, the infant is ready to start eating "table food." Initially, table foods add to—rather than replace—formula or human milk. In the first attempts to introduce solid foods, just getting the food into the infant's mouth may prove to be a challenge. By the end of the first year, though, the infant should be eating a variety of meats, vegetables, fruits, and grains so that the diet begins to resemble a balanced pattern (Table 14-2). Throughout the process of expanding the infant's mealtime choices, it is essential to allow the infant to control the situation—the caregiver must proceed slowly and respond to the infant's cues that he or she is hungry or has had enough to eat.

Recognizing the Infant's Readiness for Solid Foods

How does the caregiver know it is time to introduce solid foods? Infant size can serve as a rough indicator of readiness—reaching a weight of at least 13 pounds (6 kilograms) is a preliminary sign of readiness for solid foods. Another physiological cue is frequency of feeding, such as consuming more than 32 ounces (1 liter) of formula daily or breastfeeding more than 8 to 10 times within 24 hours. Underlying these noticeable signals are several important developmental factors:

1. *Nutritional need.* Before the infant is 6 months old, nutritional needs can generally be met with human milk and/or formula. After 6 months of age, however, many infants need the additional calories supplied by solid foods. In terms of individual

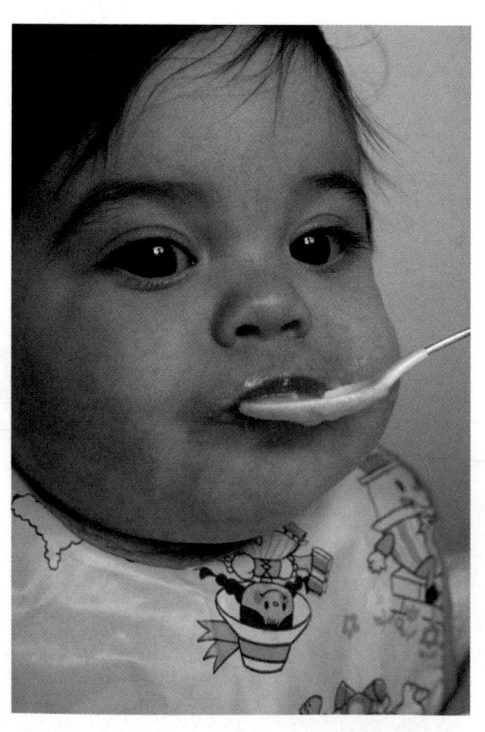

In the early stages of solid food introduction, these foods complement rather than replace human milk or infant formula in the diet.

nutrients, iron stores are exhausted by about 6 months of age. Either solid foods or iron supplements are then needed to supply iron if the child is breastfed or fed a low-iron or iron-free formula. (As previously mentioned, a vitamin D supplement should also be given to breastfed infants.)

2. *Physiological capabilities*. As the infant ages, the ability to digest and metabolize a wider range of food components improves. Before about 3 months of age, an infant's digestive tract cannot readily digest starch. Also, kidney function is quite limited until about 4 to 6 weeks of age. Until then, waste products from excessive amounts of dietary protein or minerals are difficult to excrete.

3. *Physical ability*. Three physical markers indicate that a child is ready for solid foods: (1) the disappearance of the extrusion reflex (thrusting the tongue forward and pushing food out of the mouth), (2) head and neck control, and (3) the ability to sit up with support. These usually occur around 4 to 6 months of age, but they vary with each infant.

4. *Allergy prevention*. An infant's intestinal tract is "leaky"—whole proteins can readily be absorbed from birth until 4 to 5 months of age. If the infant is exposed too early to some kinds of proteins—particularly those in cow's milk and egg whites—the infant may be predisposed to future allergies and other health problems, such as diabetes. For this reason, it is best to minimize the number of different types of proteins in an infant's diet, especially during the first 3 months (see the Looking Further section on food allergies in this chapter for details).

With these considerations in mind—nutritional need, physiological and physical readiness, and allergy prevention—the American Academy of Pediatrics recommends that solid foods not be introduced until about 6 months of age and that infants receive no unaltered cow's milk before 1 year.

Another Bite

Parents may believe that the early addition of solid foods will help an infant sleep through the night. Actually, this achievement is a developmental milestone, and the amount of food consumed by the infant is of little relevance to the achievement of a good night's sleep. Before 4 to 6 months of age, infants are not physically mature enough to consume much solid food. Only occasionally does a rapidly growing infant need solid foods to meet calorie and nutrient needs before 6 months of age.

Foods to Match Needs and Developmental Abilities During the First Year

If solid foods are introduced before 6 months of age, the primary goal of the food should be to meet iron needs. Therefore, the first solid foods should be iron-fortified cereals. Some pediatricians may recommend lean ground (strained) meats for more absorbable forms of iron. Rice is the best cereal to begin with because it is least likely to cause allergies.

When starting solid foods it is important to start with a teaspoon serving size of a single-ingredient food item, such as rice cereal, and increase the serving size gradually. Once the new food has been fed for about a week without ill effects, another food can be added to the infant's diet. At first, this can be another type of cereal or perhaps a cooked and strained (or mashed) vegetable, meat, fruit, or egg yolk.

Waiting about 7 days between the introduction of each new food is important because it can take that long for evidence of an allergy or intolerance to develop. Allergy symptoms to look for include diarrhea, vomiting, a rash, or wheezing. If one or more of these symptoms appear, the suspected problem food should be avoided for several weeks and then reintroduced in a small quantity. If the problem continues, a physician should be consulted.

Typical Solid Food Progression, Starting at 6 Months*

Week 1	Rice cereal
Week 2	Add strained carrots
Week 3	Add applesauce
Week 4	Add oat cereal
Week 5	Add cooked egg yolk
Week 6	Add strained chicken
Week 7	Add strained peas
Week 8	Add plums

*Extending the rice cereal step for a month or so is advised if solid food introduction begins at 4 months of age. Note also that, if at any point signs of allergy or intolerance develop, substitute another similar food item.

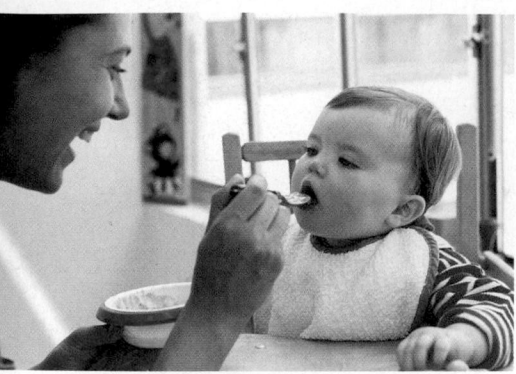

Rice cereal is recommended as the first solid food to be fed to infants.

early childhood caries Tooth decay that results from formula or juice (and even human milk) bathing the teeth as the child sleeps with a bottle in his or her mouth. The upper teeth are mostly affected as the lower teeth are protected by the tongue; formerly called *nursing bottle syndrome* and *baby bottle tooth decay*.

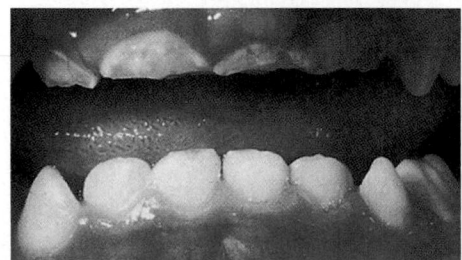

Figure 14-3 Early childhood caries. An extreme example of tooth decay probably resulting from frequently putting the child to bed with a bottle. The upper teeth have decayed almost all the way to the gum line.

Some foods that commonly cause an allergic response in infants are egg whites, chocolate, nuts, and cow's milk. It is best not to introduce these foods during infancy. Also, it is important to avoid introducing mixed foods until each component of the combination dish has been given separately. Otherwise, if an allergy or intolerance develops, it will be difficult to identify the offending food. Note that many babies outgrow food allergies during childhood.

Many strained foods for infant feeding are available at the supermarket. Single food items are more desirable than mixed dinners and desserts, which are less nutrient-dense. Most brands have no added salt, but some fruit desserts contain a lot of added sugar.

As an alternative, plain, unseasoned cooked foods—vegetables, fruits, and meats—can be ground up in an inexpensive plastic baby food grinder/mill. Another option is to puree a larger amount of food in a blender, freeze it in ice-cube portions, store in plastic bags, and defrost and warm as needed. Careful attention to cleanliness is necessary. Seasonings that may please the rest of the family should not be added to infant foods made at home. The infant doesn't notice the difference if salt, sugar, or spices are omitted. It is best to introduce infants to a variety of foods, so that at the end of the first year, the infant is consuming many foods—milk, meats, fruits, vegetables, and grains.

Self-feeding skills require coordination and can develop only if the infant is allowed to practice and experiment. By 6 to 7 months of age, the infant has learned to handle finger foods and transfer objects from one hand to the other with some dexterity. At about this time, teeth also begin to appear. Dry toast, sliced in strips, offers hours of enjoyment. By age 7 to 8 months, infants can push food around on a plate, play with a drinking cup, hold a bottle, and self-feed a cracker or a piece of toast. Through mastery of these manipulations, infants develop confidence and self-esteem. It is important that parents be patient and support these early feeding attempts, even though they appear inefficient.

At 9 to 10 months of age, the infant's desire to explore, experience, and play with foods may actually hinder feeding. Food is used as a means to explore the environment, and therefore feeding time is often very messy—a bowl of macaroni may end up in the child's hair. Presenting a new food on several consecutive days can aid in an infant's acceptance of that food. Caregivers need to relax and take this phase of infant development in stride. Sloppy, friendly mealtimes actually make for good memories. By the end of the first year, finger-feeding becomes more efficient and chewing is easier as more teeth erupt. Still, experimentation and unpredictability are to be expected.

To ease the efforts in feeding solid foods, consider the following tips:

- Use a baby-sized spoon; a small spoon with a long handle is best.
- Hold the infant comfortably on the lap, as for breastfeeding or bottle feeding, but a little more upright to ease swallowing. When in this position, the infant expects food.
- Put a small dab of food on the spoon tip and gently place it on the infant's tongue.
- Convey a calm and casual approach to the infant, who needs time to get used to food.
- Expect the infant to take only two or three bites of the first meals.

■ Weaning from the Breast or Bottle

Around the age of 6 months, juices can be offered in a sippy cup with a wide, flat bottom. Drinking from a cup rather than from a bottle helps prevent **early childhood caries** (Fig. 14-3). If an infant drinks continuously from a bottle, the carbohydrate-rich fluid bathes the teeth, providing an ideal growth medium for bacteria adhering to the teeth. These bacteria then make acids, which dissolve tooth enamel. To avoid dental caries, infants should not be put to bed with a bottle or placed in an infant seat with a bottle propped up.

By about 10 months of age, infants are learning to self-feed and likewise to drink independently from a cup. As children drink from a cup more frequently, fewer bottle feedings and/or breastfeedings are necessary. The added mobility of crawling and walking should naturally lead to gradual weaning from the bottle or breast. Even so, getting a baby out of the bedtime-bottle habit can be difficult. Determined caregivers can either wince through a few nights of their baby's crying or slowly wean the baby away from the bottle with either a pacifier or water (for a week or so).

■ Dietary Guidelines for Infant Feeding

In response to various controversies surrounding infant feeding, the American Academy of Pediatrics has issued a number of statements concerning infant diets. The following guidelines are based on these statements:

- *Build to a variety of foods.* For the first months of life, human milk (or infant formula) is all an infant needs. (Vitamin D needs of breastfed infants is an exception.) When the infant is ready, start adding new foods, one at a time. During the first year, the goal is to teach an infant to enjoy a variety of nutritious foods. A lifetime of healthy eating habits begins with this important first step.
- *Pay attention to your infant's appetite to avoid overfeeding or underfeeding.* Feed infants when they are hungry. Never force an infant to finish an unwanted serving of food. Watch for signs that indicate hunger or fullness.
- *Infants need fat.* Although fat is the cause of many adult health problems, it's an essential source of calories for growing infants. Fat also helps the nervous system develop.
- *Choose fruits, vegetables, and grains, but don't overdo high-fiber foods.* Although many adults benefit from high-fiber diets, they are not good for infants. They are bulky, filling, and often low in calories. The natural amounts of fiber and nutrients in fruits, vegetables, and grains are appropriate as part of a healthy infant diet.
- *Infants need sugars in moderation.* Sugars are an additional source of calories for active, rapidly growing infants. Foods such as human milk, fruits, and juices are natural sources of sugars and other nutrients as well. Foods that contain artificial sweeteners should be avoided; they don't provide the calories growing infants need.
- *Infants need sodium in moderation.* Sodium is a necessary mineral found naturally in almost all foods. As part of a healthy diet, infants need sodium for their bodies to work properly.
- *Choose foods containing iron, zinc, and calcium.* Infants need good sources of iron, zinc, and calcium for optimum growth in the first 2 years. These minerals are important for healthy blood, proper growth, and strong bones.

In essence, there is no evidence that very restrictive diets during infancy have positive effects, whereas their hazards are well documented.

What Not to Feed an Infant

Following are several foods and practices to avoid when feeding an infant:

- *Honey.* This product may contain spores of *Clostridium botulinum*. The spores can eventually develop into bacteria in the stomach and lead to a foodborne illness known as *botulism*. This can be fatal, especially in children under 1 year old (see Chapter 16).
- *Excessive infant formula or human milk.* After 6 to 8 months, solid foods should play a greater role in satisfying an infant's increasing appetite. The main reason to switch is that solid foods contain considerably more bioavailable iron than do human milk and low-iron formulas. About 24 to 32 ounces (¾ to 1 liters) of human milk or formula daily is ideal after 6 months, with food supplying the rest of the infant's calorie needs.
- *Foods that tend to cause choking.* These foods include hot dogs (unless finely cut into sticks, not coin shapes), candy, whole nuts, grapes, coarsely cut meats, raw carrots, popcorn, and peanut butter. Caregivers should not allow younger children to gobble snack foods during playtime and should supervise all meals.
- *Cow's milk, especially low-fat or fat-free cow's milk.* The American Academy of Pediatrics strongly urges parents not to give children under age 2 fat-reduced, 1%, or fat-free milk. Before age 2, the amount of this milk needed for calorie needs

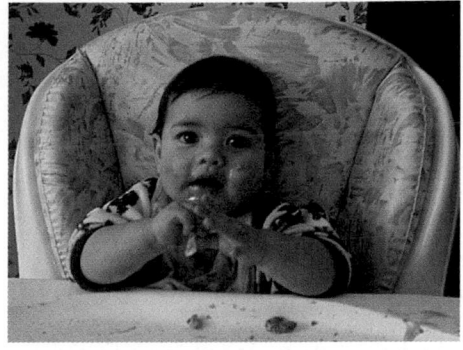

Early feeding attempts should be encouraged, even though they can be messy.

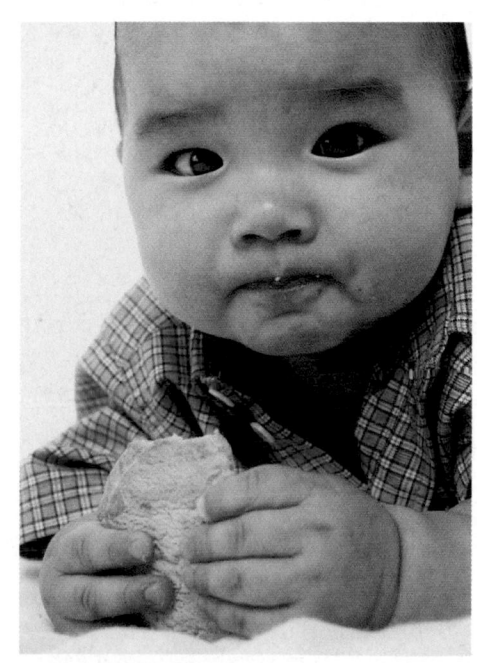

The older infant enjoys finger-feeding.

gg whites also should not be fed to children before 1 year of age to help prevent the development of allergies.

A Summary of Infant Feeding Recommendations

Breastfed Infants

- Breastfeed for 6 months or longer, if possible. Then introduce infant formula if and when breastfeeding declines or ceases. (Breast milk can also be pumped and placed in a bottle for later use.)
- Provide a vitamin D supplement (200 IU per day).
- Investigate the need for vitamin B-12, fluoride, and iron supplementation to prevent deficiencies.

Formula-Fed Infants

- Use infant formula for the first year of life, preferably an iron-fortified type.
- Investigate the need for a fluoride supplement if the water supply is not fluoridated.

All Infants

- Add iron-fortified cereal at about 6 months of age.
- Provide a variety of basic, soft foods after 6 months of age, advancing to a varied diet.

Critical Thinking

Tatiana has been breastfeeding her baby exclusively since he was born 7 months ago. When she and her husband took the baby for his checkup, they were told that he was anemic. They were very surprised, since they thought that human milk contained all the nutrients the baby needed for the first year of life. How might you explain the baby's anemia?

would supply too many minerals and in turn could overwhelm the kidneys' ability to excrete the excess. The lower fat intake might also harm nervous system development. Beyond 2 years, children can drink fat-reduced, 1%, or fat-free milk, because by this age they are consuming enough solid foods to supply calorie and fat needs.

- *Feeding excessive amounts of apple or pear juice.* The fructose and sorbitol contained in these juices can lead to diarrhea because they are slowly absorbed. Also, if fruit juice or related drink products are replacing formula or milk in the diet, the infant may not be receiving adequate amounts of calcium and other minerals that are essential for bone growth. In fact, studies have shown a link between excessive amounts of fruit juice and failure to thrive, GI tract complications, obesity, short stature, and poor dental health. Thus, these substances should be used sparingly. Infants over the age of 6 months can usually safely consume up to 6 ounces of juice in the course of a day, with no more than 2 to 4 ounces at a time.

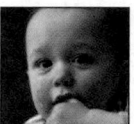

Real Life Scenario Follow-Up

Damon's diet is inadequate for a 10-month-old infant because it lacks enough of the nutritious foods his growing body needs to support weight gain. These foods include iron-fortified cereal, puréed infant foods, and appropriate table foods. Damon should continue to consume the infant formula until 1 year of age. Sugary drinks should be avoided except for small amounts of fruit juices served in a cup. Sugary drinks especially should not be fed by bottle. Damon needs a diet containing a healthful variety of solid foods to provide him with enough calories and essential nutrients to grow and develop.

∎ Inappropriate Infant Feeding Practices

Parents and other caregivers should be aware of a variety of potential health problems related to infant nutrition, so that corrective action can be taken quickly. In some cases, such problems stem from inappropriate feeding practices and inadequate nutrient intakes, including the following:

- Diet providing insufficient iron
- Absence from the diet of an entire food group in MyPyramid as solid foods are introduced and become the main source of nutrients
- Use of cow's milk
- Introduction of potential allergy-causing foods, such as egg whites and nuts
- Drinking raw (unpasteurized) milk, which may be contaminated with bacteria or viruses
- Drinking goat's milk, which is low in folate, iron, vitamin C, and vitamin D
- Failure to begin drinking from a cup by 1 year of age
- Continuing to feed from a bottle past 18 months of age
- Intake of supplemental vitamins or minerals above 100% of the appropriate RDA or other nutrient standard
- Drinking large amounts of fruit juice after 6 months of age, especially as a substitute for infant formula or human milk. (Recall that fruit juice is not to be fed at all before 6 months of age.)

The website of the American Academy of Pediatrics (www.aap.org) can also provide useful information on these and other nutrition-related problems in infancy.

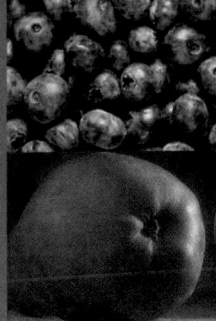

Adverse reactions to foods—indicated by sneezing, coughing, nausea, vomiting, diarrhea, hives, and other rashes—are broadly classed as food allergies (also called *hypersensitivities*) or **food intolerances.** Allergies involve responses of the immune system designed to eliminate foreign proteins, called **allergens.** The symptoms experienced by susceptible people, such as rapid increase in heart rate and shortness of breath, are the result of this battle. In contrast, the symptoms of food intolerances do not result from a true allergic reaction. Rather, food intolerances are caused by an individual's inability to digest certain food components or by the direct effect of a food component or contaminant on the body. Let's examine each process, first allergies and then intolerances.

Food Allergies: Symptoms and Mechanism

Allergic reactions to foods are common and occur more frequently in females than males. Food allergies occur most often during infancy and young adulthood. Experts estimate that up to about 2% of adults and up to about 8% of children are allergic to certain foods. Three types of reactions may occur after the ingestion of problem foods by susceptible people:

- *Classic*—itching, reddening skin, asthma, swelling, choking, and a runny nose
- *GI tract*—nausea, vomiting, diarrhea, intestinal gas, bloating, pain, constipation, and indigestion
- *General*—headache, skin reactions, tension and fatigue, tremors, and psychological problems

Any reaction that is milder than these distinct allergic ones is referred to as a **food sensitivity.**

Allergic reactions vary not only in the body system affected but also in their duration, ranging from seconds to a few days. A generalized, all-systems reaction is called **anaphylactic shock.** This severe allergic response results in low blood pressure and distress of the respiratory system and GI tract. It can be fatal. Overall, allergic reactions result in 30,000 emergency room visits and 150 to 200 deaths per year. A person who is extremely sensitive to a food may not be able to touch the food or even be in the same room where it is being cooked without reacting to it. Although any food can trigger anaphylactic shock, the most common culprits are peanuts (actually a legume, not a nut), tree nuts (walnuts, pecans, etc.), shellfish, milk (look for the protein casein on the label), eggs (look for the protein albumin on the label), soybeans, wheat, and fish. Other foods frequently identified with adverse reactions include meat and meat products, fruits, and cheese. For a small number of people, avoiding foods such as peanuts or shellfish is a matter of life and death. Almost all food allergies are caused by proteins in these foods that act as **antigens.**

Testing for a Food Allergy

The diagnosis of a food allergy can often be a difficult task (Table 14-3). It requires the participation of a skilled physician. The first step in determining whether a food allergy is present is to record in detail a history of symptoms, including the time from ingestion to onset of symptoms, duration of symptoms, most recent reaction, food suspected of causing a reaction, and quantity and nature of food needed to produce a reaction. A family history of allergic diseases can also help, as allergic reactions tend to run in families. A physical examination may reveal evidence of an allergy, such as skin diseases and asthma. Various diagnostic tests can rule out other conditions.

The diagnostic first step is to eliminate from the diet—for 1 to 2 weeks—all tested compounds that appear to cause allergic symptoms, plus all other foods suspected of causing an

food intolerance An adverse reaction to food that does not involves an allergic reaction.

allergen A foreign protein, or antigen, that induces excess production of certain immune system antibodies; subsequent exposure to the same protein leads to allergic symptoms. Whereas all allergens are antigens, not all antigens are allergens.

food sensitivity A mild reaction to a substance in a food that might be expressed as slight itching or redness of the skin.

anaphylactic shock A severe allergic response that results in lowered blood pressure and respiratory and gastrointestinal distress. This can be fatal.

People with a history of serious allergic reactions should carry a self-administered form of epinephrine, such as EpiPen, to subside an episode of anaphylactic shock, should it occur.

antigen Any substance that induces a state of sensitivity and/or resistance to microorganisms or toxic substances after a lag period; substance that stimulates a specific aspect of the immune system.

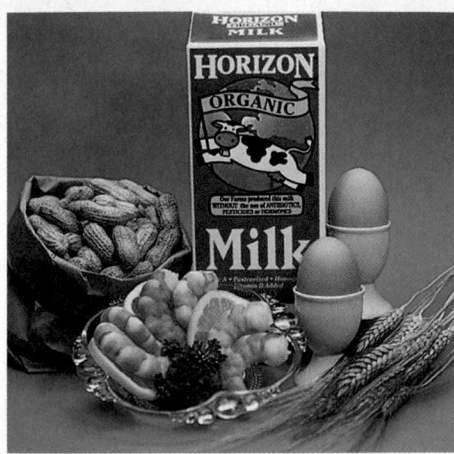

Eggs, wheat, milk, peanuts, tree nuts, soybeans, and seafood pose the greatest risk for food allergies in childhood.

Table 14-3 Assessment Strategies for Food Allergies

History	Include description of symptoms, time between food ingestion and onset of symptoms, duration of symptoms, most recent allergic episode, quantity of food required to produce reaction, suspected foods, and allergic diseases in other family members.
Physical examination	Look for signs of an allergic reaction (rash, itching, intestinal bloating, etc.).
Elimination diet	Establish a diet lacking the suspected offending foods and stay on it for 1 to 2 weeks or until symptoms clear.
Food challenge	Add back small amounts of excluded foods, one at a time, as long as anaphylactic shock is not a possible consequence.
Skin test	Place a sample of the suspected allergen under the skin and watch for an inflammatory reaction.
RAST test	Determine presence of antibodies in blood that bind to food antigens tested.

elimination diet A restrictive diet that systematically tests foods that may cause an allergic response by first eliminating them for 1 to 2 weeks and then adding them back, one at a time.

allergy based on the person's food history. The person generally starts out eating foods to which almost no one reacts, such as rice, vegetables, noncitrus fruits, and fresh meats and poultry. If symptoms are still present, the person can more severely restrict the diet or even use special formula diets that are hypoallergenic.

Once a diet is found that causes no symptoms, called an **elimination diet,** foods can be added back one at a time. This type of food challenge is an option only when the culprit foods are known to pose no risk of anaphylactic shock in the person. Doses of ½ to 1 teaspoon (2.5 to 5 milliliters) are given at first. The amount is increased until the dose approximates usual intake. Any reintroduced food that causes significant symptoms to appear is identified as an allergen for the person.

The best laboratory test for determining which compounds a person is allergic to is the RAST test. This test estimates the blood concentration of antibodies that bind certain foodborne antigens. Skin tests can also be used; a drop of a suspected antigen is placed under the skin where it has been scratched or punctured. If a person is allergic to the test antigen, a red eruption will develop.

■ Treating Food Allergies

Once potential allergens are identified, the best treatment is to avoid them, especially for people with zero tolerance. Careful reading of food labels is especially essential for many allergic people. A major challenge when treating a person with a food allergy is to make sure that what remains in the diet can still provide essential nutrients. The small food intake of children permits less leeway in removing offending foods that may contain numerous nutrients. A registered dietitian can help guide the diet-planning process to ensure that the remaining food choices still meet nutrient needs or to guide supplement use, if that is necessary.

If an allergy-prone woman is pregnant or breastfeeding, she should avoid offending foods—such as eggs, shellfish, and peanuts—because allergens can cross the placenta during pregnancy. Allergens are also secreted via her milk. She should work with her physician and registered dietitian to make sure she still consumes an adequate diet. In addition, when food allergies are common in the family, women are advised to breastfeed their infants exclusively for 6 months. Human milk contains factors that play a role in the maturation of the small intestine. Formula-fed infants, especially those on cow's milk–based formulas, have a greater risk for developing food allergies. Breastfeeding, thus, should continue for as long as possible, preferably to 1 year.

About 80% of young children with food allergies outgrow them before 3 years. Parents should be made aware of this and not assume the allergy will be long-lived. Food allergies diagnosed after 3 years of age are often more long-lived, but not always. In these cases, about 33% of people outgrow their food allergies within 3 years. For others, the condition may be prolonged; some food allergies can last a lifetime, such as those for peanuts, tree nuts, and shellfish. Periodic reintroduction of offending foods can be tried every 6 to 12 months or so to see whether the allergic reaction has decreased. If no symptoms appear, tolerance to the food has developed.

Food Intolerances

Food intolerances are adverse reactions to foods that do not involve allergic mechanisms. Generally, larger amounts of an offending food are required to produce the symptoms of an intolerance than to trigger allergic symptoms. Common causes of food intolerances include:

- Constituents of certain foods (e.g., red wine, tomatoes, pineapples) that have a druglike activity, causing physiological effects such as changes in blood pressure
- Certain synthetic compounds added to foods, such as sulfites, food-coloring agents, and monosodium glutamate (MSG)
- Food contaminants, including antibiotics and other chemicals used in the production of livestock and crops, as well as insect parts not removed during processing
- Toxic contaminants, which may be ingested with improperly handled and prepared foods containing *Clostridium botulinum*, *Salmonella* bacteria, or other foodborne microorganisms (see Chapter 16)
- Deficiencies in digestive enzymes, such as lactase (review Chapter 4)

Almost everyone is sensitive to one or more of these causes of food intolerance, many of which produce GI tract symptoms.

Sulfites, which are added to foods and beverages as antioxidants, cause flushing, spasms of the airway, and a loss of blood pressure in susceptible people. Wine, dehydrated potatoes, dried fruits, gravy, soup mixes, and restaurant salad greens commonly contain sulfites. A reaction to MSG may include an increase in blood pressure, numbness, sweating, vomiting, headache, and facial pressure. MSG is commonly found in Chinese food and many processed foods (e.g., soups). A reaction to tartrazine, a food-coloring additive, includes spasm of the airway, itching, and reddening skin. Tyramine, a derivative of the amino acid tyrosine, is commonly found in "aged" foods, such as cheeses and red wines. This natural food constituent can cause high blood pressure in people taking monoamine oxidase (MAO) inhibitor medications, which may be prescribed for clinical depression.

The basic treatment for food intolerances is to avoid specific offending components. However, total elimination often is not required because people generally are not as sensitive to compounds causing food intolerances as they are to allergens.

The American Academy of Allergy and Immunology has a 24-hour toll-free hot line (800-822-2762) to answer questions about food allergies and to help direct people to specialists who treat the problem. Free information on food allergies is available by contacting The Food Allergy & Anaphylaxis Network. The telephone number is (703-691-3179); the website is www.foodallergy.org.

Concept Check

Infant formulas generally contain lactose or sucrose, heat-treated proteins from cow's milk, and vegetable oil. Formulas may or may not be fortified with iron. Sanitation is very important in preparing and storing formula. Solid foods should not be added to an infant's diet until the child is both ready for and needs solid food, usually at about 6 months of age. The first solid food can be iron-fortified infant cereals, with very gradual additions of other foods—one at a time each week. Some foods to avoid giving to infants in the first year are honey, cow's milk (particularly fat-reduced, 1%, or fat-free milk), foods that may cause the child to choke, and excessive amounts of fruit juice or related products (e.g., fruit drinks).

Preschool Children: Nutrition Concerns

The rapid growth rate that characterizes infancy tapers off quickly during the subsequent few years. The average annual weight gain is only 4.5 to 6.6 pounds (2 to 3 kilograms), and the average annual height gain is only 3 to 4 inches (7.5 to 10 centimeters) between the ages of 2 and 5. As a toddler's growth rate tapers off, eating behavior

Carbohydrate requirements to supply energy for the central nervous system and prevent ketosis in childhood are 130 grams per day, the same as for adults. Protein requirements to allow for growth vary from 13 to 19 grams per day for children 1 to 3 years, to 34 to 52 grams per day for older children. No specific needs for total fat intake have been set, but the diet must contain at least 5 grams per day of essential fatty acids (see the inside cover for details). The general recommendation is that total fat intake gradually fall so as to eventually fit into the adult range of 20% to 35% of total calorie intake by 19 years of age.

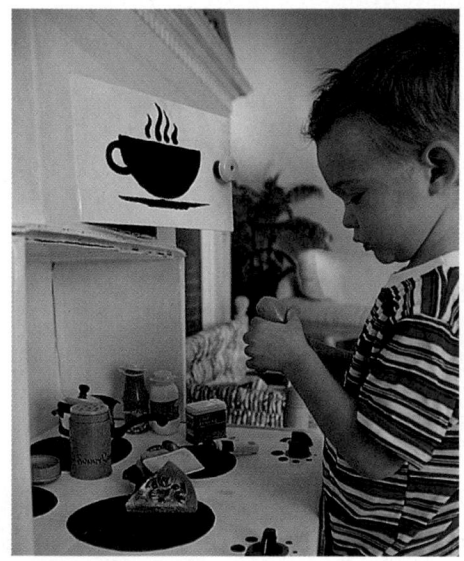

Interest in food starts early in life.

Two-year-olds commonly prefer particular foods, but parents needn't worry about this. A child may switch from one specific food focus (often called a *jag*) to another with equal intensity (older infants may also act this way). If the caregiver continues to offer choices, the child will soon begin to eat a wider variety of foods again, and the specific food focus will disappear as suddenly as it appeared.

changes. For example, the decreased growth rate leads to a decreased appetite, often called "picky eating," compared with infants.

Because of the reduced appetite of preschool children, planning a diet that meets their nutrient needs poses a challenge to caregivers. Choosing nutrient-dense foods is particularly important with children who eat relatively little. This is a good time to emphasize some whole grains, fruits, and vegetables without increasing fat and simple sugar intake. A whole-grain ready-to-eat breakfast cereal with limited fat and sugar is an excellent choice. There is no need to decrease fat or simple sugar intake severely, but fatty and sweet food choices should not overwhelm more nutritious ones.

The preschool years are the best time for a child to start a healthful pattern of living and eating, focusing on regular physical activity and nutritious foods (Fig. 14.4). Parents and other caregivers are role models: If they eat a variety of foods, the children will eat a variety of foods. One possible policy is the one-bite rule: Within reason, children should take at least one bite or taste of the foods presented to them. For snacks, parents should select several possibilities of acceptable choices and allow children to choose one; responsibility for food choice by the child ideally should start early.

▮ How to Help a Child Choose Nutritious Foods

One way adults can encourage young children to eat nutritious, well-balanced meals is to serve new foods and repeat exposure to them. The dinner hour is a good time for children to experience new foods and to develop their own food preferences. Preschool children especially tend to be wary of new foods. One reason is that they have more taste buds, and their taste buds are more sensitive than those of adults. In addition, they have a general distrust of unfamiliar foods. If adults can be patient and persevere, children will build good food habits. Above all, the dinner table should not become a battleground, and using one food as a bribe to eat another—for example, a piece of pie for peas—is strongly discouraged.

Certain food characteristics, such as crisp textures and mild flavors, are very appealing to children. Familiarity also plays an important role in food acceptance. In contrast, young children are especially wary of hot-temperature foods and tend to reject them.

Preschoolers eventually develop skill with spoons and forks and can even use dull knives. However, it's still a good idea to serve some finger foods. A goal should be to make mealtime a happy, social time to share and enjoy healthful foods.

▮ Childhood Feeding Problems

Tensions between parents, or between parents and children, especially during mealtime, often contribute to eating problems. Getting to the root of family problems and creating a more harmonious family atmosphere are important steps toward resolving many childhood feeding problems. In addition, many parents must be educated as to what to expect of a preschool child and what food-related goals to set. Let's consider some typical complaints and concerns of parents, the causes of the problems, and suggestions for correcting them.

"My Child Won't Eat as Much or as Regularly as He Did as an Infant"

This behavior is typical of preschoolers, because their growth rate slows after infancy; thus, they don't need as much food. Parents often need reminding that a 3-year-old can't be expected to eat as voraciously as an infant or to eat adult-size portions. Table 14-4 shows a general food plan, based on MyPyramid, that is appropriate for preschool and school-age children. Until about 5 years of age, portion sizes in the vegetables group, fruits group, and meat & beans group should be about 1 tablespoon per year of life, and can be increased as needed. The same advice does not apply to the grains or milk groups, but note that consuming too much milk can leave the diet short on iron. Luckily, normal-weight children have a built-in feeding mechanism, which adjusts hunger to regulate food intake at each stage of growth. If a child is developing and growing normally and the caregiver is providing a variety of healthful foods, all can be confident of the child's well-being.

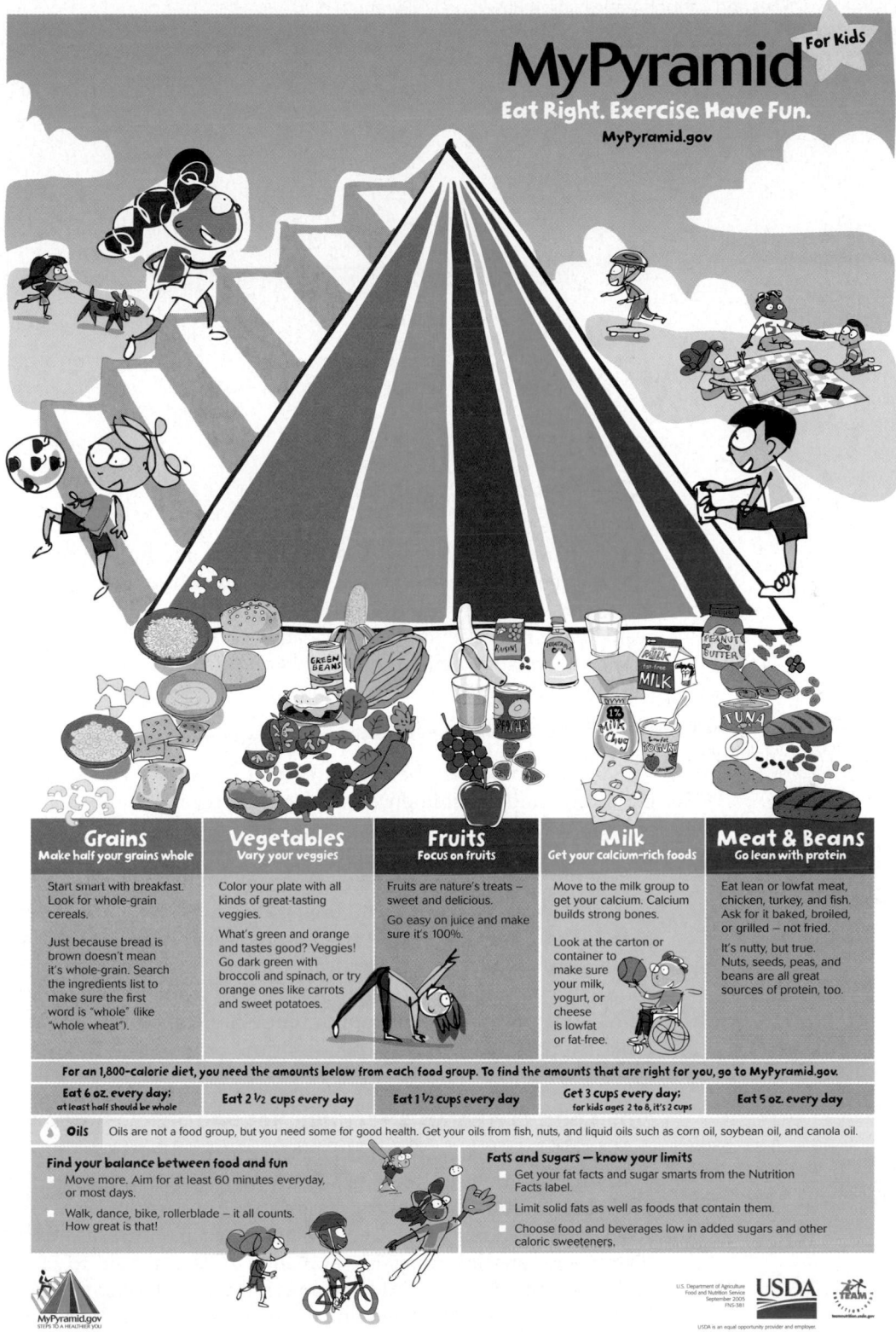

Figure 14-4 The USDA has created a version of MyPyramid for children aged 6–11. The accompanying web site (http://mypyramid.gov/kids/index.html) also features kid-friendly resources, such as an interactive MyPyramid Blast Off Game and a meal tracking worksheet, designed to encourage children to make healthier eating and activity choices. This site also contains information and resources that adults can use in educating children about proper nutrition.

Table 14-4 Food Plans for Preschool and School-Age Children Based on MyPyramid

Food Group	Serving Size	Approximate Number of Servings[1]			
		Age 2[2]	Age 5[3]	Age 8[3]	Age 12[3, 4]
Grains	ounce	3	5	5	6–7
Vegetables	cup	1	1.5	2	2.5–3
Fruits	cup	1	1.5	1.5	2
Milk	cup	2	2	3	3
Meat & Beans	ounce	2	4	5	5.5–6
Oils	teaspoon	3	4	5	6
Discretionary calories	kcal	up to 165	up to 170	up to 130	up to 265–290

[1]Log on to www.mypyramid.gov for other ages and other physical activity levels.
[2]Based on less than 30 minutes of physical activity.
[3]Based on 30–60 minutes of physical activity.
[4]The lower amounts refer to girls.

Choking is a very preventable hazard for young children. Some suggestions for caregivers include:

- Set a good example at the table by taking small bites and chewing foods thoroughly.
- Have children sit at the table, take their time, and focus on the food during meals and snacks.
- Avoid giving children any foods that are round, firm, sticky, or cut into large chunks. Some examples of foods to avoid are nuts, grapes, raisins, popcorn, peanut butter, and hard pieces of raw fruits or vegetables.

A pattern of picky eating is usually just another expression of independence for children, who have a strong desire to establish a self-determined routine. Caregivers should avoid nagging, forcing, and bribing children to encourage eating. Indirectly, these tactics reinforce picky-eating behaviors due to the added attention given to them. Overall, parents should focus on offering a variety of healthy choices, allowing the child to exert some autonomy over the specific type of food and the amount eaten. A child's sudden loss of appetite, however, may be reason for concern, as a poor appetite may be a sign of underlying illness.

Parents should also be reminded that food likes and dislikes change rapidly in childhood and are influenced by food temperature, appearance, texture, and taste. Sometimes children object to having foods mixed, as in stews and casseroles, even if they normally like the ingredients separately.

In addition, parents should recognize that this is an important age for children to explore the world around them. Even good eaters are sometimes more interested in exploring than eating. There's room for occasional indulgences, a skipped meal or two, or once in a while "less than ideal" choices. It's eating and lifestyle habits over the course of a month (and lifetime) that matter. Children master their eating when adults set a good example, provide opportunities to learn, give support for exploration, and limit inappropriate behavior.

"My Child Is Always Snacking, Yet She Never Finishes Her Meal"

Children have small stomachs. Offering them six or so small meals succeeds better than limiting them to three meals each day. Sticking to three meals a day offers no special nutritional advantages; it's just a social custom. Snacking is fine, as long as good dental habits are practiced. When we eat isn't nearly as important as what we eat. If nutritious snacks are readily available, these are good to offer at midmorning or midafternoon when the child becomes hungry. Fruits and vegetables (fresh, frozen, or juice) and whole-grain breads and crackers are good snack choices. It is important that these snack choices be planned ahead in order to have healthy choices available. Working parents should make sure their children are provided with nutritional snacks to tide them over until dinnertime.

When a child refuses to eat, it's best not to overreact. Doing so may give the child the idea that not eating is a means of getting attention or manipulating a scene. Most children don't starve themselves to any point approaching physical harm. When children refuse to eat, have them sit at the table for a while; if they still aren't interested in eating, remove the food and wait until the next scheduled meal or snack.

"My Child Never Eats Vegetables"

Children generally eat enough fruit but not an adequate amount of vegetables. Everyone dislikes certain foods. Again, the one-bite policy can be used, including vegetable servings. It takes time for a child to become enthusiastic about a new food; however, with continual exposure and a positive role model, chances are the child may even grow to like it.

Children cannot and should not be forced to eat. They need to develop independence and identities separate from their parents. As stated earlier, children have to choose for themselves—a practice that should be encouraged. No one food is an essential part of a diet. Hunger is still the best means for getting a child to eat. It may be effective to feed children vegetables at the start of a meal, when they are hungriest. Offer new foods with familiar ones. A platter of raw or lightly cooked carrots, broccoli, green and red peppers, cabbage, and mushrooms eaten as a snack with friends may be accepted. A 4- or 5-year-old child can safely eat raw vegetables without fear of choking. Recall that children often are more sensitive than adults to strong flavors and odors. Nutritious dips, such as Ranch dressing, "sell" vegetables to many children. Vegetables may acquire more appeal when children help prepare them. And, as with any food, it is important to remember that children are entitled to their own likes and dislikes, too.

■ Do Children Need a Multivitamin and Mineral Supplement?

Major scientific groups, such as the American Dietetic Association and the American Society for Clinical Nutrition, believe that multivitamin and mineral supplements are generally unnecessary for healthy children; it's better to emphasize good foods. Fortified ready-to-eat breakfast cereals with milk are especially helpful in closing any gap between current micronutrient intake and needs, such as for vitamin E, folate, and vitamin D. Two micronutrients of particular concern are iron and zinc. These may be lacking in children's diets because they consume such small portions of rich sources, such as animal protein foods. In addition, since the 2005 Dietary Guidelines for Americans suggest that children over age 2 years follow a diet low in saturated fat and cholesterol, rich sources of iron and zinc may be lacking in their diets. To compensate, parents can search for a whole-grain breakfast cereal that the child likes that also has about 50% of the Daily Value for iron and 25% of the Daily Value for zinc. (This will supply sufficient amounts of both nutrients since the Daily Values are based on the higher needs of adults.) If that's not possible, especially for a child who is ill, has a very erratic food preference pattern or appetite, or is on weight-loss diet, the American Academy of Pediatrics states that the child may benefit from a children's multivitamin and mineral supplement not exceeding 100% of Daily Values on the label, especially if these conditions persist. Still, as mentioned many times in this textbook, such a practice does not substitute for an otherwise healthy diet—children included.

If current childhood feeding practices are to become more healthful, the focus should be on whole-grain breads and cereals, fruits, vegetables, and low-fat milk and milk products. Children do not need to be severely restricted but, rather, should modify food habits with small changes. Some easy diet changes to begin with are bagels instead of doughnuts, fat-free frozen yogurt instead of ice cream, fat-reduced or 1% milk instead of whole milk, fruit instead of crackers and cheese for snacks, and air-popped popcorn instead of chips.

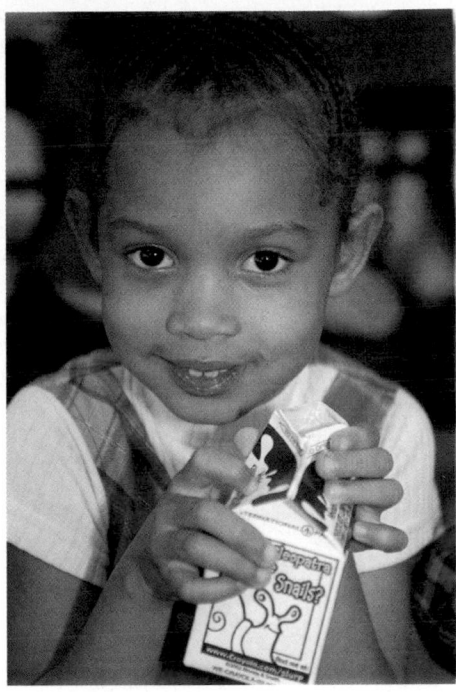

Milk is a nutrient-dense source of protein, calcium, zinc, and other nutrients to support growth. It is especially challenging to meet calcium needs in childhood without regular dairy product consumption (see Chapter 9 for alternative sources of calcium).

For children who follow a totally vegetarian diet, attention should also focus on protein and vitamin B-12 intake.

Chapter 4 noted that it's unlikely that the use of sugar is the cause of hyperactivity or antisocial behavior in most children.

■ Nutritional Problems in Preschool Children

Three nutrition-related problems found in preschool children are iron-deficiency anemia, constipation, and dental caries. Proper diet can help correct or relieve these conditions. Vegetarian diets can also pose problems.

Iron-Deficiency Anemia

The best way to prevent iron-deficiency anemia in children is to provide foods that are adequate sources of iron. Iron-fortified breakfast cereals and a few ounces of lean meat are convenient means of increasing iron in a child's diet. The high proportion of heme iron in many animal foods allows the iron to be more readily absorbed than is iron from plant foods. Consuming a vitamin C source along with the less readily absorbed iron in plants and supplements aids absorption.

Childhood iron-deficiency anemia is most likely to appear in children between the ages of 6 and 24 months. It can lead to decreases in both stamina and learning ability because the oxygen supply to cells decreases. Another effect is lowered resistance to disease. Fortunately, childhood anemia is not common today in North America, probably because of children's use of iron-fortified breakfast cereals. Also deserving of credit in the United States is the Special Supplemental Nutrition Program for Women, Infants, and Children (WIC), sponsored by the U.S. federal government. This program emphasizes the importance of iron-fortified formulas and cereals and distributes these foods—along with nutrition education—to low-income parents of infants and preschool children considered to be at nutritional risk.

Constipation

Constipation may be associated with a more serious disease, yet some young children experience constipation that is unrelated to any medical condition. When presented with a constipated child, a physician first has to rule out a medical cause, such as intestinal blockage. And, although the most common GI tract symptom that reflects intolerance to cow's milk is diarrhea, chronic constipation may also result. Treatment for constipation generally consists of first evacuating the bowels, generally with an enema. The promotion of regular bowel habits then follows, with laxative use as directed by the physician. Several months to years of supportive intervention may be required for effective treatment.

Dietary interventions include eating more fiber and drinking more fluids. Soy milk may also be substituted for cow's milk in the initial stages of treatment. Foods to emphasize for fiber are fruits, vegetables, whole-grain breads and cereals, and beans. The current daily fiber goal for children varies by age: 1 to 3 years, 19 grams per day; 4 to 8 years, 25 grams per day; 9 to 13 years, 31 grams per day for boys and 25 grams per day for girls. After age 13 years, typical adult recommendations are appropriate (review Chapter 4). Currently, few children meet these goals.

Accompanying fluid recommendations are 4 cups (900 milliliters) per day for toddlers and about 5 cups (1200 milliliters) per day for older children.

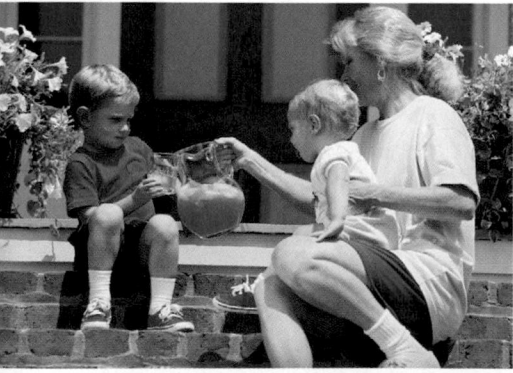

Excessive fruit drink and fruit juice use is another potential problem in preschool (and later adolescent) years. The American Academy of Pediatrics recommends no more than 4 to 6 ounces per day for children 1 to 6 years (and 8 to 12 ounces per day for ages 7 to 18 years). Sweetened soft drinks should also be limited.

Dental Caries

A proper diet goes a long way in reducing the risk for dental caries in young children. The following tips can help reduce dental problems in children:

- Begin oral hygiene when teeth start to appear.
- Seek early pediatric dental care.
- Drink fluoridated water.

- Use small amounts of fluoridated toothpaste twice daily.
- Snack in moderation.
- Have a dentist apply tooth sealants if needed.
- Avoid sticky, high-sugar snacks, especially between meals.
- If toddlers or preschoolers are chewing gum, sugarless gum is the best choice, as this has been shown to reduce the incidence of dental caries.

Vegetarianism in Childhood

Vegetarian diets can pose several risks for young children. These include the possibility of developing iron-deficiency anemia, a deficiency of vitamin B-12, and rickets from a vitamin D deficiency. During the first few years of life, children also may not consume enough calories when following a bulky vegetarian diet. But these known pitfalls are easily avoided by informed diet planning (see the Looking Further, "Vegetarian Diets" in Chapter 6). Diets for children who eat totally vegetarian fare should focus on protein, vitamin B-12, iron, and zinc content, with additional emphasis on vitamin D (or regular sun exposure) and calcium. Some of these dietary inadequacies can be compensated for by increasing oils, nuts, seeds, ready-to-eat breakfast cereals, and fortified soy milk in the diet.

Concept Check

The rapid growth rate of an infant's first year slows during the toddler and preschool years (ages 1 to 5). As a child's appetite decreases, adults need to serve nutrient-dense foods and allow the child to decide how much to eat. Sudden shifts in food preferences are to be expected. Snacking is fine if attention is given to the selection of healthful foods and good dental hygiene. Although a children's multivitamin and mineral supplement is usually not needed—a plan following MyPyramid that includes a serving of fortified ready-to-eat breakfast cereal should meet nutrient needs—use of such a supplement is a reasonable practice. Children need plenty of iron-rich food to prevent iron-deficiency anemia, as well as zinc for growth. Adequate fiber and fluid help prevent constipation. Diets for children who eat totally vegetarian fare should focus on meeting needs for protein, vitamin D (or regular sun exposure), vitamin B-12, calcium, iron, and zinc.

School-Age Children: Nutrition Concerns

In general, the nutritional concerns and goals applicable to school-age children are the same as those discussed in relation to preschoolers. MyPyramid continues to be a good basis for diet planning, with an emphasis on moderating fat and sugar intake and ensuring adequate iron, zinc, and calcium intake. The only difference is that the number of servings increases as calorie needs increase (review Table 14-4). Now let's look at several nutritional issues of particular concern during the school-age years.

▌ Breakfast, Fat Intake, and Snacks

Once children enter school, their eating patterns become more scheduled, and the consumption of regular meals—especially breakfast—becomes an important focus. A fortified ready-to-eat breakfast cereal is typically the greatest source of iron, vitamin A, and

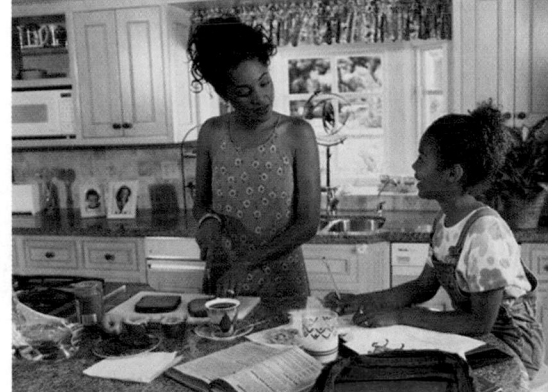

Nutrition education ideally begins in the home as parents and other caregivers provide a healthy, well-balanced diet.

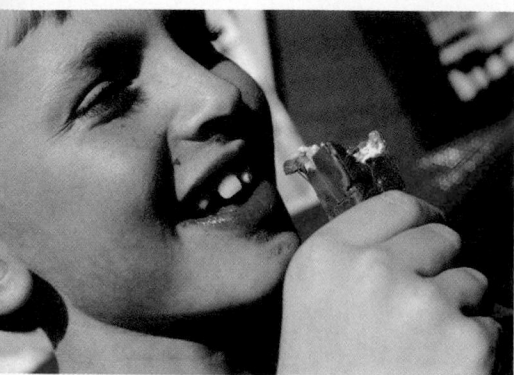

Sweets should be consumed in moderation in childhood, but do not have to be avoided altogether.

folic acid for children ages 2 to 18. Although there is controversy over the true benefit of breakfast for cognitive ability, children who eat breakfast are more likely to meet their needs for vitamins and minerals compared to children not eating breakfast. To influence morning test performance, it currently appears that breakfast must be eaten within a few hours of a test; the subsequent rise in blood glucose is thought to enhance performance.

Breakfast menus need not be limited to traditional fare. A little imagination can spark the interest of even the most reluctant child. Instead of conventional breakfast foods, parents can offer leftovers from dinner, such as pizza, spaghetti, soups, yogurt topped with trail mix, chili with beans, or sandwiches.

Diets of school-age children should include a variety of foods from each major group, not necessarily excluding any specific food because of its fat content. Overemphasis on fat-reduced diets during childhood has been linked to an increase in eating disorders and encourages an inappropriate "good food, bad food" attitude.

Steering children toward healthful foods, in school and at home, is likely to be more successful if children are exposed to nutrition education. Since children spend much of their younger years in school, it is a great place to learn about positive, healthy eating habits. Such education can help children understand why eating a proper diet will make them feel more energetic, look better, and work more efficiently. One survey of U.S. schoolchildren highlighted the need for nutrition education. On the day of the survey, 40% of the children ate no vegetables, except for potatoes or tomato sauce; 20% ate no fruits. Another study showed that only 2% of about 3300 children 2 to 19 years old had met their recommended servings from all six MyPyramid groups. Clearly, the diets of many school-age students can stand general improvement, particularly with regard to fruit, vegetable, whole grain, and dairy choices. Drinking minimal amounts of sugared soft drinks is also advised.

With regard to snacks, such as for after school, good choices include:

- Fruit smoothies
- Fruit salad (or cut-up fruit)
- Mini-pizzas
- Yogurt with granola
- Pasta salad
- Peanuts
- Veggies with dip
- Fruit-juice popsicles
- Leftovers (pizzas, macaroni and cheese, lasagna)
- Quick breads, such as banana bread
- Cheese and whole-wheat crackers
- Dried fruit
- Trail mix
- Bean and cheese burritos
- Cereal
- Hummus with veggie sticks

■ Type 2 Diabetes

Type 2 diabetes is generally thought to be an adult condition. As reviewed in the second Looking Further, "When Blood Glucose Regulation Fails" in Chapter 4, it frequently occurs in overweight people who are older than 40. However, physicians have recently noted an alarming increase in the frequency of the disease among children (and teenagers). This is primarily due to the rise in obesity in this age group, coupled with minimal physical activity. Up to 85% of children with the disease are overweight at diagnosis. Experts are currently calling for screening for diabetes in at-risk children every 2 years, starting at age 10 or at the onset of puberty. Besides obesity and a sedentary lifestyle, other risk factors include having a first- or second-degree relative

Critical Thinking

Tim refuses to eat breakfast before school. He doesn't like cereal, toast, or any of the other usual breakfast foods. What can Tim's parents do to ensure that he eats nutritious foods before leaving for school?

with the disease, or belonging to a non-White population. Appropriate diet and lifestyle intervention should be implemented, along with the use of diabetes medications when necessary. A regular intake of low-glycemic-load fruits, vegetables, and whole-grain breads and cereals is especially recommended.

■ Overweight and Obesity

In the United States, about 15% of school-age children are overweight or obese. The number of cases is currently increasing, especially in minority populations. In the short run, ridicule, embarrassment, possibly depression, and short stature linked to early puberty are the main consequences of such obesity. In the long run, significant health problems associated with obesity, such as cardiovascular disease, type 2 diabetes, and hypertension, usually will appear in adulthood. However, an increase in these health-related complications has been noted in children. Childhood obesity is a serious health threat, since about 40% of obese children (and about 80% of obese adolescents) become obese adults. Significant weight gain generally begins between ages 5 and 7, during puberty, or during the teenage years.

Current research points to many potential causes of childhood obesity. Recall the nature versus nurture discussion in Chapter 10. Some infants are born with lower metabolic rates; they use calories more efficiently and in turn can more easily produce fat stores. Studies also suggest, though, that this genetic link accounts for only one-third of individual differences in body weight.

Researchers believe that, although diet is an important factor, inactivity is also a contributor to the increase in childhood obesity. Today's generation of children now glues itself to the TV for an average of 24 hours a week; many children spend another 10 hours or so playing computer and video games. The American Academy of Pediatrics recommends a limit of 14 hours of TV and video time per week. In addition, excessive snacking, overreliance on fast-food restaurants, parental neglect, lack of safe areas to play, and the abundant availability of high-calorie food choices contribute to childhood obesity. Note that sugared soft drinks are especially implicated.

The initial approach in treating an obese child is to assess how much physical activity he or she engages in. If a child spends much free time in sedentary activities (such as watching television or playing video games), more physical activities should be encouraged. Both the U.S. federal government and health professionals recommend 60 minutes or more of moderate to intense physical activity per day for children and adolescents. Learning to engage in and enjoy regular physical activity will help children not only to attain a healthy body weight but also to keep a similar body weight later in life. An increase in physical activity won't just happen; parents and other caregivers need to plan for it. Two good ideas are getting the family together for a brisk walk after dinner and finding an after-school sport the child enjoys.

Moderation in calorie intake is important, especially the limitation of high-calorie foods, such as sugared soft drinks and whole milk. The focus should be on more vitamin and mineral-dense foods and healthy snacks.

Resorting to a weight-loss diet is usually not necessary—it's best to emphasize changing habits that allow for weight maintenance. Children have an advantage over adults in dealing with obesity; their bodies can use stored energy for growth. Thus, if weight gain can be moderated, increases in height and resulting lean body tissue may reduce the percentage of body weight accounted for as stored fat, yielding a more healthful weight-to-height ratio. This is one reason it's desirable to treat obesity in childhood. Further growth can contribute to success. If weight loss is necessary in younger children, it should be gradual, about ½ to 1 pound per week. In addition, the child should be watched closely to ensure that the rate of growth continues to be normal. The child's calorie intake shouldn't be so low that gains in height diminish. In addition, medications may be prescribed under a physician's care to reduce food intake (sibutramine [Meridia]) and/or fat absorption (orlistat [Xenical]).

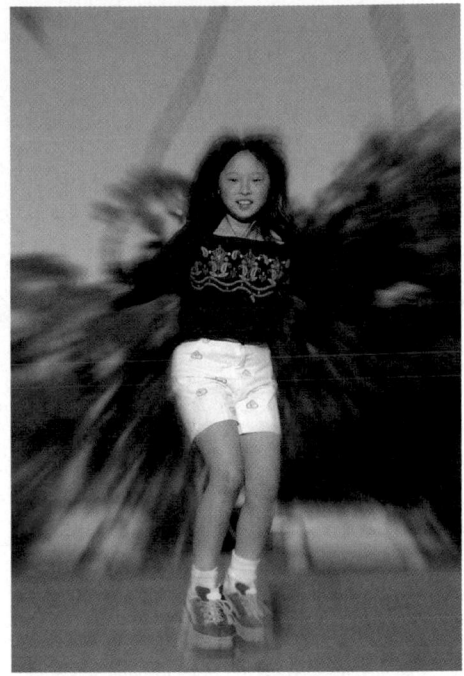

Regular physical activity is an important part of prevention and treatment of weight problems in childhood. The current goal is about 60 minutes of such activity each day. Many children do not meet this goal.

To get kids involved in exercise, new physical education classes have been introduced into schools. These classes provide lifelong fitness lessons in such activities as rock climbing, in-line skating, and recreational jogging. These classes help promote activity because they take the focus away from teams and competition, which often discourage and embarrass kids who lack athletic talent.

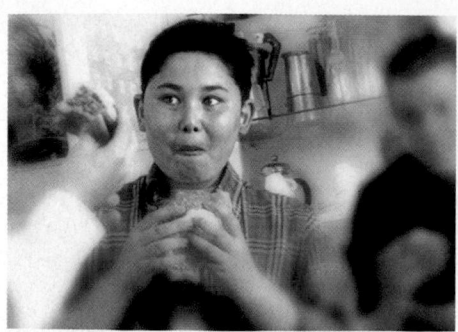

Super-sized portions of foods such as hamburgers and sugared soft drinks served to children are contributing to the obesity and type 2 diabetes epidemics they are experiencing.

Drinking soft drinks in place of milk causes many teenagers to have inadequate calcium intake. Over the last 20 years, soft drinks have been replacing milk as the preferred beverage of adolescents. This trend has been linked to decreased bone mass and increased bone fractures in this age group.

A strictly vegetarian diet must be monitored for adequate energy, protein, iron, vitamin B-12, calcium, and vitamin D (the latter if sun exposure is not sufficient). These nutrients become particularly important in teenagers, as their diets are often already compromised.

Concept Check

The school-age child is advised to follow MyPyramid, and especially moderate choices high in fat and simple sugars. Breakfast is an important meal to refuel the body for a new school day and to help ensure fulfilling nutrient needs for the day. Attention to regular physical activity and healthy diet should help prevent/treat childhood obesity and build a desirable lifestyle pattern for later life.

Teenage Years: Nutrition Concerns

Most girls begin a rapid growth spurt between the ages of 10 and 13, and most boys experience rapid growth between the ages of 12 and 15. Nearly every organ in the body grows during these periods. Most noticeable are increases in height and weight and the development of secondary sexual characteristics. Girls usually begin menstruating (reach menarche) during this growth spurt, and they grow very little beyond 2 years after menarche. Early-maturing girls may begin their growth spurt as early as age 7 to 8, whereas early-maturing boys may begin growing by age 9 to 10.

During the growth spurt, girls gain about 10 inches (25 centimeters) in height, and boys gain about 12 inches (30 centimeters). Girls also tend to accumulate both lean and fat tissue, whereas boys tend to gain mostly lean tissue. This growth spurt provides about 50% of ultimate adult weight and about 15% of ultimate adult height (review Fig. 14-1).

As the growth spurt begins, teenagers begin to eat more. If teens choose nutritious food, they can take advantage of their increased hunger and easily satisfy their nutrient needs. As discussed for younger age groups, MyPyramid can provide the basis for meeting these nutrient needs (Table 14-5). Following such a plan will meet carbohydrate needs (130 grams per day) and protein needs (52 grams per day for males and 46 grams per day for females).

Table 14-5 Food Plan for Teenagers Based on MyPyramid[1, 2]

Food Group	Serving Size	Approximate Number of Servings		
		13 Age	**16 Age**	**18 Age**
Grains	ounce	6–7	6–10	6–10
Vegetables	cup	2.5–3	2.5–3.5	2.5–3.5
Fruits	cup	2	2–2.5	2–2.5
Milk	cup	3	3	3
Meat & Beans	ounce	5.5–6	5.5–7	5.5–7
Oils	teaspoon	6	6–8	6–8
Discretionary calories	kcal	up to 265–290	up to 265–425	up to 265–425

[1]Assumes 3-–60 minutes of physical activity per day. Log on to mypyramid.gov for other ages and levels of physical activity.
[2]The larger amounts refer to boys.

▪ Nutritional Problems and Concerns of Teens

Anorexia nervosa and bulimia nervosa are nutritional concerns of the teen years, as covered in detail in Chapter 12. Other nutritional problems are more common during the teen years. A survey of high school students showed that only a little over 25% had eaten five servings of fruits and vegetables on the previous day, and they are consuming approximately 25% more sodium than recommended. Another concern is that many teenage girls stop drinking milk, so they may not consume enough calcium to allow for maximal mineralization of bones through their early twenties. Many young women who don't consume enough calcium are likely to develop osteoporosis later.

Many teenagers are not meeting their needs for calcium. The Adequate Intake for calcium for both males and females between ages 9 and 18 years is 1300 milligrams per day, compared with only 800 milligrams per day for younger children. Three servings per day from the milk, yogurt, and cheese group are recommended for all teenagers and young adults to meet calcium needs. Figure 2-1 in Chapter 2 shows the stark contrast between milk and typical soft drinks with respect to calcium and other nutrients. If dairy products are not consumed alternative calcium sources need to be included.

A further concern is iron deficiency. Iron-deficiency anemia sometimes appears in girls after they start menstruating (menarche) and in boys during their growth spurt. About 10% of teenagers have low iron stores or related anemia. Teens who strive to forge an identity by adopting dietary patterns unfamiliar to their families—vegetarianism, for example—may not know enough about the alternate diet pattern to keep from developing health problems, such as iron-deficiency anemia. It's important that teenagers choose good food sources of iron, such as lean meats, whole grains, and enriched cereals. Teenage girls, particularly those with heavy menstrual flows, need to eat good sources of iron (or regularly consume an iron supplement). Iron-deficiency anemia is a highly undesirable condition for a teen. It can produce increased fatigue and decreased ability to concentrate and learn. School and physical performance may suffer.

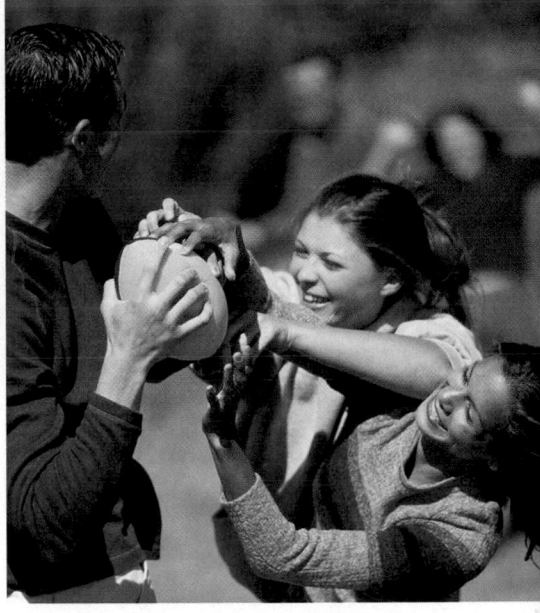

An active lifestyle coupled with a healthy diet should be part of the teen years. Both habits contribute to bone development and bone strength.

▪ Helping Teens Eat More Nutritious Foods

Teenagers face a variety of challenges. They pursue their independence, experience identity crises, seek peer acceptance, and worry about physical appearance. All of these factors affect food choice. Advertisers take advantage of this by pushing a vast array of products—candy, gum, soft drinks, and snacks—at the teenage market. Potato chips and French fries make up more than one-third of the vegetable servings consumed by teens. Additionally, many schools offer French fries on a regular basis, and soft drink machines can be found in school hallways and cafeterias, in turn competing with the school lunch.

Alcoholism, a significant health problem that may have its roots in the teen years, is covered in detail in Chapter 7. Smoking—another habit that compromises health—also often begins in teen years. Some of the impetus for smoking is the desire to control body weight—but this obviously is not an advisable method.

Obesity is a growing problem among teenagers, and about 30% of these teenagers have the metabolic syndrome (Syndrome X) discussed in Chapters 4 and 5. If a teen attains ultimate adult height and is still obese, a weight-loss regimen may be necessary. This is especially appropriate after the adolescent growth spurt. Weight loss should be gradual, perhaps 1 pound per week, and generally follow the advice in Chapter 10. Weight loss medications may also be prescribed.

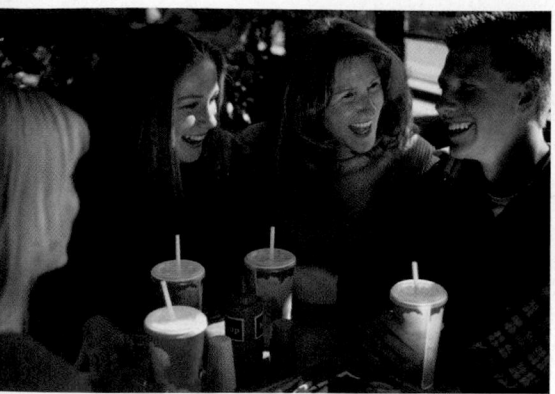

One way to reduce calorie intake in a restaurant is to choose diet soft drinks in place of regular soft drinks. This will greatly reduce sugar and overall calorie intake in the meal or snack, especially considering the large serving sizes typically offered.

Teens often do not think about the long-term benefits of good health. They have a hard time relating today's actions to tomorrow's health outcomes. Many teenagers tend to think they can just change habits later; there's no hurry.

Still, healthful teen food habits do not require giving up favorite foods. Small portions of fatty foods can complement larger portions of fat-free and reduced-fat dairy products, lean meats, vegetable proteins, fruits, vegetables, and whole-grain products. An example of this type of meal is a plain hamburger with a garden salad (minimize the amount of regular dressing or use a low-fat variety), small order of French fries or chili, and a medium diet soft drink or reduced-fat or fat-free milk.

■ Are Teenage Snacking Practices Harmful?

Teens often obtain one-fourth to one-third of all their calories and major nutrients from snacks. Unfortunately, studies have found just what you might expect—that teens snack mostly on potato and corn chips, cookies, candies, and ice cream. Key reasons for snacking include an opportunity to get out and socialize with friends, accessibility, hunger, and celebration of a special event. Teenagers can obtain many nutrients from snacking. Even fast-food restaurants offer some good food choices. By choosing wisely and eating in moderation, teens can eat at fast-food restaurants occasionally and still consume a very healthful diet. Snacks and fast-food restaurants themselves are not the problem; poor food choices in terms of type and quantity are.

Lack of exercise and poor dietary habits formed during teenage years often continue into adulthood, and may increase risk of chronic diseases, such as cardiovascular disease, osteoporosis, and some types of cancer. Getting this message across to teenagers is an important and challenging task for parents.

Concept Check

A second period of rapid growth occurs during the teen years. Girls generally start this growth spurt earlier than boys. MyPyramid can direct meal planning. Common nutritional problems in these years arise from poor food choices and include inadequate calcium intake in girls and iron-deficiency anemia. Because changes occur so rapidly during these years, and in so many areas—psychological, social, and physical— it may be difficult to stress the relevance of nutrition to teenagers. Moderation in fat and sugar intake are important goals to consider when choosing snacks.

Summary

1. Growth is very rapid during infancy; birth weight doubles in 4 to 6 months, and length increases by 50% in the first year. An adequate diet, especially in terms of calories, as well as the nutrients protein and zinc, is essential to support normal growth. Undernutrition can cause irreversible changes in growth and development. Growth in infants and children can be assessed by measuring body weight, height (or length), and head circumference over time. Growth charts have recently been revised to include a more valid measurement for determining children's growth, body mass index (BMI).

2. Nutrient needs in the first 6 months can be met by human milk or iron-fortified infant formula. Supplementary vitamin D is needed for breastfed infants, and many infants may need supplemental iron and fluoride.

3. Infant formulas generally contain lactose or sucrose, heat-treated proteins from cow's milk, and vegetable oil. These formulas may or may not be fortified with iron. Sanitation is very important when preparing and storing formula.

4. Most infants do not need solid foods before 6 months of age. Solid food should not be added to an infant's diet until the nutrients are needed, the GI tract can digest complex foods, the infant has the physical ability to control tongue thrusting, and the risk of developing food allergies has decreased.

5. The first solid food given should be iron-fortified infant cereals or ground meats. Other single foods can be added gradually, at the rate of about one each week. Some foods to avoid giving infants in the first year include honey, cow's milk (especially fat-reduced varieties), very salty or sweet foods, and foods that may cause choking.

6. Introducing iron-containing solid food at the appropriate time and not offering cow's milk until 1 year of age can generally prevent iron-deficiency anemia in late infancy.

7. A slower growth rate in preschool years underlies the importance of children's eating nutrient-dense foods and reducing their food serving sizes. Choosing iron-rich foods, such as lean red meats, is important at this age. Portion sizes of 1 tablespoon of each food for each year of life is a good starting point for the vegetables, fruits, and meats & beans groups of MyPyramid. Preschoolers also should be given some leeway in determining serving size and should be encouraged to try new foods.

8. Obese children and adolescents are more likely to become obese adults and, so, incur greater health risks. Parents can provide healthful food choices, and children should control portion sizes. When controlled early through diet and exercise interventions, the problem of obesity may correct itself as the child continues to grow in height.

9. During the adolescent growth spurt, both boys and girls have increased needs for iron and calcium. Inadequate calcium intake by teenage girls is a major concern because it can set the stage for the development of osteoporosis later in life. Teenagers generally should moderate their intake of high-fat and sugar-rich foods—especially snacks and fast-food, which they often consume in abundance—and perform regular physical activity.

Study Questions

1. List two factors that limit "catch-up" growth in adulthood when a nutrient-deficient diet has been consumed throughout childhood.

2. Describe how you would assess whether an 8-month-old infant is consuming a healthful diet.

3. Outline three key factors that help determine when to introduce solid foods into an infant's diet.

4. A 3-month-old infant is taken to a clinic with failure to thrive. What are two possible explanations?

5. List three reasons why preschoolers are noted for "picky" eating. For each, describe an appropriate parent response.

6. What three factors are likely to contribute to obesity in a typical 10-year-old child?

7. Compare the guidelines for infant feeding summarized in Chapter 14 with the 2005 Dietary Guidelines for Americans for children over age 2 and adults discussed in Chapter 2. Which guidelines are similar? Do any contradict each other? If so, why?

8. Describe three pros and cons of snacking. What is the basic advice for healthful snacking from childhood through the teenage years?

9. Which two nutrients are of particular concern in planning diets for teenagers? Why does each deserve to be singled out?

10. List three nutrients of concern for a teenage vegetarian.

Further Readings

1. Affenito SG and others: Breakfast consumption by African-American and white adolescent girls correlates positively with calcium and fiber intake and negatively with body mass index. *Journal of the American Dietitic Association* 105: 938, 2005.

   Eating breakfast on a regular basis contributes to the overall health of adolescent girls in this study. This includes helping meet calcium and fiber needs, while also contributing to weight control.

2. AHA Scientific Statement: American Heart Association guidelines for primary prevention of atherosclerotic cardiovascular disease beginning in childhood. *Circulation* 107:1562, 2003.

   It is clear that cardiovascular disease begins in childhood. A healthy diet, regular physical activity, and not smoking are three key ways to forestall the development of cardiovascular disease beginning in childhood. After age 2 it is important to limit saturated fat, trans fat, and cholesterol intake, while especially emphasizing intake of fruits, vegetables, and whole-grain breads and cereals. Rich protein sources such as dairy products, lean meats, fish, and legumes (beans) also deserve attention.

3. American Academy of Pediatrics: Policy statement of the Committee on Nutrition: Prevention of pediatric overweight and obesity. *Pediatrics* 112:424, 2003.

   Prevention of pediatric overweight and obesity is of prime importance. Once overweight and obesity develop, educating the family about proper dietary and physical activity habits is important. Parents can encourage moderation rather than overconsumption of specific foods and limitation of television and video time to a maximum of 2 hours per day.

4. Bounds W and others: The relationship of dietary and lifestyle factors to bone mineral indexes in children. *Journal of the American Dietetic Association* 105: 735, 2005.

   A primary influence on healthy bone mass parameters in this study were a nutritious diet-one ample in protein, phosphorus, vitamin K, magnesium, zinc, iron, and calories. Height and weight were also positively correlated to bone status.

5. Butte N and others: The Start Healthy Feeding Guidelines for Infants and Toddlers. *Journal of the American Dietetic Association* 104:442, 2004.

   Comprehensive guide to the what, when, and how of infant and toddler feeding. A colorful and informative guide to the timing of feeding skills and solid food introduction is included. The general guideline is to introduce solid foods to infants at 6 months of age.

6. Centers for Disease Control and Prevention: Physical activity levels among children ages 9–13 years—United States, 2002. *Journal of the American Medical Association* 290:1308, 2003.

   Most children do not participate in sufficient free-time physical activity, especially African-American and Hispanic children. Insufficient physical activity increases the risk for overweight and obesity and other chronic diseases. Physical activity habits that begin in childhood are likely to carry over into adulthood.

7. Dietz WH and Robinson TN: Overweight children and adolescents. *The New England Journal of Medicine* 352:2100, 2005.

   This article summarizes the possible diagnostic and treatment approaches for overweight children and adolescents. For the 7-year-old girl described in the article, three key recommendations were to reduce sugared-soft drink consumption and computer and television screen time, with a corresponding increase in active play.

8. Douglas KM and others: A practical guide to infant health. *American Family Physician* 70: 2113, 2004.

If an infant's diet does not provide fluoride (e.g., formula is not mixed with fluoridated water), fluoride should be given after six months of age. This article outlines how to do that safely. The authors do not recommend fluoride therapy for breastfed infants.

9. Fitch C: Preventing iron deficiency in infants and toddlers. *Today's Dietitian* p.32 December 2004.

The author stresses the need to prevent iron deficiency in infants and toddlers. After 4 to 6 months of age it is important to have a rich source of iron in an infant's diet, such as iron-fortified cereals. Any infant formula used should be iron fortified. Prevention of iron deficiency in toddlers includes limiting cow's milk to 3 cups per day, as it is a poor source of iron.

10. Harnack L and others: Dietary intake and food sources of whole grains among children and adolescents: Data from the 1994–1996 continuing survey of food intakes by individuals. *Journal of American Dietetic Association* 103:1015, 2003.

Few children are currently meeting the Healthy People 2010 goal of consuming three or more whole grains daily. The average intake is closer to one serving per day.

11. Hatun S and others: Vitamin D deficiency in early infancy. *Journal of Nutrition* 135: 279, 2005.

Prevention of vitamin D deficiencies in infants is essential. This includes supplementing the diet of all breastfed infants with vitamin D soon after birth.

12. Hellekson K: Report on the diagnosis, evaluation, and treatment of high blood pressure in children and adolescents. *American Family Physician* 71: 1014, 2005.

Screening for high blood pressure is an important part of regular checkups of children by the child's physician. The latest recommendations for treating high blood pressure if found includes a diet rich in vegetables, fruit, and low fat dairy products; low in salt; and moderate in high-calorie foods and drinks. Regular physical activity is also important, as is weight loss if needed.

13. Kazal LA: Prevention of iron deficiency in infants and toddlers. *American Family Physician* 66:1217, 2002.

Anemia is a possible problem during childhood. Anemia is most often caused by iron deficiency, and less often by deficiencies in folate and vitamin B-12. Screening for anemia in children occurs between ages 6 and 12 months for infants at high-risk for developing this disorder. Nutrition-related habits

that increase risk are use of infant formula that is not fortified with iron, breastfeeding without iron supplementation, and excessive milk consumption in toddlers.

14. Kirk S and others: Pediatric obesity epidemic: Treatment options. *Journal of the American Dietetic Association* 105: S44, 2005.

Reducing calorie intake and increasing energy expenditure are important for treating pediatric obesity. Medications and obesity-related surgery may also be employed. The authors stress the importance of involving the family to create a supportive environment as part of the overall therapeutic approach.

15. Kleinmam RE (ed): Pediatric Nutrition Handbook Chicago, Ill. American Academy of Pediatrics 2004.

Comprehensive review of issues surrounding pediatric nutrition. This reference was frequently consulted in the revision of this chapter.

16. Koplan JP and others: Preventing childhood obesity: Health in the balance: Executive Summary. *Journal of the American Dietetic Association* 105: 131, 2005.

Preventing children obesity involves a healthy eating pattern and regular physical activity. The goal should be achieving and maintaining a healthy body weight. The authors note that many social factors will have to be altered to facilitate this goal, such as providing more outlets for physical activity.

17. Kranz S and others: Dietary fiber intake by American preschoolers is associated with more nutrient-dense diets. *Journal of the American Dietetic Association* 105: 21 221, 2005.

Children in general would benefit from diets higher in fiber. Improving diet choices in general will allow for this, including increasing whole grain, fruit and vegetable content. The healthier the overall diet, the greater number of fiber-rich foods.

18. Lytle L: Nutritional issues for adolescents. *Journal of the American Dietetic Association* 102:S8, 2002.

Data from large, population-based studies suggest that the typical adolescent's diet places them at increased risk for cardiovascular disease, cancer, osteoporosis, diabetes, and obesity in adulthood. The typical adolescent's diet contains too much total fat, saturated fat, sodium, and soft drinks, and not enough fruits, vegetables, fiber, and calcium.

19. Mrdjenovic G, Levitsky, DA: Nutritional and energetic consequences of sweetened drink consumption in 6- to 13-year-old children. *Journal of Pediatrics* 142:604, 2003.

Children are not good at regulating overall calorie consumption in order to compensate for the increased calories coming from sweetened drinks. This lack of regulation results in excess calorie intake and overall poor nutrition. Children should have restrictions on sweetened drinks at home and at school, and should be encouraged to drink more water.

20. Patrick H, Nicklas TA: A review of family and social determinants of children's eating patterns and diet quality. *Journal of the American College of Nutrition* 24(2): 83, 2005.

The physical environment has a big influence on the quality of the diets of children. Adding to this is the influence of the parents. To improve the diets of children then, the authors note that many parameters must be addressed: child, parents, school, and community.

21. Rajeshwari R and others: Longitudinal changes in intake and food sources of calcium from childhood to young adulthood: The Bogalusa Heart Study. *Journal of the American College of Nutrition* 23 (4): 341, 2005.

Many children are not meeting their calcium needs, as shown in this study. Despite a gradual increase in calorie intake as children age, calcium intake does not generally increase appreciably. Overall, a greater focus on calcium-rich food choice needs to be made in this age group.

22. Rocchini A: Childhood obesity and a diabetes epidemic. *The New England Journal of Medicine* 346:854, 2002.

Obesity has been named the most serious nutritional disorder affecting children in the United States. Over the past thirty years, rates of obesity have more than doubled in the United States, and there has been a similar increase worldwide. Childhood obesity is a concern because it can lead to increased risk for cardiovascular disease, insulin resistance, and diabetes.

23. Schardt D: Food allergies. *Nutrition Action Healthletter*, p. 10, April 2001.

Since there is no treatment or cure for food allergies, the only way to avoid allergic reactions is to avoid the offending foods. Allergies to peanuts, nuts, and seafood seldom disappear. Food intolerances on the other hand—except for those caused by sulfites— are not as serious a health problem.

24. Wang MC and others: Diet in midpuberty and sedentary activity in prepuberty predict peak bone mass. *American Journal of Clinical Nutrition* 77:495, 2003.

Meeting calcium needs and performing regular physical activity are two keys to attaining peak bone mass in children. Many children do not meet calcium needs nor participate in sufficient physical activity in order to attain these benefits.

25. Yoo S and others: Comparison of dietary intakes associated with metabolic syndrome risk factors in young adults: the Bogalusa Heart Study. *American Journal of Clinical Nutrition* 80:841, 2004.

Low fruit and vegetable intake and high sweetened beverage consumption were associated with the metabolic syndrome in this study. Low-fat dairy products were found to be protective.

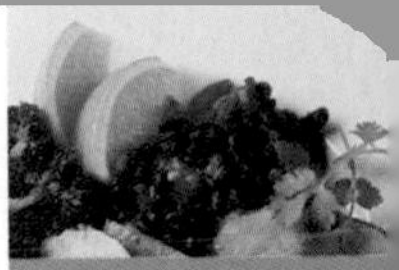

I. Getting Young Bill to Eat

Bill is 3 years old, and his mother is worried about his eating habits. He absolutely refuses to eat vegetables, meat, and dinner in general. Some days he eats very little food. He wants to eat snacks most of the time. Mealtime is a battle because Bill says he isn't hungry, and his mother wants him to eat a sit-down lunch and dinner to make sure he gets all the nutrients he needs and to eat everything served on his plate. He drinks five or six glasses of whole milk per day because that is the one food he likes.

When his mother prepares dinner, she makes plenty of vegetables, boiling them until they are soft, hoping this will appeal to Bill. Bill's dad waits to eat his vegetables last, regularly telling the family that he eats them only because he has to. He also regularly complains about how dinner has been prepared. Bill saves his vegetables until last and usually gags when his mother orders him to eat them. Bill has been known to sit at the dinner table for an hour until the war of wills ends. Bill's mother serves casseroles and stews regularly because they are convenient. Bill likes to eat breakfast cereal, fruit, and cheese and regularly requests these foods for snacks. However, his mother tries to deny his requests, so that he will have an appetite for dinner. Bill's mother comes to you and asks you what she should do to get Bill to eat.

Analysis

1. List four mistakes Bill's parents are making that contribute to Bill's poor eating habits.

_____

_____

_____

_____

2. List four strategies they might try to promote good eating habits in Bill.

_____

_____

_____

_____

II. Evaluating a Teen Lunch

  The following are two typical teen lunches and nutritional information for each:

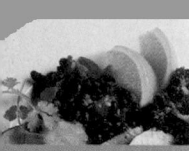

Meal 1	Meal 2
2 pieces cheese pizza 1 milk chocolate candy bar 20 fluid ounces cola	1 large hamburger sandwich with condiments 30 French fries 20 Fluid ounces cola

	Meal 1	Meal 2	Nutrient Needs for Teens
Energy (kcal)	990	1000	Males: 3000 Females: 2200
Protein	32	20	Males: 59 Females: 44
Vitamin C (milligrams)	5	18	Both genders: 45 to 75
Vitamin A (micrograms RAE)	300	10	Males: 900 Females: 700
Iron (milligrams)	3	4	Males: 11 Females: 15
Calcium (milligrams)	545	100	Both genders: 1300

1. Keeping in mind that meals should meet about one-third of nutrient needs, what are the shortcomings and excesses of these meals (i.e., given the nutritional information, compare these meals with one-third the RDA for protein, vitamin C, vitamin A, and iron and the Adequate Intake for calcium)?

   _____

   _____

   _____

2. How would you change these meals to improve balance and to meet the nutrient needs above? (Hint: Use NutritionCalc Plus or Appendix J.)

   _____

   _____

   _____

3. Reflect on your food choices as a teenager. Do you think your meal choices were balanced and varied? Why or why not? What could you have done to improve your nutritional habits at that time?

   _____

   _____

   _____

Nutrition during Adulthood

15

Real Life Scenario

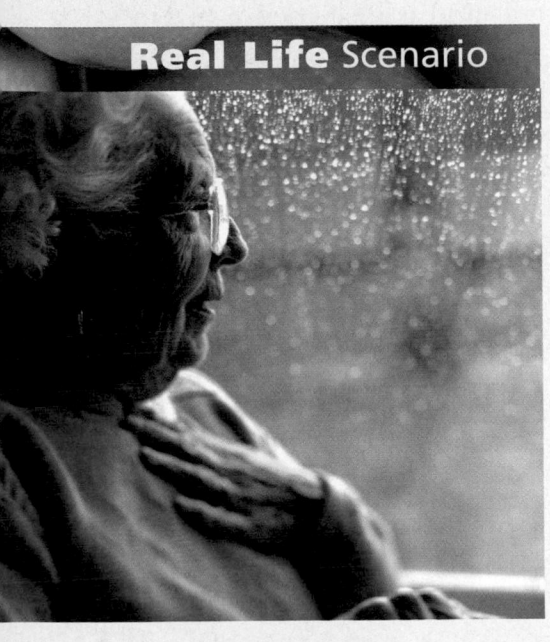

Frances is a 78-year-old woman who suffers from macular degeneration, osteoporosis, and arthritis. Since her husband died a year ago, she has moved from their family house to a small one-bedroom apartment. Her eyesight is progressively getting worse, making it hard to go to the grocery store or even to cook (for fear of burning herself). She is often lonely; her only son lives 1 hour away and works two jobs, but he visits her as often as he can. Frances has lost her appetite and, as a result, often skips meals during the week. She has resorted to eating mostly cold foods, which are simple to prepare but are seriously limiting diet variety and palatability in her diet. She is slowly losing weight as a result of her dietary changes and loss of appetite.

Her typical diet usually consists of a breakfast that may include 1 slice of wheat toast with margarine, honey, and cinnamon, and 1 cup of hot tea. If she has lunch, she normally has ½ can of peaches, half of a turkey and cheese sandwich, and ½ glass of water. For dinner, she might have half of a tuna fish sandwich made with mayonnaise and 1 cup of iced tea. She usually includes one or two cookies at bedtime.

What are the potential consequences of such a poor dietary pattern? What services are available that could help Frances improve her diet and possibly increase her appetite? What other convenience foods could be included in her diet to make it more healthful and more varied?

Chapter 15 Objectives

Chapter 15 is designed to allow you to:

1. Discuss the causes of the principal nutrition-related problems seen in adults.

2. List biological changes that occur during the aging process, and discuss how these changes affect nutrient needs of older adults.

3. Make recommendations for dietary changes in the prevention and treatment of nutritional problems in older adults.

4. List several nutritional programs that are available to help meet nutritional needs of older adults.

Check out the **Contemporary Nutrition Online Learning Center** **www.mhhe.com/wardlawcont6** for quizzes, flash cards, other activities, and web links designed to further help you learn about nutrient needs in adulthood.

Eating is one of our great pleasures. Guided by common sense and moderation, eating well is also a means to good health. Most of us want a long, productive life, free of illness, yet many people from early middle age onward suffer from obesity, cardiovascular disease, hypertension and strokes, type 2 diabetes, osteoporosis, and other chronic diseases. We can slow the development of, and in some cases even prevent, these diseases by consuming a diet that works against them. The effect of such a diet is most profitable if we begin early and continue throughout adulthood. We serve ourselves best—as individuals and as a nation—by striving to maintain vitality even in the later decades of life. This concept was first explored in Chapter 1 and is discussed again in this Chapter, along with the special nutrition needs of older persons.

Keep in mind that present day-to-day health practices can significantly influence health during later life. Although genetics does play a role, as discussed in Chapter 3, many of the health problems that occur with age are not inevitable; they result from diet-related disease processes that influence physical health. Much can be learned from healthy older people whose attention to a healthy diet and physical activity—along with a little luck—keeps them active and vibrant well beyond typical retirement years. Successful aging is the goal. Age quickly or slowly—it is partly your choice.

Refresh Your Memory

As you begin your study of adult nutrition issues in Chapter 15, you may want to review:

- Implications of the 1994 Dietary Supplement Health and Education Act in Chapter 1
- The effect of genetics on health in Chapter 3
- The various body systems covered in Chapter 3
- The sources of fiber and sugar in Chapter 4
- Guidelines for alcohol intake in Chapter 7
- The dietary sources of vitamin D, the various B vitamins, and calcium in Chapters 8 and 9
- Recommendations for salt intake in Chapter 9
- Definition of healthy body weight in Chapter 10
- The benefits of regular physical activity in Chapter 11

THE MIDDLETONS

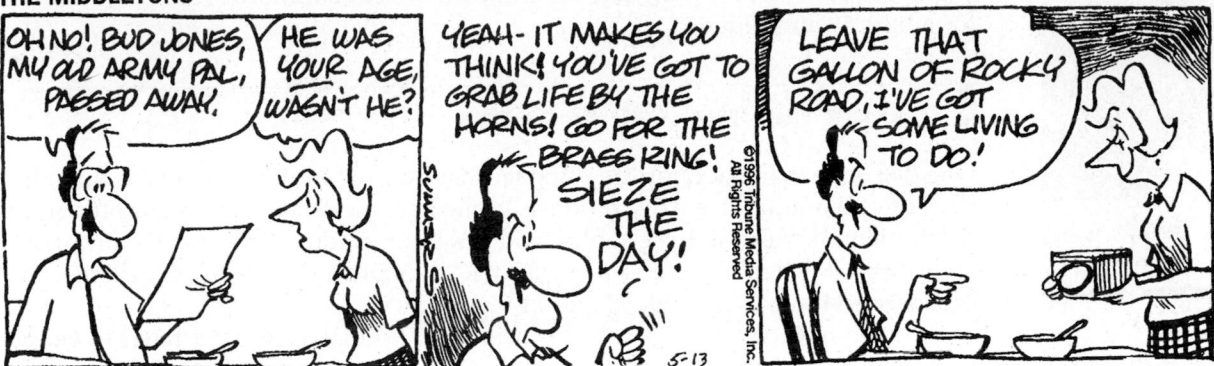

Is a decline in health inevitable as we age? Which diet and lifestyle interventions have been shown to slow (or reverse) the aging process? Which nutrition problems are typically seen in older adults? How should one compensate for these? Chapter 15 provides some answers.

Nutrition and Adulthood—An Introduction

Health conscious adults in North America today are typically doing what is within their control to achieve a healthy lifestyle, such as a consuming healthful diet, maintaining a healthy body weight, and following a regimen of regular physical activity. Coupled with avoidance of tobacco products; limitation of or adaptation to stress; adequate sleep; adequate fluid intake; maintaining friendships and optimism; lifelong learning; keeping blood cholesterol, blood glucose, and blood pressure under control; and consultation with health care professionals on a regular basis, these actions contribute to a healthful, long life. Overall, the key to maximizing health throughout life is to establish harmony among one's physical, mental, psychological, and social states (see Part I in the Rate Your Plate section at the end of this Chapter).

Based on the needs for various nutrients set by the Food and Nutrition Board, one's adult years can be divided into four stages: ages 19 to 30, 31 to 50, 51 to 70, and beyond 70 years of age. The two intervals encompassing ages 19 through 50 can be seen as young adulthood; 51 to 70 is middle-age adulthood; and beyond 70 years of age is older adulthood. Some examples of the dynamic in the nutrition needs of aging are:

- *Calcium.* Needs for this bone-related mineral increase after age 50 for males and females to help counter the harmful effects of accelerated bone loss.
- *Vitamin B-12.* After age 50, one should consume foods fortified with vitamin B-12 or take a balanced multivitamin and mineral supplement containing vitamin B-12. Recall from Chapter 8 that about 10% to 30% of older people may have decreased absorption of food-bound vitamin B-12 in part because of reduced acid production by the stomach.
- *Vitamin D.* Compared to the amount of vitamin D needed by individuals of ages 19 to 50, needs increase by 50% for the 51 to 70 age group. Adults over age 70 need *three times more* vitamin D than they did when they were ages 19 to 50. Attention to these differing needs for vitamin D is especially important if a person does not receive regular sun exposure, such as those residing the winter months in northern United States or Canada. Experts recommend that these older adults be checked yearly for vitamin D status.

Overall, attention to healthy nutrition and overall lifestyle habits is important at all ages. Providing dietary advice for adults ages 19 to 50 years is the focus of the

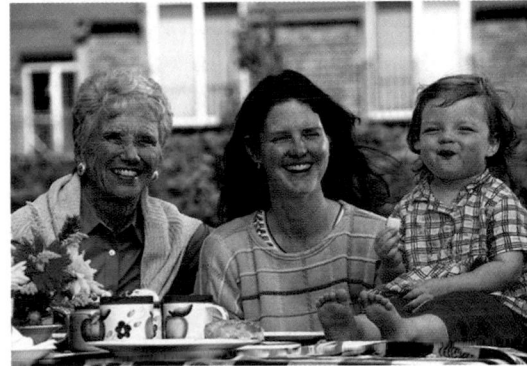

As we age, our nutrient needs change. For example, vitamin D needs are higher for older stages of adulthood.

Keep in mind that extending life without delaying onset of chronic disease prolongs suffering in many cases. In addition, the greater number of disabled years is very costly to all North Americans. For these reasons, prolonging life without compressing the number of disabled years is called the "failure of success."

503

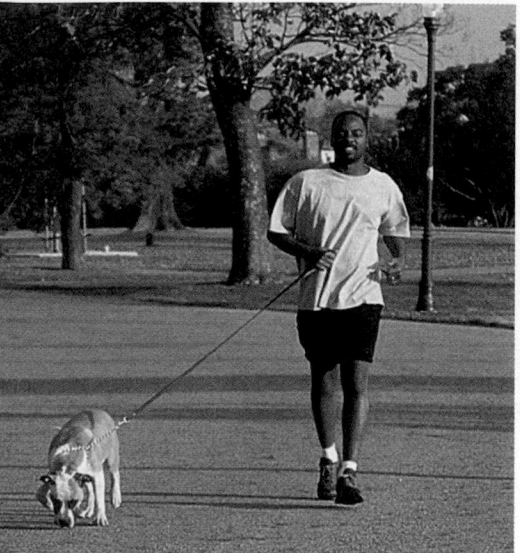

Many adults find that regular physical activity adds an important dimension to their lives. The Dietary Guidelines for Americans recommend that men over 40 and women over 50 years of age obtain physician approval before beginning a program of vigorous physical activity. This is especially important for people with evidence of cardiovascular disease, hypertension, or diabetes.

Appendix B reviews diet planning guidelines issued by the Canadian government for Canadians. In addition, Chapter 1 discussed *Healthy People 2010*, a U.S. federal agenda aimed at disease prevention and health promotion.

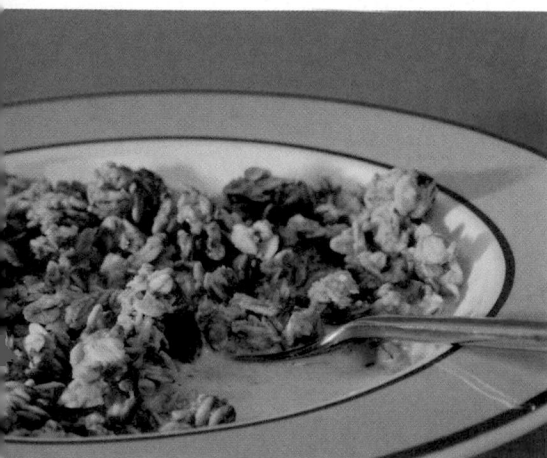

A daily serving of a whole-grain breakfast cereal provides a rich source of vitamins, minerals, and fiber for a diet.

beginning of Chapter 15; the chapter will then look at additional recommendations for adults 51 and older.

A Diet for the Adult Years

One diet approach that optimizes long-term nutritional health in adulthood emphasizes low-fat and fat-free dairy products, some lean meats and fish, plant proteins, a rich variety of fruits and vegetables, and generous amounts of whole-grain breads and cereals. MyPyramid, combined with the 2005 Dietary Guidelines for Americans discussed in Chapter 2, is one blueprint for this diet.

As noted in Chapter 2, the advice provided in those two resources refers to people two years and older:

- Consume a variety of nutrient-dense foods and beverages within and among the basic food groups of MyPyramid, while choosing foods that limit the intake of saturated and *trans* fats, cholesterol, added sugars, salt, and alcohol (if used). Foods to emphasize are vegetables, fruits, legumes (beans), whole-grain breads and cereals, and fat-free or low-fat milk or equivalent milk products.
- Maintain body weight in a healthy range by balancing calorie intake from foods and beverages with calories expended. For the latter, engage in at least 30 minutes of moderate-intensity physical activity, above usual activity, at work or home on most days of the week.
- Practice safe food handling when preparing food. This includes cleaning hands, food contact surfaces, and fruits and vegetables before preparation, and cooking foods to a safe temperature to kill microorganisms.

Beyond those general recommendations, here are a few specific nutrition tips to help promote successful aging:

- Women of childbearing age need to eat iron-rich foods, primarily to avoid developing iron-deficiency anemia. In addition, women who could become pregnant are advised to consume foods fortified with folic acid (total of 400 micrograms per day) or to take a supplement containing it, in addition to consuming folate-rich foods. Recall from Chapter 8 that this practice reduces the risk of some serious birth defects.
- Adults who seldom eat dairy products or other rich sources of calcium need a calcium supplement.
- Adults who eat no animal foods may need to take a supplement containing vitamin B-12.
- All adults could benefit from limiting their use of cured and smoked foods (see the Looking Further section on cancer in this chapter), obtaining adequate fluoride to promote dental health, and drinking plenty of fluids.

Some younger adults may benefit from a balanced multivitamin and mineral supplement to meet specific nutrient needs especially if on relatively low calorie diets (i.e., less than 1600 kcals per day). In addition, sometimes vitamins or minerals are prescribed to meet nutrient needs for various medical purposes. For example, pregnant women or those with heavy menstrual periods may be advised to take an iron supplement. Still, supplements of some nutrients, such as vitamin A and selenium, can be harmful if taken in large amounts. Because foods contain many phytochemical substances that promote health, one should use MyPyramid as a starting point when planning a diet, rather than depending mostly on supplements to meet nutrient needs.

Are Adults Following Current Dietary Recommendations?

In general, adults in North America are trying to follow many of the diet recommendations listed. Since the mid-1950s, they have consumed less saturated fat as more people substitute fat-free and low-fat milk for cream and whole milk. They eat more cheese, however, which is usually a concentrated form of saturated fat. Since 1963, they have eaten less butter, fewer eggs, less animal fat, and more vegetable oils and fish. These changes generally follow the recommendations to reduce the intake of saturated fat and cholesterol in favor of unsaturated fat choices. Today, animal breeders are raising much leaner cattle and hogs than those produced in 1950, which also helps reduce saturated fat intake.

Other aspects of the average adult diet are less promising. The latest nutrition survey of eating habits in the United States shows that the major contributors of calories to the adult diet are white bread, beef, doughnuts, cakes and cookies, soft drinks, milk, chicken, cheese, alcoholic beverages, salad dressing, mayonnaise, potatoes, and sugars/syrups/jams. If the trend in diets were truly toward decreasing sugar and saturated fat intake, and increasing fiber intake, many of these foods would not appear at the top of the list.

The overriding consideration should be quality and length of life and the impact dietary changes might have on them. Adults in general should learn more about risk factors for chronic diseases and do something about each one, when possible.

Concept Check

A basic plan to promote health and prevent disease includes eating a balanced, varied diet; performing regular physical activity; and limiting or abstaining from alcohol intake. Other recommendations are to maintain healthy weight; choose a diet low in saturated fat, *trans* fat, and cholesterol; choose a diet with plenty of vegetables, fruits, and whole-grain products; and limit use of sugars and salt. In addition, do not rely primarily on nutrient supplements to meet nutrient needs, but in some cases nutrient supplements can provide a useful addition to a diet.

Critical Thinking

The "fountain of youth" remains a mystery. Many people believe a source exists that can stop the aging process, allowing youth to remain. However, Neil, a history student, asserts that the fountain of youth is not a place or a particular thing but, rather, a combination of diet and lifestyle. How can he justify this claim?

A Closer Look at Middle Age and Older Adulthood

How long do your family members generally live? Of those who died early in adulthood, can you pinpoint some causes? Do you plan to live longer than your parents did or will? How long will that be? Some basic statistics can help you predict this.

■ Life Span

Life span refers to the maximum number of years a human can live. As far as we know, this hasn't changed in recorded time. The longest human life documented to date is 122 years for a woman and 114 years for a man. One's genes play a key role in determining longevity, but environment is also important. Note also by comparison that the domestic dog has a life span of 20 years; a rat, 5 years.

life span The potential oldest age a person can reach.

■ Life Expectancy

Life expectancy is the time an average person born in a specific year, such as 2005, can expect to live. Currently, life expectancy in North America is about 74 years for men and about 80 years for women, with a span of "healthy years" of about 64. Furthermore, if you survive to the age of 80, you can tack on another 7 to 10 years of life expectancy.

Worldwide, the highest average life expectancy is in Japan, 82 years for women and 76 years for men, especially on the island of Okinawa. Researchers suggest that their traditional Okinawan diet based on rice, fish, vegetable protein sources, fruits, vegetables, tea, herbs for seasonings, and small amounts of meat, as well as a generally low

life expectancy The average length of life for a given group of people born in a specific year (such as this year).

Besides having other long-lived family members, people who live to 100 years generally:

- Do not smoke, nor drink heavily
- Gain little weight in adulthood
- Eat many fruits and vegetables
- Perform daily physical activity
- Challenge their minds
- Have a positive outlook
- Maintain close friendships
- Are (or were) married (especially true for men)
- Have blood lipoproteins with a large particle size

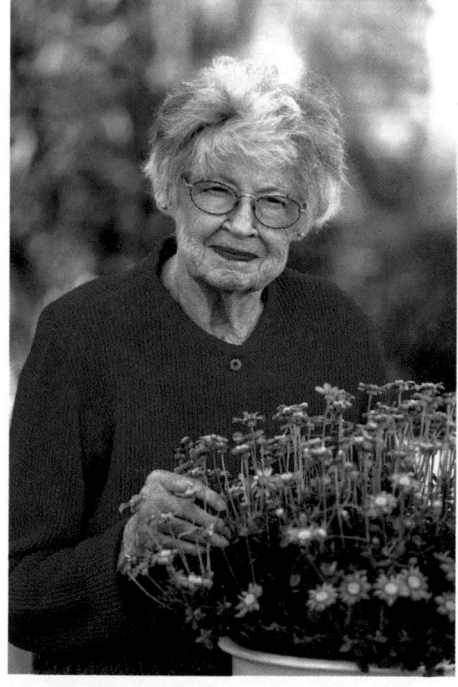

Of all North Americans who have lived to age 65, more than half are now alive.

reserve capacity The extent to which an organ can preserve essentially normal function despite decreasing cell number or cell activity.

calorie intake (BMI remains ≈ 21), contributes to this record longevity. Alcohol and salt intake is also minimal.

Life expectancy hasn't always been this long; for primitive humans, it was about 20 to 35 years. It increased to 40 years in Medieval England and increased to 49 years by the turn of the twentieth century. During the last 80 years, life expectancy for nearly all people has increased, mainly because of changes in the principal causes of death.

In the early 1900s, infectious diseases were the first three causes of death. Vaccines and antibiotics have tremendously lowered the rate of death from these causes. The decline in infant and childhood deaths, coupled with better diets and health care, has allowed more people to age first into maturity and then into older years. Now the principal causes of death in Western societies are related to cardiovascular diseases and cancer diseases that typically surface in middle age (review Table 1-2).

Historically, the trend in the United States, Canada, and other developed nations has been toward an ever older population. For example, during Colonial times, half of the U.S. population was over 16 years of age. By 1990, half were over 33. By 2050, half of the U.S. population could be over 43, and approximately 20% will be 65 years and older, twice as many as reach 65 today. This age—65 years—is arbitrarily listed as a dividing line for the beginning of later life because at this age one can currently qualify for full Social Security benefits in the United States. The time at which old age occurs, however, varies for each person, according to health and independence.

Among the older population, the group constituting those aged 85+ years is the fastest growing segment. Between 1997 and 2050, the population aged 85+ years in the United States is expected to increase from 3.4 million to 19 million. This is the first time in history North America and other Western nations will need to accommodate such a large population of older people. The associated expense will be enormous if a large percentage need special care because of ill health. Even more amazing, 1 million or more people in the United States alone could be over 100 years old in 2050.

■ The Graying of North America

This "graying" of North America poses some problems. Today, although people older than age 65 account for 13% of the U.S. population, they account for more than 25% of all prescription medications used, 40% of acute care hospital stays, and 50% of the federal health budget. Hip fractures alone cost the nation about $12 billion per year. (Note that regular physical activity reduces such risk.) Of older persons, 65% or more have nutrition-related problems, such as cardiovascular disease, type 2 diabetes, hypertension, and osteoporosis.

Postponing these chronic diseases for as long as possible will help control health care costs. The more independent, healthy years people live, the better life can be for them and the less they burden the health care system, which will be increasingly burdened by a growing older population. Keep in mind that aging is not a disease. Furthermore, diseases that commonly accompany old age—osteoporosis and atherosclerosis, for example—are not an inevitable part of aging. Many can be prevented or managed. Some people do die of old age, not as a direct result of disease.

■ What Actually Is Aging?

One view of aging describes it as processes of slow cell death, beginning soon after fertilization. When we are young, aging is not apparent because the major metabolic activities are geared toward growth and maturation. We produce plenty of active cells to meet physiological needs. During late adolescence and adulthood, the body's major task is to maintain cells. Inevitably, though, cells age and die. Eventually, as more cells die, the body can't adjust to meet all physiological demands, and body functioning begins to decrease (Fig. 15-1). Still, organs usually retain enough **reserve capacity** that,

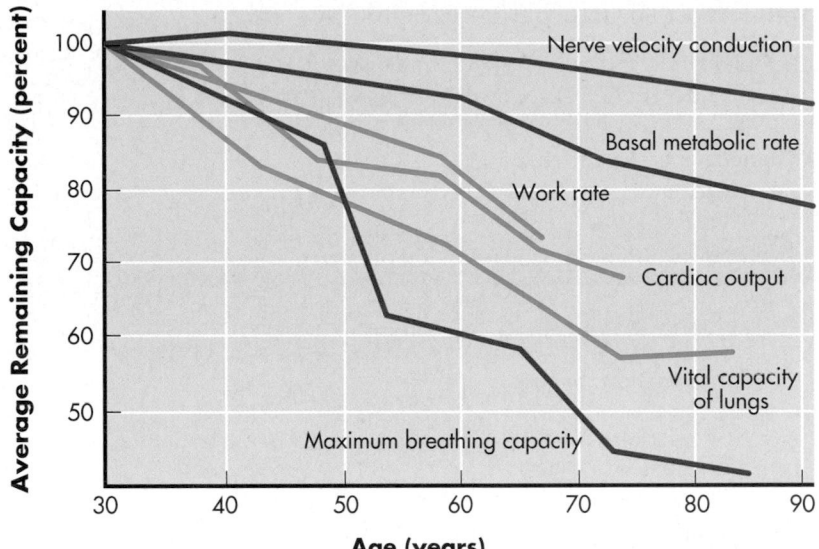

Figure 15-1 Declines in physiological function seen with aging. The decline in many body functions is especially evident in sedentary people.

for a long time, the body shows no outward disease. Although no symptoms appear, subclinical disease may develop, and, if the disease is allowed to progress unchecked, organ function and then body function eventually deteriorate noticeably.

The aging process is clearly illustrated by changes for many people in the function of the enzyme lactase. For some people, lactase activity in the small intestine slows during childhood. Generally, however, clear symptoms of this decline—gas and bloating after milk consumption—do not appear until adulthood. Although lactase output decreases in these cases, perhaps from birth, enough enzyme is present to digest the lactose consumed until adulthood.

Cells age probably because of automatic cellular changes and environmental influences. Even in the most supportive of environments, cell structure and function inevitably change with time. Eventually, cells lose their ability to regenerate the internal parts they need, and they die. This inevitable dying off of deteriorating cells is actually beneficial, as researchers have concluded it likely prevents diseases such as cancer.

Unfortunately, there are negative consequences to this natural cell progression, because as more and more cells in an organ system die, organ function decreases. For example, **kidney nephrons** are continually lost as we age. In some people, this loss leads to eventual kidney failure, but most of us maintain sufficient kidney cells to allow the organ to function throughout life. Again, in aging, there is first a reduction in reserve capacity. Only after the reserve capacity is exhausted does actual organ function noticeably decrease.

The causes of aging are still a mystery. Most likely, the physiological changes of aging are the sum of natural processes, as listed in Table 15-1, and lifestyle practices. Even very healthy people have a shortened life expectancy if they are exposed to sufficient environmental stress, such as radiation and certain chemical agents (e.g., industrial solvents). Because cell aging and diseases such as cancer are aggravated by environmental factors, it makes good sense to avoid such risks as excessive sunlight exposure and hazardous chemicals. Adopting diet and lifestyle practices that minimize a decline in body function in the adult years is an investment in your future health. You can obtain a free fact sheet from the website for the National Institute on Aging at www.nia.nih.gov or by calling (800) 222-2225. The first Rate Your Plate activity in this chapter outlines a comprehensive approach to healthful aging.

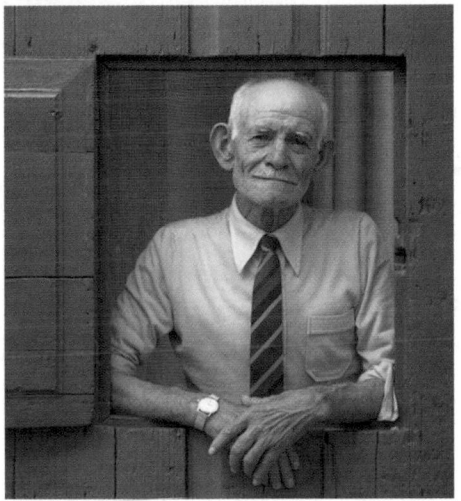

A diet based on vegetables, fruits, pasta, and olive oil as a source of fat—with a small amount of alcohol in the form of red wine—contributes to the many healthy years of life of southern Italians. Their active lifestyle is an additional contributing factor.

kidney nephrons The units of kidney cells that filter wastes from the bloodstream and deposit them into the urine.

Table 15-1 Current Hypotheses about the Causes of Aging

Errors occur in copying the genetic blueprint (DNA).

Once sufficient errors in DNA copying accumulate, a cell can no longer synthesize the major proteins needed to function, and it therefore dies.

Connective tissue stiffens.

Parallel protein strands, found mostly in connective tissue, cross-link to each other. This decreases flexibility in key body components.

Electron-seeking compounds damage cell parts.

Electron-seeking free radicals can break down cell membranes and proteins. One way to prevent some damage from these compounds is to consume adequate amounts of vitamins E and C, selenium, and carotenoids.

Hormone function changes.

The blood concentration of many hormones, such as testosterone in men, falls during the aging process. Replacement of these and other hormones is possible, but the resulting risks and benefits are largely unknown.

Glycosylation of proteins.

Blood glucose, when chronically elevated, attaches to (glycates) various blood and body proteins. This decreases protein function and can encourage immune system attack on such altered proteins.

The immune system loses some efficiency.

The immune system is most efficient during childhood and young adulthood, but with advancing age it is less able to recognize and counteract foreign substances, such as viruses, that enter the body. Nutrient deficiencies, particularly of protein, vitamin E, vitamin B-6, and zinc, also hamper immune function.

Autoimmunity develops.

Autoimmune reactions occur when white blood cells and other immune system components begin to attack body tissues in addition to foreign proteins. Many diseases, including some forms of arthritis, involve this autoimmune response.

Death is programmed into the cell.

Each human cell can divide only about 50 times. Once this total number of divisions occurs, the cell automatically succumbs.

Excess calorie intake speeds body breakdown.

Underfed animals, such as spiders, mice, and rats, live longer. Usual calorie intake must be reduced by about 30% to see this effect.

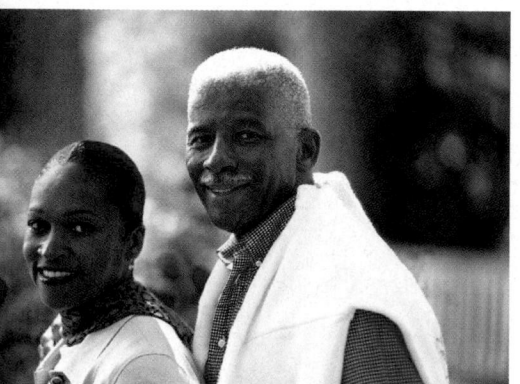

Many older adults are healthy. The goal is to remain that way as long as possible.

Concept Check

Although life span has not changed, life expectancy has increased dramatically over the past century. In many societies, this means an increasing proportion of the North American population is over 65 years of age and will live for decades longer. Avoiding continually rising health care costs and maximizing satisfaction with life require postponing and minimizing chronic illness. Aging begins early in life and probably results from both automatic cellular changes and environmental influences. Diet and regular physical activity can play a role in slowing such processes.

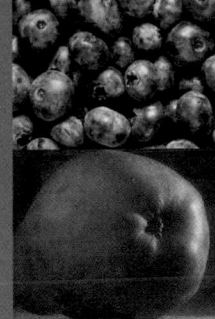

Cancer is currently the second leading cause of death for North American adults. It is further estimated that more than 1500 people die each day of cancer in the United States alone. Cancer-related expenses exceed $100 billion each year. The top four cancers, causing more than 50% of cancer deaths, are lung, colorectal, breast, and prostate cancers. Of those, lung cancer in female smokers is the only form that is increasing on a yearly basis.

Cancer is actually many diseases; these differ in the types of cells affected and, in some cases, in the factors contributing to cancer development (Fig. 15-2). For example, the factors leading to skin cancer differ from those leading to breast cancer. Similarly, the treatments for the different types of cancer often vary.

Cancer essentially represents abnormal and uncontrollable division of cells that results from mutations in DNA. This initiates the cancer process. The cells then go through a variety of steps (called promotion and progression). A cancer cell is the final result. Without effective treatment, cancer then typically leads to death. Most cancers take the form of tumors, although not all tumors are cancers. A **tumor** is simply spontaneous new tissue growth that serves no physiological purpose. It can be **benign,** like a wart, or **malignant,** like most lung cancers. The terms *malignant tumor* and *malignant neoplasm* are synonymous with cancer.

Whereas benign tumors are only dangerous if their presence interferes with normal body functions, malignant (cancerous) tumors are capable of invading surrounding structures, including blood vessels, the lymph system, and nervous tissue. Cancer can also spread, or **metastasize,** to distant sites via the blood and lymphatic circulation, thereby producing

benign Noncancerous; tumors that do not spread.

malignant Malicious; in reference to a tumor, the property of spreading locally and to distant sites.

metastasize The spreading of disease from one part of the body to another, even to parts of the body that are remote from the site of the original tumor. Cancer cells can spread via blood vessels, the lymphatic system, or direct growth of the tumor.

Estimated % of Cancer Deaths for 2004		
Male		**Female**
<1%	Brain	2%
4%	Esophagus and stomach	<1%
32%	Lung	25%
	Breast	15%
3%	Liver	<1%
5%	Pancreas	6%
9%	Leukemia and lymphomas	9%
10%	Colon and rectum	10%
6%	Urinary	
	Ovary	6%
10%	Prostate	
	Uterus and cervix	3%
25%	All others (e.g., oral and skin) (e.g., oral, skin, and bladder)	24%

Figure 15-2 Cancer is actually many diseases. Numerous types of cells and organs are its target. Note that about one-third of all cancers arise from smoking (primarily lung cancer).

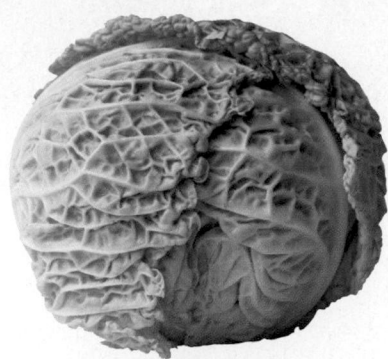

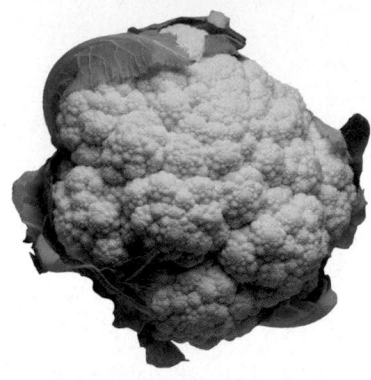

Cruciferous vegetables such as cabbage and cauliflower are rich in cancer-preventing phytochemicals.

endometrium The membrane that lines the inside of the uterus. It increases in thickness during the menstrual cycle until ovulation occurs. The surface layers are shed during menstruation if conception does not take place.

invasive tumors in almost any part of the body. Metastasis then makes the cancer much more difficult to treat. The fact that cancer can spread explains why early detection of cancer is so important. Cancers that can be diagnosed in the early stages are those in the colon, breast, and cervix.

Both genetics and lifestyle are potent forces that influence the risk for developing cancer. A genetic predisposition is especially important in development of colon cancer, some types of breast cancer (e.g., mutated BRCA1 or BRCA2 gene) and prostate cancer (35%, 27%, and 42%, respectively). About 30 cancer-susceptibility genes have been identified. However, experts estimate that only 1% to 5% of most cancers can be explained by the inheritance of a cancer gene. Overall, lifestyle is also a critical factor in most forms of cancer, as evidenced by the variation in cancer rates from country to country. In fact, diet likely accounts for 30% to 40% or more of all cancers.

Although we have little control over our genetic risks for cancer, we can exert a great deal of authority when making decisions about lifestyle risks, especially with regard to smoking, alcohol abuse, physical activity, and nutrient intake (food choice). It is well established that one-third of all cancers in North America are due directly to tobacco use. About half of the cancers of the mouth, pharynx, and larynx are associated with heavy use of alcohol. A combination of alcohol use and smoking increases cancer risks even higher.

A Closer Look at Diet and Cancer

Some food constituents may contribute to cancer development, whereas others have a protective effect (Table 15-2). First the association between fat/calorie intake and cancer risk is discussed, and then some of the food constituents that may reduce the risk for cancer are presented.

■ Contribution of Calorie and Fat Intakes to Cancer Risk

An excess calorie intake, leading eventually to obesity, is related to all major forms of cancer, except of lung cancer. This is the main diet-cancer risk factor. This includes cancer of the breast (especially in postmenopausal women), pancreas, kidney, gallbladder, colon, **endometrium,** and prostate gland. The link probably occurs between adipose tissue and the synthesis of estrogen. High concentrations of circulating estrogen in the blood over time promote cancer. Excess insulin output resulting from an obese, insulin-resistant state is also implicated.

The National Cancer Institute (NCI) also believes there is sufficient evidence for a link between dietary fat and cancer to encourage North Americans to reduce fat intake. It recommends initially decreasing dietary fat to about 30% of total calorie intake and eventually to 20% or less of total calories if the person is at high risk and can follow such a dietary pattern.

Some scientists, however, believe that the NCI has overreacted to the fat and cancer issue. Although epidemiological evidence does link fat and certain forms of cancer, the evidence is not strong. A stronger link actually exists between cancer and total calories in the diet. In animal experiments, restricting total calorie intake to about 70% of usual intake results in about a 40% reduction in tumor development, regardless of the amount of fat in the diet. Calorie restriction is currently the most effective technique for preventing cancer in laboratory animals.

Unfortunately, it is very difficult for humans to reduce dietary calories to 70% of usual intake. So while the data obtained from laboratory animal studies are interesting, nutritionists do not see any practical way to make recommendations on the basis of these studies. In addition, once cancer is present, calorie restriction is no longer helpful.

■ Cancer-Inhibiting Food Constituents

Many single nutrients may have cancer-inhibiting properties. These anticarcinogens include antioxidants and certain phytochemicals (review Table 15-2).

Table 15-2 Some Food Constituents Suspected of Having a Role in Cancer

Constituent	Dietary Sources	Action
Possibly Protective*		
Vitamin A	Liver, fortified milk, fruits, vegetables	Encourages normal cell development.
Vitamin D	Fortified milk	Increases production of a protein which suppresses cell growth, such as in the colon.
Vitamin E	Whole grains, vegetable oils, green, leafy vegetables	Prevents formation of nitrosamines and general antioxidant properties.
Vitamin C	Fruits, vegetables	Can block conversion of nitrites and nitrates to potent carcinogens and likely has general antioxidant properties.
Folate	Fruits, vegetables, whole grains	Encourages normal cell development; especially reduces the risk of colon cancer.
Selenium	Meats, whole grains	Part of antioxidant system that inhibits tumor growth and kills developing cancer cells.
Carotenoids, such as lycopene	Fruits, vegetables	Likely act as antioxidants; some of these possibly influence cell metabolism. Lycopene in particular may reduce the risk of prostate cancer.
Indoles, phenols, and other phytochemical substances	Vegetables, especially cabbage, cauliflower, broccoli, brussels sprouts, garlic, onions, tea	May reduce cancer in the stomach and other organs.
Calcium	Milk products, green vegetables	Slows cell division in the colon, binds bile acids and free fatty acids, thus reducing colon cancer risk.
Omega-3 fatty acids	Cold-water fish, such as salmon and tuna	May inhibit tumor growth.
Soy products	Tofu, soy milk, tempeh, soy nuts	Phytic acid present possibly binds carcinogens in the intestinal tract; the genistein component possibly reduces growth and metastasis of malignant cells.
Conjugated linoleic acid	Milk products, meats	May inhibit tumor development and act as an antioxidant.
Fiber-rich foods	Fruits, vegetables, whole-grain breads and cereals, beans, nuts	Colon and rectal cancer risk may be decreased by accelerating intestinal transit of binding carcinogens such that they are excreted.
Possibly Carcinogenic		
Excessive calorie intake	All macronutrients can contribute.	Excess fat mass leading to obesity; linked to increased synthesis of estrogen and other sex hormones, which in excess may themselves increase the risk for cancer. Resulting excess insulin output from creation of an insulin-resistant state is also implicated.
Total fat	Meats, high-fat milk and milk products, animal fats and vegetable oils	The strongest evidence is for excessive saturated and polyunsaturated fat intake. Saturated fat is linked to an increased risk of prostate cancer.
High glycemic load carbohydrates	Cookies, cakes, sugared soft drinks, candy	Insulin surges associated with these foods may increase tumor growth, such as in the colon.
Alcohol	Beer, wine, liquor	Contributes to cancers of the throat, liver, bladder, breast, and colon (especially if the person does not consume enough folate).
Nitrites, nitrates	Cured meats, especially ham, bacon, and sausages	Under very high temperatures will bind to amino acid derivatives to form nitrosamines, potent carcinogens.
Multi-ring compounds: Aflatoxin	Formed when mold is present on peanuts or grains	May alter DNA structure and inhibit its ability to properly respond to physiologic controls; aflatoxin in particular is linked to liver cancer.
Benzo(a)pyrene and other heterocyclic amines	Charcoal-broiled foods, especially meats	Linked to stomach and colon cancer. To limit this risk, trim fat from meat before cooking, cut barbecuing time by partially cooking meat (such as in a microwave oven), and don't consume blackened parts.

*Many of the actions listed for these possibly protective agents are speculative and have been verified only by experimental animal studies. The best evidence supports obtaining these nutrients and other food constituents from foods. Recently the U.S. Preventive Services Task Force (USPSTF) supported this statement, noting there is no clear evidence that nutrient supplements provide the same benefits.

nitrosamine A carcinogen formed from nitrates and breakdown products of amino acids; can lead to stomach cancer.

The antioxidant activity of vitamin C and vitamin E helps to prevent formation of **nitrosamines** in the GI tract, thus preventing formation of a potent carcinogen. Vitamin E also helps protect unsaturated fatty acids from damage by free radicals. Overall, carotenoids, vitamin E, vitamin C, and selenium function as or contribute to antioxidant protection for the body. Some of these antioxidant systems help prevent DNA mutations by electron-seeking compounds, which is the main way that cancer develops in the first place.

In addition, phytochemicals from fruits and vegetables, and even tea, block cancer development in some types of cells. Numerous studies suggest that fruit and vegetable intake reduces the risk of nearly all types of cancer. These foods are normally rich in carotenoids, vitamin C, and vitamin E. Adequate vitamin D intake is suspected of reducing breast, colon, prostate, and other forms of cancer. Calcium is also linked to a decreased risk for developing colon cancer. In sum, a diet that follows MyPyramid, so that fruits, vegetables, whole grains, low-fat and fat-free dairy products, and some plant oils are eaten daily, is aimed at cancer prevention. It is likely that all of these foods have a "cocktail" effect, and that no one particular food can make as strong a claim.

The Bottom Line

A variety of dietary changes will reduce your risk for cancer. Start by making sure that your diet is moderate in calorie and fat content and that you consume many fruits and vegetables, whole-grain breads and cereals, beans, some fish, and low-fat or fat-free milk products. In addition, remain physically active, avoid obesity, consume alcohol in moderation (if at all), and limit intake of animal fat and salt-cured, smoked, and nitrate-cured foods.

Remember also that if a cancer is left untreated, it can spread quickly throughout the body. When this happens, it is much more likely to lead to death. Thus early detection is critical. Aids to early detection include the following warning signs (acronym is CAUTION):

- A change in bowel or bladder habits
- A sore that does not heal
- Unusual bleeding or discharge
- A thickening or lump in the breast or elsewhere
- Indigestion or difficulty in swallowing
- An obvious change in a wart or mole
- A nagging cough or hoarseness

Unexplained weight loss is an additional warning sign.

There are still other ways to detect cancer early. Colonoscopy examinations for middle-age and older adults, PSA (prostate-specific antigen) tests for middle-age and older men, and Papanicolaou tests (Pap smears) and regular breast examinations (and mammograms starting about age 40) for women are recommended by the American Cancer Society. Finally, to learn still more about cancer, review these sources of credible cancer information on the Internet:

American Cancer Society
www.cancer.org
CancerNet
www.icic.nci.nih.gov
Oncolink
cancer.med.upenn.edu
Harvard University Center for Cancer Prevention
www.yourcancerrisk.harvard.edu

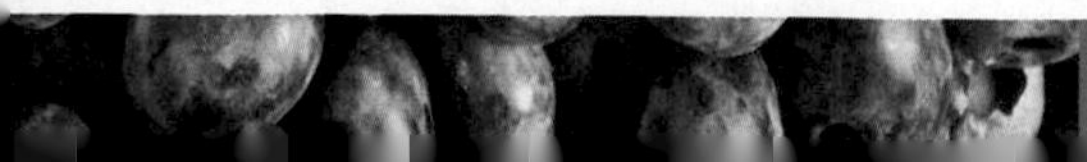

Nutritional Implications of Aging

There is more variation in health status among adults over age 50 than in any other age group. This means that chronological age is not useful in predicting physical health status (physiological age). Among people age 70 and over, some are totally "independent, healthy people, whereas others are frail and require almost total care. To predict the nutritional problems of an older person, it is necessary to know the extent of physiological change caused by aging and whether the person shows early warning signs for long-term poor nutrition. As you examine how aging affects body systems and how these changes contribute to nutritional health, note the suggested ways to lessen health risks (Table 15-3).

Table 15-3 Typical Physiological Changes of Aging and Recommended Diet and Lifestyle Responses

Physiological Changes	Recommended Responses
Appetite (↓)	• Monitor weight and strive to eat enough to maintain healthy weight. • Use meal replacement products, such as Boost® and Ensure Plus®.
Sense of taste and smell (↓)	• Vary the diet. • Experiment with herbs and spices.
Chewing ability (↓)	• Work with a dentist to maximize chewing ability. • Modify food consistency as necessary. • Eat calorie-rich snacks.
Sense of thirst (↓)	• Consume plenty of fluid each day. • Stay alert for evidence of dehydration (e.g., minimal output or dark-colored urine) Note that dehydration can lead to many problems, especially in older adults.
Bowel function (↓)	• Consume enough fiber daily, choosing primarily fruits, vegetables, and whole-grain breads and cereals. • Meet fluid needs.
Lactase production (↓)	• Limit milk serving size at each use. • Substitute yogurt or cheese for milk. • Use reduced-lactose or lactose-free products. • Seek nondairy calcium sources.
Iron status (↓)	• Include some lean meat and iron-fortified foods in the diet. • Ask physician to monitor blood iron status.
Liver function (↓)	• Consume alcohol in moderation, if at all. • Avoid consuming excess vitamin A.
Insulin function (↓)	• Maintain healthy body weight. • Perform regular physical activity.
Kidney function (↓)	• If necessary, work with physician and registered dietitian to modify protein and other nutrients in diet.
Immune function (↓)	• Meet nutrient needs, especially protein, vitamin E, vitamin B-6, and zinc. • Perform regular physical activity.
Lung function (↓)	• Avoid tobacco products. • Perform regular physical activity.

(Continued)

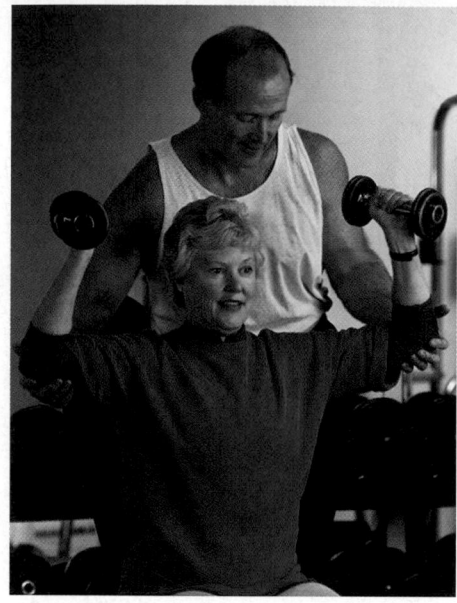

Older people benefit from both aerobic and strength-training (resistance) exercises. Strength-training especially helps reverse some of the decline in daily function associated with the muscle loss typically seen in older adulthood.

Table 15-3 *(continued)*

Physiological Changes	Recommended Responses
Vision (↓)	• Regularly consume sources of carotenoids, vitamin C, vitamin E, and zinc (e.g., fruits, vegetables and whole-grain breads and cereals). • Moderate total fat intake. • Wear sunglasses in sunny conditions. • Avoid tobacco products. • Perform regular physical activity (to lessen insulin resistance). • In the case of diagnosed moderate macular degeneration, talk with a physician about following a protocol of zinc, copper, vitamin E, vitamin C, and beta-carotene supplementation.
Lean tissue (↓)	• Meet nutrient needs, especially protein and vitamin D. • Perform regular physical activity, including strength training.
Cardiovascular function (↓)	• Use diet modifications or physician-prescribed medications to keep blood lipids and blood pressure within desirable ranges. • Stay physically active. • Achieve and maintain a healthy body weight.
Bone mass (↓)	• Meet nutrient needs, especially calcium and vitamin D (regular sun exposure helps meet needs for vitamin D). • Perform regular physical activity, especially weight-bearing exercise. • Women should consider use of approved osteoporosis medications at menopause. • Remain at a healthy weight (especially avoid unneeded weight loss).
Mental function (↓)	• Meet nutrient needs, especially for vitamin E, vitamin C, vitamin B-6, folate, and vitamin B-12. • Strive for lifelong learning. • Perform regular physical activity. • Obtain adequate sleep. • Follow a healthy dietary pattern.
Fat stores (↑)	• Avoid overeating. • Perform regular physical activity.

Registered dietitians, physicians, and pharmacists can help with any needed adjustments arising from these and other drug-related problems.

■ Medications Influence Nutrient Needs

Medications and old age often go together. Medications can improve health and quality of life, but some of them also profoundly affect nutrient needs at all ages, including the later years. Two-thirds of older adults take prescription drugs; one-half of the older adult population regularly take multiple prescription drugs. Many drugs affect appetite or the absorption of nutrients. Often, people must take medications for long periods. They should make sure to work with their physician and pharmacist to coordinate all medications taken. Pharmacists can advise when to take drugs—with or between meals—for maximum effectiveness.

Drug-related nutritional problems include:

- Increased need for potassium when certain types of diuretics increase its excretion from the body
- Changes in appetite caused by certain antidepressant agents and antibiotics
- Increased iron needs due to blood loss from the long-term use of aspirin or aspirin-like medications

■ Alternative Medicine and Aging

Adults in general and older adults in particular may be interested in using various herbal remedies. Recall from Chapter 1 that these products are not evaluated by FDA for effectiveness or safety since they fall under the regulation of the 1994 Dietary Supplement Health and Education Act (DSHEA). Purity and quantity of the product in the bottle are also suspect. Table 15-4 reviews some popular herbal remedies. Note from the table that these products can pose health risks in certain people. In addition, they may be expensive, ($100.00 per month or more in some cases) and are not covered by health insurance plans. Because of expense and questionable benefits, use of many herbal products has declined. In 2003, sales of ginseng and St. John's wort declined by 30% and 38%, respectively.

A rational approach to the use of herbal products is to use only one product at a time, keep a diary of symptoms, and check with one's physician first before discontinuing a prescribed medication. In addition, FDA advises anyone who experiences adverse side effects from an herbal remedy to contact a physician. Physicians are then encouraged to report such adverse events to FDA, state and local health departments, and consumer protection agencies.

For additional information about herbal remedies, access the following websites. These are regularly updated and cover the herbals listed in Table 15-4, as well as many others.

Alternative Medicine Foundation
www.amfoundation.org/
The NCCAM Complementary and Alternative Medicine (CAM) Citation Index (CI)
nccam.nih.gov/nccam/resources/cam-ci/
American Botanical Council
www.herbalgram.org/
Complementary and Alternative Medicine Program at Stanford (CAMPS)
scrdp.stanford.edu/camps.html
Center for Complementary and Alternative Medicine Research in Asthma, located at
   the University of California, Davis
www.camra.ucdavis.edu/
National Institutes of Health Office of Dietary Supplements
ods.od.nih.gov/
Natural Medicine Comprehensive Database
www.naturaldatabase.com

■ Depression in Older Adults

Depression occurs in about 12% to 30% of nursing home residents and 17% to 37% of older adults who reside outside of nursing homes. Depression can be a downward spiral in which poor appetite produces weakness, which leads to even poorer appetite (Fig. 15-3). Depression—combined with isolation and loneliness as family and friends die, move away, or become less mobile—frequently contributes to apathetic eating and weight loss. People living alone do not necessarily make poor food choices, but they often consume too few calories, in part by skipping meals. Older men are especially prone to this habit. In older adults, the resulting poor nutritional state can produce further mental confusion and increased isolation and loneliness.

If depression is left untreated, it is estimated that 15% of the cases may be fatal (suicide). Depression may signal an underlying illness and can also impair recovery from existing illnesses or injuries. For these reasons, early detection of depression is important in older adults. Depression is often treatable, but medication alone will not help those who are experiencing major life changes, such as the death of a spouse. Adequate social support also is essential.

Numerous reports have documented significant health risks associated with the use of some herbal and alternative remedies, sometimes resulting in death. Studies especially implicate germander, pokeroot, sassafras, mandrake, pennyroyal, comfrey, chaparral, yohimbe, lobelia, jin bu huan, kava kava, products containing stephanie and magnolia, senna, hai gen fen, paraguay tea, kombucha tea, tung shueh (Chinese black balls), and willow bark.

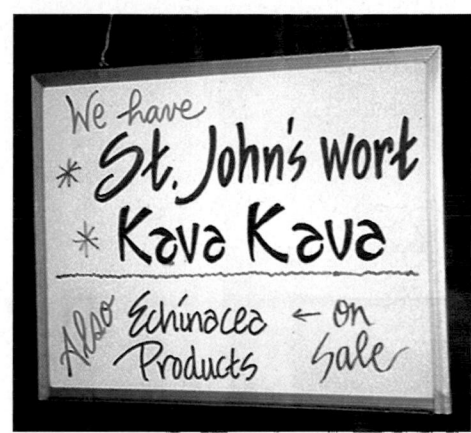

Some herbal products are effective for treating specific medical problems. Follow label instructions carefully. Note potential side effects listed, as well as who should not use the product. The best advice is to only use these substances under strict supervision of a physician.

Critical Thinking

Jamila went to her local pharmacy yesterday to look for a product to help her stay awake while studying. On the shelves she found a dietary supplement claiming to be a Chinese herbal remedy for sleepiness and fatigue. She thought that since a pharmacy carried the product, it should be safe, and work as indicated on the label.

Is she correct in these assumptions? Are there specific risks associated with taking such herbal remedies?

Table 15-4 A Close Look at Some Popular Herbal Remedies

Product	Purported Effects	Side Effects	Who Should Especially Seek Physician Guidance Before Use
Black cohosh	• Reduction of postmenopausal symptoms (shown to be effective in some but not all women; use should not go beyond 6 months in general)	• Nausea • Fall in blood pressure	• Women who have had breast cancer • Women who are pregnant • Anyone taking estrogen, hypertension medications, or blood-thinning medications*
Cranberry	• Prevention or treatment of urinary tract infections (some evidence of efficacy)	• Use of concentrated tablets may increase risk of kidney stones	• People who are susceptible to kidney stones • Anyone taking antidepressants or prescription painkillers
Echinacea	• Stimulation of the immune system • Prevention or treatment of colds or other infections (mild effect at best)	• Nausea • Skin irritation • Allergic reactions • Minor GI tract upset • Increased urination	• Anyone with an autoimmune disease • Pre- or postsurgical patients • Anyone with allergies to daisies
Garlic	• Antibiotic properties • Slight reduction of blood cholesterol or blood pressure in some, but not all, studies	• GI tract upset (e.g., heartburn, flatulence) • Unpleasant odor	• Pre- or postsurgical patients • Perinatal women • People with a history of gallstones • Anyone taking blood-thinning medications or AIDS medications
Ginkgo biloba	• Increased circulation • Improvement of memory (especially for people with Alzheimer's disease; effect is mild at best)	• Mild headache • GI tract upset • Irritability • Reduced blood clotting • Seizures (if contaminated with toxic ginkgo seeds)	• People with bleeding disorders • Pre- or postsurgical patients • Anyone with allergies to the plant • Concurrent use of feverfew, garlic, ginseng, dong quai, or red clover • Anyone taking diabetes medications, blood-thinning medications or vitamin E supplements, antidepressants, or diuretics
Ginseng	• Increased energy • Stress relief • Decreased weakness and fatigue (efficacy largely unknown)	• Hypertension • Asthma attacks • Irregular heartbeat • Insomnia • Headache • Nervousness • GI tract upset • Reduced blood clotting • Menstrual irregularities and breast tenderness	• In general, anyone who takes a prescription drug should consult a physician before using ginseng. • Women on hormone replacement therapy • Women who have had breast cancer • Anyone with chronic GI tract disease • Anyone with uncontrolled hypertension • Anyone taking blood-thinning medications, diabetes medications, antidepressants, or heart failure medications

Figure 15-3 The decline of health often seen in older adults. This decline needs to be prevented whenever possible.

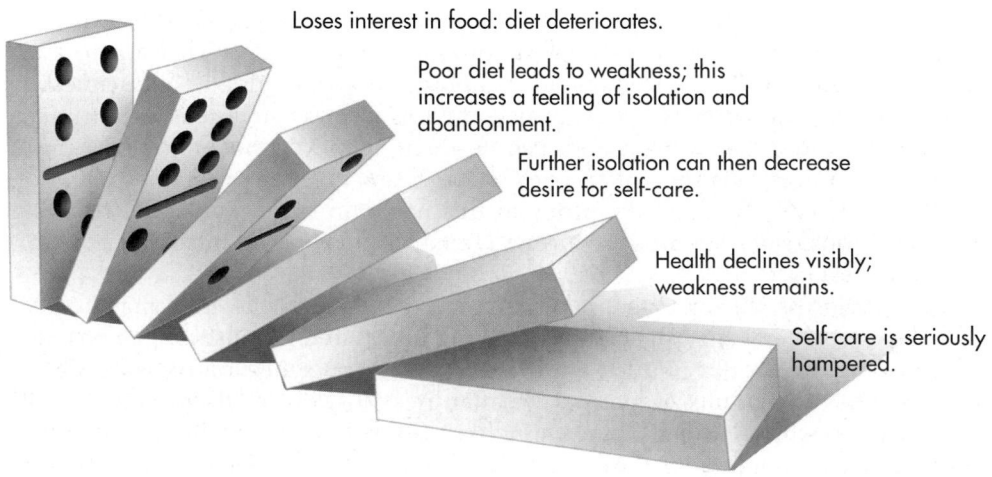

Social isolation; perhaps spouse has died.

Loses interest in food: diet deteriorates.

Poor diet leads to weakness; this increases a feeling of isolation and abandonment.

Further isolation can then decrease desire for self-care.

Health declines visibly; weakness remains.

Self-care is seriously hampered.

Table 15-4 *(continued)*

Product	Purported Effects	Side Effects	Who Should Especially Seek Physician Guidance Before Use
Glucosamine	• May decrease joint inflammation and pain associated with osteoarthritis	• GI tract discomfort, which may disappear after 2 weeks	• May disrupt blood glucose regulation in people with diabetes
Saw palmetto	• Reduction of symptoms of enlarged prostate gland (shown to be effective in some people)	When taken in large doses: • Mild GI tract upset • Headache • Feminization	• People with bleeding disorders • Pre- or postsurgery patients • People with chronic GI tract diseases • Anyone taking blood-thinning medications, vitamin E supplements, or medications to treat benign prostate hypertrophy
St. John's wort	• Alleviation of depression (mild effect at best)	• Mild GI tract upset • Rash • Tiredness • Restlessness • Increased sensitivity to sunlight	• In general, anyone who takes a prescription drug • People with UV sensitivity, including that induced by medications or other treatments** • People with bipolar disorder • Anyone recovering from a graft or organ transplant • Anyone taking ritalin, caffeine, HIV medications, heart failure medications, cholesterol-lowering medications, blood-thinning medications, chemotherapy, oral contraceptives, antidepressants, antipsychotic medications, or asthma medications
Valerian	• Alleviation of restlessness and other sleeping disorders that stem from nervous conditions • Reduction of anxiety (some evidence of effect)	• Impaired attention • Headache • Morning grogginess • Irregular heartbeat • GI tract upset • Disagreeable odor • Withdrawal delerium	• Anyone taking central nervous system depressants*** • Anyone who drinks alcohol • People about to operate heavy machinery or drive

Note that pregnant or breastfeeding women, children under 2 years of age, anyone over the age of 65 years, and anyone with a chronic disease should never take supplements unless under the guidance of a physician. A recent concern also has been raised with regard to patients who abruptly end alternative medicines at the start of hospital treatments or simply deny that they are involved in alternative therapy. Interactions between alternative therapies and pharmaceutical drugs can be drastic and include complications such as delirium, clotting abnormalities, and rapid heartbeat, resulting in the need for intensive care. If these patients had disclosed their treatments, many of the complications could have been prevented. Experts recommend that, if time permits, patients stop taking herbal products for about a week before a scheduled surgery or otherwise take all original supplement containers to the hospital, so that the anesthesiologist can evaluate what was taken.

*Coumadin, aspirin, Heparin, Lovenox, or Fragmin

**Sulfa medications, anti-inflammatory medications, or acid-reflux medications

***Valium, halcion, seconal

■ Alcoholism in Older Adults

Alcoholism is a pervasive problem in our society, including the older population. Approximately two-thirds of alcohol abusers turn to alcohol much earlier in life and simply continue the habit. About one-third begin later in life, due to a variety of factors—more free time, social events centered around drinking, loneliness, or depression. Some of the symptoms of alcoholism in older persons include trembling hands, slurred speech, sleep problems, memory loss, and unsteady gait; these can be easily overlooked simply because they are similar to symptoms of old age.

Older adults become intoxicated from a smaller amount of alcohol than when they were younger because they metabolize alcohol more slowly and have lower amounts of body water than young adults in which to dilute the alcohol. As well, even small amounts of alcohol can react negatively with various medications that many older persons take routinely. And in addition to having adverse effects on the liver, drinking

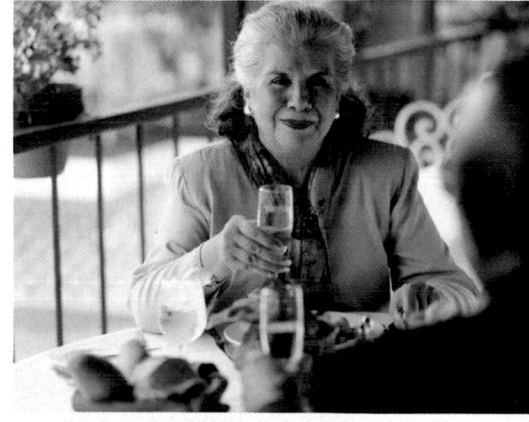

The limit for alcohol intake for older adults is one drink per day.

large amounts of alcohol increases the risk of hemorrhagic stroke and may worsen hypertension in older adults. Since drinking large amounts of alcohol produces adverse effects, people over the age of 65 should limit alcohol consumption to no more than one drink per day. Recall from Chapter 7 that one drink is defined as 5 ounces of wine, 12 ounces of beer, or 1.5 ounce shot of 80-proof liquor.

Ten Warning Signs of Alzheimer's Disease

1. Recent memory loss that affects job performance
2. Difficulty performing familiar tasks
3. Problems with language
4. Disorientation to time and place
5. Faulty or decreased judgment
6. Problems with abstract thinking
7. Tendency to misplace things
8. Changes in mood or behavior
9. Changes in personality
10. Loss of initiative

Aging is no reason to withdraw from life. Learning and practicing new skills throughout life is important. This can include perhaps volunteering services to the community or helping one's friends.

Another Bite

Alzheimer's disease often takes a terrible toll on the mental and eventual physical health of older people. About 4.5 million adults in the United States have the disease. In general terms, Alzheimer's disease is a type of dementia best described as a progressive brain disorder marked by an inability to remember, reason, or comprehend. Age is the primary risk factor. Scientists propose causes, including alterations in cell development or protein production in the brain, strokes, altered composition of lipoproteins in the blood (e.g., apo E4), as well as poor blood glucose regulation (e.g., diabetes), high blood pressure, and high blood cholesterol. Meeting needs for vitamin E, vitamin C, vitamin B-6, folate, and vitamin B-12 is especially important. For caregivers, several nutrition recommendations should be considered in meal preparation. Food intake should be monitored to ensure maintenance of a healthy weight and nutritional state. Other tips are consuming fruits and vegetables in abundance, including fish in meals twice per week, minimizing saturated and *trans* fat intake, and making sure meal habits do not pose a health risk (e.g., holding food in one's mouth or forgetting to swallow). Regular physical activity has also been shown to improve mental status in people afflicted by this disease. Four medications (e.g. donepezil [Aricept]) have been approved to treat the disease; their effects are modest at best.

The ten warning signs of Alzheimer's disease are listed in the margin. Preventive measures for Alzheimer's disease focus on maintaining brain activity through lifelong learning. Experimental therapies include regular use of ibuprofen. Recent studies cast doubt on other popular approaches, such as megadose vitamin E use. To find out more about Alzheimer's disease, you can go to the website for the Alzheimer's Association at www.alz.org, or call (800) 272-3900. You can also call the Alzheimer's Disease Education and Referral Center of the National Institute of Aging at (800) 428-4380.

Concept Check

Nutritional problems common to aging adults relate to both the process of chronic diseases and the normal decrease in organ function that occurs with time. All of these organ systems and functions can decrease as we age: appetite; sense of taste, smell, thirst, hearing, and sight; digestion and absorption; liver, gallbladder, pancreatic, kidney, lung, and heart function; and the immune system. In addition, bone mass and muscle mass gradually decrease, the latter largely because of a deficient diet and inactivity. Appropriate dietary changes and regular physical activity can often help reduce the impact of these results of aging.

Nutrient Needs in Middle Age and Older Adulthood

The latest RDAs and related standards for nutrients and calories include categories for both men and women who are 51 to 70 years of age and more than 70 years of age. Macronutrient needs do not change from young adults' needs, but needs for some micronutrients do. In addition, because the lifestyle of an active older person can differ considerably from that of a nursing home resident, establishing nutrient needs during these wide age ranges is problematic.

A well-planned diet that follows MyPyramid can meet all nutrient needs for healthy older people within about 1600 to 1800 kcal, except for probably vitamin D, vitamin B-12, and folate. Meeting the folate and vitamin B-12 standard is aided by use of fortified foods, such as ready-to-eat breakfast cereals. The use of a balanced multivitamin and mineral supplement is especially helpful for meeting vitamin D needs if the person does not receive regular sun exposure. Any supplement used should be low in or free of iron, as it may have a pro-oxidant effect. Currently, many nutrition experts recommend a daily balanced multivitamin and mineral supplement for older adults, especially for those 70 years of age and older. If rich calcium sources advised by MyPyramid are not consumed, the person would also need a calcium supplement, as typical multivitamin and mineral supplements contain little calcium (about 200 milligrams). As noted in Chapter 8, providing more calcium than that would greatly increase the pill size.

Another Bite

Postmenopausal women have iron needs that are the same as men, as they no longer lose iron in menstruation. Recall from Chapter 9 that men should not take a supplement containing iron unless they have evidence of iron-deficiency anemia, as they consume enough iron from foods and it can easily accumulate to toxic amounts in the body. This advice now applies to women, as they experience minimal iron loss in the postmenopausal state.

Sodium needs for older adults are 1200 to 1300 milligrams per day. Older adults routinely consume at least this much sodium. Potassium needs are 4700 milligrams per day. Many older adults do not meet this goal.

■ Planning a Diet for People in Their Later Years

Recommended dietary practices for later years would be to increase the diet's nutrient density and to make sure fiber intake is adequate. In addition, some protein should come from lean meats to help meet protein, vitamin B-6, vitamin B-12, and zinc needs. Fluid needs are about 13 cups (3 liters) for older men and 9 cups (2.2 liters) for older women per day. A fiber-rich diet especially requires attention to fluid needs.

Singles of all ages face logistical problems with food: Purchasing, preparing, storing, and using food with minimal waste are challenging. Economy packages of meats and vegetables are normally too large to be useful for a single person. Many singles live in small dwellings, some without kitchens and freezers. Creating a diet to accommodate a limited budget and facilities and a single appetite requires special considerations. Following are some practical suggestions for diet planning for singles:

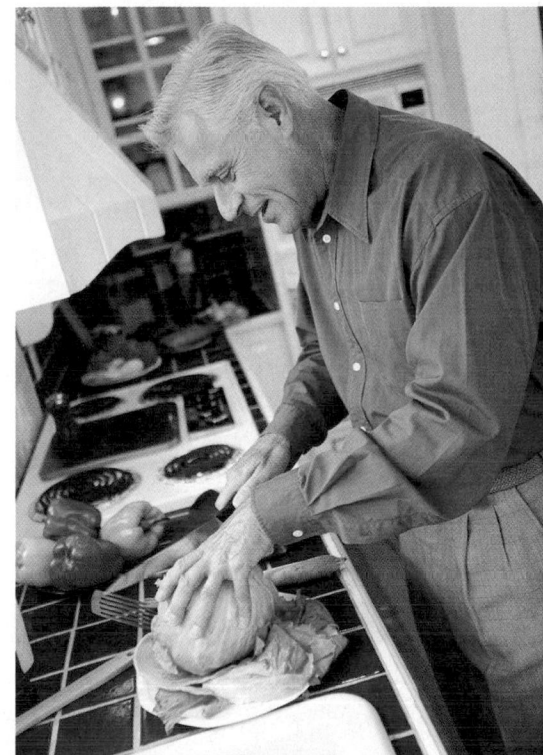

- If one owns a freezer, cook large amounts, divide into portions, and freeze.
- Buy only what one uses; small containers may be expensive, but letting food spoil is also costly.
- Ask the grocer to break open a family-sized package of wrapped meat or fresh vegetables and separate it into smaller units.
- Buy only several pieces of fruit—perhaps a ripe one, a medium-ripe one, and an unripe one—so that the fruit can be eaten over a period of several days.
- Keep a box of dry milk handy to add nutrients to recipes for baked foods and other foods for which this addition is acceptable.

Table 15-5 provides even more ideas.

Nutritional deficiencies and protein-calorie undernutrition have been identified among some aging populations, particularly those in nursing homes or long-term care facilities and those who are hospitalized. These nutritional problems increase the risk for many diseases, including bed sores (pressure ulcers), and compromise recovery from illness and surgery. Friends, relatives, and health care personnel should look for poor nutrient intake in all older people, including those who live

Great attention to food safety is also important for older adults. Chapter 16 provides advice on this topic, such as washing one's hands and work surface before preparing food.

To learn about meal programs for senior citizens in your area, call the *Administration on Aging's Elder Care Locator*, (800) 677-1116. For general information on programs for older persons, visit the following websites: *National Institute on Aging*, www.nih.gov/nia/; *American Geriatrics Society*, www.americangeriatrics.org/; and *Administration on Aging*, www.aoa.dhhs.gov/.

Table 15-5 Guidelines for Healthful Eating in Later Years

- Eat regularly; small, frequent meals may be best. Use nutrient-dense foods as a basis for menu(es).
- Use convenience foods and labor-saving devices.
- Try new foods, new seasonings, and new ways of preparing foods. Don't use just convenience foods and canned goods.
- Keep easy-to-prepare foods on hand for times when you feel tired.
- Have a treat occasionally, perhaps an expensive cut of meat or a favorite fresh fruit.
- Eat in a well-lit or sunny area; serve meals attractively; use foods with different flavors, colors, shapes, textures, and smells.
- Arrange kitchen and eating area so that food preparation and clean-up are easier.
- Eat with friends, relatives, or at a senior center when possible.
- Share cooking responsibilities with a neighbor.
- Use community resources for help in shopping and other daily care needs.
- Stay physically active.
- If possible, take a walk before eating to stimulate appetite.
- When necessary, chop, grind, or blend hard-to-chew foods. Softer, protein-rich foods can be substituted for meat when poor dental function limits normal food intake. Prepare soups, stews, cooked whole-grain cereals, and casseroles.
- If your feeding movements are limited, cut the food ahead of time, use utensils with deep sides or handles, and obtain more specialized utensils if needed.

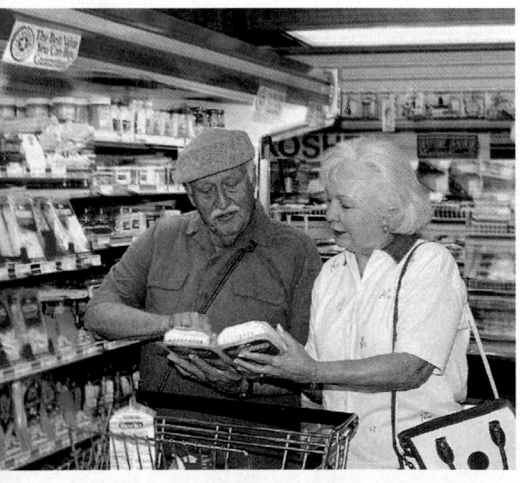

Grocery shopping can become more difficult in one's older years. Often assistance from others is very helpful.

in nursing home settings. Family members have a unique opportunity to make sure nutrient needs are met by looking for weight maintenance based on regular, healthful meal patterns. If problems arise in consuming a healthful diet, registered dietitians can offer professional and personalized advice.

Overall, good nutrition benefits older adults in many ways. Meeting nutrient needs delays the onset of some diseases; improves the management of some existing diseases; hastens recovery from many illnesses; increase(s) mental, physical, and social well-being; and often decreases the need for and length of hospitalization.

Obtaining enough food may be difficult for some older persons, especially if they are unable to drive and relatives do not live close enough to help with cooking or shopping. For an older person, a request for help may be equated to a loss of independence. Pride, or fear of being victimized by those they hire, may stand in

Another Bite

Strength training recommendations for older adults:

- Exercises should be performed at least two days per week.
- If weights are used, start with 1 to 2 pounds and gradually increase this amount over time.
- Perform exercises that involve the major muscle groups (e.g., arms, shoulders, chest, abdomen, back, hips, and legs) and exercises that enhance grip strength.
- Perform 8 to 15 repetitions of each exercise, then perform a second set.
- Breathe during strength exercises.
- Rest between sets.
- Avoid locking joints in arms and legs.
- Stretch after completing all exercises.
- Stop exercising if pain begins.

Source: National Institute on Aging.

the way of much needed help. In these cases, friends can be a big help. Special transportation arrangements may also be available through a local transit company or taxi service.

Many eligible older people are missing meals and are poorly nourished simply because they don't know of available programs to help them. Irregular meal patterns and weight loss, often caused by difficulties in preparing food, are warning signs that undernutrition may be developing. An effort should be made to identify poorly nourished people and inform them of community services.

Community Nutrition Services for Older People

Health care advice and services for older people can come from clinics, private practitioners, hospitals, and health maintenance organizations. Home health care agencies, adult day-care programs, adult overnight-care programs, and **hospice units** (for the terminally ill) can provide daily care.

The Nutrition Screening Initiative, a nutrition checklist for health care workers, family members, and older persons, can be used as a tool to increase health and nutrition awareness and to plan related education of older persons (Fig. 15-4). The

hospice units A facility offering care that emphasizes comfort and dignity in death.

A Nutrition Test for Older Adults

Here's a nutrition check for anyone over age 65. Circle the number of points for each statement that applies. Then compute the total and check it against the nutritional score.

Points	
2	1. The person has a chronic illness or current condition that has changed the kind or amount of food eaten.
3	2. The person eats fewer than two full meals per day.
2	3. The person eats few fruits, vegetables, or milk products.
2	4. The person drinks 3 or more servings of beer, liquor, or wine almost every day.
2	5. The person has tooth or mouth problems that make eating difficult.
4	6. The person does not have enough money for food.
1	7. The person eats alone most of the time.
1	8. The person takes three or more different prescription or over-the-counter drugs each day.
2	9. The person has unintentionally lost or gained 10 pounds within the last 6 months.
2	10. The person cannot always shop, cook, or feed himself or herself.
Total	

Nutritional score:

0–2: Good. Recheck in 6 months.

3–5: Marginal. A local agency on aging has information about nutrition programs for the elderly. The National Association of Area Agencies on Aging can assist in finding help; call (800) 677-1116. Recheck in 6 months.

6 or more: High risk. A doctor should review this test and suggest how to improve nutritional health.

Figure 15-4 A nutrition checklist for older adults.

Reprinted with permission by the Nutrition Screening Initiative, a project of the American Academy of Family Physicians, the American Dietetic Association, and the National Council on Aging, Inc., and funded in part by a grant from Ross Products Division, Abbott Laboratories.

DETERMINE:

- **D**isease
- **E**ating poorly
- **T**ooth loss or mouth pain
- **E**conomic hardship
- **R**educed social contact and interaction
- **M**ultiple medications
- **I**nvoluntary weight loss or gain
- **N**eed for assistance with self-care
- **E**lder at an advanced age

Nutrition Screening Initiative uses the acronym "DETERMINE" (see margin) to help identify older people whose health needs require extra attention.

Nutrition programs for those age 60 and over in the United States include congregate meal programs, which provide lunch at a central location, and home-delivered meals (often known as Meals on Wheels if sponsored by the local private or public agencies). About 2.6 million older adults are served each year. Currently about half of the meals use the home-delivered method.

The U.S. federal government sets specific standards for home-delivered meals and for those served in congregate feeding centers. The meals are designed to provide one-third of RDA/AI. The social aspect often improves appetite and general outlook on life.

Still, congregate meal programs generally provide one meal a day (some provide more) and usually just 5 days per week. Another problem with home-delivered meals is that the one or two meals delivered may never be eaten, and, if not eaten on delivery and left at room temperature, they may become unsafe to eat later. Thus, these programs can help older adults but probably don't meet all their nutritional needs.

In addition to congregate and home-delivered meals, federal commodity distribution is available in some areas of the United States to low-income older people. Food stamps can benefit older people whose incomes are below the poverty level (see Chapter 17 for details on these programs). Food cooperatives and a variety of clubs, religious, and social organizations provide additional aid.

Concept Check

Specific nutrient requirements for older adults are only now being extensively studied. Diet plans should be modified for decreased physical abilities, the presence of drug-nutrient interactions, possible depression, and economic constraints. Particular attention should be paid to the opportunity for sun exposure and intake of the vitamins D, B-6, E, folate, and B-12, as well as the minerals calcium and zinc and fiber. A nutrient-dense diet helps meet these needs. Carefully planned multivitamin and mineral supplement use can also help, especially for adults 70 years of age and older. In the United States, many nutrition services—such as congregate and home-delivered meals—are available to help the aging population obtain a healthful diet.

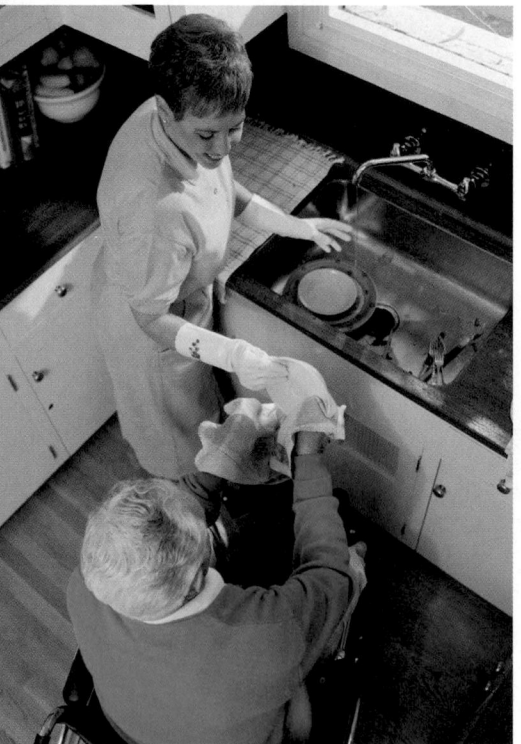

Help is available in most communities to assist older adults in daily tasks. This, in turn, helps older adults meet nutrient needs.

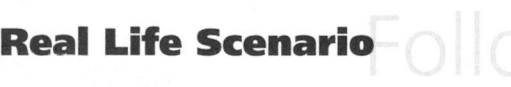

Real Life Scenario Follow-Up

Frances could contact a local government office that offers congregate meal programs at a central location. She could inquire about location and available transportation to the site. This would give her social contact with other older persons, which is probably an important element that is missing in her life. This could help alleviate her loneliness. She could also request Meals on Wheels (if available) to provide one hot meal a day. One hot meal a day that is prepared for her may be just what she needs to help stimulate her appetite. She could also have groceries delivered to her home if her budget could withstand the extra cost. Other convenience foods that could be included in her diet include milk, assorted nuts, peanut butter, breakfast cereals, canned chicken or deli meats, yogurt, sliced cheese, cottage cheese, calcium-fortified orange juice, canned or frozen fruits and vegetables, and some fresh fruits and vegetables that do not require preparation, such as prewashed lettuce and bananas. A further possibility is a nutrition bar or a liquid nutritional supplement, such as a can of Ensure® Plus. The resulting increase in her nutrient intake would help prevent disease in the future and increase her sense of well-being.

Summary

1. Most scientists agree upon diet recommendations for the general public, including those provided by MyPyramid and 2005 Dietary Guidelines for Americans. Such authorities recommend that individuals eat a variety of foods; balance the food eaten with physical activity to maintain or improve weight; choose a diet with plenty of grain products, vegetables, and fruits; choose a diet low in saturated fat, *trans* fat, and cholesterol; limit sugars and salt; and moderate or avoid alcoholic beverage intake. Regular physical activity is also important. In addition, recommendations to reduce cancer risk also emphasize moderation in the use of cured and smoked meats.

2. Although maximum life span hasn't changed, life expectancy has increased dramatically over the past century. For many societies, this means that an increasing proportion of the population is over 65 years of age. As health care costs rise, the goal of delaying disease becomes ever important.

3. Aging begins before birth. Cell aging probably results from automatic cellular changes and environmental influences, such as DNA damage. Add to this list damage caused by electron-seeking free-radical compounds, high blood glucose, hormonal changes, and alterations in the immune system as possible causes.

4. Nutritional problems of older adults are related to the presence of chronic diseases and to the normal decreases in organ function that occur with time. These include loss of teeth, lessened sensitivity to taste and smell, changes in GI tract function, and deterioration in cardiovascular and bone health. Although disease affects nutritional state, the reverse is also true. Undernutrition adversely affects immune function, allowing for infection.

5. Scientists are only now beginning extensive study of specific nutrient needs for older people. Diet plans should be based on a nutrient-dense approach and individualized for existing health problems, decreased physical abilities, presence of drug-nutrient interactions, possible depression, and economic constraints. Specific nutrients, such as protein, vitamin D, vitamin B-6, folate, vitamin B-12, zinc, and calcium, along with fiber, often deserve special attention in diet planning. A balanced multivitamin and mineral supplement can be used to help meet needs, especially for adults age 70 years and older.

6. Health care workers and family members should use available options for the procurement of food for older adults, especially for those who are nutritionally compromised. Most communities have congregate or home-delivered meal systems, food stamps, and other provisions for those who qualify.

Study Questions

1. List ten of the 2005 Dietary Guidelines for Americans for the general population and give an example of why each one may be difficult for older adults to implement. What are some solutions to these barriers?

2. What is the difference between life span and life expectancy?

3. List five general guidelines for cancer prevention.

4. Describe two hypotheses proposed to explain the causes of aging, and note evidence for each in your daily life experiences.

5. List four organ systems that can decline in function in later years, along with a diet/lifestyle response to help cope with the decline.

6. Defend the recommendation for regular physical activity during older adulthood, including some resistance activity (weight training).

7. How might the nutritional needs of older people differ from those of younger people? How are their needs similar? Be specific.

8. What three resources in a community are widely available to aid older adults in maintaining nutritional health?

9. Describe some warning signs of depression and note a possible nutritional implication as this problem advances.

10. List four warning signs of undernutrition in older people that are part of the acronym DETERMINE. Briefly justify the inclusion of each.

Further Readings

1. ADA Reports: Position of the American Dietetic Association: Nutrition across the spectrum of aging. *Journal of the American Dietetic Association* 105: 616, 2005.

   Behaviors such as a healthful diet, being physically active, and not using tobacco in any form are three keys to healthful aging. The American Dietetic Association supports these practices, as well as encourages older adults to seek medical and nutritional care to treat ongoing health problems, such as diabetes and hypertension.

2. Aging: Living to 100: What's the secret? *Harvard Health Letter* 27(3):1, 2002.

   Staying healthy is the goal in aging. Physical activity and a healthy diet are two keys, as shown by the lifestyle of the people on the island of Okinawa who typically are long-lived.

3. Birrer RB and Vermuri SP: Depression in later life: A diagnostic and therapeutic challenge. *American Family Physician* 69:2375, 2004.

   Depression is a common problem in older adulthood. It needs to be addressed as it raises the risk for suicide. Diagnosis and treatment of depression are reviewed in detail in this article.

4. Byers T and others: American Cancer Society guidelines on nutrition and physical activity for cancer prevention: Reducing the risk of cancer with healthy food choices and physical activity. *CA: Cancer Journal for Clinicians* 52:92, 2002.

   A diet low in red and processed meats and rich in fruits, vegetables, and whole grains is advocated as a strategy for reducing cancer risk. Regular physical activity is also important to include.

5. Cancer-fighting foods. *Mayo Clinic Health Letter* 22(12):1, 2004

   There are many foods, particularly plant-based foods, that might help lower the risk of certain cancers. Unlike individual supplements, foods offer a unique mix of vitamins and minerals, multiple phytochemicals, fiber and—not least of all—the pleasure of eating.

6. Coughlin L: American Cancer Society releases annual guidelines for the early detection of cancer. *American Family Physician* 71(11):2202, 2005.

   The American Cancer Society recommends that breast cancer screening should begin when women are 20 years old, with clinical breast examinations every 3 years until the age of 39. Thereafter, women at average risk should get an annual mammography.

Cervical cancer screening should begin three years after the onset of vaginal intercourse but no later than 21 years of age. Adults at average risk of developing colorectal cancer should begin screening at 50 years of age. Men at high risk for prostate cancer should begin testing at the age of 45.

7. Cummings JL: Alzheimer's disease. *The New England Journal of Medicine* 351:56, 2004.

   Detailed review of the latest findings on Alzheimer's disease. The author notes that delaying the disease should be the main focus, as current medications are not very effective.

8. Dickerson LM, Gibson MV: Management of hypertension in older persons. *American Family Physician* 71: 469, 2005.

   Hypertension is a too common result of the aging process, especially elevated systolic blood pressure. The authors suggest older people try to combat this trend by following a healthy diet low in sodium and alcohol (if consumed), and as well perform regular physical activity. Typical medications used to treat hypertension in the population are also reviewed.

9. DiMaria-Ghalili RA, Amella E: Nutrition in older adults. *American Journal of Nursing* 105(3): 40, 2005.

   Malnutrition in older persons is important to prevent, as it is a bigger risk than overweight to the health of this population. Risk factors that contribute to this state of malnutrition include a poor diet, as well as limited income, isolation, chronic illness, and various physiological changes that result from aging. These in turn can be addressed by appropriate lifestyle interventions reviewed in the article.

10. Fragalis AS: *Popular dietary supplements.* American Dietetic Association, 2nd edition, Chicago, Ill, 2003.

    This book provides a comprehensive review of nutrient and herbal supplements. Any use of herbal remedies especially deserves caution; potential benefits and risks in this regard are described.

11. Getting smart about Alzheimer's. *Tufts University Health & Nutrition Letter* 23(3):1, 2005.

    As many as 4.5 million Americans suffer from Alzheimer's disease. Consuming a diet rich in brightly colored fruits and vegetables contains many phytochemicals that may prevent the disease. Consuming fish on a regular basis is also important, as well as avoiding obesity, exercising regularly and keeping mentally active. Meeting B vitamin needs is also crucial, as many contribute to brain health, such as niacin

12. Heilbronn JK, Ravussin E: Calorie restriction and aging: Review of the literature and implications for studies in humans. *American Journal of Clinical Nutrition* 78:361, 2003.

    Calorie restriction has been long known to extend the life span and retard related chronic diseases of rats, mice, fish, flies, and other species. This may be due to a reduction in metabolic rate and oxidative stress, improved insulin sensitivity, and altered nervous system and hormonal activities. Trials are underway to test whether prolonged caloric restriction increases life span or retards the aging process in humans.

13. Keeping your mind strong as you age. *Tufts University Health & Nutrition Letter* (suppl), February 2003.

    Keeping your mind strong as you age can be accomplished using a variety of health practices. These include performing regular aerobic exercise, keeping blood glucose and blood pressure under control, re-maining socially engaged, challenging one's mind, reducing stress and anxiety, getting enough sleep, treating depression, and reviewing use of multiple medicines with a physician.

14. Litchford MD: Declining nutritional status in older adults. *Today's Dietitian* p.12, July 2004.

    The most common causes of declining nutritional status in older adults are poor food choices, failing cognitive status, oral health problems, loss of appetite, and dehydration. Implementing an action plan to treat these problems is important; a registered dietitian can help develop of such a plan.

15. Liu RH: Potential synergy of phytochemicals in cancer prevention: mechanism of action. *Journal of Nutrition* 134:347S, 2004.

    No single antioxidant can replace the combination of natural phytochemicals in fruits and vegetables to achieve the health benefits. Antioxidants or bioactive compounds are best acquired through whole-food consumption, not from dietary supplements. Consumption of 5-10 servings daily of a wide variety of fruits and vegetables is an appropriate strategy for significantly reducing the risk of chronic diseases, such as cancer, and to meet nutrient requirements for optimum health.

16. Mozaffarian D and others: Cereal, fruit, and vegetable fiber intake and the risk of cardiovascular disease in elderly individuals. *Journal of the American Medical Association* 289:1659, 2003.

    An adequate cereal fiber intake by older adults is associated with a lower risk of developing cardiovascular disease. This study supports the typical recommendation for older adults to increase consumption of fiber, such as from whole-grain cereals.

17. Patel JD and others: Lung cancer in U.S. women. *Journal of the American Medical Association* 291:1763, 2004.

    Lung cancer is the leading cause of cancer death in the United States, including women, and much more so than female breast cancer. It is important that the women that smoke cigarettes (25% of all women) not continue to do so if this health problem is to be conquered.

18. Petersen RC and others: Vitamin E and donepezil for the treatment of mild cognitive impairment. *The New England Journal of Medicine* 352: 2379, 2005.

    Megadose vitamin E therapy did not slow development of mild cognitive impairment in this study. This result questions earlier studies that showed a modest, but short-lived effect of such therapy. The medication donepezil was somewhat effective, but even this therapy only led to a modest benefit.

19. Rao SS: Prevention of falls in older persons. *American Family Physician* 72: 81, 2005.

    Risk factors for falls in older persons, such as muscular weakness, heavy use of medications, old age, impairment of gait and balance, and poor vision, are reviewed in this article. Prevention of falls especially should focus on physical exercise to improve muscular strength and gait, as well as a review of all medications used. Having a home inspection by a professional is also helpful to identify physical hazards that can be corrected, such as lack of hand rails on stairs.

20. Robertson RG, Montagnini M: Geriatric failure to thrive. *American Family Physician* 70:343, 2004.

    The many factors related to failure to thrive in older adults are reviewed. Use of multiple medications and depression are two common causes that often need to be addressed.

21. Schardt D: Are your supplements safe? *Nutrition Action Healthletter* 30(9):1, 2003.

    This article provides a comprehensive review of popular herbal supplements. Herbs and other substances to avoid because of a high potential for toxicity are also covered.

22. Staying well—at your age. *Consumer Reports on Health.* 17(9): 1, 2005.

    A detailed plan of health promotion and disease prevention as one ages is presented in the article. This includes dietary recommendations (e.g. meeting calorie, calcium, iron and vitamin D needs), as well a plan for aerobic and strength-training physical activities, and appropriate medical screening tests for each decade of adult life.

23. Sisk J: Aging & fit—The shape of things to come. *Today's Dietitian* p.34, July 2004.

    Regular physical activity is vital to prevent age-related declines in many aspects of health. A key point is that one is never too old to start an exercise program and achieve health benefits.

24. Szulc P and others: Hormonal and lifestyle determinants of appendicular skeletal muscle mass in men: the MINOS study. *American Journal of Clinical Nutrition* 80: 496, 2004.

    In older men, low physical activity, tobacco smoking, thinness, low blood testosterone, and poor vitamin D status were found to be risk factors for reduced muscle mass, termed sarcopenia. Lack of physical activity is especially important to address in order to maintain healthy amount of muscle mass as one ages.

25. Torpy J: Integrating complementary therapy into care. *Journal of the American Medical Association* 287:306, 2002.

    Nontraditional therapies such as herbal therapies can be combined with traditional Western medicine. Caution must be exercised when initiating herbal preparations, however, because herbal products are not evaluated by FDA for safety or efficacy.

26. Trichopoulou A and others: Modified Mediterranean diet and survival: EPIC-elderly prospective cohort study. *British Medical Journal* 330:991, 2005.

    A diet characterized by high intakes of vegetables, legumes, fruits, cereals, and unsaturated fats; moderate amounts of fish and alcohol; and low-to-moderate amounts of dairy products and meats lessened the risk of developing cardiovascular disease in people in this study. Total mortality was also reduced, especially so in people who closely adhered to this diet pattern.

27. Tucker KL and others: The combination of high fruit and vegetable and low saturated fat intakes is more protective against mortality in aging men than is either alone: The Baltimore longitudinal study of aging. *Journal of Nutrition* 135: 556, 2005.

    A diet rich in fruits and vegetables and low in saturated fat intakes reduced mortality in aging men in this study. Putting all three recommendations into practice was especially helpful in this regard.

28. Willett WC: Diet and cancer: an evolving picture. *Journal of the American Medical Association* 293(2):233, 2005.

    The relation between red meat consumption and colorectal cancer may not be conclusive, but prudence would suggest that red meat, and processed meats in particular, should be eaten sparingly to minimize risk. When this advice is combined with other healthful diet and lifestyle factors, it appears that approximately 70% of colon cancer can be avoided.

I. Am I Aging Healthfully?

Take Control of Your Aging by Dr. William B. Malarkey (Wooster Book Co., Wooster OH, 1999) includes a plan that incorporates various diet and lifestyle factors that are associated with successful aging. Indicate the degree to which you are following such a plan (or alternatively fill this out with a parent or another older relative in mind).

Physical: Do you eat a well-balanced diet, exercise on a regular basis, remain free of illness, abstain from smoking, refrain from drinking alcohol excessively, and experience refreshing sleep?

_____

_____

_____

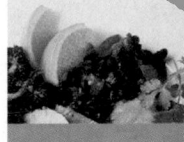

Intellectual: Are you analytical, do you read regularly, do you learn new things each day, do you engage your mental ability at work (or at school), and do you often reflect on your life?

_____

_____

_____

Emotional: Are you at peace, do you like who you are, are you optimistic, and do you laugh and relax regularly?

_____

_____

_____

Relational: Are you a good listener, do you feel supported by friends, do you attend social functions, do you talk with family members often, and do you feel close to coworkers (or fellow students)?

_____

_____

_____

Spiritual: Do you appreciate nature, give to or serve others, meditate or seek religious worship, and feel life has meaning?

_____

_____

_____

The more of these factors that you include in your life, the more well rounded your plan is for maintaining overall health. Any one of the five areas in which you are not achieving success should show you characteristics to work on in the future.

II. Helping Older Adults Eat Better

During their lifetimes, most people usually eat meals with families or loved ones. As people reach their older ages, many of them are faced with living and eating alone. In a study of the diets of 4400 older adults in the United States, one man in every five living alone and over age 55 ate poorly. One of four women between the ages of 55 and 64 years followed a low-quality diet. These poor diets can contribute to deteriorating mental and physical health. Consider the following example of the living situation of an older adult.

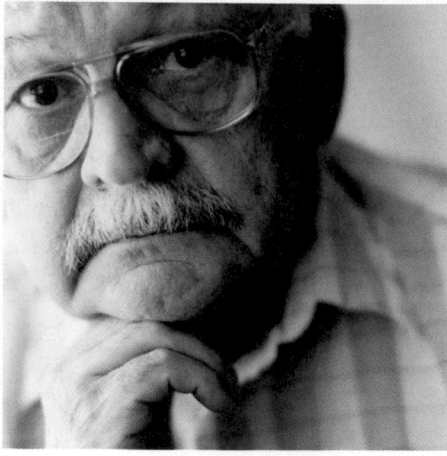

Neal, a 70-year-old man, lives alone in a home in a local suburban area. His wife died one year ago. He doesn't have many friends; his wife was his primary confidante. His neighbors across the street and next door are friendly, and Neal used to help them with yard projects in his spare time. Neal's health has been good, but he has had trouble with his teeth recently. His diet has been poor, and in the past 3 months his physical and mental vigor have deteriorated. He has been slowly lapsing into a depression and, so, keeps the shades drawn and rarely leaves his house. Neal keeps very little food in the house because his wife did most of the cooking and shopping, and he just isn't that interested in food.

If you were one of Neal's relatives and learned of Neal's situation, what six things could you do or suggest to help improve his nutritional status and mental outlook? Look back into this Chapter to get some ideas.

1. _____
2. _____
3. _____
4. _____
5. _____
6. _____

Food Safety

16

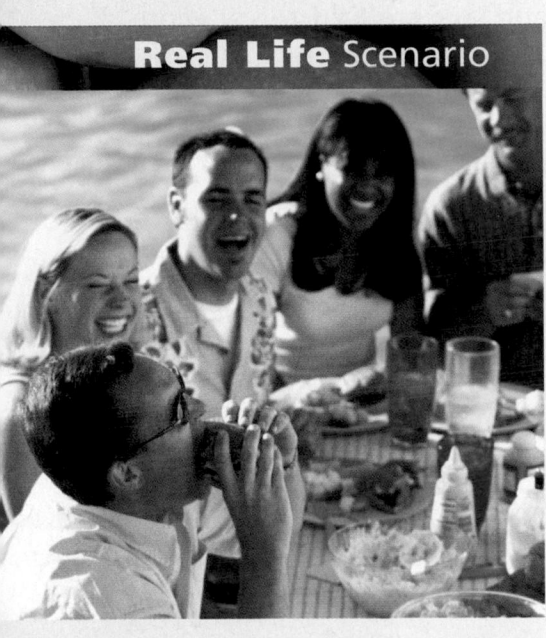

Aaron attended a gathering of his officemates on a warm July Saturday. The theme was international dining, and he and his wife were told to bring Argentine beef, a stewlike dish. They followed the recipe and cooking time carefully, removing the dish from the oven at 1 P.M. and keeping it warm by wrapping the pan in a towel. They traveled in their car to the party and set the dish out on the buffet table at 3 P.M. Dinner was to be served at 4 P.M. However, the guests were enjoying themselves so much lounging around the host's pool and drinking ginger beer (also on the menu) that no one began to eat until 6 P.M. Aaron made sure he sampled the Argentine beef that he and his wife made, while his wife did not. He also had some salad, garlic bread, and a sweet dessert made with coconut.

The couple returned home at 11 P.M. and went to bed. About 2 A.M., Aaron knew something was wrong. He had severe abdominal pain and had to make a mad dash to the bathroom. He spent most of the next 3 hours in the bathroom with severe diarrhea. By dawn, the diarrhea had subsided and he had started feeling better. After a few cups of tea and a light breakfast, he was feeling like himself by noon.

What type of foodborne illness did Aaron contract? What precautions for avoiding foodborne illness were ignored by Aaron and the rest of the people at the party? How could this scenario be rewritten to substantially reduce the risk of foodborne illness?

Chapter 16 Objectives

Chapter 16 is designed to allow you to:

1. List some of the types and common sources of viruses, bacteria, fungi, and parasites that can make their way into food.

2. Describe the procedures that can be used to limit the risk of foodborne illness.

3. Compare and contrast food-preservation methods.

4. Describe the main reasons for using chemical additives in foods, the general classes of additives, and the functions of each class.

5. Identify sources of toxic environmental contaminants in food, and the related complications of ingestion.

6. Understand the reasons behind pesticide use, the possible long-term health complications, and the safety limits set for their use.

Check out the **Contemporary Nutrition Online Learning Center** www.mhhe.com/wardlawcont6 *for quizzes, flash cards, other activities, and web links designed to further help you learn about issues surrounding food safety.*

At the turn of the twentieth century, conditions in Chicago's meat-packing industry were sickening. Moldy, spoiled meat was commonly doused with borax to cover up the smell, and glycerine was added to make it look fresh. By 1906, increasing public pressure forced the passage of the first Food and Drug Act in the United States. Federal inspection then safeguarded the public from worm-infested and diseased meat and generally improved food preparation standards.

Today, food safety warnings appear everywhere. Attention has turned to more contemporary food safety concerns, such as microbial and chemical contamination. On the one hand, we are told to eat more fruits, vegetables, fish, and poultry; on the other hand, we are warned that these foods may contain dangerous substances, so we still must ask, "How safe is our food?"

Scientists and health authorities agree that North Americans enjoy a relatively safe food supply especially if foods are stored and prepared properly. Over the past 100 or so years, tremendous progress has been made in food safety. Nonetheless, microorganisms and certain chemicals in foods still can pose a health risk. Thus the nutritional and health benefits of a food must be balanced against any food-related hazards. Chapter 16 focuses on these food-related hazards—how real they are and how you can minimize their effect on your life. Note that you bear much responsibility for this—government agencies and industry can only do so much. Recall from Chapter 2 that the 2005 Dietary Guidelines for Americans encourage us to prepare and store foods safely. A goal of *Healthy People 2010* is to reduce by 50% the number of cases of foodborne illness from typical bacterial causes.

Refresh Your Memory

As you begin your study of food safety in Chapter 16, you may want to review:

- Alternative sweeteners in Chapter 4
- The disease phenylketonuria (PKU) in Chapter 4
- Fat substitutes in Chapter 5
- The special food safety precautions recommended during pregnancy in Chapter 13
- The causes of cancer in Chapter 15

Garfield ®
by Jim Davis

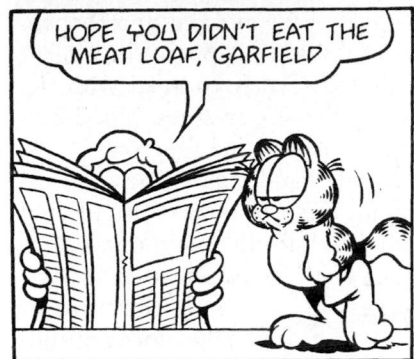 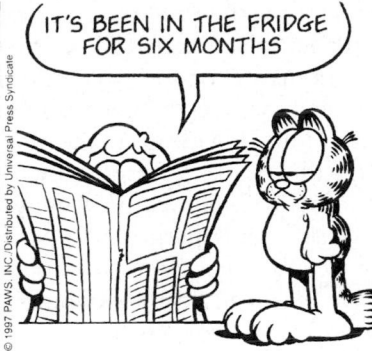 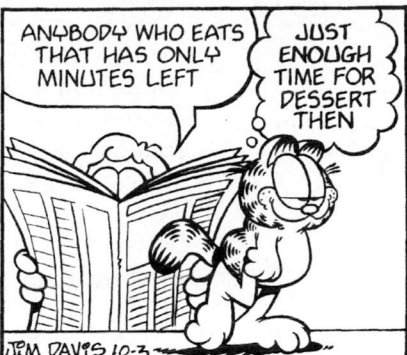

Which foods pose the greatest risk for foodborne illness? Is any food safe after being stored in the refrigerator for 6 months? Are food additives and pesticides an even greater day-to-day concern? Chapter 16 provides some answers.

Food Safety: Setting the Stage

During the early stages of urbanization in North America, contaminated water and food—notably, milk—were responsible for many large outbreaks of typhoid fever, septic sore throat, scarlet fever, diphtheria, and other devastating human diseases. These experiences led to the development of processes for purifying water, treating sewage, and **pasteurizing** milk. Since that time, safe water and milk have become universally available, with only occasional problems from either.

The greatest health risk from food today is contamination by **viruses** and **bacteria** and, to a lesser extent, by various forms of **fungi** and **parasites.** These microorganisms can all cause **foodborne illness.** For example, in one recent case a child died and 50 others became ill from *Escherichia coli (E. coli)* bacteria, found in apple juice. In another case, 170 children became ill when their school lunch contained strawberries contaminated by hepatitis A virus.

Even though microbial contamination is the cause of most incidents of foodborne illness, North Americans seem more concerned about health risks from chemicals in foods. Of U.S. consumers surveyed in a Gallup poll, about 75% said that pesticide contamination was a major concern to them. In the long run, this concern has some merit. On a day-to-day basis, however, food additives cause only about 4% of all cases of foodborne illness in North America.

Since microbial contamination of food is by far the more important issue for our day-to-day health, it will be discussed first. Chapter 16 will then cover the use and safety of food additives, and discuss the risks of pesticides in foods.

■ Effects of Foodborne Illness

According to the U.S. Centers for Disease Control and Prevention, foodborne illness caused 76 million illnesses, 325,000 hospitalizations, and 5000 deaths in the United States in 2002. Hospital costs for foodborne illnesses are estimated at more than $3 billion per year; costs from related lost productivity are estimated at $8 billion per year. Some people are particularly susceptible to foodborne illness, including the following:

- Infants and children
- Older adults
- Those with liver disease, diabetes, or HIV infection (and AIDS), or cancer

pasteurizing The process of heating food products to kill pathogenic microorganisms and reduce the total number of bacteria.

virus The smallest known type of infectious agent, many of which cause disease in humans. They do not metabolize, grow, or move by themselves. They reproduce only with the aid of a living cellular host. A virus is essentially a piece of genetic material surrounded by a coat of protein.

bacteria Single-cell microorganisms; some produce poisonous substances, which cause illness in humans. They contain only one chromosome and lack many organelles found in human cells. Some can live without oxygen and survive by means of **spore** formation.

spores Dormant reproductive cells capable of turning into adult organisms without the help of another cell. Various bacteria and fungi form spores.

fungi Simple parasitic life forms, including molds, mildews, yeasts, and mushrooms. They live on dead or decaying organic matter. Fungi can grow as single cells, like yeast, or as a multicellular colony, as seen with molds.

parasite An organism that lives in or on another organism and derives nourishment from it.

foodborne illness Sickness caused by the ingestion of food containing toxic substances produced by microorganisms.

- Pregnant women
- People taking immunosuppressant agents (e.g., transplant patients)

As you can see, foodborne illness has the greatest effect on the most vulnerable people in terms of health status (estimated to be about 30 million people in the United States alone). Some bouts of foodborne illness, especially when coupled with the ongoing health problems, are lengthy and lead to food allergies, seizures, blood poisoning (from **toxins** or microorganisms in the bloodstream), or other illnesses.

Because foodborne illnesses often result from the unsafe handling of food at home, we each bear some responsibility for preventing them. Since you can't usually tell by taste, smell, or sight that a particular food contains harmful microorganisms, you might not even be aware that food has caused your distress. In fact, your last case of diarrhea may have been caused by foodborne illness (Table 16-1). Government agencies are also at work on the problems regarding food safety, but this does not substitute for individual safety efforts (Table 16-2).

toxins Poisonous compounds produced by an organism that can cause disease.

Table 16-1 Some Examples of Cases of Foodborne Illness. We generally have a safe food supply, but there are occasional instances of foodborne illnesses, such as those listed below.

Viruses

- An estimated 6 million oysters from Louisiana were bathed with the *Norovirus* after ships with ill crew members dumped their sewage overboard. By the time the outbreak was recognized, an estimated 20,000 to 30,000 people had become ill. Another outbreak of the virus was attributed to an infected bakery worker, who stirred a vat full of buttercream frosting with his bare hand and arm. In Florida, 83 fraternity members caught the virus from the fraternity house ice machine. During the Gulf War, Norovirus was one of the most common causes of gastroenteritis among U.S. troops. Recently passengers on cruise ships have also contracted Norovirus illness.
- Over 500 adults in the United States contracted hepatitis A after eating raw green onions in a Mexican restaurant. These were contaminated during growth in Mexico and not properly washed by food service workers.

Bacteria

- A previously healthy 5-month-old girl suddenly died at home from contact with a pet iguana infected with *Salmonella*. Unpasteurized juice products were recalled after 57 cases of *Salmonella* illness were reported in California and Colorado. Eight people became ill from *Salmonella* after consuming tiramisu, a dessert that contains raw eggs.
- Six persons were reported ill from a *Shigella* infection after eating chopped, uncooked parsley that was served on chicken sandwiches and in coleslaw. A cruise ship had to return to port when more than 600 people developed shigellosis and one person died.
- The first documented foodborne illness caused by *Listeria* organisms in North America occurred in commercially prepared coleslaw. Later, 48 deaths were associated with soft, Mexican-style cheeses. A listeriosis outbreak associated with undercooked hot dogs and cold cuts resulted in more than 82 illnesses and 17 deaths in 19 states. Another outbreak of *Listeria* sickened at least 120 people and killed 20 in the northeastern United States. Recently 14.5 million pounds of ready-to-eat meat and poultry products were recalled because of possible *Listeria* contamination. A meat-packing firm recalled 27.4 million pounds of turkey and chicken after finding *Listeria* bacteria at the plant.
- The first community outbreak in the United States of *E. coli* 0111:H8 sickened 58 teenagers at a cheerleading camp in Texas. The camp salad bar and a communal water barrel were suspected sources of infection. One of the largest *E. coli* 0157:H7 outbreaks on record infected more than 1000 people in upstate New York at a county fair. The bacterium was found in infected well water. It killed a 79-year-old man and a 4-year-old girl, and it caused 10 other children to undergo kidney dialysis. Six adults and a 2-year-old child were killed after an *E. coli* outbreak from contaminated drinking water in Canada. The bacteria entered the water supply from animal manure after flooding from a heavy storm. In northeastern Oklahoma, five children were infected with *E. coli* after consuming unpasterized apple cider. Recently 25 million pounds of hamburger had to be recalled because of potential *E. coli* 0157:H7 contamination. A woman died in Columbus, Ohio after she was infected with *E. coli* 0157:H7 bacteria.
- A man in Arkansas developed botulism after eating stew that was cooked and then kept at room temperature for 3 days. He spent 49 days in the hospital—42 of them on mechanical ventilation. Another recent case involved a man who ate hard-boiled eggs that were left in a pickling solution at room temperature for 7 days.
- Since 1992, 17 people in Florida died of *Vibrio vulnificus* infections after eating raw oysters.
- A teenage boy and his father experienced abdominal pain, vomiting, and diarrhea within 30 minutes of eating 4-day-old homemade pesto. The pesto had been reheated and left out a number of times during the 4-day period. It was apparently contaminated with *Bacillus cereus*. As a result, the boy died of liver failure.

Parasites

- A group attending a dinner banquet developed diarrhea 3 to 9 days after eating green onions, which was the likely cause of the outbreak. Eight of 10 stool specimens obtained from the group with foodborne illness were positive for *Cryptosporidium*. Food workers at the restaurant reported they did not consistently wash green onions before using them.

Risks from Seafood

- Four adults became ill with scombroid fish poisoning after eating tuna-spinach salad at a restaurant in Pennsylvania.
- An outbreak of ciguatera fish poisoning involved 17 crew members of a cargo ship that caught, cooked, and ate a barracuda in the Bahamas. All 17 men became ill with nausea, vomiting, abdominal cramps, and diarrhea within hours of eating the fish. Within 2 days, all of the men suffered from muscle pain and weakness, dizziness, and numb or itchy feet, hands, and mouth.

Table 16-2 U.S. Agencies Responsible for Monitoring the Food Supply

Agency Name	Responsibilities	Methods	How to Contact
United States Department of Agriculture (USDA)	• Enforces wholesomeness and quality standards for grains and produce (while in the field), meat, poultry, milk, eggs, and egg products	• Inspection • Grading • "Safe Handling Label"	www.usda.gov/fsis or www.nal.usda.gov/fnicfoodborne/foodborn.htm or call 1-800-535-4555
Bureau of Alcohol, Tobacco, and Firearms and Explosives (ATF)	• Enforces laws on alcoholic beverages	• Inspection	www.atf.treas.gov
Environmental Protection Agency (EPA)	• Regulates pesticides • Establishes water quality standards	• Approval required for all U.S. pesticides • Sets pesticide residue limits in food	www.epa.gov
Food and Drug Administration (FDA)	• Ensures safety and wholesomeness of all foods in interstate commerce (except meat, poultry, and processed egg products) • Regulates seafood • Controls product labels	• Inspection • Food sample studies • Sets standards for specific foods	www.fda.gov or call 1-800-FDA-4010
Centers for Disease Control and Prevention (CDC)	• Promotes food safety	• Responds to emergencies concerning foodborne illness • Surveys and studies environmental health problems • Directs/enforces quarantines • National programs for prevention and control of foodborne and other diseases	www.cdc.gov
National Marine Fisheries Service or NOAA Fisheries	• Domestic and international conservation and management of living marine resources	• Voluntary seafood inspection program • Can use mark to show federal inspection	www.nmfs.noaa.gov
State and local governments	• Milk safety • Monitors food industry within their borders	• Inspection of food-related establishments	Government pages of telephone book

Government agencies responsible for monitoring food safety in Canada and the specific laws followed are listed in Appendix B.

■ Why Is Foodborne Illness So Common?

Foodborne illness is carried or transmitted to people by food. Most foodborne illnesses are transmitted through food in which microorganisms are able to grow rapidly. These foods are generally moist, rich in protein, and have a neutral or slightly acidic pH. Unfortunately, this describes many of the foods we eat every day, such as meats, eggs, and dairy products.

The risk of contracting foodborne illness also is high because of recent consumer trends. First, there is greater consumer interest in eating raw or undercooked animal products. In addition, more people receive medication that suppresses their ability to combat foodborne infectious agents. Another factor is the continuing increase in the number of older adults in the population.

Furthermore, the food industry tries whenever possible to increase the shelf life of food products; however, a longer shelf life at room temperature allows more time for bacteria in foods to multiply. Some bacteria grow even at refrigeration temperatures. Partially cooked—and some fully cooked—products pose a particular risk because refrigerated storage may only slow, not prevent, bacterial growth.

The risk of illness from foodborne microorganisms increases as more of our foods are prepared in kitchens outside the home. Supermarkets have become major food

Note that restaurants that will serve requested undercooked food are now warning patrons (on the menu) of the health risks of ordering such foods, particularly with undercooked eggs and meats.

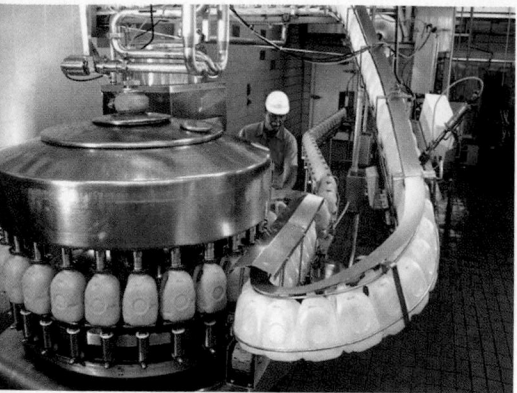

Food contaminated in a central plant can go on to produce illness in people in surrounding states or even across the nation. In the case of juices, it is important that they are pasteurized to reduce risk of foodborne illness, especially for the more susceptible of us.

A new tool in the battle against foodborne illness is HACCP, or Hazard Analysis Critical Control Point. Rather than treating the cause after a foodborne illness outbreak has occurred, by applying the principles of HACCP, food handlers critically analyze how they approach food preparation and what conditions may exist that might allow pathogenic microorganisms to enter and thrive in the food system. Once specific hazards and critical control points (potential problems) are identified, preventive measures can be used to reduce specific sources of contamination.

processors over the past decade and now offer a variety of prepared foods from specialty meat shops, salad bars, and bakeries. With the increasing number of two-income families, more people are looking for convenient, easy-to-prepare, nutritious foods. Supermarkets offer entrées that can be served immediately or reheated. The foods are usually prepared in central kitchens or processing plants and shipped to individual stores.

The centralization of food production by the food-processing and restaurant industry also adds to the risk of foodborne illness. If a food product is contaminated in a processing plant, consumers over a wide area can suffer foodborne illness. For example, a malfunction in an ice cream plant in Minnesota resulted in 224,000 suspected cases of *Salmonella* bacterial infections, linked to use of contaminated ice cream mix. At least 4 people died and 700 became ill in Washington and surrounding western states after eating at a chain of fast-food restaurants. The source of the problem was undercooked hamburger contaminated with the bacterium *E. coli* 0157:H7. Note that generally restaurants encounter only inspection by local health departments about every 6 months. We must primarily rely on each restaurant to practice good food safety.

Greater consumption of ready-to-eat foods imported from foreign countries is still another cause of increased foodborne illness in North America. In the past, food imports were mostly raw products processed here under strict sanitation standards. Now, however, we import more ready-to-eat processed foods—such as cheese from France and seafood from Asia—some of which are contaminated. U.S. authorities are currently reexamining inspection procedures for these imports.

The use of antibiotics in animal feeds is also increasing the severity of cases of foodborne illness. This antibiotic use encourages bacteria to develop antibiotic-resistant strains, those that can grow even if exposed to typical antibiotic medicines. This issue currently is receiving considerable attention by scientists in the field.

Finally, more cases of foodborne disease are reported now because scientists are more aware of the roles of various players in the process. Every decade the list of microorganisms suspected of causing foodborne illness lengthens. In addition, physicians are more likely to suspect foodborne contaminants as a cause of illness. Furthermore, we now know that food, besides serving as a good growth medium for some microorganisms, simply transmits many others as well. Seafood is receiving greater scrutiny and surveillance by FDA as a cause of foodborne illness. In addition, FDA is conducting a $500,000 campaign to educate U.S. consumers about the risks of eating raw oysters. For more information about these risks, contact FDA's Seafood Hotline at 1-800-FDA-4010 or log on to www.safefood.gov.

Food Preservation—Past, Present, and Future

For centuries, salt, sugar, smoke, fermentation, and drying have been used to preserve food. Ancient Romans used sulfites to disinfect wine containers and preserve wine. In the age of exploration, European adventurers traveling to the New World preserved their meat by salting it. Most preserving methods work on the principle of decreasing water content. Bacteria need abundant stores of water to grow; yeasts and molds can grow with less water, but some is still necessary. Adding sugar or salt binds water and so decreases the water available to these microbes. The process of drying evaporates off free water.

Decreasing the water content of some high-moisture foods, however, would cause them to lose essential characteristics. To preserve such foods—cucumber pickles, sauerkraut, milk (yogurt), and wine—fermentation has been a traditional alternative. Selected bacteria or yeast are used to ferment or pickle foods. The fermenting bacteria or yeast make acids and alcohol, which minimize the growth of other bacteria and yeast.

Today we can add pasteurization, sterilization, refrigeration, freezing, food **irradiation,** canning, and chemical preservation to the list of food preservation techniques. An additional method of food preservation—**aseptic processing**—simultaneously sterilizes the food and package separately before the food enters the package. Liquid foods, such as fruit juices, are especially easy to process in this manner. With aseptic packaging, boxes of sterile milk and juices can remain on supermarket shelves, free of microbial growth, for many years.

Food irradiation uses minimal doses of radiation in order to control pathogens such as *E. coli* 0157:H7 and *Salmonella*. Even though FDA has permitted irradiation of certain food products for more than a decade, the history of the technology goes back nearly a century, including scientific research, evaluation, and testing. The radiation energy used does not make the food radioactive. The energy essentially passes through the food, as in microwave cooking, and no radioactive residues are left behind. However, the energy is strong enough to break chemical bonds, destroy cell walls and cell membranes, break down DNA, and link proteins together. Irradiation thereby controls growth of insects, bacteria, fungi, and parasites in foods.

FDA recently approved the use of irradiation for raw red meat to reduce risk of *E. coli* and other infectious microorganisms. Some food processors are now doing so. Other additions to the approved list are shell eggs and seeds. Prior to this, the only animal products so treated were pork and chicken. Irradiation also extends the shelf life of spices, dry vegetable seasonings, meats, and fresh fruits and vegetables.

Irradiated food, except for dried seasonings, must be labeled with the international food irradiation symbol, the Radura, and a statement that the product has been treated by irradiation. Foods treated in this way are safe in the opinion of FDA and many other health authorities, including the American Academy of Pediatrics. Although the demand for irradiated foods is still low in the United States, other countries, including Canada, Japan, Italy, and Mexico, all use food irradiation technology widely. Certain consumer groups continually try to block its use in the United States, claiming that irradiation diminishes the nutritional value of food and that it can lead to the formation of harmful compounds, such as carcinogens. Future research should be able to sort out this controversy, but in any case the risk is very low. Keep in mind also that, even when foods, especially meats, have been irradiated, it is still important to follow basic food-safety procedures, as later contamination in food preparation is possible.

irradiation A process in which **radiation** energy is applied to foods, creating compounds (free radicals) within the food that destroy cell membranes, break down DNA, link proteins together, limit enzyme activity, and alter a variety of other proteins and cell functions of microorganisms that can lead to food spoilage. This process does not make the food radioactive.

aseptic processing A method by which food and container are separately and simultaneously sterilized; it allows manufacturers to produce boxes of milk that can be stored at room temperature.

This is the Radura, the international label denoting prior irradiation of the food product.

Foodborne Illness: When Undesirable Microorganisms Alter Foods

Most cases of foodborne illness are caused by specific viruses, bacteria, and other microorganisms. Bacteria specifically cause health problems either directly by invading the intestinal wall and producing an *infection* via a toxin contained in the organism, or indirectly by producing a toxin that is secreted into the food, which later harms us (called an *intoxication*). The main way to distinguish an infectious route from an intoxication is time: If symptoms appear in 4 hours or less, it is an intoxication.

Many types of bacteria cause foodborne illness, including *Bacillus, Campylobacter, Clostridium, Escherichia, Listeria, Vibrio, Salmonella,* and *Staphylococcus* (Table 16-3). Because each teaspoon of soil contains about 2 billion bacteria, we are constantly at risk for foodborne illness. Luckily, only a small number of all bacteria actually pose a threat. In addition, experts speculate that about 70% of cases of foodborne illness go undiagnosed because they result from viral causes, such as Norovirus, and there is no easy way to test for these pathogens. A website coordinating the U.S. efforts on food safety is the www.foodsafety.gov site mentioned earlier. Other useful websites are www.ama-assn.org/foodborne and www.homefoodsafety.org.

A goal of *Healthy People 2010* is to reduce the number of cases of foodborne illness from *Campylobacter, E. coli, Listeria,* and *Salmonella* by 50%.

Table 16-3 Important Microorganisms and Related Factors That Cause Foodborne Illness: Their Sources, Symptoms, and Prevention

Microorganism	Sources	Symptoms	Prevention Methods
Viruses			
Norovirus (Norwalk and Norwalk-like virus), human rotavirus	Found in the human intestinal tract and feces. Contamination occurs: (1) when sewage is used to enrich garden/farm soil (2) by direct hand-to-food contact during the preparation of meals (3) when shellfish are harvested from waters contaminated by sewage.	Onset: 1–2 days Severe diarrhea, nausea, and vomiting. Respiratory symptoms. Usually lasts 4–5 days but may last for weeks.	• Sanitary handling of foods • Use of pure drinking water • Adequate sewage disposal • Adequate cooking of foods • Good personal hygiene
Hepatitis A virus	Fecal-oral route that contaminates food, beverages, or shellfish.	Onset: 15–50 days Anorexia, diarrhea, fever, jaundice, and fatigue. May cause liver damage and death.	• Sanitary handling of foods • Use of pure drinking water • Adequate sewage disposal • Thorough cooking of foods
Bacteria			
Campylobacter jejuni	Found on poultry, beef, and lamb and can contaminate meat and milk. Chief food sources are raw poultry and meat and unpasteurized milk.	Onset: 2–5 days after eating, or longer Diarrhea, abdominal cramping, fever, and sometimes bloody stools. Lasts 2–7 days.	• Thorough cooking of foods • Sanitary food-handling practices • Avoidance of unpasteurized milk
Salmonella species	Found in raw meats, poultry, eggs, fish, sprouts, unpasteurized milk, and products made with these items. Multiplies rapidly at room temperature. The bacteria themselves are toxic.	Onset: 1–3 days after eating Nausea, fever, headache, abdominal cramps, diarrhea, and vomiting Can be fatal in infants, the elderly, and the sick.	• Sanitary food-handling practices • Avoidance of any use of unpasteurized raw eggs or undercooked eggs • Thorough cooking of foods • Prompt refrigeration of foods
Shigella species	Transmitted via fecal-oral route and somewhat in food and water.	Onset: 1–3 days Abdominal cramps, diarrhea, fever, bloody stools	• Handwashing and sanitary food production
Escherichia coli (0157:H7 and other strains)	Undercooked beef, especially ground beef. Fruits, vegetables, sprouts, and yogurt are also possible sources.	Onset: 1–8 days Bloody diarrhea, abdominal cramps, kidney failure	• Thorough cooking, especially of beef • Avoidance of unpasteurized milk, untreated apple cider
Clostridium perfringens	Found throughout the environment. Generally found in meat and poultry dishes. Multiply rapidly in anaerobic conditions when foods are left for extended time at room temperature.	Onset: 8–24 hours after eating (usually 12 hours) Abdominal pain and diarrhea Symptoms last a day or less, usually mild. Can be more serious in older or ill people.	• Sanitary handling of foods, especially meat and meat dishes, gravies, and leftovers • Thorough cooking and reheating of foods, especially leftovers • Prompt and proper refrigeration
Listeria monocytogenes	Found in soft cheeses made with unpasteurized milk and unpasteurized milk itself. Resists acid, heat, salt, nitrate, and refrigeration temperatures.	Onset: 9–48 hours for early symptoms; 14–42 days for severe symptoms. Fever, headache, vomiting, and sometimes more severe symptoms. May be fatal.	• Thorough cooking of foods • Sanitary food-handling practices • Avoidance of unpasteurized milk
Staphylococcus aureus	Found in nasal passages and in cuts on skin. Toxin is produced when food contaminated by bacteria is left for extended time at room temperature. Meats, poultry, egg products, pose the greatest risk.	Onset: 2–6 hours after eating Diarrhea, vomiting, nausea, and abdominal cramps Mimics flu Lasts 24–36 hours Rarely fatal	• Sanitary food-handling practices • Prompt and proper refrigeration of foods • Covering cuts on skin
Clostridium botulinum	Found throughout the environment. However, bacteria produce toxin only in a low-acid, anaerobic environment, such as in canned green beans, mushrooms, spinach, olives, and beef. Honey may carry spores.	Onset: 12–72 hours after eating Neurotoxic symptoms include double vision, inability to swallow, speech difficulty, and progressive paralysis of the respiratory system. OBTAIN MEDICAL HELP IMMEDIATELY. BOTULISM CAN BE FATAL.	• Use proper methods for canning low-acid foods • Avoidance of commercial cans of low-acid foods that have leaky seals or are bent, bulging, or broken • Discard if toxin is suspected (off odors are a sign)
Vibrio vulnificus	Raw seafood, especially raw oysters.	Onset: 1–7 days Diarrhea, fever, weakness, blood infection, death	• Thorough cooking of seafood

Table 16-3 (continued)

Microorganism	Sources	Symptoms	Prevention Methods
Bacteria (continued)			
Vibrio cholerae	Human carriers, infected shellfish, contaminated water and food.	Onset: 2–3 days Vomiting, severe watery diarrhea, which can lead to dehydration and cardiovascular collapse; death	• Handwashing after using the bathroom
Parasites			
Trichinella spiralis	Pork and wild game.	Onset: weeks to months Muscle weakness, fluid retention in face, fever, flulike symptoms	• Thorough cooking of pork and wild game
Anisakis	Raw fish.	Onset: 12 hours Stomach infection, severe stomach pain	• Thorough cooking of fish
Tapeworms	Raw beef, pork, and fish.	May cause abdominal discomfort, diarrhea	• Thorough cooking of all animal products • Avoidance of raw fish dishes, such as sushi
Cyclospora cayetanensis	Carried to food via contaminated water; Guatemalan raspberries suspected in recent outbreaks.	Onset: 1–11 days Prolonged diarrhea, vomiting, muscle aches, fatigue	• Irradiation (not yet in practice)
Cryptosporidium	Contaminated water (especially fecal material). Large outbreaks have been caused by such contamination of municipal water in Milwaukee, Wisconsin.	Onset: 1–12 days Diarrhea, vomiting, fever	• Handwashing • Consume clean or treated water • Boil water if at high risk, such as one who is on immune suppression drugs or has AIDS
Toxoplasma gondii	Raw or undercooked meat, unwashed fruits and vegetables, cat feces.	Onset: 5–20 days Fever, headache, sore muscles, diarrhea (can be deadly to the fetus of pregnant women)	• Cook meats thoroughly • Wash raw fruits and vegetables • Wash hands after changing cat litter (avoid cat litter when pregnant)
Fungi			
Mycotoxins are a group of toxic compounds produced by molds, such as aflatoxin B-1	Found in foods that are relatively high in moisture. Chief food sources are beans and grains that have been stored in a moist place.	May cause liver and/or kidney disease	• Discard foods with visible mold • Proper storage of susceptible foods
Ciguatera	Large tropical fish, especially grouper, snapper, and barracuda.	Onset: generally within 6 hours Diarrhea, abdominal pain, nausea, vomiting, and nerve disorders	• Avoid grouper, amberjack, and barracuda from Caribbean waters, especially larger fish
Paralytic shellfish poisoning	Shellfish that have consumed large amounts of dinoflagellate algae (i.e., red tide).	Onset: within 4 hours Respiratory difficulty	• Observe local precautions when harvesting shellfish
Scombroid poisoning	Spoiled fish, especially tuna, mackerel, and mahi-mahi.	Onset: 1–180 minutes Facial flushing, burning sensation in the mouth, intestinal distress, and headache	• Avoid spoiled fish • Refrigerate fresh fish and use as soon as possible
Prions			
Proteins that help maintain nerve cells. These can turn into infectious prions, likely leading to diseases such as mad cow disease (bovine spongiform encephalopathy).	Cows, goats, and sheep harboring infectious prions. These are spread from one animal to another if certain by-products of the infected animal (e.g., brains) are used to feed other animals (this process is banned in the U.S. and Canada). Cooking does not destroy prions.	Onset: 2–30 years Dementia and psychosis, leading eventually to seizures, blindness, paralysis, and death, Once symptoms begin, death usually occurs within 1 year. At autopsy the person shows numerous holes in the brain.	• Isolated cases of mad cow disease have been confirmed in U.S. cattle, some of which were imported from Canada. (These animals were infected before strict preventive actions were put in place in Canada.) The biggest risk is consumption of meat, from cows, goats, and sheep in Europe or Asia. FDA and USDA have banned imports of such animals from Europe. There is a possibility that the prion also may be present in foods or dietary supplements containing brain tissue from cattle.

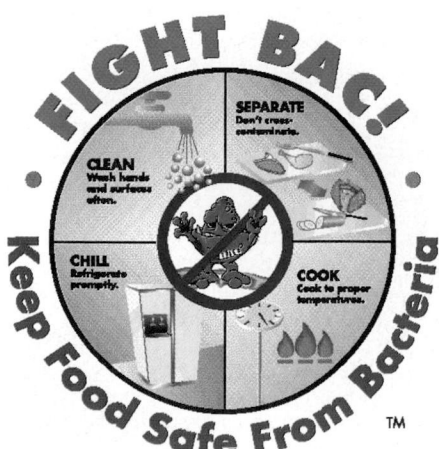

Food safety logo of USDA.

■ General Rules for Preventing Foodborne Illness

You can greatly reduce the risk of foodborne illness by following some very important rules. It's a long list, because many risky habits need to be addressed.

Purchasing Food

- When shopping, select frozen foods and perishable foods, such as meat, poultry, or fish, last. Always have these products put in separate plastic bags, so that drippings don't contaminate other foods in the shopping cart. Don't let groceries sit in a warm car; this allows bacteria to grow. Get the perishable foods such as meat and egg and dairy products home and promptly refrigerate or freeze them.
- Don't buy or use food from damaged containers that leak, bulge, or are severely dented or from jars that are cracked or have loose or bulging lids. Don't taste or use food that has a foul odor or spurts liquid when the can is opened; the deadly *Clostridium botulinum* toxin may be present.
- Purchase only pasteurized milk and cheese (check the label). This is especially important for pregnant women because highly toxic bacteria and viruses that can harm the fetus thrive in unpasteurized milk.
- Purchase only the amount of produce needed for a week's time. The longer you keep fruits and vegetables, the more time is available for bacteria to grow.
- When purchasing precut produce or salads, avoid those that look slimy, brownish, or dry; these are signs of improper holding temperatures.

Preparing Food

- Thoroughly wash your hands for 20 seconds with hot, soapy water before and after handling food. This practice is especially important when handling raw meat, fish, poultry, and eggs, after using the bathroom, after playing with pets, or after changing diapers.
- Make sure counters, cutting boards, dishes, and other equipment are thoroughly sanitized and rinsed before use. Be especially careful to use hot, soapy water to wash surfaces and equipment that have come in contact with raw meat, fish, poultry, and eggs as soon as possible to remove *Salmonella* bacteria that may be present. In addition, replace sponges and wash kitchen towels frequently.
- If possible, cut foods to be eaten raw on a clean cutting board reserved for that purpose. Then clean this cutting board using hot, soapy water. If the same board must be used for both meat and other foods, cut any potentially contaminated items, such as meat, last. After cutting the meat, wash the cutting board thoroughly.

FDA recommends cutting boards with unmarred surfaces made of easy-to-clean, nonporous materials, such as plastic, marble, or glass. If you prefer a wooden board make sure it is made of a nonabsorbent hardwood, such as oak or maple, and has no obvious seams or cracks. Then reserve it for a specific purpose; for example, set it aside for cutting raw meat and poultry. Keep a separate wooden cutting board for chopping produce and slicing bread to prevent these products from picking up bacteria from raw meat. Note that many foods are served raw, so any bacteria clinging to them are not destroyed.

Furthermore, FDA recommends that all cutting boards be replaced when they become streaked with hard-to-clean grooves or cuts, which may harbor bacteria. In addition, cutting boards should be sanitized once a week in a solution of 2 teaspoons chlorine bleach per quart of water. Flood the board with the solution, let it sit a few minutes, then rinse thoroughly.

- When thawing foods, do so in the refrigerator for 1 to 3 days, or under cold running water, or in a microwave oven. Also, cook foods immediately after thawing under cold water or in the microwave. Never let frozen foods thaw unrefrigerated all day or night. Also, marinate food in the refrigerator.
- Avoid coughing or sneezing over foods, even when you're healthy. Cover cuts on hands with a sterile bandage. This helps stop *Staphylococcus* from entering food.

- Carefully wash fresh fruit and vegetables under running water to remove dirt and bacteria clinging to the surface, using a vegetable brush if the skin is to be eaten. People have become ill from *Salmonella* that was introduced from melons used in making a fruit salad and from oranges used for fresh-squeezed orange juice. The bacteria were on the outside of the melons and oranges.
- Completely remove moldy portions of food or don't eat the food. *When in doubt, throw the food out.* Mold growth is prevented by properly storing food at cold temperatures and using the food promptly.
- Use refrigerated ground meat and patties in 1 to 2 days and frozen meat and patties within 3 to 4 months. The 6 month interval mentioned in the comic at the beginning of this chapter is too long a time to be safe.

Cooking Food

- Cook food thoroughly using a bimetallic thermometer to check for doneness, especially for beef and fish (145°F [63°C]), pork (160°F [71°C]), and poultry (165°F [74°C]) (Fig. 16-1). Eggs should be cooked until the yolk and white are hard. Alfalfa sprouts and other types of sprouts should be cooked until they are steaming. Cooking is by far the most reliable way to destroy foodborne viruses and bacteria, such as Norovirus and toxic strains of *E. coli*. Freezing only halts viral and bacterial growth. FDA does not recommend that eggs be prepared sunny-side-up or

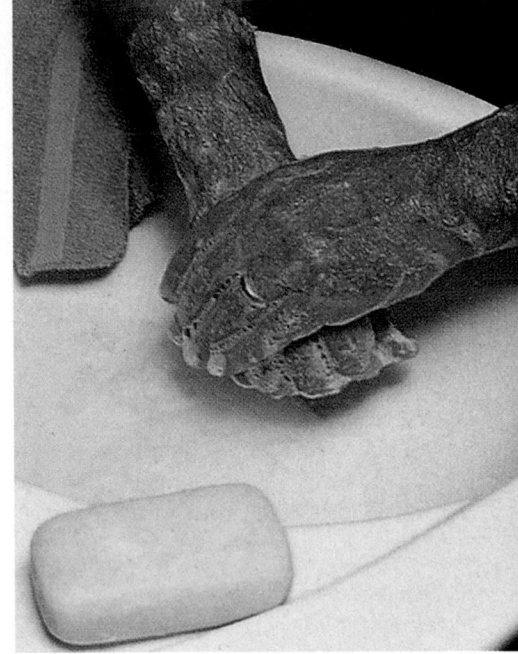

Washing hands thoroughly (for at least 20 to 30 seconds) with hot water and soap should be the first step in food preparation. The 4 "F's" of food contamination are fingers, foods, feces, and flies. Handwashing especially combats the fecal and finger routes.

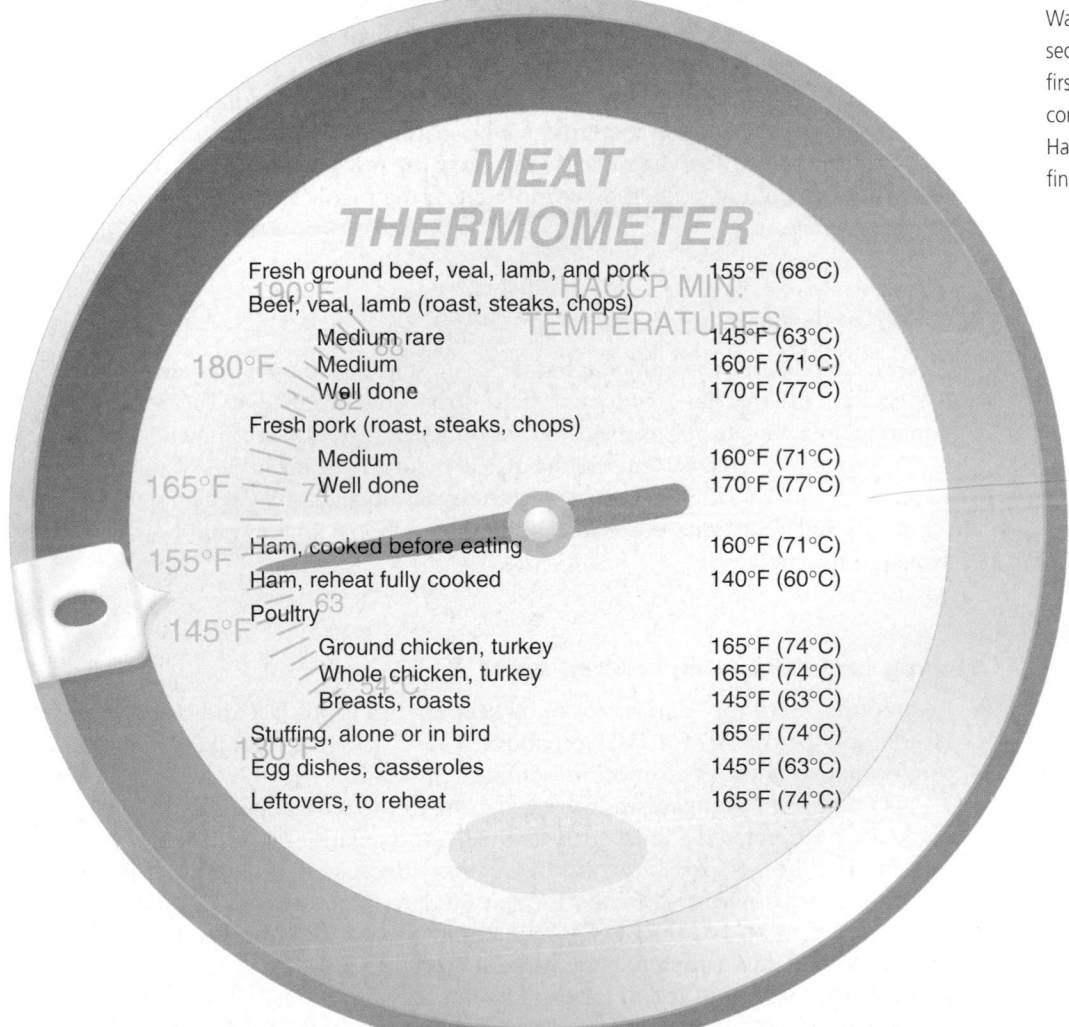

MEAT THERMOMETER

HACCP MIN. TEMPERATURES

	°F (°C)
Fresh ground beef, veal, lamb, and pork	155°F (68°C)
Beef, veal, lamb (roast, steaks, chops)	
Medium rare	145°F (63°C)
Medium	160°F (71°C)
Well done	170°F (77°C)
Fresh pork (roast, steaks, chops)	
Medium	160°F (71°C)
Well done	170°F (77°C)
Ham, cooked before eating	160°F (71°C)
Ham, reheat fully cooked	140°F (60°C)
Poultry	
Ground chicken, turkey	165°F (74°C)
Whole chicken, turkey	165°F (74°C)
Breasts, roasts	145°F (63°C)
Stuffing, alone or in bird	165°F (74°C)
Egg dishes, casseroles	145°F (63°C)
Leftovers, to reheat	165°F (74°C)

Figure 16-1 Minimum internal temperatures when cooking or reheating foods.

Current Safe Handling Instructions Issued by USDA for Labeling Meat and Poultry Products

This product was prepared from inspected and passed meat and/or poultry. Some food products may contain bacteria that could cause illness if the product is mishandled or cooked improperly. For your protection, follow these handling instructions.

Keep refrigerated or frozen.

Thaw in refrigerator or microwave.

Keep raw meat and poultry separate from other foods.

Wash working surfaces (including cutting boards), utensils, and hands after touching raw meat or poultry.

Cook thoroughly.

Keep hot foods hot. Refrigerate leftovers immediately or discard.

Safe Handling Instructions for Eggs

To prevent illness from bacteria: keep eggs refrigerated, cook eggs until yolks are firm, and cook foods containing eggs thoroughly.

over-easy for consumption. As noted earlier, restaurants must now include an advisory on menus stating that an increased risk of foodborne illness is associated with eating undercooked eggs. As long as restaurants provide this warning on their menus, however, they are allowed to cook eggs to any temperature requested by the consumer. FDA warns us not to consume homemade ice cream, eggnog, and mayonnaise if made with unpasteurized, raw eggs because of the risk of *Salmonella* foodborne illness. It is safer to use eggs or egg products that have been pasteurized, which kills *Salmonella* bacteria. Overall, a good general precaution is to eat no raw animal products. USDA answers questions about the safe use of animal products (800-535-4555, 10 A.M. to 4 P.M. weekdays, Eastern time).

Seafood also poses a risk of foodborne illness, especially oysters. Properly cooked seafood should flake easily and/or be opaque or dull and firm. If it's translucent or shiny, it's not done.

- Cook stuffing separately from poultry (or wash poultry thoroughly, stuff immediately before cooking, and then transfer the stuffing to a clean bowl immediately after cooking). Make sure the stuffing reaches 165°F (74°C). *Salmonella* is the major concern with poultry.
- Once a food is cooked, consume it right away, or cool it to 41°F (5°C) within 2 hours. If it is not to be eaten immediately, in hot weather (80°F and above) make sure this cooling is done within 1 hour. Do this by separating the food into as many shallow pans as needed to provide a large surface area for cooling. Be careful not to recontaminate cooked food by contact with raw meat or juices from hands, cutting boards, dirty utensils, or in other ways.
- Serve meat, poultry, and fish on a clean plate—never the same plate that was used to hold the raw product. For example, when grilling hamburgers, don't put cooked items on the same plate that was used to carry the raw product out to the grill.
- For outdoor cooking, cook food completely at the picnic site, with no partial cooking in advance.

Another Bite

Raw fish dishes, such as sushi, can be safe for most people to eat if they are made with very fresh fish that has been commercially frozen and then thawed. The freezing is important to eliminate potential health risks from parasites. FDA recommends that the fish be frozen to an internal temperature of −10°F for 7 days. If you choose to eat uncooked fish, purchase the fish from reputable establishments that have high standards for quality and sanitation. People at high risk for foodborne illness would be wise to avoid raw fish products.

Storing and Reheating Cooked Food

- Keep foods out of the "danger zone" by keeping hot foods hot and cold foods cold. Hold food below 41°F (5°C) or above 135°F (57°C) (Fig. 16-2). Foodborne microorganisms thrive in more moderate temperatures (60°F to 110°F [16°C to 43°C]). Some microorganisms can even grow in the refrigerator. Again, don't leave cooked or refrigerated foods, such as meats and salads, at room temperature for more than 2 hours (or 1 hour in hot weather) because that gives microorganisms an opportunity to grow. Store dry food at 60°F to 70°F (16°C to 21°C).
- Reheat leftovers to 165°F (74°C); reheat gravy to a rolling boil to kill *Clostridium perfringens* bacteria, which may be present. Merely reheating to a good eating temperature isn't sufficient to kill harmful bacteria.
- Store peeled or cut-up produce, such as melon balls, in the refrigerator.
- Make sure the refrigerator stays below 41°F (5°C). Either use a refrigerator thermometer or keep it as cold as possible without freezing milk and lettuce.

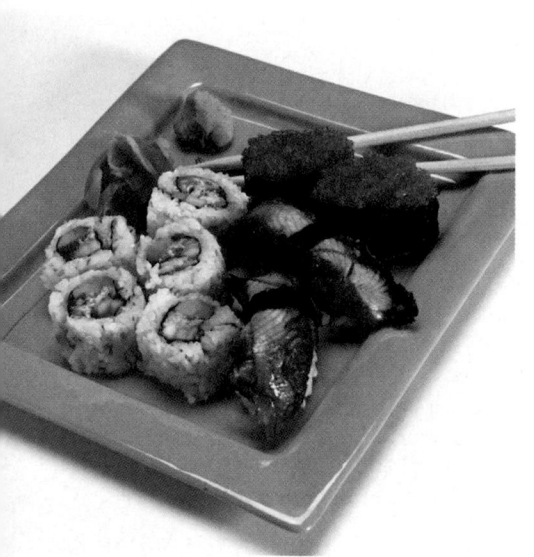

Sushi, like all raw fish or meat dishes, is a high-risk food. For maximum protection from foodborne illness, animal foods should be cooked thoroughly before eating.

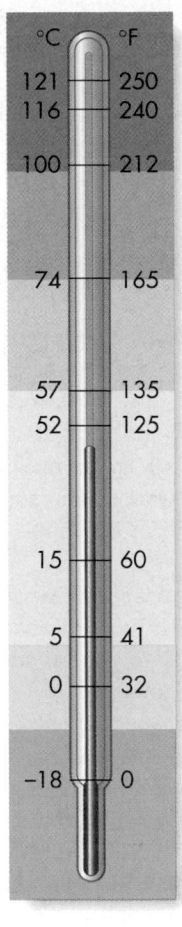
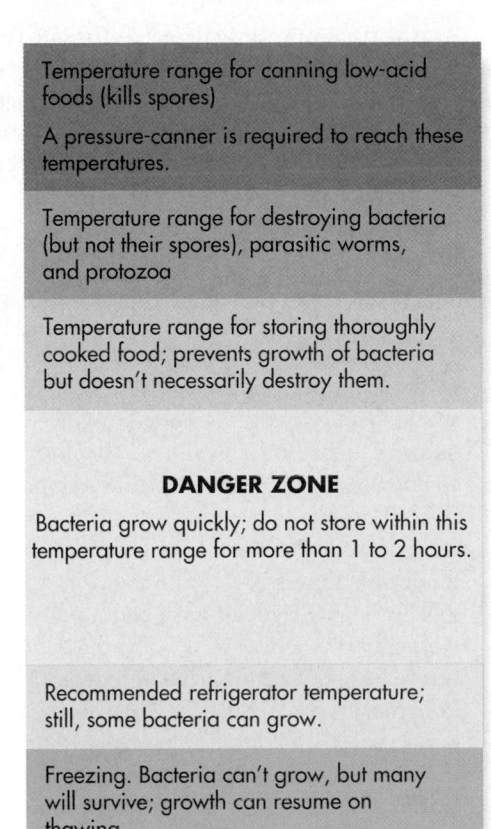

°C | °F
121 — 250 | Temperature range for canning low-acid foods (kills spores)
116 — 240 | A pressure-canner is required to reach these temperatures.
100 — 212 |
| Temperature range for destroying bacteria (but not their spores), parasitic worms, and protozoa
74 — 165 |
| Temperature range for storing thoroughly cooked food; prevents growth of bacteria but doesn't necessarily destroy them.
57 — 135 |
52 — 125 |
| **DANGER ZONE**
| Bacteria grow quickly; do not store within this temperature range for more than 1 to 2 hours.
15 — 60 |
5 — 41 |
0 — 32 | Recommended refrigerator temperature; still, some bacteria can grow.
–18 — 0 | Freezing. Bacteria can't grow, but many will survive; growth can resume on thawing.

Figure 16-2 Effects of temperature on microbes that cause foodborne illness.
Adapted from *Temperature Guide to Food Safety: Food and Home Notes.* No. 25, Washington DC, June 20, 1977, USDA.

Cross-contamination is not only a threat during food preparation; it can also become a problem during food storage. Make sure all foods, including leftovers, are contained and covered in the refrigerator to prevent drippings from uncooked and potentially hazardous foods from tainting other foods. It is a good idea to store foods that are likely to pose risk of foodborne illness on lower shelves of the refrigerator, beneath other foods that are to be eaten raw.

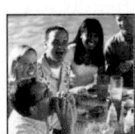

Real Life Scenario Follow-Up

Aaron likely contracted *Clostridium perfringens,* based on the fact that he had diarrhea but did not vomit, and the symptoms occurred about 8 hours after consuming the contaminated food (review Table 16-3). Spores of *Clostridium perfringens* are typically present in meat. Thorough cooking will kill any of the live bacteria present, but the product may still contain spores. These can later develop into bacteria if the food is kept in a warm setting for a few hours. The Argentine beef was likely the bearer of the spores, and they likely germinated and produced a toxin as the beef sat in the car and on the buffet table. Ideally, this cooked food should have remained at room temperature for no longer than 1 hour. Thus, soon after Aaron and his wife took it out of the oven, it should have been separated into a few smaller pans to speed cooling and then refrigerated because they knew it was not going to be served within 1 to 2 hours. Before leaving, they could have recombined the dish into one clean pan. Once they arrived at the party, the dish should have been refrigerated again, and then thoroughly reheated when it was time to eat. Overall, it is risky to leave perishable items such as meat, fish, poultry, eggs, and dairy products at room temperature for more than 1 to 2 hours.

To reduce the risk of bacteria surviving during microwave cooking,

- Cover food with glass or ceramic when possible to decrease evaporation and heat the surface.
- Stir and rotate food at least once or twice for even cooking. Then, allow microwaved food to stand, covered, after heating is completed to help cook the exterior and equalize the temperature throughout.
- Use the oven temperature probe or a meat thermometer to check that food is done. Insert it at several spots.
- If thawing meat in the microwave, use the oven's defrost setting. Ice crystals in frozen foods are not heated well by the microwave oven and can create cold spots, which later cook more slowly.

Critical Thinking

Diana had a party at her house for her son's birthday. While cleaning up after the kids went home, she realized she had forgotten to put away the potato salad and coleslaw and decided to discard it. However, her husband, Tim, wanted her to just refrigerate it. "After all," he reasoned, "it was only left out for a couple of hours." Why was Diana right in wanting to throw the leftover unrefrigerated food away?

As one final precaution, watch for safe food-handling techniques when you eat out. Check that foods in a salad bar are iced; custard and pudding pies are chilled; hot foods served on a hot food bar are, in fact, hot; and vending machines are checked regularly, especially those containing sandwiches and milk. Send back any meat, poultry, seafood, or fish that does not appear thoroughly cooked, including in dormitory cafeterias.

Concept Check

Viruses and bacteria and the toxins they produce pose the greatest risk for food-borne illness. In the past, the addition of sugar and salt to foods, as well as smoking and drying, were used to prevent the growth of microorganisms. Today, we know that ensuring cleanliness, keeping hot foods hot and cold foods cold, and cooking foods thoroughly offer additional protection from foodborne illness. Commercial processes, such as pasteurization and irradiation, do the same. Treat all raw animal products, cooked food, and raw fruits and vegetables as potential sources of foodborne illness.

Thoroughly cook all meat and poultry to reduce the risk of foodborne illness from Norovirus, *Campylobacter*, *E. coli*, and *Salmonella*. In addition, always separate raw meats and poultry products from cooked foods. To prevent foodborne intoxication from *Staphylococcus* organisms, cover cuts on hands and avoid sneezing on foods. To avoid intoxication from *Clostridium perfringens*, rapidly cool leftover foods and thoroughly reheat them. To avoid intoxication from *Clostridium botulinum*, carefully examine canned foods. Overall, don't allow cooked food to stand for more than 1 to 2 hours at room temperature. For other causes of foodborne illness, precautions already mentioned generally apply as well. In addition, thoroughly cook fish and other seafood; consume only pasteurized dairy products; wash all fruits and vegetables; and thoroughly wash your hands with soap and water before and after preparing food and after using the bathroom.

additives Substances added to foods, such as preservatives.

When buying food products, especially perishables, check the product date for safety. Four types of dates are commonly used. The pack date is the day the product was manufactured. The pull or sell date indicates the last date the product should be sold. It allows some time for storing food at home before eating. Check the expiration date of foods stored at home, because that is the last date the food can safely be consumed. Last, baked goods may have a freshness date, indicating that the product may be eaten safely for a short time after the date but may not taste the same.

Food Additives

By the time you see a food on the market shelf, it usually contains substances added to make it more palatable or increase its nutrient content or shelf life. Manufacturers also add some substances to foods to make them easier to process. Other substances may have accidentally found their way into the foods you buy. All of these extraneous substances are known as **additives**, and, although some may be beneficial, others, such as sulfites, may be harmful for some people. All purposefully added substances must be evaluated by FDA.

■ Why Are Food Additives Used?

Most additives are used to limit food spoilage. Food additives, such as potassium sorbate are used to maintain the safety and acceptability of foods by retarding the growth of microbes implicated in foodborne illness.

Additives are also used to combat some enzymes that lead to undesirable changes in color and flavor in foods but don't cause anything as serious as foodborne illness. This second type of food spoilage occurs when enzymes in a food react to oxygen—for example, when apple and peach slices darken or turn rust color as they are exposed to air. Antioxidants are a type of preservative that slow the action of oxygen-requiring enzymes on food surfaces. These preservatives are not necessarily novel chemicals. They include vitamins E and C and a variety of sulfites.

Without the use of some food additives, it would be impossible to produce massive quantities of foods and safely distribute them nationwide or worldwide, as is now done. Despite consumer concerns about the safety of food additives, many have been extensively studied and proven safe when FDA guidelines for their use are followed.

■ Intentional versus Incidental Food Additives

Food additives are classified into two types: **intentional food additives** (directly added to foods) and **incidental food additives** (indirectly added as contaminants). Both types of agents are regulated by FDA in the United States. Currently, more than 2800 different substances are intentionally added to foods. As many as 10,000 other substances enter foods as contaminants. This includes substances that may reasonably be expected to enter food through surface contact with processing equipment or packaging materials.

■ The GRAS List

In 1958, all food additives used in the United States and considered safe at that time were put on a **generally recognized as safe (GRAS)** list. The U.S. Congress established the GRAS list because it believed manufacturers did not need to prove the safety of substances that had been used for a long time and were already generally regarded as safe. Since that time, FDA has been responsible for proving that a substance does not belong on the GRAS list.

Since 1958, some substances on the list have been reviewed. A few, such as cyclamates, failed the review process and were removed from the list. The additive red dye #3 was removed because it is linked to cancer. Many chemicals on the GRAS list have not yet been rigorously tested, primarily because of expense. These chemicals have received a low priority for testing, mostly because they have long histories of use without evidence of toxicity or because their chemical characteristics do not suggest they are potential health hazards.

■ Are Synthetic Chemicals Always Harmful?

Nothing about a natural product makes it inherently safer than a synthetic product. Many synthetic products are simply laboratory copies of chemicals that also occur in nature (see the discussion in Chapter 17 on biotechnology for some examples). Moreover, although human endeavors contribute some toxins to foods, such as synthetic pesticides and industrial chemicals, nature's poisons are often even more potent and widespread. Some cancer researchers suggest that we ingest at least 10,000 times more (by weight) natural toxins produced by plants than we do synthetic pesticide residues. This comparison does not make synthetic chemicals any less toxic, but it does put them in a more accurate perspective.

Consider vitamin E, which is often added to food to prevent rancidity of fats. This chemical is safe when used within certain limits. However, high doses have been associated with health problems, such as interfering with vitamin K activity in the body (review Chapter 8). Thus, even well-known chemicals we are comfortable using can be toxic in some circumstances and at some concentrations.

■ Tests of Food Additives for Safety

Food additives are tested by FDA for safety on at least two animal species, usually rats and mice. Scientists determine the highest dose of the additive that produces *no observable effects* in the animals. These doses are proportionately much higher than humans are ever exposed to. The maximum dosage that produced no observable effects is then divided by at least 100 to establish a margin of safety for human use. This 100-fold margin is used because it is assumed that we are at least 10 times more sensitive to food additives than are laboratory animals and that any one person might

---

intentional food additives Additives knowingly (directly) incorporated into food products by manufacturers.

incidental food additives Additives that appear in food products indirectly, from environmental contamination of food ingredients or during the manufacturing process.

generally recognized as safe (GRAS) A list of food additives that in 1958 were considered safe for consumption. Manufacturers were allowed to continue to use these additives, without special clearance, when needed for food products. FDA bears responsibility for proving they are not safe, but can remove unsafe products from the list.

Some important definitions:

toxicology	The scientific study of harmful substances
safety	The relative certainty that a substance won't cause injury
hazard	The chance that injury will result from use of a substance
toxicity	The capacity of a substance to produce injury or illness at some dosage

---

Note that the 100-fold margin of safety is 25 times less than that for vitamin A, when you compare the RDA to a potentially harmful dose of vitamin A for pregnant women.

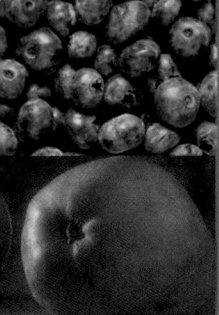

Looking *Further*

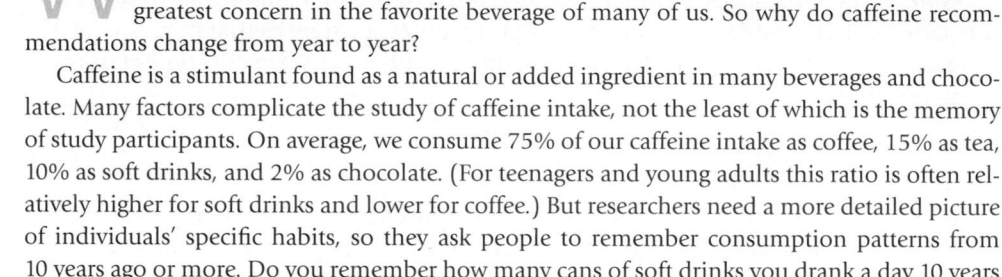

Why all the controversy over a cup of coffee? Can't we come to one definite conclusion? Researchers have spent a great deal of time on the study of caffeine, the substance of greatest concern in the favorite beverage of many of us. So why do caffeine recommendations change from year to year?

Caffeine is a stimulant found as a natural or added ingredient in many beverages and chocolate. Many factors complicate the study of caffeine intake, not the least of which is the memory of study participants. On average, we consume 75% of our caffeine intake as coffee, 15% as tea, 10% as soft drinks, and 2% as chocolate. (For teenagers and young adults this ratio is often relatively higher for soft drinks and lower for coffee.) But researchers need a more detailed picture of individuals' specific habits, so they ask people to remember consumption patterns from 10 years ago or more. Do you remember how many cans of soft drinks you drank a day 10 years ago, or how many cups of regular versus decaf coffee you drank 3 years ago?

Another factor that complicates research is that heavy coffee drinkers often have other deleterious health habits such as heavy alcohol consumption and smoking. In addition, smokers are likely to drink more coffee than nonsmokers because the blood of smokers is quickly cleared of caffeine. Are the health consequences found in heavy coffee drinkers due to caffeine, or is it possible that these other harmful habits are the true cause? In addition, caffeine is not often consumed by itself. With the recent popularity of trendy coffee shops that serve everything from mocha java to flavored lattes, it is difficult to separate caffeine intake from cream, sugar, alternative sweeteners, and flavorings. So what is the conscientious coffee drinker to think? Let's explore the myths and facts of caffeine intake as it is known today.

Caffeine does not accumulate in the body and is normally excreted within several hours following consumption. Caffeine can cause anxiety, increased heart rate, insomnia, increased urination (possibly resulting in dehydration), diarrhea, and gastrointestinal upset in high doses. In addition, those already suffering from ulcers may experience irritation due to increased acid production; those who have anxiety or panic attacks may find that caffeine worsens their symptoms; and those prone to heartburn may find that caffeine worsens this symptom because it relaxes sphincter muscles in the esophagus. Some people need very little caffeine to feel such effects, and the dosage for children is likely even lower than that for adults.

Withdrawal symptoms are also very real. Former coffee drinkers may experience headache, nausea, and depression for a short time after discontinuing use. These symptoms can be expected to peak at 20 to 48 hours following the last intake of caffeine. Symptoms hold true even for those trying to quit as little as one cup of coffee a day. Slow tapering of use over a few days is recommended to avoid these problems.

Are there more serious consequences of consuming caffeine regularly? It has been hypothesized that caffeine consumption can lead to certain types of cancer, such as pancreatic and bladder cancers. The association of caffeine with cancer has not been supported in recent literature. If fact, regular coffee consumption has been linked to a decreased risk of colon cancer.

The limelight also has been drawn away from caffeine with regard to cardiovascular disease and moderate coffee consumption. Heavy use does increase blood pressure for a short period of time. Coffee consumption also has been linked to increased LDL-cholesterol and triglycerides in the blood. This association was found to be caused by cafestol and kahweol, two oils in ground coffee. However, filtered and instant coffees do not contain the harmful oils. When researchers correct for tobacco use in coffee drinkers, no distinct correlation is seen between moderate use of filtered or instant coffee consumption and increased risk for cardiovascular

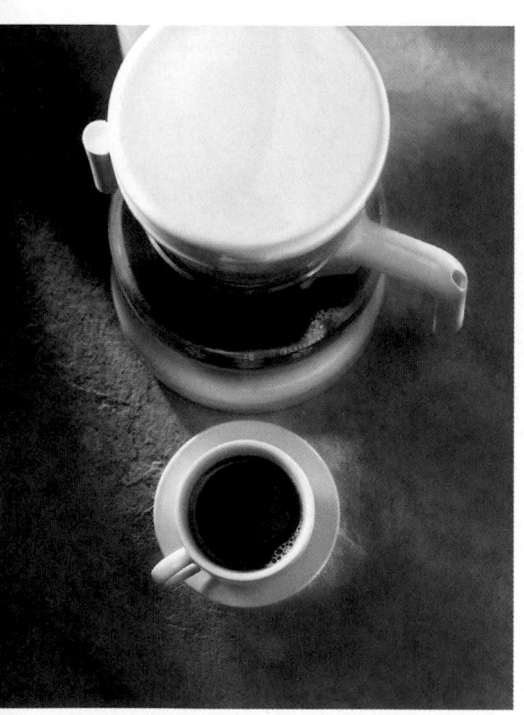

Coffee is a common source of caffeine for many adults.

disease. It is prudent, though, to limit the amount of coffee in general, especially from French coffee presses and from espresso as these beverages are not filtered.

Women are thought to be at higher risk for a variety of deleterious effects with caffeine consumption, including miscarriages, osteoporosis, and birth defects in their offspring. It is true that heavy caffeine use mildly increases the amount of calcium excreted in urine. For this reason, it is important that heavy coffee drinkers check their diets for adequate calcium sources. Some studies do show a higher likelihood for miscarriages in women consuming more than 500 milligrams of caffeine per day (about five 8 ounce cups of coffee). FDA warns women to consume caffeine in moderation (no more than the equivalent of one to two 8 ounce cups of coffee per day).

In contrast to these possibly harmful effects of caffeine consumption, many people are convinced of the benefits of a "cup of joe." Though some women testify to the idea that caffeine improves premenstrual symptoms, currently no study proves this theory. Some weight-loss drugs previously contained caffeine, under the assumption that it made the drugs more effective. FDA has since banned this use as it was found to be ineffective. Some newer research findings suggest caffeine may reduce the risk of developing headaches, cirrhosis of the liver, some forms of kidney stones, gallbladder stones, some nerve-related diseases, and aids in blood glucose regulation. You may have heard that caffeine can improve physical performance. This has been shown in highly trained athletes; recall that use of large amounts of caffeine is banned by the NCAA (review Chapter 11). For those who are below professional status, though, no benefit has been shown. Also keep in mind that coffee will not "sober up" a person who is drunk.

Though the debate over caffeine will likely continue as long as North Americans drink coffee, current research does not support many of the concepts previously thought of as fact. These studies are, in fact, reinforcing the idea of moderation—the equivalent of about two to three 8 ounce cups of coffee per day. A prudent dose of caffeine is 200 to 300 milligrams per day. Table 16-4 lists the caffeine content of typical sources, as does Appendix J.

Table 16-4 Caffeine Content of Common Sources

Item	Milligrams of Caffeine	
	Typical	Range*
Coffee (8 fl oz cup)		
Brewed, drip method	85	65–120
Brewed, percolator	75	60–85
Decaffeinated, brewed	3	2–4
Espresso (1 fl oz serving)	40	30–50
Teas (8 fl oz cup)		
Brewed	40	20–90
Instant	28	24–31
Iced (8 fl oz glass)	25	9–50
Some soft drinks (8 fl oz)	24	20–40
"Energy drinks" such as Red Bull	80	0–80
Cocoa beverage (8 fl oz)	6	3–32
Chocolate milk beverage (8 fl oz)	5	2–7
Milk chocolate (1 oz)	6	1–15
Dark chocolate, semi-sweet (1 oz)	20	5–35
Baker's chocolate (1 oz)	26	26
Chocolate-flavored syrup (1 fl oz)	4	4

*For the coffee and tea products, the range varies due to brewing method, plant variety, brand of product, etc.

Source: International Food Information Council. *Caffeine and women's health,* August 2002.

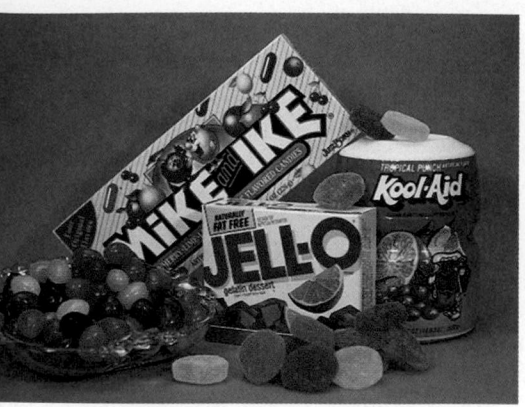

Color additives make some foods more desirable. Their use must be noted on the label so people sensitive to certain varieties can avoid that substance.

be 10 times more sensitive than another. This very broad margin essentially ensures that the food additive in question will cause no harmful health effects in humans. In fact, many synthetic chemicals are probably less dangerous at these low doses than some of the natural compounds in common foods such as apples or celery.

One important exception applies to the schema for testing intentional food additives: If an additive is shown to cause cancer, even though only in very high doses, no margin of safety is allowed. The food additive cannot be used, because it would violate the **Delaney Clause** in the 1958 Food Additives Amendment. This clause prohibits intentionally adding to foods a compound that was introduced after 1958 and causes cancer at any level of exposure. Evidence for cancer could come from either laboratory animal or human studies. Very few exceptions to this clause are allowed; exceptions are discussed regarding curing and pickling agents in Table 16-5.

Incidental food additives are another matter altogether. FDA cannot simply ban various industrial chemicals, pesticide residues, and mold toxins from foods, even though some of these contaminants can cause cancer. These products are not purposely added to foods. FDA sets an acceptable level for these substances. Basically, an incidental substance found in a food cannot contribute to more than one cancer case during the lifetimes of 1 million people. If a higher risk exists, the amount of the compound in a food must be reduced until the guideline is met.

■ Approval for a New Food Additive

Today, before a new food additive can be added to foods, FDA must approve its use. Besides rigorously testing an additive to establish its safety margins, manufacturers must give FDA information that (1) identifies the new additive, (2) gives its chemical composition, (3) states how it is manufactured, and (4) specifies laboratory methods used to measure its presence in the food supply at the amount of intended use.

Manufacturers must also offer proof that the additive will accomplish its intended purpose in a food, that it is safe, and that it is to be used in no higher amount than needed. Additives cannot be used to hide defective food ingredients, such as rancid oils; to deceive customers; or replace good manufacturing practices. A manufacturer must establish that the ingredient is necessary for producing a specific food product.

Common Food Additives

Common food additives serve the general function of **preservatives,** including acidic or alkaline agents, antioxidants, antimicrobial agents, curing and pickling agents, and

Delaney Clause A clause to the 1958 Food Additives Amendment of the Pure Food and Drug Act in the United States that prevents the intentional (direct) addition to foods of a compound that has been shown to cause cancer in laboratory animals or humans.

preservatives Compounds that extend the shelf life of foods by inhibiting microbial growth or minimizing the destructive effect of oxygen and metals.

Sugar, salt, corn syrup, and citric acid constitute 98% of all additives (by weight) used in food processing.

Table 16-5 Types of Food Additives—Sources and Related Health Concerns

Food Additive Class	Attributes	Health Risks
Acidic or alkaline agents, such as citric acid, calcium lactate, and sodium hydroxide	Acids impart a tart taste to soft drinks, sherbets, and cheese spreads; inhibit mold growth; lessen discoloration and rancidity. They also reduce the risk of botulism in naturally low-acid vegetables, such as canned green beans. Alkaline agents neutralize acids produced during fermentation, and so improve flavor.	No known health risks when used properly
Alternative low-calorie sweeteners, such as saccharin, sucralose, ascesulfame potassium, aspartame neotame, and tagatose	Sweeten foods without adding more than a few calories	Moderate use of these alternative sweeteners is considered safe (except for use of aspartame by people with the disease PKU)

Table 16-5 (continued)

Food Additive Class	Attributes	Health Risks
Anticaking agents, such as calcium silicate, magnesium stearate, and silicon dioxide	Absorb moisture to keep table salt, baking powder, or powdered sugar and powdered food products free-flowing and prevent caking and lumping	No known health risks when used properly
Antimicrobial agents, such as salt, sodium benzoate, sorbic acid, and calcium propionate	Inhibit mold and fungal growth	Salt increases the risk of developing hypertension, especially in some individuals. No known health risks from other agents when used properly
Antioxidants, such as BHA (butylated hydroxyanisole), BHT (butylated hydroxytoluene), alpha-tocopherol (vitamin E), ascorbic acid (vitamin C), and sulfites	Delay food discolorations from oxygen exposure Reduce rancidity from the breakdown of fats Maintain the color of luncheon meats Prevent the formation of cancer-causing nitrosamines	Sulfites can cause an allergic reaction in about 1 in every 100 people. Symptoms include difficulty breathing, wheezing, hives, diarrhea, abdominal pain, cramps, and dizziness. Salad bars, dried fruit, and wine are typical sources of sulfites.
Color additives, such as tartrazine	Make foods more appealing	Tartrazine (FD&C yellow number 5) can cause allergic symptoms such as hives and nasal discharge in some people, especially those allergic to aspirin. FDA requires manufacturers to list all forms of synthetic colors on the labels of foods that contain them.
Curing and pickling agents, such as salt, nitrates, and nitrites	Nitrates and nitrites act as preservatives, especially to prevent the growth of *Clostridium botulinium;* often used in conjunction with salt.	Salt increases the risk of developing hypertension, especially in some individuals. Nitrate and nitrite consumption from both cured foods and that found naturally in some vegetables has been associated with synthesis of nitrosamines. (An adequate vitamin C intake may reduce this synthesis.) Some nitrosamines are cancer-causing agents, particularly for the stomach, esophagus, and colon, but the risk is quite low. The National Cancer Institute advises consuming these foods in moderation.
Emulsifiers, such as monoglycerides and lecithins	Suspend fat in water to improve uniformity, smoothness, and body of foods, such as baked goods, ice cream, and mayonnaise	No known health risks when used properly
Fat replacements, such as Paselli SA2, Dur-Low, Oatrim, Sta-Slim 143, Stellar, and Olean	Limit calorie content of foods by reducing some of the fat content	Generally no known health risks when used properly.

Soft drinks are typical sources of alternative sweeteners for many of us. Moderate use of these products generally poses no health risk in most people.

You might wonder why, if nitrates and nitrites form chemical substances that can cause cancer, they aren't banned by the Delaney Clause. In the United States, USDA regulates the use of chemicals in meats. The laws that govern USDA regulation of foods are separate from those that govern FDA regulation. Because of this, the Delaney Clause does not apply to USDA actions. Currently USDA sees no clear threat to public safety from the regulated use of nitrates and nitrites in meats, so no action has been taken.

(Continued)

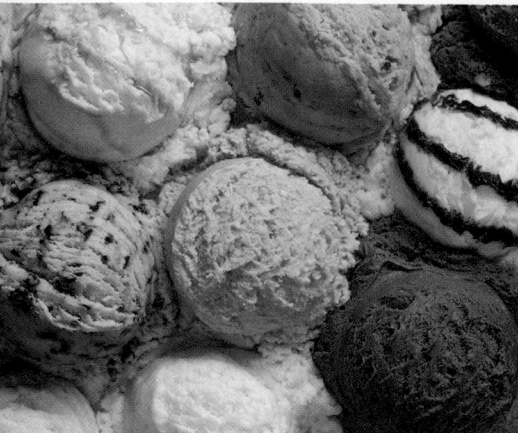

Emulsifiers improve the texture of foods such as ice cream, baked goods, and cookies.

Critical Thinking

Recognizing that Joseph is taking a nutrition class, his roommate asks him, "What is more risky: the bacteria that can be present in food or the additives listed on the label of my favorite snack cake?" How should Joseph respond? On what information should he base his conclusions?

Table 16-5 (concluded)

Food Additive Class	Attributes	Health Risks
Flavor and flavoring agents (such as natural and artificial flavors), sugar, and corn syrup	Impart more or improve flavor of foods	Sugar and corn syrup can increase risk for dental caries. Generally no known health risks for flavoring agents when used properly.
Flavor enhancers, such as monosodium glutamate (MSG) and salt	Help bring out the natural flavor of foods, such as meats	Some people (especially infants) are sensitive to the glutamate portion of MSG and after exposure experience flushing, chest pain, facial pressure, dizziness, sweating, rapid heart rate, nausea, vomiting, increase in blood pressure, and headache. Those so affected should look for the word glutamate on food labels, as well as isolated protein, yeast extract, bullion, and soup stock. Salt increases the risk of developing hypertension, especially in some people.
Humectants, such as glycerol, propylene glycol, and sorbitol	Retain more moisture, texture, and fresh flavor in foods such as candies, shredded coconut, and marshmallows	No known health risk when used properly
Leavening agents, such as yeast, baking powder, and baking soda	Introduce carbon dioxide into food products	No known health risk when used properly
Maturing and bleaching agents, such as bromates, peroxides, and ammonium chloride	Shorten the time needed for maturation of flour to become usable for baking products	No known health risk when used properly
Nutrient supplements, such as vitamin A, vitamin D, and potassium iodide	Enhance the nutrient content of foods such as margarine, milk, and ready-to-eat breakfast cereals	No known health risk if intake from such supplemental sources combined with other natural food sources of a nutrient does not exceed the Upper Level set for a particular nutrient (iron may be one exception; review Chapter 9)
Stabilizers and thickeners, such as pectins, gums, gelatins, and agars	Impart a smooth texture and uniform color and flavor to candies, ice cream and other frozen desserts, chocolate milk, and beverages containing alternative sweeteners. Prevent evaporation and deterioration of flavorings used in cakes, puddings, and gelatin mixes	No known health risk when used properly
Sequestrants, such as EDTA and citric acid	Bind free ions, helping preserve food quality by reducing ability of ions to cause rancidity in products containing fat	No known health risk when used properly

sequestrants. Table 16-5 helps you to understand exactly why these are used and to learn more about the specific substances used.

In general, if you consume a variety of foods in moderation, the chances of food additives jeopardizing your health are minimal. Pay attention to your body. If you suspect an intolerance or a sensitivity, consult your physician for further evaluation. Remember that in the short run, you are more likely to suffer either from foodborne illness due to poor food-handling practices that allow viral and bacterial contamination in food, or from the consumption of raw animal foods, than from consuming additives. Excess calories, saturated fat, cholesterol, *trans* fat, salt, and other potential "problem" nutrients in our diets pose the greatest long-term health risk.

sequestrants Compounds that bind free metal ions. By so doing, they reduce the ability of ions to cause rancidity in foods containing fat.

Another Bite

If you are bewildered or concerned about all the additives in your diet, you can easily avoid most of them by consuming unprocessed whole foods (Fig. 16-3). However, no evidence shows that this will necessarily make you healthier, nor can you avoid all additives, since some are used even on whole foods, such as with pesticides. It amounts to a personal decision. Do you have confidence that FDA and food manufacturers are adequately protecting your health and welfare, or do you want to take more personal control by minimizing your intake of compounds not naturally found in foods?

Concept Check

Food additives are used to reduce spoilage from microbial growth, oxygen, metals, and other compounds. Additives are also used to adjust acidity, improve flavor and color, leaven, provide nutritional fortification, thicken, and emulsify food components. Additives are classified as intentional (direct), which are purposely added to foods, and incidental (indirect), which turn up in foods from environmental contamination or various manufacturing practices. The amount of an additive allowed in a food is limited to one-one-hundredth of the highest amount that has no observable effect when fed to animals. The Delaney Clause allows FDA to limit intentional addition of cancer-causing compounds to food in the United States under its jurisdiction. Also set by law in the United States are the permissible amounts of carcinogens that incidentally enter foods.

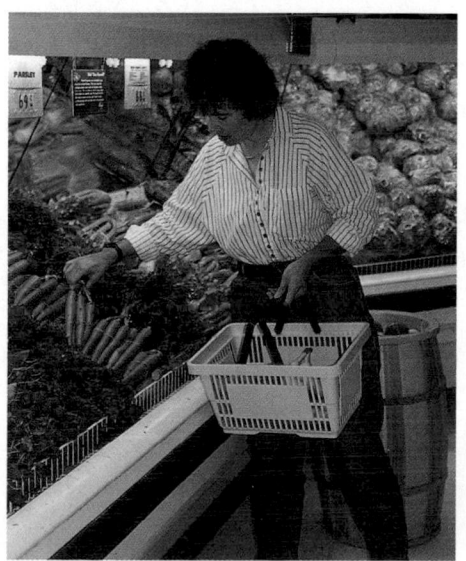

(a)

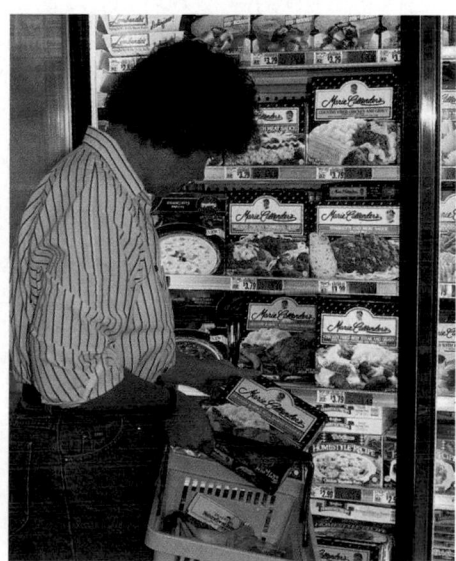

(b)

Figure 16-3 Depending on food choices, fresh vs. processed a diet can be either (a) essentially free of or (b) contain food additives. For most of us, this specific concern regarding food choice is not worth worrying about.

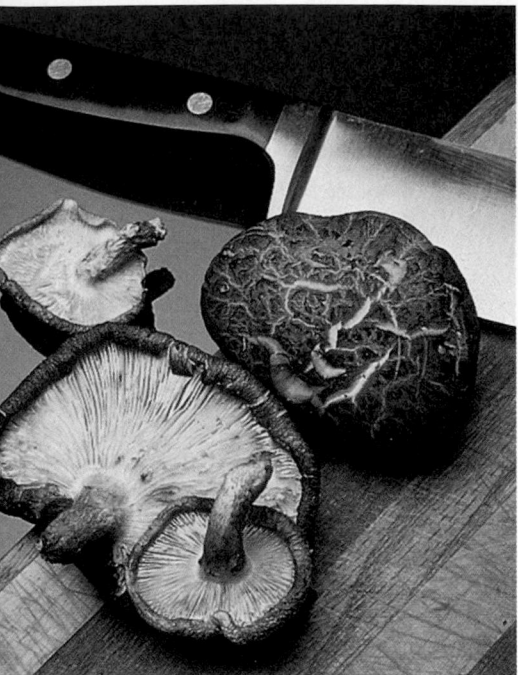

When hunting wild mushrooms, know what you are looking for. Many varieties contain deadly toxins.

Substances That Occur Naturally in Foods and Can Cause Illness

Foods contain a variety of naturally occurring substances that can cause illness. Here are some of the more important examples:

Safrole—found in sassafras, mace, and nutmeg; causes cancer when consumed in high doses

Solanine—found in potato shoots and green spots on potato skins; inhibits the action of neurotransmitters

Mushroom toxins—found in some species of mushrooms such as aminita; can cause stomach upset, dizziness, hallucinations, and other neurological symptoms. The more lethal varieties can cause liver and kidney failure, coma, and even death. FDA regulates commercially grown and harvested mushrooms. These are cultivated in concrete buildings or caves. However, there are no systematic controls on individual gatherers harvesting wild species, except in Michigan and Illinois.

Avidin—found in raw egg whites (cooking destroys avidin); binds the vitamin biotin in a way that prevents its absorption, so a biotin deficiency may ultimately develop over the long term

Thiaminase—found in raw fish, clams, and mussels; destroys the vitamin thiamin

Tetrodotoxin—found in puffer fish; causes respiratory paralysis

Oxalic acid—found in spinach, strawberries, sesame seeds, and other foods; binds calcium and iron in the foods, and so limits absorption of these nutrients

Herbal teas—containing senna or comfrey; can cause diarrhea and liver damage

People have coexisted for centuries with these naturally occurring substances and have learned to avoid some of them and limit intake of others. Today, they pose little health risk. Farmers know potatoes must be stored in the dark, so that solanine won't be synthesized. Furthermore, we've developed cooking and food-preparation methods to limit the potency of other substances, such as thiaminase. Spices are used in such small amounts that health risks don't result. Nevertheless, it's important to understand that some potentially harmful chemicals in foods occur naturally.

Genetic alteration of foods such as corn and soybeans has recently created concern, especially in Europe. FDA considers genetically altered products safe if approval for human use has been granted (see Chapter 17 for details).

Environmental Contaminants in Food

A variety of environmental contaminants can be found in foods. The second Looking Further section in this chapter looks at risks of pesticide residues in the diet. Aside from pesticide residues, other potential contaminants that deserve attention are listed in Table 16-6.

Protection from Environmental Toxins in Foods

To reduce exposure to environmental toxins present in our foods that cause disease, find out which foods pose a risk. In addition, emphasize variety and moderation in food selection. Note also that tips provided in Table 16-7 in the Looking Further, "Pesticides in Food," also apply to reducing exposure to environmental contaminants.

Concept Check

A general program to minimize exposure to environmental contaminants includes knowing which foods pose greater risks and consuming a wide variety of foods in moderation.

Table 16-6 Potential Environmental and Other Contaminants in Our Food Supply

Chemical Substance	Sources	Toxic Effects	Preventive Measures
Lead	Lead-based paint chips and related dust in older homes Occupational exposure (e.g., radiator repair) Lead caps on wine bottles Fruit juices and pickled vegetables stored in galvanized or tin containers or leaded glass Some types of solder used in joining copper pipes (mostly in older homes) Mexican pottery dishes Koo Soo herbal remedies Leaded glass containers	Anemia Kidney disease Nervous system damage (tiredness and changes in behavior are symptoms) Reduced learning capacity in childhood (even from mild lead exposure)	Avoid paint chips and related dust in older homes; regular cleaning of these homes is also important (see www.hud.gov/offices/lead/index.cfm). Meet iron and calcium needs to reduce lead absorption. Wipe the inside and outside neck of wine bottles before use if the bottle has a lead cap. Store fruit juices and pickled vegetables in glass or plastic or waxed paper containers. Let water run 1 minute or so if off for more than 2 hours, and use only cold water for cooking; do not soften drinking water. Do not store alcoholic beverages in leaded glass containers.
Dioxin	Trash-burning incinerators Bottom-feeding fish from the Great Lakes Animal fats from animals exposed to such contamination via water or soil	Abnormal reproduction and fetal/infant development Immune suppression Cancer (to date only clearly shown in laboratory animals)	Pay attention to warnings of dioxin risks from local fish; if risk exists, limit intake as suggested on the fishing license. Consume a variety of fish from local waters rather than mostly one specific species.
Mercury	Swordfish, shark, king mackerel, and tilefish. Fresh and canned albacore tuna also is a possible source. (In contrast, the more typical light chuck tuna is very low in mercury.)	Reduced fetal/child development and birth defects; toxic to nervous system	Consume these sources no more than once per week, no more than two times per week for albacore tuna. Pregnant women should avoid these species of fish, but some albacore tuna consumption is fine. Two to three fish meals per week is appropriate for pregnant (and nursing) women if different types of fish are eaten.
Cadmium	Plants in general if much cadmium is in the soil Clams, shellfish, tobacco smoke (occupational exposure) in some cases	Kidney disease Liver disease Prostate cancer (debatable) Bone deformaties Lung disease (when inhaled)	Consume a wide variety of foods, including seafood sources.
Urethane	Alcoholic beverages such as sherry, bourbon, sake, and fruit brandies	Cancer (to date only clearly shown in laboratory animals)	Avoid generous amounts of typical sources.
Polychlorinated biphenyls (PCBs)	Fish from the Great Lakes and Hudson River Valley (e.g., coho salmon) Farmed salmon are a possible source, but less so.	Cancer (to date only clearly shown in laboratory animals), as well as a potential for liver, immune, and reproductive disorders	Pay attention to warnings of PCB contamination from local fish; if risk exists, limit intake as suggested on the fishing license or on state advisories. Vary the type of fish eaten during a specific week.
Acrylamide	Fried foods rich in carbohydrate cooked at high temperatures for extended periods of time, such as French fries and potato chips	Potential neurotoxin and carcinogen. Known carcinogen for laboratory animals; however, studies have not clearly proven the relationship between acrylamide ingestion and the development of cancer in humans.	Limit intake of deep-fat fried foods rich in carbohydrate.

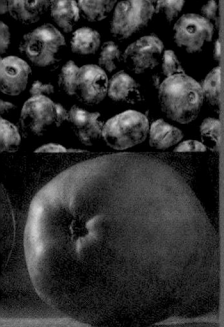

Looking Further

Pesticides in Food

One of the problems with pesticides is that they create new pests because they destroy the predators (spiders, wasps, and beetles) that naturally keep most plantfeeding insect populations in check. The brown plant hopper, which recently plagued Indonesian rice fields, was not a serious problem before heavy pesticide use began to kill its predators in the early 1970s. In the United States, such major pests as spider mites and the cotton bollworm were merely nuisances until pesticides decimated their predators.

Pesticides used in food production produce both beneficial and unwanted effects. Most health authorities believe that the benefits outweigh the risks. Pesticides help ensure a safe and adequate food supply and help make foods available at reasonable cost. However, sentiment is growing nationwide that pesticides pose avoidable health risks. Consumers have come to assume that synthetic is dangerous and organic is safe. Some researchers believe this sentiment is grounded in fear and fueled by unbalanced reports. Other researchers say concern about pesticides is valid and overdue.

Most concern about pesticide residues in food appropriately focuses on chronic rather than acute toxicity because the amounts of residue present, if any, are extremely small. These low concentrations found in foods are not known to produce adverse effects in the short term, although harm has been caused by the high amounts that occasionally result from accidents or misuse. For humans, pesticides pose a danger mainly in their cumulative effects, so their threats to health are difficult to determine. However, growing evidence, including the problems of the contamination of underground water supplies and destruction of wildlife habitats, indicates that North Americans would probably be better off if we could reduce our use of pesticides. Both the U.S. federal government and many farmers are working toward that end. Chapter 17 discusses the lastest use of biotechnology to reduce pesticide use.

What Is a Pesticide?

Federal law defines a pesticide as any substance or mixture of substances intended to prevent, destroy, repel, or mitigate any pest. The built-in toxic properties of pesticides lead to the possibility that other, nontarget organisms, including humans, might also be harmed. The term *pesticide* tends to be used as a generic reference to many types of products, including insecticides, herbicides, fungicides, and rodenticides. A pesticide product may be chemical or bacterial, natural or synthetic. For agriculture, EPA allows about 10,000 pesticides to be used, containing some 300 active ingredients. About 1.2 billion pounds of pesticides are used each year in the United States, much of which is applied to agricultural crops.

Once a pesticide is applied, it can turn up in a number of unintended and unwanted places. It may be carried in the air and dust by wind currents, remain in soil attached to soil particles, be taken up by organisms in the soil, decompose to other compounds, be taken up by plant roots, enter groundwater, or invade aquatic habitats. Each is a route to the food chain; some are more direct than others.

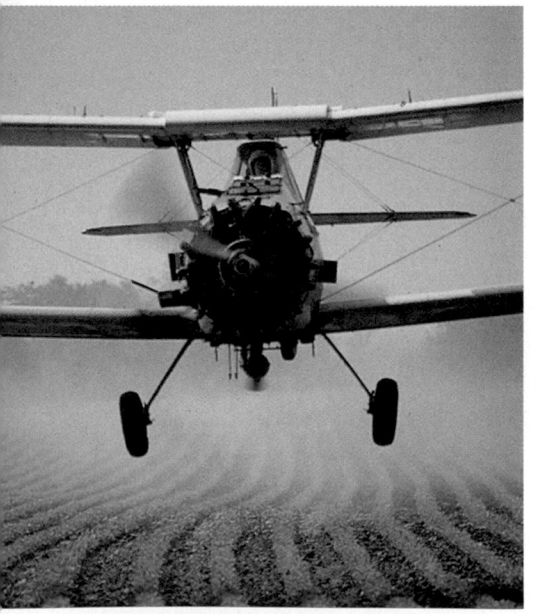

Pesticide use poses a risk-versus-benefit question. Each side has points that deserve to be considered. Rural communities, where exposure is more direct, experience the greatest short-term risk.

Why Use Pesticides?

In the United States alone, pests destroy nearly $20 billion of food crops yearly, despite extensive pesticide use. The primary reason for using pesticides is economic—the use of agricultural chemicals increases production and lowers the cost of food, at least in the short run. Many farmers believe that it would be impossible to stay in business without pesticides, which help protect farmers from ruinous losses.

Consumer demands also have changed over the years. At one time, we wouldn't have thought twice about buying an apple with a worm hole; we simply took it home, cut out the wormy part, and ate the apple. Today, consumers find worm holes less acceptable, so farmers rely more and more on pesticides to produce cosmetically attractive fruits and vegetables. On the practical side, pesticides can protect against the rotting and decay of fresh fruits and vegetables. This is helpful because our food distribution system doesn't usually permit consumer purchase within hours of harvest. Also, food grown without pesticides can contain naturally occurring organisms that produce carcinogens at concentrations far above current standards for pesticide residues. For example, fungicides help prevent the carcinogen aflatoxin (caused by growth of a fungus) from forming on some crops. Thus, although some pesticides may do little more than improve the appearance of food products, others help keep foods fresher and safer to eat.

Regulation of Pesticides

The responsibility for ensuring that residues of pesticides in foods are below amounts that pose a danger to health is shared by FDA, EPA, and the Food Safety and Inspection Service of USDA in the United States. Table 16-2 listed the roles of various food protection agencies. FDA is responsible for enforcing pesticide tolerances in all foods except meat, poultry, and certain egg products, which are monitored by USDA. A newly proposed pesticide is exhaustively tested, perhaps over 10 years or more, before it is approved for use. EPA must decide both that the pesticide causes no unreasonable adverse effects on people and the environment and that benefits of use outweigh the risks of using it. However, there is concern about older chemicals registered before 1970, when less stringent testing conditions were permitted. EPA is now asking chemical companies to retest the old compounds using more rigorous tests. Unfortunately, inadequate funding at EPA has hampered the review of older pesticides. The slow pace of this retesting has angered the critics of pesticide use. When weighing whether to approve or cancel a pesticide, EPA considers how much more it would cost the farmer to use an alternative pesticide or process and whether cancellation would decrease productivity. After determining the dollar cost to the farmer, EPA then looks at costs to processors and consumers. Once a pesticide is approved for use, it must follow the margin of safety provisions required of food additives (see a previous section, "Tests of Food Additives for Safety").

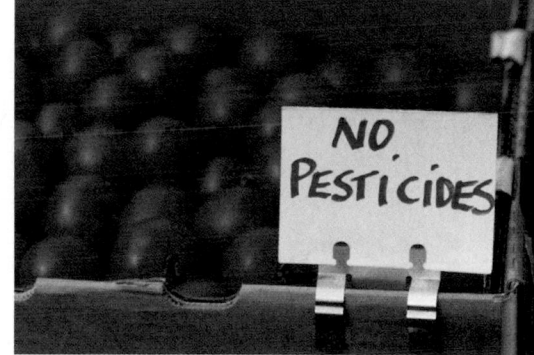

How Safe Are Pesticides?

Dangers from exposure to pesticides through food depend on how potent the chemical toxin is, how concentrated it is in the food, how much and how frequently it's eaten, and the consumer's resistance or susceptibility to the substance. Accumulating information links pesticide use to increased cancer rates in farm communities. For rural counties in the United States, the incidence of lymph, genital, brain, and digestive tract cancers increases with higher-than-average pesticide use. Respiratory cancer cases increase with greater insecticide use. In tests using laboratory animals, scientists have found that some of the chemicals present in pesticide residues cause birth defects, sterility, tumors, organ damage, and injury to the central nervous system. Some pesticides persist in the environment for years.

Fruits and vegetables grown without use of pesticides are available and may bear an "organic" label (see Table 2-9 in Chapter 2 for rules regarding the use of the term "organic" on food labels). These products generally are more expensive than those grown using pesticides. Consumers need to decide if the potential benefits of the products are worth the extra cost.

Still, some researchers argue that the cancer risk from pesticide residues is hundreds of times less than the risk from eating such common foods as peanut butter, brown mustard, and basil. Plants manufacture their own toxic substances to defend themselves against insects, birds, and grazing animals (including humans). When plants are stressed or damaged, they produce even more of these toxins. Because of this, many foods contain naturally occurring chemicals considered toxic, and some are even carcinogenic. Other scientists argue that if natural carcinogens are already in the food supply, then we should reduce the number of added carcinogens whenever possible. In other words, we should do what we can to decrease the problem.

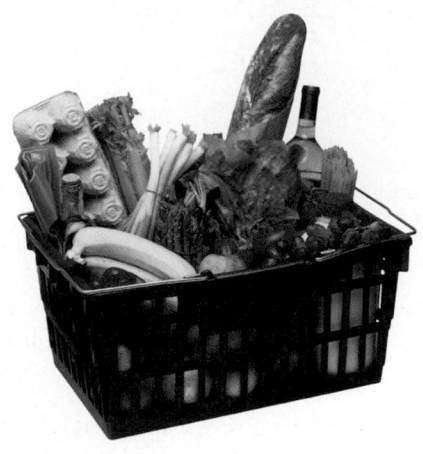

FDA's yearly evaluation of a "market basket" of typical foods shows that pesticide content is minimal in most foods.

Tests of the Amounts of Pesticides in Foods

FDA tests thousands of raw products each year for pesticide residues. (A pesticide is considered illegal in this case if it is not approved for use on the crop in question or if the amount used exceeds the allowed tolerance.) The latest FDA studies show no residues in about 60% of samples. Less than 1% of domestic and about 3% of import samples have residues that are continually over tolerance. These findings continue to support previous FDA studies over the past 10 years that pesticide residues in food are generally well below EPA tolerances, and they confirm the safety of the food supply relative to pesticide residues.

Personal Action

We often take risks in our own lives, but we prefer to have a choice in the matter after weighing the pros and cons. With regard to pesticides in food, however, someone else is deciding what is acceptable and what is not. Our only choice is whether to buy or avoid pesticide-containing foods. In reality it's almost impossible to avoid pesticides entirely, because even organic produce often contains traces of pesticides, probably as the result of cross-contamination from nearby farms.

Short-term studies of the effects of pesticides on laboratory animals cannot precisely pinpoint long-term cancer risks in humans. It should be clearly understood, however, that the presence of minute traces of an environmental chemical in a food does not mean that any adverse effect will result from eating that food.

FDA and other scientific organizations believe that the hazards are comparatively low and in the short run are less dangerous than the hazards of foodborne illness created in our own kitchens. We can not avoid pesticide risks entirely, but we can limit exposure by following some simple advice (Table 16-7).

We can also encourage farmers to use fewer pesticides to reduce exposure to our foods and water supplies, but we'll have to settle for produce that isn't perfect in appearance or that has been grown with the aid of biotechnology (again, see Chapter 17 for details). Are you concerned enough about pesticides on food to change your shopping habits or take more political action?

Table 16-7 What You Can Do to Reduce Exposure to Pesticides

FDA's sampling and testing show that pesticide residues in foods do not pose a health hazard. Nevertheless, if you want to reduce dietary exposure to pesticides, follow this advice from the Environmental Protection Agency:

- Consume a wide variety of foods, especially regarding fruits, vegetables, and fish.
- Thoroughly rinse and scrub (with a brush if possible) fruits and vegetables. Peel them, if appropriate—although some nutrients will be peeled away.
- Remove the outer leaves of leafy vegetables, such as lettuce and cabbage.
- Since residues of some pesticides in animal feed concentrate in the animals' fat, trim fat from meat, poultry, and fish, remove skin (which contains most of the fat) from poultry and fish, and discard fats and oils in broths and pan drippings.
- When fishing, throw back the big fish—the little ones have had less time to take up and concentrate pesticides and other harmful residues. In addition, pay attention to any warnings by local authorities (and on the fishing license) about the high risk for contamination in specific waters or species of fish.
- Avoid lawns, gardens, and flower beds that have recently been treated with pesticides and herbicides.

Rinsing fruits and vegetables under running water is advised to reduce pesticide exposure.

Adapted from Food and Drug Administration: Safety first: Protecting America's food supply, *FDA Consumer*, p. 26, November 1988.

Summary

1. Viruses, bacteria, and other microorganisms in food pose the greatest risk for foodborne illness. In the past, salt, sugar, smoke, fermentation, and drying were used to protect against foodborne illness. Today, careful cooking, pasteurization, keeping hot foods hot and cold foods cold, and thorough handwashing provide additional insurance.

2. Major causes of foodborne illness are Norovirus and the bacteria *Campylobacter jejuni*, *Salmonella*, *Staphylococcus aureus*, and *Clostridium perfringens*. In addition, such bacteria as *Clostridium botulinum*, *Listeria monocytogenes*, *Yersinia enterocolitica*, and *Escherichia coli* have been found to cause illness.

3. To protect against viruses and bacteria, cook susceptible foods thoroughly. In addition, cover cuts on the hands, do not sneeze or cough on foods, avoid contact between raw meat or poultry products and other food products, rapidly cool and thoroughly reheat leftovers, and use pasteurized dairy products. Overall, be careful when foods are in the "danger zone" (41°F to 135°F).

4. Cross-contamination commonly causes foodborne illness. It occurs particularly when bacteria on raw animal products contact foods that can support bacterial growth. Because of the risk of cross-contamination, no perishable food should be kept in the "danger zone" for more than 1 to 2 hours (depending on the environmental temperature), especially if it may have come in contact with raw animal products.

5. Treatment for foodborne illness usually requires drinking lots of fluids, avoiding touching food while diarrhea is present, washing hands thoroughly, and getting bed rest. Avoid preparing food for yourself or others and wash hands thoroughly and frequently while foodborne illness symptoms persist. Botulism and hepatitis A infections are types of foodborne illness that require prompt medical attention.

6. Food additives are used primarily to extend shelf life by preventing microbial growth and the destruction of food components by oxygen, metals, and other substances. Food additives are classified as those intentionally added to foods and those that incidentally appear in foods. An intentional additive is limited to no more than one-one-hundredth of the greatest amount that causes no observed symptoms in animals. The Delaney Clause allows FDA to ban the use of any intentional food additive under its jurisdiction in the United States that causes cancer.

7. Antioxidants, such as BHA, BHT, vitamins E and C, and sulfites, prevent oxygen and enzyme destruction of food products. Emulsifiers suspend fat in water, improving the uniformity, smoothness, and body of foods such as ice cream. Common preservatives include salt, sodium benzoate, and sorbic acid, which prevent bacterial growth. Sequestrants bind metals and thus prevent spoilage of food from metal contamination. Various natural products such as natural flavors, sugar, and corn syrup, as well as artificial flavors and sweeteners, such as aspartame, improve the flavor of food.

8. Toxic substances occur naturally in a variety of foods, such as green potatoes, raw fish, mushrooms, and raw egg whites. Cooking foods limits their toxic effects in some cases; others are best to avoid altogether, such as toxic mushroom species and the green parts of potatoes.

9. A variety of environmental contaminants and pesticide residues can be found in foods. It is helpful to know which foods pose the greatest risks and act accordingly to reduce exposure, such as washing fruits and vegetables before use.

Study Questions

1. Identify three major classes of microorganisms that are responsible for foodborne illness.

2. Which kinds of foods are most likely to be involved in foodborne illness? Why are they targets for contamination?

3. What three trends in food purchasing and production have led to a greater number of cases of foodborne illness in recent years?

4. Why is thoroughly cooking food an important practice for reducing the risk of foodborne illness?

5. List four techniques other than thorough cooking that are important in preventing foodborne illness.

6. Define the term *food additive*, and give examples of four intentional food additives. What are their specific functions in foods? What is their relationship to the GRAS list?

7. Describe the federal process that governs the use of food additives, including the Delaney Clause.

8. Put into perspective the benefits and risks of using additives in food. Point out an easy way to reduce the consumption of food additives. Do you think this is worth the effort in terms of maintaining health? Why or why not?

9. Describe four recommendations for reducing the risk of toxicity from environmental contaminants.

10. How do various U.S. federal agencies work together to maintain the safety of food?

Further Readings

1. Acheson DWK: Emerging food pathogens. *Nutrition & the M.D.* 29(3):1, 2003.

   Many diseases known to be transmitted via food have been identified, including illnesses caused by microorganisms, toxins, chemicals, and prions. The actual list of important agents is relatively short. Many of these agents can be considered emerging because they were not recognized until recent times.

   The article reviews in detail the major agents responsible for foodborne illness.

2. Acheson DWK and Fiore AE: Preventing foodborne illness—what clinicians can do. *The New England Journal of Medicine* 350:437, 2004.

   The food supply in the United States is mostly safe, but more could be done to lessen the risk for developing foodborne illness. This article discusses strategies to do so, as well as summarizes the characteristics of the major organisms that cause foodborne illness.

3. ADA Reports: Position of the American Dietetic Association: Food and water safety. *Journal of the American Dietetic Association* 103:1203, 2003.

It is the position of the American Dietetic Association that the public has a right to a safe food and water supply. Still, it is estimated that on an annual basis there are 76 million cases of foodborne illness in the United States, with significant economic cost. Thus more work needs to be done with regard to food safety. The safety of drinking water is a lesser concern in general for most consumers, but still deserves consideration as a potential source of illness.

4. Anderson JB and others: A camera's view of consumer food-handling behaviors. *Journal of the American Dietetic Association* 104:186, 2004.

    Improper food handling practices were common in the households studied in this survey. Implementing the Fight BAC! Campaign recommendations, such as using a thermometer to test for doneness in meats, would improve food handling practices.

5. Atreya CD: Major foodborne illness causing viruses and current status of vaccines against the disease. *Foodborne Pathogens and Disease* 1(2): 89, 2004 (Summer)

    As many as 67% of cases of foodborne illnesses are caused by viruses. Except for hepatitis A virus, no vaccines are available for the major players, but may be available in the near future. This article reviews the current progress in this area.

6. Bren L: Turning up the heat on acrylamide. *FDA Consumer*, p. 10, January-February, 2003.

    FDA is currently investigating the risks of acrylamide in our diets, but does not consider the evidence sufficient to warn people about the proposed risk. FDA instead is re-emphasizing its traditional advice to eat a balanced diet, choosing a variety of low-fat and high-fiber grains, fruits, and vegetables.

7. Calvert GM: Health effects of pesticides. *American Family Physician* 69: 1613, 2004.

    Clear cases of disease from pesticide exposure are seen from acute exposures with high amounts. The true effects of low dose, chronic exposure has been hard to quantify, but most adults have detectable pesticide levels in their blood. Thus, efforts should be made to reduce pesticide exposure when possible, especially with use in and around the house.

8. Foodborne Illness primer Work Group: Foodborne illness primer for physicians and other healthcare professionals. *Nutrition in Clinical Care* 7:131, 2004.

    Foodborne illness is a serious health problem, primarily for the very young, older adults, and those using immunosuppressive medications. This article provides practical advice on the diagnosis, treatment, and prevention of foodborne illness.

9. Gerner-Smidt P and others: Invasive listeriosis in Denmark 1994-2003: A review of 299 cases with special emphasis on risk factors for mortality. *Clinical Microbiological Infections* 11: 618, 2005.

    Listeria infections lead to death primarily in older people and those with underlying cases of cancer. It

is therefore especially important for these people to careful of exposure to Listeria.

10. Hillers VN and others: Consumer food-handling behaviors associated with prevention of 13 foodborne illnesses. *Journal of Food Protection* 66:1893, 2003.

    Handwashing is highly recommended by experts for the prevention of foodborne illness. The importance of not eating certain foods, such as raw seafood, is another important habit to consider. The use of a thermometer in cooking is also an important practice, as is avoidance of cross-contamination of food products.

11. How now mad cow? *Tufts University Health & Nutrition Letter* p. 4, May 2004.

    After the recent case of mad cow disease in the United States, FDA expanded regulations regarding the feeding and slaughter of cattle. This goes beyond the already strict regulations put in place in 1997 to limit risk of mad cow disease. Overall, the risk of contracting mad cow disease from meat in the United States remains very low. Still one could consider avoiding ground meat products, such as hot dogs, and cow brains to further reduce risk as these are most likely to contain the agent that is linked to the disease.

12. Kline DA: Naturally occurring food contaminants. *Today's Dietitian*, p. 10, December 2001.

    A variety of naturally occurring toxins are present in our food supply. The mycotoxins from mold are common, as well as a variety of toxins present in mushrooms. The article discusses these and other naturally occurring toxins, and provides advice for minimizing such exposure.

13. McCabe-Sellers BJ, Beattie SF: Food safety: emerging trends in foodborne illness survreilance and prevention. *Journal of the American Dietetic Association* 104: 1708, 2004.

    Detailed discussion of prevention of foodborne illness, such as paying attention to fresh produce as a source of the primary causative agents—viruses and bacteria. Recommendations for consumers and food handlers are given to reduce risk of foodborne illness, with proper personal hygiene being a major focus.

14. Musher DM, Musher BL: Contagious acute bacterial infections. *The New England Journal of Medicine* 351: 2417, 2004.

    Detailed discussion of the viruses and bacteria associated with foodborne illness. Hand washing is one important method mentioned to reduce exposure. Use of diluted bleach solutions (1:10) on surfaces is also recommended when possible¡ .

15. New findings on caffeine and your health. *Tufts University Health & Nutrition Letter* 19(1) (March), 2001.

    Coffee use has been linked to a decreased risk of headaches, colon cancer, and some nerve disorders. Up to three cups of coffee per day is a safe intake for men and women.

16. Roche SJ, Keenan MJ: Should we be eating organically grown foods? *Today's Dietitian*, p. 50, September 2003.

    Probably the most valid reason for consuming organically grown foods instead of conventionally grown foods is the protection of the environment, farmers, and wildlife from pesticide exposure. Promotion of organic foods, however, must be balanced by the observation that use of pesticides by farmers increases efficiency and is a key reason for the abundance of food available in the United States.

17. Osterholm MT, Norgan AP: The role of food irradiation in food safety. *The New England Journal of Medicine* 350:1898, 2004.

    Irradiation of certain foods such as hamburger greatly reduces the risk for related foodborne illness, and so should be employed when useful for a specific food in question. Many government and professional organizations support use of irradiation. Still, proper food handling by manufacturers and consumers remains important, especially since some agents that cause foodborne illness are not susceptible to the radiation doses used.

18. Schardt D: Fishing for mercury. Who is at risk? *Nutrition Action Healthletter*, p. 9, March 2003.

    People should avoid eating swordfish and shark regularly or at all (since these fish are often high in mercury) and eat a variety of fish. People who eat locally caught fish should take into account any state and local advisories regarding the fish that are caught in mercury-contaminated lakes, rivers, and streams.

19. Schardt D: Get the lead out—What you don't know can hurt you. *Nutrition Action Healthletter* p. 1, March 2005.

    Reducing lead exposure as much as possible is important to protect one's health. There is evidence that hypertension, kidney disease, declines in brain function, and cataracts are linked to lead exposure. Testing your water supply for lead as outlined in the article is one inexpensive way to be alerted to a possible source. Using only cold tap water for cooking is also advised.

20. Sivapalasingam S and others: Fresh produce: a growing cause of outbreaks of foodborne illness in the United States. *Journal of Food Protection* 67: 2342, 2004.

    Fresh produce such as lettuce juices, melons, sprouts, and berries have recently been highlighted as sources of agents that lead to foodborne illness. Caution should be used with these items, just as one would with raw meat and dairy products.

21. Widdowson MA and others: Norovirus and foodborne disease, United States, 1991-2000. *Emerging Infectious Diseases* 11: 95, 2005.

    The norovirus leads to more causes of foodborne illness than any other agent. What is now needed is better surveillance for this organism so better estimates of actual cases can be made.

I. Can You Spot the Improper Food Safety Practices?

In this chapter you learned the following facts: (1) foodborne illness strikes up to 76 million U.S. citizens each year; (2) about 5000 deaths each year in the United States are caused by foodborne organisms.

Carefully preparing foods to prevent foodborne illness can minimize its occurrence for most of us. Read the following excerpt and find the food safety violations that could lead to illness.

A Local Health Department Inspector Gives the Following Account of His Visit to a Local Diner

As I walked through the kitchen of the Morningside Diner, I noticed that all food handlers washed their hands thoroughly with hot, soapy water before handling the food, especially after handling raw meat, fish, poultry, or eggs. Before preparing raw foods, they also thoroughly washed the cutting boards, dishes, and other equipment. As they used their cutting boards after cutting foods, they wiped them with a damp rag and used them again to cut more food.

When preparing fresh fruits and vegetables, they washed them but were careful to leave a little dirt on for fear of washing important nutrients from the outside. The cooks generally cooked meats to an internal temperature of 180°F (82°C). However, to preserve the flavor, pork was cooked to an internal temperature of 140°F (60°C). Some cooked foods to be served later were cooled to below 41°F (5°C) within 2 hours, and foods like beef stew were cooled in shallow pans.

The diner served canned foods, even when the cans were dented. When leftovers were reheated, they were raised to an internal temperature of 130°F (55°C) and served immediately. Food handlers took great care to remove moldy portions of food. The cooks prepared stuffing separately from the poultry. The temperature of refrigerators was approximately 45°F (7°C).

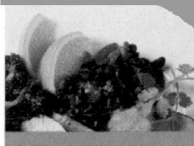

1. List the violations of food safety practices that could contribute to foodborne illness.

   _____

   _____

   _____

   _____

2. If you were writing a report describing ways to correct these practices, what would you say?

   _____

   _____

   _____

   _____

   _____

3. List the food safety practices that follow the general rules for preventing foodborne illness.

   _____

   _____

   _____

   _____

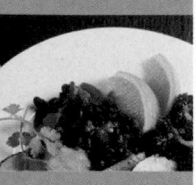

II. *Take a Closer Look at Food Additives*

Evaluate a food label of a convenience food (e.g., frozen entree, ready-to-eat baked good) item either in the supermarket or one you have available.

1. Write out the list of ingredients.

   _____

   _____

   _____

   _____

2. Identify the ingredients that you think may be food additives.

   _____

   _____

   _____

   _____

   _____

3. Based on the information available in this chapter, what are the functions of these food additives?

   _____

   _____

   _____

   _____

4. How might this food product differ without these ingredients?

   _____

   _____

   _____

   _____

Undernutrition throughout the World

Real Life Scenario

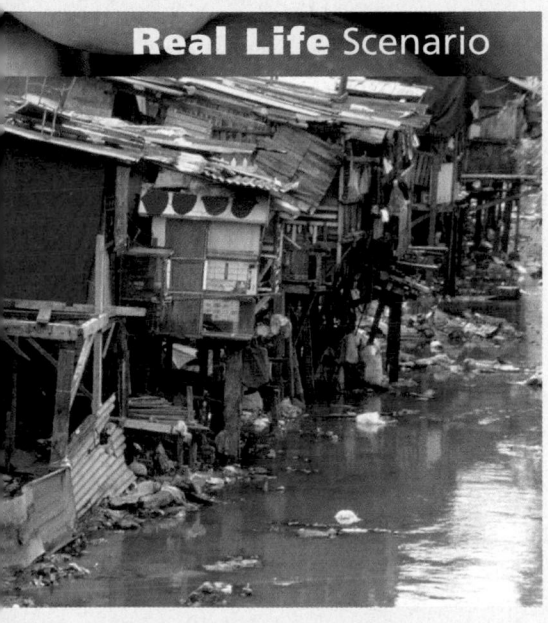

Jamal traveled to the Philippines with his church group during summer break. During their stay, they were to help build shelters for people in the village where a few weeks before a storm had destroyed most of the housing. Jamal noticed that many of the children in the village were short, much shorter than the children in his neighborhood. Mothers in the village stated that their children often had diarrhea and were ill. Jamal also noticed that the children were not as lively as he would expect.

A Filipino nurse at the local health clinic pointed out that these children generally did not have enough to eat and that health problems were rampant. She hoped that the recent storm would spur the Philippine government to send supplies to the village, particularly food and medicines.

Should Jamal have been surprised by widespread disease and general listlessness of the Philippine children? What nutrients are likely to be deficient in the diets of these children, in turn contributing to their poor health status?

Chapter 17 Objectives

Chapter 17 is designed to allow you to:

1. Define and characterize the terms *hunger*, *malnutrition*, and *undernutrition*.

2. Evaluate the consequences of undernutrition during critical periods in a person's life.

3. Examine undernutrition in the United States and highlight several programs established to combat this problem.

4. Examine undernutrition in the developing world and evaluate the major obstacles that hinder a solution.

5. Outline some possible solutions to undernutrition in the developing world.

6. List the worldwide effects of AIDS.

7. Consider how biotechnology may help solve the food shortage/distribution problem in the developing world.

Check out the **Contemporary Nutrition Online Learning Center**
www.mhhe.com/wardlawcont6 *for quizzes, flash cards, other activities, and web links designed to further help you learn about issues surrounding world hunger.*

Chapter 17 Outline

The images are vivid and appalling. Emaciated children with haunting eyes and distended stomachs, and too weak to cry, stare at us from news photos and television screens. Nearly 12 million children under age 5 die each year in developing countries; 55% of the deaths are attributable to undernutrition.

Today, nearly one in six people worldwide is chronically undernourished—too hungry to lead a productive, active life. Over the past 10 years, this problem has worsened. Throughout the world, the problems of poverty and undernutrition are widespread and growing—despite the fact that there is enough food available to sufficiently feed all of us.

The majority (two-thirds) of undernourished people live in Asia. However, the largest increase in numbers of chronically hungry people have recently occurred in eastern Africa, particularly in Ethiopia, Sudan, Rwanda, Burundi, Sierra Leone, Kenya, Somalia, Eritrea, and Tanzania.

Chapter 17 examines the problem of undernutrition, the conditions that create it, and some possible solutions. If we are to eradicate undernutrition, we all have to understand the problem and assume responsibility for supplying solutions. It is important to recognize that many political, economic, and social factors worldwide contribute directly and indirectly to the hunger problem.

Refresh Your Memory

As you begin your study of world hunger in Chapter 17, you may want to review:

- The health effects of protein-calorie malnutrition in Chapter 6
- The role of vitamin A and rich food sources in Chapter 8
- The roles and rich food sources of iron, zinc, and iodide in Chapter 9
- The advantages of breastfeeding for infants in Chapter 13
- Methods to monitor the adequacy of growth in Chapter 14

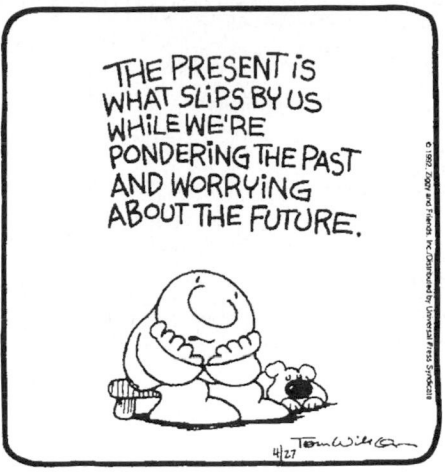

THE PRESENT iS WHAT SLiPS BY US WHiLE WE'RE PONDERING THE PAST AND WORRYING ABOUT THE FUTURE.

Millions of people worldwide die each year from health problems related to undernutrition. War and environmental catastrophe combine today with the global threat of AIDS as important causes. Why must we act today to stem this tide of undernutrition? Why is Ziggy's concern an important one? Chapter 17 provides some answers.

World Hunger: A Continuing Plague

In November 1974, the United Nations World Food Conference proclaimed its bold objective "that within a decade no child will go to bed hungry, that no family will fear for its next day's bread, and that no human being's future and capacities will be stunted by malnutrition." Today, this promise remains unfulfilled: Uncertainty regarding the source of one's next meal remains a daily experience for one in six people in the developing world (800 million to 1.1 billion) and one in ten households in North America.

We must face the reality that the United Nations' members have yet to meet their current pledge to elevate 3 billion people (half of the world's population) out of poverty (living on less than $2 per day). We also have to consider that 45% of the world's income currently goes to the 12% of the world's people who live in the rich industrial nations such as the United States and Canada.

World Hunger Today

Let's begin our look at the problem of world hunger and malnutrition today by defining some key terms.

Hunger is the physiological state that results when not enough food is eaten to meet energy needs. It also describes an uneasiness, a discomfort, a weakness, or a pain caused by lack of food. The medical and social costs of the undernutrition that can result from hunger are high—preterm births, mental disabilities, inadequate growth and development in childhood, poor school performance, decreased work output in adulthood, and chronic disease (Table 17-1). Although malnutrition does occur in North America, it is not due to extreme poverty over a large section of the population. Instead, there are usually specific causes such as an eating disorder, alcoholism, problems in nursing home settings, or homelessness. There is also some degree of moderate malnutrition in some of the poorer segments of North American society. Fortunately, there are resources such as food banks and food stamps that are available to many such people, though sometimes there are bureaucratic obstacles to getting these resources to the people who need them. In addition, there is also a problem known as **food insecurity** that is used to categorize individuals who have anxiety about running out of food or running out of money to buy more food. In 2002, over 11% of households in the United States reported that they experienced food insecurity.

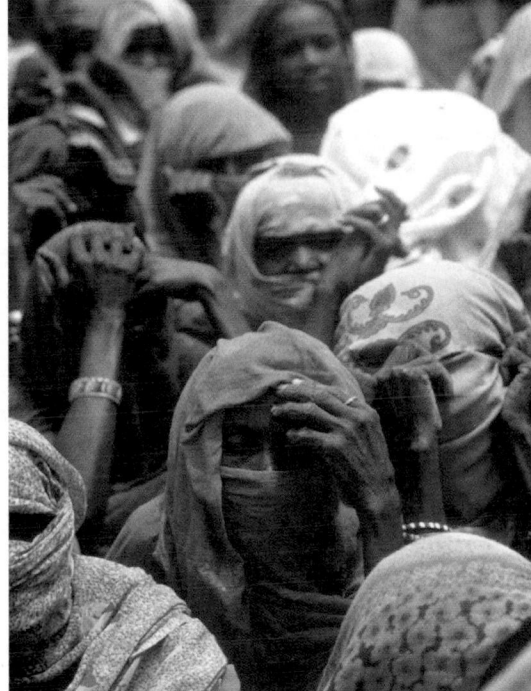

Every year crises that develop worldwide put many people at risk of undernutrition.

hunger The primarily physiological (internal) drive to find and eat food.

food insecurity A condition of anxiety regarding running out of either food or money to buy more food.

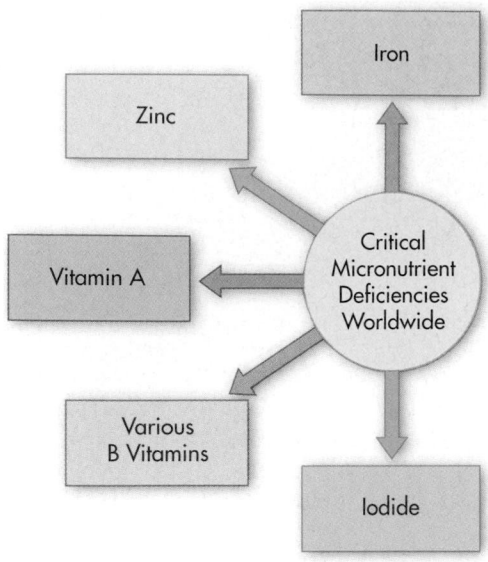

Table 17-1 The Realities of Undernutrition

- Nearly one in six people worldwide is chronically undernourished—too hungry to lead a productive, active life. This includes one-third of the world's children.
- About 55,000 people die of hunger each day—two-thirds of them are children.
- About 2 billion people in the world suffer from a micronutrient deficiency.
- About 1 billion people in the world have iron deficiency. The same is true for zinc deficiencies.
- Up to 500,000 children are permanently blinded each year simply from lack of vitamin A. About 100 million to 140 million children are deficient in vitamin A.
- About 50 million people worldwide have developed brain damage from maternal iodide deficiency; currently, 2 billion people are at risk for iodide deficiency.
- Residents in developed countries spend more money on pet food, perfumes, and cosmetics than it would take to provide basic education, water, sanitation, health care, and nutrition for all those now deprived of it.
- Every day the world produces enough food to provide about 2400 kcal for each person, generally meeting average calorie needs. A daily intake less than 2100 kcal would not likely sustain an older child or adult, depending on workload.
- Poor women in developing countries face a 50- to 200-fold increased risk of death in pregnancy, compared with women in North America.
- In many developing countries, life expectancy of the population is one-half to two-thirds of North Americans.
- Almost half of the world's people earn less than $200 a year—many use 80% to 90% of that income to obtain food. About $2000 to $3000 of income each year is needed for a person to reach the life expectancy seen in North America.
- Of the 6.2 billion people in the world, about 1.1 billion drink contaminated water. In India alone, 300,000 children die each year from drinking polluted water.
- About 2 billion people in the world live without proper sanitation, such as reliable toilet facilities.
- Developing countries have 95% of the **acquired immune deficiency syndrome (AIDS)** cases worldwide.
- Developing countries bear 93% of the world's disease burden but use only 11% of the world's health care resources.

acquired immunodeficiency syndrome (AIDS) A disorder in which a virus (human immunodeficiency virus [HIV]) infects specific types of immune system cells. This leaves the person with reduced immune function and, in turn, defenseless against numerous infectious agents; typically contributes to the person's death.

malnutrition Failing health that results from longstanding dietary practices that do not coincide with nutritional needs.

undernutrition Failing health that results from a longstanding dietary intake that is not enough to meet nutritional needs.

Of these, 3% reported that they experienced hunger at least one time during that year. Food insecurity is also a problem in Canada.

According to UNICEF (United Nations Children's Fund), the United States ranks eleventh out of sixteen industrialized countries for child poverty. Fortunately, the United States does have food assistance programs for low-income families, and therefore most children in the United States are shielded from hunger.

Malnutrition is a condition of impaired development or function caused by either a long-term deficiency or excess in calorie and/or nutrient intake. When food supplies are low and the population is large, **undernutrition** is common, leading to nutritional deficiency diseases, such as goiter (from an iodide deficiency) and xerophthalmia (eye problems caused by poor vitamin A intake). However, when the food supply is ample or overabundant, incorrect food choices coupled with an excessive intake can lead to overnutrition-related chronic diseases, such as type 2 diabetes.

Undernutrition is the most common form of malnutrition among the poor in both developing and developed countries. Currently, about half of the 4 million African children under 5 years of age who die annually are undernourished. Undernutrition is also the primary cause of specific nutrient deficiencies that can result in muscle wasting, blindness, scurvy, pellagra, beriberi, anemia, rickets, goiter, and a host of other problems (Table 17-2).

The most critical micronutrients missing from diets worldwide are iron, vitamin A, iodide, zinc, and various B vitamins (e.g., folate), as well as selenium and vitamin C. About 1 billion people, mostly in the developing world, are affected by iron deficiency.

Table 17-2 Nutrient-Deficiency Diseases That Commonly Accompany Undernutrition

Disease and Key Nutrient Involved	Typical Effects	Foods Rich in Deficient Nutrient	Target Populations for Intervention
Xerophthalmia Vitamin A	Blindness from chronic eye infections, restricted growth, dryness and keratinization of epithelial tissues	Liver, fortified milk, sweet potatoes, spinach, greens, carrots, cantaloupe, apricots	Asia, Africa
Rickets Vitamin D	Poorly calcified bones, bowed legs, other bone deformities	Fortified milk, fish oils, sun exposure	Asia, Africa, and parts of the world where religious dress codes prevent women and children from receiving adequate sun exposure; older adults in developed nations
Beriberi Thiamin	Nerve degeneration, altered muscle coordination, cardiovascular problems	Sunflower seeds, pork, whole and enriched grains, dried beans	Victims of famine in Africa
Ariboflavinosis Riboflavin	Inflammation of tongue, mouth, face and oral cavity, nervous system disorders	Milk, mushrooms, spinach, liver, enriched grains	Victims of famine in Africa
Pellagra Niacin	Diarrhea, dermatitis, dementia	Mushrooms, bran, tuna, chicken, beef, peanuts, whole and enriched grains	Victims of famine in Africa, survivors of war-torn Eastern Europe
Megaloblastic anemia Folate	Enlarged red blood cells, fatigue, weakness	Green leafy vegetables, legumes, oranges, liver	Asia, Africa
Scurvy Vitamin C	Delayed wound healing, internal bleeding, abnormal formation of bones and teeth	Citrus fruits, strawberries, broccoli	Victims of famine in Africa
Iron-deficiency anemia Iron	Reduced work output, retarded growth, increased health risk in pregnancy	Meats, seafood, broccoli, peas, bran, whole-grain and enriched breads	Worldwide
Goiter Iodide	Enlarged thyroid gland in teenagers and adults, possible mental retardation, cretinism	Iodized salt, saltwater fish	South America, Eastern Europe, Africa

Although the nutrients are listed separately to illustrate the important role of each one, often two or more nutrition-deficiency diseases are found in an undernourished person in the developing world.

The same is true for zinc deficiencies. With poor iron status, cognitive development will likely be impaired, particularly if prolonged deficiency occurs during early infancy. An estimated 50 million people worldwide also suffer brain damage from preventable maternal iodide deficiency. Although severe vitamin A deficiency, which causes blindness, is on the decline, up to 500,000 preschool-age children are still blinded by it each year. UNICEF reports that the lives of 1 million to 3 million children could be saved annually in the developing world if vitamin A supplements were provided a few times each year. The annual cost per child would be about 6 cents.

Of the 6.2 billion people in the world, about 2 billion may experience episodes of food shortages and be affected by some form of micronutrient malnutrition. Death and disease from infections, particularly those causing acute and prolonged diarrhea or respiratory disease, increase dramatically when the infections occur during a state of chronic undernutrition. Chronic undernutrition leaves many people in the developing world in a continual state of depressed immune function, in turn greatly increasing the risk of death, especially in childhood.

Blood loss caused by intestinal and bloodborne parasite infections is another common cause of anemia among poor populations, especially when people do not wear shoes. Parasites, such as hookworms, can easily penetrate the soles of the feet and legs and enter the bloodstream. Although hookworm disease has been largely eradicated through improved sanitation in the United States and other industrialized nations, it continues to plague more than one-eighth of the world's population, mostly in tropical regions.

famine An extreme shortage of food, which leads to massive starvation in a population; often associated with crop failures, war, and political unrest.

The Irish potato famine of 1840 to 1850 caused an estimated 2 million deaths and resulted in nearly as many people emigrating to other countries, such as the United States and Canada. More than 3 million people may have perished in the great famine of 1943 in Bengal, India. In 1974, another 1.5 million starved in the country of Bangladesh. China suffered a famine from 1959 to 1961—estimates of mortality range from 16 million to 64 million.

Protein-calorie malnutrition (PCM) is a form of undernutrition caused by an extremely deficient intake of calories or protein generally accompanied by an illness. The dramatic results of PCM—kwashiorkor and marasmus—were described in Chapter 6. This chapter focuses on the more subtle effects of a chronic lack of food.

Famine is the extreme form of chronic hunger. Periods of famine are characterized by large-scale loss of life, social disruption, and economic chaos that slows food production. As a result of these extreme events, the affected community experiences a downward spiral characterized by human distress; sales of land, livestock, and other farm assets; migration; division and impoverishment of the poorest families; crime; and the weakening of customary moral codes, as seen in Sudan and Rwanda. In the midst of all this, undernutrition rates soar; infectious diseases, such as cholera, spread; and many people die.

Special efforts are needed to eradicate the fundamental causes of famine. Causes vary by region and decade, but the most common is crop failure. The most obvious reasons for crop failure are bad weather, war, and civil strife. War deserves a special focus and will be specifically addressed in a separate section on war and political/civil unrest.

■ Critical Life Stages When Undernutrition Is Particularly Devastating

Prolonged undernutrition is detrimental to many aspects of human health (Fig. 17-1). It is particularly damaging during some periods of growth and old age.

Pregnancy

Undernutrition poses the greatest health risk during pregnancy. Currently about 500,000 women worldwide die each year from complications of pregnancy and

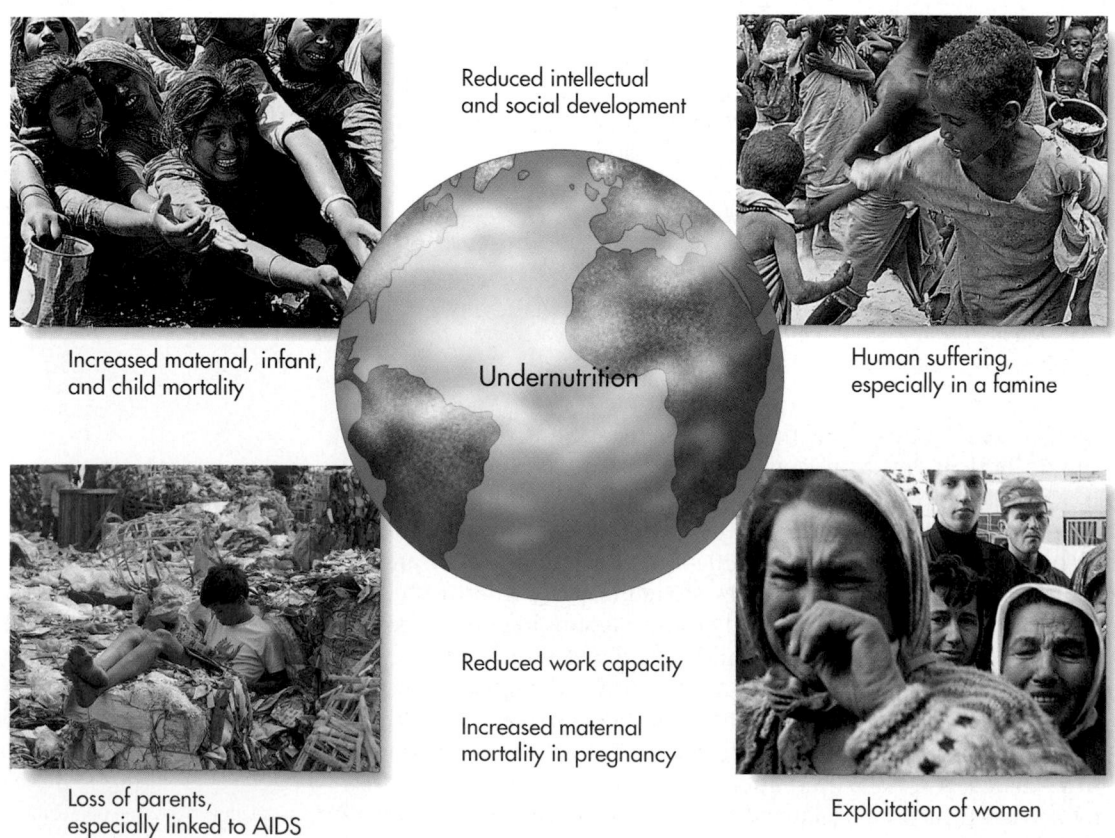

Reduced intellectual and social development

Increased maternal, infant, and child mortality

Human suffering, especially in a famine

Undernutrition

Reduced work capacity

Increased maternal mortality in pregnancy

Loss of parents, especially linked to AIDS

Exploitation of women

Figure 17-1 Undernutrition affects many aspects of human health and humanity.

childbirth. A pregnant woman needs extra nutrients to meet both her own needs and those of her developing offspring. Nourishing the fetus may deplete maternal stores of nutrients. Maternal iron deficiency anemia is one possible consequence (review Chapter 13).

In Africa, women in their lifetimes give birth, on average, to more than six live babies. Coupled with chronic undernutrition, these high birth rates result a 1 in 20 chance that a woman will die from pregnancy-related causes. In contrast, North American women only face a risk of 1 death in about 8000 births from pregnancy-related causes. Pregnancy-related death is the social indicator with the biggest difference between the developing and industrialized worlds. Smaller differences exist for literacy, life expectancy, and infant mortality.

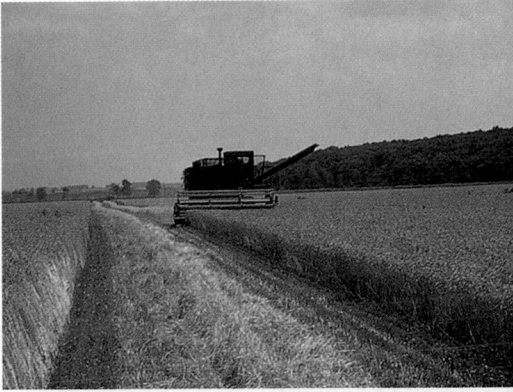

Fetal and Infant Stages

The fetus faces major health risks from undernutrition during gestation. To support growth and development of the brain and other body tissues, a growing fetus requires a rich supply of protein, vitamins, and minerals. When these needs are not met, the infant is often born before 37 weeks of gestation, well before the 40 weeks of gestation that is considered ideal. The consequences of this preterm birth include reduced lung function and a weakened immune system. These conditions not only compromise health but also increase the likelihood of premature death. Long-term problems in growth and development can result if the infant survives. In extreme cases, low-birth-weight infants (about 5.5 pounds [2.5 kilograms] or less) face 5 to 10 times the normal risk of dying before the age of 1 year, primarily because of reduced lung development. When low birth weight is accompanied by other physical abnormalities, medical intervention can cost $200,000 or more. These costs can be met only in developed countries.

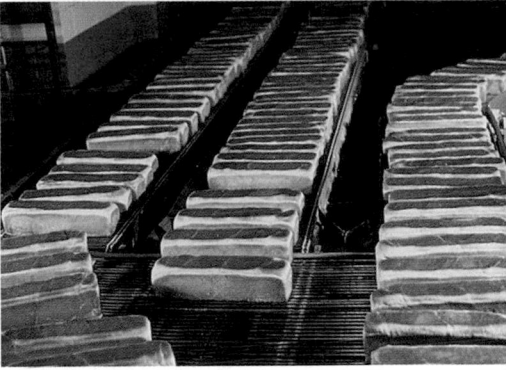

The bounty of food enjoyed in North America relies on rich agricultural resources. Many developing countries do not have such resources to employ.

Worldwide, more than 30 million infants are born each year with low birth weight. Currently, about 7% of infants born in the United States and 6% in Canada have low birth weights. In the United States, low birth weight accounts for more than half of all infant deaths and 75% of deaths of infants younger than 1 month old. Whereas undernutrition is a major contributor to low birth weight in developing countries, the primary cause for this problem in industrialized countries is cigarette smoking. Pregnancy during the teenage years, while a girl's body is still growing, contributes to low birth weight in developing and industrialized countries alike.

The percentage of infants born with low birth weight in the United States has been increasing steadily during the past 20 years. One reason is that more twins, triplets, and higher-order multiple births are being born because of improvements in medicine and fertility procedures. Rates of low birth weight vary by race. About 13% of infants born to African-American women have low birth weights. Among Hispanics in the United States, infants of Mexican origin have the lowest rate of low birth weight (6%), while infants of Puerto Rican heritage have the highest (9%). Among Asian subgroups, low-birth-weight rates range from 5% for infants of Chinese heritage to nearly 9% for Filipino infants.

Childhood

Early childhood, when growth is rapid, is another period when undernutrition is extremely risky. The central nervous system—including the brain—continues to be vulnerable because of rapid growth through early childhood. After the preschool years, brain growth and development slow dramatically until maturity. Nutritional deprivation, especially in early infancy, can lead to permanent brain impairment. Without an effective intervention, it is projected that ongoing undernutrition could leave more than 1 billion children with mental impairment by 2020.

In general, poor children are at the greatest risk for nutritional deprivation and subsequent illness. Stunted growth is an obvious effect, seen in about one-third of children under 5 years of age worldwide. In addition, iron-deficiency anemia is much more

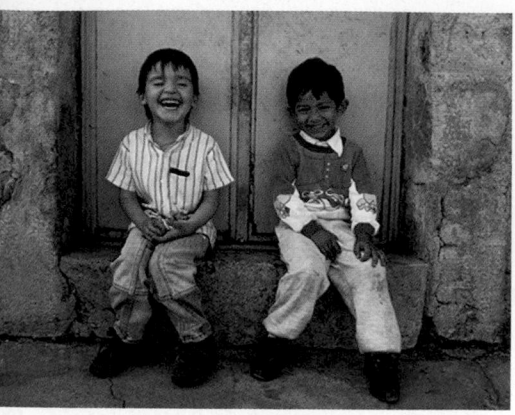

Minimal intakes of protein and zinc limit the growth of children worldwide. About 30% of children in developing countries show evidence of poor growth rates.

The effects of hunger are widespread:

- Reduced energy and strength
- Diminished concentration
- Impaired ability to learn
- Lowered productivity
- Worsening of chronic health conditions
- Increased susceptibility to infectious diseases
- Deterioration of mood
- Slowed recovery from illness and injury

common among low-income children than children from less deprived families. This deficiency can lead to fatigue upon exertion, reduced stamina, stunted growth, impaired motor development, and learning problems. Undernutrition in childhood can also weaken resistance to infection because immune function decreases when nutrients such as protein, vitamin A, and zinc are very low in a diet. Clearly, undernutrition and illness have a cyclical relationship. Not only does undernutrition lead to illness, but illness, particularly diarrhea and infectious diseases, worsens undernutrition. For this reason, many children in developing countries are dying from the combination of malnutrition and infection. Conversely, when missing nutrients such as vitamin A and zinc are restored to children's diets, improvements in health can be obvious.

Later Years

Older adults, especially older women living alone in poverty, are also at risk for undernutrition. Older adults in general require nutrient-dense foods, in amounts dependent on their state of health and degree of physical activity. Because many of them have fixed incomes and incur significant medical costs, food often becomes a low-priority item. In addition, depression, social isolation, and declining physical and mental health can compound the problem of undernutrition in older adults (review Chapter 15).

■ General Effects of Semistarvation

In the initial stages, the results of undernutrition from semistarvation are often so mild that physical symptoms are absent and blood tests do not usually detect the slight metabolic changes. Even in the absence of clinical symptoms, however, undernourishment may affect reproductive capacity, resistance to and recovery from disease, physical activity and work output, and lead to fatigue and behavior problems. Recall from Chapter 2 that, as tissues continue to be depleted of nutrients, blood tests eventually detect biochemical changes, such as a drop in blood hemoglobin concentration. Physical symptoms, such as body weakness, appear with further depletion. Finally, the full-blown symptoms of the predominating deficiency are recognizable, such as when blindness accompanies a vitamin A deficiency.

When a few people in a population develop a severe deficiency, this may represent only the "tip of the iceberg." Typically, a much greater number have milder degrees of undernutrition. These deficiencies should not, therefore, be dismissed as trivial, especially in the developing world. It is becoming clear that combined deficiencies of specific vitamins and the minerals iron and zinc can seriously reduce work performance, even when they do not cause obvious physical symptoms. This resulting state of ill health, in turn, diminishes the ability of individuals, communities, and even whole countries to perform at peak levels of physical and mental capacity (Fig. 17-2).

Figure 17-2 The downward spiral of poverty and illness can ultimately end in death (based on World Food Program graphic).

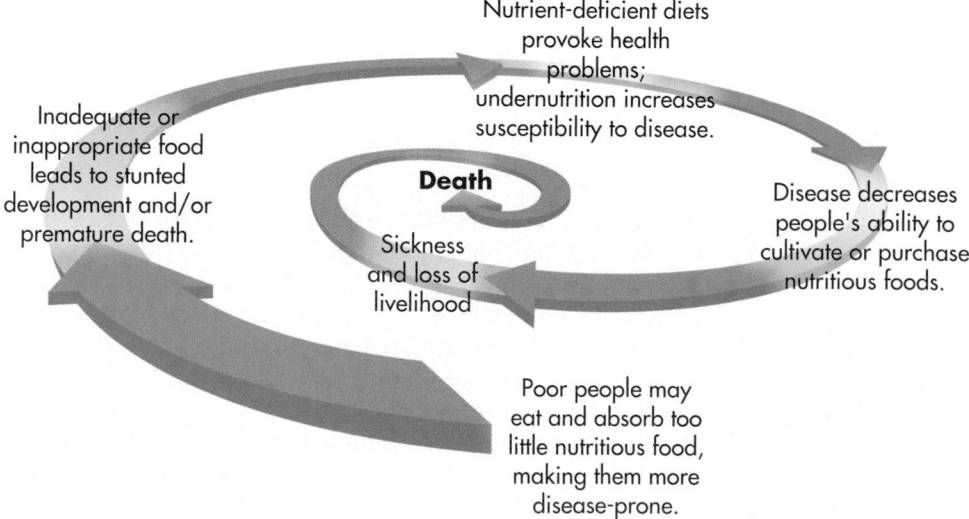

Nutrient-deficient diets provoke health problems; undernutrition increases susceptibility to disease.

Inadequate or inappropriate food leads to stunted development and/or premature death.

Death

Sickness and loss of livelihood

Disease decreases people's ability to cultivate or purchase nutritious foods.

Poor people may eat and absorb too little nutritious food, making them more disease-prone.

Added to their lack of nourishment, the inhabitants of poorer countries must also contend with recurrent infections, poor sanitation, extreme weather conditions, and regular exposure to infectious diseases. They require greater amounts of certain nutrients—especially iron—to combat rampant parasite and other infections. Deficiencies in both iron and zinc can lead to reduced immune function and thereby increase the risk of diseases, such as diarrhea and pneumonia.

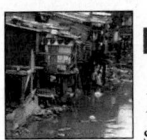 ## Real Life Scenario Follow-Up

Jamal should not be surprised that the children in the village were often sick and listless. Protein, vitamin A, iron, iodide, and zinc deficiencies contribute to poor growth and depressed immune function. One or more of these deficiencies is likely present in many children in the village. The diets of these children may also be marginal in calorie content, further depressing growth and overall health. We know from many nutrition intervention studies that the provision of calories, protein, vitamin A, iron, iodide, and zinc—along with other micronutrients—can reverse some of this disease pattern and improve health. Still, many children throughout the world exist in a stunted and immune-depressed state associated with their chronically deficient diets.

In the 1940s a group of researchers led by Dr. Ansel Keys examined the general effects of undernutrition on adults. The researchers maintained 32 previously healthy men on a diet averaging about 1800 kcal daily for 6 months. During this time, the men lost an average of 24% of their body weight. After about 3 months, the participants complained of fatigue, muscle soreness, irritability, intolerance to cold, and hunger pains. They exhibited a lack of ambition, self-discipline, and concentration, and were often moody, apathetic, and depressed. Their heart rate and muscle tone decreased and they developed edema. When the men were permitted to eat normally again, feelings of recurrent hunger and fatigue persisted even after 12 weeks of rehabilitation. Full recovery required about 8 months. This study tells us a lot about the general state of undernourished adults worldwide.

Concept Check

Hunger provokes uneasiness and pain when insufficient food is eaten to meet calorie needs. Food insecurity is anxiety about running out of food or money to buy more food. Chronic hunger leads to undernutrition, which can cause growth failure in children and physical weakness in adults. Risk of infection increases, and nutrient-deficiency diseases result. The primary cause of undernutrition is poverty. The critical periods for undernutrition occur during pregnancy, infancy, childhood, and old age. Chronic undernutrition decreases work performance, motivation, and immune function. The adverse effects in pregnancy and infancy are quite dramatic, as evidenced by mortality rates much higher than those of healthy populations. Irreversible developmental damage in surviving children is also common.

Undernutrition in the United States

About 33 million (12%) people in the United States live at or below the poverty level, currently estimated at about $18,400 annually for a family of four (Table 17-3). Of those 33 million, 12 million (37%) are children.

Currently, 8% of Caucasians, 24% of African-Americans, and 23% of Hispanics live in poverty. Many Native Americans are also poor, as are 11% of Asian Americans. (Many Native Americans in Canada also live in poverty.)

The poor often face difficult choices: whether to buy groceries for the family or pay this month's rent; whether to have dental work done or pay the current utility bill; whether to replace clothes the children have outgrown or pay for transportation to apply for a job. Food is one of the few flexible items in a poor person's budget. Whereas housing and utility costs, medical care, and transportation fares are non-negotiable, a person can always eat less. The short-term consequences of eating less may be less dramatic than getting evicted, but the long-term cumulative effects are significant.

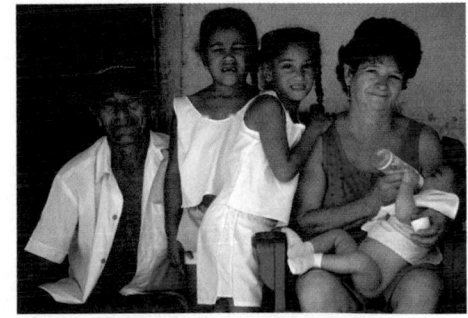

Food insecurity is part of the North American landscape. A "safety net" of programs exists, but it is "porous."

Undernutrition in North America is a much more subtle problem than in developing countries. To the untrained eye, undernourished children may just seem skinny, when, in fact, their growth is being stunted by insufficient nutrients. More likely, though, children from food-insecure households are prone to be overweight. This may be the result of considerable reliance on convenience foods that provide mostly fat and sugar. Also, food-insecure families may buy candies and snack foods as treats when expensive toys and clothing aren't affordable.

Table 17-3 The Realities of Poverty and Undernutrition in the United States

- About 7% of infants born in the United States are low birth weight. This accounts for more than half of all infant deaths and for 75% of deaths of babies under 1 month of age.

- The infant mortality rate in the United States is higher than that of 26 other industrialized countries. Teenage pregnancy contributes to infant mortality in part because young mothers frequently don't meet their nutrient needs.

- Single-parent families constitute about 25% of all families with children. The poverty rate (40%) for the approximately 19 million children in such families is five times higher than that for children in two-parent families.

- About 33 million people in the United States live at or below the poverty level. These poor include about 16% of all children; children, in fact, comprise 37% of the poor. Hunger frequently accompanies poverty.

- A family of four in the United States at the bottom 20% of households has an average income one-fifth of that of the average income of the top 20% of households.

- In the United States, an estimated 12 million people, or 6.5% of all adults, have experienced homelessness sometime during their lives. An episode of homelessness nearly always lasts for at least 1 week and often for a month or more.

- The Food Stamp Program for low-income people provides each household with $190 per month. About 1 person in 16 currently participates in this program.

- Second Harvest, the largest U.S. food bank, estimates that more than 23 million people, or more than 1 person in 10, rely on food depositories and soup kitchens to feed themselves and their families. Most of these people, the organization reports, are workers who have lost their jobs.

- Food thrown out in U.S. cafeterias, supermarkets, and restaurants could feed 49 million people per year.

Critical Thinking

While studying early childhood development, Nakia was surprised to learn that some children in the United States are undernourished. What evidence might Nakia observe in children that would suggest undernourishment?

■ Helping the Hungry in the United States

Until the twentieth century, individuals and a wide variety of charitable, often church-related organizations, provided most of the help to poor, undernourished people in the United States. Early programs rarely distributed direct cash payments to poor people because these were thought to reduce recipients' motivation to improve their circumstances or change behaviors, such as excessive drinking, that contributed to their poverty. Beginning in the early 1900s, the involvement of local, county, and state governments in providing assistance to the poor has steadily increased.

After observing extensive hunger and poverty during his presidential campaign in the 1960s, John F. Kennedy revitalized the Food Stamp Program, which actually had begun two decades earlier, and expanded commodity distribution programs. Today the Food Stamp Program for low-income people allows recipients to use an Electronic Benefit Transfer (EBT) card to purchase food and garden seeds—but not tobacco, cleaning items, alcoholic beverages, and nonedible products—at stores authorized to accept them. Each participating household receives about $190 per month, on average. Currently about 21 million people in the United States participate in this program (Table 17-4).

The U.S. Congress established the School Breakfast Program in 1965 as politicians became aware of the number of hungry children coming to school. School breakfast and lunch programs still enable low-income students—8.4 million for breakfast and 27 million for lunch—to receive meals free or at reduced cost if certain income guidelines are met (under $23,920 to $34,040, respectively, for annual income of a family of four). In the same year, the U.S. Congress funded group noontime (called *congregate*) meals and home-delivered meals for all citizens over 60 years of age, regardless of income (donations are requested, however). Both remain active programs, serving about 1 million meals each day, but they still do not reach all who need help. In addition, in 1972 the Special Supplemental Nutrition Program for Women, Infants,

Table 17-4 Some Current Federally Subsidized Programs That Supply Food for People in the United States

Program	Eligibility	Description
Food Stamp Program	Low-income families	Electronic Benefit Transfer (debit) cards are given to purchase food at grocery stores; the amount is based on size of household and income.
The Emergency Food Assistance Program (TEFAP)	Low-income families	Provides nutrition assistance to needy Americans through distribution of USDA food commodities.
Commodity Supplemental Food Program	Certain low-income populations, such as pregnant women, children until the age of 6 years, and seniors	USDA surplus foods are distributed by county agencies; not found in all states; may be based on nutritional risk.
Special Supplemental Nutrition Program for Women, Infants, and Children (WIC)	Low-income pregnant/lactating women, infants, and children less than 5 years old at nutritional risk	Coupons are given to purchase milk, cheese, fruit juice, cereal, infant formula, and other specific food items at grocery stores; includes nutrition education component.
National School Lunch Program	Low-income children of school age	Free or reduced-price lunch is distributed by the school; meal follows USDA pattern based on MyPyramid; cost for the child depends on family income. For students who do not participate in the lunch program, special milk program may be available.
School Breakfast Program	Low-income children of school age	Free or reduced-price breakfast is distributed by the school; meal follows USDA pattern; cost for the child depends on family income.
Child and Adult Care Food Program	Child enrolled in organized child-care program and seniors in adult-care programs; income guidelines are the same as those for the School Lunch Program	Reimbursement is given for meals supplied to children at the site; meals must follow USDA guidelines based on MyPyramid.
Congregate Meals for the Elderly	Age 60 or over (no income guidelines)	Free noon meal is furnished at a site; meal follows specific pattern based on one-third of nutrient needs.
Home-Delivered Meals	Age 60 or over, homebound	Noon meal is delivered at no cost or for a donation at least 5 days a week. Sometimes additional meals for later consumption are delivered at the same time; often referred to as "Meals on Wheels."
Summer Food Service Program	Residence in a low-income neighborhood or participation in a program	Free, nutritious meals and snacks are given to children in a low-income area at a central site, such as a school or a community center during long school vacations.
Food Distribution Program on Indian Reservations	Low-income American Indian and non-Indian households on reservations; members of federally recognized tribes	Alternative to Food Stamp Program, distribution of monthly food packages; includes nutrition education component.

and Children (WIC) was authorized. This program provides food vouchers and nutrition education to low-income pregnant and lactating women and their young children. Today, it serves about 7.6 million people.

Between 1969 and 1971, some already large federal food programs were expanded and others were created. For example, the Food Stamp Program served only 2 million people in 1968, but by 1971 it was serving 11 million. The National School Lunch Program, which served only 2 million poor children before 1970, was serving 8 million children by 1971. Soon after, the School Breakfast Program, a pilot program for children living in impoverished areas, became available nationally. And, as just mentioned, in 1972 the Special Supplemental Nutrition Program for Women, Infants, and Children (WIC) began.

Sometimes, severe undernutrition due to involuntary hunger does occur in the United States. More often, though, Americans experience periodic episodes of hunger and food insecurity. Unemployment, medical and housing expenses, and even occasional holiday shopping can cause a household to be hungry or food insecure.

Government food assistance programs are like a "safety net"—they are strong, yet porous. Privately funded programs have stepped in to also take an important role in

The availability of cooking facilities affects nutrient intake among the poor. Without cooking facilities, people may buy expensive convenience foods that require no preparation. These are typically highly processed snack foods, which provide calories but are often lacking in nutrients.

add to state and federal efforts to combat hunger and related food insecurity in the United States. There are currently more than 150,000 charitable food providers (such as food banks and food pantries) helping to cope with this problem. They serve about 23 million Americans. Many low-income U.S. households rely on food pantries, and a recent survey found that slightly more than two of every three people requesting such emergency food assistance being members of families—children and their parents.

■ Socioeconomic Factors Related to Undernutrition

In the United States, persistent hunger and food insecurity are largely associated with two interrelated conditions: poverty and homelessness. Thus, the economic, social, and political changes that lead to an increase in the number of poor or homeless people also tend to intensify the problem of undernutrition.

Poverty

Unemployment is a major contributor to poverty. Although highly trained people are quite competitive in the increasingly global economy, there is an overabundance of unskilled manual laborers available throughout North America. Many such people (and families) suffer hardships when layoffs occur seasonally or because of changes in the economy. Furthermore, underemployment is a hardship that leads to poverty. Contrary to common perceptions, the parents in most poor families are working— nearly two in three families contain at least one worker. Often, the jobs available to untrained adults are in the service sector, such as the food service and retail industries, which pay minimum wage and may not offer health and other benefits to employees. Even when one or both parents work at these low-paying jobs, their families may still be left with the choice of either paying rent or buying groceries.

Another primary factor contributing to poverty has been the dramatic increase in the number of single-parent families in the United States, the result of high rates of divorce and out-of-wedlock births. Currently, there are about 4 million single-parent families. The poverty rate (40%) for the approximately 19 million children in single-parent families is five times higher than the rate for children in two-parent families.

Homelessness

Homelessness is much more evident now than in 1980 as the economics of poverty and undernutrition has changed in an important way. The economic status of the working poor has declined because affordable housing is harder for them to find. Due to the nation's rising affluence, higher-income tenants have bid up the prices of the apartments in some cities beyond the financial resources of poorer tenants. The U.S. government considers housing costs, which include rent and utilities, to be affordable if they make up no more than 30% of a family's income. A recent U.S. government report stated that 1 in 8 low-income families pay more than half their incomes for housing or live in dilapidated units. These families, although not homeless, are likely to experience undernutrition without direct food assistance. Families with children currently account for about 43% of the homeless. An estimated 12 million people in the United States, or 1 in 15 of all adults, have experienced homelessness sometime during their lives. This statistic rises to about 1 in 7 when it includes people who have moved into someone else's residence during periods when they had nowhere else to live. Moreover, the continuing changes in the economic circumstances they face could force such low-income families into homelessness, at least temporarily.

Other important causes of homelessness include unemployment, personal crises, and widespread release of mentally ill patients from mental institutions in the 1980s. The abuse of alcohol and crack cocaine is another notable cause. Up to 85% of all homeless people in large cities in the United States abuse alcohol or drugs or have a

Homeless children suffer higher rates of many medical problems than do other children, some of which include:

Upper respiratory tract infections

Scabies and lice

Tooth decay

Ear and skin infections

Diaper rash

Eye infections

Developmental delays

Trauma-related injuries

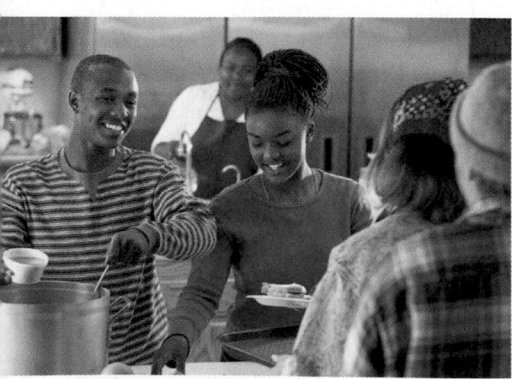

Food pantries and soup kitchens are important sources of nutrients for a growing number of people in the United States. Consider volunteering some of your time to a local program.

mental illness. Most people with such problems are unable to find and hold employment; without support from family or friends, they and their dependents will probably become homeless.

■ Possible Solutions to Poverty and Hunger in the United States

Few would dispute the importance of supporting physically and mentally challenged adults and the multitude of poor children in the United States. The debate begins when able-bodied adults are receiving public aid. Many of these people have extenuating circumstances or have dug such a deep financial hole for themselves that it is difficult to get out. The United States has enough resources to feed every citizen; government-funded food assistance programs have helped to alleviate some problems of undernutrition in the United States. The question is, *Can government programs provide a permanent solution to poverty and undernutrition . . . and should they?*

Private emergency food network systems are also important to consider, but are not sufficient to meet all food needs in the United States. Furthermore, most of the donated items are limited in nutritional value. By necessity, processed and canned grocery items predominate, rather than fresh or frozen fruits and vegetables, or protein-rich foods such as milk.

Some observers believe that publicly funded assistance programs have self-propagated—that they provide an incentive for poor, single women to have more children, since more children entitle a family to more benefits. New welfare reform laws have addressed this issue by requiring able-bodied adults to get jobs and by limiting future direct support to 5 years in a lifetime. It is up to each state to determine how to implement this work requirement and establish exceptions for such situations, as in the case of disability, short-term downturns in the economy, or other overwhelming hardships.

Many states are improving child care, teaching parenting skills, and expanding job opportunities as they help people end their dependence on welfare payments. Nationwide, the number of people on welfare has fallen 60% since 1992, but recently the number has stabilized, and in some states has increased slightly.

Despite even the highest motivation, the outlook is bleak for many people who attempt to gain independence from assistance programs. Teen pregnancy may have cut short the education or vocational training of one or both parents, thwarting efforts to earn adequate income. Often, the expense of reliable and safe child care far exceeds the meager income from a minimum-wage job. Illness of either the parents or children may prevent the adults from holding steady employment. Poor communication skills, inability to relocate, and a lack of economic reserves also complicate financial independence. Moreover, many of the poor, particularly older adults, sick and disabled people, and young single mothers with children, are unable to meet the demands of a modern, dynamic society. Regardless of how wasteful government assistance appears to some people, it will probably always be necessary to some extent.

Many in the United States consider an increase in individual responsibility as a critical goal. Government programs cannot easily fix poverty and the resulting hunger that stem from irresponsible individual behavior. Government programs can, however, help reduce or prevent the poverty that results largely from lack of education or opportunity.

Because long-term undernutrition—especially among children—has both individual and societal consequences, everyone in the United States is affected by this problem, either directly or indirectly. The next few years are likely to bring further changes in both government and private assistance programs, demanding new initiatives. As the welfare system is reformed and government programs are redesigned, it is likely that some will suffer. The hope is that these new approaches will lead to long-term progress and the eventual relief of poverty and hunger.

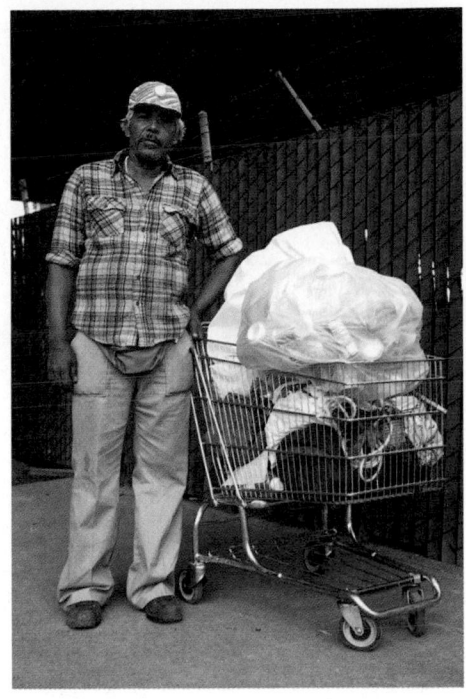

Homelessness can be the result of many problems, including poverty.

One goal of *Healthy People 2010* is to increase food security among U.S. households from the current 88% to 94%. Another is to reduce growth retardation to 5% among low-income children under age 5.

Concept Check

In response to reports of widespread poverty and hunger during the 1960s, the U.S. Congress established several food assistance programs and substantially increased funding for already existing programs. Largely as a result of these federal programs, undernutrition had decreased substantially by the mid-1970s. The presence of poverty, homelessness, and undernutrition is influenced by economic, cultural, and individual factors, as well as government policies. The serious questions about the long-term effectiveness of many government assistance programs are causing major changes in their program design. All citizens can help reduce the problem of undernutrition.

Undernutrition in the Developing World

Undernutrition in the developing world is also tied to poverty, and any true solution must address this problem. However, these countries have a multitude of problems so complex and interrelated that they cannot be treated separately. Programs that have proved immensely helpful in the United States (and throughout the rest of North America) are only a starting point in this context. The following major obstacles challenge those seeking a solution:

- Extreme imbalances in the food/population ratio in different regions of a country
- War and political/civil unrest, especially in Africa
- The rapid depletion of natural resources, such as farmland, fish, and water
- The disease AIDS, especially in sub-Saharan Africa and Asia
- High external debt, much of which is owed to developed nations
- Poor **infrastructure**, especially poor housing, sanitation and storage facilities, education, communications, and transportation systems

Each problem deserves individual consideration (Fig. 17-3).

infrastructure The basic framework of a system of organization. For a society, this includes roads, bridges, telephones, and other basic technologies.

Food/Population Ratio

The world has 6.2 billion inhabitants. Currently, population growth exceeds economic growth in much of the developing world, and as a result, poverty is increasing. This disrupts the balance in the food/population ratio, tipping it toward food

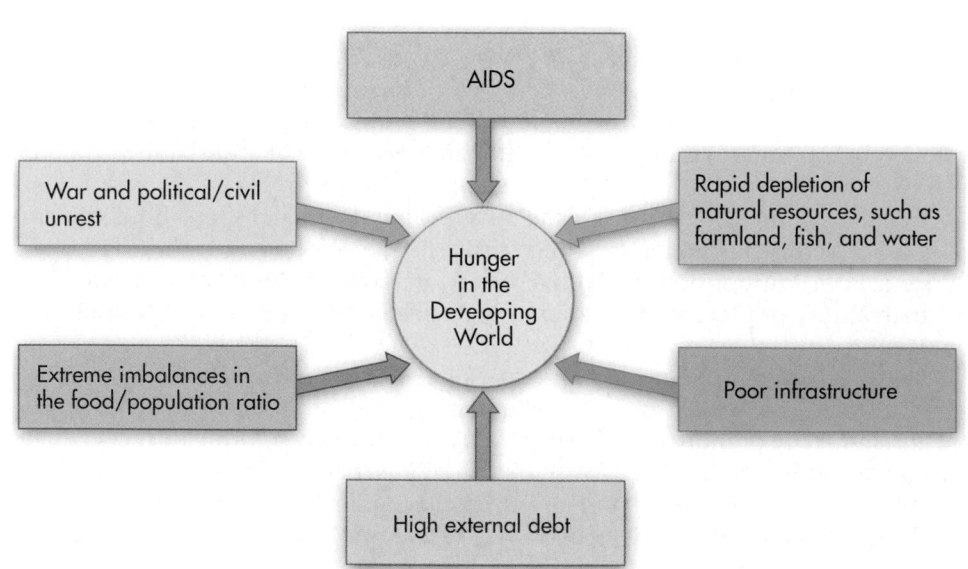

Figure 17-3 Many factors contribute to undernutrition in the developing world. Any solutions to the problem must take these factors into consideration.

shortages. If we want to ensure a decent life for a widening segment of humanity, many experts suggest that the growth in the earth's most vulnerable populations should slow. If not, by 2050 the world may have 1 to 3 billion more people than it does today—most of them in countries where the average person earns less than $2 per day. Currently in Africa's poorest countries, nearly 65% of people live on less than $1 per day. Unless a catastrophe occurs, more than 9 of 10 infants in the next generation will be born in the poorest parts of the world.

More than three-quarters of people in the world live in developing countries, and more than half live in Asia. A recent United Nations report on worldwide hunger revealed that almost two-thirds of the world's undernourished live in Asia and the Pacific Rim. The world's food supplies also are not distributed equally among consumers. Gross disparities exist between developed and developing countries, among the rich and the poor within countries, and even within families (males may be fed before females).

Still, economists estimate that world food production will, in fact, continue to increase more rapidly than world population in the near future, allowing the food/population ratio to increase through the year 2020. This will come at a high cost, however, in terms of the water, fertilizer, and pesticides needed to allow for this production. Overall, in the short run, the primary problem appears not to be food production *but* distribution and use, especially in poverty-stricken areas of the developing nations.

Eventually, though, food production will begin to lag behind population growth. Most good farmland in the world is already in use, and because of poor farming practices or competing land-use demands, the number of farmable acres worldwide decreases annually. For many reasons, sustainable world food output—an amount that doesn't deplete the earth's resources—is now running well behind food consumption. This discrepancy suggests that food production in less-developed countries will barely keep up with population growth and will soon lag behind.

Birth control programs, an obvious brake on population expansion, have been effective in developed countries but relatively ineffective in many developing countries that could really benefit from them. Among women, family planning and contraceptive use worldwide has increased to 60% today, up from 10% in 1969. If the United Nations, voluntary organizations, and governments had not started promoting family planning and contraceptive use, the population today might be as high as 7 or 8 billion. However, women (and men) in many developing countries are still lacking adequate access to contraceptives. Organizations such as Population Services International are trying to keep distribution costs low and make the products available to as many people as possible by subsidizing condoms and oral contraceptives to areas such as Bangladesh.

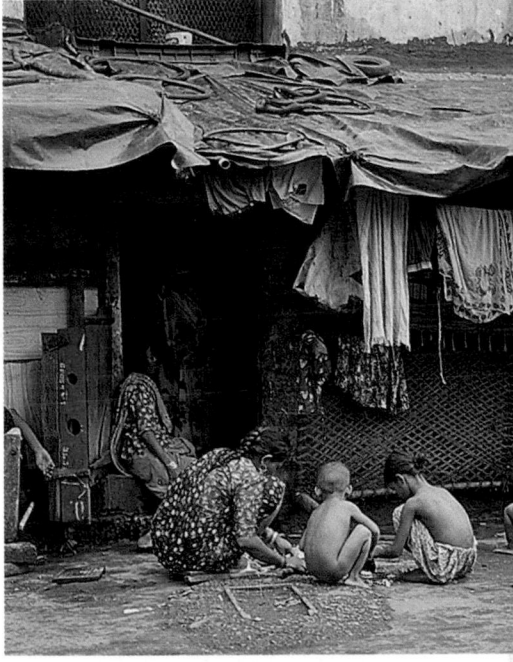

Poverty aggravates the problem of hunger in the developing world.

Another Bite

In addition to its many other benefits, breastfeeding contributes to the goal of birth control. Although it is not a completely reliable method of contraception, exclusively breastfeeding an infant lessens ovulation, thereby lowering the likelihood of fertilization, for an average of six months. (Women who do not breastfeed generally begin to ovulate within a month or so after giving birth.) When childbirths are more widely spaced, not only do fewer total births occur, but the mother has a longer chance to recover from pregnancy, and the infant receives feeding priority for a longer time.

One possible exception to the healthful nature of breastfeeding occurs when mothers are infected with the **human immunodeficiency virus (HIV)**. The risk of transferring the virus through human milk is about 10%. Depending on the circumstances, this may outweigh the benefits of breastfeeding. However, in areas with contaminated sources of water, the risk of HIV transmission may be eclipsed by the threat of infant death due to diarrheal disease.

human immunodeficiency virus (HIV)
The virus that leads to acquired immune deficiency syndrome (AIDS).

Experience with family planning programs in developing countries and historical changes in birth rates in many developed countries suggest an important conclusion: Generally, only when people have enough to eat and are financially secure do they feel confident that having fewer children will still result in enough surviving sons and/or daughters to provide for their care in later years. Increasing per capita income and improving education, especially for women in developing nations, are currently considered to be the most likely long-term solutions to excessive population growth. In the last few years this effort has led to a decline in family size in Brazil, Egypt, India, and Mexico. A major concern is whether there are enough resources worldwide to raise per capita income and provide enough education to slow population growth.

Concept Check

Currently, world food production is sufficient to meet the calorie needs of the world's population. Despite these adequate food resources, undernutrition continues to exist because of poverty, politics, and unequal food distribution. In addition, projected population growth may soon overwhelm food production. Most scientists and world leaders recommend limiting population growth, especially in developing countries where birth rates are high.

■ War and Political/Civil Unrest

The Millennium Summit of the United Nations pledged to "spare no effort to free our peoples from the scourge of war." Against that background stands the reality that worldwide military spending has doubled over the past 20 years. In the twentieth century, deadly weapons of war took an enormous toll on civilians living in poor, politically vulnerable, war-torn nations. Although Africa has been ravaged by economic decay and famine for years, military spending in Africa more than doubled in the 1970s and held firm through the 1990s. Currently, less than one-half of 1% of the world's yearly production of goods and services is devoted to economic development assistance, whereas approximately 6% goes to military expenditures.

Aside from the economic impact of military spending, civil disruptions and wars are setting back the progress of the poor and contributing to massive undernutrition. All but two of the major conflicts in 2000 took place in the developing world. War-related famine affects at least 20 million people in southern and northeastern Africa. The border war between Ethiopia and neighboring Eritrea has had a tremendous negative impact on food resources. A World Bank official stated that the food shortage in Ethiopia is a problem that will persist until political changes are made. Currently, 12.4 million people in Ethiopia, Eritrea, Djibouti, Kenya, Somalia, and Zimbabwe are at risk for food shortages. Other conflicts continue between Congo (formerly Zaire) and the Republic of Congo, as well as in Angola and Sudan, where millions have been put at risk of starvation. In the capitol city of war-torn Iraq, Baghdad, child malnutrition nearly doubled between 2002 and 2003. Disruptions in infrastructure from bombing and looting limit the safety of water, and as a result, health officials have observed a 250% increase in cases of diarrhea. Furthermore, health facilities needed to cope with undernutrition and dehydration have been damaged and looted throughout the area. Overall, most people in war-torn areas are without sufficient shelter, clothing, food, or means of obtaining them. Worldwide, this entire problem is projected to worsen over the next 15 years.

Even when food is available, political divisions may impede its distribution to the point that undernutrition will plague many people for years to come. Especially during emergencies, programs designed to help the poor have been undermined by

The recent conflicts in the Darfur region of Sudan have led to high rates of death and undernutrition among people displaced by war.

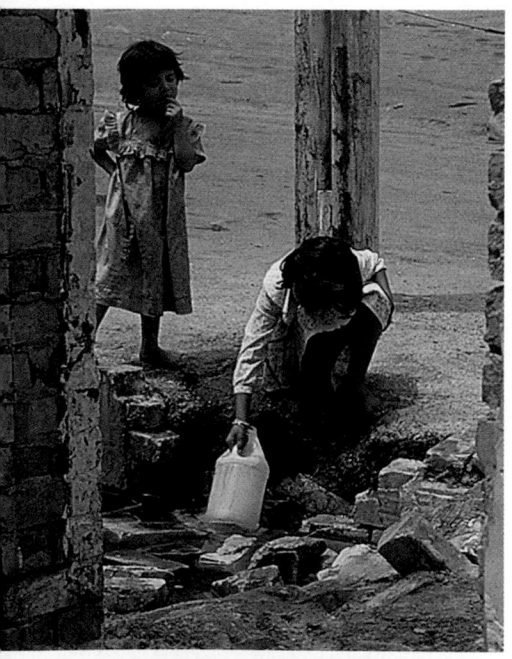

Homes and infrastructure are often damaged during times of war and political unrest.

unstable administration, corruption, and political influence. During such political chaos, relief agencies are often caught between warring factions and those they are trying to help. This was the case in the mid-1990s in Zaire, where Rwandan refugee camps fell under the control of a militant group. The rebels controlled the food coming into the camps and would not allow relief agencies to do their work.

During the 1960s and 1970s, the problem of undernutrition in developing countries was perceived as a technical one: how to produce enough food for the growing world population. The problem is now seen as largely political: how to achieve cooperation among and within nations, so that gains in food production and infrastructure are not wiped out by war. The best answer lies in a combination of approaches—finding technical solutions to help with the problems of chronic hunger and poverty and resolving political crises that have pushed developing nations into a state of acute hunger and chaos.

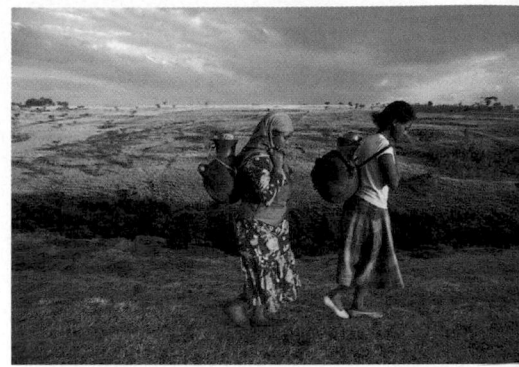

Lasting gains have come slowly in the worlds battle against undernutrition.

▪ Rapid Depletion of Natural Resources

As we quickly deplete the earth's resources, population control grows increasingly critical. Agriculture production is approaching its limits in many areas worldwide. Environmentally unsustainable farming methods are undermining food production, especially in developing countries.

The **green revolution** was a phenomenon that began in the 1960s when crop yields rose dramatically in some countries, such as the Philippines, India, and Mexico (countries in Africa did not benefit because climates were not compatible with the crops used). The increased use of fertilizers, irrigation, and the development of superior crops through careful plant breeding made this boost in agricultural production possible. Many of the technologies associated with the green revolution have now achieved their potential. Rice yields, for example, have not increased significantly since the release of superior varieties in 1966. (Actually, the green revolution was intended as a stopgap measure until world leaders could control population growth.)

Future gains in productivity may be much harder to accomplish because of the existence of less productive farmland. Until the introduction of another superior strain of rice or other grain, developing countries will not benefit greatly from recent, more modest breakthroughs in biotechnology (see the Looking Further section on use of biotechnology).

Areas of the world that remain uncultivated or ungrazed are mostly too rocky, steep, infertile, dry, wet, or inaccessible to sustain farming. Nearly all irrigation water available worldwide is currently being used, and groundwater supplies are becoming depleted at rapid rates in many regions. An eventual water shortage is projected to increase war and civil unrest in arid areas of the world, such as Northern Africa and the Middle East. China, which has more than 20% of the world's irrigated land, is also plagued with a growing scarcity of fresh water. In the future, billions of people will face ongoing water shortages.

The prospects of obtaining substantially more food from the oceans are also poor. In recent years, the amount of fish caught worldwide has leveled off. Fish was once considered the poor person's protein, but this is not likely to continue since farming of fish currently does not fully compensate for the reduction in wild fish populations.

Clearly, we can exploit the earth's resources only so far—the world population probably cannot continue to expand as it does today without the potential for serious famine and death. The Food and Agriculture Organization (FAO) of the United Nations works on this principle: "The fight to ensure that all people have enough nutritious food to eat is worthy of our greatest efforts, but it must be fought with the full recognition that it cannot be won unless agricultural, fishery, and forestry production returns to the earth as much as—or more than—it takes." Thus, if food production is to keep up with the expanding population, immediate action is needed to protect the earth's already deteriorated environment from further destruction.

green revolution This refers to increases in crop yields that accompanied the introduction of new agricultural technologies in less-developed countries, beginning in the 1960s. The key technologies were high-yielding, disease-resistant strains of rice, wheat, and corn; greater use of fertilizer and water; and improved cultivation practices.

In Brazil, migrants displaced by multinational land developers have flooded from the north and northeast into Rio de Janeiro and São Paulo, attracted by the prospect of jobs. There they have built shantytowns next to apartment towers and affluent suburbs, but the jobs do not materialize, and urban poverty simply replaces rural impoverishment.

■ Inadequate Shelter and Sanitation

When people die from undernutrition in developing countries, other factors, such as inadequate shelter and sanitation, almost always contribute. Poor sanitation along with undernutrition particularly raises the risk of infection. For example, the 1994 plague in Surat (in northwest India) that killed almost 5000 people, sparked the panicked exodus of another half a million, and was linked mainly to unsanitary housing conditions.

Inadequate and deteriorating shelters threaten the lives of more than 500 million people today. Many of the 15 million annual deaths of children—half of them under 5 years old—in developing countries could be prevented by improving the standards of environmental hygiene. Urban populations of some developing countries are currently growing at an annual rate of 5% to 7%. Such a skewed population distribution will result in more poverty. The current urban explosion is the result of both high birth rates and continuing migration of people to the cities from rural areas. People go to the cities to find employment and resources the countryside can no longer provide. Worldwide, 38% of people lived in urban areas in 1975. The figure is now about 50%, and is expected to reach 70% by 2050. Nine of the 10 largest cities will be in poor countries 20 years from now. Currently 12 of the 15 most polluted cities are in Asia alone.

In developing countries, the poor make up most of the urban population, and their needs for housing and community services often go beyond available governmental resources. Most of these urban poor live in overcrowded, self-made shelters, which lack a safe and adequate water supply and are only partially served by public utilities. The shantytowns and ghettos of the developing world are often worse than the rural areas the people left behind. Because the urban poor need cash to purchase food, they often subsist on diets that are even more meager than the homegrown rural fare. Making matters worse, haphazard shelters often lack facilities to protect food from spoilage or damage by insects and rodents. The inability to protect food supplies in some developing countries leads to the loss of as much as 40% of all perishable foods.

The shift from rural to urban life takes its greatest toll on infants and children. Infants are often weaned early from the breast to infant formula, partly because the mother must find employment and partly because she may be influenced by advertisements depicting images of sophisticated, formula-feeding women. Unfortunately, because infant formulas are relatively expensive, poor parents may try to conserve the formula by either overdiluting the mixture or using too little to meet the infant's needs. Because the water supply may not be safe, the prepared formula is also likely to be contaminated with bacteria. Human milk, in contrast, is much more hygienic, readily available, and nutritious. It also provides infants with immunity to some ailments. Promoting breastfeeding is important when it is safe for the infant (review the earlier discussion of AIDS, HIV, and breastfeeding).

Overall, the single most effective health advantage for people, wherever they live, is a safe and convenient water supply. Inadequate sanitation and the consumption of contaminated water cause 75% of all diseases and more than one-third of all deaths in developing countries. The World Health Organization (WHO) estimates that 1.1 billion people, about one-sixth of all people, have an unsafe and inadequate water supply. In addition, up to 90% of the diseases seen in developing countries may be attributed to contaminated water.

Poor sanitation, another example of inadequate infrastructure in the developing world, creates a critical public health problem. Human feces, rotting garbage, and associated insect and rodent infestations are potent sources of disease organisms commonly seen in urban areas of the developing world. Two of the most dangerous substances encountered in routine daily living are human urine and feces. The inability to dispose of the massive numbers of dead people (and dead animals) resulting from civil wars causes additional sanitation problems. In some developing countries, diarrheal diseases account for as many as one-third of all deaths in children under 5 years of age. WHO estimates that even with improvements in housing, 2 billion people in the world still lack proper sanitation facilities.

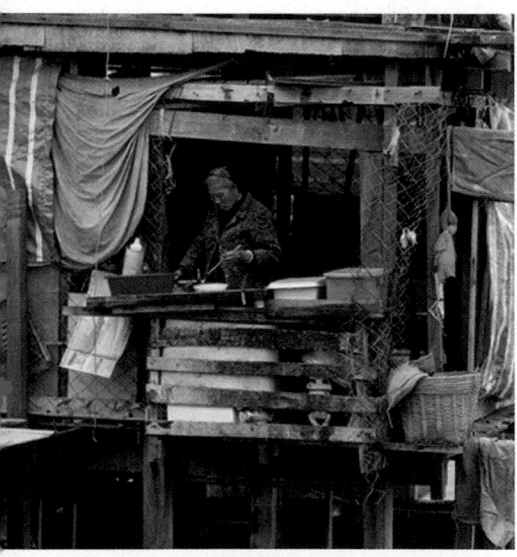

Inadequate sanitation facilities and the consumption of contaminated water cause the majority of all diseases. About 1 billion people in developing countries often lack access to a safe water supply.

■ High External Debt

Since the 1970s many developing countries have become trapped in a cycle of borrowing repeatedly from foreign countries and international banks. Servicing these external debts, which now total about $2.5 trillion, has brought several countries to the verge of economic collapse. About $6 billion is owed to the United States. The external debt of Latin America represents 45% of the region's gross regional output of goods and services.

Many African nations also carry large debt burdens—currently, $350 billion. This problem is made worse by recent drops in prices for the raw commodities they export, higher prices for imported oil, and embezzlement of funds by high-ranking officials. To make up the difference between export income and import expenses, countries have been forced to borrow millions of dollars from international banks. Although the African debts are much smaller in absolute terms than those of Brazil, Argentina, and Mexico, for example, the actual burden is greater when national incomes and export earnings are considered. Nearly half the money African nations earn from exports goes to paying off the continent's multibillion-dollar debt. Much of the rest goes to fund imports of machinery, concrete, trucks, and consumer goods from developed countries. This leaves little for domestic programs, necessitating cutbacks that translate into fewer resources to counter already widespread undernutrition.

The Group of Eight most industrialized nations is planning to forgive some external debt owed by developing countries. $40 billion has been promised; this should be able to end the external debt of 18 countries, including some in Africa and South America. The debt repayment depends on the developing country's agreement to practice good governance, and to use the money saved to support health care, education, and infrastructure improvements.

Concept Check

War and civil strife, along with a decline in the world's natural resources, contribute to the difficulty of ending undernutrition in many developing countries. In addition, substandard housing conditions, impure water, and inadequate sanitation worldwide increase the risk for infection and disease. Infection then combines with undernutrition to compromise further the health of impoverished people. Finally, many developing countries are burdened by extremely high external debts, which severely limit their ability to implement programs to reduce undernutrition.

■ The Impact of AIDS Worldwide

Currently, up to 46 million people around the world are infected with the human immunodeficiency virus (HIV) or have gone on to develop acquired immune deficiency syndrome (AIDS) from the infection. The male to female ratio is about 1:1. About 20 million people worldwide have died from AIDS.

An individual can be infected with HIV through contact with bodily fluids including blood, semen, vaginal secretions, and human milk. Thus the virus can be transmitted through sexual contact, through blood-to-blood contact, as well as from a mother to an infant during pregnancy, delivery, or breastfeeding. The virus has a very limited ability to exist outside the body.

Once infected with HIV, the individual is said to be HIV-positive. If untreated, the viral disease progresses over the next few years, and the individual develops symptoms of opportunistic infections such as diarrhea, lung disease, weight loss, and a form of cancer. Once the individual has developed these symptoms, they are said to have AIDS. Without treatment, an individual will likely die from AIDS within 4 to 5 years.

In Africa, particularly sub-Saharan countries, HIV is rampant throughout the entire population, both men and women. This region contains nearly 70% of the world's HIV-positive people. In most areas of sub-Saharan Africa, AIDS is reducing life expectancy by one-half, especially if the person also has tuberculosis. In many countries, AIDS is also creating orphans, an estimated 3.7 million worldwide (660,000 in South Africa alone).

The face of AIDS is quickly becoming the face of a child. About 500,000 deaths of children in subsaharan Africa in 2004 were linked to AIDS. (Compare that to about 300 deaths of children linked to AIDS in deveoped countries during the same year.)

North America also has an AIDS problem. In the United States alone, it is estimated that about 900,000 people (1 in every 320 persons) are infected with HIV, many of whom are unaware of their infections. (Recent reports show 1 in every 100 persons in New York City are infected with HIV.) About 450,000 people in the United States have died from the disease since it surfaced in the early-1980s, and each year, about 50,000 new cases are reported. HIV affects a greater percentage of minority populations in the United States.

Although no vaccine is available to prevent AIDS, the latest antiviral drugs can significantly slow the progression of the disease. However, there are many barriers to the use of these drugs in the developing world. For example, the newest therapies require a person to take at least three different drugs in the form of about 14 pills each day. Just a few missed doses can significantly reduce the effectiveness of the drugs and result in faster disease progression. Another barrier is economic: a typical drug regimen can cost approximately $14,000 per year, not including unforeseen hospital stays. Certain drug companies and governments are working to lower the cost of AIDS drugs for developing nations. Still, in most cases, the drugs will remain out of reach to those who need them. It has been suggested that developed nations should step in and cover most or all of the costs. The United Nations is spearheading an effort to raise the $8 to $10 billion needed to fight the disease.

Another Bite

Can eating a balanced diet prevent AIDS? The answer, unfortunately, is no. Healthy eating does not cure the disease, but it can help to lessen the impact of infections associated with AIDS. Poor nutritional status contributes to a quicker onset of symptoms such as body wasting and fever, and a more rapid demise. This explains why daily use of a balanced vitamin and mineral supplment was shown to slow health declines in such people in a recent study. Overall, maintenance of nutritional status should be an integral part of the treatment for AIDS.

The main goal for addressing the problem of AIDS in the developing world is prevention of new cases through education regarding safer sex and the importance of clean needles, and other behavior-linked approaches. Providing AIDS drugs to pregnant women is also important. If a woman begins taking AIDS drugs such as zidovudine (AZT) by the fourteenth week of pregnancy, the risk of transferring the virus to her offspring is greatly reduced. Providing the drug immediately before birth also helps.

The devastating effects of AIDS on our civilization have been very rapid when measured by earth's scale of time. And the true costs to society—other than the cost of human lives—have yet to emerge. The very nature of the disease is likely to inflict significant human devastation worldwide. This is partly because its primary route of transmission—sexual activity—is basic human behavior. A recent study warns us that 57 countries risk major HIV outbreaks. Reported HIV cases are increasing rapidly in Africa, the Indian subcontinent, Southeast Asia, China, the Caribbean, Russia, and much of Eastern Europe.

Behind the mind-boggling statistics on AIDS are less obvious costs to businesses, families, schools and universities, and society in general. For example, worker productivity will plummet because AIDS victims produce less and demand more, especially in the latter stages of the disease. Business productivity drops even further when relatives take time away from work and school to care for family members afflicted with AIDS. Furthermore, AIDS demands a considerable amount of family income. Hard-pressed families, who have to devote much of their income to doctors and medicines, have little left for living expenses. Other family members must struggle to keep up with daily duties because they must care for orphans left behind in the disease's wake. To learn more about AIDS, check out the website www.unaids.org.

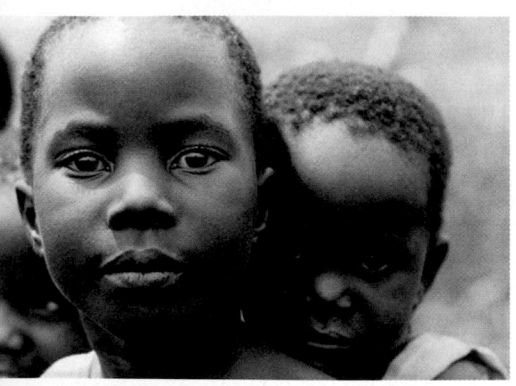

A particularly sad consequence of AIDS in Africa is the number of AIDS orphans, children whose parents have both died of AIDS. The United Nations has estimated that there will be 20 million AIDS orphans in Africa by the year 2010.

■ Reducing Undernutrition in the Developing World

As you have probably guessed, greatly reducing undernutrition in the developing world will be complicated and will take considerable time to accomplish (Fig. 17-4). Today, it is a common practice for the more affluent nations to supply famine areas with direct food aid. However, direct food aid is not a long-term solution. Although it reduces the number of deaths from famine, it can also reduce incentives for local production by driving down prices. In addition, the affected countries may have little or no means of transporting the food to those who need it most, and the donated foods may not be culturally acceptable.

In the short run, there is no choice—aid must be given because people are starving. Still, improving the infrastructure for poor people, especially rural people, needs to be the long-term focus. This future-minded approach is necessary because the most

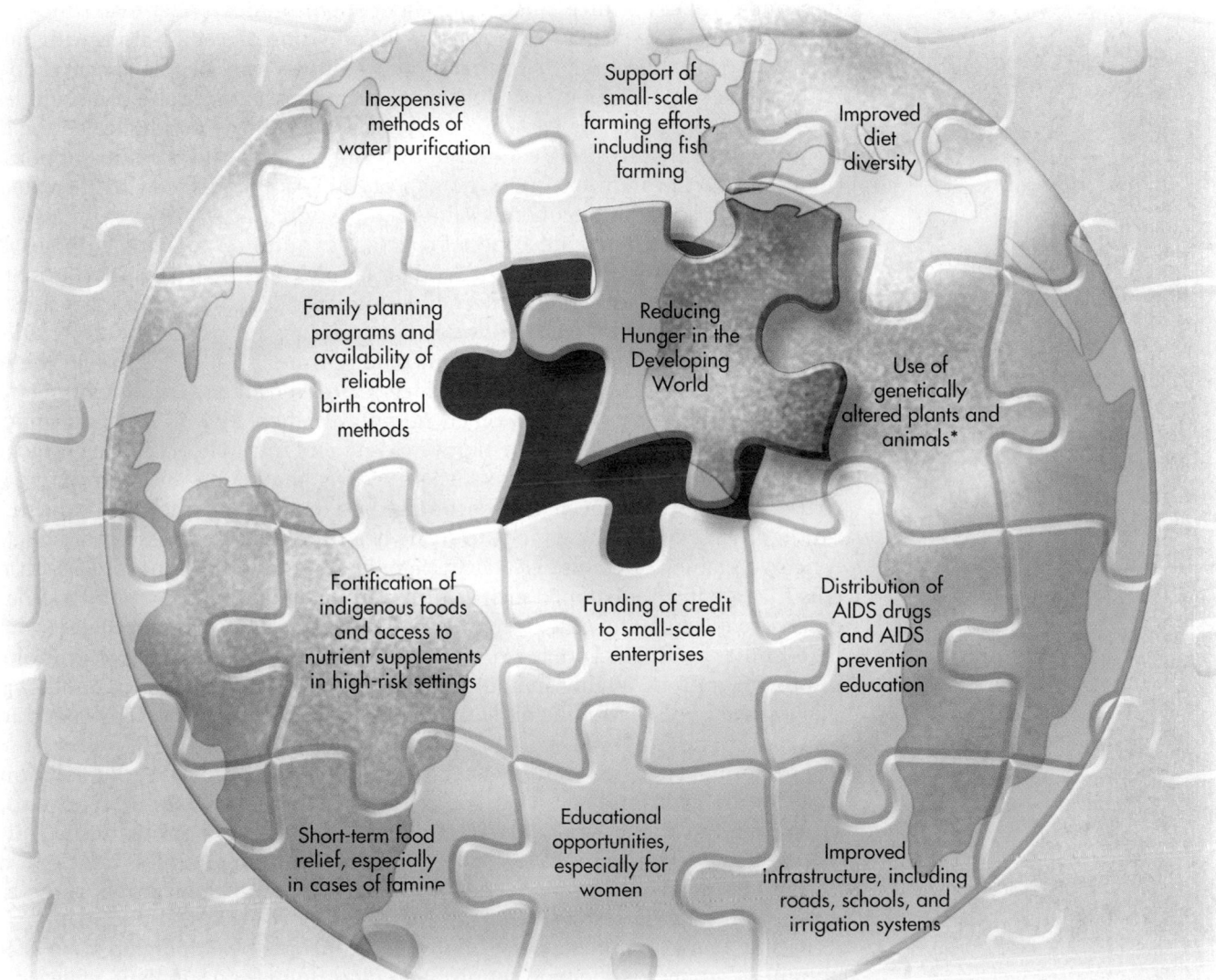

Figure 17-4 Possible solutions to the puzzle of hunger in the developing world. Putting all the pieces together employs the action steps that contribute to meeting the overall goal. *Note that the Looking Further section in this chapter discusses the genetic alteration of plants and animals in detail.

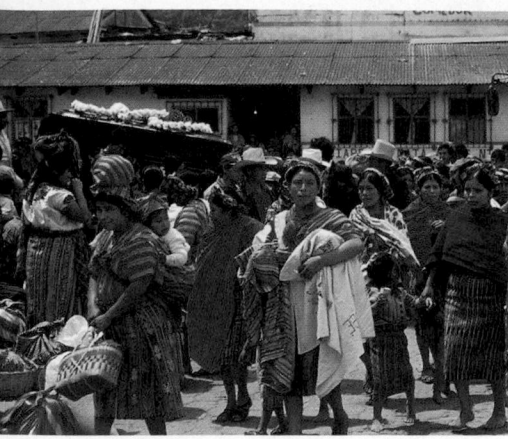

Food security is fostered by communities raising and distributing locally grown food.

Critical Thinking

Stan has read about various relief efforts to help undernourished people in developing countries, especially the emergency food aid programs for famine-ravaged areas. Many of these efforts appear to be only temporary, and he wonders what long-range approaches might help alleviate the problem of undernutrition. What suggestions would you give Stan about possible long-term solutions for undernutrition in developing countries?

significant factor affecting the undernutrition of people in impoverished areas of the world is their reliance on outside sources for basic needs. Their dependence makes them constantly vulnerable.

Three basic approaches to counteract micronutrient deficiencies are suggested by the World Bank: increase diversity of the food supply; fortify specific foods with nutrients; and provide nutrient supplementation for individuals when necessary.

Development Tailored to Local Conditions Is Important

Recall that, in the past 40 years, world food supplies have grown faster than the population. Thus, the increase in undernutrition during this period has been caused by an increase in the number of people cut off from their share of this supply. Millions of farmers are losing access to resources they need to be self-reliant. There is a growing realization that unless economic opportunities can be created as part of a plan for sustainable development, rural people who own no land will flock to the overcrowded cities. In response, careful, small-scale regional development is one option.

For the most part, the solution lies in helping people meet their own needs and directing them to resources and employment opportunities, rather than simply giving them resources. Experience has shown that the provision of credit—along with training, food storage facilities, and marketing support—allows rural people to actively participate in their own development, which will benefit their families and communities.

One U.S. program, the Peace Corps, has helped improve conditions in the developing nations by providing education, distributing food and medical supplies, and building structures for local use. The aim of the Peace Corps is to help create independent, self-sustaining economies around the world.

Impoverished women are a special concern. In addition to working longer hours than men do, they grow most of the food for family consumption and make up three-fourths of the labor force in the informal sector of the economy and an increasing proportion in the formal sector. Economic opportunities for women and education regarding family planning must be augmented. Of the 3 billion people in the world living on less than $2 a day, 70% are women. Moreover, among the developing world's 900 million illiterate people, women outnumber men 2 to 1. Thus, an important means of propelling nations out of poverty is to end the cycle of female neglect.

Suitable technologies for processing, preserving, marketing, and distributing nutritious local staples also need to be encouraged, so that small farmers can flourish. Education on how to use these foods to create healthful diets, such as preparing vitamin A-rich vegetables, adds further benefit. Supplementing indigenous foods with nutrients that are in short supply, such as iron, various B vitamins, zinc, and iodide, also deserves consideration. One current program involves adding iron to sugar in various parts of the world. The Looking Further section examines the role of biotechnology in improving nutrient quality and other plant and animal characteristics, another possible positive step in lessening undernutrition. In addition, advances in water purification need to be employed.

Promoting extensive land ownership may also be one part of the solution. Increasing the availability of food is one of its many advantages. If food resources are concentrated among a minority of people, as often happens with unequal land ownership, food is not likely to be equally distributed unless efficient transportation systems are in place. Inequitable distribution then proves to be a very difficult problem to resolve.

Raising the economic status of impoverished people by employing them is as important as expanding the food supply. If an increase in food supply is achieved without an accompanying rise in employment, there may be no long-term change in the number of undernourished people. Although food prices may fall with increased mechanization, use of fertilizers, and other modern technologies, it needs to be realized that these advances can also displace people from jobs, a result that worsens rather than helps the population.

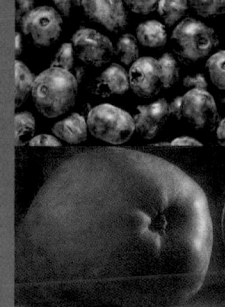

The ability of humans to manipulate nature has enabled us to improve the production and yield of many important foods. Traditional **biotechnology** is almost as old as agriculture. The first farmer to improve his stock by selectively breeding the best bull with the best cows was implementing biotechnology in a simple sense. The first baker to use yeast to make bread rise took advantage of biotechnology.

By the 1930s, biotechnology made possible the selective breeding of better plant hybrids. As a result, corn production in the United States quickly doubled. Through similar methods, agricultural wheat was crossed with wild grasses to confer more desirable properties, such as greater yield, increased resistance to mildew and bacterial diseases, and tolerance to salt or adverse climatic conditions.

Another type of biotechnology uses hormones rather than breeding. In the last decade, Canadian salmon have been treated with a hormone that allows them to mature three times faster than normal—without changing the fish in any other way. In general terms, biotechnology can be understood as the use of living things—plants, animals, bacteria—to manufacture products.

biotechnology A collection of processes that involve the use of biological systems for altering and, ideally, improving the characteristics of plants, animals, and other forms of life.

genetic engineering Manipulation of the genetic makeup of any organism with recombinant DNA technology.

The New Biotechnology

The new biotechnology used in agriculture includes several methods that directly modify products. It differs from traditional methods because it more directly changes some of the genetic material (DNA) of organisms to improve characteristics. Crossbreeding plants or animals is no longer the only tool. Development of the new process, called **genetic engineering,** began in the 1970s. The field now features a wide range of cell and subcell techniques for the synthesis and placement of genetic material in organisms (Fig. 17-5).

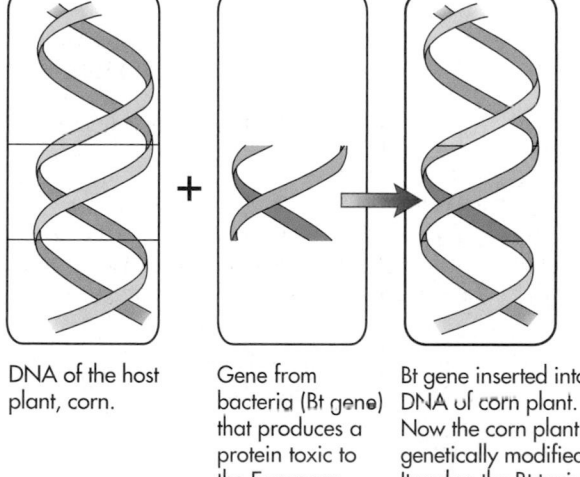

DNA of the host plant, corn.

Gene from bacteria (Bt gene) that produces a protein toxic to the European corn borer.

Bt gene inserted into DNA of corn plant. Now the corn plant is genetically modified. It makes the Bt toxin and, so, is resistant to the European corn borer.

Figure 17–5 Biotechnology involves various techniques for transferring foreign DNA into an organism. In this diagram, a sample of DNA is cleaved out of a larger DNA fragment and inserted into the DNA of a host cell. Thus, the host cell contains new genetic information, with the potential of providing the cell with new capabilities. For corn, this could mean resistance to the European corn borer. The corn plant is now referred to as a genetically modified organism (GMO). In another application, bacteria can be engineered to produce the human form of the hormone insulin.

recombinant DNA technology A test tube technology that rearranges DNA sequences in an organism by cutting the DNA, adding or deleting a DNA sequence and rejoining DNA molecules with a series of enzymes.

genetically modified organism (GMO) Any organism created by genetic engineering.

transgenic Organism that contains genes originally present in another organism.

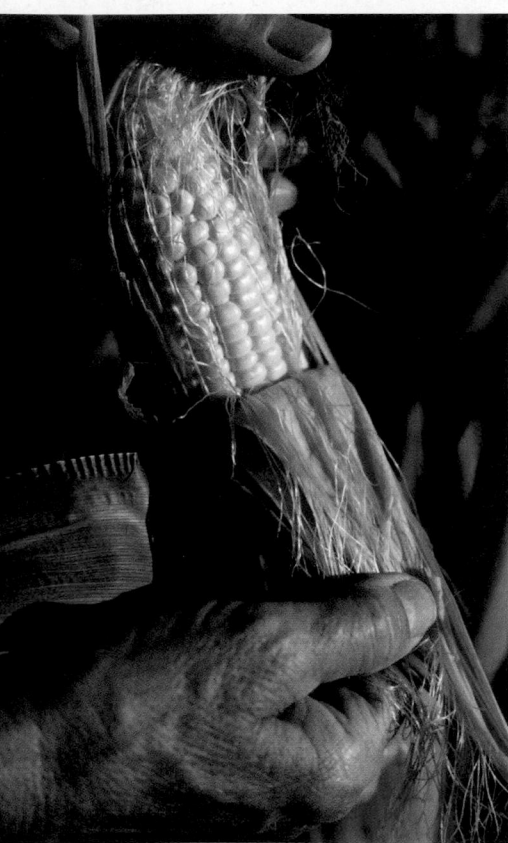

Both traditional plant breeding and biotechnology have produced high-yielding and disease-resistant plant varieties, such as with corn.

This process of **recombinant DNA technology** allows access to a wider gene pool, and it permits faster and more accurate production of new and more useful microbial, plant, and animal species. Conventional breeding is inefficient and has inconsistent results; biotechnology utilizes genetic material more precisely. Scientists select the traits they want and genetically engineer or introduce the gene that produces the desired trait into plants or animals (now called a **genetically modified organism [GMO]** or **transgenic**). It is important to note, however, that the genetic engineering does not replace conventional breeding practices; both work together.

Already, genetic engineering of agricultural products has allowed us to make use of new types of seeds, growth hormones, and microbial inoculants to stop pests and frost damage. Biotechnology is also used to develop drought-tolerant crops, as well as to detect *Listeria* and other microorganisms that cause foodborne illness. Scientists are engineering plants that grow with the use of less pesticides and new forms of potatoes that can be stored longer without preservatives. In addition, biotechnology can allow scientists to create fruits and grains with greater amounts of nutrients such as beta-carotene (e.g. "golden rice") and vitamins E and C. Researchers are also examining ways to modify the fatty-acid makeup of vegetable oils. Because biotechnology is being used cautiously and conservatively, these early benefits of the new biotechnology will strike us as only subtly different. The ultimate benefits, however, could be important if foods eaten by people in the developing world can be so enhanced.

Few consumers in the United States realize that currently about 40% of all corn and 90% of all soybeans produced in the United States have been genetically engineered to either resist certain insects, thereby reducing pesticide use, and/or survive when sprayed with herbicides that kill surrounding weeds. Some papaya plants have been genetically engineered for viral resistance.

Another Bite

GMO products are so widely distributed in our food supply that 70% of processed foods contain at least one GMO ingredient. Thus it is not surprising that when Gerber Products Co. tried to introduce a line of GMO-free baby foods, they found that they could not produce products from raw materials currently available.

Genetic modification of corn has received a lot of media attention. Corn can be genetically altered by inserting a gene from the bacterium *Bacillus thuringiensis,* usually referred to as the Bt gene, into the corn DNA. The gene allows the corn plant to make a protein that is lethal to certain caterpillars that destroy the plant. The Bt protein in the corn, however, is present in the plant in very low concentrations and has no effect on humans—it is digested along with the other proteins in corn. For many years organic farmers have used the Bt bacteria as a dust on plants in order to destroy pests. (Dusting crops, however, does not change the DNA of the plant.)

FDA is confident that currently approved varieties of genetically engineered foods are safe to consume. A controversy arose over use of StarLink corn in 2000. In this case, the GMO corn variety was approved for animal feed but not human consumption, yet it found its way into some corn products, such as taco shells. Food manufacturers are not currently required to disclose the GMO content on food labels. Some manufacturers however have promoted their products as being "GMO-free" on labels. A recent study showed that even these foods typically have GMO content. FDA does not feel labeling of GMO products is needed because they pose no health risk.

Public response to use of GMO biotechnology has been mixed. Even the scientific community has conflicting opinions about this technology, with supporters as convinced about the benefits as opponents are of the risks. The biggest debate in the United States surrounds the potential environmental hazards of introducing genes from one species to another. Some challengers even question the actual reduction in pesticide use that accompanies the cultivation of GMO crops. Although the use of GMOs may reduce the need for environmentally harmful activities, such as spraying crops with pesticides, critics point out that seeds produced with additional insecticide potential will lead to rapid insect resistance because the insecticides are continuously emitted. Use of traditional pesticides involves prudent application, in part to avoid insect resistance. In addition, accidental release of genetically modified animals, such as fish, may go on to harm wild varieties.

Although the risks of biotechnology may appear to be momentarily negligible, they may be cumulative and therefore of concern in the long run. In addition, will allergens, such as those found in peanuts, eggs, milk, wheat, and shellfish, be added to genetically engineered foods that previously did not contain them? Evidence that this can happen has been seen in soybeans. Note, however, that FDA carefully examines all products developed using this technology and will enforce labeling of potential allergens that may be newly present in food altered by biotechnology.

The public has long been opposed to processes perceived as harmful to the environment, such as producing unnatural products. Because food reserves are high in the United States, Canada, and Europe, some question the need to increase food production. Skepticism surrounds unnatural products, as exemplified by Western Europe's ban of hormones used in beef and milk production, and also almost all GMO foods. Some North Americans support this stance. Citizens believe the increase in the food supply is not worth the perceived risks associated with the products.

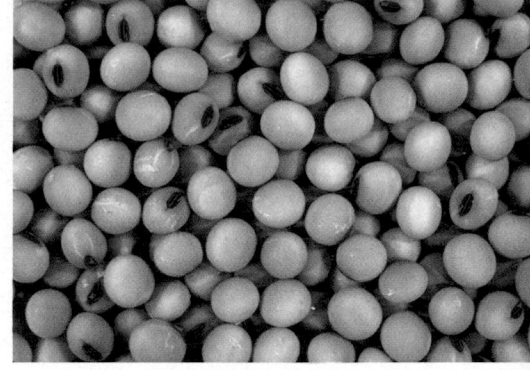

Soybeans are a common GMO food in the marketplace (80% of the total).

Role of the New Biotechnology in the Developing World

Whether applications of genetic engineering will help to significantly reduce undernutrition in the developing world remains to be seen. Unless price cuts accompany the increased production, only landowners and suppliers of biotechnology will enjoy the benefits. Small farmers may benefit if they can afford to purchase the GMO seeds. This point deserves emphasis: The person who cannot afford to buy enough food today will still face that same predicament in the future.

As with most innovations, the more successful farmers—often those with larger farms—will adopt the new biotechnology first. Because of this, the present trend toward fewer and larger farms will continue in the developing world, a movement that undermines the solution to one of the most pressing undernutrition issues there. Furthermore, biotechnology does not promise dramatic increases in the production of most grains and cassava, the primary food resources in developing parts of the world.

With the introduction of drought- and pest-resistant, as well as self-fertilizing crops, agricultural biotechnology may help to lessen world hunger. Perhaps the most promising potential of genetically modified foods today lies within the realm of plant breeding for micronutrients. Developing countries will then have a tool to treat and prevent selected nutrient deficiencies among their populations if they have access to farming resources to augment the micronutrient composition of crops. In addition, greater yields for indigenous plants, such as tomatoes that tolerate high soil salinity, are another hopeful outcome. Biotechnology will likely be a useful tool against the complex scourge of world undernutrition. Improved crops produced by this technology, together with political and other efforts, can contribute to the battle of worldwide undernutrition.

Ultimately, the depletion of world resources, the massive debt incurred by poorer countries, the threat of danger to more prosperous countries nearby, and the toll taken in human lives does affect the world economy and well-being. The resulting instability can go on to affect the developing world, as has been apparent in recent years.

▮ Some Concluding Thoughts

Today, the economic loss from undernutrition is staggering, and the amount of human pain and suffering is incalculable. With all the international relief efforts and assistance from governments and private organizations combined, we are still failing in our battle against undernutrition.

Life is not necessarily fair, but the aim of civilization should be to make it more so. The world has both enough food and the technical expertise to end hunger. What is lacking is the political will to do so.

Concept Check

Overall, one important solution to reducing undernutrition in the developing world lies in providing sufficient employment, so that people can purchase the food their families need. Providing access to land and other food production resources will also counteract undernutrition. Development programs must be sensitive to regional conditions to ensure that the new technologies introduced do not intensify existing problems for the poorest people.

Summary

1. Poverty is commonly linked to chronic or periodic undernutrition. Malnutrition can occur when the food supply is either scarce or abundant. The resulting deficiency conditions and degenerative diseases contribute to poor health.

2. Undernutrition is the most common form of malnutrition in developing countries. It results from inadequate intake, absorption, or use of nutrients or food energy. Many deficiency conditions consequently appear, and infectious diseases thrive because the immune system cannot function properly.

3. The greatest risk of undernutrition occurs during critical periods of growth and development: gestation, infancy, and childhood. Low birth weight is a leading cause of infant deaths worldwide. Many developmental problems are caused by nutritional deprivation during critical periods of brain growth. People in their later years are also at great risk.

4. Undernutrition diminishes both physical and mental capabilities. In poor countries, this is worsened by recurrent infections, unsanitary conditions, extreme weather, inadequate shelter, and exposure to diseases.

5. In the United States, famine is not seen but food insecurity and undernutrition remain problems. Soup kitchens, food stamps, the school lunch and breakfast programs, and the Special Supplemental Nutrition Program for Women, Infants, and Children (WIC) have focused on improving the nutritional health of poor and at-risk people. When adequately funded, these programs have proved effective in reducing undernutrition. The need to reduce out-of-wedlock pregnancies remains a national priority because single parents and their children are much more likely to live in poverty.

6. Multiple factors contribute to the problem of undernutrition in the developing world. In densely populated countries, food resources, as well as the means for distributing food, may be inadequate. Farming methods often encourage erosion, which deprives the soil of valuable nutrients and thereby hampers future efforts to grow food. Limited water availability hinders food production. Naturally occurring devastation from droughts, excessive rainfall, fire, crop infestation, and human causes—such as urbanization, war and civil unrest, debt, poor sanitation, and AIDS—all contribute to the major problem of undernutrition.

7. Proposed solutions to world undernutrition must consider multiple interacting factors, many of which are thoroughly embedded in cultural traditions. Family planning efforts, for example, may not succeed until life expectancy increases. Through education, efforts should be made to upgrade farming methods, improve crops, limit pregnancies, encourage breastfeeding when it is safe to do so, and improve sanitation and hygiene. Direct food aid is only a short-term solution. In what may appear to be a step backward, many experts recommend more sustainable subsistence-level farming. Small-scale industrial development is another way to create meaningful employment and purchasing power for vast numbers of the rural poor. Various biotechnology applications may also prove beneficial.

Study Questions

1. Describe the difference between malnutrition and undernutrition.
2. Describe in a short paragraph any evidence of undernutrition that you saw while you were growing up, such as on television. What are/were the likely roots of these problems?
3. What do you believe are the major factors contributing to undernutrition in wealthy nations, such as the United States? What are some solutions to this problem?

4. What three points would you make to a group of seventh grade girls concerning the economic perils of teen pregnancy and parenting?

5. Personal responsibility is a common theme in political circles. How does this relate to the problem of undernutrition in the United States? Does it apply to all causes of the problem?

6. Outline how war and civil unrest in developing countries have worsened problems of chronic hunger over the past few years.

7. How important is population control in addressing the problem of world hunger now and in the future? Support your answer with three main points.

8. Why is solving the problem of undernutrition a key factor in the development of the full potential of developing countries?

9. Discuss how infrastructure could influence the causes and solutions of chronic hunger in a developing nation.

10. Name three nutrients that are often lacking in the diets of undernourished people. What effects can be expected with each deficiency?

Further Readings

1. ADA Reports: Position of the American Dietetic Association: Assessing world hunger, malnutrition and food security. *Journal of the American Dietetic Association* 103:1046, 2003.

   It is the position of the American Dietetic Association that access to adequate amounts of safe, nutritious, and culturally appropriate foods is a fundamental human right. Still, hunger continues to be a worldwide problem of staggering proportions. In response, it is important to encourage programs and practices that combat hunger and malnutrition, increase food security, promote self-sufficiency, and are environmentally and economically sustainable.

2. ADA Reports: Position of the American Dietetic Association: Child and adolescent food and nutrition programs. *Journal of the American Dietetic Association* 103:887, 2003.

   The current food programs targeted to low-income households, such as the Food Stamp Program, have gone a long way to increasing the nutrient intake of children and adolescents. It is important that these food programs are supported by adequate funding since the health of many children and adolescents is dependent upon these resources to provide sufficient nutrients to promote optimal physical, social, and cognitive growth and development.

3. Ash DM and others: Randomized efficacy trial of a micronutrient-fortified beverage in primary school children in Tanzania. *American Journal of Clinical Nutrition* 77:891, 2003.

   Fortifying beverages with micronutrients is one strategy to help reduce micronutrient deficiencies in developing countries. Such practices have been shown to reduce the risk of nutrient deficiencies. (Other recent studies also support the efficacy of this practice: Journal of Nutrition 133:1834, 2003 and Journal of Nutrition 133:1339, 2003.)

4. Black RE and others: Why are 10 million children dying each year? *The Lancet* 361:2226, 2003.

   More than 10 million children die each year, mostly from preventable causes. Undernutrition is the underlying cause of a substantial portion of these childhood deaths.

5. Brown KH: Diarrhea and malnutrition. *Journal of Nutrition* 133:328S, 2003.

   Undernutrition increases the risk of severe diarrheal disease, which can lead to undernutrition. Prevention strategies include promotion of breastfeeding to prevent diarrheal disease, continued feeding during illness, and supplementation with selected micronutrients to prevent infections and reduce their severity.

6. Darton-Hill I and others: Micronutrient deficiencies and gender: social and economic costs. *American Journal of Clinical Nutrition* 81:1198S, 2005.

   Micronutrient deficiencies in developing countries, such as for vitamin A, iodine, iron, and zinc, lead to health problems, especially in females. Addressing these micronutrient deficiencies is important in order to economic status at the personal, community, and national level in developing countries.

7. Davies PW: Historical perspective from the green revolution to the gene revolution. *Nutrition Reviews* 61(6):S124, 2003.

   Improved strains of plants can be achieved through traditional plant breeding and direct genetic manipulation. Greater application of both technologies is needed to attain the full benefits with regard to an increase in food production.

8. Dunford M: The GM food debate. *Today's Dietitian*, p. 12, June 2004.

   The genetic engineering of foods has both risks and benefits, and these are described in this article. The potential to improve the quality of individual foods is especially exciting, but has yet to be a major factor in reducing micronutrient deficiencies worldwide.

9. Fawzi W and others: Studies of vitamins and minerals and HIV transmission and disease progression. *Journal of Nutrition* 135:938, 2005.

   Nutrient deficiencies, such as for vitamin A and vitamin E, are related to faster disease progression in HIV infections and AIDS. Daily use of a multivitamin and mineral supplement has been shown to be helpful in a few studies, and may be especially helpful to reduce disease progression since nutrient deficiencies are common in people with HIV infections and AIDS.

10. Grandesso F and others: Mortality and malnutrition among populations living in South Darfur, Sudan. *Journal of the American Medical Association* 293: 1490, 2005.

    The recent conflicts in the Darfur region of Sudan have lead to high rates of death and undernutrion among people displaced by war. This article describes what has been seen numerous time in the last 50 years—undernutitrition and related death is a typical casualty of war.

11. Hoetz PJ and others: Hookworm infection. *The New England Journal of Medicine* 351:799, 2004.

    An estimated 740 million cases of hookworm infections exist in the world, primarily in the tropics and subtropics. Excellent medications are available to treat the disease and these should be made widely available.

12. Kalm LM, Semba RD: They starved so that others be better fed: Remembering Ancel Keys and the Minnesota experiment. *Journal of Nutrition* 135: 1347, 2005.

    Detailed and interesting account of the semi-starvation studies conducted in the 1940's by Ancel Keys and colleagues. These experiments were conducted to better understand the effects of semi-starvation that many peoples in World War II were experiencing, as well as to determine how best to safely refeed semi-starved individuals.

13. Palmer S: GE foods under the microscope. *Today's Dietitian* p. 34, May 2005.

    About 70% of all processed foods sold in the U.S. have contents that that have undergone some genetic alteration. This article explores some of the benefits and concerns regarding using this fairly recent technology in our food supply.

14. Pelletier DL, Frongillo EA: Changes in child survival are strongly associated with changes in malnutrition in developing countries. *Journal of Nutrition* 133:107, 2003.

    Considerable evidence suggests that undernutrition affects human performance, overall health and survival, physical growth, cognitive development, reproduction, physical work capacity, and risks for many chronic diseases. Efforts to reduce undernutrition worldwide are important if we are to reduce overall mortality.

15. Scrimshaw NS: Historical concepts of interactions, synergism, and antagonism between nutrition and infection. *Journal of Nutrition* 133:316S, 2003.

    Maintaining nutritional health is important for proper functioning of the immune system and thereby reducing the risk of infectious diseases.

16. Steinbrook R: After Bangkok—Expanding the global response to AIDS. *The New England Journal of Medicine* 351:738, 2004.

    The advances in treatment of AIDS have largely benefited developed countries. There is an urgent need to provide the benefits to those infected with AIDS in the developing world.

17. Yach D and others: The global burden of chronic diseases: Overcoming impediments to prevention and control. *Journal of the American Medical Association* 291:2616, 2004.

    Nutrient deficiencies are common in the developing world. Such areas also experience the greatest burden of deaths from diarrhea, HIV and AIDS, and various childhood diseases. There needs be more attention to this enormous problem in the developing world.

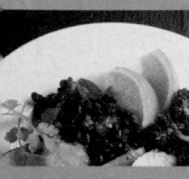

I. Fighting World Undernutrition on a Personal Level

If you want to do something about world and domestic undernutrition, consider the following activities. It is a noble act to try to make a difference, even if you make just one small step. As with any change in behavior, do not try to do too many things at once. Try one or two activities that represent your commitment to solving this problem.

1. Volunteer at a local soup kitchen or homeless shelter for a period of time (1 month, for example). What insights did you gain?

2. Coordinate the efforts of a campus organization to donate some money to a voluntary agency that does antihunger work, such as the following:

Bread for the World
802 Rhode Island Ave., NE
Washington, DC 20018

Oxfam America
115 Broadway
Boston, MA 02116

Save the Children Foundation
P.O. Box 970
Westport, CT 06881

Earth Save Foundation
1509 Suite B1 Seabright Ave.
Santa Cruz, CA 95062

Catholic Relief Services
209 W. Fayette St.
Baltimore, MD 21201

CARE
650 First Ave.
New York, NY 10016

Second Harvest
116 Michigan Ave., Suite #4
Chicago, IL 60603

3. Make a contribution of nonperishable foods to the ongoing offering at a place of worship near you. If such an offering does not exist, start one.

4. Get on a food recovery program's mailing list, read its newsletters for information on upcoming fund-raisers and other activities, become involved.

5. Participate in food drives organized by local grocery stores by contributing food or services. Food-drive organizers may need volunteers to transport the donations from the store to a food pantry. Pay special attention to events around World Food Day, October 16.

6. Point, click, and fight hunger. Internet users can find information on hunger at several sites, including the following:

- Someone somewhere dies of hunger every 3.6 seconds. You can help stop the clock: go to www.thehungersite.com and click on Donate Free Food to send a meal to a needy someone. This site is affiliated with the UN World Food Program, which tracks the number of clicks and then sends a bill to one of its corporate or nonprofit sponsors.

- HungerWeb, at Brown University, offers information on hunger research, programs, mailing lists, education, advocacy, and an overview of the Alan Shawn Feinstein World Hunger Program at Brown. This site contains web links to Internet sites run by the UN, U.S. AID, and the World Bank. www.brown.edu/Departments/World_Hunger_Program/

- The Food and Agriculture Organization of the United Nations has worked to alleviate poverty and hunger by promoting agricultural development, improved nutrition, and the pursuit of food security. This website will keep you up-to-date on recent issues and provides an extensive list of publications related to food security: www.fao.org

- America's Second Harvest, the largest domestic hunger-relief organization, shows you how to help online and has information about the latest updates. www.secondharvest.org

- Bread for the World is a nationwide Christian citizens' movement seeking justice for the world's hungry people by lobbying our nation's decision makers. www.bread.org

- CARE is one of the world's largest private international relief and development organizations, with the goal of saving lives, building opportunity, and bringing hope to people in need. www.care.org

II. Joining the Battle Against Undernutrition

Imagine that you recently spent your summer vacation in a developing country and saw evidence of undernutrition and hunger. Then imagine that you are now asking a large corporation to support your efforts to ease hunger and suffering in this area. Develop a two-paragraph statement outlining why addressing hunger issues in this area is important. Include how you think a large corporation could assist you in your efforts.

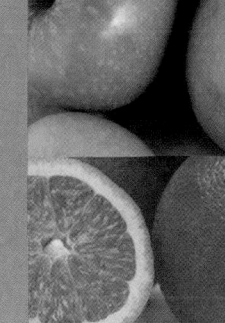
The Daily Values Used on Food Labels in the United States, with a Comparison to the Latest RDAs and Other Nutrient Standards*

Dietary Constituent	Unit of Measure	Current Daily Values for People Over 4 Years of Age	RDA or Other Current Dietary Standard	
			Males 19 Years Old	Females 19 Years Old
Total Fat‡	g	<65	—	—
Saturated fatty acids‡	"	<20	—	—
Protein‡	"	50	56	46
Cholesterol§	mg	<300	—	—
Carbohydrate‡	g	300	130	130
Fiber	"	25	38	25
Vitamin A	μg Retinol activity equivalents	1000	900	700
Vitamin D	International units	400	200	200
Vitamin E	"	30	22–33	22–33
Vitamin K	μg	80	120	90
Vitamin C	mg	60	90	75
Folate	μg	400	400	400
Thiamin	mg	1.5	1.20	1.10
Riboflavin	"	1.7	1.30	1.10
Niacin	"	20	16	14
Vitamin B-6	"	2	1.30	1.30
Vitamin B-12	μg	6	2.40	2.40
Biotin	mg	0.3	0.03	0.03
Pantothenic acid	"	10	5	5
Calcium	"	1000	1000	1000
Phosphorus	"	1000	700	700
Iodide	μg	150	150	150
Iron	mg	18	8	18
Magnesium	"	400	400	310
Copper	"	2	0.9	0.9
Zinc	"	15	11	8
Sodium†	"	<2400	1500	1500
Potassium†	"	3500	4700	4700
Chloride†	"	3400	2300	2300
Manganese	"	2	2.3	1.8
Selenium	μg	70	55	55
Chromium	"	120	35	25
Molybdenum	"	75	45	45

Abbreviations: g = gram, mg = milligram, μg = microgram

*Daily Values are generally set at the highest nutrient recommendation in a specific age and gender category. Many Daily Values exceed current nutrient standards. This is in part because aspects of the Daily Values were originally developed in the early 1970s using estimates of nutrient needs published in 1968. The Daily Values have yet to be updated to reflect the current state of knowledge.

†The considerably higher Daily Values for sodium and chloride are there to allow for more diet flexibility, but the extra amounts are not needed to maintain health.

‡These Daily Values are based on a 2000 kcal diet, instead of RDAs, with a caloric distribution of 30% from fat (and one-third of this total from saturated fat), 60% from carbohydrate, and 10% from protein.

§Based on recommendations of U.S. federal agencies.

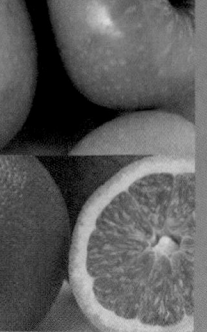

Appendix B

Dietary Advice for Canadians

Recommended Nutrient Intake (RNI) The Canadian version of RDA published in 1990.

The information in this appendix includes advice on dietary patterns, as well as regulations that apply to food labeling. Previous **RNIs** for nutrients have been replaced by the Dietary Reference Intakes (DRIs) that apply to Canadian and U.S. citizens. These are listed on the inside cover. Both Canadian and American scientists worked on the various DRI committees, coming up with a set of harmonized Dietary Reference Intakes for both countries.

Summary of the Nutrition Recommendations for Canadians

The latest Nutrition Recommendations of the Scientific Review Committee of the Office of Nutrition Policy and Promotion suggest that the Canadian diet should supply:

Excellent World Wide Web resources for Canadians are Health Canada (www.hc-sc.gc.ca), Dietitians of Canada (www.dietitians.ca), and the National Institute of Nutrition (www.nin.ca).

- Essential nutrients in the amounts specified in the updated Recommended Nutrient Intakes (RNIs);
- Sufficient energy to maintain a healthy weight when balanced with physical activity (energy intakes for adults should not be lower than 1800 kilocalories in order to meet RNIs);
- No more than 30% of energy as fat and no more than 10% of energy as saturated fat;
- At least 55% energy as carbohydrates;
- Less sodium than is now used;
- No more than 5% of energy as alcohol, or 2 drinks per day (whichever is less), with no alcohol during pregnancy;
- No more caffeine than the equivalent of four regular cups of coffee per day; and
- Water containing no less than 1 mg/litre of fluoride.

In essence, suggested actions toward healthful eating as listed in Canada's Guidelines for Healthy Eating include the following:

- Enjoy a VARIETY of foods.
- Emphasize cereals, breads, other grain products, vegetables, and fruit.
- Choose lower-fat dairy products, leaner meats, and foods prepared with little or no fat.
- Achieve and maintain a healthful body weight by enjoying regular physical activity and healthy eating.
- Limit salt, alcohol, and caffeine.

The Canadian Food Guide is a guide to help Canadians make wise food choices (Fig. B-1). The rainbow side of the Food Guide places foods into four groups: grain products; vegetables and fruit; milk products; and meat and meat alternatives. The rainbow includes information about the types of foods to choose from each food group for healthy eating.

The bar side of the Food Guide helps Canadians decide how much they need from each group every day. The guide gives a range for the number of servings for each food group, since different people need different amounts of food. The Food Guide also shows serving sizes for different foods.

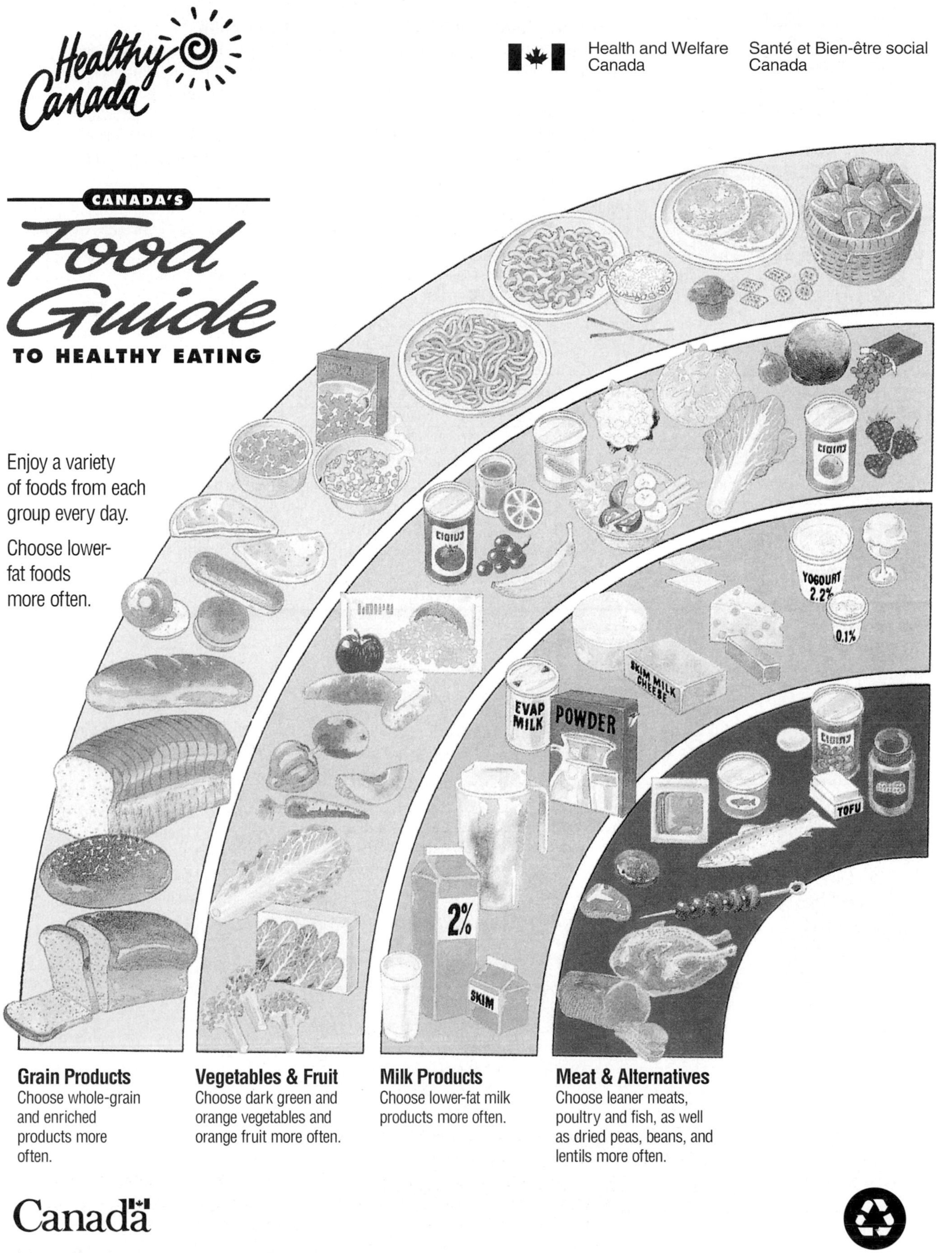

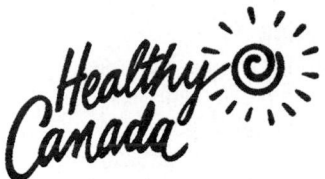

▌✦▌ Health and Welfare
Canada

Santé et Bien-être social
Canada

CANADA'S
Food Guide
TO HEALTHY EATING

Enjoy a variety
of foods from each
group every day.

Choose lower-
fat foods
more often.

Grain Products
Choose whole-grain
and enriched
products more
often.

Vegetables & Fruit
Choose dark green and
orange vegetables and
orange fruit more often.

Milk Products
Choose lower-fat milk
products more often.

Meat & Alternatives
Choose leaner meats,
poultry and fish, as well
as dried peas, beans, and
lentils more often.

Canadä

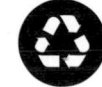

Figure B-1 Canadian Food Guide to Healthy Eating.

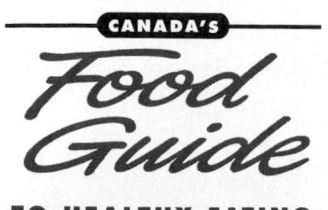

Different People Need Different Amounts of Food

The amount of food you need every day from the four food groups and other foods depends on your age, body size, activity level, whether you are male or female and if you are pregnant or breastfeeding. That's why the Food Guide gives a lower and higher number of servings for each food group. For example, young children can choose the lower number of servings, while male teenagers can go to the higher number. Most other people can choose servings somewhere in between.

Grain Products
5–12 SERVINGS PER DAY

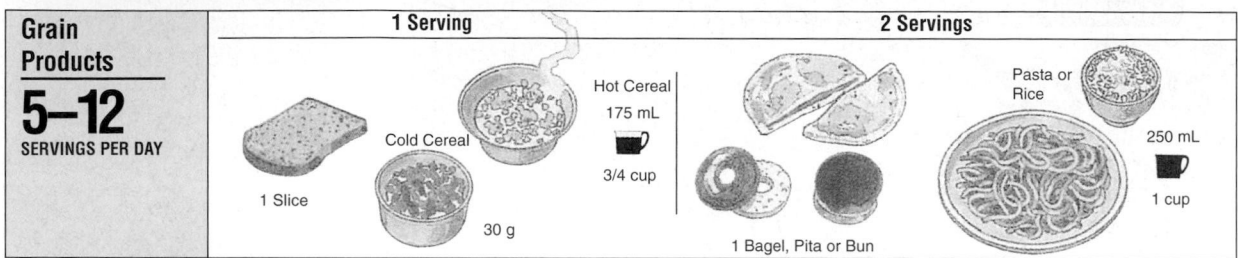

Vegetables & Fruit
5–10 SERVINGS PER DAY

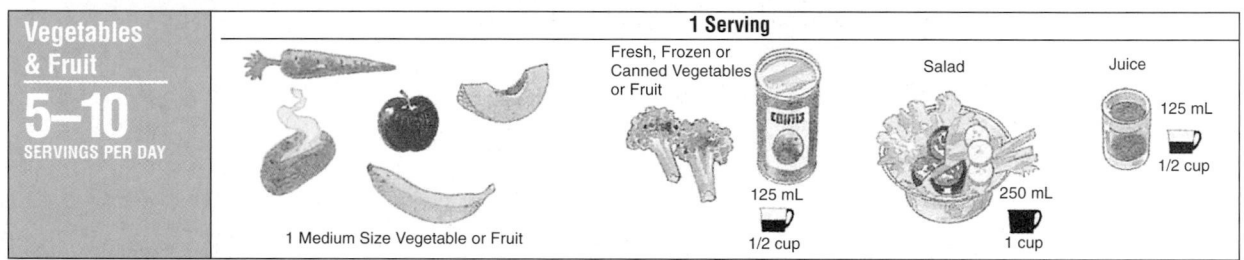

Milk Products
SERVINGS PER DAY
Children 4–9 years: 2-3
Youth 10–16 years: 3–4
Adults: 2-4
Pregnant & Breast-feeding Women: 3-4

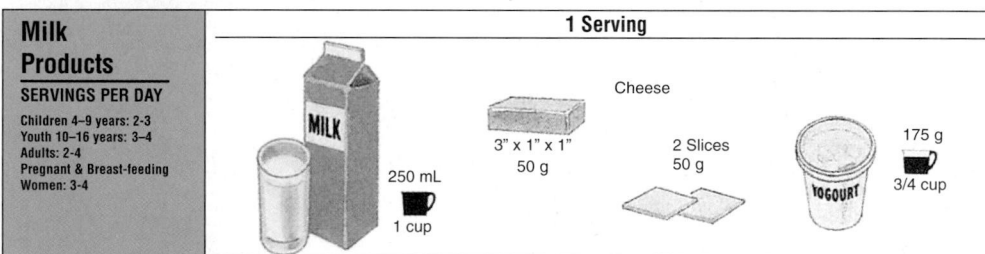

Other Foods

Taste and enjoyment can also come from other foods and beverages that are not part of the four food groups. Some of these foods are higher in fat or Calories, so use these foods in moderation.

Meat & Alternatives
2–3 SERVINGS PER DAY

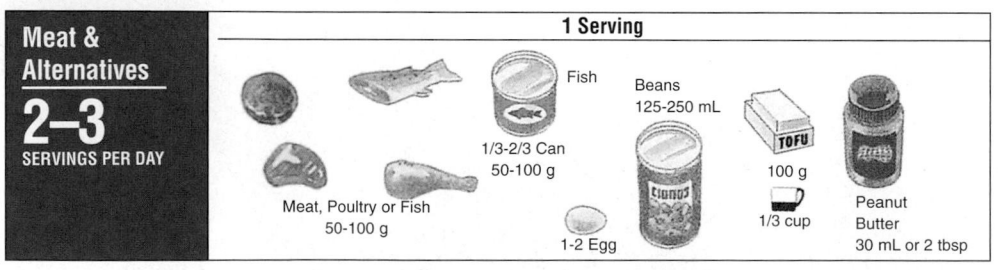

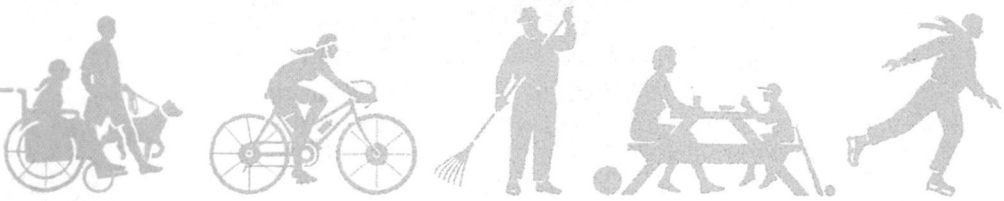

Enjoy eating well, being active, and feeling good about yourself. That's

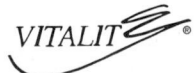

VITALIT ®

© Minister of Supply and Services Canada 1992   Cat. No. H39-252 / 1992E   No changes permitted. Reprint permission not required.
ISBN 0-662-19648-1

Figure B-1 *(concluded)*

The bar side of the Food Guide also tells how other foods that are not part of the four food groups can have a role in healthy eating. Since some of these "other foods" are higher in fat or calories, the Food Guide recommends using these foods in moderation.

Nutrition Labels

The current Canadian Nutrition Label is shown below. Consumers will soon start to see more information about the nutritional value of most prepackaged food under new labeling requirements that were published on January 1, 2003. The new regulations require most food labels to carry a mandatory Nutrition Facts table listing Calories and 13 key nutrients.

HOW TO READ THE ORIGINAL CANADIAN NUTRITION LABEL

Nutrition information is expressed per **suggested serving.** The serving size will vary according to food type and brand. Consider this fact when comparing foods.

Gives the calorie content (Cal)

Indicates the quantity of naturally occurring and added sugars as well as dietary fibre

Indicates the level of sodium from salt and all other sources

Vitamins and minerals are expressed as a percentage of the highest recommended amount

millilitres:
5 mL = 1 teaspoon

kilojoules:
metric unit of energy
1 Cal = 4.18kJ

grams: 28 g = 1 ounce

LASAGNA
Nutrition Information
per 275 g serving
(1 cup/250 mL)

Energy	275	Cal
	1140	kJ
Protein	19	g
Fat	7	g
Polyunsaturates	0.8	g
Monounsaturates	1.9	g
Saturates	2.5	g
Cholesterol	46	mg
Carbohydrate	34	g
Starch	29	g
Sugars	5	g
Dietary Fibre	0.2	g
Sodium	850	mg
Potassium	675	mg

Percentage of Recommended
Daily Intake

Thiamine	20%
Riboflavin	19%
Niacin	18%
Calcium	12%
Iron	28%

▪ The New Canadian Nutrition Facts Label

As noted on page A-5, new regulations published on January 1, 2003 make nutrition labelling mandatory on most food labels using a new format. The regulations also update requirements for nutrient content claims and permit, for the first time in Canada, diet-related health claims for foods.

How to Read the New Canadian Nutrition Label

The Regulations provide for the optional declaration of the number of Calories both from fat and from saturates plus *trans*. Recommendations on the % of Calories from fat apply to the total diet rather than to an individual food. Therefore, inclusion of the % of Calories from fat in the Nutrition Facts table may be confusing and is not permitted.

The Nutrition Facts table provides information on saturated and *trans* fatty acids which have been shown to raise serum cholesterol levels. The declaration of the other groups of fatty acids, mono-unsaturates, omega-3 and omega-6 polyunsaturates, is optional unless claims are made, in which case all three must be declared.

Potassium is not included as a mandatory nutrient of the Nutrition Facts table because it is not considered to be a nutrient of general public health importance. The declaration of potassium, however, is mandatory when a claim is made for the sodium or salt content of a food which contains an added potassium salt.

Daily Value is a comparison standard comprised of
(*a*) vitamin or mineral amounts referred to in the definition of a recommended daily intake for that vitamin or mineral
(*b*) nutrient amounts referred to in the definition of reference standard for that nutrient

Serving size is stipulated for various foods.

The amount of vitamins and minerals is expressed as a percentage of the Daily Value per serving of stated size.

Nutrition Facts
Per 1 cup (264g)

Amount	% Daily Value
Calories 260	
Fat 13g	**20%**
Saturated Fat 3g + *Trans* Fat 2g	**25%**
Cholesterol 30mg	
Sodium 660mg	**28%**
Carbohydrate 31g	**10%**
Fibre 0g	**0%**
Sugars 5g	
Protein 5g	
Vitamin A 4%	Vitamin C 2%
Calcium 15%	Iron 4%

New Canadian Nutrition Facts Label for Children Under Two Years of Age

Nutrition Facts
Per 1 jar (126 mL)

	Amount
Calories	110
Fat	0g
Sodium	10 mg
Carbohydrate	27g
Fibre	4g
Sugars	18g
Protein	0g

% Daily Value

Vitamin A	6%	Vitamin C	45%
Calcium	2%	Iron	2%

■ Recommended Daily Intakes and Reference Standards

Below are the Recommended Daily Intakes and Reference Standards used on Nutrition Labels for persons 2 years of age and older.*†‡

Dietary Constituent	Amount	Dietary Constituent	Amount
Fat	**65 g**	Folacin	220 μg
The sum of saturated fatty acids and *trans* fatty acids	**20 g**	Vitamin B$_{12}$	2 μg
Cholesterol	**300 mg**	Pantothenic acid or pantothenate	7 mg
Carbohydrate	**300 g**	Vitamin K	**80 mg**
Fibre	**25 g**	Biotin	**30 μg**
Sodium	**2400 mg**	Calcium	1100 mg
Chloride	**3400 μg**	Phosphorus	1100 mg
Potassium	**3500 mg**	Magnesium	250 mg
Vitamin A	1000 RE	Iron	14 mg
Vitamin D	5 μg	Zinc	9 mg
Vitamin E	10 mg	Iodide	160 μg
Vitamin C	60 mg	Selenium	**50 μg**
Thiamin, thiamine or vitamin B$_1$	1.3 mg	Copper	**2 mg**
Riboflavin or vitamin B$_2$	1.6 mg	Manganese	**2 mg**
Niacin	23 NE	Chromium	**120 μg**
Vitamin B$_6$	1.8 mg	Molybdenum	**75 μg**

*RE = retinol equivalents
†NE = niacin equivalents
‡Together these constitute the Daily Values used on the new Canadian Nutrition Facts Label. Note that Reference Standards are bolded.

■ Approved Nutrient Content Claims

Below is a sample of approved nutrient content claims for food labels (for the complete list of regulations see the website http://canadagazette.gc.ca/partII/2003/20030101/html/sor11-e.html).

Energy

- *Free of energy:* The food provides less than 5 Calories or 21 kilojoules per reference amount and serving of stated size.
- *Low in energy:* The food provides 40 Calories or 167 kilojoules or less per reference amount and serving of stated size.
- *Reduced in energy:* The food is processed, formulated, reformulated or otherwise modified so that it provides at least 25% less energy per reference amount of a similar food.
- *Lower in energy:* The food provides at least 25% less energy per reference amount of a similar food.
- *Source of energy:* The food provides at least 100 Calories or 420 kilojoules per reference amount and serving of stated size.
- *More energy:* The food provides at least 25% more energy, totalling at least 100 more Calories or 420 more kilojoules per reference amount of a similar food.

Protein

- *Low in protein:* The food contains no more than 1 g of protein per 100 g of the food.
- *Source of protein:* The food has a protein rating of 20 or more, as determined by official method FO-1, *Determination of Protein Rating*, October 15, 1981, (*a*) per reasonable daily intake;

or (*b*) per 30 g combined with 125 mL of milk, if the food is a breakfast cereal.

- *Excellent source of protein:* The food has a protein rating of 40 or more, as determined by official method FO-1, *Determination of Protein Rating,* October 15, 1981, (*a*) per reasonable daily intake; or (*b*) per 30 g combined with 125 mL of milk, if the food is a breakfast cereal.
- *More protein:* The food (*a*) has a protein rating of 20 or more, as determined by official method FO-1, *Determination of Protein Rating,* October 15, 1981, (i) per reasonable daily intake, or (ii) per 30 g combined with 125 mL of milk, if the food is a breakfast cereal; and (*b*) contains at least 25% more protein, totalling at least 7 g more, per reasonable daily intake compared to the reference food of the same food group or the similar reference food.

Fat

- *Free of fat:* The food contains less than 0.5 g of fat per reference amount and serving of stated size.
- *Low in fat:* The food contains 3 g or less of fat per reference amount and serving of stated size and, if the reference amount is 30 g or 30 mL or less, per 50 g.
- *Reduced in fat:* The food is processed, formulated, reformulated or otherwise modified so that it contains at least 25% less fat than the reference amount of a similar food.
- *Lower in fat:* The food contains at least 25% less fat per reference amount of the food, than the reference amount of the reference food of the same food group.
- *100% fat-free:* The food (*a*) contains less than 0.5 g of fat per 100 g; (*b*) contains no added fat.
- *No added fat:* The food contains no added fats or oils set out in Division 9, or added butter or ghee, or ingredients that contain added fats or oils, or butter or ghee.
- *Free of saturated fatty acids:* The food contains less than 0.2 g saturated fatty acids and less than 0.2 g *trans* fatty

acids per reference amount and serving of stated size.

- *Low in saturated fatty acids:* (1) The food contains 2 g or less of saturated fatty acids and *trans* fatty acids combined per reference amount and serving of stated size. (2) The food provides 15% or less energy from the sum of saturated fatty acids and *trans* fatty acids.
- *Reduced in saturated fatty acids:* The food is processed, formulated, reformulated or otherwise modified, without increasing the content of *trans* fatty acids, so that it contains at least 25% less saturated fatty acids per reference amount of the food than the reference amount of the similar reference food.
- *Lower in saturated fatty acids:* The food contains at least 25% less saturated fatty acids and the content of *trans* fatty acids is not higher per reference amount of the food, than the reference amount of the reference food of the same food group.
- *Free of trans fatty acids:* The food contains less than 0.2 g of *trans* fatty acids per reference amount and serving of stated size.
- *Reduced in trans fatty acids:* The food is processed, formulated, reformulated or otherwise modified, without increasing the content of saturated fatty acids, so that it contains at least 25% less *trans* fatty acids per reference amount of the food than the reference amount of the similar reference food.
- *Lower in trans fatty acids:* The food contains at least 25% less *trans* fatty acids and the content of saturated fatty acids is not higher per reference amount of the food compared to the reference amount of a similar food.
- *Source of omega-3 polyunsaturated fatty acids:* The food contains 0.3 g or more of omega-3 polyunsaturated fatty acids per reference amount and serving of stated size.
- *Source of omega-6 polyunsaturated fatty acids:* The food contains 2 g or more of omega-6 polyunsaturated fatty acids per reference amount and serving of stated size.

Cholesterol

- *Free of cholesterol:* The food contains less than 2 mg of cholesterol per reference amount and serving of stated size.
- *Low in cholesterol:* The food contains 20 mg or less of cholesterol per reference amount and serving of stated size (if the reference amount is 30 g or 30 mL or less, per 50 g).
- *Reduced in cholesterol:* The food is processed, formulated, reformulated or otherwise modified so that it contains at least 25% less cholesterol per reference amount of a similar food.
- *Lower in cholesterol:* The food contains at least 25% less cholesterol per reference amount of a similar food.

Sodium or Salt

- *Free of sodium or salt:* The food contains less than 5 mg of sodium per reference amount and serving of stated size.
- *Low in sodium or salt:* The food contains 140 mg or less of sodium per reference amount and serving of stated size.
- *Reduced in sodium or salt:* The food is processed, formulated, reformulated or otherwise modified so that it contains at least 25% less sodium per reference amount of a similar food.
- *Lower in sodium or salt:* The food contains at least 25% less sodium per reference amount of the food.
- *No added sodium or salt:* The food contains no added salt, other sodium salts, or ingredients that contain sodium that functionally substitute for added salt.
- *Lightly salted:* The food contains at least 50% less added sodium than the sodium added to a similar reference food.

Sugars

- *Free of sugars:* The food contains less than 0.5 mg of sugars per reference amount and serving of stated size.
- *Reduced in sugars:* The food is processed, formulated, reformulated or otherwise modified so that it contains at least 25% less sugars, totalling at least 5 g less, per reference amount of the food.

- *Lower in sugars:* The food contains at least 25% less sugars, totalling at least 5 g less, per reference amount of the food.
- *No added sugars:* The food contains no added sugars, no ingredients containing added sugars or ingredients that contain sugars that functionally substitute for added sugars.

Fibre

- *Source of fibre:* The food contains 2 g or more (*a*) of fibre per reference amount and serving of stated size, if no fibre or fibre source is identified in the statement or claim; or (*b*) of each identified fibre or fibre from an identified fibre source per reference amount and serving of stated size, if a fibre or fibre source is identified in the statement or claim.
- *High source of fibre:* The food contains 4 g or more (*a*) of fibre per reference amount and serving of stated size, if no fibre or fibre source is identified in the statement or claim; or (*b*) of each identified fibre or fibre from an identified fibre source per reference amount and serving of stated size, if a fibre or fibre source is identified in the statement or claim.
- *Very high source of fibre:* The food contains 6 g or more (*a*) of fibre per reference amount and serving of stated size, if no fibre or fibre source is identified in the statement or claim; or (*b*) of each identified fibre or fibre from an identified fibre source per reference amount and serving of stated size, if a fibre or fibre source is identified in the statement or claim.
- *More fibre:* The food contains at least 25% more fibre, totalling at least 1 g more, if no fibre or fibre source is identified in the statement or claim, or at least 25% more of an identified fibre or fibre from an identified fibre source, totalling at least 1 g more, if a fibre or fibre source is identified in the statement or claim compared to reference amount of a similar food.

Light and Lean

- *Light in energy or fat:* The food meets the conditions set out for the subject "reduced in energy" or "reduced in fat."
- *Lean:* The food (*a*) is meat or poultry that has not been ground, a marine or fresh water animal or a product of any of these; and (*b*) contains 10% or less fat.
- *Extra lean:* The food (*a*) is meat or poultry that has not been ground, a marine or fresh water animal or a product of any of these; and (*b*) contains 7.5% or less fat.

▮ Approved Health Claims for Nutrition Labels

If a manufacturer follows specific guidelines addressing both the nutrients noted in the claim as well as guidelines pertaining to other nutrients in a food, the following health claims can be made.

- A healthy diet containing foods high in potassium and low in sodium may reduce the risk of high blood pressure, a risk factor for stroke and heart disease.
- A healthy diet with adequate calcium and vitamin D, and regular physical activity, help to achieve strong bones and may reduce the risk of osteoporosis.
- A healthy diet low in saturated and *trans* fats may reduce the risk of heart disease.
- A healthy diet rich in a variety of vegetables and fruit may help reduce the risk of some types of cancer.
- Foods very low in starch and fermentable sugars can make the following health claims:
  - Won't cause cavities;
  - Does not promote tooth decay;
  - Does not promote dental caries; or is
  - Non-cariogenic.

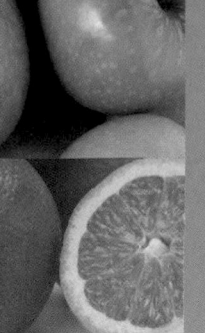

Appendix C

The Exchange System: A Helpful Menu-Planning Tool

Exchange System A system for classifying foods into numerous lists based on the foods' macronutrient composition and establishing serving sizes, so that one serving of each food on a list contains the same amount of carbohydrate, protein, fat, and calorie content.

exchange The serving size of a food on a specific exchange list.

The Exchange System

The **Exchange System** is a valuable tool for roughly estimating the calorie, protein, carbohydrate, and fat content of a food or meal. This tool organizes many details of the nutrient composition of foods into a manageable framework. By using the Exchange System, you can plan daily menus to fall roughly within specific percentages of macronutrients without having to look up or memorize the nutrient values of numerous foods, so the time you spend now becoming familiar with the Exchange System will pay off in the future.

In the Exchange System, individual foods are placed into three broad groups: carbohydrate, meat and meat substitutes, and fat. Within these groups are lists that contain foods of similar macronutrient composition: various types of milk, fruit, vegetables, starch, other carbohydrates, meat and meat substitutes, and fat. These lists are designed so that, when the proper serving size is observed, each food on a list provides about the same amount of carbohydrate, protein, fat, and calories. This equality allows the exchange of foods on each list, hence the term *Exchange System*.

The Exchange System was originally developed for planning diabetic diets. Diabetes is easier to control if the person's diet has about the same composition day after day. If a certain number of **exchanges** from each of the various lists is eaten each day, that regularity is easier to achieve. However, because the Exchange System provides a quick way to estimate the calorie, carbohydrate, protein, and fat content in any food or meal, it is a valuable menu-planning tool.

Becoming Familiar with the Exchange System

To use the Exchange System, you must know which foods are on each list and the serving sizes for each food.

Table C-1 gives the serving sizes for foods on each exchange list, as well as the carbohydrate, protein, fat, and calorie content per exchange. Note that the meat and milk lists are divided into subclasses, which vary in fat content and, hence, in the amount of calorie they provide. Foods on the meat and fat lists contain essentially no carbohydrate; those on the fruit and fat lists lack appreciable amounts of protein; and those on the vegetable, fruit, and other carbohydrates lists contain essentially no fat. You need to study Table C-1 and Figure C-1 to become familiar with the exchange lists, the sizes of the exchanges (that is, serving sizes) on each list, and the amounts of carbohydrate, protein, fat, and calories per exchange.

Before you can turn a group of exchanges into a daily meal plan, you must be aware of which foods are on each exchange list (Figure C-1). The entire U.S. Exchange System (2003) is presented in Appendix D, which you should consult frequently while exploring the system to discover its various peculiarities. For example, the starch list includes not only bread, dry cereal, cooked cereal, rice, and pasta, but also baked beans, corn on the cob, and potatoes. These foods are not identical to those composing the bread, cereal, rice, and pasta group in MyPyramid. The Exchange System is not concerned with the origin of a food, whether animal or vegetable. It is primarily concerned with the macronutrients carbohydrate, protein, and fat in each food on a specific list. For example, the carbohydrate composition of potatoes resembles that of bread more than that of broccoli, although potatoes are vegetables. In addition, several

Table C-1 Nutrient Composition of Exchange System Lists (2003 Edition)

Groups/Lists	Household Measures*	Carbohydrate (g)	Protein (g)	Fat (g)	Energy (kcal)
Carbohydrate Group					
Starch	1 slice, ¾ cup raw, or ½ cup cooked	15	3	1 or less[†]	80
Fruit	1 small/medium piece	15	—	—	60
Milk	1 cup				
Fat-free/very low-fat		12	8	0–3[†]	90
Reduced-fat		12	8	5	120
Whole		12	8	8	150
Other carbohydrates	Varies	15	Varies	Varies	Varies
Nonstarchy vegetables	1 cup raw or ½ cup cooked	5	2	—	25
Meat and Meat Substitutes Group	1 ounce				
Very lean		—	7	0–1	35
Lean		—	7	3	55
Medium-fat		—	7	5	75
High-fat		—	7	8	100
Fat Group	1 teaspoon	—	—	5	45

*Just an estimate; see exchange lists for actual amounts.

[†]Calculated as 1 gram for purposes of calorie contribution.

Reproduction of the exchange lists in whole or in part, without permission of The American Dietetic Association or the American Diabetes Association, Inc. is a violation of federal law. This material has been modified from *Exchange Lists for Meal Planning,* which is the basis of a meal planning system designed by a committee of the American Diabetes Association and The American Dietetic Association. While designed primarily for people with diabetes and others who must follow special diets, the exchange lists are based on principles of good nutrition that apply to everyone. Copyright © 2003 by the American Diabetes Association and the American Dietetic Association.

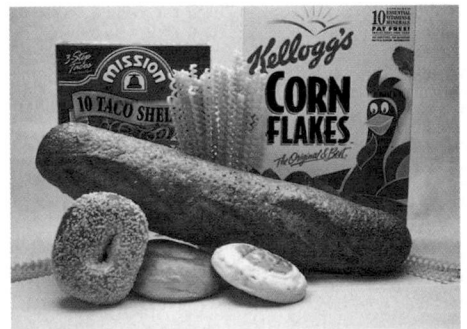

Starch exchange choices

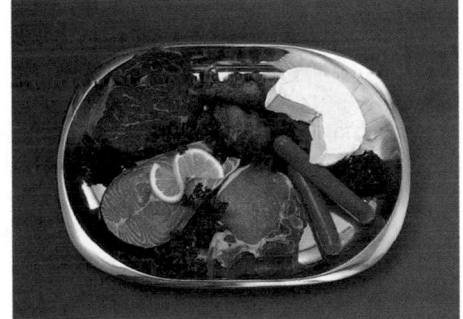

Meat and meat substitutes exchange choices

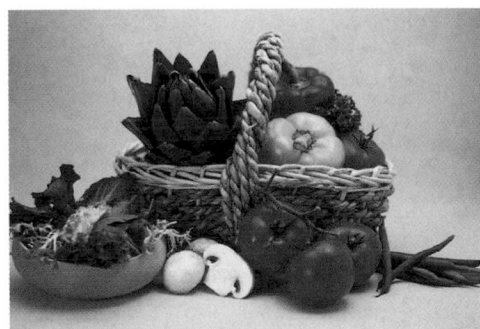

Vegetable exchange choices

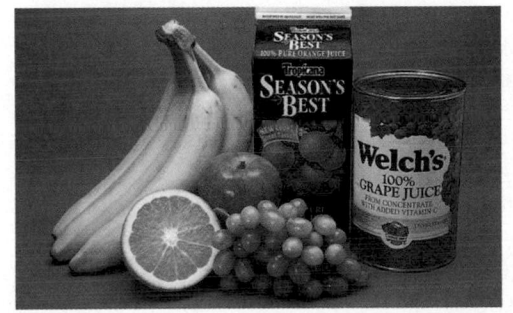

Fruit exchange choices

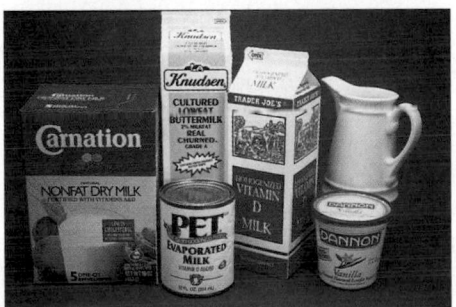

Milk exchange choices

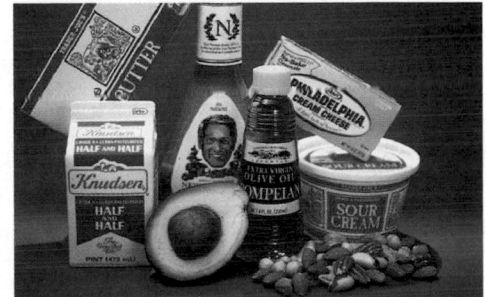

Fat exchange choices

Figure C-1 Foods arranged according to the Exchange System lists.

Table C-2 Possible Exchange Patterns for Calorie Intakes Greater Than 2000 kcal That Yield 55% of Calories as Carbohydrate, 30% as Fat, and 15% as Protein

kcal/Day Exchange List	1200*	1600*	2000	2400	2800	3200	3600
Milk (reduced-fat)	2	2	2	2	2	2	2
Vegetable	3	3	3	4	4	4	4
Fruit	3	4	5	6	8	9	9
Starch	5	8	11	13	15	18	21
Meat (lean)	4	4	4	5	6	7	8
Fat	2	4	6	8	10	11	13

This is just one set of options. More meat could be included if less milk were used, for example.
*Calorie intakes of 1200 and 1600 kcal contain 20% of calories as protein and 50% calories as carbohydrate to allow for greater flexibility in diet planning.

foods on the meat and meat substitutes list are not meats. The list of other carbohydrates includes jam, angel food cake, fat-free frozen yogurt, and foods such as frosted cake that count as both other carbohydrate exchanges and fat exchanges. Bacon appears in the fat list, rather than the high-fat meat category.

Free foods (essentially calorie-free) include bouillon, diet soda, coffee, tea, dill pickles, and vinegar, as well as herbs and spices. Most vegetables, such as cabbage, celery, mushrooms, lettuce, and zucchini, also can be considered free foods; their minimal energy contribution need not count in the calculations when they are eaten in moderation (1 to 2 servings per meal or snack).

■ Using the Exchange System to Develop Daily Menus

Now let's use the Exchange System to plan a 1-day menu. Let's target a calorie content of 2000 kcal, with 55% derived from carbohydrates (1100 kcal), 15% from protein (300 kcal), and 30% from fat (600 kcal). This can be translated into 2 reduced-fat milk exchanges, 3 vegetable exchanges, 5 fruit exchanges, 11 starch exchanges, 4 lean meat exchanges, and 6 fat exchanges (Table C-2). Note that this is only one of many possible combinations; the Exchange System offers great flexibility.

Table C-3 arbitrarily separates these exchanges into breakfast, lunch, dinner, and a snack. Breakfast includes 1 reduced-fat milk exchange, 2 fruit exchanges, 2 starch exchanges, and 1 fat exchange. This total corresponds to ¾ cup of a ready-to-eat breakfast cereal, 1 cup of reduced-fat milk, 1 slice of bread with 1 teaspoon margarine, and 1 cup of orange juice.

Lunch consists of 2 fat exchanges, 4 starch exchanges, 1 vegetable exchange, 1 reduced-fat milk exchange, and 2 fruit exchanges. This translates into one slice of bacon with 1 teaspoon mayonnaise on two slices of bread, with tomato—in other words, a bacon and tomato sandwich. You can also add lettuce to the sandwich. This can be considered a free vegetable choice. Add to this meal a 9-inch banana (1 exchange = 1 small banana), 1 cup of reduced-fat milk, and 6 graham crackers (2½ inches by 2½ inches). Later add a snack of ¾ ounce of pretzels for another starch exchange.

Dinner consists of 4 lean meat exchanges, 1 fruit exchange, 2 vegetable exchanges, 1 fat exchange, and 2 starch exchanges. This total corresponds to a 4-ounce broiled steak (meat only, no bone), 1 medium baked potato (1 exchange = 1 small baked potato) with 1 teaspoon of margarine, 1 cup of broccoli, and 1 kiwi fruit. Coffee (if desired) is not counted, since it contains no appreciable calories.

Finally, we have a snack containing 2 starch exchanges and 2 fat exchanges. This translates into 1 bagel with 2 tablespoons of regular cream cheese.

Table C-3 Sample 1-Day 2000 kcal Menu Based on the Exchange System Plan*

Breakfast

1 reduced-fat milk exchange	1 cup reduced-fat milk (some on cereal)
2 fruit exchanges	1 cup orange juice
2 starch exchanges	¾ cup ready-to-eat breakfast cereal, 1 piece whole-wheat toast
1 fat exchange	1 teaspoon soft margarine on toast

Lunch

4 starch exchanges	2 slices whole-wheat bread, 6 graham crackers (2½ inches by 2½ inches)
2 fat exchanges	1 slice bacon, 1 teaspoon mayonnaise
1 vegetable exchange	1 sliced tomato
2 fruit exchanges	1 banana (9 inches)
1 reduced-fat milk exchange	1 cup reduced-fat milk

Snack

1 starch exchange	¾ ounce pretzels

Dinner

4 lean meat exchanges	4 ounces lean steak (well trimmed)
2 starch exchanges	1 medium baked potato
1 fat exchange	1 tsp soft margarine
2 vegetable exchanges	1 cup cooked broccoli
1 fruit exchange	1 kiwi fruit
	Coffee (if desired)

Snack

2 starch exchanges	1 bagel
2 fat exchanges	2 tablespoons regular cream cheese

*The target plan was a 2000 kcal intake, with 55% of calories from carbohydrate, 15% from protein, and 30% from fat. Computer analysis indicates that this menu yielded 2040 kcal, with 53% of calories from carbohydrate, 16% from protein, and 31% from fat—in close agreement with the targeted goals.

This 1-day menu is only one of many that are possible with the exchange lists. Apple juice could replace the orange juice; two apples could be exchanged for the banana. The choices are endless. Notice that an exchange diet is much easier to plan if you use individual foods, as was done here; however, the Exchange System tables list some combination foods to help you (see Appendix D). Using combination foods, such as pizza or lasagna, however, makes it more difficult to calculate the number of exchanges in a serving. For instance, lasagna typically has meat exchanges, vegetable exchanges, and starch exchanges. With practice, you will be able to tackle such complex foods (Fig. C-2). For now, using individual foods makes learning the Exchange System much easier. Finally, you might want to prove to yourself that the food choices listed in Table C-3 really meet the Exchange plan. This demonstration will give you practice turning exchanges into actual food servings.

Figure C-2 Record the Exchange System pattern you have chosen in the left-hand column. Then distribute the exchanges throughout the day, noting the food to be used and the serving size.

Exchange List	Total Exchanges to Be Consumed Daily	Exchanges Consumed at Each Meal		
		Breakfast	Lunch	Dinner
MILK				
VEGETABLE				
FRUIT				
STARCH				
MEAT AND SUBSTITUTES				
FAT				

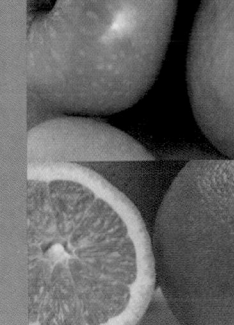

Milk Exchange List**

Fat-Free and Low-Fat Milk

(12 g carbohydrate, 8 g protein, 0–3 g fat, 90 kcal)

1 cup	fat-free, ½%, and 1% milk and buttermilk
⅓ cup	powdered (fat-free dry, before adding liquid)
½ cup	canned, evaporated fat-free milk
1 cup	buttermilk made from fat-free or low-fat milk
1 cup	soy milk (low-fat or fat-free)
⅔ cup (6 oz)	yogurt made from fat-free milk (plain, unflavored)
⅔ cup (6 oz)	yogurt, fat-free, flavored, sweetened with nonnutritive sweetener and fructose

Reduced-Fat Milk

(12 g carbohydrate, 8 g protein, 5 g fat, 120 kcal)

1 cup	2% milk
1 cup	soy milk
¾ cup	yogurt plain, low-fat (added milk solids)
1 cup	sweet acidophilus milk

Whole Milk

(12 g carbohydrate, 8 g protein, 8 g fat, 150 kcal)

1 cup	whole milk
½ cup	evaporated whole milk
1 cup	goat's milk
1 cup	kefir
1 cup	yogurt, plain (made from whole milk)

Vegetable Exchange List

(5 g carbohydrate, 2 g protein, 0 g fat, 25 kcal)
1 vegetable exchange equals:

½ cup cooked vegetables or vegetable juice
1 cup raw vegetables

artichoke	bean sprouts	cabbage
artichoke hearts	beets	carrots
asparagus	broccoli	cauliflower
beans (green, wax, Italian)	brussels sprouts	celery

*The exchange lists are the basis of a meal planning system designed by a committee of the American Diabetes Association and the American Dietetic Association. While designed primarily for people with diabetes and others who must follow special diets, the exchange lists are based on principles of good nutrition that apply to everyone. Copyright © 2003 by the American Diabetes Association and the American Dietetic Association.
**g = gram

cucumber	mushrooms	spinach
eggplant	okra	squash (summer)
green onions or scallions	onions	tomato (fresh, canned, sauce)
greens (e.g., collard)	pea pods	tomato/vegetable juice
kohlrabi	peppers (all varieties)	turnips
leeks	radishes	water chestnuts
mixed vegetables (without corn, peas, or pasta)	salad greens (all varieties)	watercress
	sauerkraut	zucchini

Fruit Exchange List

■ Fruit

(15 g carbohydrate, 0 g protein, 0 g fat, 60 kcal)
1 fruit exchange equals:

1 (4 oz)	apple, unpeeled (small)		1 (4 oz)	peach, fresh (medium)
4 rings	apple, dried		½ cup	peaches, canned
½ cup	applesauce (unsweetened)		½ (4 oz)	pear, fresh
4 (5½ oz)	apricots, fresh		½ cup	pear, canned
8 halves	apricots, dried		¾ cup	pineapple, fresh
½ cup	apricots, canned		½ cup	pineapple, canned
1 (4 oz)	banana (small)		2 (5 oz)	plums (small)
¾ cup	blackberries		½ cup	plums, canned
¾ cup	blueberries		3	plums dried (prunes)
⅓ melon (11 oz)	cantaloupe (small)		2 tbsp	raisins
1 cup cubes	cantaloupe		1 cup	raspberries
12 (3 oz)	cherries		1¼ cup	strawberries (raw, whole)
½ cup	cherries, canned		2 (8 oz)	tangerines (small)
3	dates		1 slice (13½ oz)	watermelon (or 1¼ cups cubes)
2 (3½ oz)	figs, fresh (large)			
1½	figs, dried		**■ Fruit Juice**	
½ cup	fruit cocktail			
½ (11 oz)	grapefruit (large)		½ cup	apple juice/cider
¾ cup	grapefruit sections, canned		⅓ cup	cranberry juice cocktail
17 (3 oz)	grapes (small)		1 cup	cranberry juice cocktail, reduced-calorie
1 slice (10 oz)	honeydew melon (or 1 cup cubes)		⅓ cup	fruit juice blends, 100% juice
1 (3½ oz)	kiwi		⅓ cup	grape juice
¾ cup	mandarin orange sections		½ cup	grapefruit juice
½ (5½ oz)	mango (or ½ cup)		½ cup	orange juice
1 (5 oz)	nectarine (small)		½ cup	pineapple juice
1 (6½ oz)	orange (small)		⅓ cup	prune juice
½ (8 oz)	papaya (or 1 cup cubes)			

Starch Exchange List

(15 g carbohydrate, 3 g protein, 0–1 g fat, 80 kcal)
1 starch exchange equals:

■ Bread

¼ (1 oz)	bagel		1 slice (1 oz)	bread, white, whole-wheat, pumpernickel, or rye
2 slices (1½ oz)	bread, reduced-calorie			

4 (⅔ oz)	bread sticks, crisp, 4 inch × ½ inch
½	English muffin
½ (1 oz)	hot dog or hamburger bun
¼	naan, 8 inch × 2 inch
1	pancake, 4 inch across × ¼ inch thick
½	pita, 6 inches across
1 slice (1 oz)	raisin bread, unfrosted
1 (1 oz)	roll, plain (small)
1	tortilla, corn, 6 inches across
1	tortilla, flour, 6 inches across
⅓	tortilla, flour, 10 inches across
1	waffle, 4 inches square or across, reduced-fat

■ Cereals and Grains

½ cup	bran cereal
½ cup	bulgur
½ cup	cereal, cooked
¾ cup	cereal, unsweetened, ready-to-eat
3 tbsp	cornmeal (dry)
⅓ cup	couscous
3 tbsp	flour (dry)
¼ cup	granola, low-fat
¼ cup	Grape-Nuts®
½ cup	grits
½ cup	kasha
⅓ cup	millet
¼ cup	muesli
½ cup	oats
⅓ cup	pasta
1½ cups	puffed cereal
⅓ cup	rice, white or brown
½ cup	Shredded Wheat
½ cup	sugar-frosted cereal
3 tbsp	wheat germ

■ Starchy Vegetables

⅓ cup	baked beans
½ cup	corn
½ (5 oz)	corn on the cob (large)
1 cup	mixed vegetables with corn, peas, or pasta
½ cup	peas, green
½ cup	plantain
½ cup or ½ medium (3 oz)	potato, boiled
¼ large (3 oz)	potato, baked with skin
½ cup	potato, mashed
1 cup	squash, winter (acorn, butternut, pumpkin)
½ cup	yam, sweet potato, plain

■ Crackers and Snacks

8	animal crackers
3	graham crackers, 2½-inch square
¾ oz	matzoh
4 slices	melba toast
24	oyster crackers
3 cups	popcorn (popped, no fat added or low-fat microwave)
¾ oz	pretzels
2	rice cakes, 4 inches across
6	saltine-type crackers
15–20 (¾ oz)	snack chips, fat-free (tortilla, potato)
2–5 (¾ oz)	whole-wheat crackers, no fat added

■ Dried Beans, Peas, and Lentils

(Counts as 1 starch exchange plus 1 very lean meat exchange)

½ cup	beans and peas (garbanzo, pinto, kidney, white, split, black-eyed)
⅔ cup	lima beans
½ cup	lentils
3 tbsp	miso

■ Starchy Foods Prepared with Fat

(Counts as 1 starch exchange, plus 1 fat exchange)

1	biscuit, 2½ inches across
½ cup	chow mein noodles
1 (2 oz)	corn bread, 2-inch cube
6	crackers, round butter type
1 cup	croutons
1 cup (2 oz)	French-fried potatoes (oven-baked) (see also the fast-foods list)
¼ cup	granola
⅓ cup	hummus
⅕ (1 oz)	muffin, 5 oz
3 cups	popcorn, microwaved
3	sandwich crackers, cheese or peanut butter filling
9–13 (3/4 oz)	snack chips (potato, tortilla)
⅓ cup	stuffing, bread (prepared)
2	taco shell, 6 inches across
1	waffle, 4-inch square or across
4–6 (1 oz)	whole-wheat crackers, fat added

Other Carbohydrates Exchange List

One exchange equals 15 g carbohydrate, or 1 starch, or 1 fruit, or 1 milk.

■ Exchanges per Serving

1/12th cake (about 2 oz)	angel food cake, unfrosted	2 carbohydrates
2-inch square (about 1 oz)	brownie, unfrosted (small)	1 carbohydrate, 1 fat
2-inch square (about 1 oz)	cake, unfrosted	1 carbohydrate, 1 fat
2-inch square (about 2 oz)	cake, frosted	2 carbohydrates, 1 fat
2	cookies, fat-free (small)	1 carbohydrate
2 (about 2/3 oz)	cookies or sandwich cookies with creme filling (small)	1 carbohydrate, 1 fat
1/4 cup	cranberry sauce, jellied	1 1/2 carbohydrates
1 (about 2 oz)	cupcake, frosted (small)	2 carbohydrates, 1 fat
1 (1 1/2 oz)	doughnut, plain cake (medium)	1 1/2 carbohydrates, 2 fats
3 3/4 inches across (2 oz)	doughnuts, glazed	2 carbohydrates, 2 fats
1 bar (1 1/3 oz)	Energy, sport or breakfast bar	2 carbohydrates, 1 fat
1 bar (2 oz)	Energy, sport or breakfast bar	3 carbohydrates, 1 fat
1/2 cup (3 1/2 oz)	fruit cobbler	3 carbohydrates, 1 fat
1 bar (3 oz)	fruit juice bars, frozen, 100% juice	1 carbohydrate
1 roll (3/4 oz)	fruit snacks, chewy (puréed fruit concentrate)	1 carbohydrate
1 tbsp	honey	1 carbohydrate
1 tbsp	sugar	1 carbohydrate
1 1/2 tbsp	fruit spread, 100% fruit	1 carbohydrate
1/2 cup	gelatin, regular	1 carbohydrate
3	gingersnaps	1 carbohydrate
1 bar (1 oz)	granola or snack bar (regular and low-fat)	1 1/2 carbohydrates
1/2 cup	ice cream, low-fat	1 1/2 carbohydrates
1/2 cup	ice cream	1 carbohydrate, 2 fats
1/2 cup	ice cream, light	1 carbohydrate, 1 fat
1/2 cup	ice cream, fat-free, no sugar added	1 carbohydrate
1 tbsp	jam or jelly, regular	1 carbohydrate
1 cup	milk, chocolate, whole	2 carbohydrates, 1 fat
1/6 pie	pie, fruit, 2 crusts (8 inches across)	3 carbohydrates, 2 fats
1/8 pie	pie, pumpkin or custard (8 inches across)	2 carbohydrates, 2 fats
1/2 cup	pudding, regular (made with reduced-fat milk)	2 carbohydrates
1/2 cup	pudding, sugar-free (made with fat-free milk)	1 carbohydrate
1 can (10–11 oz)	reduced-calorie meal replacement (shake)	1 1/2 carbohydrates, 0–1 fat
1 cup	rice milk, low-fat or fat-free, plain	1 carbohydrate
1 cup	rice milk, low-fat, flavored	1 1/2 carbohydrates
1/4 cup	salad dressing, fat-free	1 carbohydrate
1/2 cup	sherbet, sorbet	2 carbohydrates
1/2 cup	spaghetti or pasta sauce, canned	1 carbohydrate, 1 fat
1 cup (8 oz)	sports drinks	1 carbohydrate
1 tbsp	sugar	1 carbohydrate
1 (2 1/2 oz)	sweet roll or Danish	2 1/2 carbohydrates, 2 fats
2 tbsp	syrup, light	1 carbohydrate
1 tbsp	syrup, regular	1 carbohydrate
5	vanilla wafers	1 carbohydrate, 1 fat
1/3 cup	yogurt, frozen, fat-free	1 carbohydrate
1 cup	yogurt, low-fat with fruit	3 carbohydrates, 0–1 fat

■ Meat and Meat Substitutes Exchange List

■ Very Lean Meat and Substitutes List

(0 g carbohydrate, 7 g protein, 0–1 g fat, and 35 kcal)
One very lean meat exchange equals:

	Poultry
1 oz	chicken or turkey (white meat, no skin), Cornish hen (no skin)
	Fish
1 oz	fresh or frozen cod, flounder, haddock, halibut, trout; tuna, fresh or canned in water
	Shellfish
1 oz	clams, crab, lobster, scallops, shrimp, imitation shellfish
	Game
1 oz	duck or pheasant (no skin), venison, buffalo, ostrich
	Cheese with 1 g or less fat per oz
¼ cup	fat-free or low-fat cottage cheese
1 oz	fat-free cheese

	Other
1 oz	processed sandwich meats with 1 g or less fat per oz, such as deli thin, shaved meats, chipped beef, turkey, ham
2	egg whites
¼ cup	egg substitute, plain
1 oz	hot dogs with 1 g or less fat per oz
1 oz	kidney (high in cholesterol)
1 oz	sausage with 1 g or less fat per oz

Counts as one very lean meat and one starch exchange:

½ cup	dried beans, peas, lentils (cooked)

■ Lean Meat and Substitutes List

(0 g carbohydrate, 7 g protein, 3 g fat, and 55 kcal)
One lean meat exchange equals:

	Beef
1 oz	USDA Select or Choice grades of lean beef trimmed of fat, such as round, sirloin, and flank steak; tenderloin; roast (rib, chuck, rump); steak (T-bone, porterhouse, cubed), ground round
	Pork
1 oz	lean pork, such as fresh ham; canned, cured, or boiled ham; Canadian bacon; tenderloin, center loin chop
	Lamb
1 oz	roast, chop, leg
	Veal
1 oz	lean chop, roast
	Poultry
1 oz	chicken, turkey (dark meat, no skin), chicken white meat (with skin), domestic duck or goose (well drained of fat, no skin)

	Fish
1 oz	herring (uncreamed or smoked)
6	oysters (medium)
1 oz	salmon (fresh or canned), catfish
2	sardines (canned, medium)
1 oz	tuna (canned in oil, drained)
	Game
1 oz	goose (no skin), rabbit
	Cheese
¼ cup	4.5%–fat cottage cheese
2 tbsp	grated Parmesan
1 oz	cheeses with 3 g or less fat per oz

	Other
1½ oz	hot dogs with 3 g or less fat per oz
1 oz	processed sandwich meat with 3 g or less fat per oz, such as turkey pastrami or kielbasa
1 oz	liver, heart (high in cholesterol)

■ Medium-Fat Meat and Substitutes List

(0 g carbohydrate, 7 g protein, 5 g fat, and 75 kcal)
One medium-fat meat exchange equals:

	Beef
1 oz	most beef products (ground beef, meatloaf, corned beef, short ribs, prime grades of meat trimmed of fat, such as prime rib)
	Pork
1 oz	top loin, chop, Boston butt, cutlet

	Lamb
1 oz	rib roast, ground
	Veal
1 oz	cutlet (ground or cubed, unbreaded)
	Poultry
1 oz	chicken dark meat (with skin), ground turkey or ground chicken, fried chicken (with skin)

	Fish			**Other**
1 oz	any fried fish product		1	egg (high in cholesterol, limit to 3 per week)
	Cheese (with 5 g or less fat per oz)		1 oz	sausage with 5 g or less fat per oz
1 oz	feta		¼ cup	tempeh
1 oz	mozzarella		4 oz (½ cup)	tofu
¼ cup (2 oz)	ricotta			

■ High-Fat Meat and Substitutes List

(0 g carbohydrate, 7 g protein, 8 g fat, and 100 kcal)
One high-fat meat exchange equals:

	Pork			**Other**
1 oz	spareribs, ground pork, pork sausage		1 oz	processed sandwich meats with 8 g or less fat per oz, such as bologna, pimento loaf, salami
	Cheese		1 oz	sausage, such as bratwurst, Italian, knockwurst, Polish, smoked
1 oz	all regular cheeses, such as American, cheddar, Monterey Jack, Swiss		1	hot dog (turkey or chicken) (10 per pound)
			3 slices	bacon (20 slices per pound)

Counts as one high-fat meat plus one fat exchange:

1	hot dog (beef, pork, or combination) (10 per pound)

Fat Exchange List

■ Monounsaturated Fats List

(5 g fat and 45 kcal)
One exchange equals:

2 tbsp (1 oz)	avocado (medium)		6 nuts	mixed (50% peanuts)
1 tsp	oil (canola, olive, peanut)		10 nuts	peanuts
	olives:		4 halves	pecans
8	ripe, black (large)		½ tbsp	peanut butter, smooth or crunchy
10	green, stuffed (large)		1 tbsp	sesame seeds
6 nuts	almonds, cashews		2 tsp	tahini or sesame paste

■ Polyunsaturated Fats List

(5 g fat and 45 kcal)
One exchange equals:

	margarine:			salad dressing:
1 tsp	stick, tub, or squeeze		1 tbsp	regular
1 tbsp	lower-fat (30% to 50% vegetable oil)		2 tbsp	reduced-fat
	mayonnaise:			Miracle Whip Salad Dressing®:
1 tsp	regular		2 tsp	regular
1 tbsp	reduced-fat		1 tbsp	reduced-fat
4 halves	nuts, walnuts, English		1 tbsp	seeds: pumpkin, sunflower
1 tsp	oil (corn, safflower, soybean)			

■ Saturated Fats List

(5 g fat and 45 kcal)
One exchange equals:

1 slice	bacon, cooked (20 slices per pound)			butter:
1 tsp	bacon, grease		1 tsp	stick
			2 tsp	whipped
			1 tbsp	reduced-fat

2 tbsp (½ oz)	chitterlings, boiled			sour cream:
	cream cheese:	2 tbsp		regular
1 tbsp (½ oz)	regular	3 tbsp		reduced-fat
2 tbsp (1 oz)	reduced-fat			
1 tsp	shortening or lard			

Free Foods List

A *free food* is any food or drink that contains less than 20 kcal or less than 5 g of carbohydrate per serving. Foods with a serving size listed should be limited to three servings per day. Foods listed without a serving size can be eaten as often as you like.

■ Fat-Free or Reduced-Fat Foods

1 tbsp (½ oz)	cream cheese, fat-free	1 tbsp		salad dressing, fat-free
1 tbsp	creamers, nondairy, liquid			nonstick cooking spray
2 tsp	creamers, nondairy, powdered	1 tbsp		salad dressing, fat-free or low-fat, Italian
1 tbsp	mayonnaise, fat-free	2 tbsp		salad dressing, fat-free, Italian
1 tsp	mayonnaise, reduced-fat	1 tbsp		sour cream, fat-free, reduced-fat
4 tbsp	margarine, fat-free	1 tbsp		whipped topping, regular
1 tsp	margarine, reduced-fat	2 tbsp		whipped topping, light or fat-free
1 tbsp	Miracle Whip®, fat-free			
1 tsp	Miracle Whip®, reduced-fat nonstick cooking spray			

■ Sugar-Free Foods

1 candy	candy, hard, sugar-free	2 tsp		jam or jelly, light
	gelatin dessert, sugar-free			sugar substitutes*
	gelatin, unflavored	2 tbsp		syrup, sugar-free
	gum, sugar-free			

■ Drinks

	bouillon, broth, consommé		coffee
	bouillon or broth, low-sodium		diet soft drinks, sugar-free
	carbonated or mineral water		drink mixes, sugar-free
	club soda		tea
1 tbsp	cocoa powder, unsweetened		tonic water, sugar-free

■ Condiments

1 tbsp	catsup	2 slices		pickles, sweet (bread and butter)
	horseradish	¾ oz		pickles, sweet (gherkin)
	lemon juice	¼ cup		salsa
	lime juice	1 tbsp		soy sauce, regular or light
	mustard	1 tbsp		taco sauce
1 tbsp	pickle relish			vinegar
1½	pickles, dill (medium)	2 tbsp		yogurt

*Sugar substitutes, alternatives, or replacements that are approved by the Food and Drug Administration (FDA) are safe to use. Common brand names include:

Equal® (aspartame)

Splenda® (sucralose)

Sprinkle Sweet® (saccharin)

Sweet One® (acesulfame K)

Sweet-10® (saccharin)

Sugar Twin® (saccharin)

Sweet 'N Low® (saccharin)

Cannot display

▮ Seasonings

flavoring extracts
garlic
herbs, fresh or dried
pimento

spices
Tabasco® or hot pepper sauce
wine, used in cooking
Worcestershire sauce

▮ Combination Foods List

	Entrées	Exchanges per Serving
1 cup (8 oz)	tuna noodle casserole, lasagna, spaghetti with meatballs, chili with beans, macaroni and cheese	2 carbohydrates, 2 medium-fat meats
2 cups (16 oz)	chow mein (without noodles or rice)	1 carbohydrate, 2 lean meats
½ cup (3½ oz)	tuna or chicken salad	½ carbohydrate, 2 lean meats, 1 fat
	Frozen Entrées and Meals	
generally 14–17 oz	dinner-type meal	3 carbohydrates, 3 medium-fat meats, 3 fats
3 oz	meatless burger, soy-based	½ carbohydrate, 2 lean meats
3 oz	meatless burger, vegetable and starch-based	1 carbohydrate, 1 lean meat
¼ of 12-inch (6 oz)	pizza, cheese, thin crust	2 carbohydrates, 2 medium-fat meats, 1 fat
¼ of 12-inch (6 oz)	pizza, meat topping, thin crust	2 carbohydrates, 2 medium-fat meats, 2 fats
1 (7 oz)	pot pie	2½ carbohydrates, 1 medium-fat meat, 3 fats
8–11 oz	entrée or meal with less than 340 kcal	2–3 carbohydrates, 1–2 lean meats
	Soups	
1 cup	bean	1 carbohydrate, 1 very lean meat
1 cup (8 oz)	cream (made with water)	1 carbohydrate, 1 fat
6 oz prepared	instant	1 carbohydrate
8 oz prepared	instant with beans/lentils	2½ carbohydrates, 1 very lean meat
½ cup (4 oz)	split pea (made with water)	1 carbohydrate
1 cup (8 oz)	tomato (made with water)	1 carbohydrate
1 cup (8 oz)	vegetable beef, chicken noodle, or other broth-type	1 carbohydrate

▮ Fast-Foods

		Exchanges per Serving
1 (5–7 oz)	burritos with beef	3 carbohydrates, 1 medium-fat meat, 1 fat
6	chicken nuggets	1 carbohydrate, 2 medium-fat meats, 1 fat
1 each	chicken breast and wing, breaded and fried	1 carbohydrate, 4 medium-fat meats, 2 fats
1	chicken sandwich, grilled	2 carbohydrates, 3 very lean meats
6 (5 oz)	chicken wings, hot	1 carbohydrate, 3 medium-fat meats, 4 fats
1	fish sandwich/tartar sauce	3 carbohydrates, 1 medium-fat meat, 3 fats
1 medium serving (5 oz)	French fries	4 carbohydrates, 4 fats
1	hamburger (regular)	2 carbohydrates, 2 medium-fat meats
1	hamburger (large)	2 carbohydrates, 3 medium-fat meats, 1 fat
1	hot dog with bun	1 carbohydrate, 1 high-fat meat, 1 fat
1	individual pan pizza	5 carbohydrates, 3 medium-fat meats, 3 fats
¼ 12-inch (about 6 oz)	pizza, cheese, thin crust	2½ carbohydrates, 2 medium-fat meats
¼ 12-inch (about 6 oz)	pizza, meat, thin crust	2½ carbohydrates, 2 medium-fat meats, 1 fat
1 (5 oz)	soft-serve cone (small)	2½ carbohydrates, 1 fat
1 sub (6 inches)	submarine sandwich	3 carbohydrates, 1 vegetable, 2 medium-fat meats, 1 fat
1 (3–3½ oz)	taco, hard or soft shell	1 carbohydrate, 1 medium-fat meat, 1 fat

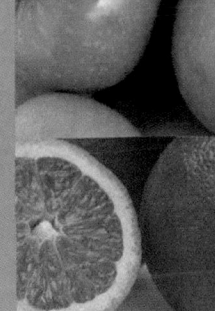

Although it may seem overwhelming at first, it is actually very easy to track the foods you eat. One tip is to record foods and beverages consumed as soon as possible after the actual time of consumption.

I. **Fill in the food record form that follows.** Appendix E contains a blank copy (see the completed example in Table E-1). Then, to estimate the nutrient values of the foods you are eating, consult food labels and the food composition table in this book (Appendix J), or use the NutritionCalc Plus software (CD or online) available with this book. If these resources do not have the serving size you need, adjust the value. If you drink ½ cup of orange juice, for example, but a table has values only for 1 cup, halve all values before you record them. Then, consider pooling all the same food to save time; if you drink a cup of 1% milk three times throughout the day, enter your milk consumption only once as 3 cups. As you record your intake for use on the nutrient analysis form that follows, consider the following tips:

- Measure and record the amounts of foods eaten in portion sizes of cups, teaspoons, tablespoons, ounces, slices, or inches (or convert metric units to these units).
- Record brand names of all food products, such as "Quick Quaker Oats."
- Measure and record all those little extras, such as gravies, salad dressings, taco sauces, pickles, jelly, sugar, catsup, and margarine.
- For beverages
  - List the type of milk, such as whole, fat-free, 1%, evaporated, chocolate, or reconstituted dry.
  - Indicate whether fruit juice is fresh, frozen, or canned.
  - Indicate type for other beverages, such as fruit drink, fruit-flavored drink, Kool-Aid, and hot chocolate made with water or milk.
- For fruits
  - Indicate whether fresh, frozen, dried, or canned.
  - If whole, record number eaten and size with approximate measurements (such as 1 apple—3 in. in diameter).
  - Indicate whether processed in water, light syrup, or heavy syrup.
- For vegetables
  - Indicate whether fresh, frozen, dried, or canned.
  - Record as portion of cup, teaspoon, or tablespoon, or as pieces (such as carrot sticks—4 in. long, ½ in. thick).
  - Record preparation method.
- For cereals
  - Record cooked cereals in portions of tablespoon or cup (a level measurement after cooking).
  - Record dry cereal in level portions of tablespoon or cup.
  - If margarine, milk, sugar, fruit, or something else is added, measure and record amount and type.
- For breads
  - Indicate whether whole wheat, rye, white, and so on.
  - Measure and record number and size of portion (biscuit—2 in. across, 1 in. thick; slice of homemade rye bread—3 in. by 4 in., ¼ in. thick).
  - Sandwiches: list all ingredients (lettuce, mayonnaise, tomato, and so on).

- For meat, fish, poultry, and cheese
  - Give size (length, width, thickness) in inches or weight in ounces after cooking for meat, fish, and poultry (such as cooked hamburger patty—3 in. across, ½ in. thick).
  - Give size (length, width, thickness) in inches or weight in ounces for cheese.
  - Record measurements only for the cooked, edible part—without bone or fat that is left on the plate.
  - Describe how meat, poultry, or fish was prepared.
- For eggs
  - Record as soft or hard cooked, fried, scrambled, poached, or omelet.
  - If milk, butter, or drippings are used, specify kinds and amount.
- For desserts
  - List commercial brand or "homemade" or "bakery" under brand.
  - Purchased candies, cookies, and cakes: specify kind and size.
  - Measure and record portion size of cakes, pies, and cookies by specifying thickness, diameter, and width or length, depending on the item.

Table E-1 One Day's Food Record—This Activity Can Help You Understand More about Your Food Habits

Time	Minutes Spent Eating	M or S*	H† (0–3)	Activity While Eating	Place of Eating	Food and Quantity	Others Present	Reason for Choice
7:10 A.M.	15	M	2	Standing, fixing lunch	Kitchen	Orange juice, 1 cup Crispix, 1 cup Reduced-fat milk, ½ cup Sugar, 2 tsp Black coffee	—	Health Habit Health Taste Habit
10:00 A.M.	4	S	1	Sitting, taking notes	Classroom	Diet cola, 12 oz	Class	Weight control
12:15 P.M.	40	M	2	Sitting, talking	Student union	Chicken sandwich with lettuce and mayonnaise (3 oz chicken, 2 slices of bread, 2 tsp mayonnaise) Pear, 1 Reduced-fat milk, 1 cup	Friends	Taste Health Health
2:30 P.M.	10	S	1	Sitting, studying	Library	Regular cola, 12 oz	Friend	Hunger
6:30 P.M.	35	M	3	Sitting, talking	Kitchen	Pork chop, 1 Baked potato, 1 Margarine, 2 tbsp Lettuce and tomato salad Ranch dressing, 2 tbsp Peas, ½ cup Whole milk, 1 cup Cherry pie, 1 piece Iced tea, 12 oz	Boyfriend	Convenience Health Taste Health Taste Health Habit Taste Health
9:10 P.M.	10	S	2	Sitting, studying	Living room	Apple, 1 Glass mineral water, 1	—	Weight control Weight control

*M or S: Meal or snack

†H: Degree of hunger (0 = none; 3 = maximum)

Time	Minutes Spent Eating	M or S*	H† (0–3)	Activity While Eating	Place of Eating	Food and Quantity	Others Present	Reason for Choice

*M or S: Meal or snack
†H: Degree of hunger (0 = none; 3 = maximum)

II. Now complete the nutrient analysis form as shown, using your food record. A blank copy of this form for your use is on A–28–A–29. NutritionCalc Plus will create such a table for you if you simply enter all food eaten.

Nutrient Analysis Form (Sample)

Name	Quantity	kcal	Protein (g)	Carbohydrates (g)	Fiber (g)	Total fat (g)	Monounsaturated fat (g)	Polyunsaturated fat (g)	Saturated fat (g)	Cholesterol (g)	Calcium (mg)	Iron (mg)
Egg bagel, 3.5-in. diameter	1 ea.	180	7.45	34.7	0.748	1.00	0.286	0.400	0.171	44.0	20.0	2.10
Jelly	1 tbsp	49.0	0.018	12.7	—	0.018	0.005	0.005	0.005	—	2.00	0.120
Orange juice, prepared fresh or frozen	1½ cup	165	2.52	40.2	1.49	0.210	0.037	0.045	0.025	—	33.0	0.411
Cheeseburger, McDonald's	2 ea.	636	30.2	57.0	0.460	32.0	12.2	2.18	13.3	80.0	338	5.68
French fries, McDonald's	1 order	220	3.00	26.1	4.19	11.5	4.37	0.570	4.61	8.57	9.10	0.605
Cola beverage, regular	1½ cup	151	—	38.5	—	—	—	—	—	—	9.00	0.120
Pork loin chop, broiled, lean	4 oz	261	36.2	—	—	11.9	5.35	1.43	4.09	112	5.67	1.04
Baked potato with skin	1 ea.	220	4.65	51.0	3.90	0.200	0.004	0.087	0.052	—	20.0	2.75
Peas, frozen, cooked	½ cup	63.0	4.12	11.4	3.61	0.220	0.019	0.103	0.039	—	19.0	1.25
Margarine, regular or soft, 80% fat	20 g	143	0.160	0.100	—	16.1	5.70	6.92	2.76	—	5.29	—
Iceberg lettuce, chopped	2 cup	14.6	1.13	2.34	1.68	0.212	0.008	0.112	0.028	—	21.2	0.560
French dressing	2 oz	300	0.318	3.63	0.431	32.0	14.2	12.4	4.94	—	7.10	0.227
Reduced-fat (i.e., 2%) milk	1 cup	121	8.12	11.7	—	4.78	1.35	0.170	2.92	22.0	297	0.120
Graham crackers	2 ea.	60.0	1.04	10.8	1.40	1.46	0.600	0.400	0.400	—	6.00	0.367
Totals		2584	99.0	300	17.9	112	44.1	24.8	33.4	266	792	15.4
RDA or related nutrient standard*		2900	58	130	38						1000	8
% of nutrient needs			89	170	230	47					79	193

Abbreviations: g = grams, mg = milligrams, μg = micrograms

*Values from inside cover. The values listed are for a male age 19 years. Note that number of kcal is just a rough estimate. It is better to base energy needs on actual energy output.

†In RAE units. Table values generally are in RE units today since the food values have not been updated to reflect the latest vitamin A standards. RAE equal RE for foods with preformed vitamin A, such as for the pork chop, but RAE are only about half the RE listed for foods with provitamin A carotenoids, such as for the peas (see Chapter 8 for details).

‡Amounts refer to actual folate content, rather than dietary folate equivalents (DFE). This difference is important to consider if the food contains added synthetic folic acid as part of enrichment or fortification. Any such folic acid is absorbed about twice as much as the folate present naturally in foods. So the total contribution of folate in the food in comparison to human needs will be greater than if all the folate was naturally in the food product. Nutrient analysis tables have yet to be updated to reflect the dietary folate equivalents of products (see Chapter 8 for more details).

Nutrient Analysis Form (Sample) cont'd

Magnesium (mg)	Phosphorus (mg)	Potassium (mg)	Sodium (mg)	Zinc (mg)	Vitamin A (RE)	Vitamin C (mg)	Vitamin E (mg)	Thiamin (mg)	Riboflavin (mg)	Niacin (mg)	Vitamin B-6 (mg)	Folate (µg)	Vitamin B-12 (µg)
18.0	61.0	65.0	300	0.612	7.00	—	1.80	2.58	0.197	2.40	0.030	16.3	0.065
0.720	1.00	16.0	4.00	—	0.200	0.710	0.016	0.002	0.005	0.036	0.005	2.00	—
36.0	60.0	711	3.00	0.192	28.5	145	0.714	0.300	0.060	0.750	0.165	163	
45.8	410	314	1460	5.20	134	4.10	0.560	0.600	0.480	8.66	0.230	42.0	1.82
26.7	101	564	109	0.320	5.00	12.5	0.203	0.122	0.020	2.26	0.218	19.0	0.027
3.00	46.0	4.00	15.0	0.049	—	—	—	—	—	—	—	—	—
34.0	277	476	88.2	2.54	3.15	0.454	0.405	1.30	0.350	6.28	0.535	6.77	0.839
55.0	115	844	16.0	0.650	—	26.1	0.100	0.216	0.067	3.32	0.701	22.2	—
23.0	72.0	134	70.0	0.750	53.4	7.90	0.400	0.226	0.140	1.18	0.090	46.9	—
0.467	4.06	7.54	216	0.041	199	0.028	2.19	0.002	0.006	0.004	0.002	0.211	0.017
10.1	22.4	177	10.1	0.246	37.0	4.36	0.120	0.052	0.034	0.210	0.044	62.8	—
5.81	3.63	7.03	666	0.045	0.023	—	15.9	—	—	—	0.006	—	—
33.0	232	377	122	0.963	140	2.32	0.080	0.095	0.403	0.210	0.105	12.0	0.888
6.00	20.0	36.0	86.0	0.113	—	—	—	0.020	0.030	0.600	0.011	1.80	—
298	1425	3732	3165	11.7	607	204	22.5	5.52	1.79	25.9	2.14	395	3.65
400	700	4700	1500	11	900[†]	90	15	1.2	1.3	16	1.3	400[‡]	2.4
75	204	80	210	106	67	226	150	450	138	162	160	99	152

Nutrient Analysis Form

Name	Quantity	kcal	Protein (g)	Carbohydrates (g)	Fiber (g)	Total fat (g)	Monounsaturated fat (g)	Polyunsaturated fat (g)	Saturated fat (g)	Cholesterol (g)	Calcium (mg)	Iron (mg)
Totals												
RDA or related nutrient standard*												
% of nutrient needs												

*Values from inside cover. Note that number of kcals is just a rough estimate. It is better to base energy needs on actual energy output.

†Use RAE values, even though food table is based on RE units.

‡Use DFE values, even though the food is based on total folate content, irrespective of natural or synthetic source.

Nutrient Analysis Form cont'd

Magnesium (mg)	Phosphorus (mg)	Potassium (mg)	Sodium (mg)	Zinc (mg)	Vitamin A (RE)	Vitamin C (mg)	Vitamin E (mg)	Thiamin (mg)	Riboflavin (mg)	Niacin (mg)	Vitamin B-6 (mg)	Folate (μg)	Vitamin B-12 (μg)
					†							‡	

III. Complete the following table as you summarize your dietary intake.

Percentage of kcal from Protein, Fat, Carbohydrate, and Alcohol

Intake

Protein (P): _____ g/day × 4 kcal per gram = (P) _____ kcal per day

Fat (F): _____ g/day × 9 kcal per gram = (F) _____ kcal per day

Carbohydrate (C): _____ g/day × 4 kcal per gram = (C) _____ kcal per day

Alcohol (A): (A) _____ kcal per day*

Total kcal (T)/day = (T) _____ kcal per day

Percentage of kcal from protein:

$$\frac{(P)}{(T)} \times 100 = \underline{\hspace{1cm}} \%$$

Percentage of kcal from fat:

$$\frac{(F)}{(T)} \times 100 = \underline{\hspace{1cm}} \%$$

Percentage of kcal from carbohydrate:

$$\frac{(C)}{(T)} \times 100 = \underline{\hspace{1cm}} \%$$

Percentage of kcal from alcohol:

$$\frac{(A)}{(T)} \times 100 = \underline{\hspace{1cm}} \%$$

NOTE: The four percentages can total 99, 100, or 101, depending on the way in which figures were rounded off earlier.

*To calculate how many kcal in a beverage are from alcohol, first look up the beverage in Appendix J. Then determine how many kcal are from carbohydrate (multiply carbohydrate grams times 4), fat (fat grams times 9), and protein (protein grams times 4). The remaining kcal are from alcohol.

IV. Use the table on the following page to again record your food intake for one day, placing each food item in the correct category of MyPyramid, with the correct number of servings (see Chapter 2). A food such as toast with soft margarine contributes to two categories—namely, to the grains group and to the oils group. You can expect that many food choices will contribute to more than one group. Indicate the number of servings from MyPyramid that each food yields.

Indicate the Number of Servings from MyPyramid That Each Food Yields

Food or Beverage	Amount Eaten	Milk	Meat & Beans	Fruits	Vegetables	Grains	Oils
Group totals							
Recommended servings from www.mypyramid.gov							
Shortages in numbers of servings							

V. Evaluation. Are there weaknesses suggested in your nutrient intake that correspond to missing servings in MyPyramid? Consider replacing the missing servings to improve your nutrient intake.

VI. For the same day you keep your food record, also keep a 24-hour record of your activities. Include sleeping, sitting, and walking, as well as the obvious forms of exercise. Calculate your energy expenditure for these activities using Table 10-6 in Chapter 10 or the diet analysis software available with this book. Try to substitute a similar activity if your particular activity is not listed. Calculate the total kcal you used for the day (total for column 3). Following is an example of an activity record. A blank form follows for your use. Ask your professor whether you are to turn in the form or the activity printout from NutritionCalc Plus.

Weight (kg)*: 70 kg

| Activity | Time (Minutes): Convert to Hours | Energy Cost | | |
		Column 1 kcal/kg/hr (from Table 10-6)	Column 2 (Column 1 × Time)	Column 3 (Column 2 × Weight in kg)
Brisk walking	(60 min) 1 hr	4.4	(× 1) = 4.4	(× 70) = 308

*lb/2.2

Weight (kg)*:

| Activity | Time (Minutes): Convert to Hours | Energy Cost | | |
		Column 1 kcal/kg/hr (from Table 10-6)	Column 2 (Column 1 × Time)	Column 3 (Column 2 × Weight in kg)

Total kcal used (from adding all of column 3)

*lb/2.2

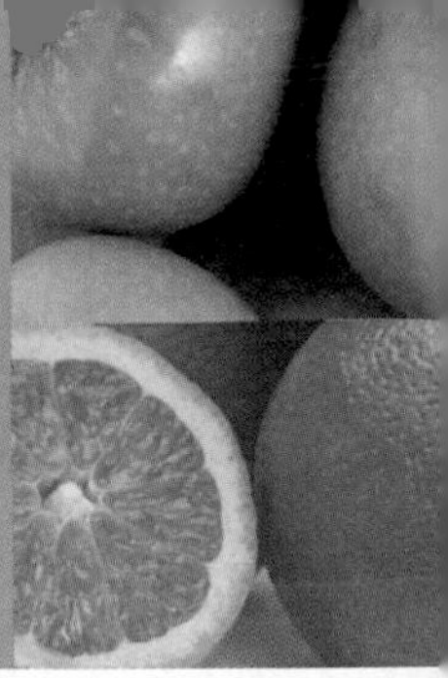

Amino Acids

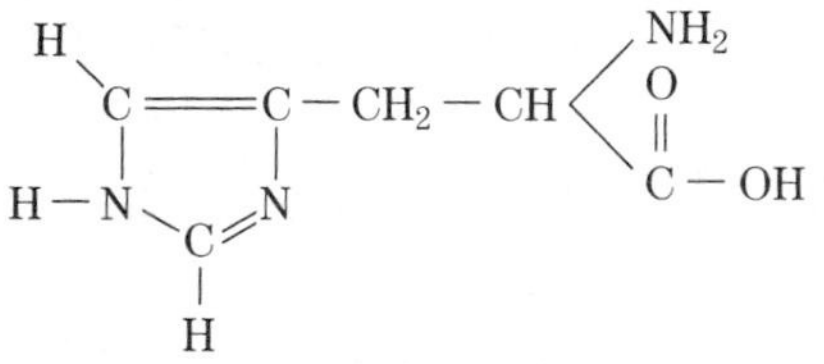

Histidine (His)
(essential)

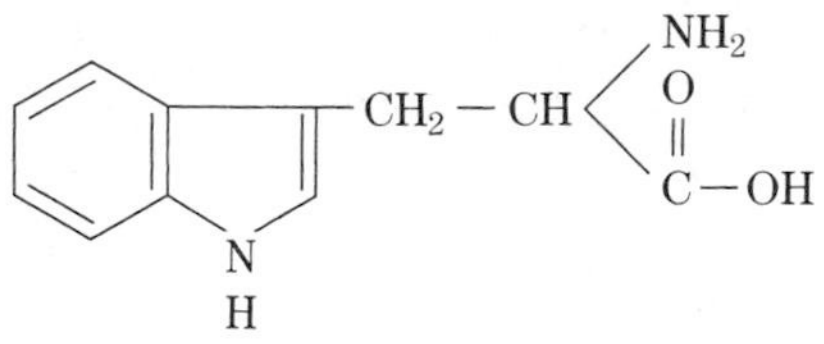

Tryptophan (Trp)
(essential)

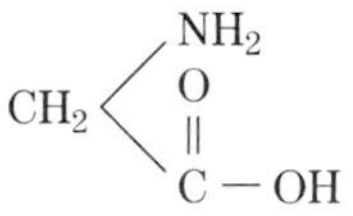

Glycine (Gly)

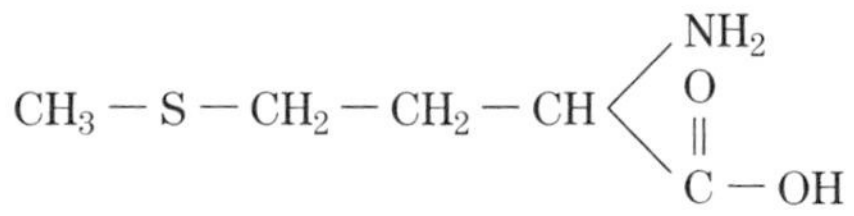

$CH_3 - S - CH_2 - CH_2 - CH$

Methionine (Met)
(essential)

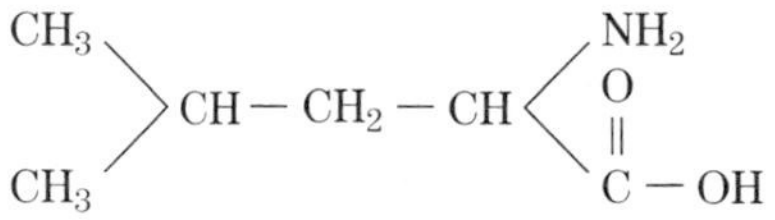

Leucine (Leu)
(essential)

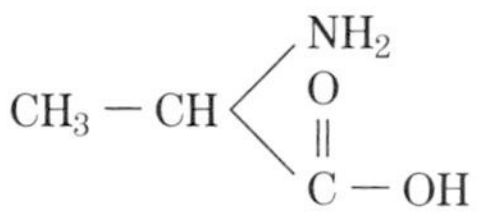

$CH_3 - CH$

Alanine (Ala)

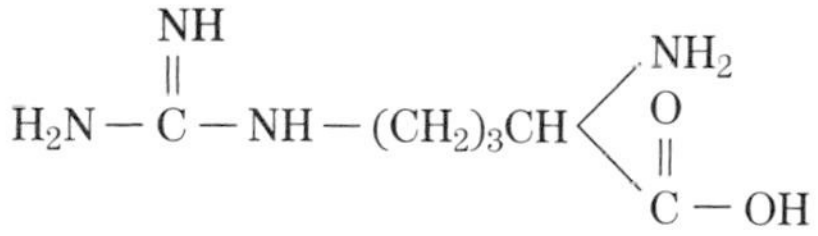

Arginine (Arg)
(essential in infancy)

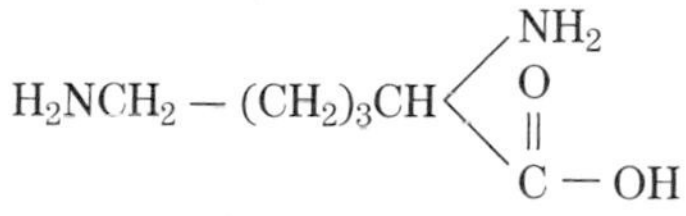

Lysine (Lys)
(essential)

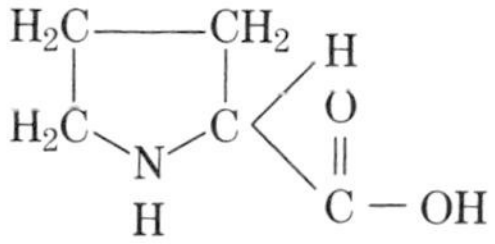

Proline (Pro)

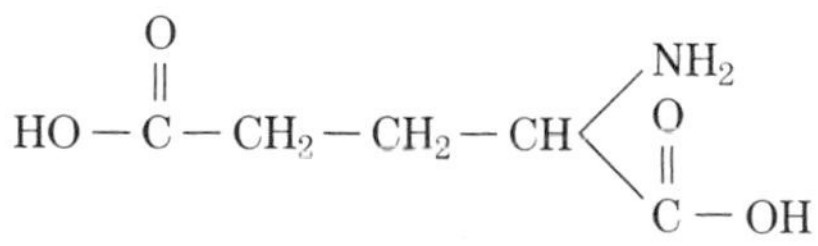

Glutamic Acid (Glu)

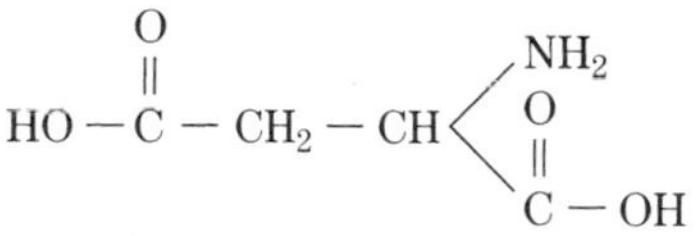

Aspartic Acid (Asp)

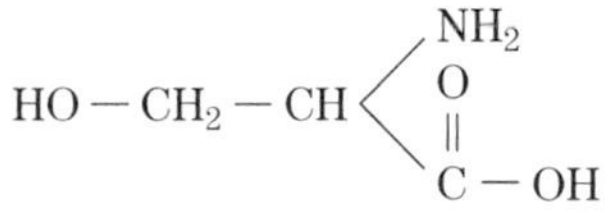

$HO - CH_2 - CH$

Serine (Ser)

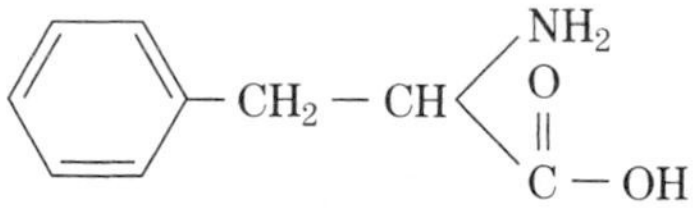

Phenylalanine (Phe)
(essential)

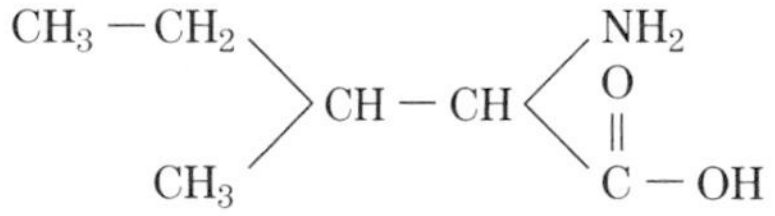

Isoleucine (Ile)
(essential)

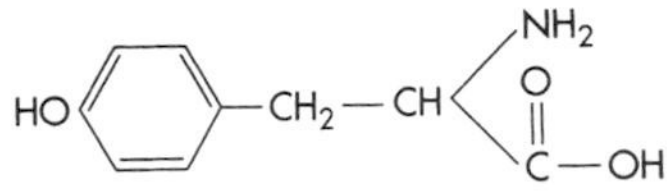

Tyrosine (Tyr)

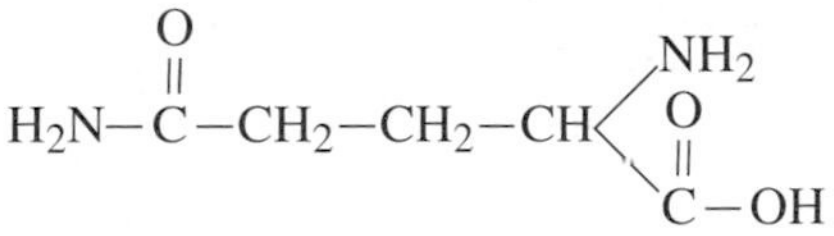

Glutamine (Gln)

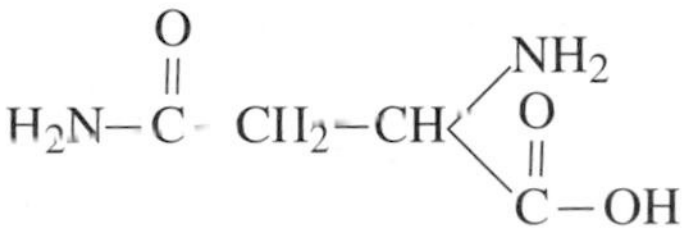

Asparagine (Asn)

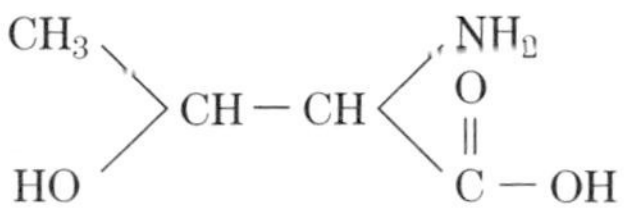

Threonine (Thr)
(essential)

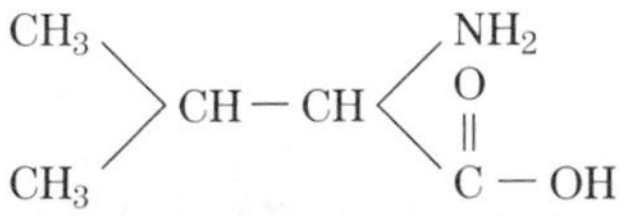

Valine (Val)
(essential)

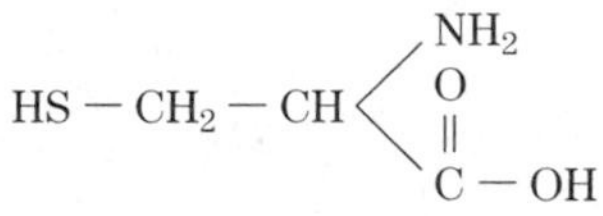

Cysteine (Cys)

Vitamins

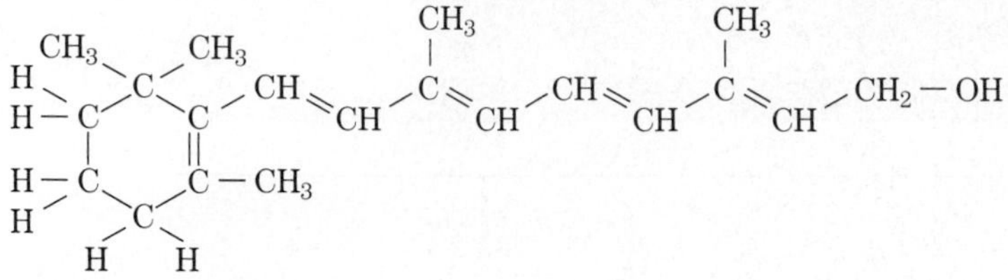

Vitamin A: retinol

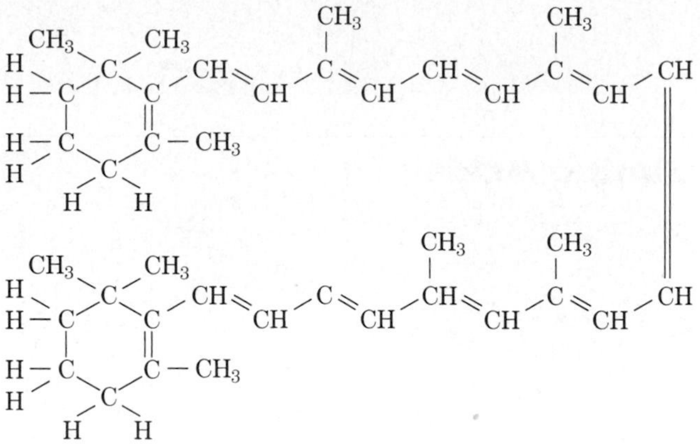

Beta-carotene

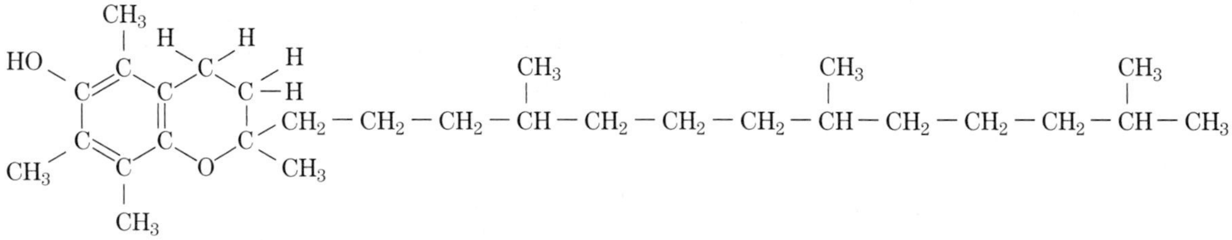

Vitamin E

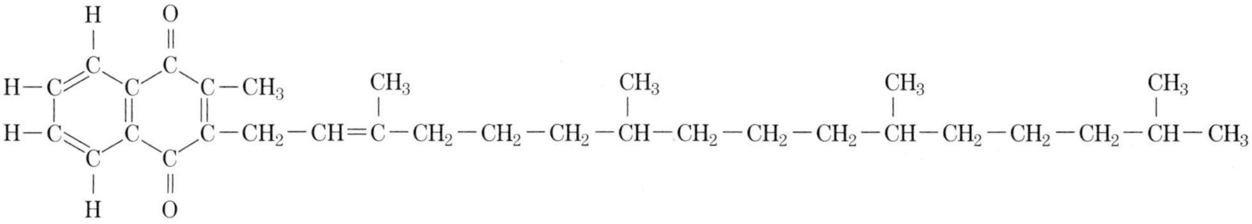

Vitamin K

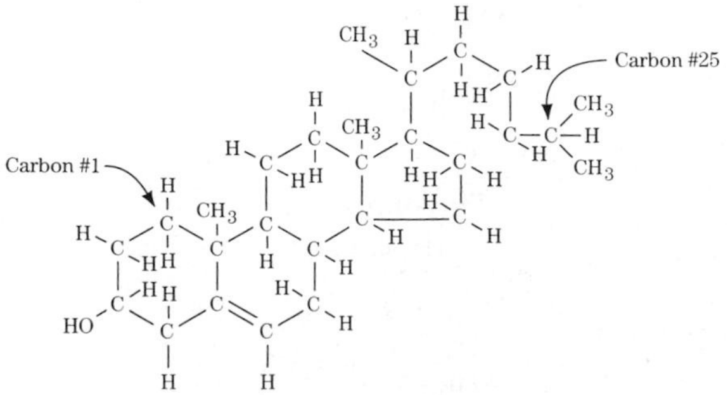

7-dehydrocholesterol

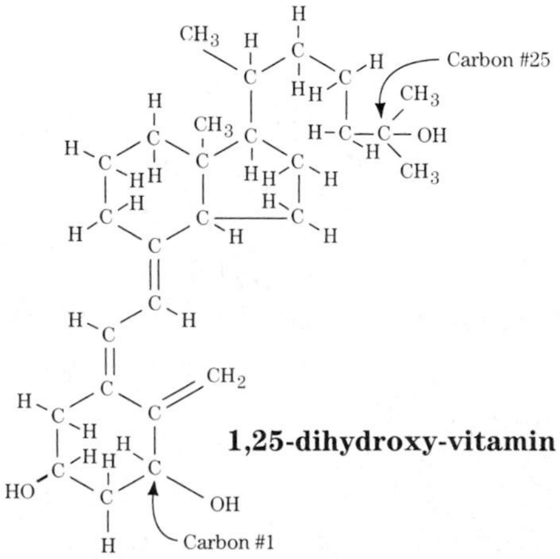

1,25-dihydroxy-vitamin D₃ (calcitriol)

Active vitamin D (calcitriol) and its precursor 7-dehydrocholesterol

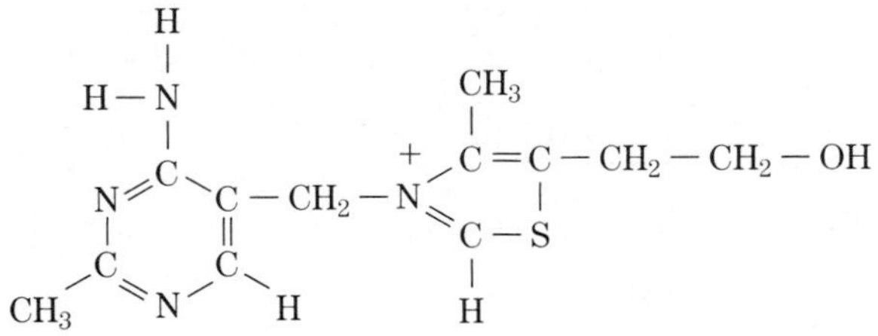

Thiamin

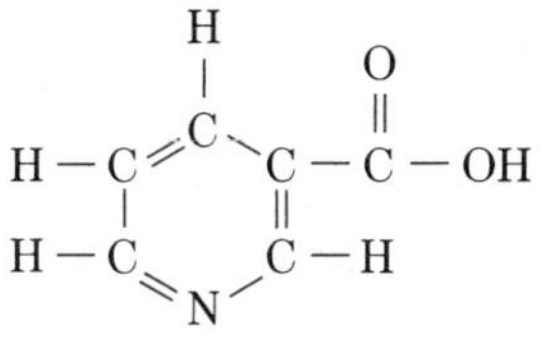

Niacin (nicotinic acid and nicotinamide)

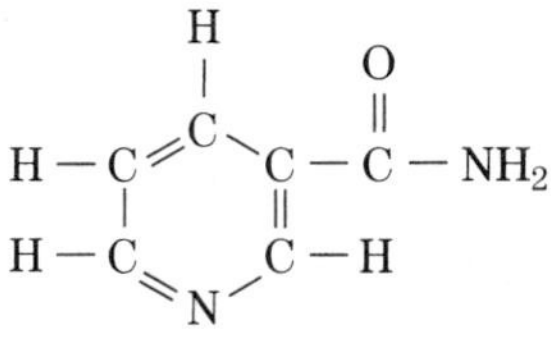

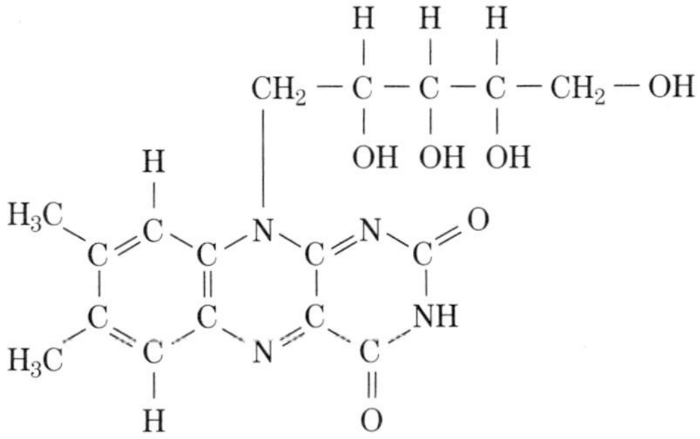

Nicotinic acid

Nicotinamide

Riboflavin

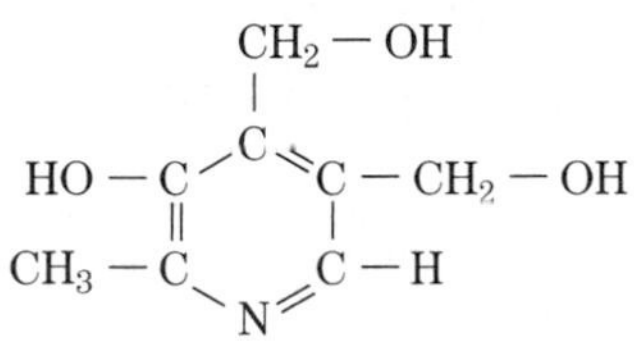

Vitamin B-6 (a general name for three compounds—pyridoxine, pyridoxal, and pyridoxamine)

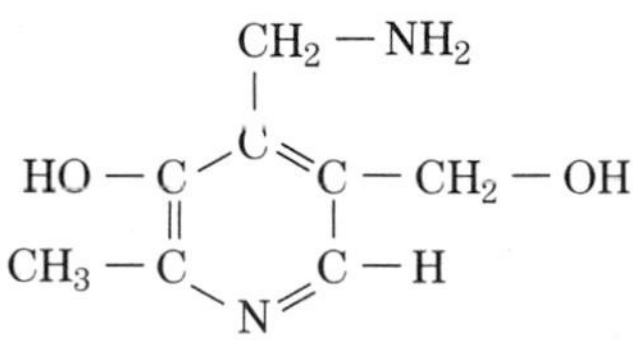

Pyridoxine

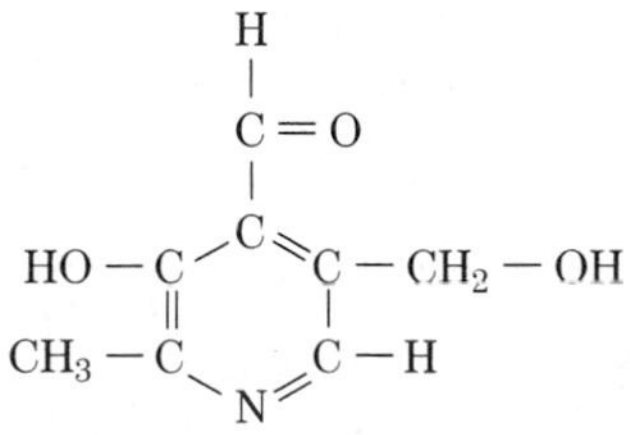

Pyridoxal

Pyridoxamine

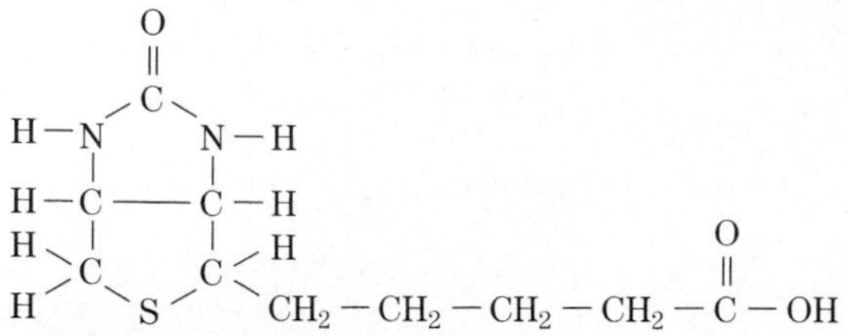

Biotin

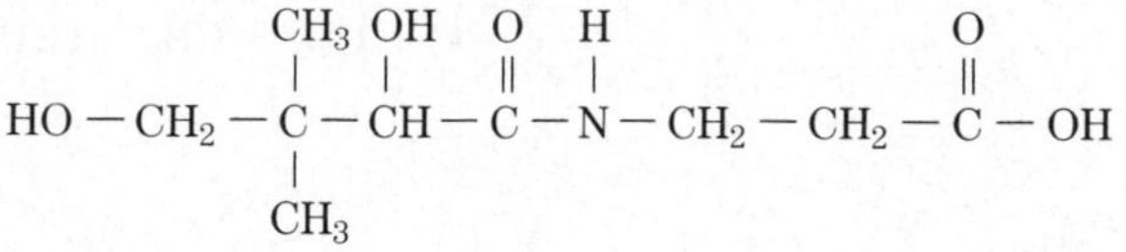

Pantothenic acid

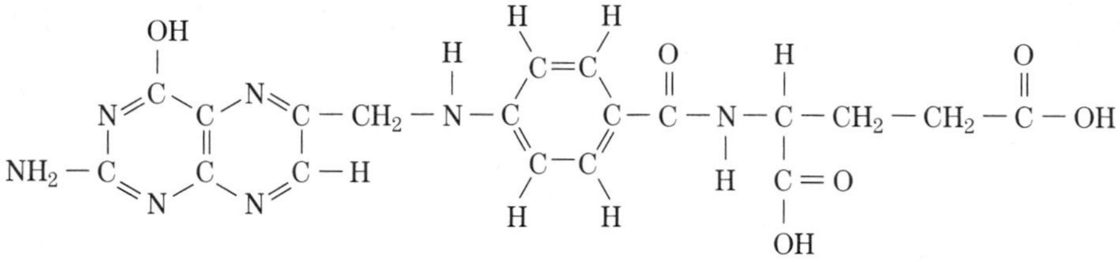

Folate (folic acid form)

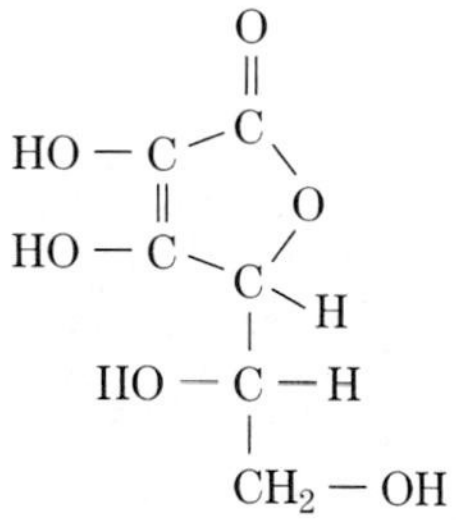

Vitamin C (ascorbic acid)

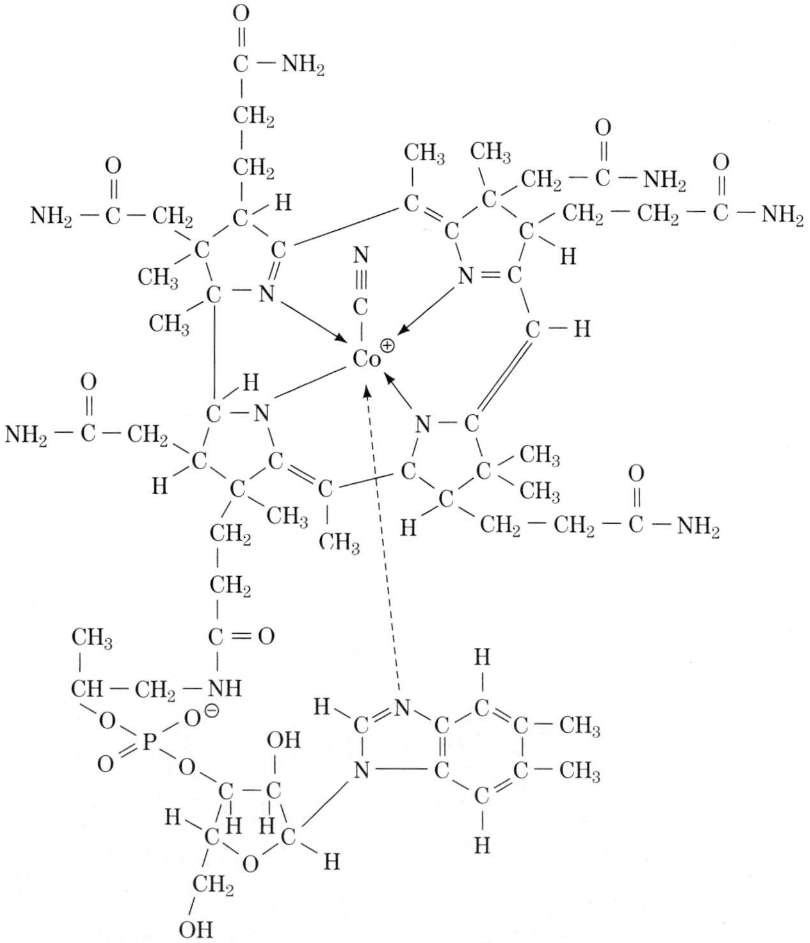

Vitamin B-12 (cyanocobalamin) The arrows in this diagram indicate that the spare electrons on the nitrogens attract them to the cobalt atom.

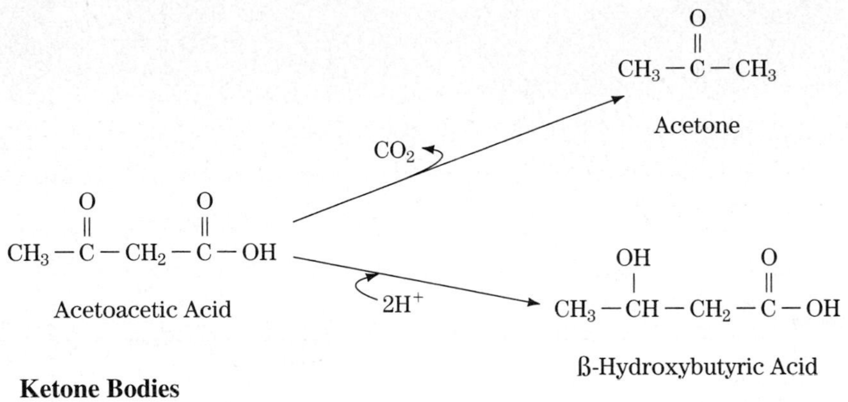

$$CH_3 - \overset{\overset{\displaystyle O}{\|}}{C} - CH_3$$

Acetone

$$CH_3 - \overset{\overset{\displaystyle O}{\|}}{C} - CH_2 - \overset{\overset{\displaystyle O}{\|}}{C} - OH$$

Acetoacetic Acid

CO_2

$2H^+$

$$CH_3 - \overset{\overset{\displaystyle OH}{|}}{CH} - CH_2 - \overset{\overset{\displaystyle O}{\|}}{C} - OH$$

ß-Hydroxybutyric Acid

Ketone Bodies

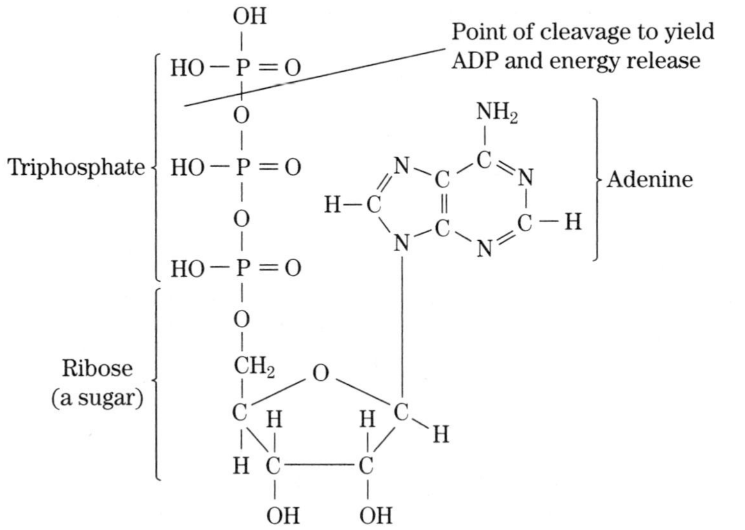

Triphosphate

$$\overset{\overset{\displaystyle OH}{|}}{HO - P = O}$$

Point of cleavage to yield
ADP and energy release

$$HO - P = O$$

$$HO - P = O$$

Adenine

Ribose
(a sugar)

CH_2

**Adenosine Triphosphate
(ATP)**

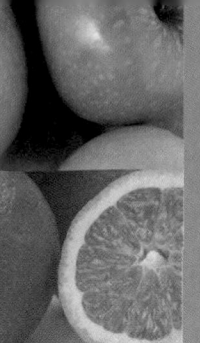

Appendix G

The 1983 Metropolitan Life Insurance Company Height-Weight Table and Determination of Frame Size

1983 Metropolitan Life Insurance Company Height-Weight Table*†

Women					Men				
Height		Frame			Height		Frame		
Ft.	In.	Small	Medium	Large	Ft.	In.	Small	Medium	Large
4	10	102–111	109–121	118–131	5	2	128–134	131–141	138–150
4	11	103–113	111–123	120–134	5	3	130–136	133–143	140–153
5	0	104–115	113–126	122–137	5	4	132–138	135–145	142–156
5	1	106–118	115–129	125–140	5	5	134–140	137–148	144–160
5	2	108–121	118–132	128–143	5	6	136–142	139–151	146–164
5	3	111–124	121–135	131–147	5	7	138–145	142–154	149–168
5	4	114–127	124–138	134–151	5	8	140–148	145–157	152–172
5	5	117–130	127–141	137–155	5	9	142–151	148–160	155–176
5	6	120–133	130–144	140–159	5	10	144–154	151–163	158–180
5	7	123–136	133–147	143–163	5	11	146–157	154–166	161–184
5	8	126–139	136–150	146–167	6	0	149–160	157–170	164–188
5	9	129–142	139–153	149–170	6	1	152–164	160–174	168–192
5	10	132–145	142–156	152–173	6	2	155–168	164–178	172–197
5	11	135–148	145–159	155–176	6	3	158–172	167–182	176–202
6	0	138–151	148–162	158–179	6	4	162–176	171–187	181–207

Reprinted courtesy of Metropolitan Life Insurance Company, *Statistical Bulletin.*

Permission granted courtesy of Metropolitan Life Insurance Company, *Statistical Bulletin.*

*Based on a weight-height mortality study conducted by the Society of Actuaries and the Association of Life Insurance Medical Directors of America, Metropolitan Life Insurance Medical Directors of America, Metropolitan Life Insurance Company, revised 1983.

†Weights in pounds (lb) at ages 25 to 59 based on lowest mortality. Height includes 1-in. heel. Weight for women includes 3 lb for indoor clothing. Weight for men includes 5 lb for indoor clothing.

Using the Metropolitan Life Insurance Table to Estimate Healthy Weight

The Metropolitan Life Insurance table is a common method for estimating healthy weight. The table lists for any height the weight that is associated with a maximum life span. The table does not tell the healthiest weight for a living person; it simply lists the weight associated with longevity.

There are many criticisms of this table. These stem from the inclusion of some people and the exclusion of others. For example, only policyholders of life insurance are included. In addition, smokers are included, but anyone over the age of 60 is excluded. Weight is only measured at the time of purchase of insurance, and there is no follow-up. All of these factors contribute to the fact that this table is to be used only as a rough screening tool; not meeting the exact recommendations should not be cause for alarm.

To diagnose overweight or obesity using the table, calculate the percentage of the Metropolitan Life Insurance table weight. Use the midpoint of a weight range for a specific height.

Equation: $$\frac{(\text{Current wt.} - \text{wt. from table})}{\text{Weight from table}} \times 100$$

Example: $$\frac{140 - 120}{120} \times 100 = 17\% \text{ over standard}$$

Overweight can be defined as weighing at least 10% more than the weight listed on the table. Determination of obesity is 20% more than that listed on the table. Moreover, this measure of obesity comes in degrees. Whereas mild obesity carries little health risk, severe obesity raises overall health risk twelvefold.

Degrees of Obesity	
% Over Healthy Body Weight	**Form of Obesity**
20–40%	Mild
41–99%	Moderate
100%+	Severe

Determining Frame Size

Method 1

Height is recorded without shoes.

Wrist circumference is measured just beyond the bony (styloid) process at the wrist joint on the right arm, using a tape measure.

The following formula is used:

$$r = \frac{\text{Height (cm)}}{\text{Wrist circumference (cm)}}$$

Frame size can be determined as follows:[†]

Males	Females
$r > 10.4$ small	$r > 11$ small
$r = 9.6{-}10.4$ medium	$r = 10.1{-}11$ medium
$r < 9.6$ large	$r < 10.1$ large

Method 2

The person's right arm is extended forward, perpendicular to the body, with the arm bent so the angle at the elbow forms 90 degrees, with the fingers pointing up and the palm turned away from the body. The greatest breadth across the elbow joint is measured with a sliding caliper along the axis of the upper arm, on the two prominent bones on either side of the elbow. This is recorded as the elbow breadth. The following tables give elbow breadth measurements for medium-framed men and women of various heights. Measurements lower than those listed indicate a small frame size; higher measurements indicate a large frame size.[‡]

Men		Women	
Height in 1″ Heels	**Elbow Breadth**	**Height in 1″ Heels**	**Elbow Breadth**
5′2″–5′3″	2½–2⅞″	4′10″–4′11″	2¼–2½″
5′4″–5′7″	2⅝–2⅞″	5′0″–5′3″	2¼–2½″
5′8″–5′11″	2¾–3″	5′4″–5′7″	2⅜–2⅝″
6′0″–6′3″	2¾–3¼″	5′8″–5′11″	2⅜–2⅝″
6′4″ and over	2⅞–3¾″	6′0″ and over	2½–2¾″

[†]From Grant JP: *Handbook of Total Parenteral Nutrition.* Philadelphia: WB Saunders, 1980.
[‡]From Metropolitan Life Insurance Co., 1983.

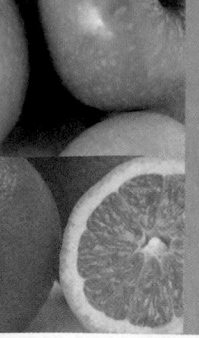

Appendix H

Sources of Nutrition Information

Consider the following reliable sources of food and nutrition information:

Journals That Regularly Cover Nutrition Topics

American Family Physician*
American Journal of Clinical Nutrition
American Journal of Epidemiology
American Journal of Medicine
American Journal of Nursing
American Journal of Obstetrics
  and Gynecology
American Journal of Physiology
American Journal of Public Health
American Scientist
Annals of Internal Medicine
Annual Reviews of Medicine
Annual Reviews of Nutrition
Archives of Disease in Childhood
Archives of Internal Medicine
British Journal of Nutrition
BMJ (British Medical Journal)
Cancer
Cancer Research
Circulation
Diabetes

Diabetes Care
Disease-a-Month
FASEB Journal
FDA Consumer*
Food Chemical Toxicology
Food Engineering
Gastroenterology
Geriatrics
Gut
Human Nutrition: Applied Nutrition
Human Nutrition: Clinical Nutrition
Journal of the American College of
  Nutrition*
Journal of the American Dietetic
  Association*
Journal of the American Geriatric Society
JAMA (Journal of the American Medical
  Association)
Journal of Applied Physiology
Journal of the Canadian Dietetic
  Association*
Journal of Clinical Investigation
Journal of Food Service

Journal of Food Technology
JNCI (Journal of the National Cancer
  Institute)
Journal of Nutrition
Journal of Nutritional Education*
Journal of Nutrition for the Elderly
Journal of Nutrition Research
Journal of Pediatrics
Lancet
Mayo Clinic Proceedings
Medicine & Science in Sports & Exercise
Nature
The New England Journal of Medicine
Nutrition
Nutrition Reviews
Nutrition Today*
Pediatrics
The Physician and Sports Medicine
Postgraduate Medicine*
Proceedings of the Nutrition Society
Science
Science News*
Scientific American*

The majority of these journals are available in college and university libraries or in a specialty library on campus, such as one designated for health services or home economics. As indicated, a few journals will be filed under their abbreviations, rather than the first word in their full name. A reference librarian can help you locate any of these sources. The journals with an asterisk (*) are ones you may find especially interesting and useful because of the number of nutrition articles presented each month or the less technical nature of the presentation.

Magazines for the Consumer That Cover Nutrition Topics

Men's Health
Better Homes and Gardens

Good Housekeeping
Health

Parents
Self

Textbooks and Other Sources for Advanced Study of Nutrition Topics

Brody T: Nutritional biochemistry. 2nd ed. San Diego: Academic Press, 1999.
Groff JL, Gropper SS: Advanced human nutrition and metabolism. Belmont, CA: Wadsworth, 2005.

International Life Sciences Institute: Present knowledge in nutrition. 8th ed. Washington DC: The Nutrition Foundation, 2001.
Mahan LK, Escott-Stump S: Krause's food, nutrition, and diet therapy. 11th ed. Philadelphia: W.B. Saunders, 2004.

Murray RK and others: Harper's biochemistry. 26th ed. New York: McGraw-Hill, 2003.
Schils ME, Olson JA, Shike M, Ross AC: Modern nutrition in health and disease. 9th ed. Philadelphia: Lippincott, 1999.

Stipanuk MH: *Biochemical and physiological aspects of human nutrition.* Philadelphia: W.B. Saunders, 2000.

Newsletters That Cover Nutrition Issues on a Regular Basis

American Institute for Cancer Research Newsletter
American Institute for Cancer Research (AICR) Washington, DC 20069
www.icr.ac.uk/

Dairy Council Digest
National Dairy Council
10255 West Higgins Road, Suite 900
Rosemont, IL 60018
(inexpensive)
www.nationaldairycouncil.org

Dietetic Currents
Ross Laboratories
Director of Professional Services
625 Cleveland Ave.
Columbus, OH 43216
(free)
www.ross.com

Nutrition Close-Up
Egg Nutrition Center
1819 H St. N.W., No. 510
Washington, DC 20009
(free)
www.enc-online.org/

ENVIRONMENTAL NUTRITION
Environmental Nutrition
52 Riverside Dr.
New York, NY 10024
www.environmentalnutrition.com

Food and Nutrition News
National Cattlemen's Beef Association
444 Michigan Ave.
Chicago, IL 60611
(free)
www.beef.org

Harvard Medical School Health Letter
Department of Continuing Education
25 Shattuck St.
Boston, MA 02115
www.hms.harvard.edu/news/index.html

Mayo Clinic Health Letter
P.O. Box 53889
Boulder, CO 80322-3889
mayohealth.org

National Council Against Health Fraud Newsletter (NCAHF)
P.O. Box 1276
Loma Linda, CA 92354
www.ncahf.org/

Nutrition Action Healthletter
1875 Connecticut Ave.
Washington, DC 20009-5728
www.cspinet.org

Nutrition Forum
George Stickley Co.
210 Washington Square
Philadelphia, PA 19106
www.quackwatch.com

Nutrition Research Newsletter
P.O. Box 700
Pallisades, NY 10964
www.biz-lib.com/ZTINR.html

Soy Connection
United Soybean Board
16305 Swingley Ridge Drive
Suite 110
Chesterfield, MO 63017
(free)
smartsoy.ag.uiuc.edu/usb/speced.html/

Tufts University Diet & Nutrition Letter
P.O. Box 420235
Palm Coast, FL 32142
www.healthletter.tufts.edu/

University of California at Berkeley Wellness Letter
P.O. Box 420148
Palm Coast, FL 32142
magazines.enews.com/magazines/vcbw

Professional Organizations with a Commitment to Nutrition Issues

American Academy of Pediatrics
P.O. Box 1034
Evanston, IL 60204
www.aap.org

American Cancer Society
90 Park Ave.
New York, NY 10016
www.cancer.org

American College of Sports Medicine
P.O. Box 1440
Indianapolis, IN 46204
www.acsm.org

American Dental Association
211 E. Chicago Ave.
Chicago, IL 60611
www.ada.org

American Diabetes Association
2 Park Ave.
New York, NY 10016
www.diabetes.org

American Dietetic Association
120 S. Riverside Plaza
Suite 2000
Chicago, IL 60606
www.eatright.org

American Geriatrics Society
770 Lexington Ave.
Suite 400
New York, NY 10021
www.americangeriatrics.org

American Heart Association
7272 Greenville Ave.
Dallas, TX 75231
www.americanheart.org

American Home Economics Association
2010 Massachusetts Ave. N.W.
Washington, DC 20036
www.orst.edu

American Medical Association
Nutrition Information Section
535 N. Dearborn St.
Chicago, IL 60610
www.ama-assn.org/

American Public Health Association
1015 Fifteenth St. N.W.
Washington, DC 20005
www.apha.org

American Society for Clinical Nutrition
9650 Rockville Pike
Bethesda, MD 20014
www.faseb.org/ajcn

American Society for Nutritional Sciences
9650 Rockville Pike
Bethesda, MD 20014
www.asns.org

The Canadian Diabetes Association
15 Toronto St.
Suite 1001
Toronto, Ontario M5C 2E3 Canada
www.diabetes.ca

The Canadian Dietetic Association
480 University Ave.
Suite 601
Toronto, Ontario M5G 1V2 Canada
www.dietitians.ca

The Canadian Society for Nutritional
   Sciences
Department of Foods and Nutrition
University of Manitoba
Winnipeg, Manitoba, R3T 2N2 Canada
www.hc-sc.gc.ca

Environmental Working Group (EWG)
1718 Connecticut Ave., N.W. Suite 600
Washington, DC 20009
www.ewg.org

Food and Nutrition Board
National Research Council
National Academy of Sciences
2101 Constitution Ave. N.W.
Washington, DC 20418
www.nas.edu

Institute of Food Technologies
221 N. LaSalle St.
Chicago, IL 60601
www.ift.org

National Council on the Aging
1828 L St. N.W.
Washington, DC 20036
www.ncoa.org

National Institute of Nutrition
1335 Carling Ave.
Suite 210
Ottawa, Ontario K1Z OL2 Canada
www.nin.ca/En/home.html

National Osteoporosis Foundation
1150 Seventeenth St. N.W., Suite 500
Washington, DC 20036
www.nof.org

Society for Nutrition Education
2001 Killebrew Dr., Suite 340
Minneapolis, MN 55425
www.sne.org

Professional or Lay Organizations Concerned with Nutrition Issues

Bread for the World Institute
50 F Street, N.W., Suite 500
Washington, DC 20001
www.bread.org

California Council Against Health
   Fraud, Inc.
P.O. Box 1276
Loma Linda, CA 92354
www.ncahf.org

Children's Foundation
1420 New York Ave. N.W.
Suite 800
Washington, DC 20005
www.childrenfoundation.com

Food Research and Action Center
   (FRAC)
1875 Connecticut Ave. N.W. #540
Washington, DC 20009
www.frac.org

Institute for Food and Development
   Policy
1885 Mission St.
San Francisco, CA 94103
www.foodfirst.org

La Leche League International, Inc.
9616 Minneapolis Ave.
Franklin Park, IL 60131
www.lalecheleague.org

March of Dimes Birth Defects
   Foundation
(National Headquarters)
1275 Mamaroneck Ave.
White Plains, NY 10605
www.modimes.org

National WIC Association (NWA,
   formerly the National Association
   of WIC Directors)
2001 S Street, N.W., Suite 580
Washington, DC 20009
www.nwica.org

Overeaters Anonymous (OA)
2190 190th St.
Torrance, CA 90504
www.overeatersanonymous.org

Oxfam America
26 West St.
Boston, MA 02111
www.oxfamamerica.org

Local Resources for Advice on Nutrition Issues

Registered dietitians (R.D.s or in Canada
   also RDNs) in health care, city,
   county, or state agencies, as well as in
   private practice

Cooperative extension agents in county
   extension offices
Nutrition faculty affiliated with
   departments of food and
   nutrition, home economics, and
   dietetics

Government Agencies Concerned with Nutrition Issues or That Distribute Nutrition Information

United States
The Consumer Information
   Center
Department 609K
Pueblo, CO 81009
www.pueblo.gsa.gov

Food and Drug Administration (FDA)
5600 Fishers Lane
Rockville, MD 20852
www.fda.gov

Food and Nutrition Information and
   Education Resources Center
National Library of Congress
Beltsville, MD 20705
www.nal.usda.gov

Human Nutrition Research Division
Agricultural Research Center
Beltsville, MD 20705
www.usda.gov

National Center for Health Statistics
3700 East-West
Hyattsville, MD 20782
www.cdc.gov/nchs

National Heart, Lung, and Blood
   Institute
9000 Rockville Pike, Building 31,
   Room 4A21
Bethesda, MD 20892
www.nhlbi.nih.gov

National Institute on Aging
Information Office
Building 31, Room 5C35
Bethesda, MD 20205
www.nih.gov/nia/

Office of Cancer Communications
National Cancer Institute
Building 31, Room 10A18
90 Rockville Pike
Bethesda, MD 20205
www.nci.nih.gov

MyPyramid
USDA, Center for Nutrition Policy
    and Promotion
www.mypyramid.gov

USDA, Agricultural Research Service
6505 Belcrest Rd., Room 344
Hyattsville, MD 20782
www.usda.gov

USDA, Food Safety & Inspection Service
Room 1180 South, 14th and
    Independence Ave. S.W.
Washington, DC 20250
www.usda.gov

U.S. Government Printing Office
The Superintendent of Documents
Washington, DC 20402
www.gpo.gov/

Canada
Canadian Food Inspection Agency
59 Camelot Dr.
Nepean, Ontario K1A OY9
www.inspection.gc.ca/

Health and Welfare Canada
Canadian Government Publishing
    Center
Minister of Supply and Services
Ottawa, Ontario K1A 0S9
www.hc-sc.gc.ca

Nutrition Programs
446 Jeanne Mance Building
Tunney's Pasture
Ottawa, Ontario K1A 1B4
www.hc-sc.gc.ca

Nutrition Services
P.O. Box 488
Halifax, Nova Scotia B3J 3R8
www.fns.usda.gov

United Nations
Food and Agriculture Organization
North American Regional Office
1001 22nd St. N.W.
Washington, DC 20437
www.fao.org

World Health Organization (WHO)
1211 Geneva 27
Switzerland
www.who.org

Trade Organizations and Companies That Distribute Nutrition Information

American Institute of Baking
P.O. Box 1148
Manhattan, KS 66502
www.aibonline.org

American Meat Institute
P.O. Box 3556
Washington, DC 20007
www.meatami.com

Beech-Nut Nutrition Corporation
Booth 1414
Checkerboard Square
St. Louis, MO 63164
www.beech-nut.com/index.htm

Best Foods
Consumer Service Department
Division of CPC International
International Plaza
Englewood Cliffs, NJ 07632
www.bestfoods.com

Campbell Soup Co.
Food Service Products Division
Campbell Plaza
Camden, NJ 08103
www.campbellsoups.com

The Dannon Company, Inc.
120 White Plains Rd.
Tarrytown, NY 10591-5536
www.dannon.com

Del Monte Foods
One Market Plaza
San Francisco, CA 94105
www.delmonte-international.com

General Mills
P.O. Box 1113
Minneapolis, MN 55440
www.generalmills.com

Gerber Products Co.
445 State St.
Fremont, MI 49413
www.gerber.com

H.J. Heinz
Consumer Relations
P.O. Box 57
Pittsburgh, PA 15230
www.heinzbaby.com

Idaho Potato Commission
P.O. Box 1968
Boise, ID 83701
www.idahopotatoes.com

Kellogg Company
Department of Home Economics
    Services
Battle Creek, MI 49016
www.kellog.com

Kraft General Foods
Three Lakes Dr.
Northfield, IL 60093
www.kraftfoods.com

Mead Johnson Nutritionals
2404 Pennsylvania Ave.
Evansville, IN 47721
www.meadjohnson.com

National Dairy Council
10255 W. Higgins Rd.
Rosemont, IL 60018-4233
www.natdairycoun.org

The NutraSweet Kelco
    Company
1751 Lake Cook Rd.
Deerfield, IL 60015
www.nutrasweetkelco.com/
    default.htm

Pillsbury Company
1177 Pillsbury Building
608 Second Ave. S.
Minneapolis, MN 55402
www.pillsbury.com

Ross Laboratories
Director of Professional
    Services
625 Cleveland Ave.
Columbus, OH 43216
www.ross.com

Sunkist Growers, Inc.
14130 Riverside Dr.
Sherman Oaks, CA 91423
www.sunkist.com/index.html

Vitamin Nutrition Information Service
    (VNIS)
Hoffmann-LaRoche
340 Kingsland Ave.
Nutley, NJ 07110
www.rocheusa.com

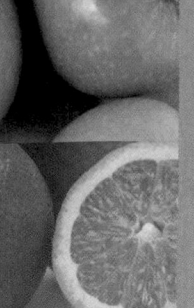

Appendix I

Metric-English Conversions

Length

English (USA)	Metric
inch (in)	= 2.54 cm, 25.4 mm
foot (ft)	= 0.30 m, 30.48 cm
yard (yd)	= 0.91 m, 91.4 cm
mile (statute) (5280 ft)	= 1.61 km, 1609 m
mile (nautical)	
(6077 ft, 1.15 statute mi)	= 1.85 km, 1850 m

Metric	English (USA)
millimeter (mm)	= 0.039 in (thickness of a dime)
centimeter (cm)	= 0.39 in
meter (m)	= 3.28 ft, 39.37 in
kilometer (km)	= 0.62 mi, 1091 yd, 3273 ft

Weight

English (USA)	Metric
grain	= 64.80 mg
ounce (oz)	= 28.35 g
pound (lb)	= 453.60 g, 0.45 kg
ton (short—2000 lb)	= 0.91 metric ton (907 kg)

Metric	English (USA)
milligram (mg)	= 0.002 grain (0.000035 oz)
gram (g)	= 0.04 oz ($\frac{1}{28}$ of an oz)
kilogram (kg)	= 35.27 oz, 2.20 lb
metric ton (1000 kg)	= 1.10 tons

Volume

English (USA)	Metric
cubic inch	= 16.39 cc
cubic foot	= 0.03 m^3
cubic yard	= 0.765 m^3
teaspoon (tsp)	= 5 ml
tablespoon (tbsp)	= 15 ml
fluid ounce	= 0.03 liter (30 ml)*
cup (c)	= 237 ml
pint (pt)	= 0.47 liter
quart (qt)	= 0.95 liter
gallon (gal)	= 3.79 liters

Metric	English (USA)
milliliter (ml)	= 0.03 oz
liter (L)	= 2.12 pt
liter	= 1.06 qt
liter	= 0.27 gal

1 liter ÷ 1000 = 1 milliliter or 1 cubic centimeter (10^{-3} liter)
1 liter ÷ 1,000,000 = 1 microliter (10^{-6} liter)
*Note: 1 ml = 1 cc

Metric and Other Common Units

Unit/Abbreviation	Other Equivalent Measure
milligram/mg	$\frac{1}{1000}$ of a gram
microgram/µg	$\frac{1}{1,000,000}$ of a gram
deciliter/dl	$\frac{1}{10}$ of a liter (about ½ cup)
milliliter/ml	$\frac{1}{1000}$ of a liter (5 ml is about 1 tsp)
International Unit/IU	Crude measure of vitamin activity generally based on growth rate seen in animals

Fahrenheit-Celsius Conversion Scale

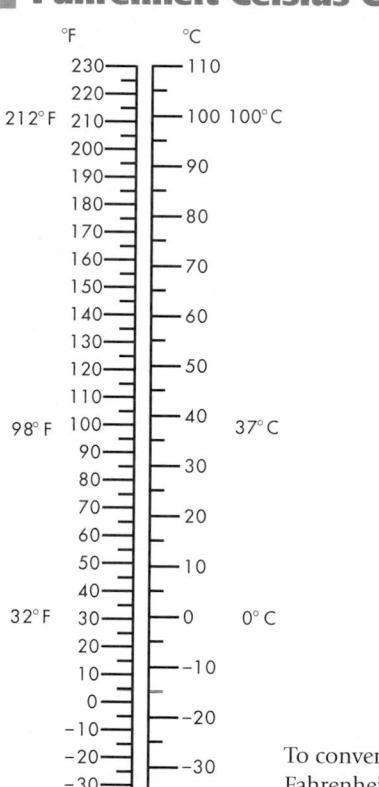

To convert temperature scales:
Fahrenheit to Celsius °C = (°F − 32) × 5/9
Celsius to Fahrenheit °F = 9/5 (°C) + 32

Household Units

3 teaspoons	= 1 tablespoon
4 tablespoons	= ¼ cup
5⅓ tablespoons	= ⅓ cup
8 tablespoons	= ½ cup
10⅔ tablespoons	= ⅔ cup
16 tablespoons	= 1 cup
1 tablespoon	= ½ fluid ounce
1 cup	= 8 fluid ounces
1 cup	= ½ pint
2 cups	= 1 pint
4 cups	= 1 quart
2 pints	= 1 quart
4 quarts	= 1 gallon

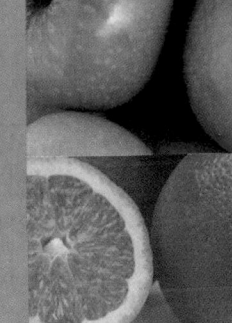

The following table of nutrient values of foods represents a small portion of the database found in the NutritionCalc Plus diet analysis program available from McGraw-Hill. The nutrient data in the software and in Appendix J comes from the ESHA Research database. (*Note:* Due to space constraints, Appendix J contains fewer nutrient categories, such as soluble and insoluble fiber, than are included in NutritionCalc Plus reports.)

The following is a list of abbreviations used in the Food Composition Table:

Note: Some nutrient or food component values for some foods are not included in the database because no *accurate* data values exist. The nutrient or component may in fact be present in the food, but insufficient laboratory analyses have been performed to establish an accurate value. These are indicated by a – (dash) in the appropriate nutrient columns.

Name brand foods often have missing values because manufacturers are only required to analyze for nutrients that must appear on Nutrition Facts labels and only to the level of accuracy required by the nutrition labeling regulations. All missing nutrient or food component values are clearly marked in the table.

Abbreviation Key

Unit/Amt = Unit Amount
Wt (g) = Weight in grams
Energy (kcal) = kilocalories
Prot (g) = Protein
Carb (g) = Carbohydrate
Fiber (g) = Dietary fiber
Fat (g) = Total fat
Sat (g) = Saturated fat
Mono (g) = Monounsaturated fat
Poly (g) = Polyunsaturated fat
Chol (mg) = Cholesterol
Vit A (RE) = Vitamin A
Thia (mg) = Thiamin
Ribo (mg) = Riboflavin
Niac (mg NE) = Niacin
Vit B-6 (mg) = Vitamin B-6
Vit B-12 (µg) = Vitamin B-12
Fol (µg) = Folate
Vit C (mg) = Vitamin C
Vit D (IU) = Vitamin D
Vit E (mg AT) = Vitamin E
Cal (mg) = Calcium

Iron (mg) = Iron
Magn (mg) = Magnesium
Phos (mg) = Phosphorus
Pota (mg) = Potassium
Sodi (mg) = Sodium
Zinc (mg) = Zinc
Wat (%) = Water
Alco (g) = Alcohol
Caff (g) = Caffeine

g = gram
mg = milligram
µg = microgram
mg AT = milligrams of alpha-
  tocopheral
mg NE = milligrams of Niacin
  Equivalents
oz = ounce
lb = pound
Tbs = tablespoon
tsp = teaspoon

Code	Food Name	Unit/ Amt	Wt (g)	Energy (kcal)	Prot (g)	Carb (g)	Fiber (g)	Fat (g)	Sat (g)	Mono (g)	Poly (g)	Chol (mg)	Vit A (RE)
BEVERAGE AND BEVERAGE MIXES													
Carbonated Drinks													
4794	Lemonade, cnd, Country Time	1 cup	247	90	0	23	0	0	0.0	0.0	0.0	—	0
20055	Soda, 7 Up	1 cup	240	100	0	26	0	0	0.0	0.0	0.0	0	0
20207	Soda, 7 Up, diet	1 cup	240	0	0	0	0	0	0.0	0.0	0.0	0	0
20006	Soda, club	1 cup	237	0	0	0	0	0	0.0	0.0	0.0	0	0
20147	Soda, Coca Cola/Coke	1 cup	246	103	0	27	0	0	0.0	0.0	0.0	0	0
443	Soda, cola, caff free	12 fl-oz	372	156	0	40	0	0	0.0	0.0	0.0	0	0
4796	Soda, Dr Pepper	1 cup	246	100	0	27	0	0	0.0	0.0	0.0	—	0
4797	Soda, Dr Pepper, diet	1 cup	246	0	0	0	0	0	0.0	0.0	0.0	—	0
20530	Soda, fruit punch	1 cup	251	117	0	32	0	0	0.0	0.0	0.0	—	0
20031	Soda, grape	1 cup	248	107	0	28	0	0	0.0	0.0	0.0	0	0
20032	Soda, lemon lime	1 cup	246	98	0	26	0	0	0.0	0.0	0.0	0	0
20271	Soda, Mountain Dew	1 cup	240	113	0	31	0	0	0.0	0.0	0.0	0	0
20272	Soda, Mountain Dew, diet	1 cup	240	0	0	0	0	0	0.0	0.0	0.0	0	0
20161	Soda, Mr Pibb	1 cup	249	97	0	26	0	0	0.0	0.0	0.0	0	0
20029	Soda, orange	1 cup	248	119	0	31	0	0	0.0	0.0	0.0	0	0
20166	Soda, Pepsi	1 cup	240	100	0	27	0	0	0.0	0.0	0.0	0	0
20167	Soda, Pepsi, diet	1 cup	240	0	0	0	0	0	0.0	0.0	0.0	0	0
20009	Soda, root beer	1 cup	246	101	0	26	0	0	0.0	0.0	0.0	0	0
20454	Soda, root beer, diet, w/nutrasweet	1 cup	240	0	0	0	0	0	0.0	0.0	0.0	0	—
20163	Soda, Sprite	1 cup	249	96	0	26	0	0	0.0	0.0	0.0	0	0
4815	Soda, Squirt	1 cup	246	100	0	27	0	0	0.0	0.0	0.0	—	0
Coffee and Substitutes													
20312	Coffee Substitute, inst, dry	1 tsp	3	10	0	3	—	0	0.0	0.0	0.0	0	0
20592	Coffee, cappuccino, w/lowfat milk, tall	1.5 cup	244	110	8	11	0	4	2.5	—	—	15	80
20639	Coffee, cappuccino, w/whole milk, tall	1.5 cup	244	140	7	11	0	7	4.5	—	—	30	60
20439	Coffee, espresso, prep at restaurant	1 cup	237	5	0	0	0	0	0.2	0.0	0.2	0	0
20659	Coffee, latte, iced, w/lowfat milk, tall	1.5 cup	392	90	7	10	0	3	2.0	—	—	15	60
20023	Coffee, reg, inst, prep w/water	1 cup	238	5	0	1	0	0	0.0	0.0	0.0	0	0
Dairy Mixed Drinks and Mixes													
44	Drink, carob, prep f/dry mix w/milk	1 cup	256	192	8	22	1	8	4.6	2.0	0.5	26	69
14	Drink, chocolate, dry mix	2.5 tsp	22	75	1	20	1	1	0.4	0.2	0.0	0	0
40	Drink, strawberry, dry mix	2.5 tsp	22	85	0	22	0	0	0.0	0.0	0.0	0	0
12	Hot Cocoa, dry mix	3 tsp	28	113	2	24	1	1	0.7	0.4	0.0	2	0
48	Hot Cocoa, prep f/dry mix w/water	1 cup	275	151	2	32	1	2	0.9	0.5	0.0	3	1
62057	Instant Breakfast, French vanilla, dry mix, pkt	1 ea	36	130	4	27	0	0	0.0	0.0	0.0	3	350
101	Instant Breakfast, prep w/1% milk	1 cup	281	233	15	36	0	3	1.8	—	—	14	469
25	Instant Breakfast, prep w/2% milk, pwd	1 cup	281	253	15	36	0	5	3.1	—	—	24	469
26	Instant Breakfast, prep w/whole milk	1 cup	281	280	15	36	0	9	5.3	—	—	38	630
30	Malted Milk, chocolate, dry mix	3 tsp	21	79	1	18	1	1	0.5	0.2	0.1	0	1

PAGE KEY: A-96 Granola Bars, Cereal Bars, Diet Bars, Scones, and Tarts   A-96 Meals and Dishes   A-100 Meats   A-106 Nuts, Seeds, and Products   A-108 Poultry   A-110 Salad Dressings, Dips, and Mayonnaise   A-110 Salads   A-110 Sandwiches   A-114 Sauces and Gravies   A-114 Snack Foods—Chips, Pretzels, Popcorn   A-116 Soups, Stews, and Chilis   A-118 Spices, Flavors, and Seasonings   A-120 Sports Bars and Drinks   A-120 Supplemental Foods and Formulas   A-122 Sweeteners and Sweet Substitutes   A-122 Vegetables and Legumes   A-136 Weight Loss Bars and Drinks   A-138 Miscellaneous

Thia (mg)	Ribo (mg)	Niac (mg NE)	Vit B6 (mg)	Vit B12 (µg)	Fol (µg)	Vit C (mg)	Vit D (IU)	Vit E (mg AT)	Cal (mg)	Iron (mg)	Magn (mg)	Phos (mg)	Pota (mg)	Sodi (mg)	Zinc (mg)	Wat (%)	Alco (g)	Caff (g)
—	—	—	—	—	—	0.0	—	—	—	—	—	—	—	90	—	91	0.00	0.00
—	—	—	—	0.00	—	0.0	—	—	—	—	—	45	—	50	—	89	0.00	0.00
0.00	0.00	—	0.00	0.00	—	0.0	—	—	—	—	—	—	—	35	—	100	0.00	0.00
0.00	0.00	0.00	0.00	0.00	0.0	0.0	—	0.0	12	0.01	2.4	0	5	50	0.2	100	0.00	0.00
0.00	0.00	0.00	0.00	0.00	0.0	0.0	0.0	0.0	7	0.07	2.5	36	2	5	0.0	89	0.00	30.67
0.00	0.00	0.00	0.00	0.00	0.0	0.0	—	0.0	11	0.07	3.7	48	4	15	0.0	89	0.00	0.00
—	—	—	—	—	—	0.0	—	—	—	—	—	—	—	35	—	89	0.00	27.20
—	—	—	—	—	—	0.0	—	—	—	—	—	—	—	35	—	—	0.00	27.20
—	—	—	—	—	—	0.0	—	—	0	0.00	—	0	13	10	—	—	0.00	0.00
0.00	0.00	0.00	0.00	0.00	0.0	0.0	—	0.0	7	0.20	2.5	0	2	37	0.2	89	0.00	0.00
0.00	0.00	0.03	0.00	0.00	0.0	0.0	—	0.0	5	0.17	2.5	0	2	27	0.1	90	0.00	0.00
—	—	—	—	0.00	—	0.0	—	—	0	0.00	—	0	—	47	—	87	0.00	36.66
—	—	—	—	0.00	—	0.0	—	—	0	0.00	—	0	—	23	—	100	0.00	36.66
0.00	0.00	0.00	0.00	0.00	0.0	0.0	0.0	0.0	—	—	—	29	14	7	—	90	0.00	27.00
0.00	0.00	0.00	0.00	0.00	0.0	0.0	—	0.0	12	0.15	2.5	2	5	30	0.2	88	0.00	0.00
—	—	—	—	0.00	—	0.0	—	—	0	0.00	—	35	—	23	—	88	0.00	24.67
—	—	—	—	0.00	—	0.0	—	—	0	0.00	—	27	5	23	—	—	0.00	24.00
0.00	0.00	0.00	0.00	0.00	0.0	0.0	—	0.0	12	0.11	2.5	0	2	32	0.2	89	0.00	0.00
—	—	—	—	0.00	—	—	—	—	—	—	—	—	—	30	—	100	0.00	0.00
—	—	—	—	—	—	0.0	—	—	—	—	—	0	0	23	—	89	0.00	0.00
—	—	—	—	—	—	0.0	—	—	—	—	—	—	—	15	—	89	0.00	0.00
—	—	—	—	—	—	0.0	—	—	0	0.00	—	—	—	0	—	0	0.00	0.00
—	—	—	—	—	—	2.4	—	—	250	0.00	—	—	—	110	—	—	0.00	90.00
—	—	—	—	—	—	2.4	—	—	250	0.00	—	—	—	105	—	—	0.00	90.00
0.00	0.41	12.34	0.00	0.00	2.4	0.5	—	0.0	5	0.31	189.6	17	273	33	0.1	98	0.00	502.44
—	—	—	—	—	—	1.2	—	—	250	0.00	—	—	—	100	—	—	0.00	90.00
0.00	0.00	0.56	0.00	0.00	0.0	0.0	—	0.0	10	0.10	7.2	7	72	5	0.0	99	0.00	61.97
0.10	0.44	0.34	0.10	1.08	12.8	0.0	—	0.1	251	0.63	25.6	205	335	118	0.9	84	0.00	0.00
0.00	0.02	0.10	0.00	0.00	1.5	0.2	—	0.0	8	0.68	21.2	28	128	45	0.3	1	0.00	7.78
0.00	0.01	0.01	0.00	0.00	0.0	0.1	0.0	0.0	1	0.10	0.2	1	1	8	0.0	0	0.00	0.00
0.02	0.15	0.17	0.02	0.37	0.0	0.5	—	0.2	40	0.34	23.5	89	202	143	0.4	2	0.00	5.09
0.03	0.20	0.21	0.03	0.49	0.0	0.5	—	0.2	60	0.46	33.0	118	269	195	0.6	86	0.00	5.48
0.30	0.14	5.00	0.40	0.60	99.7	27.0	0.0	6.8	250	4.50	79.7	100	249	95	3.0	—	0.00	0.00
0.40	0.47	5.48	0.52	1.53	117.7	30.9	100.0	5.4	406	4.86	118.5	392	731	267	4.1	79	0.00	0.00
0.40	0.47	5.48	0.52	1.50	117.7	30.9	100.0	5.5	403	4.86	118.5	390	726	264	4.1	78	0.00	0.00
0.40	0.46	5.46	0.51	1.50	117.7	30.7	100.0	5.5	396	4.86	117.1	386	721	262	4.1	77	0.00	0.00
0.03	0.03	0.41	0.02	0.03	10.7	0.3	1.0	0.0	13	0.47	14.7	37	130	53	0.2	1	0.00	7.76

PAGE KEY: A-46 Beverage and Beverage Mixes A-48 Other Beverages A-48 Beverages, Alcoholic A-50 Candies and Confections, Gum A-54 Cereals, Breakfast Type A-58 Cheese and Cheese Substitutes A-60 Dairy Products and Substitutes A-62 Desserts A-68 Dessert Toppings A-68 Eggs, Substitutes, and Egg Dishes A-70 Ethnic Foods A-74 Fast Foods/Restaurants A-88 Fats, Oils, Margarines, Shortenings, and Substitutes A-88 Fish, Seafood, and Shellfish A-90 Food Additives A-90 Fruit, Vegetable, or Blended Juices A-92 Grains, Flours, and Fractions A-92 Grain Products, Prepared and Baked Goods

Code	Food Name	Unit/Amt	Wt (g)	Energy (kcal)	Prot (g)	Carb (g)	Fiber (g)	Fat (g)	Sat (g)	Mono (g)	Poly (g)	Chol (mg)	Vit A (RE)
Fruit Flavored Drinks													
20004	Drink, breakfast, orange, prep f/pwd	1 cup	248	122	0	31	0	0	0.0	0.0	0.0	0	191
20385	Drink, cherry, swtnd, prep	8 fl-oz	254	60	0	16	0	0	0.0	0.0	0.0	0	0
20737	Drink, fruit punch	8 fl-oz	252	110	0	29	—	0	0.0	0.0	0.0	0	—
20176	Drink, fruit punch, non carbonated	12 fl-oz	360	200	0	50	0	0	0.0	0.0	0.0	0	—
20761	Drink, Island Punch	1 cup	252	110	0	27	—	0	0.0	0.0	0.0	0	—
20045	Drink, lemonade, prep f/pwd	1 cup	266	112	0	29	0	0	0.0	0.0	0.0	0	0
20746	Drink, pink lemonade	8 fl-oz	252	110	0	26	—	0	0.0	0.0	0.0	0	—
20123	Juice Drink, citrus fruit, calc fort	1 cup	240	112	1	28	0	0	0.0	0.0	0.0	0	1
20744	Juice Drink, raspberry peach	1 cup	252	120	0	29	—	0	0.0	0.0	0.0	0	—
793	Juice, apple	8 fl-oz	236	110	0	29	0	0	0.0	0.0	0.0	0	—
1853	Juice, grape	8 fl-oz	236	150	0	38	0	0	0.0	0.0	0.0	0	—
794	Juice, grapefruit	8 fl-oz	236	120	0	29	0	0	0.0	0.0	0.0	0	—
1854	Juice, orange	8 fl-oz	236	120	0	29	0	0	0.0	0.0	0.0	0	—
3128	Juice, prune, cnd	1 cup	256	182	2	45	3	0	0.0	0.1	0.0	0	1
6504	Juice, tomato, cnd	1 cup	243	50	2	10	2	0	0.0	0.0	0.0	0	100
6507	Juice, vegetable, cnd	1 cup	243	50	2	10	2	0	0.0	0.0	0.0	0	400
OTHER BEVERAGES													
38405	Drink, atole, cornmeal	1 cup	245	206	4	40	1	4	2.2	1.1	0.3	14	33
38362	Drink, horchata de arroz, rice beverage, Mexican	1 cup	245	100	0	25	0	0	0.0	0.0	0.0	0	0
20589	Drink, sugar cane, Puerto Rico	1 cup	240	164	0	42	0	0	0.0	0.0	0.0	0	0
Teas													
20495	Tea, bag	1 ea	2	0	0	0	0	0	0.0	0.0	0.0	0	0
20014	Tea, brewed w/tap water	1 cup	237	2	0	1	0	0	0.0	0.0	0.0	0	0
20538	Tea, Cool Drink, can/btl	1 cup	248	82	0	22	0	0	0.0	0.0	0.0	0	0
20681	Tea, green, sweetened, btl	1 cup	252	100	0	25	—	0	0.0	0.0	0.0	0	—
20894	Tea, herbal, Cranberry Cove, brewed	1 cup	237	0	0	0	0	0	0.0	0.0	0.0	0	0
20853	Tea, herbal, Echinacea Complete Care, brewed	1 cup	237	0	0	0	0	0	0.0	0.0	0.0	0	0
20899	Tea, herbal, Sleepytime, brewed	1 cup	237	0	0	0	0	0	0.0	0.0	0.0	0	0
30451	Tea, iced, 100%, inst, pwd	2 tsp	1	0	0	0	0	0	0.0	0.0	0.0	0	0
20724	Tea, iced, w/lemonade	8 fl-oz	252	110	0	28	0	0	0.0	0.0	0.0	0	—
Water													
20051	Water, btld	1 cup	237	0	0	0	0	0	0.0	0.0	0.0	0	0
20041	Water, municipal	1 cup	237	0	0	0	0	0	0.0	0.0	0.0	0	0
BEVERAGES, ALCOHOLIC													
34066	Beer, amber ale	12 fl-oz	356	169	2	14	—	0	0.0	0.0	0.0	0	—
22500	Beer, can/btl, 12 fl oz	12 fl-oz	356	139	1	11	0	0	0.0	0.0	0.0	0	0
34053	Beer, Light	12 fl-oz	353	105	1	5	0	0	0.0	0.0	0.0	0	—
22685	Beer, non alcoholic, Near	12 fl-oz	356	32	1	5	0	0	0.0	0.0	0.0	0	0
22671	Bourbon, 80 proof	1 fl-oz	28	64	0	0	0	0	0.0	0.0	0.0	0	0
22513	Brandy, 80 proof	1 fl-oz	28	64	0	0	0	0	0.0	0.0	0.0	0	0
22514	Gin, 80 proof	1 fl-oz	28	64	0	0	0	0	0.0	0.0	0.0	0	0
22547	Liqueur, Amaretto, 1 shot	1 ea	30	106	0	13	0	0	0.0	0.0	0.0	0	0
34052	Malt Beverage, Zima	12 fl-oz	353	185	0	21	0	0	0.0	0.0	0.0	0	—
22555	Mixed Drink, Bacardi cocktail	1 ea	63	117	0	6	0	0	0.0	0.0	0.0	0	0

PAGE KEY: A-96 Granola Bars, Cereal Bars, Diet Bars, Scones, and Tarts   A-96 Meals and Dishes   A-100 Meats   A-106 Nuts, Seeds, and Products   A-108 Poultry   A-110 Salad Dressings, Dips, and Mayonnaise   A-110 Salads   A-110 Sandwiches   A-114 Sauces and Gravies   A-114 Snack Foods—Chips, Pretzels, Popcorn   A-116 Soups, Stews, and Chilis   A-118 Spices, Flavors, and Seasonings   A-120 Sports Bars and Drinks   A-120 Supplemental Foods and Formulas   A-122 Sweeteners and Sweet Substitutes   A-122 Vegetables and Legumes   A-136 Weight Loss Bars and Drinks   A-138 Miscellaneous

Thia (mg)	Ribo (mg)	Niac (mg NE)	Vit B6 (mg)	Vit B12 (μg)	Fol (μg)	Vit C (mg)	Vit D (IU)	Vit E (mg AT)	Cal (mg)	Iron (mg)	Magn (mg)	Phos (mg)	Pota (mg)	Sodi (mg)	Zinc (mg)	Wat (%)	Alco (g)	Caff (g)
0.00	0.21	2.53	0.25	0.00	0.0	73.2	—	0.0	126	0.01	2.5	47	60	10	0.0	87	0.00	0.00
—	—	—	—	0.00	—	6.0	—	—	0	0.00	—	0	0	0	—	94	0.00	0.00
—	—	—	—	—	—	0.0	—	—	—	—	—	—	—	10	—	88	0.00	0.00
—	—	—	—	0.00	—	65.0	—	—	—	—	—	0	0	45	—	—	0.00	0.00
—	—	—	—	—	—	—	—	—	—	—	—	—	—	10	—	89	0.00	0.00
0.00	0.00	0.00	0.00	0.00	0.0	34.0	—	0.0	29	0.05	2.7	3	3	19	0.1	89	0.00	0.00
—	—	—	—	—	—	0.0	—	—	—	—	—	—	—	10	—	90	0.00	0.00
0.05	0.02	0.31	0.05	0.00	5.2	79.8	0.0	0.1	316	0.21	16.7	20	196	4	0.1	88	0.00	0.00
—	—	—	—	—	—	0.0	—	—	—	—	—	—	—	10	—	88	0.00	0.00
—	—	—	—	—	—	—	—	—	—	—	—	—	—	10	—	88	0.00	0.00
—	—	—	—	—	—	—	—	—	—	—	—	—	—	10	—	84	0.00	0.00
—	—	—	—	—	—	—	—	—	—	—	—	—	—	0	—	87	0.00	0.00
—	—	—	—	—	—	—	—	—	—	—	—	—	—	0	—	—	0.00	0.00
0.03	0.18	2.00	0.56	0.00	0.0	10.5	—	0.3	31	3.01	35.8	64	707	10	0.5	81	0.00	0.00
—	—	—	—	—	—	72.0	—	—	20	0.72	—	—	430	750	—	94	0.00	0.00
—	—	—	—	—	—	60.0	—	—	40	0.72	—	—	520	620	—	94	0.00	0.00
0.12	0.23	0.81	0.07	0.36	6.4	0.9	—	0.1	140	0.67	24.2	117	185	55	0.6	80	0.00	0.00
0.00	0.00	0.14	0.00	0.00	0.4	0.1	—	0.0	12	0.34	3.5	5	6	7	0.1	89	0.00	0.00
0.07	0.03	0.05	0.00	0.00	0.0	0.0	—	0.0	12	2.25	8.0	5	39	42	0.2	81	0.00	0.00
—	—	—	—	—	—	0.0	—	—	0	0.00	—	—	25	0	—	—	0.00	55.00
0.00	0.02	0.00	0.00	0.00	11.8	0.0	—	0.0	0	0.05	7.1	2	88	7	0.0	100	0.00	47.36
—	—	—	—	—	—	0.0	—	—	0	0.00	—	73	38	33	—	—	0.00	11.00
—	—	—	—	—	—	0.0	—	—	—	—	—	—	—	10	—	90	0.00	18.00
—	—	—	—	—	—	0.0	—	—	0	0.00	—	—	30	0	—	100	0.00	0.00
—	—	—	—	—	—	35.0	—	—	0	0.00	—	—	—	0	7.5	100	0.00	0.00
—	—	—	—	—	—	0.0	—	—	0	0.00	—	—	30	0	—	100	0.00	0.00
—	—	—	—	—	—	0.0	—	—	0	0.00	—	—	45	0	—	—	0.00	40.00
—	—	—	—	—	—	0.0	—	—	—	—	—	—	—	10	—	89	0.00	18.00
0.00	0.00	0.00	0.00	0.00	0.0	0.0	—	0.0	2	0.01	2.4	0	0	2	0.0	100	0.00	0.00
0.00	0.00	0.00	0.00	0.00	0.0	0.0	—	0.0	5	0.00	2.4	0	0	5	0.0	100	0.00	0.00
—	—	—	—	—	—	—	—	—	—	—	—	—	—	44	—	—	18.65	0.00
0.01	0.09	1.83	0.15	0.07	21.4	0.0	—	0.0	14	0.07	21.4	50	96	14	0.0	93	12.82	0.00
0.03	0.03	1.40	—	—	—	—	—	—	11	—	—	—	59	11	—	98	14.11	0.00
0.01	0.09	1.61	0.18	0.07	21.4	0.0	—	0.0	25	0.03	32.1	110	89	18	0.0	98	1.07	0.00
0.00	0.00	0.00	0.00	0.00	0.0	0.0	—	0.0	0	0.00	0.0	1	1	0	0.0	67	9.28	0.00
0.00	0.00	0.00	0.00	0.00	0.0	0.0	—	0.0	0	0.00	0.0	1	1	0	0.0	67	9.28	0.00
0.00	0.00	0.00	0.00	0.00	0.0	0.0	—	0.0	0	0.00	0.0	1	1	0	0.0	67	9.28	0.00
0.00	0.00	0.01	0.00	0.00	0.0	0.0	0.0	0.0	0	0.01	0.5	1	4	2	0.0	30	7.73	0.00
0.03	0.03	0.87	—	—	—	—	—	—	38	—	—	—	51	20	—	—	16.94	0.00
0.00	0.00	0.02	0.00	0.00	1.2	1.0	0.0	0.0	2	0.05	1.2	3	12	11	0.0	68	13.72	0.00

PAGE KEY: A-46 Beverage and Beverage Mixes A-48 Other Beverages A-48 Beverages, Alcoholic A-50 Candies and Confections, Gum A-54 Cereals, Breakfast Type A-58 Cheese and Cheese Substitutes A-60 Dairy Products and Substitutes A-62 Desserts A-68 Dessert Toppings A-68 Eggs, Substitutes, and Egg Dishes A-70 Ethnic Foods A-74 Fast Foods/Restaurants A-88 Fats, Oils, Margarines, Shortenings, and Substitutes A-88 Fish, Seafood, and Shellfish A-90 Food Additives A-90 Fruit, Vegetable, or Blended Juices A-92 Grains, Flours, and Fractions A-92 Grain Products, Prepared and Baked Goods

Code	Food Name	Unit/ Amt	Wt (g)	Energy (kcal)	Prot (g)	Carb (g)	Fiber (g)	Fat (g)	Sat (g)	Mono (g)	Poly (g)	Chol (mg)	Vit A (RE)
34057	Mixed Drink, bloody mary, prep f/recipe	1 ea	209	46	1	7	1	0	0.0	—	—	0	117
22538	Mixed Drink, daiquiri, 6.8 fl oz can	1 ea	207	259	0	33	0	0	0.0	0.0	0.0	0	0
34058	Mixed Drink, gin & tonic, prep f/recipe	1 ea	232	160	0	8	0	0	0.0	0.0	0.0	0	0
22556	Mixed Drink, high ball	1 ea	160	105	0	0	0	0	0.0	0.0	0.0	0	0
22569	Mixed Drink, Irish coffee, 1 fl oz	1 ea	26	26	0	1	0	1	0.8	0.4	0.0	5	15
22568	Mixed Drink, Long Island iced tea	1 ea	125	119	0	9	0	0	0.0	0.0	0.0	0	0
22566	Mixed Drink, Mai Tai	1 ea	126	305	0	29	0	0	0.0	0.0	0.1	0	0
22557	Mixed Drink, margarita	1 ea	77	170	0	11	0	0	0.0	0.0	0.0	0	0
22571	Mixed Drink, Mexican eggnog/rompope	4 fl-oz	122	203	5	19	0	7	2.8	2.3	0.7	184	102
22561	Mixed Drink, pina colada	1 ea	141	245	1	32	0	3	2.3	0.1	0.0	0	0
22683	Mixed Drink, screwdriver cocktail	1 ea	213	182	1	18	0	0	0.0	0.0	0.0	0	14
22567	Mixed Drink, tequila sunrise	1 ea	172	189	1	15	0	0	0.0	0.0	0.0	0	17
22534	Mixed Drink, whiskey sour mix, btld	4 fl-oz	124	108	0	26	0	0	0.0	0.0	0.0	0	0
22593	Rum, 80 proof	1 fl-oz	28	64	0	0	0	0	0.0	0.0	0.0	0	0
22515	Tequila, 80 proof	1 fl-oz	28	64	0	0	0	0	0.0	0.0	0.0	0	0
22594	Vodka, 80 proof	1 fl-oz	28	64	0	0	0	0	0.0	0.0	0.0	0	0
22670	Whiskey, 80 proof	1 fl-oz	28	64	0	0	0	0	0.0	0.0	0.0	0	0
22577	Wine, all table types	6 fl-oz	177	136	0	6	0	0	0.0	0.0	0.0	0	0
22608	Wine, cooking, red	1 fl-oz	30	20	0	3	0	0	0.0	0.0	0.0	0	0
22609	Wine, cooking, white	1 fl-oz	30	20	0	3	0	0	0.0	0.0	0.0	0	0
22681	Wine, cooler	1 cup	227	113	0	13	0	0	0.0	0.0	0.0	0	0
22509	Wine, dry, sherry	1 fl-oz	29	20	0	0	—	0	0.0	0.0	0.0	0	0
20076	Wine, non alcoholic	4 fl-oz	116	7	1	1	0	0	0.0	0.0	0.0	0	0
22501	Wine, red	6 fl-oz	177	127	0	3	0	0	0.0	0.0	0.0	0	0
22600	Wine, rice, Japanese	1 fl-oz	29	39	0	1	0	0	0.0	0.0	0.0	0	0
22511	Wine, Sweet Vermouth	1 fl-oz	30	46	0	4	—	0	0.0	0.0	0.0	0	0
CANDIES AND CONFECTIONS, GUM													
23017	Baking Chips, milk chocolate	1.5 oz	43	228	3	25	1	13	6.1	5.6	0.3	10	21
90704	Candy Bar, 3 Musketeers, 0.8 oz bar	1 ea	23	94	1	17	0	3	1.5	1.0	0.1	2	3
23125	Candy Bar, 5th Avenue, 2 oz bar	1 ea	57	273	5	36	2	14	3.8	6.0	1.9	3	8
23049	Candy Bar, Almond Joy, 1.7 oz	1 ea	48	231	2	29	2	13	8.5	2.5	0.6	2	4
90678	Candy Bar, Baby Ruth, 1.2 oz bar	1 ea	34	158	2	21	1	9	4.2	2.2	1.1	1	1
90653	Candy Bar, Butterfinger, 1.6 oz bar	1 ea	45	216	3	33	1	9	4.6	2.2	1.1	0	0
23116	Candy Bar, Caramello, 1.6 oz bar	1 ea	45	210	3	29	1	10	5.8	2.4	0.3	12	28
23118	Candy Bar, carob, 3 oz bar	1 ea	85	459	7	48	3	27	24.7	0.4	0.3	3	0
23099	Candy Bar, crisped rice, chocolate chip, 1 oz bar	1 ea	28	115	1	21	1	4	1.5	1.1	1.0	0	100
4196	Candy Bar, dark chocolate, 1.5 oz bar	0.5 ea	42	230	2	25	4	14	9.0	—	—	3	0
4198	Candy Bar, dark chocolate, w/almonds, 1.5 oz bar	0.5 ea	42	230	3	23	4	15	8.0	—	—	3	0
91519	Candy Bar, Heath, bites	15 pce	39	207	2	25	1	12	6.1	3.4	1.0	7	18
23060	Candy Bar, Kit Kat, 1.5 oz bar	1 ea	43	220	3	27	0	11	7.6	2.5	0.4	5	10
23061	Candy Bar, Krackel, 1.5 oz bar	1 ea	43	218	3	27	1	11	6.8	2.7	0.2	5	9
23037	Candy Bar, Mars almond, 1.76 oz bar	1 ea	50	234	4	31	1	12	3.6	5.3	2.0	8	8
92633	Candy Bar, milk chocolate, 0.6 oz bar	1 ea	17	90	1	10	0	5	3.5	—	—	5	0
90687	Candy Bar, Milky Way, 1.9 oz bar	1 ea	54	228	2	39	1	9	4.2	3.2	0.3	8	10
23035	Candy Bar, Mounds, 1.9 oz bar	1 ea	54	262	2	32	2	14	11.1	0.2	0.1	1	0
23062	Candy Bar, Mr. Goodbar, 1.75 oz bar	1 ea	50	267	5	27	2	16	7.0	4.1	2.2	5	17
23133	Candy Bar, Nestle Crunch, 1.4 oz bar	1 ea	40	207	2	26	1	10	6.0	3.4	0.3	5	6

PAGE KEY: A-96 Granola Bars, Cereal Bars, Diet Bars, Scones, and Tarts   A-96 Meals and Dishes   A-100 Meats   A-106 Nuts, Seeds, and Products   A-108 Poultry
A-110 Salad Dressings, Dips, and Mayonnaise   A-110 Salads   A-110 Sandwiches   A-114 Sauces and Gravies   A-114 Snack Foods—Chips, Pretzels, Popcorn
A-116 Soups, Stews, and Chilis   A-118 Spices, Flavors, and Seasonings   A-120 Sports Bars and Drinks   A-120 Supplemental Foods and Formulas
A-122 Sweeteners and Sweet Substitutes   A-122 Vegetables and Legumes   A-136 Weight Loss Bars and Drinks   A-138 Miscellaneous

Thia (mg)	Ribo (mg)	Niac (mg NE)	Vit B6 (mg)	Vit B12 (µg)	Fol (µg)	Vit C (mg)	Vit D (IU)	Vit E (mg AT)	Cal (mg)	Iron (mg)	Magn (mg)	Phos (mg)	Pota (mg)	Sodi (mg)	Zinc (mg)	Wat (%)	Alco (g)	Caff (g)
0.00	0.00	0.03	0.00	0.00	2.4	23.6	0.0	0.0	19	1.07	2.2	4	52	558	0.0	94	1.38	0.00
0.00	0.00	0.02	0.00	0.00	2.1	2.7	0.0	0.0	0	0.01	2.1	4	23	83	0.1	75	19.90	0.00
0.00	0.00	0.00	0.00	0.00	0.0	0.0	0.0	0.0	3	0.03	0.9	2	1	7	0.1	88	18.56	0.00
0.00	0.00	0.00	0.00	0.00	0.0	0.0	0.0	0.0	6	0.02	1.2	2	3	25	0.1	90	15.09	0.00
0.00	0.00	0.03	0.00	0.00	0.1	0.0	1.8	0.0	3	0.00	1.1	3	12	2	0.0	86	1.63	—
0.00	0.00	0.02	0.00	0.00	1.3	3.2	0.0	0.0	4	0.05	1.8	12	14	6	0.0	83	12.14	0.00
0.00	0.00	0.05	0.00	0.00	1.2	1.0	0.0	0.0	3	0.09	2.4	6	24	11	0.1	54	27.56	0.00
0.00	0.00	0.03	0.00	0.00	1.2	1.0	0.0	0.0	2	0.05	1.4	4	15	4	0.0	62	18.50	0.00
0.03	0.20	0.07	0.07	0.55	18.0	0.6	43.7	0.5	106	0.54	11.1	136	125	42	0.7	69	7.48	0.00
0.03	0.02	0.17	0.05	0.00	16.5	6.9	0.0	0.1	11	0.27	10.6	10	100	9	0.2	65	13.89	0.00
0.14	0.02	0.34	0.07	0.00	74.9	66.5	0.0	0.3	15	0.18	17.1	29	326	2	0.1	83	15.10	0.00
0.07	0.02	0.33	0.09	0.00	18.2	33.3	0.0	0.1	10	0.46	11.7	17	179	7	0.1	80	18.68	0.00
0.01	0.00	0.00	0.00	0.00	0.0	3.3	—	0.0	2	0.14	1.2	7	35	126	0.1	78	0.00	0.00
0.00	0.00	0.00	0.00	0.00	0.0	0.0	—	0.0	0	0.02	0.0	1	1	0	0.0	67	9.28	0.00
0.00	0.00	0.00	0.00	0.00	0.0	0.0	—	0.0	0	0.00	0.0	1	1	0	0.0	67	9.28	0.00
0.00	0.00	0.00	0.00	0.00	0.0	0.0	—	0.0	0	0.00	0.0	1	0	0	0.0	67	9.28	0.00
0.00	0.00	0.00	0.00	0.00	0.0	0.0	—	0.0	0	0.00	0.0	1	1	0	0.0	67	9.28	0.00
0.00	0.02	0.12	0.03	0.01	1.8	0.0	—	0.0	14	0.62	15.9	23	149	11	0.1	87	16.45	0.00
0.30	0.30	0.30	—	0.00	—	0.3	—	—	2	0.30	—	4	24	180	—	88	3.59	0.00
0.30	0.30	0.30	—	0.00	—	0.3	—	—	2	0.30	—	4	26	180	—	88	3.59	0.00
0.00	0.01	0.10	0.02	0.00	2.7	4.1	0.0	0.0	13	0.62	11.9	15	102	19	0.1	90	8.81	0.00
0.00	0.00	0.01	0.00	0.00	0.3	0.0	—	0.0	2	0.11	2.9	4	26	2	0.0	89	2.72	0.00
0.00	0.00	0.11	0.01	0.00	1.2	0.0	—	0.0	10	0.46	11.6	17	102	8	0.1	98	0.00	0.00
0.00	0.05	0.14	0.05	0.01	3.5	0.0	—	0.0	14	0.75	23.0	25	198	9	0.2	88	16.45	0.00
0.00	0.00	0.00	0.00	0.00	0.0	0.0	—	0.0	1	0.02	1.7	2	7	1	0.0	78	4.69	0.00
0.00	0.00	0.05	0.00	0.00	0.1	0.0	—	0.0	2	0.07	2.7	3	28	3	0.0	72	4.59	0.00
0.05	0.12	0.15	0.01	0.25	5.1	0.0	—	0.9	80	1.00	26.8	88	158	34	0.9	2	0.00	8.51
0.00	0.02	0.05	0.00	0.03	0.0	0.1	—	0.2	19	0.17	6.6	21	30	44	0.1	6	0.00	1.80
0.07	0.05	2.21	0.05	0.10	20.4	0.2	—	1.5	41	0.68	35.2	80	197	128	0.6	2	0.00	2.83
0.00	0.07	0.23	0.02	0.05	—	0.3	—	0.0	31	0.61	31.8	54	122	68	0.4	8	0.00	—
0.02	0.02	0.94	0.01	0.00	10.5	0.0	—	0.6	15	0.23	24.8	47	121	73	0.4	5	0.00	1.36
0.05	0.02	1.39	0.05	0.00	15.0	0.0	—	0.8	16	0.34	37.6	61	179	97	0.5	1	0.00	2.26
0.01	0.18	0.51	0.01	0.28	—	0.8	0.0	0.1	97	0.49	19.1	68	155	55	0.4	7	0.00	1.80
0.09	0.15	0.87	0.10	0.85	17.9	0.4	—	1.0	258	1.10	30.6	107	538	91	3.0	2	0.00	0.00
0.15	0.17	2.00	0.20	0.00	39.7	0.0	—	0.0	6	1.78	13.6	38	48	79	0.2	7	0.00	—
—	—	—	—	—	—	0.0	—	—	0	1.08	—	—	—	0	—	—	0.00	—
—	—	—	—	—	—	0.0	—	—	20	1.08	—	—	—	0	—	—	0.00	—
0.00	0.03	0.03	0.00	—	0.4	0.3	—	0.0	34	0.30	7.3	28	82	96	0.0	1	0.00	0.00
0.05	0.09	0.20	0.00	0.23	6.0	0.0	—	0.1	53	0.43	15.7	57	98	23	0.0	2	0.00	5.94
0.01	0.07	0.10	0.01	0.25	2.6	0.3	—	0.0	67	0.44	5.5	52	138	83	0.2	1	0.00	—
0.01	0.15	0.46	0.02	0.18	4.5	0.3	—	3.9	84	0.55	36.0	117	162	85	0.6	4	0.00	2.00
—	—	—	—	—	—	0.0	—	—	32	0.14	—	—	—	15	—	5	0.00	3.96
0.01	0.11	0.18	0.02	0.17	3.2	0.5	—	0.7	70	0.40	18.3	78	130	129	0.4	6	0.00	4.30
0.00	0.00	0.00	0.00	0.00	0.0	0.4	—	0.1	11	1.12	0.0	0	173	78	0.0	9	0.00	9.15
0.07	0.07	1.71	0.02	0.15	18.9	0.4	—	1.6	55	0.68	23.3	81	195	20	0.5	0	0.00	8.93
0.12	0.21	1.57	0.15	0.15	31.4	0.1	—	0.4	67	0.20	23.0	80	137	53	0.6	1	0.00	9.52

PAGE KEY: A-46 Beverage and Beverage Mixes A-48 Other Beverages A-48 Beverages, Alcoholic A-50 Candies and Confections, Gum A-54 Cereals, Breakfast Type A-58 Cheese and Cheese Substitutes A-60 Dairy Products and Substitutes A-62 Desserts A-68 Dessert Toppings A-68 Eggs, Substitutes, and Egg Dishes A-70 Ethnic Foods A-74 Fast Foods/Restaurants A-88 Fats, Oils, Margarines, Shortenings, and Substitutes A-88 Fish, Seafood, and Shellfish A-90 Food Additives A-90 Fruit, Vegetable, or Blended Juices A-92 Grains, Flours, and Fractions A-92 Grain Products, Prepared and Baked Goods

Code	Food Name	Unit/ Amt	Wt (g)	Energy (kcal)	Prot (g)	Carb (g)	Fiber (g)	Fat (g)	Sat (g)	Mono (g)	Poly (g)	Chol (mg)	Vit A (RE)
92654	Candy Bar, Payday, snack size, 0.7 oz bar	1 ea	20	90	2	10	—	5	0.5	—	—	0	—
23137	Candy Bar, peanut, 1.4 oz bar	1 ea	40	207	6	19	2	13	1.9	6.6	4.2	0	0
91513	Candy Bar, Reese's Nutrageous, 0.6 oz bar	2 ea	34	176	4	18	1	11	3.0	4.3	2.8	1	2
23036	Candy Bar, Skor, toffee bar, 1.4 oz bar	1 ea	40	212	1	24	1	13	7.5	3.7	0.5	21	57
23040	Candy Bar, Snickers, 2 oz bar	1 ea	57	265	5	37	1	11	4.2	4.7	1.5	8	22
23146	Candy Bar, Symphony, milk chocolate, 1.5 oz bar	1 ea	43	226	4	25	1	13	7.8	3.4	0.3	10	20
90705	Candy Bar, Twix, caramel, 2.06 oz two bar pkg	1 ea	58	291	3	38	1	14	5.2	7.8	0.5	3	15
92221	Candy Bar, Twix, chocolate fudge cookie bar, 3.6 oz bar	1 ea	100	550	7	56	3	33	5.0	14.3	12.5	6	11
23151	Candy Bar, Whatchamacallit, 1.7 oz bar	1 ea	48	238	4	30	1	11	8.2	1.8	0.4	6	19
92658	Candy Bar, Zero, 0.6 oz bar	1 ea	17	70	1	12	—	2	1.5	—	—	0	—
23085	Candy, Almond Roca	1 pce	11	48	1	7	0	2	1.1	0.6	0.2	1	2
4148	Candy, Bit O Honey, Nestle	6 pce	40	160	1	32	0	3	2.0	0.8	0.2	0	0
92707	Candy, caramel, Sugar Daddy, lrg	1 ea	48	200	1	43	0	2	1.0	—	—	0	0
23015	Candy, caramels	1 pce	10	39	0	8	0	1	0.7	0.1	0.0	1	0
92374	Candy, cotton	2.1 oz	60	220	3	56	—	0	0.0	0.0	0.0	0	—
23078	Candy, fondant, chocolate cvrd	2 pce	28	102	1	22	0	3	1.5	0.9	0.1	0	1
92647	Candy, Good N Plenty, snack size box	1 ea	17	60	0	14	0	0	0.0	0.0	0.0	0	0
23409	Candy, gumdrops	1.5 oz	43	168	0	42	0	0	0.0	0.0	0.0	0	0
23412	Candy, gummy worms, pces	10 pce	74	293	0	73	0	0	0.0	0.0	0.0	0	0
23031	Candy, hard, all flvrs	1 pce	6	24	0	6	0	0	0.0	0.0	0.0	0	0
92653	Candy, hard, lollipop	1 ea	17	60	0	16	0	0	0.0	0.0	0.0	0	0
23472	Candy, jawbreakers, Everlasting Gobstoppers, Willy Wonka	6 pce	16	59	0	15	—	0	0.0	0.0	0.0	—	—
23033	Candy, jellybeans, sml	10 pce	11	41	0	10	0	0	0.0	0.0	0.0	0	0
23063	Candy, Kisses, milk chocolate	6 pce	28	145	2	17	1	9	5.2	2.8	0.3	6	16
52154	Candy, licorice, black, vines/ropes	4 pce	40	140	1	33	0	0	0.0	0.0	0.0	0	0
52155	Candy, licorice, red, vines/ropes	4 pce	40	140	1	34	0	0	0.0	0.0	0.0	0	0
92644	Candy, malt choc, Whoppers	9 ea	20	90	1	15	0	4	3.0	—	—	0	0
23047	Candy, milk chocolate peanut	1.5 oz	43	219	4	26	1	11	4.4	4.7	1.8	4	11
92642	Candy, Milk Duds	7 ea	21	90	1	15	0	4	1.0	—	—	0	—
23193	Candy, mints, After Eight	5 pce	41	147	1	31	1	6	3.4	1.8	0.2	0	1
23225	Candy, mints, peppermint, Breath Saver	1 pce	2	10	0	2	0	0	0.0	0.0	0.0	0	0
92657	Candy, Nibs, licorice	9 ea	12	35	0	9	—	0	0.0	0.0	0.0	0	0
92201	Candy, nougat, 0.5 oz pce	1 ea	14	56	0	13	0	0	0.2	0.0	0.0	0	0
23021	Candy, peanuts, milk chocolate cvrd	1.5 oz	43	221	6	21	2	14	6.2	5.5	1.8	4	14
23088	Candy, peanuts, yogurt cvrd	1.5 oz	43	230	6	18	2	16	6.9	4.8	3.1	0	0
90803	Candy, pralines, prep f/recipe	1 pce	40	174	1	22	1	10	2.7	—	—	10	30
23517	Candy, raisins, chocolate cvrd	35 pce	40	160	1	27	2	7	4.0	—	—	0	2
23089	Candy, raisins, yogurt cvrd	1.5 oz	43	167	2	31	1	5	4.3	0.1	0.1	0	0
92643	Candy, Sixlets	6 ea	38	170	1	29	0	7	5.0	—	—	0	0
23485	Candy, Skittles, original bite size candies, 2.17 oz pkg	1 ea	62	249	0	56	0	3	0.5	1.8	0.1	0	0
23144	Candy, Starburst, fruit chews	1 pce	5	20	0	4	0	0	0.1	0.2	0.2	0	0
92705	Candy, Sugar Babies	30 ea	44	180	0	41	0	2	0.0	—	—	0	0
4149	Candy, SweeTarts, reg	8 pce	15	60	0	14	0	0	0.0	0.0	0.0	0	0
90806	Candy, taffy, prep f/recipe	1 pce	34	99	1	17	0	3	1.0	—	—	4	—
92769	Candy, Tootsie Roll	6 pce	40	155	1	35	0	1	0.4	0.8	0.1	1	0

Thia (mg)	Ribo (mg)	Niac (mg NE)	Vit B6 (mg)	Vit B12 (µg)	Fol (µg)	Vit C (mg)	Vit D (IU)	Vit E (mg AT)	Cal (mg)	Iron (mg)	Magn (mg)	Phos (mg)	Pota (mg)	Sodi (mg)	Zinc (mg)	Wat (%)	Alco (g)	Caff (g)
—	—	—	—	—	—	—	—	—	—	—	—	—	—	65	—	13	0.00	0.00
0.03	0.05	3.14	0.05	0.00	29.8	0.0	—	1.6	31	0.37	43.7	122	162	62	1.6	2	0.00	0.00
0.05	0.02	1.77	0.02	—	19.0	0.2	—	0.4	23	0.41	23.1	60	124	48	0.4	2	0.00	—
0.00	0.03	0.05	0.00	0.10	1.2	0.2	—	0.0	52	0.23	4.0	24	61	126	0.1	2	0.00	—
0.02	0.07	2.03	0.05	0.09	15.3	0.0	—	0.9	60	0.68	40.8	108	183	129	1.4	6	0.00	4.53
0.03	0.15	0.14	0.01	0.17	—	0.9	0.0	0.1	107	0.38	23.4	88	186	43	0.5	1	0.00	28.06
0.07	0.10	0.43	0.01	0.17	11.1	0.2	—	1.1	53	0.46	18.7	64	110	113	0.6	4	0.00	1.75
0.14	0.20	1.11	0.03	0.33	9.0	1.0	—	2.7	130	1.30	46.0	147	309	266	0.9	2	0.00	10.00
0.05	0.10	1.19	0.01	0.18	8.7	0.4	—	0.6	57	0.54	13.5	67	146	144	0.2	3	0.00	4.82
—	—	—	—	—	—	—	—	—	—	—	—	—	—	35	—	—	0.00	—
0.00	0.01	0.15	0.00	0.00	3.3	0.0	—	0.2	16	0.10	4.9	19	34	20	0.1	5	0.00	—
0.00	0.10	0.01	0.00	0.07	1.6	0.0	—	0.4	20	0.11	2.8	18	50	120	0.1	8	0.00	0.00
—	—	—	—	—	—	0.0	—	—	20	0.00	—	—	—	65	—	—	0.00	0.00
0.00	0.02	0.02	0.00	0.00	0.5	0.1	—	0.3	14	0.00	1.7	12	22	25	0.0	8	0.00	0.00
—	—	—	—	—	—	—	—	—	—	—	—	—	—	0	—	—	0.00	0.00
0.00	0.01	0.15	0.00	0.00	0.3	0.0	—	0.1	5	0.43	17.6	27	47	7	0.1	8	0.00	1.12
—	—	—	—	—	—	0.0	—	—	0	0.11	—	—	—	40	—	—	0.00	0.00
0.00	0.00	0.00	0.00	0.00	0.0	0.0	—	0.0	1	0.17	0.4	0	2	19	0.0	1	0.00	0.00
0.00	0.00	0.00	0.00	0.00	0.0	0.0	—	0.0	2	0.30	0.7	1	4	33	0.0	1	0.00	0.00
0.00	0.00	0.00	0.00	0.00	0.0	0.0	—	0.0	0	0.01	0.2	0	0	2	0.0	1	0.00	0.00
—	—	—	—	—	—	0.0	—	—	0	0.00	—	—	—	10	—	5	0.00	0.00
—	—	—	—	—	—	—	—	—	—	—	—	—	—	1	—	8	0.00	0.00
0.00	0.00	0.00	0.00	0.00	0.0	0.0	—	0.0	0	0.00	0.2	0	4	6	0.0	6	0.00	0.00
0.01	0.09	0.09	0.00	0.10	2.3	0.1	—	0.4	54	0.38	17.0	61	109	23	0.4	1	0.00	6.96
—	—	—	—	—	—	0.0	—	—	0	0.00	—	—	—	60	—	15	0.00	0.00
—	—	—	—	—	—	0.0	—	—	0	0.00	—	—	—	20	—	12	0.00	0.00
—	—	—	—	—	—	0.0	—	—	40	0.18	—	—	—	65	—	—	0.00	—
0.03	0.07	1.74	0.03	0.07	16.2	0.2	—	1.1	43	0.49	32.3	99	148	20	1.0	2	0.00	4.67
—	—	—	—	—	—	0.0	—	—	—	—	—	—	—	40	—	6	0.00	—
0.01	0.01	0.11	0.00	0.00	0.4	0.0	—	0.2	9	0.62	18.5	23	69	5	0.2	6	0.00	8.19
—	—	—	—	—	—	—	—	—	—	—	—	—	0	—	—	0	—	—
—	—	—	—	—	—	0.0	—	—	0	0.00	—	—	—	60	—	25	0.00	0.00
0.00	0.01	0.07	0.00	0.00	0.7	0.0	—	0.4	4	0.07	4.5	8	15	5	0.1	2	0.00	0.00
0.05	0.07	1.80	0.09	0.18	3.4	0.0	—	1.5	44	0.56	40.8	90	213	17	1.0	2	0.00	9.35
0.14	0.09	2.48	0.07	0.18	49.9	0.1	—	2.3	64	0.93	35.0	113	202	24	0.8	4	0.00	0.00
0.05	0.02	0.11	0.01	0.02	2.5	0.2	4.8	0.4	20	0.34	13.4	33	67	40	0.4	17	0.00	0.00
—	—	—	—	—	—	1.0	—	—	16	3.00	—	—	—	40	—	10	0.00	—
0.05	0.07	0.33	0.07	0.12	3.9	0.9	—	0.6	48	0.50	10.3	55	236	19	0.2	10	0.00	0.00
—	—	—	—	—	—	0.0	—	—	40	0.00	—	—	—	55	—	1	0.00	—
0.00	0.00	0.00	0.00	0.00	0.0	41.2	—	0.3	0	0.00	0.6	1	6	10	0.0	4	0.00	0.00
0.00	0.00	0.00	0.00	0.00	0.0	2.6	—	0.0	0	0.00	0.1	0	0	3	0.0	7	0.00	0.00
—	—	—	—	—	—	0.0	—	—	20	0.00	—	—	—	40	—	—	0.00	0.00
—	—	—	—	—	—	0.0	—	—	0	0.00	—	—	—	0	—	—	0.00	0.00
0.00	0.01	0.10	0.00	0.00	1.3	0.0	1.0	0.6	9	0.01	9.1	16	19	152	0.1	34	0.00	0.00
0.01	0.02	0.07	0.00	0.00	3.6	0.0	—	0.3	14	0.31	8.8	23	46	18	0.2	7	0.00	2.79

Code	Food Name	Unit/Amt	Wt (g)	Energy (kcal)	Prot (g)	Carb (g)	Fiber (g)	Fat (g)	Sat (g)	Mono (g)	Poly (g)	Chol (mg)	Vit A (RE)
4144	Candy, Treasures, peanut butter	4 pce	43	240	3	22	1	16	7.0	—	—	5	0
4143	Candy, Treasures, w/caramel	3 pce	35	170	1	22	0	9	5.0	—	—	5	0
23082	Chewing Gum, stick	1 pce	3	7	0	2	0	0	0.0	0.0	0.0	0	0
23369	Fruit Leather, cherry	1 oz	28	105	0	23	0	2	0.7	0.9	0.0	0	—
91256	Fudge, plain	1.5 oz	43	188	0	27	0	9	6.0	—	—	11	10
23007	Marshmallows	4 ea	29	92	1	23	0	0	0.0	0.0	0.0	0	0
92226	Snack, crisped rice, peanut butter, 3.6 oz bar	1 ea	100	443	6	71	2	16	5.3	6.0	3.0	3	250

CEREALS, BREAKFAST TYPE

Cereals, Cooked and Dry

Code	Food Name	Unit/Amt	Wt (g)	Energy (kcal)	Prot (g)	Carb (g)	Fiber (g)	Fat (g)	Sat (g)	Mono (g)	Poly (g)	Chol (mg)	Vit A (RE)
40055	Cereal, hot, breakfast pilaf, ckd	0.5 cup	140	170	6	30	6	3	—	—	—	0	0
40179	Cereal, hot, Cream Of Rice, ckd w/water & salt	1 cup	244	127	2	28	0	0	0.0	0.1	0.1	0	0
38497	Cereal, hot, Farina, enrich, prep w/water & salt	1 cup	233	119	4	26	1	0	0.0	0.1	0.0	0	0
40186	Cereal, hot, Maltex, ckd w/water & salt	1 cup	249	189	6	39	2	1	0.2	0.1	0.4	0	0
40239	Cereal, hot, Maypo, ckd w/water & salt	1 cup	240	170	6	32	5	2	0.4	0.6	0.5	0	701
40138	Cereal, hot, multigrain, ckd	1 cup	246	202	7	40	4	2	0.3	0.5	1.1	0	116
38500	Cereal, hot, oat bran, prep w/water & salt	1 cup	219	94	4	16	4	2	0.4	0.7	0.8	0	4
40072	Cereal, hot, oatmeal, plain, inst, fort, prep w/water	0.75 cup	177	97	4	17	3	2	0.3	0.5	0.6	0	285
40190	Cereal, hot, Roman Meal, plain, ckd w/water & salt	1 cup	241	147	7	33	8	1	0.1	0.1	0.4	0	0
40188	Cereal, hot, wheat, plain, ckd w/water & salt	1 cup	240	122	4	26	1	0	0.0	0.1	0.0	0	0
40191	Cereal, hot, Wheatena, ckd w/water & salt	1 cup	243	143	5	29	5	1	0.2	0.2	0.6	0	1
40089	Grits, corn, inst, plain, prep w/water f/pkt	1 ea	137	93	2	21	1	0	0.0	0.0	0.1	0	0
38455	Grits, corn, white, dry	0.25 cup	42	150	3	33	1	0	0.0	0.0	0.0	0	20
38571	Grits, hominy, yellow, quick, dry	0.25 cup	37	125	3	29	2	1	0.2	0.2	0.3	0	21

Cereals, Ready To Eat

Code	Food Name	Unit/Amt	Wt (g)	Energy (kcal)	Prot (g)	Carb (g)	Fiber (g)	Fat (g)	Sat (g)	Mono (g)	Poly (g)	Chol (mg)	Vit A (RE)
54234	Cereal, 100% Bran	0.33 cup	29	83	4	23	8	1	0.1	—	—	0	150
40095	Cereal, All-Bran	0.5 cup	30	78	4	22	9	1	0.2	0.2	0.6	0	158
40258	Cereal, Alpha-Bits, 1.1 oz svg	1 ea	32	130	3	27	1	2	0.0	—	—	0	150
40098	Cereal, Apple Jacks	1 cup	30	117	1	27	1	1	0.1	0.2	0.3	0	42
40278	Cereal, Banana Nut Crunch	1 cup	59	249	5	44	4	6	0.8	—	—	0	150
40394	Cereal, Basic 4	1 cup	55	202	4	42	3	3	0.4	1.0	1.1	0	118
61203	Cereal, bran flakes	0.75 cup	30	96	3	24	5	1	0.1	0.1	0.3	0	225
40032	Cereal, Cap'N Crunch	0.75 cup	27	108	1	23	1	2	0.4	0.3	0.2	0	4
40297	Cereal, Cheerios	1 cup	30	111	4	22	4	2	0.4	0.6	0.2	0	150
40325	Cereal, Chex, corn	1 cup	30	112	2	26	1	0	0.1	0.1	0.1	0	140
40333	Cereal, Chex, rice	1.25 cup	31	117	2	27	0	0	0.1	0.1	0.1	0	155
40335	Cereal, Chex, wheat	1 cup	30	104	3	24	3	1	0.1	0.1	0.2	0	90
40414	Cereal, Cinnamon Grahams	0.75 cup	30	113	2	26	1	1	0.2	0.3	0.3	0	150
40126	Cereal, Cinnamon Toast Crunch	0.75 cup	30	127	2	24	1	3	0.5	1.5	1.0	0	150
61272	Cereal, Coco Roos, chocolate	0.75 cup	30	122	1	26	1	1	0.3	0.6	0.1	0	397
40102	Cereal, Cocoa Krispies	0.75 cup	31	118	2	27	1	1	0.6	0.1	0.1	0	153
40257	Cereal, Cocoa Pebbles	0.75 cup	29	115	1	25	0	1	1.1	—	—	0	150
40425	Cereal, Cocoa Puffs	1 cup	30	117	1	26	1	1	0.2	0.5	0.2	0	0
40103	Cereal, Complete Oat Bran Flakes	0.75 cup	30	105	3	23	4	1	0.2	0.5	0.3	0	235
40324	Cereal, Cookie Crisp	1 cup	30	117	1	26	0	1	0.2	0.4	0.2	0	145
61214	Cereal, corn flakes, plain	1 cup	28	101	2	24	1	0	0.0	0.0	0.0	0	216
40206	Cereal, Corn Pops	1 cup	31	118	1	28	0	0	0.1	0.1	0.1	0	144

Thia (mg)	Ribo (mg)	Niac (mg NE)	Vit B6 (mg)	Vit B12 (µg)	Fol (µg)	Vit C (mg)	Vit D (IU)	Vit E (mg AT)	Cal (mg)	Iron (mg)	Magn (mg)	Phos (mg)	Pota (mg)	Sodi (mg)	Zinc (mg)	Wat (%)	Alco (g)	Caff (g)
—	—	—	—	—	—	0.0	—	—	40	0.36	—	—	—	80	—	—	0.00	—
—	—	—	—	—	—	0.0	—	—	40	0.00	—	—	—	60	—	—	0.00	—
0.00	0.00	0.00	0.00	0.00	0.0	0.0	0.0	0.0	0	0.00	0.0	0	0	0	0.0	3	0.00	0.00
0.00	0.00	0.00	—	—	—	—	—	—	7	0.07	—	—	46	56	—	—	0.00	0.00
—	—	—	—	—	—	0.0	—	—	0	0.18	—	—	—	42	—	—	0.00	0.00
0.00	0.00	0.01	0.00	0.00	0.3	0.0	—	0.0	1	0.07	0.6	2	1	23	0.0	16	0.00	0.00
0.43	0.44	6.90	0.52	—	119.0	14.9	—	—	344	5.17	28.0	102	185	406	0.5	4	0.00	0.00
—	—	—	—	—	—	0.0	—	—	20	1.44	—	—	—	15	—	—	0.00	0.00
0.00	0.00	0.98	0.07	0.00	7.3	0.0	0.0	0.0	7	0.49	7.3	41	49	422	0.4	88	0.00	0.00
0.15	0.10	1.80	0.01	0.00	53.6	0.0	0.0	0.0	9	11.00	7.0	30	33	128	0.2	87	0.00	0.00
0.25	0.10	2.36	0.07	0.00	29.9	0.0	0.0	1.1	22	1.78	57.3	177	266	189	1.9	81	0.00	0.00
0.70	0.79	9.35	0.93	2.77	12.0	28.3	0.0	0.2	130	8.38	52.8	247	211	259	1.5	83	0.00	0.00
0.38	0.46	4.42	0.46	0.00	17.2	0.0	0.0	3.4	69	5.40	66.4	184	138	2	0.9	79	0.00	0.00
0.25	0.07	0.20	0.02	0.00	11.0	0.0	0.0	0.1	24	2.11	65.7	180	151	101	1.2	89	0.00	0.00
0.25	0.31	3.59	0.37	0.00	76.1	0.0	0.0	0.2	99	7.67	40.7	96	94	80	0.8	86	0.00	0.00
0.23	0.11	3.07	0.10	0.00	24.1	0.0	0.0	0.4	29	2.11	108.5	214	301	198	1.8	83	0.00	0.00
0.47	0.23	5.76	0.01	0.00	4.8	0.0	0.0	0.0	5	9.60	4.8	24	31	324	0.2	88	0.00	2.40
0.02	0.05	1.33	0.05	0.00	21.9	0.0	0.0	1.3	15	1.36	51.0	146	187	578	1.7	85	0.00	0.00
0.15	0.18	2.21	0.05	0.00	46.6	0.0	0.0	0.0	8	7.96	9.6	29	38	288	0.2	82	0.00	0.00
—	—	—	—	—	—	0.0	—	—	0	0.36	—	—	35	0	—	14	0.00	0.00
0.18	0.14	1.59	0.09	0.00	57.0	0.0	—	0.1	1	1.51	14.8	46	62	1	0.3	12	0.00	0.00
0.37	0.43	5.00	0.50	0.00	100.0	0.0	0.0	—	22	8.10	80.6	236	275	121	3.7	3	0.00	0.00
0.68	0.81	4.44	3.59	5.63	393.0	6.0	51.0	0.4	117	5.28	108.6	345	306	73	3.7	2	0.00	0.00
—	—	—	—	—	—	0.0	—	—	100	2.70	—	—	—	210	—	—	0.00	0.00
0.50	0.38	4.61	0.44	1.37	93.0	13.8	38.1	0.0	8	4.17	16.5	38	36	142	1.5	3	0.00	0.00
0.37	0.41	5.00	0.50	1.50	99.7	0.1	40.1	—	21	16.20	48.4	183	171	253	1.5	4	0.00	0.00
0.30	0.34	3.90	0.38	1.14	78.7	0.0	31.4	0.6	196	3.51	40.2	232	155	316	3.0	7	0.00	0.00
0.37	0.43	5.00	0.50	1.50	99.9	0.0	39.9	0.3	17	8.10	64.2	152	185	220	1.5	4	0.00	0.00
0.43	0.47	5.71	0.56	0.00	420.1	0.0	0.0	0.2	4	5.15	15.1	45	54	202	4.3	2	0.00	0.00
0.54	0.50	5.76	0.66	1.42	200.1	6.0	39.9	0.1	122	10.31	39.3	132	209	213	4.6	4	0.00	0.00
0.37	0.43	5.01	0.50	1.50	200.1	6.0	0.0	0.1	100	9.00	8.4	22	25	288	3.8	2	0.00	0.00
0.38	0.43	5.17	0.51	1.54	206.8	6.2	41.2	0.0	103	9.30	9.3	35	30	292	3.9	3	0.00	0.00
0.23	0.25	3.00	0.30	0.89	240.0	3.6	24.0	0.2	60	8.69	24.0	90	113	267	2.4	2	0.00	0.00
0.37	0.43	5.01	0.50	1.50	99.9	6.0	39.9	0.1	100	4.50	8.1	20	44	237	3.8	3	0.00	0.00
0.37	0.43	5.01	0.50	1.50	99.9	6.0	39.9	0.3	100	4.50	8.1	80	43	206	3.8	3	0.00	0.00
0.40	0.44	5.28	0.52	1.59	105.9	15.9	—	0.1	21	4.76	10.8	42	53	201	0.2	3	0.00	1.20
0.46	0.69	4.96	1.01	2.15	197.5	15.0	40.3	0.1	40	6.88	11.8	32	61	197	1.5	3	0.00	1.54
0.37	0.43	5.00	0.50	1.50	100.0	0.0	40.0	—	3	1.79	10.7	23	42	157	1.5	3	0.00	—
0.37	0.43	5.01	0.50	1.50	99.9	6.0	0.0	0.1	100	4.50	8.1	20	50	171	3.8	3	0.00	0.60
1.64	1.79	21.00	2.09	6.03	403.5	63.0	42.0	12.7	16	18.89	45.0	105	120	210	15.6	3	0.00	0.00
0.37	0.43	5.01	0.50	1.50	99.9	6.0	39.9	0.1	100	4.50	8.4	40	27	178	3.8	2	0.00	0.60
0.37	0.43	5.00	0.50	1.50	100.0	0.0	40.0	0.1	1	5.40	4.5	15	33	266	0.1	4	0.00	0.00
0.37	0.43	4.98	0.50	1.51	102.0	6.0	50.2	0.0	5	1.91	2.2	10	26	120	1.5	3	0.00	0.00

PAGE KEY: A-46 Beverage and Beverage Mixes A-48 Other Beverages A-48 Beverages, Alcoholic A-50 Candies and Confections, Gum A-54 Cereals, Breakfast Type
A-58 Cheese and Cheese Substitutes A-60 Dairy Products and Substitutes A-62 Desserts A-68 Dessert Toppings A-68 Eggs, Substitutes, and Egg Dishes A-70 Ethnic Foods
A-74 Fast Foods/Restaurants A-88 Fats, Oils, Margarines, Shortenings, and Substitutes A-88 Fish, Seafood, and Shellfish A-90 Food Additives
A-90 Fruit, Vegetable, or Blended Juices A-92 Grains, Flours, and Fractions A-92 Grain Products, Prepared and Baked Goods

Code	Food Name	Unit/ Amt	Wt (g)	Energy (kcal)	Prot (g)	Carb (g)	Fiber (g)	Fat (g)	Sat (g)	Mono (g)	Poly (g)	Chol (mg)	Vit A (RE)
40205	Cereal, Cracklin' Oat Bran	0.75 cup	55	225	5	39	6	8	2.3	4.6	1.2	0	252
4354	Cereal, Cranberry Almond Crunch	1 cup	55	210	4	43	3	3	0.0	—	—	0	150
40017	Cereal, crispy rice	1 cup	28	111	2	25	0	0	0.0	0.0	0.0	0	372
40040	Cereal, Crispy Wheaties 'N Raisins	1 cup	55	183	4	45	5	1	0.2	0.1	0.4	0	150
61179	Cereal, Familia	1 cup	122	473	12	90	10	8	0.9	3.9	2.0	0	2
61303	Cereal, Fiber 7	3.6 oz	100	353	14	78	14	1	0.3	0.2	0.6	0	106
40130	Cereal, Fiber One	0.5 cup	30	59	2	24	14	1	0.1	0.1	0.4	0	0
40218	Cereal, Froot Loops	1 cup	30	118	2	26	1	1	0.5	0.1	0.2	0	142
61306	Cereal, frosted flakes	0.75 cup	30	116	1	27	1	0	0.1	0.0	0.1	0	218
40043	Cereal, Frosted Mini Wheats	1 cup	51	173	5	41	5	1	0.2	0.1	0.5	0	0
60932	Cereal, Frosted Oats	0.75 cup	28	111	2	23	1	2	0.4	0.5	0.3	0	178
40256	Cereal, Fruit & Bran, peaches raisins & almonds, svg	1 cup	55	190	4	42	6	3	0.0	—	—	0	150
40266	Cereal, Fruity Pebbles	0.75 cup	27	108	1	24	0	1	0.2	—	—	0	150
60964	Cereal, Go Lean	0.75 cup	40	114	10	23	8	1	0.2	0.2	0.4	0	1
40245	Cereal, Golden Crisp	0.75 cup	27	107	1	25	0	0	0.1	—	—	0	150
40299	Cereal, Golden Grahams	0.75 cup	30	112	2	25	1	1	0.2	0.4	0.4	0	150
40009	Cereal, granola, 100% Natural, honey raisin oats	0.5 cup	51	225	5	34	3	9	3.6	3.8	1.1	1	1
40048	Cereal, granola, homemade, w/oats & wheat germ	0.5 cup	61	299	9	32	5	15	2.8	4.7	6.5	0	1
40277	Cereal, Grape Nuts	0.5 cup	58	208	6	47	5	1	0.2	0.2	0.7	0	150
40265	Cereal, Grape Nuts Flakes	0.75 cup	29	106	3	24	3	1	0.2	0.2	0.5	0	150
60969	Cereal, Harmony	3.6 oz	100	365	11	79	4	2	0.5	0.8	0.6	0	273
40004	Cereal, Harvest Oat Flakes	0.75 cup	29	109	3	23	2	1	0.2	0.4	0.4	0	2
61344	Cereal, Healthy Fiber, multigrain flakes	0.75 cup	28	100	3	23	4	0	0.0	0.0	0.0	0	20
60958	Cereal, Heart to Heart	1 oz	28	99	4	22	4	1	0.3	0.3	0.3	0	323
40293	Cereal, Honey Bunches Of Oats, almond	0.75 cup	31	126	2	24	1	3	0.3	—	—	0	150
40427	Cereal, Honey Graham Oh!s	0.75 cup	27	111	1	23	1	2	0.5	0.4	0.2	0	177
40264	Cereal, Honeycomb	1.33 cup	29	115	2	26	1	1	0.2	—	—	0	150
40134	Cereal, Just Right	1 cup	43	160	3	36	2	1	0.1	0.2	0.8	0	294
40410	Cereal, Kaboom	1.25 cup	30	115	3	24	2	1	0.3	0.3	0.4	0	150
40010	Cereal, Kix	1.33 cup	30	113	2	26	1	1	0.2	0.2	0.2	0	154
40011	Cereal, Life, plain	0.75 cup	32	120	3	25	2	1	0.3	0.5	0.5	0	1
40300	Cereal, Lucky Charms	1 cup	30	114	2	25	2	1	0.2	0.3	0.3	0	150
40124	Cereal, Mueslix, five grain muesli	1 cup	82	289	6	63	6	5	0.7	2.0	1.8	0	747
40449	Cereal, Oat Bran O's	0.75 cup	28	100	3	23	3	0	0.0	0.0	0.0	0	20
40302	Cereal, Oatmeal Raisin Crisp	1 cup	55	204	5	45	4	2	0.4	0.7	0.6	0	0
54233	Cereal, Oreo O's	0.75 cup	27	112	1	22	1	2	0.4	—	—	0	150
40216	Cereal, Product 19	1 cup	30	100	2	25	1	0	0.1	0.1	0.2	0	216
40018	Cereal, puffed rice	1 cup	14	54	1	12	0	0	0.0	0.0	0.0	0	0
40209	Cereal, raisin bran	1 cup	61	195	5	47	7	2	0.3	0.3	0.9	0	155
40210	Cereal, Rice Krispies	1.25 cup	33	119	2	28	0	0	0.1	0.1	0.1	0	153
40420	Cereal, Rice Krispies Treats	0.75 cup	30	122	1	26	0	2	0.4	0.9	0.2	0	152
40020	Cereal, Shredded Wheat, biscuits	1 ea	21	72	2	17	2	0	0.1	0.1	0.2	0	0
40068	Cereal, Smacks	0.75 cup	27	104	2	24	1	0	0.1	0.2	0.2	0	153
40211	Cereal, Special K	1 cup	31	117	7	22	1	0	0.1	0.1	0.2	0	230
40413	Cereal, Toasty O's	1 cup	30	112	3	22	3	2	0.4	0.7	0.6	0	375
40412	Cereal, Tootie Fruities	1 cup	32	125	2	28	1	1	0.3	0.3	0.2	0	218

PAGE KEY: A-96 Granola Bars, Cereal Bars, Diet Bars, Scones, and Tarts   A-96 Meals and Dishes   A-100 Meats   A-106 Nuts, Seeds, and Products   A-108 Poultry   A-110 Salad Dressings, Dips, and Mayonnaise   A-110 Salads   A-110 Sandwiches   A-114 Sauces and Gravies   A-114 Snack Foods—Chips, Pretzels, Popcorn   A-116 Soups, Stews, and Chilis   A-118 Spices, Flavors, and Seasonings   A-120 Sports Bars and Drinks   A-120 Supplemental Foods and Formulas   A-122 Sweeteners and Sweet Substitutes   A-122 Vegetables and Legumes   A-136 Weight Loss Bars and Drinks   A-138 Miscellaneous

Thia (mg)	Ribo (mg)	Niac (mg NE)	Vit B6 (mg)	Vit B12 (µg)	Fol (µg)	Vit C (mg)	Vit D (IU)	Vit E (mg AT)	Cal (mg)	Iron (mg)	Magn (mg)	Phos (mg)	Pota (mg)	Sodi (mg)	Zinc (mg)	Wat (%)	Alco (g)	Caff (g)
0.41	0.47	5.67	0.56	1.71	112.8	17.6	45.0	0.8	23	2.03	67.7	179	248	157	1.7	3	0.00	0.00
—	—	—	—	—	—	0.0	—	—	0	1.79	—	—	—	190	—	—	0.00	0.00
0.51	0.58	6.92	0.68	0.07	88.2	14.8	—	0.0	5	0.69	11.8	31	27	206	0.5	2	0.00	0.00
0.75	0.85	10.01	1.00	3.02	200.2	0.0	40.2	0.3	0	7.48	42.4	140	227	251	7.5	7	0.00	0.00
0.38	0.67	2.20	0.11	0.34	19.5	0.7	—	1.4	211	3.39	386.7	411	603	61	2.3	2	0.00	0.00
0.52	0.60	7.05	0.69	2.11	141.0	4.2	—	1.0	71	2.53	144.0	327	460	53	2.9	3	0.00	0.00
0.37	0.43	5.01	0.50	1.50	99.9	6.0	0.0	0.2	100	4.50	60.0	150	232	129	3.8	4	0.00	0.00
0.68	0.57	7.26	1.10	2.11	105.6	14.1	37.5	0.1	4	6.11	9.9	34	36	150	5.7	3	0.00	0.00
0.73	0.81	9.68	0.97	1.45	96.9	14.5	38.7	0.0	0	4.36	2.4	10	20	194	0.1	3	0.00	0.00
0.37	0.41	5.00	0.50	1.50	100.0	0.0	0.0	0.3	16	14.78	60.2	150	173	5	1.6	6	0.00	0.00
0.28	0.50	5.90	0.58	0.00	448.0	7.1	0.0	0.1	7	5.32	17.4	68	52	242	4.4	2	0.00	0.00
—	—	—	—	—	—	0.0	—	—	20	5.40	—	—	—	260	—	—	0.00	0.00
0.37	0.41	5.00	0.50	1.50	99.9	0.0	40.0	—	1	1.79	5.1	16	30	158	1.5	3	0.00	0.00
0.14	0.05	1.29	0.12	0.00	25.6	0.0	—	0.2	56	2.00	66.0	190	370	66	0.3	2	0.00	0.00
0.37	0.41	5.00	0.50	1.50	99.9	0.0	40.0	—	4	1.79	16.5	37	34	40	1.5	3	0.00	0.00
0.37	0.43	5.01	0.50	1.50	99.9	6.0	39.9	0.1	350	4.50	8.1	200	50	268	3.8	3	0.00	0.00
0.12	0.11	0.80	0.07	0.10	14.1	0.4	0.0	0.5	59	1.24	48.9	152	250	19	1.0	4	0.00	0.00
0.44	0.18	1.28	0.18	0.00	50.6	0.7	0.0	3.6	48	2.58	106.8	279	328	13	2.5	5	0.00	0.00
0.37	0.41	5.00	0.50	1.50	99.8	0.0	40.0	—	20	16.20	58.0	139	178	354	1.2	4	0.00	0.00
0.37	0.43	5.00	0.50	1.50	100.0	0.0	40.0	0.1	11	8.10	29.9	88	99	140	1.2	3	0.00	0.00
2.73	1.54	18.20	1.82	7.59	727.0	55.0	73.0	24.5	1091	16.39	44.0	182	166	645	13.6	3	0.00	0.00
0.07	0.10	0.69	0.05	0.00	11.1	0.0	0.0	0.5	16	0.87	32.4	102	99	204	0.8	2	0.00	0.00
0.15	0.17	2.00	0.20	0.60	40.0	0.0	—	—	0	0.72	—	—	100	15	—	5	0.00	0.00
0.15	0.05	0.51	1.73	5.15	343.6	25.8	—	11.6	15	1.84	85.1	25	85	1	1.3	3	0.00	0.00
0.37	0.41	5.00	0.50	1.50	100.1	0.0	40.0	—	11	8.10	21.4	60	70	187	0.3	3	0.00	0.00
0.43	0.50	5.90	0.58	0.00	420.1	7.1	0.0	0.2	3	5.30	0.0	38	42	162	4.4	3	0.00	0.00
0.37	0.43	5.00	0.50	1.50	100.0	0.0	40.0	—	5	2.70	10.7	27	35	215	1.5	2	0.00	0.00
0.30	0.34	3.91	0.38	1.15	80.0	0.0	—	1.8	11	12.68	26.7	83	95	264	0.7	3	0.00	0.00
0.37	0.43	5.01	0.50	1.50	200.1	6.0	39.9	0.1	100	8.10	15.9	80	63	285	3.8	2	0.00	0.00
0.37	0.43	5.01	0.50	1.50	200.1	6.3	42.3	0.1	150	8.10	8.1	40	35	267	3.8	2	0.00	0.00
0.40	0.46	5.50	0.55	0.00	416.0	0.0	0.0	0.2	112	8.94	30.7	133	91	164	4.1	4	0.00	0.00
0.37	0.43	5.01	0.50	1.50	200.1	6.0	39.9	0.1	100	4.50	15.9	60	57	203	3.8	2	0.00	0.00
0.75	0.83	9.84	0.99	3.27	196.8	0.8	0.0	8.9	67	8.93	82.0	215	369	107	7.5	8	0.00	0.00
0.15	0.17	2.00	0.20	0.60	40.0	0.0	—	—	0	0.72	—	—	90	90	—	3	0.00	0.00
0.37	0.41	5.01	0.50	1.49	100.1	6.1	0.0	1.4	20	4.51	40.2	100	200	216	3.8	6	0.00	0.00
0.37	0.41	5.00	0.50	1.50	99.9	0.0	40.0	—	5	1.79	14.9	32	49	128	1.5	2	0.00	
1.50	1.71	20.01	2.06	6.00	399.9	61.2	39.3	13.5	5	18.09	15.9	40	50	207	15.3	3	0.00	0.00
0.05	0.03	0.49	0.00	0.00	21.6	0.0	0.0	0.0	1	0.40	4.2	17	16	1	0.7	4	0.00	0.00
0.38	0.43	5.17	0.51	1.54	103.7	0.4	41.5	0.4	29	4.63	83.0	259	372	362	1.5	8	0.00	0.00
0.87	0.79	7.09	0.92	2.00	151.1	6.4	40.9	0.0	5	2.65	9.6	39	39	319	0.5	4	0.00	0.00
0.38	0.41	5.09	0.50	1.50	204.0	6.0	40.5	0.1	3	1.86	6.9	24	24	189	0.2	3	0.00	0.00
0.05	0.01	1.09	0.05	—	10.5	0.0	0.0	—	9	0.68	35.7	75	74	1	0.5	5	0.00	0.00
0.37	0.43	5.00	0.50	1.50	101.3	6.1	40.0	0.1	6	0.34	15.9	46	41	50	0.4	2	0.00	0.00
0.52	0.58	7.13	1.98	6.05	399.9	21.0	50.0	4.7	9	8.36	19.2	68	61	224	0.9	3	0.00	0.00
0.37	0.43	5.00	0.50	0.00	99.9	15.0	40.0	0.2	40	8.10	32.1	100	94	284	3.8	4	0.00	0.00
0.37	0.43	5.00	0.50	1.50	99.8	15.0	40.0	0.3	100	4.50	8.0	20	39	149	3.8	3	0.00	0.00

PAGE KEY: A-46 Beverage and Beverage Mixes   A-48 Other Beverages   A-48 Beverages, Alcoholic   A-50 Candies and Confections, Gum   A-54 Cereals, Breakfast Type
A-58 Cheese and Cheese Substitutes   A-60 Dairy Products and Substitutes   A-62 Desserts   A-68 Dessert Toppings   A-68 Eggs, Substitutes, and Egg Dishes   A-70 Ethnic Foods
A-74 Fast Foods/Restaurants   A-88 Fats, Oils, Margarines, Shortenings, and Substitutes   A-88 Fish, Seafood, and Shellfish   A-90 Food Additives
A-90 Fruit, Vegetable, or Blended Juices   A-92 Grains, Flours, and Fractions   A-92 Grain Products, Prepared and Baked Goods

Code	Food Name	Unit/ Amt	Wt (g)	Energy (kcal)	Prot (g)	Carb (g)	Fiber (g)	Fat (g)	Sat (g)	Mono (g)	Poly (g)	Chol (mg)	Vit A (RE)
40021	Cereal, Total, wheat	0.75 cup	30	97	3	22	3	1	0.2	0.1	0.3	0	150
40128	Cereal, Uncle Sam	1 cup	55	237	9	36	11	6	0.7	1.1	4.6	0	0
40307	Cereal, Wheaties	1 cup	30	107	3	24	3	1	0.2	0.3	0.3	0	150
40362	Cereal, whole grain, w/raisins, all nat	0.5 cup	50	195	4	41	3	3	0.7	0.8	0.5	0	1

CHEESE AND CHEESE SUBSTITUTES

Natural Cheeses

Code	Food Name	Unit/ Amt	Wt (g)	Energy (kcal)	Prot (g)	Carb (g)	Fiber (g)	Fat (g)	Sat (g)	Mono (g)	Poly (g)	Chol (mg)	Vit A (RE)
47855	Cheese, blue, 1" cube	1 ea	17	61	4	0	0	5	3.2	1.3	0.1	13	35
47859	Cheese, brie, 1" cube	1 ea	17	57	4	0	0	5	3.0	1.4	0.1	17	30
47861	Cheese, camembert, 1" cube	1 ea	17	51	3	0	0	4	2.6	1.2	0.1	12	41
47863	Cheese, cheddar, 1" cube	1 ea	17	69	4	0	0	6	3.6	1.6	0.2	18	46
1551	Cheese, cheddar, fat free, 1" cube	1 ea	28	40	8	1	0	0	0.0	0.0	0.0	3	60
1525	Cheese, cheddar, five peppercorn, 1" cube	1 ea	28	110	7	1	0	9	5.0	—	—	30	60
1008	Cheese, cheddar, shredded	0.25 cup	28	114	7	0	0	9	6.0	2.7	0.3	30	77
47864	Cheese, cheddar, slice, 1 oz	1 ea	28	114	7	0	0	9	6.0	2.7	0.3	30	77
47865	Cheese, colby, 1" cube	1 ea	17	68	4	0	0	6	3.5	1.6	0.2	16	47
1010	Cheese, colby, shredded	0.25 cup	28	111	7	0	0	9	5.7	2.6	0.3	27	77
47866	Cheese, colby, slice, 1 oz	1 ea	28	112	7	1	0	9	5.7	2.6	0.3	27	77
47871	Cheese, feta, 1" cube	1 ea	17	45	2	1	0	4	2.5	0.8	0.1	15	21
47873	Cheese, fontina, 1" cube	1 ea	15	58	4	0	0	5	2.9	1.3	0.2	17	40
1078	Cheese, goat, hard	3.6 oz	100	452	31	2	0	36	24.6	8.1	0.8	105	494
1080	Cheese, goat, soft	3.6 oz	100	268	19	1	0	21	14.6	4.8	0.5	46	293
1054	Cheese, gouda	1 oz	28	101	7	1	0	8	5.0	2.2	0.2	32	47
47881	Cheese, limburger, 1" cube	1 ea	18	59	4	0	0	5	3.0	1.5	0.1	16	61
47884	Cheese, monterey jack, 1" cube	1 ea	17	64	4	0	0	5	3.3	1.5	0.2	15	35
1017	Cheese, monterey jack, shredded	0.25 cup	28	105	7	0	0	9	5.4	2.5	0.3	25	58
47885	Cheese, monterey jack, slice, 1 oz	1 ea	28	106	7	0	0	9	5.4	2.5	0.3	25	58
1553	Cheese, mozzarella, fat free, 1" cube	1 ea	28	40	8	1	0	0	0.0	0.0	0.0	3	60
47891	Cheese, muenster, 1" cube	1 ea	18	64	4	0	0	5	3.3	1.5	0.1	17	52
1021	Cheese, muenster, shredded	0.25 cup	28	104	7	0	0	8	5.4	2.5	0.2	27	84
1075	Cheese, parmesan, grated	1 Tbs	5	22	2	0	0	1	0.9	0.4	0.1	4	6
1061	Cheese, parmesan, hard, 1" cube	1 ea	10	40	4	0	0	3	1.7	0.8	0.1	7	11
1510	Cheese, pepper jack, 1" cube	1 ea	28	110	7	1	0	9	5.0	—	—	30	60
47899	Cheese, provolone, 1" cube	1 ea	17	60	4	0	0	5	2.9	1.3	0.1	12	41
47900	Cheese, provolone, slice, 1 oz	1 ea	28	100	7	1	0	8	4.8	2.1	0.2	20	69
1064	Cheese, ricotta, whole milk	0.25 cup	62	108	7	2	0	8	5.1	2.2	0.2	32	76
13348	Cheese, string, mozzarella, sticks, 1 oz	1 ea	28	50	8	1	0	2	1.0	—	—	5	40
47911	Cheese, sweitzer, 1" cube	1 ea	15	57	4	1	0	4	2.7	1.1	0.1	14	34
47908	Cheese, Swiss, 1" cube	1 ea	15	57	4	1	0	4	2.7	1.1	0.1	14	34
1027	Cheese, Swiss, shredded	0.25 cup	27	103	7	1	0	8	4.8	2.0	0.3	25	61
47912	Cheese, Swiss, slice, 1 oz	1 ea	28	108	8	2	0	8	5.0	2.1	0.3	26	64
1508	Cottage Cheese	0.5 cup	114	100	13	4	0	4	3.0	—	—	15	60
1047	Cottage Cheese, 1% fat	0.5 cup	113	81	14	3	0	1	0.7	0.3	0.0	5	12
1014	Cottage Cheese, 2% fat	0.5 cup	113	102	16	4	0	2	1.4	0.6	0.1	9	25
47848	Cottage Cheese, fat free, small curd	0.5 cup	126	90	12	8	0	0	0.0	0.0	0.0	10	40
1015	Cream Cheese	2 Tbs	29	101	2	1	0	10	6.4	2.9	0.4	32	108
1452	Cream Cheese, fat free	2 Tbs	29	28	4	2	0	0	0.3	0.1	0.0	2	81
1083	Cream Cheese, soft	2 Tbs	30	100	2	1	0	10	7.0	—	—	30	60

Thia (mg)	Ribo (mg)	Niac (mg NE)	Vit B6 (mg)	Vit B12 (µg)	Fol (µg)	Vit C (mg)	Vit D (IU)	Vit E (mg AT)	Cal (mg)	Iron (mg)	Magn (mg)	Phos (mg)	Pota (mg)	Sodi (mg)	Zinc (mg)	Wat (%)	Alco (g)	Caff (g)
2.10	2.42	26.43	2.81	6.42	477.0	60.0	39.9	13.5	1104	22.35	39.3	89	103	192	17.5	3	0.00	0.00
1.25	1.45	8.97	0.52	0.00	29.2	33.8	—	0.4	52	2.22	113.3	206	245	113	2.1	4	0.00	0.00
0.75	0.85	9.98	1.00	3.00	200.1	6.0	39.9	0.2	0	8.10	32.1	100	111	218	7.5	3	0.00	0.00
0.15	0.09	0.93	0.07	0.05	12.0	0.3	0.0	0.9	30	1.32	42.5	134	204	118	1.0	4	0.00	0.00
0.00	0.07	0.18	0.02	0.20	6.2	0.0	—	0.0	91	0.05	4.0	67	44	241	0.5	42	0.00	0.00
0.00	0.09	0.05	0.03	0.28	11.1	0.0	—	0.0	31	0.09	3.4	32	26	107	0.4	48	0.00	0.00
0.00	0.07	0.10	0.03	0.21	10.5	0.0	2.0	0.0	66	0.05	3.4	59	32	143	0.4	52	0.00	0.00
0.00	0.05	0.00	0.00	0.14	3.1	0.0	2.0	0.0	123	0.11	4.8	87	17	106	0.5	37	0.00	0.00
—	—	—	—	—	—	—	—	—	400	—	—	—	—	220	—	63	0.00	0.00
—	—	—	—	—	—	0.0	—	—	200	0.00	—	—	—	180	—	36	0.00	0.00
0.00	0.10	0.01	0.01	0.23	5.1	0.0	3.4	0.1	204	0.18	7.9	145	28	175	0.9	37	0.00	0.00
0.00	0.10	0.01	0.01	0.23	5.1	0.0	3.4	0.1	204	0.18	7.9	145	28	176	0.9	37	0.00	0.00
0.00	0.05	0.01	0.00	0.14	3.1	0.0	—	0.0	118	0.12	4.5	79	22	104	0.5	38	0.00	0.00
0.00	0.10	0.02	0.01	0.23	5.1	0.0	—	0.1	194	0.20	7.3	129	36	171	0.9	38	0.00	0.00
0.00	0.10	0.02	0.01	0.23	5.1	0.0	—	0.1	194	0.21	7.4	130	36	171	0.9	38	0.00	0.00
0.02	0.14	0.17	0.07	0.28	5.4	0.0	—	0.0	84	0.10	3.2	57	11	190	0.5	55	0.00	0.00
0.00	0.02	0.01	0.00	0.25	0.9	0.0	—	0.0	82	0.02	2.1	52	10	120	0.5	38	0.00	0.00
0.14	1.19	2.40	0.07	0.11	4.0	0.0	—	0.3	895	1.87	54.0	729	48	346	1.6	29	0.00	0.00
0.07	0.37	0.43	0.25	0.18	12.0	0.0	—	0.2	140	1.89	16.0	256	26	368	0.9	61	0.00	0.00
0.00	0.09	0.01	0.01	0.43	6.0	0.0	2.7	0.1	198	0.07	8.2	155	34	232	1.1	41	0.00	0.00
0.00	0.09	0.02	0.01	0.18	10.4	0.0	—	0.0	89	0.01	3.8	71	23	144	0.4	48	0.00	0.00
0.00	0.07	0.01	0.00	0.14	3.1	0.0	—	0.0	128	0.11	4.6	76	14	92	0.5	41	0.00	0.00
0.00	0.10	0.02	0.01	0.23	5.1	0.0	—	0.1	211	0.20	7.6	125	23	151	0.8	41	0.00	0.00
0.00	0.10	0.02	0.01	0.23	5.1	0.0	—	0.1	211	0.20	7.7	126	23	152	0.9	41	0.00	0.00
—	—	—	—	—	—	—	—	—	400	—	—	—	—	220	—	63	0.00	0.00
0.00	0.05	0.01	0.00	0.25	2.1	0.0	—	0.0	125	0.07	4.7	82	23	110	0.5	42	0.00	0.00
0.00	0.09	0.02	0.01	0.41	3.4	0.0	—	0.1	203	0.11	7.6	132	38	177	0.8	42	0.00	0.00
0.00	0.01	0.00	0.00	0.10	0.5	0.0	—	0.0	55	0.03	1.9	36	6	76	0.2	21	0.00	0.00
0.00	0.02	0.02	0.00	0.11	0.7	0.0	2.9	0.0	122	0.07	4.5	71	9	165	0.3	29	0.00	0.00
—	—	—	—	—	—	0.0	—	—	200	0.00	—	—	—	170	—	36	0.00	0.00
0.00	0.05	0.02	0.00	0.25	1.7	0.0	—	0.0	129	0.09	4.8	84	23	149	0.5	41	0.00	0.00
0.00	0.09	0.03	0.01	0.40	2.8	0.0	—	0.1	214	0.15	7.9	141	39	248	0.9	41	0.00	0.00
0.00	0.11	0.05	0.02	0.20	7.4	0.0	—	0.1	128	0.23	6.8	98	65	52	0.7	72	0.00	0.00
—	—	—	—	—	—	0.0	—	—	200	0.00	—	—	—	220	—	58	0.00	0.00
0.00	0.03	0.00	0.00	0.50	0.9	0.0	6.6	0.1	119	0.02	5.7	85	12	29	0.7	37	0.00	0.00
0.00	0.03	0.00	0.00	0.50	0.9	0.0	6.6	0.1	119	0.02	5.7	85	12	29	0.7	37	0.00	0.00
0.01	0.07	0.01	0.01	0.89	1.6	0.0	11.9	0.1	214	0.05	10.3	153	21	52	1.2	37	0.00	0.00
0.01	0.07	0.02	0.01	0.94	1.7	0.0	12.5	0.1	224	0.05	10.8	161	22	54	1.2	37	0.00	0.00
—	—	—	—	—	—	0.0	—	—	100	0.00	—	—	—	400	—	80	0.00	0.00
0.01	0.18	0.14	0.07	0.70	13.6	0.0	—	0.0	69	0.15	5.7	151	97	459	0.4	82	0.00	0.00
0.02	0.20	0.15	0.09	0.80	14.7	0.0	—	0.0	78	0.18	6.8	171	108	459	0.5	79	0.00	0.00
—	—	—	—	—	—	0.0	—	—	80	0.00	—	—	—	450	—	—	0.00	0.00
0.00	0.05	0.02	0.00	0.11	3.8	0.0	—	0.1	23	0.34	1.7	30	35	86	0.2	54	0.00	0.00
0.00	0.05	0.05	0.00	0.15	10.7	0.0	—	0.0	54	0.05	4.1	126	47	158	0.3	76	0.00	0.00
—	0.02	—	—	0.00	—	0.0	—	—	20	0.00	0.0	40	40	100	0.0	56	0.00	0.00

PAGE KEY: A-46 Beverage and Beverage Mixes A-48 Other Beverages A-48 Beverages, Alcoholic A-50 Candies and Confections, Gum A-54 Cereals, Breakfast Type A-58 Cheese and Cheese Substitutes A-60 Dairy Products and Substitutes A-62 Desserts A-68 Dessert Toppings A-68 Eggs, Substitutes, and Egg Dishes A-70 Ethnic Foods A-74 Fast Foods/Restaurants A-88 Fats, Oils, Margarines, Shortenings, and Substitutes A-88 Fish, Seafood, and Shellfish A-90 Food Additives A-90 Fruit, Vegetable, or Blended Juices A-92 Grains, Flours, and Fractions A-92 Grain Products, Prepared and Baked Goods

Code	Food Name	Unit/ Amt	Wt (g)	Energy (kcal)	Prot (g)	Carb (g)	Fiber (g)	Fat (g)	Sat (g)	Mono (g)	Poly (g)	Chol (mg)	Vit A (RE)
Process Cheese and Cheese Substitutes													
1001	Cheese Product, American, cold pack	1 oz	28	94	6	2	0	7	4.4	2.0	0.2	18	48
1376	Cheese Product, monterey, past, proc, slice	1 pce	21	70	4	1	0	5	3.0	—	—	20	20
48288	Cheese Substitute	3.6 oz	100	141	22	9	0	1	0.8	0.4	0.0	6	10
48332	Cheese, American, past, proc, fat free, 1" cube	1 ea	16	24	4	2	0	0	0.1	0.0	0.0	2	70
48314	Cheese, American, past, proc, low fat, 1" cube	1 ea	18	32	4	1	0	1	0.8	0.4	0.0	6	11
1096	Cheese, American, past, proc, low fat, shredded	1 cup	113	203	28	4	0	8	5.0	2.3	0.3	40	67
1092	Cheese, mozzarella, imit	0.25 cup	28	70	3	7	0	3	1.0	1.8	0.5	0	123
47918	Cheese, pimento, past, proc, 1" cube	1 ea	18	66	4	0	0	5	3.4	1.6	0.2	16	46
48311	Cottage Cheese Substitute, soy	1 cup	225	340	28	16	0	18	2.6	4.0	10.3	0	9
DAIRY PRODUCTS AND SUBSTITUTES													
Creams and Substitutes													
54390	Cream Substitute, light	1 cup	242	167	2	22	0	8	2.2	4.9	1.0	0	1
506	Cream Substitute, pwd	1 tsp	2	11	0	1	0	1	0.6	0.0	0.0	0	0
500	Cream, half & half	2 Tbs	30	39	1	1	0	3	2.1	1.0	0.1	11	30
54384	Cream, half & half, fat free	1 Tbs	15	9	0	1	0	0	0.1	0.1	0.0	1	2
501	Cream, light	1 Tbs	15	29	0	1	0	3	1.8	0.8	0.1	10	28
502	Cream, whipping, heavy	2 Tbs	30	103	1	1	0	11	6.9	3.2	0.4	41	124
503	Cream, whipping, heavy, whipped	2 Tbs	15	52	0	0	0	6	3.4	1.6	0.2	20	62
54262	Creamer, non-dairy	1 Tbs	17	20	0	2	0	1	0.0	0.5	0.0	0	0
54315	Creamer, soy milk, plain	1 Tbs	15	15	0	1	0	1	0.0	—	—	0	0
504	Sour Cream, cultured	2 Tbs	29	62	1	1	0	6	3.8	1.7	0.2	13	52
54383	Sour Cream, fat free	3.6 oz	100	74	3	16	0	0	0.0	0.0	0.0	9	74
505	Sour Cream, imitation, cultured	2 Tbs	29	60	1	2	0	6	5.1	0.2	0.0	0	0
Milks and Non-Dairy Milks													
7	Buttermilk, low fat, cultured	1 cup	245	98	8	12	0	2	1.3	0.6	0.1	10	17
17	Eggnog	1 cup	254	343	10	34	0	19	11.3	5.7	0.9	150	117
81	Milk Substitute, fluid, w/hydrog veg oil	1 cup	244	149	4	15	0	8	1.9	4.9	1.2	0	0
4	Milk, 1%, w/add vit A & D	1 cup	244	102	8	12	0	2	1.5	0.7	0.1	12	142
2	Milk, 2%, w/add vit A & D	1 cup	244	122	8	11	0	5	3.1	1.4	0.2	20	134
18	Milk, chocolate, 2%, cmrcl	1 cup	250	180	8	26	1	5	3.1	1.5	0.2	18	138
59	Milk, chocolate, nonfat/skim	1 cup	250	144	9	27	1	1	0.7	0.3	0.0	4	142
173	Milk, evaporated	2 Tbs	32	40	2	3	0	2	1.5	0.4	0.1	10	0
23	Milk, goat	1 cup	244	168	9	11	0	10	6.5	2.7	0.4	27	142
1	Milk, whole, 3.25%	1 cup	244	146	8	11	0	8	4.6	2.0	0.5	24	70
66	Milk, whole, dry pwd	1 Tbs	8	40	2	3	0	2	1.3	0.6	0.1	8	21
20584	Rice Milk	1 cup	245	144	3	28	2	2	0.3	0.5	1.1	0	0
20033	Soy Milk	1 cup	245	127	11	12	3	5	0.6	0.9	1.9	0	152
20920	Soy Milk, chocolate	1 cup	250	140	5	23	0	4	0.0	—	—	0	100
20493	Tea, rice	1 cup	245	144	3	28	2	2	0.3	0.5	1.1	0	0
Yogurt													
2425	Yogurt, banana creme, lowfat, 6 oz ctn	1 ea	170	170	5	33	0	2	1.0	—	—	10	150
2836	Yogurt, cherry, fruit on the bottom, 8 oz ctn	1 ea	227	220	9	42	1	2	1.0	—	—	10	0
2574	Yogurt, coffee, nonfat, 8 oz ctn	1 ea	227	207	12	40	0	0	0.2	0.1	0.0	4	4
72088	Yogurt, fruit, nonfat	1 cup	245	230	11	47	0	0	0.3	0.1	0.0	5	7
2426	Yogurt, plain custard	1 cup	227	130	15	19	0	0	0.0	0.0	0.0	5	0

PAGE KEY: A-96 Granola Bars, Cereal Bars, Diet Bars, Scones, and Tarts   A-96 Meals and Dishes   A-100 Meats   A-106 Nuts, Seeds, and Products   A-108 Poultry   A-110 Salad Dressings, Dips, and Mayonnaise   A-110 Salads   A-110 Sandwiches   A-114 Sauces and Gravies   A-114 Snack Foods—Chips, Pretzels, Popcorn   A-116 Soups, Stews, and Chilis   A-118 Spices, Flavors, and Seasonings   A-120 Sports Bars and Drinks   A-120 Supplemental Foods and Formulas   A-122 Sweeteners and Sweet Substitutes   A-122 Vegetables and Legumes   A-136 Weight Loss Bars and Drinks   A-138 Miscellaneous

Thia (mg)	Ribo (mg)	Niac (mg NE)	Vit B6 (mg)	Vit B12 (µg)	Fol (µg)	Vit C (mg)	Vit D (IU)	Vit E (mg AT)	Cal (mg)	Iron (mg)	Magn (mg)	Phos (mg)	Pota (mg)	Sodi (mg)	Zinc (mg)	Wat (%)	Alco (g)	Caff (g)
0.00	0.12	0.01	0.03	0.36	1.4	0.0	—	0.2	141	0.23	8.5	113	103	274	0.9	43	0.00	0.00
—	—	—	—	—	—	0.0	—	—	100	0.00	—	—	—	280	—	—	0.00	0.00
0.02	0.47	0.15	0.12	1.23	8.0	0.0	—	0.0	552	0.91	35.0	499	336	1239	3.3	64	0.00	0.00
0.00	0.07	0.02	0.00	0.18	4.3	0.0	—	0.0	110	0.03	5.8	150	46	244	0.5	57	0.00	0.00
0.00	0.07	0.00	0.00	0.14	1.6	0.0	—	0.0	123	0.07	4.3	149	32	257	0.6	59	0.00	0.00
0.02	0.43	0.09	0.09	0.87	10.2	0.0	—	0.3	773	0.49	27.1	935	203	1616	3.8	59	0.00	0.00
0.00	0.12	0.09	0.00	0.23	3.1	0.0	0.6	0.6	172	0.10	11.6	165	129	194	0.5	47	0.00	0.00
0.00	0.05	0.00	0.00	0.11	1.4	0.4	—	0.1	107	0.07	3.8	130	28	250	0.5	39	0.00	0.00
0.00	0.31	1.12	0.15	0.00	49.5	0.0	—	1.4	423	12.60	513.0	500	448	45	3.9	71	0.00	0.00
0.00	0.00	0.00	0.00	0.00	0.0	0.0	—	0.7	2	1.36	0.0	182	428	145	0.1	86	0.00	0.00
0.00	0.00	0.00	0.00	0.00	0.0	0.0	—	0.0	0	0.01	0.1	8	16	4	0.0	2	0.00	0.00
0.00	0.03	0.01	0.00	0.10	0.9	0.3	—	0.1	32	0.01	3.0	29	39	12	0.2	81	0.00	0.00
0.00	0.03	0.01	0.00	0.07	0.6	0.1	—	0.0	14	0.00	2.4	23	31	22	0.1	86	0.00	0.00
0.00	0.01	0.00	0.00	0.02	0.3	0.1	—	0.1	14	0.00	1.4	12	18	6	0.0	74	0.00	0.00
0.00	0.02	0.00	0.00	0.05	1.2	0.2	15.5	0.3	19	0.00	2.1	18	22	11	0.1	58	0.00	0.00
0.00	0.01	0.00	0.00	0.02	0.6	0.1	7.8	0.2	10	0.00	1.0	9	11	6	0.1	58	0.00	0.00
—	—	—	—	—	—	0.0	—	—	0	0.00	—	—	25	0	—	82	0.00	0.00
—	—	—	—	—	—	0.0	—	—	0	0.00	—	—	—	5	—	—	0.00	0.00
0.00	0.03	0.01	0.00	0.09	3.2	0.3	—	0.2	33	0.01	3.2	24	41	15	0.1	71	0.00	0.00
0.03	0.15	0.07	0.01	0.30	11.0	0.0	—	0.0	125	0.00	10.0	95	129	141	0.5	81	0.00	0.00
0.00	0.00	0.00	0.00	0.00	0.0	0.0	—	0.2	1	0.10	1.7	13	46	29	0.3	71	0.00	0.00
0.07	0.37	0.14	0.07	0.54	12.2	2.5	—	0.1	284	0.11	27.0	218	370	257	1.0	90	0.00	0.00
0.09	0.47	0.27	0.12	1.13	2.5	3.8	—	0.5	330	0.50	48.3	277	419	137	1.2	74	0.00	0.00
0.02	0.20	0.00	0.00	0.00	0.0	0.0	—	0.7	81	0.94	14.6	181	278	190	2.9	88	0.00	0.00
0.05	0.44	0.23	0.09	1.07	12.2	0.0	126.8	0.0	290	0.07	26.8	232	366	107	1.0	90	0.00	0.00
0.10	0.44	0.21	0.09	1.12	12.2	0.5	104.8	0.1	285	0.07	26.8	229	366	100	1.0	89	0.00	0.00
0.09	0.40	0.31	0.10	0.85	12.5	2.2	100.0	0.1	285	0.60	32.5	255	422	150	1.0	84	0.00	5.00
0.09	0.34	0.28	0.10	0.87	13.6	2.3	100.0	0.1	292	0.68	45.5	265	486	121	1.2	85	0.00	7.50
0.00	0.10	0.05	0.01	0.05	2.5	0.0	25.0	0.0	80	0.00	7.6	60	95	30	0.2	76	0.00	0.00
0.11	0.34	0.68	0.10	0.17	2.4	3.2	29.3	0.2	327	0.11	34.2	271	498	122	0.7	87	0.00	0.00
0.10	0.44	0.25	0.09	1.07	12.2	0.0	98.7	0.1	276	0.07	24.4	222	349	98	1.0	88	0.00	0.00
0.01	0.10	0.05	0.01	0.25	3.0	0.7	25.0	0.0	73	0.03	6.8	62	106	30	0.3	2	0.00	0.00
0.09	0.02	1.86	0.17	0.00	3.4	0.0	—	1.3	15	0.50	53.6	96	50	86	0.8	86	0.00	—
0.15	0.11	0.70	0.23	2.99	39.2	0.0	39.2	3.3	93	2.70	61.2	135	304	135	1.1	88	0.00	0.00
—	0.50	—	—	3.00	24.0	0.0	120.0	—	300	1.44	—	—	350	75	0.6	—	0.00	—
0.09	0.02	1.86	0.17	0.00	3.4	0.0	—	1.3	15	0.50	53.6	96	50	86	0.8	86	0.00	—
—	—	—	—	—	—	0.0	80.0	—	200	0.00	—	150	260	80	—	76	0.00	0.00
—	—	—	—	—	—	0.0	—	—	300	0.00	—	—	480	150	—	77	0.00	0.00
0.10	0.47	0.25	0.10	1.24	24.7	1.8	2.3	0.0	404	0.20	38.7	318	518	155	2.0	76	0.00	0.00
0.10	0.43	0.25	0.10	1.14	22.1	1.7	—	0.1	372	0.17	36.8	292	475	142	1.8	75	0.00	0.00
0.15	0.50	—	—	—	—	0.0	—	—	400	0.00	32.0	300	550	220	—	84	0.00	0.00

Code	Food Name	Unit/ Amt	Wt (g)	Energy (kcal)	Prot (g)	Carb (g)	Fiber (g)	Fat (g)	Sat (g)	Mono (g)	Poly (g)	Chol (mg)	Vit A (RE)
2000	Yogurt, plain, low fat, 12g prot/8 oz	1 cup	245	154	13	17	0	4	2.5	1.0	0.1	15	34
71587	Yogurt, soy, vanilla, 6 oz ctn	1 ea	170	120	4	23	1	2	0.0	—	—	0	10
7546	Yogurt, tofu	1 cup	262	246	9	42	1	5	0.7	1.0	2.7	0	10
2015	Yogurt, vanilla, low fat	1 cup	245	208	12	34	0	3	2.0	0.8	0.1	12	29

DESSERTS

Brownies and Bars

Code	Food Name	Unit/ Amt	Wt (g)	Energy (kcal)	Prot (g)	Carb (g)	Fiber (g)	Fat (g)	Sat (g)	Mono (g)	Poly (g)	Chol (mg)	Vit A (RE)
47100	Bar, apple cinnamon, fruit & oatmeal, 1.3 oz pce	1 ea	37	136	2	26	1	3	0.4	1.0	0.2	0	261
23171	Bar, Rice Krispie, 1 oz pce	1 ea	28	107	1	20	0	3	0.6	1.3	0.8	0	85
62904	Brownie, cmrcl prep, square, lrg, 2 3/4" x 7/8"	1 ea	56	227	3	36	1	9	2.4	5.0	1.3	10	11
47019	Brownie, prep f/recipe, 2" square	1 ea	24	112	1	12	1	7	1.8	2.6	2.3	18	46

Cakes & Cheesecakes

Code	Food Name	Unit/ Amt	Wt (g)	Energy (kcal)	Prot (g)	Carb (g)	Fiber (g)	Fat (g)	Sat (g)	Mono (g)	Poly (g)	Chol (mg)	Vit A (RE)
46004	Cake, angel food, cmrcl prep, 1/12 pce	1 pce	28	73	2	16	0	0	0.0	0.0	0.1	0	0
46102	Cake, applesauce, w/icing	1 pce	108	399	3	69	1	13	2.7	5.9	4.0	20	39
46103	Cake, banana, w/o icing	1 pce	87	262	3	46	1	8	1.6	3.6	2.1	32	83
46262	Cake, carrot, buttercream frosted	1 pce	71	280	2	36	1	15	3.5	—	—	35	100
46062	Cake, chocolate, prep f/rec, w/o frosting 9" whl or 1/12 pce	1 pce	95	340	5	51	2	14	5.2	5.7	2.6	55	39
46120	Cake, chocolate, w/fluffy white icing, prep f/recipe, slice	1 pce	91	280	3	43	1	11	2.7	—	—	23	50
46118	Cake, chocolate, w/vanilla icing, 1/12 piece	1 pce	103	367	3	53	1	17	4.3	—	—	23	52
46005	Cake, coffee, cinnamon, w/crumb topping prep f/mix, 1/8 pce	1 pce	56	178	3	30	1	5	1.0	2.2	1.8	27	20
42721	Cake, Ding Dongs, w/cream filling, Hostess	1 ea	80	368	3	45	2	19	11.0	4.0	1.2	14	—
46205	Cake, fruit, cmrcl prep	1 pce	43	139	1	26	2	4	0.5	1.8	1.4	2	3
45562	Cake, funnel	1 pce	90	278	7	29	1	14	2.7	4.4	6.3	63	58
46000	Cake, gingerbread, prep f/rec, 1/9 of 8" square	1 pce	74	263	3	36	1	12	3.1	5.3	3.1	24	10
46108	Cake, graham cracker	1 pce	45	159	3	22	0	7	1.6	3.2	1.6	33	66
46111	Cake, lemon, w/icing	1 pce	109	385	3	71	1	11	1.9	4.8	3.4	34	62
46070	Cake, pineapple upside down, prep f/rec, 1/9th of 8" square	1 pce	115	367	4	58	1	14	3.4	6.0	3.8	25	75
71261	Cake, pound, w/butter, cmrcl prep, 1/10 pce	1 pce	30	116	2	15	0	6	3.5	1.8	0.3	66	47
46077	Cake, shortcake, biscuit type, prep f/recipe	3.6 oz	100	346	6	48	1	14	3.8	6.0	3.6	3	19
46116	Cake, spice, w/icing	1 pce	109	368	5	62	1	12	3.2	5.9	1.9	50	39
46115	Cake, sponge, chocolate, w/o icing	1 pce	66	197	5	36	1	4	1.4	1.5	0.5	139	62
46455	Cake, yellow, prep f/dry mix, 2" x 3" pce	1 pce	55	150	2	27	0	4	1.0	2.5	0.0	0	0
46012	Cake, yellow, w/chocolate icing, cmrcl prep, 1/8 of 18 oz	1 pce	64	243	2	35	1	11	3.0	6.1	1.4	35	21
62352	Cheesecake, cherry	1 ea	113	330	6	27	1	22	13.0	—	—	100	300
49001	Cheesecake, no bake, prep f/dry mix, 1/12 of 9"	1 pce	99	271	5	35	2	13	6.6	4.5	0.8	29	99
46426	Cupcake, chocolate, w/frosting, low fat	1 ea	43	131	2	29	2	2	0.5	0.8	0.2	0	0

Cookies

Code	Food Name	Unit/ Amt	Wt (g)	Energy (kcal)	Prot (g)	Carb (g)	Fiber (g)	Fat (g)	Sat (g)	Mono (g)	Poly (g)	Chol (mg)	Vit A (RE)
90634	Cookie Crumbs, chocolate wafer	1 cup	112	485	7	81	4	16	4.7	5.4	4.7	2	3
62910	Cookie Crumbs, vanilla wafer, lower fat	1 cup	80	353	4	59	2	12	3.1	5.2	3.1	41	6
47073	Cookie, almond	2 ea	20	103	2	10	1	6	1.0	3.4	1.6	9	41
47074	Cookie, applesauce	2 ea	36	132	2	23	1	4	0.9	2.0	1.2	9	42
47746	Cookie, biscotti, chocolate	1 ea	30	120	1	15	2	6	3.0	—	—	20	0
90163	Cookie, biscuit, arrowroot	1 ea	5	22	0	4	0	1	0.2	0.4	0.1	0	0
90164	Cookie, biscuit, tea	1 ea	5	22	0	4	0	1	0.2	0.4	0.1	0	0
90637	Cookie, chocolate chip bar, prep w/marg f/recipe, 2" square	1 ea	32	156	2	19	1	9	2.6	3.3	2.7	10	50
47031	Cookie, chocolate chip, enrich, higher fat, cmrcl, med 2.25"	1 ea	10	49	1	6	0	2	0.8	1.3	0.1	0	0
42726	Cookie, chocolate chip, refrig dough	1 ea	28	127	1	18	1	6	1.8	2.5	0.5	—	—

PAGE KEY: A-96 Granola Bars, Cereal Bars, Diet Bars, Scones, and Tarts   A-96 Meals and Dishes   A-100 Meats   A-106 Nuts, Seeds, and Products   A-108 Poultry   A-110 Salad Dressings, Dips, and Mayonnaise   A-110 Salads   A-110 Sandwiches   A-114 Sauces and Gravies   A-114 Snack Foods—Chips, Pretzels, Popcorn   A-116 Soups, Stews, and Chilis   A-118 Spices, Flavors, and Seasonings   A-120 Sports Bars and Drinks   A-120 Supplemental Foods and Formulas   A-122 Sweeteners and Sweet Substitutes   A-122 Vegetables and Legumes   A-136 Weight Loss Bars and Drinks   A-138 Miscellaneous

Thia (mg)	Ribo (mg)	Niac (mg NE)	Vit B6 (mg)	Vit B12 (µg)	Fol (µg)	Vit C (mg)	Vit D (IU)	Vit E (mg AT)	Cal (mg)	Iron (mg)	Magn (mg)	Phos (mg)	Pota (mg)	Sodi (mg)	Zinc (mg)	Wat (%)	Alco (g)	Caff (g)
0.10	0.51	0.28	0.11	1.37	27.0	2.0	—	0.1	448	0.20	41.7	353	573	172	2.2	85	0.00	0.00
—	—	—	—	—	—	0.0	—	—	500	0.72	—	—	—	20	—	—	0.00	0.00
0.15	0.05	0.62	0.05	0.00	15.7	6.5	—	0.8	309	2.77	104.8	100	123	92	0.8	78	0.00	0.00
0.10	0.49	0.25	0.10	1.29	27.0	2.0	—	0.0	419	0.17	39.2	331	537	162	2.0	79	0.00	0.00
0.23	0.49	5.80	0.57	0.00	116.1	0.2	0.0	0.0	10	0.46	8.2	34	49	85	0.2	15	0.00	0.00
0.10	0.10	1.30	0.12	0.00	27.5	3.9	0.0	0.4	2	0.50	4.2	12	12	123	0.1	13	0.00	0.00
0.14	0.11	0.95	0.01	0.03	26.3	0.0	—	0.1	16	1.25	17.4	57	83	175	0.4	14	0.00	1.12
0.02	0.05	0.23	0.01	0.03	7.0	0.1	—	0.7	14	0.43	12.7	32	42	82	0.2	13	0.00	—
0.02	0.14	0.25	0.00	0.01	9.9	0.0	—	0.0	40	0.15	3.4	9	26	212	0.0	33	0.00	0.00
0.11	0.11	0.99	0.05	0.05	5.2	0.9	3.5	1.8	20	1.28	10.1	45	137	163	0.2	20	0.07	0.00
0.14	0.17	1.16	0.20	0.07	11.5	2.9	3.1	1.2	26	1.11	15.5	50	168	181	0.3	33	0.10	0.00
0.05	0.07	0.40	—	—	8.0	0.0	—	—	20	0.72	—	—	—	230	—	—	0.00	0.00
0.12	0.20	1.08	0.03	0.15	25.6	0.2	—	1.5	57	1.52	30.4	101	133	299	0.7	24	0.00	—
0.10	0.12	0.82	0.01	0.07	29.3	0.1	2.9	0.9	18	0.93	10.8	41	64	207	0.3	36	0.00	—
0.12	0.12	0.94	0.01	0.09	33.4	0.2	4.6	0.9	23	1.02	11.3	47	61	232	0.3	28	0.00	—
0.09	0.10	0.85	0.02	0.07	26.9	0.1	—	0.1	76	0.80	10.1	120	63	236	0.3	30	0.00	0.00
—	—	—	—	—	—	—	—	—	3	1.84	—	—	—	241	—	12	0.00	—
0.01	0.03	0.34	0.01	0.00	8.6	0.2	—	0.4	14	0.88	6.9	22	66	116	0.1	25	0.00	0.00
0.23	0.31	1.86	0.05	0.23	13.6	0.4	—	2.4	128	1.86	17.7	137	155	117	0.6	42	0.00	0.00
0.14	0.11	1.28	0.14	0.03	24.4	0.1	—	1.8	53	2.13	51.8	40	325	242	0.3	28	0.00	0.00
0.05	0.10	0.61	0.01	0.09	5.2	0.1	7.2	1.0	51	0.75	6.9	52	50	189	0.3	28	0.07	0.00
0.07	0.11	0.73	0.03	0.11	6.0	1.5	4.4	1.6	67	0.81	5.9	154	53	359	0.2	22	0.00	0.00
0.18	0.18	1.37	0.03	0.09	29.9	1.4	—	1.5	138	1.70	14.9	94	129	367	0.4	32	0.00	0.00
0.03	0.07	0.38	0.00	0.07	12.3	0.0	—	0.2	10	0.40	3.3	41	36	119	0.1	25	0.00	0.00
0.31	0.27	2.56	0.02	0.07	53.0	0.2	—	2.0	205	2.53	16.0	143	106	506	0.5	28	0.00	0.00
0.12	0.18	1.12	0.03	0.11	9.1	0.1	8.7	2.2	76	1.50	13.4	209	136	281	0.4	27	0.17	0.00
0.10	0.20	0.73	0.05	0.25	14.2	0.9	15.8	0.4	21	1.66	19.7	89	98	42	0.6	30	0.00	4.59
—	—	—	—	—	—	0.0	—	—	12	0.54	—	90	45	240	—	—	0.00	0.00
0.07	0.10	0.80	0.01	0.10	14.1	0.0	—	1.5	24	1.33	19.2	103	114	216	0.4	22	0.00	—
—	—	—	—	—	—	1.2	—	—	60	1.08	—	—	—	250	—	—	0.00	0.00
0.11	0.25	0.49	0.05	0.31	29.7	0.5	—	1.1	170	0.46	18.8	232	209	376	0.5	44	0.00	0.00
0.01	0.05	0.31	0.00	0.00	6.5	0.0	—	0.8	15	0.66	10.8	79	96	178	0.2	23	0.00	0.86
0.23	0.30	3.20	0.05	0.10	68.3	0.0	—	0.8	35	4.48	59.4	148	235	650	1.2	4	0.00	7.84
0.21	0.25	2.48	0.05	0.10	48.0	0.0	—	0.2	38	1.89	11.2	83	78	250	0.3	5	0.00	0.00
0.05	0.07	0.50	0.00	0.01	4.1	0.0	0.8	1.0	15	0.51	14.9	35	44	47	0.2	6	0.00	0.00
0.07	0.05	0.37	0.02	0.01	3.1	0.4	1.0	0.7	27	0.72	11.4	47	74	78	0.2	19	0.00	0.00
—	—	—	—	—	—	0.0	—	—	0	0.72	—	—	—	30	—	—	0.00	0.00
0.01	0.01	0.17	0.00	0.00	5.0	0.0	—	0.0	2	0.12	0.9	6	5	19	0.0	4	0.00	0.00
0.01	0.01	0.17	0.00	0.00	5.0	0.0	—	0.0	2	0.12	0.9	6	5	19	0.0	4	0.00	0.00
0.05	0.05	0.43	0.02	0.02	10.6	0.1	—	0.9	12	0.79	17.6	32	72	116	0.3	6	0.00	5.11
0.01	0.01	0.23	0.00	0.00	6.3	0.0	—	0.2	4	0.36	4.8	12	15	30	0.1	4	0.00	1.10
—	—	—	—	—	—	—	—	—	—	—	—	—	—	88	—	10	0.00	—

PAGE KEY: A-46 Beverage and Beverage Mixes   A-48 Other Beverages   A-48 Beverages, Alcoholic   A-50 Candies and Confections, Gum   A-54 Cereals, Breakfast Type   A-58 Cheese and Cheese Substitutes   A-60 Dairy Products and Substitutes   A-62 Desserts   A-68 Dessert Toppings   A-68 Eggs, Substitutes, and Egg Dishes   A-70 Ethnic Foods   A-74 Fast Foods/Restaurants   A-88 Fats, Oils, Margarines, Shortenings, and Substitutes   A-88 Fish, Seafood, and Shellfish   A-90 Food Additives   A-90 Fruit, Vegetable, or Blended Juices   A-92 Grains, Flours, and Fractions   A-92 Grain Products, Prepared and Baked Goods

Code	Food Name	Unit/ Amt	Wt (g)	Energy (kcal)	Prot (g)	Carb (g)	Fiber (g)	Fat (g)	Sat (g)	Mono (g)	Poly (g)	Chol (mg)	Vit A (RE)
43660	Cookie, chocolate sandwich	3 ea	33	150	2	23	2	6	0.5	3.5	2.0	0	0
47041	Cookie, chocolate wafer	2 ea	12	52	1	9	0	2	0.5	0.6	0.5	0	0
50962	Cookie, chocolate, fudge stripes	3 ea	32	159	2	21	1	8	5.1	—	—	2	5
47183	Cookie, cinnamon, Teddy Grahams	22 ea	28	120	2	22	—	4	1.0	—	—	—	—
50971	Cookie, creme sandwich, sug free	3 ea	28	120	1	21	2	6	1.3	—	—	1	0
47733	Cookie, Do-Si-Dos	3 ea	36	170	3	22	1	8	1.0	—	—	0	0
47012	Cookie, fig bar	2 ea	32	111	1	23	1	2	0.4	1.0	0.9	0	3
47043	Cookie, fortune	3 ea	24	91	1	20	0	1	0.2	0.3	0.1	0	0
47324	Cookie, fudge brownie, sugar free	1 ea	24	79	1	18	0	0	0.1	0.1	0.0	0	0
47044	Cookie, fudge, cake type	1 ea	21	73	1	16	1	1	0.2	0.4	0.1	0	0
47045	Cookie, gingersnap	4 ea	28	116	2	22	1	3	0.7	1.5	0.4	0	0
47077	Cookie, granola	1 ea	13	60	1	9	1	2	1.6	0.2	0.2	0	0
47737	Cookie, lemon drop	3 ea	33	160	2	20	0	8	2.0	—	—	0	0
43676	Cookie, lemon sandwich	3 ea	33	469	2	23	2	6	0.5	3.5	2.0	0	0
47109	Cookie, molasses, med	1 ea	15	64	1	11	0	2	0.5	1.1	0.3	0	0
47161	Cookie, newton, fig	2 ea	31	116	2	19	2	3	1.0	1.0	0.0	0	—
47252	Cookie, Nutter Butter sandwich	2 ea	28	130	3	19	1	6	1.0	2.5	1.0	5	—
47496	Cookie, oatmeal raisin, home style	1 ea	26	107	1	17	1	4	0.8	1.3	0.3	3	1
47052	Cookie, oatmeal, refrig dough	2 ea	32	136	2	19	1	6	1.5	3.4	0.8	8	3
50948	Cookie, peanut butter	2 ea	28	134	2	16	1	7	1.5	—	—	0	0
47079	Cookie, pecan sandies	1 ea	15	75	1	10	0	4	0.9	2.0	0.5	3	2
47061	Cookie, raisin, soft type	2 ea	30	120	1	20	0	4	1.0	2.3	0.5	1	2
47734	Cookie, Samoas	2 ea	28	160	2	17	2	9	6.0	—	—	0	0
47665	Cookie, shortbread	1 ea	15	75	1	10	0	4	0.9	2.0	0.5	3	2
47011	Cookie, snickerdoodle, prep f/recipe	1 ea	20	80	1	12	0	3	2.1	—	—	9	25
50941	Cookie, sugar	2 ea	28	127	1	18	0	6	1.2	—	—	0	0
47738	Cookie, Tagalongs	2 ea	28	150	3	13	2	10	4.0	—	—	0	0
47739	Cookie, Thin Mints	4 ea	28	140	1	18	1	8	2.0	—	—	0	0
47740	Cookie, Trefoils	5 ea	32	160	2	20	0	8	1.0	—	—	0	0
47715	Cookie, vanilla sandwich	5 ea	43	210	2	30	1	10	2.5	—	—	5	0
47513	Cookie, wedding cake	1 ea	10	53	0	7	0	3	0.5	—	—	0	0
47026	Crackers, animal	10 ea	12	56	1	9	0	2	0.4	1.0	0.2	0	0
50966	Crackers, animal, frosted	1 ea	56	282	2	38	1	14	8.3	—	—	0	0
Doughnuts													
45630	Doughnut, buttermilk, glazed	1 ea	64	270	3	35	0	13	3.0	—	—	15	0
71335	Doughnut, cake, holes	1 ea	14	59	1	7	0	3	0.5	1.3	1.1	5	5
62914	Doughnut, cream puff, choc, custard filled, prep f/rec 3.5 x 2	1 ea	112	293	7	27	1	18	4.6	7.3	4.4	142	234
45508	Doughnut, eclair, chocolate, custard filled, prep f/rec, 5 x 2	1 ea	100	262	6	24	1	16	4.1	6.5	3.9	127	209
71343	Doughnut, glazed, enrich, lrg, 4 1/4"	1 ea	75	302	5	33	1	17	4.4	9.6	2.2	4	3
45507	Doughnut, jelly filled, 3 1/2" oval	1 ea	85	289	5	33	1	16	4.1	8.7	2.0	22	15
71856	Doughnut, plain, wheat free	1 ea	54	154	8	19	0	5	1.5	—	—	33	4
Frozen Desserts													
46110	Cake, ice cream, chocolate roll, 12 oz whl or 1/10 pce	1 pce	34	101	1	14	0	5	2.1	1.8	0.8	15	22
90721	Frozen Dessert Pop, 1.75 fl oz bar	1 ea	52	37	0	10	0	0	0.0	0.0	0.0	0	0
23050	Frozen Dessert Pop, double stick	1 ea	128	92	0	24	0	0	0.0	0.0	0.0	0	0
23051	Frozen Dessert, slushy	1 cup	193	247	1	63	0	0	0.0	0.0	0.0	0	0
23114	Frozen Dessert, snow cone	1 ea	190	243	1	62	0	0	0.0	0.0	0.0	0	0

PAGE KEY: A-96 Granola Bars, Cereal Bars, Diet Bars, Scones, and Tarts   A-96 Meals and Dishes   A-100 Meats   A-106 Nuts, Seeds, and Products   A-108 Poultry   A-110 Salad Dressings, Dips, and Mayonnaise   A-110 Salads   A-110 Sandwiches   A-114 Sauces and Gravies   A-114 Snack Foods—Chips, Pretzels, Popcorn   A-116 Soups, Stews, and Chilis   A-118 Spices, Flavors, and Seasonings   A-120 Sports Bars and Drinks   A-120 Supplemental Foods and Formulas   A-122 Sweeteners and Sweet Substitutes   A-122 Vegetables and Legumes   A-136 Weight Loss Bars and Drinks   A-138 Miscellaneous

Thia (mg)	Ribo (mg)	Niac (mg NE)	Vit B6 (mg)	Vit B12 (µg)	Fol (µg)	Vit C (mg)	Vit D (IU)	Vit E (mg AT)	Cal (mg)	Iron (mg)	Magn (mg)	Phos (mg)	Pota (mg)	Sodi (mg)	Zinc (mg)	Wat (%)	Alco (g)	Caff (g)
—	—	—	—	—	—	0.0	—	—	40	1.08	—	—	—	105	—	—	0.00	—
0.01	0.02	0.34	0.00	0.00	7.3	0.0	—	0.1	4	0.47	6.4	16	25	70	0.1	4	0.00	0.83
—	—	—	—	—	—	0.0	—	—	14	0.61	—	—	—	128	—	—	0.00	—
—	—	—	—	—	—	—	—	—	—	—	—	—	—	170	—	—	0.00	—
0.07	0.07	0.75	—	—	16.5	0.0	—	—	4	0.38	—	—	—	67	—	1	0.00	0.00
—	—	—	—	—	—	0.0	—	—	0	0.36	—	—	—	105	—	—	0.00	0.00
0.05	0.07	0.60	0.01	0.02	11.2	0.1	—	0.2	20	0.93	8.6	20	66	112	0.1	16	0.00	0.00
0.03	0.02	0.43	0.00	0.00	15.8	0.0	—	0.0	3	0.34	1.7	8	10	66	0.0	8	0.00	0.00
0.01	0.02	0.38	0.00	0.00	—	0.0	—	0.0	4	0.43	7.3	17	40	106	0.1	14	0.00	—
0.05	0.03	0.25	0.00	0.01	9.0	0.0	—	0.1	7	0.51	6.7	17	29	40	0.1	12	0.00	0.00
0.05	0.07	0.91	0.02	0.00	24.4	0.0	—	0.3	22	1.78	13.7	23	97	183	0.2	5	0.00	0.00
0.07	0.02	0.23	0.05	0.00	10.5	0.1	—	0.0	9	0.37	13.1	46	47	43	0.2	3	0.00	0.00
—	—	—	—	—	—	0.0	—	—	0	0.72	—	—	—	150	—	8	0.00	0.00
—	—	—	—	—	—	0.0	—	—	40	1.08	—	—	—	80	—	5	0.00	0.00
0.05	0.03	0.44	0.01	0.00	13.4	0.0	—	0.0	11	0.95	7.8	14	52	69	0.1	6	0.00	0.00
—	—	—	—	—	—	—	—	—	—	0.69	—	—	78	116	—	—	0.00	0.00
—	—	—	—	—	—	—	—	—	—	0.72	—	—	55	110	—	0	0.00	0.00
0.07	0.03	0.44	—	—	—	0.0	—	—	8	0.58	—	—	60	98	—	11	0.00	0.00
0.07	0.05	0.60	0.00	0.00	11.2	0.0	—	0.8	10	0.68	9.0	33	47	94	0.2	15	0.00	0.00
0.05	0.05	1.20	—	—	17.4	0.0	—	—	10	0.62	—	—	—	114	—	8	0.00	0.00
0.05	0.05	0.50	0.00	0.00	1.4	0.0	0.9	0.5	5	0.40	2.6	16	15	68	0.1	4	0.00	0.00
0.05	0.05	0.58	0.01	0.00	9.6	0.1	—	0.7	14	0.68	6.3	25	42	101	0.1	13	0.00	0.00
—	—	—	—	—	—	2.4	—	—	0	0.72	—	—	—	45	—	—	0.00	0.00
0.05	0.05	0.50	0.00	0.00	1.4	0.0	0.9	0.5	5	0.40	2.6	16	15	68	0.1	4	0.00	0.00
0.05	0.03	0.40	0.00	0.00	13.6	0.1	2.7	0.1	8	0.46	2.1	10	23	75	0.1	18	0.00	0.00
0.05	0.02	0.67	—	—	14.8	0.0	—	—	12	0.63	—	—	—	86	—	9	0.00	0.00
—	—	—	—	—	—	0.0	—	—	0	0.72	—	—	—	85	—	—	0.00	0.00
—	—	—	—	—	—	0.0	—	—	200	—	—	—	—	80	—	0	0.00	0.00
—	—	—	—	—	—	0.0	—	—	0	0.36	—	—	—	90	—	—	0.00	0.00
—	—	—	—	—	—	0.0	—	—	20	1.08	—	—	—	125	—	1	0.00	0.00
—	—	—	—	—	—	0.0	—	—	0	0.23	—	—	—	15	—	—	0.00	0.00
0.03	0.03	0.43	0.00	0.00	12.9	0.0	—	0.0	5	0.34	2.2	14	12	49	0.1	4	Alco	0.00
—	—	—	—	—	—	0.0	—	—	5	0.62	—	—	—	141	—	—	0.00	0.00
—	—	—	—	—	—	0.0	—	—	60	1.08	—	—	—	290	—	19	0.00	0.00
0.02	0.02	0.25	0.00	0.03	7.3	0.0	—	0.3	6	0.27	2.8	38	18	76	0.1	21	0.00	0.00
0.12	0.30	0.88	0.07	0.37	48.2	0.3	—	2.3	71	1.32	16.8	120	131	377	0.7	52	0.00	2.24
0.11	0.27	0.80	0.05	0.34	43.0	0.3	—	2.0	63	1.17	15.0	107	117	337	0.6	52	0.00	2.00
0.27	0.15	2.14	0.03	0.07	36.8	0.1	—	0.3	32	1.52	16.5	70	81	256	0.6	25	0.00	0.00
0.27	0.11	1.82	0.09	0.18	57.8	0.0	—	0.4	21	1.50	17.0	72	67	249	0.6	36	0.00	0.00
0.02	133.86	0.10	0.02	0.00	19.9	9.6	0.0	0.0	57	0.40	8.2	84	132	—	—	—	0.00	0.00
0.03	0.07	0.30	0.00	0.07	2.3	0.1	3.5	0.3	42	0.50	9.1	40	57	45	0.2	39	0.02	—
0.00	0.00	0.00	0.00	0.00	0.0	0.0	—	0.0	0	0.00	0.5	0	2	6	0.0	80	0.00	0.00
0.00	0.00	0.00	0.00	0.00	0.0	0.0	—	0.0	0	0.00	1.3	0	5	15	0.0	80	0.00	0.00
0.00	0.00	0.00	0.00	0.00	0.0	1.9	—	0.0	4	0.31	1.9	2	6	42	0.0	67	0.00	0.00
0.00	0.00	0.00	0.00	0.00	0.0	1.9	—	0.0	4	0.30	1.9	2	6	42	0.0	67	0.00	0.00

PAGE KEY: A-46 Beverage and Beverage Mixes   A-48 Other Beverages   A-48 Beverages, Alcoholic   A-50 Candies and Confections, Gum   A-54 Cereals, Breakfast Type   A-58 Cheese and Cheese Substitutes   A-60 Dairy Products and Substitutes   A-62 Desserts   A-68 Dessert Toppings   A-68 Eggs, Substitutes, and Egg Dishes   A-70 Ethnic Foods   A-74 Fast Foods/Restaurants   A-88 Fats, Oils, Margarines, Shortenings, and Substitutes   A-88 Fish, Seafood, and Shellfish   A-90 Food Additives   A-90 Fruit, Vegetable, or Blended Juices   A-92 Grains, Flours, and Fractions   A-92 Grain Products, Prepared and Baked Goods

Code	Food Name	Unit/ Amt	Wt (g)	Energy (kcal)	Prot (g)	Carb (g)	Fiber (g)	Fat (g)	Sat (g)	Mono (g)	Poly (g)	Chol (mg)	Vit A (RE)
2032	Frozen Dessert, sundae, hot fudge	1 ea	158	284	6	48	0	9	5.0	2.3	0.8	21	62
2045	Frozen Yogurt Cone, chocolate, sml	1 ea	78	168	4	24	1	7	4.2	2.3	0.4	1	37
2044	Frozen Yogurt Sandwich	1 ea	85	181	4	32	0	4	2.3	1.3	0.4	1	37
72125	Frozen Yogurt, chocolate	1 cup	174	221	5	38	4	6	4.0	1.7	0.2	23	70
625	Frozen Yogurt, vanilla, lowfat	0.5 cup	106	200	9	31	0	4	2.5	—	—	65	40
72188	Ice Cream Bar, Fudgsicle	1 ea	61	90	3	16	1	2	1.0	—	—	5	0
72187	Ice Cream Bar, Fudgsicle, fat free	1 ea	51	65	3	14	1	0	0.2	—	—	2	0
2113	Ice Cream Cone, chocolate, small	1 ea	78	173	3	25	1	7	4.4	2.2	0.4	18	62
2092	Ice Cream Cone, chocolate dipped	1 ea	78	187	3	24	1	10	5.7	2.9	0.5	29	77
2093	Ice Cream Cone, vanilla, small	1 ea	78	166	3	21	0	8	5.0	2.4	0.4	32	86
2087	Ice Cream Sandwich	1 ea	59	144	3	22	1	6	3.2	1.7	0.4	20	53
2051	Ice Cream, chocolate, soft serve	1 cup	173	355	6	48	1	17	10.3	4.8	0.6	43	147
71814	Ice Cream, neapolitan	0.5 cup	65	130	2	16	0	7	4.0	—	—	25	40
71810	Ice Cream, rocky road	0.5 cup	65	160	3	19	1	8	4.5	—	—	25	40
2053	Ice Cream, strawberry, imit	0.5 cup	66	132	2	16	0	7	5.9	0.4	0.1	0	0
2004	Ice Cream, vanilla	0.5 cup	66	133	2	16	0	7	4.5	2.0	0.3	29	79
72119	Ice Cream, vanilla, fat free	3.6 oz	100	138	4	30	1	0	0.0	0.0	0.0	0	202
2052	Ice Cream, vanilla, imit	0.5 cup	66	132	2	16	0	7	5.9	0.4	0.1	0	0
2020	Milk Shake, chocolate, fast food	1 cup	166	211	6	34	3	6	3.8	1.8	0.2	22	45
2482	Milk Shake, vanilla, fountain type	1 cup	166	224	5	35	0	8	4.9	2.3	0.3	32	80
2011	Sherbet, orange	0.5 cup	74	107	1	22	2	1	0.9	0.4	0.1	0	8

Fruit Desserts

Code	Food Name	Unit/ Amt	Wt (g)	Energy (kcal)	Prot (g)	Carb (g)	Fiber (g)	Fat (g)	Sat (g)	Mono (g)	Poly (g)	Chol (mg)	Vit A (RE)
49005	Apple Brown Betty	0.75 cup	155	268	4	47	3	8	4.2	—	—	16	53
49019	Cobbler, berry	1 cup	217	507	6	94	4	13	2.9	5.6	4.1	2	23
49023	Crisp, cherry	1 cup	246	704	6	113	3	27	4.7	12.3	8.6	2	250
49015	Strudel, apple	1 pce	71	195	2	29	2	8	1.5	2.3	3.8	4	5

Gelatin Desserts

Code	Food Name	Unit/ Amt	Wt (g)	Energy (kcal)	Prot (g)	Carb (g)	Fiber (g)	Fat (g)	Sat (g)	Mono (g)	Poly (g)	Chol (mg)	Vit A (RE)
23052	Gelatin, prep f/dry mix w/water	0.5 cup	135	84	2	19	0	0	0.0	0.0	0.0	0	0

Pastries and Sweet Rolls

Code	Food Name	Unit/ Amt	Wt (g)	Energy (kcal)	Prot (g)	Carb (g)	Fiber (g)	Fat (g)	Sat (g)	Mono (g)	Poly (g)	Chol (mg)	Vit A (RE)
42363	Buns, honey	1 ea	65	270	3	35	1	13	3.0	—	—	0	0
45523	Croissant, cheese, med	1 ea	57	236	5	27	1	12	6.1	3.7	1.4	32	120
71042	Danish, cinnamon nut, 4 1/4"	1 ea	65	280	5	30	1	16	3.8	8.9	2.8	30	6
71041	Danish, raisin nut, 4 1/4"	1 ea	65	280	5	30	1	16	3.8	8.9	2.8	30	6
42746	Danish, strawberry swirl	1 ea	62	254	3	37	1	11	3.0	3.6	4.4	0	0
45549	Dumpling, apple	1 ea	190	672	7	85	3	35	6.9	15.2	10.7	0	8
45515	Fritter, apple	1 ea	24	87	1	8	0	6	1.2	2.4	1.6	20	13
45593	Pastry, apple cinnamon	1 ea	52	205	2	37	1	5	0.9	3.1	1.4	0	100
45594	Pastry, brown sugar cinnamon	1 ea	50	219	3	32	1	9	1.0	3.6	4.6	0	100
45572	Pastry, cheese danish	1 ea	71	266	6	26	1	16	4.8	8.0	1.8	11	26
45595	Pastry, cherry	1 ea	52	204	2	37	1	5	0.9	3.0	1.6	0	100
45601	Pastry, chocolate fudge, frosted	1 ea	52	201	3	37	1	5	1.0	2.7	1.1	0	100
45782	Pastry, s'mores	1 ea	52	204	3	36	1	5	1.5	3.1	0.9	0	100

Pastry, Pie, Dessert Crusts, and Cones

Code	Food Name	Unit/ Amt	Wt (g)	Energy (kcal)	Prot (g)	Carb (g)	Fiber (g)	Fat (g)	Sat (g)	Mono (g)	Poly (g)	Chol (mg)	Vit A (RE)
45500	Crust, pie, graham cracker, prep f/rec, bkd, 9" or 1/8 pce	1 pce	30	148	1	19	0	7	1.6	3.4	2.1	0	61
45535	Crust, pie, rtb, enrich, fzn, 9" whl or 1/8 pce	1 pce	18	82	1	8	0	5	0.8	2.2	2.0	0	0

PAGE KEY: A-96 Granola Bars, Cereal Bars, Diet Bars, Scones, and Tarts   A-96 Meals and Dishes   A-100 Meats   A-106 Nuts, Seeds, and Products   A-108 Poultry   A-110 Salad Dressings, Dips, and Mayonnaise   A-110 Salads   A-110 Sandwiches   A-114 Sauces and Gravies   A-114 Snack Foods—Chips, Pretzels, Popcorn   A-116 Soups, Stews, and Chilis   A-118 Spices, Flavors, and Seasonings   A-120 Sports Bars and Drinks   A-120 Supplemental Foods and Formulas   A-122 Sweeteners and Sweet Substitutes   A-122 Vegetables and Legumes   A-136 Weight Loss Bars and Drinks   A-138 Miscellaneous

Thia (mg)	Ribo (mg)	Niac (mg NE)	Vit B6 (mg)	Vit B12 (µg)	Fol (µg)	Vit C (mg)	Vit D (IU)	Vit E (mg AT)	Cal (mg)	Iron (mg)	Magn (mg)	Phos (mg)	Pota (mg)	Sodi (mg)	Zinc (mg)	Wat (%)	Alco (g)	Caff (g)
0.05	0.30	1.07	0.12	0.64	9.5	2.4	19.0	0.7	207	0.57	33.2	228	395	182	0.9	60	0.00	1.58
0.07	0.18	0.68	0.05	0.18	4.7	0.5	—	0.2	99	0.97	30.8	116	197	84	0.6	53	0.00	—
0.03	0.15	0.34	0.05	0.18	7.3	0.5	—	0.1	95	0.34	12.0	98	151	57	0.4	52	0.00	0.00
0.07	0.31	0.23	0.07	0.11	20.9	11.7	—	0.2	174	0.80	43.5	155	407	110	0.5	71	0.00	5.21
—	—	—	—	—	—	0.0	—	—	250	0.00	—	—	—	55	—	—	0.00	0.00
—	—	—	—	—	—	0.0	—	—	80	0.36	—	—	—	65	—	65	0.00	—
—	—	—	—	—	—	0.5	—	—	81	0.46	—	—	—	48	—	66	0.00	—
0.03	0.12	0.36	0.02	0.27	4.3	0.4	6.2	0.3	88	0.49	17.3	83	168	46	0.4	54	0.00	2.33
0.03	0.18	0.34	0.03	0.25	3.8	0.4	3.7	0.2	88	0.46	18.2	83	161	61	0.6	52	0.00	2.33
0.03	0.18	0.28	0.03	0.28	3.9	0.4	3.7	0.1	95	0.23	11.5	82	151	65	0.5	58	0.00	0.00
0.02	0.11	0.18	0.02	0.18	4.8	0.3	2.4	0.1	60	0.28	12.7	64	122	36	0.4	48	0.00	—
0.07	0.27	0.21	0.05	0.63	9.4	1.1	6.9	0.5	206	0.66	37.3	184	384	89	1.0	58	0.00	5.19
—	—	—	—	—	—	2.0	0.0	—	60	0.00	—	—	—	55	—	61	0.00	—
—	—	—	—	—	—	0.0	0.0	—	60	0.36	—	—	—	65	—	—	0.00	—
0.02	0.15	0.07	0.03	0.38	1.3	0.3	0.0	0.1	90	0.07	10.0	71	144	49	0.7	61	0.00	0.00
0.02	0.15	0.07	0.02	0.25	3.3	0.4	22.9	0.2	84	0.05	9.2	69	131	53	0.5	61	0.00	0.00
0.05	0.25	0.14	0.05	0.44	7.0	0.0	—	0.0	149	0.00	21.0	150	302	97	1.1	64	0.00	0.00
0.02	0.15	0.07	0.03	0.38	1.3	0.3	0.0	0.1	90	0.07	10.0	71	144	49	0.7	61	0.00	0.00
0.10	0.40	0.27	0.07	0.56	8.3	0.7	57.7	0.2	188	0.51	28.3	170	333	161	0.7	72	0.00	1.65
0.05	0.25	0.20	0.05	0.49	7.4	9.0	—	0.1	172	0.38	19.6	135	247	86	0.8	70	0.00	0.00
0.01	0.07	0.05	0.01	0.09	5.2	4.3	—	0.0	40	0.10	5.9	30	71	34	0.4	66	0.00	0.00
0.23	0.14	2.01	0.07	0.01	32.4	0.3	8.2	0.3	74	1.98	16.4	51	150	309	0.4	61	0.00	0.00
0.31	0.28	2.55	0.07	0.05	12.8	12.4	—	2.8	181	2.39	19.7	134	189	260	0.5	47	0.00	0.00
0.20	0.25	1.98	0.14	0.14	16.1	2.7	—	4.3	153	3.50	19.7	323	219	836	0.4	40	0.00	0.00
0.02	0.01	0.23	0.02	0.15	19.9	1.2	—	1.0	11	0.30	6.4	23	106	191	0.1	44	0.00	
0.00	0.00	0.00	0.00	0.00	1.4	0.0	—	0.0	4	0.02	1.4	30	1	101	0.0	84	0.00	0.00
—	—	—	—	—	—	0.0	—	—	0	0.36	—	—	—	160	—	—	0.00	0.00
0.30	0.18	1.23	0.03	0.18	42.2	0.1	—	0.8	30	1.23	13.7	74	75	316	0.5	21	0.00	0.00
0.14	0.15	1.49	0.07	0.14	53.9	1.1	—	0.5	61	1.16	20.8	72	62	236	0.6	20	0.00	0.00
0.14	0.15	1.49	0.07	0.14	53.9	1.1	—	0.5	61	1.16	20.8	72	62	236	0.6	20	0.00	0.00
—	—	—	—	—	—	0.0	—	—	20	1.08	—	—	—	170	—	16	0.00	0.00
0.40	0.30	3.53	0.05	0.00	11.2	1.6	—	4.5	13	3.11	16.6	76	130	10	0.5	33	0.00	0.00
0.03	0.05	0.31	0.01	0.05	2.9	0.3	—	0.7	13	0.34	3.0	22	34	10	0.1	37	0.00	0.00
0.15	0.17	1.98	0.20	0.00	41.6	0.0	—	0.0	12	1.82	5.7	28	47	174	0.3	12	0.00	0.00
0.15	0.17	2.00	0.20	0.00	40.0	0.0	—	0.0	16	1.79	8.0	32	68	214	0.6	10	0.00	0.00
0.12	0.18	1.41	0.02	0.11	42.6	0.1	—	0.2	25	1.13	10.6	77	70	320	0.5	31	0.00	0.00
0.15	0.17	1.98	0.20	0.00	41.6	0.0	—	0.0	15	1.82	8.3	44	59	220	0.6	12	0.00	0.00
0.15	0.15	1.98	0.20	0.00	52.0	0.0	—	0.0	20	1.82	15.1	44	82	203	0.3	12	0.00	—
0.15	0.15	1.98	0.20	0.00	52.0	0.0	—	0.0	15	1.82	10.9	39	65	199	0.2	12	0.00	—
0.02	0.05	0.63	0.00	0.00	7.2	0.0	—	0.7	6	0.64	5.4	19	26	171	0.1	4	0.00	0.00
0.05	0.07	0.43	0.00	0.00	12.6	0.0	—	0.4	3	0.36	2.9	10	18	104	0.1	21	0.00	0.00

PAGE KEY: A-46 Beverage and Beverage Mixes   A-48 Other Beverages   A-48 Beverages, Alcoholic   A-50 Candies and Confections, Gum   A-54 Cereals, Breakfast Type
A-58 Cheese and Cheese Substitutes   A-60 Dairy Products and Substitutes   A-62 Desserts   A-68 Dessert Toppings   A-68 Eggs, Substitutes, and Egg Dishes   A-70 Ethnic Foods
A-74 Fast Foods/Restaurants   A-88 Fats, Oils, Margarines, Shortenings, and Substitutes   A-88 Fish, Seafood, and Shellfish   A-90 Food Additives
A-90 Fruit, Vegetable, or Blended Juices   A-92 Grains, Flours, and Fractions   A-92 Grain Products, Prepared and Baked Goods

Code	Food Name	Unit/ Amt	Wt (g)	Energy (kcal)	Prot (g)	Carb (g)	Fiber (g)	Fat (g)	Sat (g)	Mono (g)	Poly (g)	Chol (mg)	Vit A (RE)
Pies													
48004	Pie, apple, cmrcl prep, w/enrich flour, 8" whl or 1/6 pce	1 pce	117	277	2	40	2	13	4.4	5.1	2.6	0	39
48023	Pie, banana cream, no bake, prep f/mix, 9" whl or 1/8 pce	1 pce	92	231	3	29	1	12	6.4	4.2	0.7	27	92
48025	Pie, blueberry, cmrcl prep, 8" whl or 1/6 pce	1 pce	117	271	2	41	1	12	2.0	5.0	4.1	0	55
48005	Pie, cherry, cmrcl prep, 8" whl or 1/6 pce	1 pce	117	304	2	47	1	13	3.0	6.8	2.4	0	68
48031	Pie, chocolate cream, cmrcl prep, 8" whl or 1/6 pce	1 pce	113	344	3	38	2	22	5.6	12.6	2.7	6	0
71646	Pie, key lime, w/o topping, 10" whl or 1/8 pce	1 pce	113	420	6	55		20	12.0	—	—	20	40
48177	Pie, lemon, 4 oz svg	1 ea	113	320	3	50	2	12	3.0	—	—	40	0
48040	Pie, peach, 8" whl or 1/6 pce	1 pce	117	261	2	38	1	12	1.8	5.0	4.4	0	19
48012	Pie, pecan, cmrcl prep, 8" whl or 1/6 pce	1 pce	113	452	5	65	4	21	4.0	12.1	3.6	36	59
48000	Pie, pumpkin, cmrcl prep, 8" whl or 1/6 pce	1 pce	109	229	4	30	3	10	1.9	4.4	3.4	22	613
48130	Pie, rhubarb, 9" or 1/8 pce	1 pce	118	316	3	48	2	13	3.6	—	—	3	18
48185	Pie, strawberry, 3.7 oz svg	1 ea	106	310	2	50	1	12	3.0	—	—	0	0
Puddings, Custards, and Pie Fillings													
2659	Custard, chocolate, prep f/dry mix w/2% milk	0.5 cup	136	116	4	18	1	3	1.7	0.8	0.1	10	68
48001	Pie Filling, apple, cnd	0.5 cup	128	129	0	33	1	0	0.0	0.0	0.0	0	0
48015	Pie Filling, cherry, cnd	0.5 cup	132	152	0	37	1	0	0.0	0.0	0.0	0	26
48017	Pie Filling, lemon	0.5 cup	133	463	6	93	1	9	2.2	3.8	1.9	175	125
48044	Pie Filling, pumpkin, cnd	0.5 cup	135	140	1	36	11	0	0.1	0.0	0.0	0	1120
58203	Pudding, all flvrs, not choc, inst, low cal, dry mix	3.6 oz	100	342	1	82	1	1	0.2	0.2	0.3	0	0
2649	Pudding, rice, prep f/dry mix w/2% milk	0.5 cup	144	160	5	30	0	2	1.4	0.6	0.1	9	68
2653	Pudding, tapioca, prep f/dry mix w/2% milk	0.5 cup	141	148	4	28	0	2	1.4	0.6	0.1	8	68
2764	Pudding, vanilla, fat free, 4 oz snack cup	1 ea	113	104	2	23	0	0	0.2	0.0	0.0	2	35
56331	Roll, yorkshire pudding, prep f/recipe, 1.5 oz svg	1 pce	42	87	3	10	0	4	1.8	1.7	0.3	32	27
DESSERT TOPPINGS													
46037	Frosting, chocolate, creamy, 16 oz can	1.328 oz	38	149	0	24	0	7	2.1	3.4	0.8	0	0
46038	Frosting, coconut nut, rte, 16 oz can	1.328 oz	38	155	1	20	1	9	2.6	4.6	1.3	0	0
46323	Frosting, cream cheese, rte	2 Tbs	35	150	0	24	0	6	1.5	—	—	0	0
46330	Frosting, lemon creme, rte	2 Tbs	35	150	0	24	0	6	1.5	—	—	0	0
46336	Frosting, strawberry creme, rte	2 Tbs	35	150	0	24	0	6	1.5	—	—	0	0
54308	Syrup, caramel	2 Tbs	39	100	1	25	0	0	0.0	0.0	0.0	0	0
23437	Syrup, chocolate	2 Tbs	39	100	1	24	—	0	0.0	0.0	0.0	0	0
54312	Syrup, raspberry	2 Tbs	38	100	0	25	0	0	0.0	0.0	0.0	0	0
23069	Topping, butterscotch	2 Tbs	41	103	1	27	0	0	0.0	0.0	0.0	0	11
23070	Topping, caramel	2 Tbs	41	103	1	27	0	0	0.0	0.0	0.0	0	11
23014	Topping, chocolate fudge	2 Tbs	38	133	2	24	1	3	1.5	1.5	0.1	1	2
92528	Topping, hot fudge	1 Tbs	19	70	1	10	—	2	1.0	—	—	5	—
23071	Topping, marshmallow cream, 7 oz jar	1 ea	198	639	2	157	0	1	0.1	0.2	0.1	0	0
23163	Topping, pineapple	2 Tbs	42	108	0	28	0	0	0.0	0.0	0.0	0	1
23164	Topping, strawberry	2 Tbs	42	108	0	28	0	0	0.0	0.0	0.0	0	1
510	Topping, whipped cream, pressurized	2 Tbs	8	19	0	1	0	2	1.0	0.5	0.1	6	14
565	Topping, whipped, lite, Cool Whip	2 Tbs	9	20	0	2	0	1	1.0	0.0	0.0	0	0
EGGS, SUBSTITUTES, AND EGG DISHES													
19525	Egg Substitute, liquid	0.25 cup	63	53	8	0	0	2	0.4	0.6	1.0	1	23
7736	Egg Substitute, Scramblers, fzn	0.25 cup	57	39	7	2	0	0	—	—	—	2	62
19507	Egg Whites, raw	0.625 cup	152	79	17	1	0	0	0.0	0.0	0.0	0	0

PAGE KEY: A-96 Granola Bars, Cereal Bars, Diet Bars, Scones, and Tarts   A-96 Meals and Dishes   A-100 Meats   A-106 Nuts, Seeds, and Products   A-108 Poultry   A-110 Salad Dressings, Dips, and Mayonnaise   A-110 Salads   A-110 Sandwiches   A-114 Sauces and Gravies   A-114 Snack Foods—Chips, Pretzels, Popcorn   A-116 Soups, Stews, and Chilis   A-118 Spices, Flavors, and Seasonings   A-120 Sports Bars and Drinks   A-120 Supplemental Foods and Formulas   A-122 Sweeteners and Sweet Substitutes   A-122 Vegetables and Legumes   A-136 Weight Loss Bars and Drinks   A-138 Miscellaneous

Thia (mg)	Ribo (mg)	Niac (mg NE)	Vit B6 (mg)	Vit B12 (µg)	Fol (µg)	Vit C (mg)	Vit D (IU)	Vit E (mg AT)	Cal (mg)	Iron (mg)	Magn (mg)	Phos (mg)	Pota (mg)	Sodi (mg)	Zinc (mg)	Wat (%)	Alco (g)	Caff (g)
0.02	0.02	0.31	0.03	0.00	31.6	3.7	—	1.8	13	0.52	8.2	28	76	311	0.2	52	0.00	0.00
0.09	0.12	0.64	0.02	0.18	19.3	0.5	—	1.5	67	0.41	11.0	154	104	267	0.3	51	0.00	0.00
0.00	0.03	0.34	0.03	0.00	31.6	3.2	—	1.2	9	0.34	5.8	27	58	380	0.2	52	0.00	0.00
0.02	0.02	0.23	0.05	0.00	31.6	1.1	—	0.9	14	0.56	9.4	34	95	288	0.2	46	0.00	0.00
0.03	0.11	0.76	0.01	0.00	14.7	0.0	—	3.1	41	1.21	23.7	77	144	154	0.3	44	0.00	0.00
—	—	—	—	—	—	0.0	—	—	150	0.72	—	—	—	200	—	—	0.00	0.00
—	—	—	—	—	—	0.0	—	—	20	0.72	—	—	—	330	—	—	0.00	0.00
0.07	0.03	0.23	0.02	0.00	33.9	1.1	—	1.1	9	0.57	7.0	26	146	316	0.1	54	0.00	0.00
0.10	0.14	0.28	0.01	0.10	38.4	1.2	—	0.4	19	1.17	20.3	87	84	479	0.6	19	0.00	0.00
0.05	0.17	0.20	0.05	0.28	26.2	1.1	—	1.1	65	0.86	16.4	77	168	307	0.5	58	0.00	0.00
0.18	0.14	1.53	0.01	0.00	36.3	3.8	0.8	1.1	46	1.30	11.4	35	166	197	0.2	45	0.00	0.00
—	—	—	—	—	—	9.0	—	—	20	1.08	—	—	—	300	—	—	0.00	0.00
0.05	0.20	0.15	0.05	0.44	6.8	1.2	49.0	0.1	171	0.40	27.2	133	248	71	0.7	80	0.00	1.36
0.01	0.00	0.03	0.01	0.00	0.0	0.1	—	0.0	5	0.37	2.5	9	57	56	0.1	73	0.00	0.00
0.02	0.01	0.18	0.05	0.00	5.3	4.8	—	0.3	15	0.31	9.2	20	139	24	0.1	71	0.00	0.00
0.09	0.25	0.56	0.07	0.34	18.9	14.1	—	1.2	29	1.12	8.3	88	99	108	0.6	18	0.00	0.00
0.01	0.15	0.50	0.20	0.00	47.2	4.7	—	1.1	50	1.42	21.6	61	186	281	0.4	71	0.00	0.00
0.00	0.00	0.00	0.00	0.00	0.0	0.0	—	0.1	19	0.23	7.0	2179	47	4232	0.0	4	0.00	0.00
0.10	0.20	0.63	0.05	0.34	5.8	1.0	48.3	0.1	151	0.52	18.7	125	187	157	0.5	73	0.00	0.00
0.03	0.20	0.10	0.05	0.34	5.6	1.0	48.5	0.1	148	0.07	16.9	116	188	171	0.5	75	0.00	0.00
—	—	—	—	—	—	0.3	—	—	86	0.05	—	115	123	241	—	76	0.00	0.00
0.03	0.07	—	0.02	0.41	3.8	0.4	—	—	55	0.37	—	—	67	248	0.3	57	0.00	0.00
0.00	0.00	0.03	0.00	0.00	0.4	0.0	—	0.6	3	0.52	7.9	30	74	69	0.1	17	0.00	0.75
0.00	0.00	0.07	0.01	0.00	0.8	0.1	—	0.6	5	0.20	7.2	24	70	73	0.2	21	0.00	0.00
—	—	—	—	—	—	0.0	—	—	0	0.00	—	—	—	70	—	14	0.00	0.00
—	—	—	—	—	—	0.0	—	—	0	0.00	—	—	—	70	—	14	0.00	0.00
—	—	—	—	—	—	0.0	—	—	0	0.00	—	—	—	70	—	14	0.00	0.00
—	—	—	—	—	—	0.0	—	—	20	0.00	—	—	—	105	—	33	0.00	0.00
—	—	—	—	—	—	0.0	—	—	0	0.36	—	—	—	25	—	35	0.00	7.00
—	—	—	—	—	—	0.0	—	—	0	0.00	—	—	—	5	—	31	0.00	0.00
0.00	0.03	0.01	0.00	0.03	0.8	0.1	—	0.0	22	0.07	2.9	19	34	143	0.1	32	0.00	0.00
0.00	0.03	0.01	0.00	0.03	0.8	0.1	—	0.0	22	0.07	2.9	19	34	143	0.1	32	0.00	0.00
0.02	0.10	0.14	0.02	0.10	1.9	0.0	—	0.9	38	0.60	24.3	64	171	131	0.3	22	0.00	2.66
—	—	—	—	—	—	—	—	—	—	—	—	—	—	80	—	25	0.00	—
0.00	0.00	0.15	0.00	0.00	2.0	0.0	—	0.0	6	0.43	4.0	16	10	159	0.1	20	0.00	0.00
0.01	0.00	0.03	0.00	0.00	0.9	1.3	—	0.0	3	0.05	2.6	1	18	18	0.0	33	0.00	0.00
0.00	0.00	0.07	0.00	0.00	2.6	5.8	—	0.0	3	0.11	1.7	2	22	9	0.0	33	0.00	0.00
0.00	0.00	0.00	0.00	0.01	0.2	0.0	—	0.0	8	0.00	0.8	7	11	10	0.0	61	0.00	0.00
—	—	—	—	—	—	0.0	—	—	0	0.00	—	0	0	0	—	66	0.00	0.00
0.07	0.18	0.07	0.00	0.18	9.4	0.0	—	0.2	33	1.32	5.6	76	207	111	0.8	83	0.00	0.00
0.17	0.40	0.00	0.12	1.76	—	0.0	—	—	19	0.62	—	59	95	122	0.7	83	0.00	0.00
0.00	0.67	0.15	0.00	0.14	6.1	0.0	0.0	0.0	11	0.11	16.7	23	248	252	0.0	88	0.00	0.00

PAGE KEY: A-46 Beverage and Beverage Mixes   A-48 Other Beverages   A-48 Beverages, Alcoholic   A-50 Candies and Confections, Gum   A-54 Cereals, Breakfast Type
A-58 Cheese and Cheese Substitutes   A-60 Dairy Products and Substitutes   A-62 Desserts   A-68 Dessert Toppings   A-68 Eggs, Substitutes, and Egg Dishes   A-70 Ethnic Foods
A-74 Fast Foods/Restaurants   A-88 Fats, Oils, Margarines, Shortenings, and Substitutes   A-88 Fish, Seafood, and Shellfish   A-90 Food Additives
A-90 Fruit, Vegetable, or Blended Juices   A-92 Grains, Flours, and Fractions   A-92 Grain Products, Prepared and Baked Goods

Code	Food Name	Unit/ Amt	Wt (g)	Energy (kcal)	Prot (g)	Carb (g)	Fiber (g)	Fat (g)	Sat (g)	Mono (g)	Poly (g)	Chol (mg)	Vit A (RE)
19600	Egg Yolks, raw	0.25 cup	61	196	10	2	0	16	5.8	7.1	2.6	750	238
19539	Eggs, deviled	1 ea	31	63	4	0	0	5	1.2	1.7	1.5	122	50
19510	Eggs, hard bld, lrg	1 ea	50	78	6	1	0	5	1.6	2.0	0.7	212	85
19516	Eggs, scrambled, prep f/one lrg egg butter & milk	1 ea	61	101	7	1	0	7	2.2	2.9	1.3	215	89
19509	Eggs, whole, lrg, fried	1 ea	46	92	6	0	0	7	2.0	2.9	1.2	210	93
19501	Eggs, whole, raw, lrg	1 ea	50	74	6	0	0	5	1.5	1.9	0.7	212	70
19535	Omelette, one egg w/cheese & ham	1 ea	78	156	11	2	0	11	4.5	4.4	1.4	198	133
19536	Omelette, Spanish	1 ea	145	178	8	6	1	14	3.4	5.9	3.0	220	211
19544	Omelette, w/sausage, one egg	1 ea	95	167	11	2	0	13	3.9	5.2	1.9	267	149

ETHNIC FOODS

Italian Foods

Code	Food Name	Unit/ Amt	Wt (g)	Energy (kcal)	Prot (g)	Carb (g)	Fiber (g)	Fat (g)	Sat (g)	Mono (g)	Poly (g)	Chol (mg)	Vit A (RE)
16260	Dinner, chicken, alfredo, w/broccoli, fzn, Healthy Choice	1 ea	326	300	25	34	2	7	3.0	—	—	50	20
56128	Dish, ravioli, cheese, w/tomato sauce, svg	1 ea	250	341	15	38	2	15	6.4	5.0	1.9	162	236
53432	Sauce, marinara	0.5 cup	127	120	2	20	2	4	1.0	—	—	0	50

Mexican Foods

Code	Food Name	Unit/ Amt	Wt (g)	Energy (kcal)	Prot (g)	Carb (g)	Fiber (g)	Fat (g)	Sat (g)	Mono (g)	Poly (g)	Chol (mg)	Vit A (RE)
90856	Beans, refried, fat free, cnd	0.5 cup	130	110	7	21	6	0	0.0	0.0	0.0	0	0
9096	Beans, refried, original, cnd	0.5 cup	128	100	6	18	5	2	1.0	—	—	0	0
9095	Beans, refried, spicy, cnd	0.5 cup	128	100	6	18	6	2	1.0	—	—	0	0
82019	Burrito, bean & cheese, ckd	1 ea	142	300	9	46	4	9	4.5	—	—	15	40
3770	Chicle, fresh, pulp	1 cup	241	200	1	48	13	3	0.5	1.3	0.0	0	14
7931	Chili Peppers, jalapeno, fresh	1 ea	14	4	0	1	0	0	0.0	0.0	0.0	0	11
45777	Dessert, Churro	1 ea	26	116	1	12	0	7	2.0	4.1	0.9	2	6
70150	Dinner, burrito, beef & bean, w/salsa, fzn	1 ea	305	540	24	62	8	22	9.2	8.8	1.8	49	81
1753	Dinner, enchilada & tamale, beef, combination ckd f/fzn	1 ea	312	450	10	56	9	20	8.0	—	—	30	150
56124	Dish, fajitas, beef	1 ea	223	399	23	36	3	18	5.5	7.6	3.5	45	43
56123	Dish, fajitas, chicken	1 ea	223	363	20	44	5	12	2.3	5.5	3.1	39	65
3634	Guava, fresh	0.5 cup	82	56	2	12	4	1	0.2	0.1	0.3	0	51
5224	Jicama, fresh	1 cup	120	46	1	11	—	0	0.0	0.0	0.1	0	2
20122	Mixed Drink, pina colada, non alcoholic, mix	1 ea	30	32	0	7	0	1	0.5	0.0	0.0	0	0
3199	Passion Fruit, purple, fresh	1 ea	18	17	0	4	2	0	0.0	0.0	0.1	0	23
3745	Plantain, fresh, med	1 ea	179	218	2	57	4	1	0.3	0.1	0.1	0	200
56122	Quesadilla	1 ea	54	183	6	18	1	10	3.5	3.4	2.2	13	41
42185	Rolls, Mexican, bolillo	1 ea	117	307	10	61	2	2	0.5	0.2	0.6	1	4
53676	Salsa	2 Tbs	30	10	0	2	0	0	0.0	0.0	0.0	0	0
53207	Salsa, chunky, restaurant style	2 Tbs	30	10	0	1	0	0	0.0	0.0	0.0	0	0
27127	Salsa, garden pepper, med	2 Tbs	31	10	0	2	0	0	0.0	0.0	0.0	0	10
53642	Salsa, green chili, mild	2 Tbs	30	8	0	1	0	0	—	—	—	—	14
53584	Salsa, hot, cnd	2 Tbs	32	5	0	2	0	0	0.0	0.0	0.0	0	20
53645	Salsa, picante, med	2 Tbs	30	8	0	1	0	0	—	—	—	0	14
53647	Salsa, ranchera, hot	2 Tbs	30	9	0	2	0	0	—	—	—	0	36
53686	Salsa, restaurant style	62 g	62	30	2	6	2	0	0.0	0.0	0.0	0	20
4017	Salsa, rstd garlic	68 g	68	30	2	6	2	0	0.0	0.0	0.0	0	20
53643	Salsa, suprema, med	2 Tbs	30	8	0	1	0	0	—	—	—	0	10
27123	Salsa, thick 'n chunky, med	2 Tbs	30	10	0	3	0	0	0.0	0.0	0.0	0	20
53640	Salsa, thick 'n chunky, med	2 Tbs	30	8	0	1	0	0	—	—	—	0	18
53245	Salsa, verde, med	2 Tbs	29	10	0	2	—	0	0.0	0.0	0.0	0	0
53103	Sauce, enchilada, green	1 cup	250	187	4	13	4	14	8.1	3.9	1.2	43	156

PAGE KEY: A-96 Granola Bars, Cereal Bars, Diet Bars, Scones, and Tarts   A-96 Meals and Dishes   A-100 Meats   A-106 Nuts, Seeds, and Products   A-108 Poultry
A-110 Salad Dressings, Dips, and Mayonnaise   A-110 Salads   A-110 Sandwiches   A-114 Sauces and Gravies   A-114 Snack Foods—Chips, Pretzels, Popcorn
A-116 Soups, Stews, and Chilis   A-118 Spices, Flavors, and Seasonings   A-120 Sports Bars and Drinks   A-120 Supplemental Foods and Formulas
A-122 Sweeteners and Sweet Substitutes   A-122 Vegetables and Legumes   A-136 Weight Loss Bars and Drinks   A-138 Miscellaneous

Thia (mg)	Ribo (mg)	Niac (mg NE)	Vit B6 (mg)	Vit B12 (µg)	Fol (µg)	Vit C (mg)	Vit D (IU)	Vit E (mg AT)	Cal (mg)	Iron (mg)	Magn (mg)	Phos (mg)	Pota (mg)	Sodi (mg)	Zinc (mg)	Wat (%)	Alco (g)	Caff (g)
0.10	0.31	0.00	0.20	1.17	88.7	0.0	65.3	1.6	78	1.65	3.0	237	66	29	1.4	52	0.00	0.00
0.01	0.15	0.01	0.05	0.31	12.7	0.0	15.0	0.6	15	0.34	2.9	50	37	50	0.3	70	0.00	0.00
0.02	0.25	0.02	0.05	0.56	22.0	0.0	—	0.5	25	0.60	5.0	86	63	62	0.5	75	0.00	0.00
0.02	0.27	0.05	0.07	0.46	18.3	0.1	21.0	0.5	43	0.73	7.3	104	84	171	0.6	73	0.00	0.00
0.02	0.23	0.03	0.07	0.63	23.5	0.0	17.2	0.6	27	0.91	6.0	96	68	94	0.6	69	0.00	0.00
0.02	0.23	0.03	0.07	0.63	23.5	0.0	17.3	0.5	26	0.92	6.0	96	67	70	0.6	76	0.00	0.00
0.10	0.31	0.60	0.11	0.61	17.0	0.1	—	0.8	113	0.81	12.4	179	145	372	1.2	67	0.00	0.00
0.07	0.36	0.81	0.17	0.50	29.7	19.0	—	2.0	60	1.15	16.2	142	269	170	0.8	80	0.00	0.00
0.12	0.36	0.69	0.12	0.79	23.1	0.4	52.4	1.0	64	1.07	12.1	156	162	294	1.1	72	0.00	0.00
—	—	—	—	—	—	12.0	—	—	100	1.79	—	—	—	530	—	—	0.00	0.00
0.31	0.43	2.95	0.18	0.38	30.3	9.4	—	2.1	172	3.09	32.9	220	405	574	1.5	72	0.00	0.00
—	—	—	—	0.00	—	1.2	—	—	0	0.72	—	—	—	480	—	—	0.00	0.00
—	—	—	—	—	—	0.0	—	—	40	2.70	—	—	—	460	—	77	0.00	0.00
—	—	—	—	—	—	0.0	—	—	40	1.98	—	—	—	510	—	78	0.00	0.00
—	—	—	—	—	—	0.0	—	—	40	1.98	—	—	—	630	—	78	0.00	0.00
—	—	—	—	—	—	0.0	—	—	40	0.72	—	—	—	690	—	—	0.00	0.00
0.00	0.05	0.47	0.09	0.00	33.7	35.4	—	0.6	51	1.92	28.9	29	465	29	0.2	78	0.00	0.00
0.01	0.00	0.15	0.07	0.00	6.6	6.2	—	0.1	1	0.10	2.7	4	30	0	0.0	92	0.00	0.00
0.03	0.02	0.37	0.00	0.00	1.2	0.0	—	1.0	2	0.33	1.7	8	8	7	0.1	23	0.00	0.00
0.49	0.44	5.69	0.31	1.08	134.4	20.1	—	1.6	144	5.53	70.7	350	685	881	3.6	63	0.00	0.00
—	—	—	—	—	—	0.0	—	—	150	1.79	—	—	—	1530	—	—	0.00	0.00
0.38	0.30	5.40	0.37	2.05	23.0	26.8	—	1.7	84	3.75	37.6	238	479	316	3.5	65	0.00	0.00
0.43	0.33	6.11	0.37	0.10	41.8	36.8	—	1.7	101	3.31	48.2	188	534	343	1.6	65	0.00	0.00
0.05	0.02	0.88	0.09	0.00	40.4	188.3	—	0.6	15	0.20	18.1	33	344	2	0.2	81	0.00	0.00
0.01	0.02	0.23	0.05	0.00	14.4	24.2	—	0.5	14	0.72	14.4	22	180	5	0.2	90	0.00	0.00
0.00	0.00	0.03	0.00	0.00	3.5	1.5	0.0	0.0	3	0.05	2.3	2	21	2	0.0	75	0.00	0.00
0.00	0.01	0.27	0.01	0.00	2.5	5.4	—	0.0	2	0.28	5.2	12	63	5	0.0	73	0.00	0.00
0.09	0.10	1.23	0.54	0.00	39.4	32.9	—	0.3	5	1.07	66.2	61	893	7	0.3	65	0.00	0.00
0.12	0.14	1.09	0.03	0.05	5.8	14.7	—	1.0	132	1.21	13.4	107	77	230	0.6	35	0.00	0.00
0.69	0.46	6.59	0.03	0.00	41.1	0.0	0.3	0.1	14	3.80	22.1	90	98	7	0.8	37	0.00	0.00
—	—	—	—	—	—	2.4	—	—	0	0.00	—	—	55	115	—	92	0.00	0.00
—	—	—	—	—	—	0.0	—	—	0	0.00	—	—	—	140	—	95	0.00	0.00
—	—	—	—	—	—	0.0	—	—	0	0.00	—	—	—	240	—	91	0.00	0.00
—	—	—	—	—	—	4.1	—	—	5	0.28	—	—	—	175	—	92	0.00	0.00
—	—	—	—	—	—	2.4	—	—	0	0.00	—	—	95	170	—	92	0.00	0.00
—	—	—	—	—	—	2.5	—	—	4	0.01	—	—	—	150	—	92	0.00	0.00
—	—	—	—	—	—	1.3	—	—	5	0.03	—	—	—	171	—	91	0.00	0.00
—	—	—	—	—	—	1.2	—	—	0	0.36	—	—	—	420	—	85	0.00	0.00
—	—	—	—	—	—	1.2	—	—	20	0.00	—	—	—	460	—	—	0.00	0.00
—	—	—	—	—	—	1.5	—	—	3	0.01	—	—	—	166	—	92	0.00	0.00
—	—	—	—	—	—	0.0	—	—	0	0.00	—	—	—	230	—	88	0.00	0.00
—	—	—	—	—	—	4.4	—	—	6	0.05	—	—	—	160	—	92	0.00	0.00
—	—	—	—	—	—	0.0	—	—	0	0.00	—	—	—	95	—	91	0.00	0.00
0.09	0.15	2.92	0.18	0.14	13.3	23.1	0.0	0.9	77	1.17	41.4	118	540	30	0.6	87	0.00	0.00

PAGE KEY: A-46 Beverage and Beverage Mixes   A-48 Other Beverages   A-48 Beverages, Alcoholic   A-50 Candies and Confections, Gum   A-54 Cereals, Breakfast Type
A-58 Cheese and Cheese Substitutes   A-60 Dairy Products and Substitutes   A-62 Desserts   A-68 Dessert Toppings   A-68 Eggs, Substitutes, and Egg Dishes   A-70 Ethnic Foods
A-74 Fast Foods/Restaurants   A-88 Fats, Oils, Margarines, Shortenings, and Substitutes   A-88 Fish, Seafood, and Shellfish   A-90 Food Additives
A-90 Fruit, Vegetable, or Blended Juices   A-92 Grains, Flours, and Fractions   A-92 Grain Products, Prepared and Baked Goods

Code	Food Name	Unit/Amt	Wt (g)	Energy (kcal)	Prot (g)	Carb (g)	Fiber (g)	Fat (g)	Sat (g)	Mono (g)	Poly (g)	Chol (mg)	Vit A (RE)
53102	Sauce, enchilada, red	1 cup	250	321	3	10	2	31	16.7	10.1	2.8	91	349
53224	Sauce, taco, thick & smooth, med	1 Tbs	16	10	0	2	0	0	0.0	0.0	0.0	0	0
91932	Seasoning, fajita	0.25 tsp	1	0	0	0	0	0	0.0	0.0	0.0	0	—
57531	Taco, sml	1 ea	171	369	21	27	—	21	11.4	6.6	1.0	56	139
56113	Tamale, w/meat	1 ea	70	134	6	11	1	7	2.6	3.1	1.0	19	14
5445	Tomatillo, fresh, med	1 ea	34	11	0	2	1	0	0.0	0.1	0.1	0	4
42023	Tortilla, corn, med, 6"	1 ea	26	57	1	12	2	1	0.1	0.2	0.4	0	0
90646	Tortilla, flour, 6"	1 ea	32	100	3	16	1	2	0.6	1.2	0.5	0	0
66017	Tostada, bean & cheese	1 ea	144	223	10	27	—	10	5.4	3.1	0.7	30	73
56645	Tostada, beef & cheese	1 ea	163	315	19	23	—	16	10.4	3.3	1.0	41	83

Asian Foods

Code	Food Name	Unit/Amt	Wt (g)	Energy (kcal)	Prot (g)	Carb (g)	Fiber (g)	Fat (g)	Sat (g)	Mono (g)	Poly (g)	Chol (mg)	Vit A (RE)
7084	Bean Cakes, Japanese style	1 ea	32	130	2	16	1	7	1.0	2.9	2.6	0	0
6459	Bean Sprouts, cnd, svg	1 ea	83	12	1	2	1	0	0.0	—	—	0	0
5654	Broccoli, stir fried	1 cup	156	44	5	8	5	1	0.1	0.0	0.3	0	216
1717	Dinner, stir fry, chicken & veg, oriental, fzn, Healthy Choice	1 ea	337	360	19	57	5	6	2.0	—	—	25	350
70455	Dish, beef, oriental style	1 ea	227	300	10	45	2	7	3.0	—	—	51	100
56094	Dish, chop suey, beef, w/noodles	1 cup	220	421	22	31	—	24	4.7	8.3	9.2	43	103
56234	Dish, chop suey, pork, w/noodles	1 cup	220	448	22	31	4	27	4.8	7.7	12.8	48	19
57618	Dish, chow mein, pork, w/noodles	1 cup	220	448	22	31	4	27	4.8	7.7	12.8	48	19
56238	Dish, chow mein, shrimp, w/noodles	1 cup	220	272	17	24	3	13	1.9	3.1	6.9	82	15
2999	Dish, duck curry, Thai, prep f/recipe, svg	1 ea	277	316	17	5	1	25	8.3	—	—	72	77
56288	Dish, egg foo yung, pork	1 ea	86	124	8	4	1	8	2.1	3.0	2.3	167	86
1991	Dish, green curry chicken, Thai, prep f/recipe, svg	1 ea	386	614	23	18	5	54	42.6	—	—	53	846
1998	Dish, peanut chicken w/rice, Thai, prep f/recipe, svg	1 ea	309	272	19	26	3	11	2.3	—	—	36	351
2998	Dish, potstickers, veal, Thai, prep f/recipe, svg	1 ea	244	647	27	99	4	14	5.0	—	—	58	26
2995	Dish, spring roll, vegetable, Thai, prep f/recipe	1 pce	63	158	4	20	1	7	0.9	—	—	3	140
2996	Dish, sweet noodles, Thai, prep f/recipe, svg	1 ea	142	339	14	37	2	15	2.4	—	—	121	66
3249	Java Plum, fresh	3 ea	9	5	0	1	—	0	—	—	—	0	0
7503	Miso	1 cup	275	547	32	73	15	17	3.1	3.4	8.8	0	22
7508	Natto	1 cup	175	371	31	25	9	19	2.8	4.3	10.9	0	0
38048	Pasta, chow mein noodles, dry	1 cup	45	237	4	26	2	14	2.0	3.5	7.8	0	0
5121	Peas, edible pod, fresh	10 ea	34	14	1	3	1	0	0.0	0.0	0.0	0	37
5666	Peas, snow, pods, stir fried	1 cup	165	69	5	12	4	0	0.1	0.0	0.1	0	21
5665	Peas, snow, pods, stmd	1 cup	165	69	5	12	4	0	0.1	0.0	0.1	0	23
38082	Rice, brown, med grain, ckd	0.5 cup	98	109	2	23	2	1	0.2	0.3	0.3	0	0
38021	Rice, wild, ckd	1 cup	164	166	7	35	3	1	0.1	0.1	0.3	0	0
38289	Rice, wild, dry	1 cup	160	571	24	120	10	2	0.2	0.3	1.1	0	3
1985	Salad, chicken, broiled, Thai, prep f/recipe, svg	1 ea	403	257	24	25	2	7	1.9	—	—	60	139
1987	Sauce, coconut, Thai, prep f/recipe, svg	1 ea	126	65	2	13	2	1	0.1	—	—	0	207
1999	Sauce, peanut, Thai, prep f/recipe, svg	0.75 cup	199	412	18	19	4	33	6.6	—	—	0	37
53461	Sauce, plum, rts	2 Tbs	38	70	0	16	0	0	0.1	0.1	0.2	0	2
53357	Sauce, sweet & sour, rts	2 Tbs	33	40	0	8	0	1	0.1	0.2	0.4	0	5
53004	Sauce, teriyaki, rts	1 Tbs	18	15	1	3	0	0	0.0	0.0	0.0	0	0
5253	Seaweed, agar, fresh	0.5 cup	40	10	0	3	0	0	0.0	0.0	0.0	0	0
50181	Soup, won ton	1 cup	241	182	14	14	1	7	2.3	3.0	1.0	53	99
91818	Sushi, California roll	1 ea	198	292	8	49	3	3	1.0	—	—	3	90

PAGE KEY: A-96 Granola Bars, Cereal Bars, Diet Bars, Scones, and Tarts   A-96 Meals and Dishes   A-100 Meats   A-106 Nuts, Seeds, and Products   A-108 Poultry   A-110 Salad Dressings, Dips, and Mayonnaise   A-110 Salads   A-110 Sandwiches   A-114 Sauces and Gravies   A-114 Snack Foods—Chips, Pretzels, Popcorn   A-116 Soups, Stews, and Chilis   A-118 Spices, Flavors, and Seasonings   A-120 Sports Bars and Drinks   A-120 Supplemental Foods and Formulas   A-122 Sweeteners and Sweet Substitutes   A-122 Vegetables and Legumes   A-136 Weight Loss Bars and Drinks   A-138 Miscellaneous

Thia (mg)	Ribo (mg)	Niac (mg NE)	Vit B6 (mg)	Vit B12 (µg)	Fol (µg)	Vit C (mg)	Vit D (IU)	Vit E (mg AT)	Cal (mg)	Iron (mg)	Magn (mg)	Phos (mg)	Pota (mg)	Sodi (mg)	Zinc (mg)	Wat (%)	Alco (g)	Caff (g)
0.07	0.12	0.74	0.14	0.10	17.0	20.3	0.0	1.6	55	0.62	20.0	76	336	36	0.3	82	0.00	0.00
—	—	—	—	—	—	0.0	—	—	0	0.36	—	—	40	125	—	85	0.00	0.00
—	—	—	—	—	—	—	—	—	—	—	—	—	—	130	—	—	0.00	0.00
0.15	0.43	3.21	0.23	1.03	68.4	2.2	—	1.9	221	2.41	70.1	203	474	802	3.9	58	0.00	0.00
0.17	0.14	2.49	0.09	0.17	4.5	1.0	—	0.3	24	1.41	20.7	67	140	84	0.9	64	0.00	0.00
0.00	0.00	0.62	0.01	0.00	2.4	4.0	—	0.1	2	0.20	6.8	13	91	0	0.1	92	0.00	0.00
0.01	0.01	0.38	0.05	0.00	1.3	0.0	—	0.1	21	0.31	18.7	82	48	12	0.3	46	0.00	0.00
0.17	0.09	1.13	0.01	0.00	33.3	0.0	—	0.1	41	1.07	7.0	40	50	204	0.2	30	0.00	0.00
0.10	0.33	1.32	0.15	0.68	43.2	1.3	—	1.2	210	1.88	59.0	117	403	543	1.9	66	0.00	0.00
0.10	0.55	3.15	0.23	1.16	75.0	2.6	—	—	217	2.86	63.6	179	572	896	3.7	62	0.00	0.00
0.07	0.05	0.55	0.01	0.00	9.1	0.0	0.0	1.2	3	0.67	6.1	21	58	1	0.2	23	0.00	0.00
—	—	—	—	0.00	—	14.2	—	—	10	0.25	—	—	—	20	—	96	0.00	0.00
0.09	0.18	0.93	0.23	0.00	88.5	123.4	0.0	0.7	75	1.37	39.0	103	505	42	0.6	91	0.00	0.00
—	—	—	—	—	—	4.8	—	—	40	2.70	—	—	—	600	—	—	0.00	0.00
—	—	—	—	—	—	18.0	—	—	60	2.70	—	—	—	1220	—	—	0.00	0.00
0.36	0.37	5.73	0.38	1.67	43.8	20.1	—	1.8	39	4.19	54.2	262	519	950	3.5	63	0.00	0.00
0.77	0.43	6.23	0.41	0.41	41.8	20.2	—	2.7	45	3.29	52.8	249	489	848	2.6	62	0.00	0.00
0.77	0.43	6.23	0.41	0.41	41.8	20.2	—	2.7	45	3.29	52.8	249	489	848	2.6	62	0.00	0.00
0.23	0.23	4.46	0.18	0.58	45.1	9.4	—	1.3	58	3.42	51.2	220	391	710	1.3	74	0.00	0.00
0.15	0.25	4.46	0.23	0.28	8.9	5.0	10.2	0.6	72	2.94	77.8	204	742	602	1.7	80	0.00	0.00
0.12	0.25	0.79	0.14	0.40	22.3	3.2	—	1.1	27	0.81	11.9	105	157	131	0.9	75	0.00	0.00
0.15	0.17	7.65	0.49	0.23	57.0	91.5	7.1	2.0	65	7.82	140.7	331	866	889	2.6	74	0.00	0.00
0.21	0.11	8.25	0.47	0.14	66.1	67.3	5.1	1.7	42	2.66	48.0	191	344	901	1.2	81	0.00	0.00
0.87	0.72	12.23	0.21	0.57	145.1	1.8	5.1	1.4	106	6.73	50.2	238	329	1020	2.9	41	0.00	0.00
0.18	0.14	1.87	0.02	0.00	31.7	0.9	8.2	1.3	58	1.77	11.9	42	75	263	0.4	49	0.00	0.00
0.07	0.09	1.01	0.14	0.56	15.2	4.6	50.8	1.6	277	2.92	40.1	170	176	377	1.3	50	0.00	0.00
0.00	0.00	0.01	0.00	0.00	—	1.3	—	—	2	0.01	1.4	2	7	1	0.0	83	0.00	0.00
0.27	0.63	2.49	0.55	0.21	52.2	0.0	—	0.0	157	6.84	132.0	437	578	10252	7.0	43	0.00	0.00
0.28	0.33	0.00	0.23	0.00	14.0	22.8	—	0.0	380	15.05	201.2	304	1276	12	5.3	55	0.00	0.00
0.25	0.18	2.68	0.05	0.00	40.5	0.0	—	1.6	9	2.13	23.4	72	54	198	0.6	1	0.00	0.00
0.05	0.02	0.20	0.05	0.00	14.3	20.4	—	0.1	15	0.70	8.2	18	68	1	0.1	89	0.00	0.00
0.21	0.12	0.93	0.25	0.00	55.1	84.2	0.0	0.6	71	3.43	39.6	87	330	7	0.4	89	0.00	0.00
0.21	0.12	0.93	0.23	0.00	58.4	84.2	0.0	0.6	71	3.43	39.6	87	330	7	0.4	89	0.00	0.00
0.10	0.00	1.29	0.15	0.00	3.9	0.0	—	0.2	10	0.51	42.9	75	77	1	0.6	73	0.00	0.00
0.09	0.14	2.10	0.21	0.00	42.6	0.0	—	0.4	5	0.98	52.5	134	166	5	2.2	74	0.00	0.00
0.18	0.41	10.77	0.62	0.00	152.0	0.0	—	1.3	34	3.14	283.2	693	683	11	9.5	8	0.00	0.00
0.15	0.15	10.36	0.56	0.25	29.1	27.3	8.6	0.7	38	2.00	48.7	208	511	1637	1.1	85	0.00	0.00
0.05	0.05	0.85	0.02	0.00	6.9	5.0	0.0	0.1	33	0.74	17.2	27	319	82	0.2	85	0.00	0.00
0.09	0.14	10.18	0.44	0.00	55.1	2.2	0.0	6.4	40	2.13	107.8	297	544	3376	2.1	60	0.00	0.00
0.00	0.02	0.38	0.02	0.00	2.3	0.2	—	0.1	5	0.55	4.6	8	99	205	0.1	54	0.00	0.00
0.00	0.00	0.07	0.00	0.00	0.7	0.0	—	0.1	6	0.28	2.3	3	22	116	0.0	71	0.00	0.00
0.00	0.00	0.23	0.01	0.00	3.6	0.0	—	0.0	4	0.31	11.0	28	40	690	0.0	68	0.00	0.00
0.00	0.00	0.01	0.00	0.00	34.0	0.0	—	0.3	22	0.74	26.8	2	90	4	0.2	91	0.00	0.00
0.40	0.25	4.59	0.20	0.40	18.8	3.4	—	0.4	31	1.75	20.6	153	316	543	1.1	84	0.00	0.00
—	—	—	—	—	—	4.8	—	—	20	1.08	—	—	—	952	—	—	0.00	0.00

Code	Food Name	Unit/ Amt	Wt (g)	Energy (kcal)	Prot (g)	Carb (g)	Fiber (g)	Fat (g)	Sat (g)	Mono (g)	Poly (g)	Chol (mg)	Vit A (RE)
91814	Sushi, cucumber roll	6 pce	85	120	3	25	2	1	0.0	—	—	0	50
92378	Sushi, krab roll	6 pce	112	150	7	30	2	1	0.0	—	—	3	60
56313	Sushi, w/veg & fish	3 oz	85	119	5	24	1	0	0.1	0.1	0.1	6	70
6880	Sweetpotatoes, fresh, cubes	1 cup	133	114	2	27	4	0	0.0	0.0	0.0	0	1886
6206	Vegetables, Japanese style, fzn	0.5 cup	127	78	2	8	2	5	2.3	—	—	12	96
6208	Vegetables, Japanese style, stir fry, fzn	0.5 cup	116	35	2	7	2	0	0.0	—	—	0	74
57294	Vegetables, oriental style, stir fry, fzn	0.5 cup	54	41	2	7	0	1	0.1	—	—	0	38
6646	Vegetables, pepper style, stir fry, fzn	0.5 cup	54	15	0	3		0	0.0	—	—	0	23
6592	Vegetables, teriyaki, marinated/seasoned, fzn	1.25 cup	110	100	2	7	2	7	1.0	—	—	0	500
6460	Waterchestnuts, slices, cnd	100 g	100	50	1	12	5	0	0.0	—	—	0	0
5222	Watercress, fresh, chpd	1 cup	34	4	1	0	0	0	0.0	0.0	0.0	0	160
49116	Wrappers, egg roll, 7" square	1 ea	32	93	3	19	1	0	0.1	0.1	0.2	3	1

FAST FOODS/RESTAURANTS

Generic Fast Food

Code	Food Name	Unit/ Amt	Wt (g)	Energy (kcal)	Prot (g)	Carb (g)	Fiber (g)	Fat (g)	Sat (g)	Mono (g)	Poly (g)	Chol (mg)	Vit A (RE)
56654	Cheeseburger, double, double bun, reg, w/condiments & veg	1 ea	228	650	30	53	—	35	12.8	12.6	6.4	93	84
56648	Cheeseburger, lrg, plain	1 ea	185	609	30	47	—	33	14.8	12.7	2.4	96	185
66015	Cheeseburger, reg, w/condiments & veg	1 ea	154	359	18	28	—	20	9.2	7.2	1.5	52	91
6175	Dish, corn, cob, w/butter	1 ea	146	155	4	32	—	3	1.6	1.0	0.6	6	51
6185	Dish, mashed potatoes	0.5 cup	121	100	3	20	—	1	0.6	0.4	0.4	2	15
17187	Fish, fillet, brd/batter fried	3 oz	85	197	12	14	0	10	2.4	2.2	5.3	29	9
42353	French Toast, w/butter	2 pce	135	356	10	36	0	19	7.7	7.1	2.4	116	138
66007	Hamburger, reg, plain	1 ea	90	274	12	31	—	12	4.1	5.5	0.9	35	0
2022	Milk Shake, strawberry, fast food	1 cup	283	320	10	53	1	8	4.9	2.2	0.3	31	74
2024	Milk Shake, vanilla, fast food	1 cup	166	185	6	30	0	5	3.1	1.4	0.2	18	63
56639	Nachos, w/cheese	7 pce	113	346	9	36	—	19	7.8	8.0	2.2	18	154
6176	Onion Rings, breaded, fried, svg	8 pce	78	259	3	29	—	15	6.5	6.3	0.6	13	2
45122	Pancakes, w/butter & syrup	1 ea	116	260	4	45	1	7	2.9	2.6	1.0	29	41
5463	Potatoes, hash browns	0.5 cup	72	151	2	16	—	9	4.3	3.9	0.5	9	3
6173	Salad, potato	0.333 cup	95	108	1	13	—	6	1.0	1.6	2.9	57	28
56623	Salad, tossed, veg, w/o dressing	1.5 cup	207	33	3	7	—	0	0.0	0.0	0.1	0	236
56601	Sandwich, breakfast, egg bacon, w/biscuit	1 ea	150	458	17	29	1	31	8.0	13.4	7.5	352	108
56602	Sandwich, breakfast, egg ham, w/biscuit	1 ea	192	442	20	30	1	27	5.9	11.0	7.7	300	240
56600	Sandwich, breakfast, egg, w/biscuit	1 ea	136	373	12	32	1	22	4.7	9.1	6.4	245	181
56606	Sandwich, croissant, w/egg & cheese	1 ea	127	368	13	24	—	25	14.1	7.5	1.4	216	282
56607	Sandwich, croissant, w/egg, cheese & bacon	1 ea	129	413	16	24	—	28	15.4	9.2	1.8	215	142
66031	Sandwich, english muffin, w/cheese & sausage	1 ea	115	393	15	29	1	24	9.9	10.1	2.7	59	104
56604	Sandwich, ham, w/biscuit	1 ea	113	386	13	44	1	18	11.4	4.8	1.0	25	33

A&W Restaurants

Code	Food Name	Unit/ Amt	Wt (g)	Energy (kcal)	Prot (g)	Carb (g)	Fiber (g)	Fat (g)	Sat (g)	Mono (g)	Poly (g)	Chol (mg)	Vit A (RE)
81303	Cheeseburger	1 ea	191	500	28	43	3	24	9.0	—	—	90	200
81305	Cheeseburger, deluxe, w/bacon	1 ea	278	600	32	44	4	33	12.0	—	—	110	250
81319	Dish, french fries, cheese, svg	1 ea	170	390	4	50	4	19	5.0	—	—	5	0
81352	Frozen Dessert, Oreo, med, A&W Polar Swirl	1 ea	397	833	16	125	2	30	11.7	—	—	54	350
81330	Frozen Dessert, sundae, hot fudge, A&W	1 ea	189	350	8	54	1	11	6.0	—	—	30	150
81311	Hamburger	1 ea	177	460	26	39	3	22	8.0	—	—	75	40
81314	Hot Dog, cheese, w/bun	1 ea	126	320	11	25	1	20	7.0	—	—	40	20
81315	Hot Dog, chili & cheese, w/bun	1 ea	154	350	13	27	2	21	8.0	—	—	45	40

PAGE KEY: A-96 Granola Bars, Cereal Bars, Diet Bars, Scones, and Tarts   A-96 Meals and Dishes   A-100 Meats   A-106 Nuts, Seeds, and Products   A-108 Poultry
A-110 Salad Dressings, Dips, and Mayonnaise   A-110 Salads   A-110 Sandwiches   A-114 Sauces and Gravies   A-114 Snack Foods—Chips, Pretzels, Popcorn
A-116 Soups, Stews, and Chilis   A-118 Spices, Flavors, and Seasonings   A-120 Sports Bars and Drinks   A-120 Supplemental Foods and Formulas
A-122 Sweeteners and Sweet Substitutes   A-122 Vegetables and Legumes   A-136 Weight Loss Bars and Drinks   A-138 Miscellaneous

Thia (mg)	Ribo (mg)	Niac (mg NE)	Vit B6 (mg)	Vit B12 (µg)	Fol (µg)	Vit C (mg)	Vit D (IU)	Vit E (mg AT)	Cal (mg)	Iron (mg)	Magn (mg)	Phos (mg)	Pota (mg)	Sodi (mg)	Zinc (mg)	Wat (%)	Alco (g)	Caff (g)
—	—	—	—	—	—	0.0	—	—	0	0.36	—	—	—	90	—	65	0.00	0.00
—	—	—	—	—	—	0.0	—	—	0	0.36	—	—	—	240	—	—	0.00	0.00
0.14	0.03	1.51	0.07	0.17	7.9	2.0	—	0.3	13	1.19	13.7	56	112	48	0.4	65	0.03	0.00
0.10	0.07	0.74	0.28	0.00	14.6	3.2	—	0.3	40	0.81	33.2	63	448	73	0.4	77	0.00	0.00
0.05	0.09	0.37	0.10	0.00	35.4	44.4	—	—	40	0.69	21.6	50	179	320	—	—	0.00	0.00
—	—	—	—	—	—	32.4	—	—	31	0.70	15.1	42	191	439	—	—	0.00	0.00
—	—	—	—	0.00	—	5.6	—	—	33	0.27	—	—	—	281	—	—	0.00	0.00
—	—	—	—	0.00	—	9.1	—	—	3	0.10	—	—	—	9	—	—	0.00	0.00
—	—	—	—	0.00	—	21.0	—	—	20	0.00	—	—	—	510	—	—	0.00	0.00
—	—	—	—	0.00	—	0.0	—	—	3	0.27	—	—	—	12	—	86	0.00	0.00
0.02	0.03	0.07	0.03	0.00	3.1	14.6	—	0.3	41	0.07	7.1	20	112	14	0.0	95	0.00	0.00
0.17	0.11	1.74	0.00	0.00	27.5	0.0	—	0.0	15	1.08	6.4	26	26	183	0.2	29	0.00	0.00
0.56	0.43	8.34	0.27	2.06	91.2	2.7	—	2.0	169	4.71	36.5	349	390	921	4.1	47	0.00	0.00
0.47	0.56	11.17	0.28	2.52	74.0	0.0	22.2	—	91	5.46	38.9	422	644	1589	5.6	39	0.00	0.00
0.31	0.23	6.38	0.15	1.23	64.7	2.3	—	1.3	182	2.65	26.2	216	229	976	2.6	55	0.00	0.00
0.25	0.10	2.18	0.31	0.00	43.8	6.9	—	—	4	0.87	40.9	108	359	29	0.9	72	0.00	0.00
0.10	0.05	1.45	0.28	0.05	9.7	0.5	—	—	25	0.56	21.8	67	356	275	0.4	79	0.00	0.00
0.09	0.09	1.78	0.09	0.93	14.5	0.0	—	—	15	1.78	20.4	145	272	452	0.4	54	0.00	0.00
0.57	0.50	3.92	0.05	0.36	72.9	0.1	—	—	73	1.88	16.2	146	177	513	0.6	51	0.00	0.00
0.33	0.27	3.72	0.05	0.88	53.1	0.0	10.8	0.5	63	2.40	18.9	103	145	387	2.0	38	0.00	0.00
0.12	0.55	0.50	0.11	0.87	8.5	2.3	22.6	0.4	320	0.31	36.8	283	515	235	1.0	74	0.00	0.00
0.07	0.30	0.31	0.09	0.60	8.3	1.3	60.6	0.1	203	0.15	20.0	170	290	136	0.6	75	0.00	0.00
0.18	0.37	1.53	0.20	0.81	10.2	1.2	—	—	272	1.27	55.4	276	172	816	1.8	40	0.00	0.00
0.07	0.09	0.87	0.05	0.11	51.6	0.5	—	0.3	69	0.80	14.8	81	122	405	0.3	37	0.00	0.00
0.20	0.28	1.69	0.05	0.11	25.5	1.7	—	0.7	64	1.30	24.4	238	125	552	0.5	50	0.00	0.00
0.07	0.00	1.07	0.17	0.00	7.9	5.5	—	0.1	7	0.47	15.8	69	267	290	0.2	60	0.00	0.00
0.07	0.10	0.25	0.14	0.10	23.8	1.0	—	—	13	0.68	7.6	53	256	312	0.2	79	0.00	0.00
0.05	0.10	1.13	0.17	0.00	76.6	48.0	—	—	27	1.29	22.8	81	356	54	0.4	96	0.00	0.00
0.14	0.23	2.40	0.14	1.02	60.0	2.7	—	2.0	189	3.74	24.0	238	250	999	1.6	47	0.00	0.00
0.67	0.60	2.00	0.27	1.19	65.3	0.0	—	2.3	221	4.55	30.7	317	319	1382	2.2	55	0.00	0.00
0.30	0.49	2.15	0.10	0.62	57.1	0.1	—	3.3	82	2.90	19.0	388	238	891	1.0	50	0.00	0.00
0.18	0.37	1.50	0.10	0.76	47.0	0.1	—	—	244	2.20	21.6	348	174	551	1.8	45	0.00	0.00
0.34	0.34	2.19	0.11	0.86	45.1	2.2	—	—	151	2.19	23.2	276	201	889	1.9	44	0.00	0.00
0.69	0.25	4.13	0.15	0.68	66.7	1.3	—	1.3	168	2.25	24.1	186	215	1036	1.7	38	0.00	0.00
0.50	0.31	3.48	0.14	0.02	38.4	0.1	—	1.7	160	2.72	22.6	554	197	1433	1.6	28	0.00	0.00
—	—	—	—	—	—	2.4	—	—	150	4.50	—	—	—	870	—	—	0.00	0.00
—	—	—	—	—	—	6.0	—	—	200	5.40	—	—	—	1390	—	—	0.00	0.00
—	—	—	—	—	—	18.0	—	—	40	0.00	—	—	—	880	—	—	0.00	0.00
—	—	—	—	—	—	0.0	—	—	467	4.19	—	—	—	646	—	—	0.00	—
—	—	—	—	—	—	0.0	—	—	200	0.36	—	—	—	140	—	60	0.00	—
—	—	—	—	—	—	2.4	—	—	100	4.50	—	—	—	690	—	—	0.00	0.00
—	—	—	—	—	—	1.2	—	—	60	1.44	—	—	—	920	—	—	0.00	0.00
—	—	—	—	—	—	1.2	—	—	80	1.79	—	—	—	1080	—	—	0.00	0.00

Code	Food Name	Unit/ Amt	Wt (g)	Energy (kcal)	Prot (g)	Carb (g)	Fiber (g)	Fat (g)	Sat (g)	Mono (g)	Poly (g)	Chol (mg)	Vit A (RE)
81317	Hot Dog, w/bun	1 ea	90	280	11	22	1	17	6.0	—	—	35	20
81341	Ice Cream Float, root beer, med	1 ea	467	330	4	70	0	4	2.5	—	—	15	100
81348	Milk Shake, chocolate, med, A&W	1 ea	475	700	11	100	2	29	18.1	—	—	125	312
81358	Milk Shake, vanilla, med, A&W	1 ea	475	719	12	97	0	31	18.8	—	—	134	250
81343	Potatoes, french fries, sml svg	1 ea	113	313	4	45	4	13	3.3	—	—	0	0
81310	Sandwich, chicken, grilled	1 ea	262	430	37	37	4	15	3.5	—	—	90	40

Arby's

Code	Food Name	Unit/ Amt	Wt (g)	Energy (kcal)	Prot (g)	Carb (g)	Fiber (g)	Fat (g)	Sat (g)	Mono (g)	Poly (g)	Chol (mg)	Vit A (RE)
42433	Biscuit, w/butter	1 ea	82	280	5	27	0	17	4.0	—	—	0	—
9008	Cheese, mozzarella sticks, 4.8 oz svg	1 ea	137	470	18	34	2	29	14.0	—	—	60	—
9011	Chicken, finger, 4 pack	1 ea	192	640	31	42	0	38	8.0	—	—	70	—
9009	Onion, petals	4 oz	113	410	4	43	2	24	3.5	—	—	0	—
8986	Potatoes, french fries, curly, med svg	1 ea	128	400	5	50	4	19	4.5	—	—	0	0
8997	Salad, caesar	1 ea	223	90	7	8	3	4	2.5	—	—	10	—
52074	Salad, garden	1 ea	349	70	4	14	6	1	0.0	—	—	0	518
8988	Sandwich, beef melt, w/cheddar	1 ea	150	320	16	36	2	14	6.0	—	—	45	—
69045	Sandwich, beef, Arby Q	1 ea	186	360	16	40	2	14	4.0	—	—	70	—
69055	Sandwich, beef, philly & swiss cheese, submarine	1 ea	311	670	36	46	4	40	16.0	—	—	75	—
56341	Sandwich, chicken, breast fillet	1 ea	208	550	24	47	2	30	5.0	—	—	90	—
69095	Sandwich, chicken, cordon bleu	1 ea	242	630	34	47	2	35	8.0	14.4	12.6	120	—
69046	Sandwich, chicken, grilled, deluxe	1 ea	252	450	29	37	2	22	4.0	—	—	110	88
69043	Sandwich, French dip, submarine	1 ea	285	410	28	43	2	16	9.0	—	—	45	—
56342	Sandwich, ham swiss, hot	1 ea	170	340	23	35	1	13	4.5	—	—	90	40
8992	Sandwich, roast beef swiss	1 ea	360	780	37	74	6	40	14.0	—	—	80	—
56336	Sandwich, roast beef, regular	1 ea	157	330	21	35	2	14	7.0	—	—	45	0
53256	Sauce, Arbys, pkt	1 ea	14	15	0	4	0	0	0.0	0.0	0.0	0	—
9025	Sauce, honey mustard, dipping	1 oz	28	130	0	5	0	12	1.5	—	—	10	—

Boston Market

Code	Food Name	Unit/ Amt	Wt (g)	Energy (kcal)	Prot (g)	Carb (g)	Fiber (g)	Fat (g)	Sat (g)	Mono (g)	Poly (g)	Chol (mg)	Vit A (RE)
52109	Cole Slaw, svg	1 ea	430	310	7	29	10	22	3.0	—	—	20	—
57529	Dish, macaroni & cheese, svg	1 ea	192	280	13	33	1	11	6.0	—	—	30	—
7390	Dish, mashed potatoes, homestyle, svg	1 ea	173	210	4	30	2	9	5.0	—	—	25	—
57528	Dish, mashed potatoes, w/gravy, homestyle, svg	1 ea	201	230	4	32	3	9	5.0	—	—	25	—
57530	Dish, pot pie, chicken, original, svg	1 ea	425	750	26	57	2	46	14.0	—	—	110	—
53541	Gravy, chicken, 1 oz svg	1 ea	28	15	0	2	0	0	0.0	—	—	0	—
52104	Salad, caesar, svg	1 ea	269	470	14	17	3	40	9.0	—	—	35	—
1143	Sandwich, marinated grilled chicken	1 ea	284	670	42	45	2	36	6.0	—	—	105	—
50299	Soup, chicken noodle, hearty, svg	1 cup	190	100	6	8	0	4	1.5	—	—	30	—
7391	Spinach, creamed, svg	1 ea	181	260	9	11	2	20	13.0	—	—	55	—

Burger King

Code	Food Name	Unit/ Amt	Wt (g)	Energy (kcal)	Prot (g)	Carb (g)	Fiber (g)	Fat (g)	Sat (g)	Mono (g)	Poly (g)	Chol (mg)	Vit A (RE)
56352	Cheeseburger	1 ea	136	370	20	31	2	18	9.0	—	—	55	60
57001	Cheeseburger, double	1 ea	197	570	35	32	2	34	17.0	—	—	110	100
56355	Cheeseburger, Whopper	1 ea	303	780	34	55	4	47	17.0	—	—	105	150
57000	Cheeseburger, Whopper Jr	1 ea	180	460	21	33	2	27	10.0	—	—	60	80
9087	Chicken, Tenders, 4 pce svg	1 ea	62	170	11	10	0	9	3.0	—	—	25	0
42429	French Toast, sticks, svg	1 ea	112	390	6	46	2	20	4.5	—	—	0	0
56351	Hamburger	1 ea	123	320	18	30	2	14	6.0	—	—	45	20
56354	Hamburger, Whopper	1 ea	278	680	29	53	4	39	12.0	—	—	80	100

PAGE KEY: A-96 Granola Bars, Cereal Bars, Diet Bars, Scones, and Tarts   A-96 Meals and Dishes   A-100 Meats   A-106 Nuts, Seeds, and Products   A-108 Poultry   A-110 Salad Dressings, Dips, and Mayonnaise   A-110 Salads   A-110 Sandwiches   A-114 Sauces and Gravies   A-114 Snack Foods—Chips, Pretzels, Popcorn   A-116 Soups, Stews, and Chilis   A-118 Spices, Flavors, and Seasonings   A-120 Sports Bars and Drinks   A-120 Supplemental Foods and Formulas   A-122 Sweeteners and Sweet Substitutes   A-122 Vegetables and Legumes   A-136 Weight Loss Bars and Drinks   A-138 Miscellaneous

Thia (mg)	Ribo (mg)	Niac (mg NE)	Vit B6 (mg)	Vit B12 (µg)	Fol (µg)	Vit C (mg)	Vit D (IU)	Vit E (mg AT)	Cal (mg)	Iron (mg)	Magn (mg)	Phos (mg)	Pota (mg)	Sodi (mg)	Zinc (mg)	Wat (%)	Alco (g)	Caff (g)
—	—	—	—	—	—	0.0	—	—	40	1.44	—	—	—	710	—	—	0.00	0.00
—	—	—	—	—	—	0.0	—	—	150	0.36	—	—	—	120	—	—	0.00	0.00
—	—	—	—	—	—	0.0	—	—	281	1.69	—	—	—	200	—	—	0.00	—
—	—	—	—	—	—	0.0	—	—	438	1.69	—	—	—	212	—	—	0.00	0.00
—	—	—	—	—	—	19.6	—	—	0	0.00	—	—	—	465	—	—	0.00	0.00
—	—	—	—	—	—	6.0	—	—	100	3.59	—	—	—	1080	—	—	0.00	0.00
0.23	0.14	3.00	—	—	—	0.0	—	—	40	0.00	—	—	130	780	—	—	0.00	0.00
—	—	—	—	—	—	1.2	—	—	400	0.72	—	—	—	1330	—	—	0.00	0.00
—	—	—	—	—	—	0.0	—	—	20	2.70	—	—	—	1590	—	—	0.00	0.00
—	—	—	—	—	—	0.0	—	—	40	0.72	—	—	—	300	—	—	0.00	0.00
0.07	0.09	2.57	—	0.00	—	15.5	—	—	0	1.86	—	—	934	993	0.8	41	0.00	0.00
—	—	—	—	—	—	42.0	—	—	200	1.79	—	—	—	170	—	—	0.00	0.00
0.17	0.20	1.26	—	—	—	42.0	—	—	80	1.44	—	—	635	45	0.9	—	0.00	0.00
—	—	—	—	—	—	0.0	—	—	80	2.70	—	—	—	850	—	—	0.00	0.00
0.25	0.37	9.00	—	—	—	4.8	—	—	80	3.59	—	—	456	1530	—	—	0.00	0.00
0.44	0.72	13.89	—	—	—	9.0	—	—	300	2.70	—	—	646	1850	5.9	—	0.00	0.00
0.23	0.56	9.17	0.38	—	18.4	3.6	—	—	80	1.79	30.6	184	336	1160	0.2	—	0.00	0.00
0.44	0.68	10.97	—	—	—	1.2	—	—	200	0.89	—	—	499	1820	2.4	—	0.00	0.00
0.34	0.31	14.89	—	—	—	1.2	—	—	60	2.70	—	—	722	1050	—	—	0.00	0.00
0.36	0.87	15.55	—	—	—	1.2	—	—	80	4.50	—	—	679	1200	—	—	0.00	0.00
0.81	0.37	7.80	0.31	—	26.0	1.2	—	—	150	2.70	31.0	405	382	1450	0.9	—	0.00	0.00
—	—	—	—	—	—	2.4	—	—	200	2.70	—	—	—	1690	—	—	0.00	0.00
—	—	—	—	—	—	0.0	—	—	60	3.59	16.2	122	427	890	3.8	—	0.00	0.00
—	—	—	—	—	—	1.2	—	—	0	0.00	—	—	28	180	—	—	0.00	0.00
—	—	—	—	—	—	0.0	—	—	0	0.00	—	—	—	160	—	—	0.00	0.00
—	—	—	—	—	—	—	—	—	—	—	—	—	—	230	—	—	0.00	0.00
—	—	—	—	—	—	—	—	—	—	—	—	—	—	890	—	—	0.00	0.00
—	—	—	—	—	—	—	—	—	—	—	—	—	—	590	—	74	0.00	0.00
—	—	—	—	—	—	—	—	—	—	—	—	—	—	780	—	—	0.00	0.00
—	—	—	—	—	—	—	—	—	—	—	—	—	—	1530	—	—	0.00	0.00
—	—	—	—	—	—	—	—	—	—	—	—	—	—	180	—	89	0.00	0.00
—	—	—	—	—	—	—	—	—	—	—	—	—	—	1070	—	—	0.00	0.00
—	—	—	—	—	—	—	—	—	—	—	—	—	—	810	—	—	0.00	0.00
—	—	—	—	—	—	—	—	—	—	—	—	—	—	500	—	89	0.00	0.00
—	—	—	—	—	—	—	—	—	—	—	—	—	—	740	—	—	0.00	0.00
—	—	—	—	—	—	0.0	—	—	150	2.70	—	—	—	750	—	—	0.00	0.00
—	—	—	—	—	—	0.0	—	—	250	4.50	—	—	—	1020	—	—	0.00	0.00
—	—	—	—	—	—	9.0	—	—	250	5.40	—	—	—	1390	—	—	0.00	0.00
—	—	—	—	—	—	4.8	—	—	150	3.59	—	—	—	740	—	—	0.00	0.00
—	—	—	—	—	—	0.0	—	—	0	0.36	—	—	—	420	—	—	0.00	0.00
—	—	—	—	—	—	0.0	—	—	60	1.79	—	—	—	440	—	—	0.00	0.00
—	—	—	—	—	—	0.0	—	—	80	2.70	—	—	—	530	—	—	0.00	0.00
—	—	—	—	—	—	9.0	—	—	100	5.40	—	—	—	940	—	—	0.00	0.00

Code	Food Name	Unit/ Amt	Wt (g)	Energy (kcal)	Prot (g)	Carb (g)	Fiber (g)	Fat (g)	Sat (g)	Mono (g)	Poly (g)	Chol (mg)	Vit A (RE)
56999	Hamburger, Whopper Jr	1 ea	167	410	18	32	2	23	7.0	—	—	50	40
9041	Onion Rings, lrg	1 ea	137	480	7	60	5	23	6.0	—	—	0	0
56362	Sandwich, Big Fish	1 ea	263	710	24	67	4	38	14.0	—	—	50	20
56360	Sandwich, chicken	1 ea	224	660	25	53	3	39	8.0	—	—	70	20
9057	Sandwich, chicken tenders	1 ea	148	450	14	37	2	27	5.0	—	—	30	40
Carl's Junior													
91433	Burrito, breakfast	1 ea	185	480	27	26	2	30	13.0	—	—	465	150
91404	Cheeseburger, Western Bacon	1 ea	225	650	32	63	2	30	12.0	—	—	80	40
91419	Chicken, nuggets, Chicken Stars, svg	1 ea	90	280	12	15	0	19	4.5	—	—	40	0
91421	Dish, baked potato bacon cheese, Great Stuff	1 ea	411	630	20	76	6	29	7.0	—	—	35	150
91406	Hamburger, Jr	1 ea	134	330	18	34	1	13	5.0	—	—	45	0
91403	Hamburger, Super Star	1 ea	345	790	42	49	2	46	14.0	—	—	130	100
91414	Potatoes, french fries, svg	1 ea	92	290	5	37	3	14	3.0	—	—	0	0
91425	Salad, garden, Salad To Go	1 ea	137	50	3	4	2	2	1.5	—	—	10	600
91407	Sandwich, chicken, bbq, charbroiled	1 ea	199	280	25	37	2	3	1.0	—	—	60	60
91411	Sandwich, chicken, crispy, bacon swiss	1 ea	291	720	32	66	3	36	10.0	—	—	75	80
91413	Sandwich, fish, Carl's Catch	1 ea	201	510	18	50	1	27	7.0	—	—	80	60
Chick-Fil-A													
69188	Chicken, breast, fillet, brd	1 ea	105	230	23	10	0	11	2.5	—	—	60	40
52139	Salad, carrot raisin, sml	1 ea	91	130	1	22	2	5	1.0	—	—	0	1700
52135	Salad, Chick-N-Strips	1 ea	315	340	30	19	3	16	5.0	—	—	85	600
69152	Sandwich, chicken	1 ea	170	410	28	38	1	16	3.5	—	—	60	40
69183	Wrap, chicken caesar, Cool Wrap	1 ea	227	460	38	51	3	11	6.0	—	—	85	150
69182	Wrap, chicken, spicy	1 ea	225	390	31	51	3	7	3.5	—	—	70	40
Chili's Grill&Bar													
4822	Dinner, chicken, platter, Guiltless Grill	0.5 ea	326	282	19	42	2	4	1.5	—	—	29	368
4826	Salad, chicken, w/dressing	1 ea	445	272	29	27	6	5	1.0	—	—	47	416
4825	Sandwich, chicken, Guiltless Grill	1 ea	553	527	44	70	11	8	2.0	—	—	43	620
Dairy Queen													
56372	Cheeseburger, double, homestyle	1 ea	219	540	35	30	2	31	16.0	—	—	115	150
16287	Dinner, chicken, strip, basket, w/gravy	1 ea	415	1000	35	102	5	50	13.0	—	—	55	40
2131	Frozen Dessert, banana split, Royal Treats	1 ea	369	510	8	96	3	12	8.0	—	—	30	200
2352	Frozen Dessert, Misty Slush, med	1 ea	595	290	0	74	0	0	0.0	0.0	0.0	0	0
2368	Frozen Dessert, oreo, med, Dairy Queen Blizzard	1 ea	326	640	12	97	1	23	11.0	—	—	45	250
56368	Hamburger, homestyle	1 ea	138	290	17	29	2	12	5.0	—	—	45	40
56374	Hot Dog	1 ea	99	240	9	19	1	14	5.0	—	—	25	20
2222	Ice Cream Cone, chocolate, med	1 ea	198	340	8	53	0	11	7.0	—	—	30	150
2143	Ice Cream Cone, vanilla, med	1 ea	213	355	9	57	0	10	6.5	—	—	32	161
2134	Ice Cream Sandwich, Dairy Queen	1 ea	85	200	4	31	1	6	3.0	—	—	10	40
2348	Ice Cream, chocolate, soft serve, Dairy Queen	0.5 cup	94	150	4	22	0	5	3.5	—	—	15	100
2224	Milk Shake, chocolate, med, Dairy Queen	1 ea	539	770	17	130	0	20	13.0	—	—	70	400
56383	Onion Rings, svg	1 ea	113	320	5	39	3	16	4.0	—	—	0	0
71690	Sandwich, bbq beef	1 ea	142	300	16	37	2	9	3.5	—	—	35	40
Dennys													
1125	Biscuit, w/sausage gravy, svg	1 ea	198	398	8	45	0	21	6.0	—	—	12	0
25238	Breakfast, Country Slam	1 ea	510	1000	41	61	1	66	21.0	—	—	467	300
1077	Breakfast, sausage supreme skillet	1 ea	425	857	27	29	8	62	19.0	—	—	466	490

PAGE KEY: A-96 Granola Bars, Cereal Bars, Diet Bars, Scones, and Tarts   A-96 Meals and Dishes   A-100 Meats   A-106 Nuts, Seeds, and Products   A-108 Poultry   A-110 Salad Dressings, Dips, and Mayonnaise   A-110 Salads   A-110 Sandwiches   A-114 Sauces and Gravies   A-114 Snack Foods—Chips, Pretzels, Popcorn   A-116 Soups, Stews, and Chilis   A-118 Spices, Flavors, and Seasonings   A-120 Sports Bars and Drinks   A-120 Supplemental Foods and Formulas   A-122 Sweeteners and Sweet Substitutes   A-122 Vegetables and Legumes   A-136 Weight Loss Bars and Drinks   A-138 Miscellaneous

Thia (mg)	Ribo (mg)	Niac (mg NE)	Vit B6 (mg)	Vit B12 (μg)	Fol (μg)	Vit C (mg)	Vit D (IU)	Vit E (mg AT)	Cal (mg)	Iron (mg)	Magn (mg)	Phos (mg)	Pota (mg)	Sodi (mg)	Zinc (mg)	Wat (%)	Alco (g)	Caff (g)
—	—	—	—	—	—	4.8	—	—	80	3.59	—	—	—	520	—	55	0.00	0.00
—	—	—	—	—	—	0.0	—	—	150	0.00	—	—	—	690	—	—	0.00	0.00
—	—	—	—	—	—	0.0	—	—	80	3.59	—	—	—	1200	—	—	0.00	0.00
—	—	—	—	—	—	0.0	—	—	80	2.70	—	—	—	1330	—	—	0.00	0.00
—	—	—	—	—	—	3.6	—	—	60	1.79	—	—	—	680	—	—	0.00	0.00
—	—	—	—	—	—	0.0	—	—	350	2.70	—	—	—	750	—	—	0.00	0.00
—	—	—	—	—	—	1.2	—	—	200	4.50	—	—	—	1430	—	—	0.00	0.00
—	—	—	—	—	—	0.0	—	—	20	1.08	—	—	—	330	—	47	0.00	0.00
—	—	—	—	—	—	36.0	—	—	150	4.50	—	—	—	1700	—	—	0.00	0.00
—	—	—	—	—	—	2.4	—	—	60	3.59	—	—	—	480	—	—	0.00	0.00
—	—	—	—	—	—	9.0	—	—	100	5.40	—	—	—	910	—	—	0.00	0.00
—	—	—	—	—	—	21.0	—	—	0	1.08	—	—	—	170	—	36	0.00	0.00
—	—	—	—	—	—	15.0	—	—	80	0.72	—	—	—	60	—	93	0.00	0.00
—	—	—	—	—	—	4.8	—	—	80	2.70	—	—	—	830	—	—	0.00	0.00
—	—	—	—	—	—	6.0	—	—	250	3.59	—	—	—	1610	—	—	0.00	0.00
—	—	—	—	—	—	2.4	—	—	150	1.79	—	—	—	1030	—	51	0.00	0.00
—	—	—	—	—	—	0.0	—	—	40	1.08	—	—	—	990	—	—	0.00	0.00
—	—	—	—	—	—	3.6	—	—	20	0.36	—	—	—	90	—	—	0.00	0.00
—	—	—	—	—	—	6.0	—	—	150	1.08	—	—	—	680	—	—	0.00	0.00
—	—	—	—	—	—	0.0	—	—	100	2.70	—	—	—	1300	—	—	0.00	0.00
—	—	—	—	—	—	0.0	—	—	400	3.59	—	—	—	1540	—	—	0.00	0.00
—	—	—	—	—	—	4.8	—	—	200	3.59	—	—	—	1150	—	—	0.00	0.00
—	—	—	—	—	—	16.5	—	—	86	4.00	—	—	—	1642	—	—	0.00	0.00
—	—	—	—	—	—	16.0	—	—	36	4.00	—	—	—	1475	—	—	0.00	0.00
—	—	—	—	—	—	26.0	—	—	306	9.00	—	—	—	2923	—	—	0.00	0.00
—	—	—	—	—	—	3.6	—	—	250	4.50	—	—	—	1130	—	—	0.00	0.00
—	—	—	—	—	—	9.0	—	—	60	4.50	—	—	—	2510	—	—	0.00	0.00
—	—	—	—	—	—	15.0	—	—	250	1.79	—	—	—	180	—	—	0.00	—
—	—	—	—	—	—	0.0	—	—	0	0.00	—	—	—	30	—	—	0.00	0.00
—	—	—	—	—	—	1.2	—	—	400	2.70	—	—	—	500	—	—	0.00	—
—	—	—	—	—	—	3.6	—	—	60	2.70	—	—	—	630	—	56	0.00	0.00
—	—	—	—	—	—	3.6	—	—	60	1.79	—	—	—	730	—	55	0.00	0.00
—	—	—	—	—	—	1.2	—	—	250	1.79	—	—	—	160	—	—	0.00	—
—	—	—	—	—	—	2.6	—	—	269	1.94	—	—	—	172	—	—	0.00	0.00
—	—	—	—	—	—	0.0	—	—	80	1.08	—	—	—	140	—	51	0.00	—
—	—	—	—	—	—	0.0	—	—	100	0.72	—	—	—	75	—	—	0.00	—
—	—	—	—	—	—	2.4	—	—	600	2.70	—	—	—	420	—	—	0.00	—
—	—	—	—	—	—	0.0	—	—	20	1.44	—	—	—	180	—	—	0.00	0.00
—	—	—	—	—	—	0.0	—	—	60	2.70	—	—	—	610	—	—	0.00	0.00
—	—	—	—	—	—	0.0	—	—	10	0.18	—	—	—	1267	—	—	0.00	0.00
—	—	—	—	—	—	0.0	—	—	70	4.13	—	—	—	2727	—	—	0.00	0.00
—	—	—	—	—	—	22.8	—	—	180	2.88	—	—	—	1700	—	—	0.00	0.00

PAGE KEY: A-46 Beverage and Beverage Mixes   A-48 Other Beverages   A-48 Beverages, Alcoholic   A-50 Candies and Confections, Gum   A-54 Cereals, Breakfast Type
A-58 Cheese and Cheese Substitutes   A-60 Dairy Products and Substitutes   A-62 Desserts   A-68 Dessert Toppings   A-68 Eggs, Substitutes, and Egg Dishes   A-70 Ethnic Foods
A-74 Fast Foods/Restaurants   A-88 Fats, Oils, Margarines, Shortenings, and Substitutes   A-88 Fish, Seafood, and Shellfish   A-90 Food Additives
A-90 Fruit, Vegetable, or Blended Juices   A-92 Grains, Flours, and Fractions   A-92 Grain Products, Prepared and Baked Goods

Code	Food Name	Unit/ Amt	Wt (g)	Energy (kcal)	Prot (g)	Carb (g)	Fiber (g)	Fat (g)	Sat (g)	Mono (g)	Poly (g)	Chol (mg)	Vit A (RE)
17277	Chicken, breast, grilled, svg	1 ea	170	219	26	16	0	6	1.0	—	—	67	60
25249	Chicken, buffalo wings	1 ea	35	71	8	0	0	4	1.4	—	—	42	15
25248	Dish, appetizer sampler, w/chicken mozzarella onion & sauce	1 ea	482	1405	47	124	4	80	24.0	—	—	75	30
10432	Dish, fish & chips, w/tartar sauce, svg	1 ea	255	732	30	48	3	47	7.0	—	—	105	0
38655	French Toast, cinnamon swirl, w/o topping & margarine, svg	1 ea	341	1030	23	124	4	49	21.0	—	—	280	370
52144	Hamburger, classic	1 ea	312	673	37	42	3	40	15.0	—	—	106	200
12199	Hamburger, w/cheese, classic	1 ea	369	836	47	43	3	53	19.0	—	—	137	210
19548	Omelette, ham 'n cheddar, Dennys	1 ea	397	743	36	24	2	55	10.0	—	—	657	580
19547	Omelette, ultimate, Dennys	1 ea	482	780	31	29	4	62	14.0	—	—	639	540
38657	Onion Rings, basket	1 ea	255	824	11	83	1	50	12.0	—	—	14	30
25250	Quesadilla, chicken	1 ea	454	827	50	43	2	55	23.0	—	—	181	630
12195	Sandwich, club	1 ea	312	718	32	62	3	38	7.0	—	—	75	60
Dominos Pizza													
91365	Breadsticks	1 ea	37	116	3	18	1	4	0.8	—	—	0	4
91369	Chicken, buffalo wings	1 ea	25	50	6	2	0	2	0.6	—	—	26	8
56386	Pizza, cheese, hand tossed, 12"	2 pce	159	375	15	55	3	11	4.8	—	—	23	131
91360	Pizza, Hawaiian feast, hand tossed, 12"	2 pce	204	450	21	58	3	16	7.2	—	—	41	173
91361	Pizza, pepperoni feast, hand tossed, 12"	2 pce	196	534	24	56	3	25	10.9	—	—	57	175
91357	Pizza, veggie feast, hand tossed, 12"	2 pce	203	439	19	57	4	16	7.1	—	—	34	181
Dunkin' Donuts													
50720	Chowder, clam, New England, svg	1 ea	227	200	10	16	0	10	3.0	—	—	30	100
45742	Doughnut, Bismark	1 ea	80	310	4	42	1	14	4.0	—	—	0	0
45700	Doughnut, cake, chocolate	1 ea	59	210	3	19	1	14	3.0	—	—	0	0
45695	Doughnut, cake, old fash	1 ea	60	280	3	24	1	19	4.0	—	—	0	0
45708	Doughnut, raised, glazed	1 ea	46	160	3	23	1	7	2.0	—	—	0	0
42636	Fritter, apple	1 ea	95	300	5	41	2	13	3.0	—	—	0	0
69090	Sandwich, ham cheese, croissant	1 ea	192	710	33	29	0	32	13.0	—	—	85	100
50722	Soup, cream of broccoli, svg	1 ea	227	200	8	17	0	11	6.0	—	—	25	200
45749	Turnover, apple	1 ea	109	350	5	49	2	15	4.0	—	—	0	0
El Pollo Loco													
28110	Chicken, strips, svg	1 ea	213	558	41	48	2	25	5.0	—	—	76	0
49103	Frozen Dessert, banana split	1 ea	425	717	12	107	3	28	11.0	—	—	56	80
4012	Guacamole, 1.8 oz svg	1 ea	50	52	0	5	0	3	0.0	—	—	0	30
1655	Salad, garden, reg	1 ea	113	105	5	7	1	7	3.0	—	—	15	60
1656	Salad, tostada	1 ea	397	304	29	28	4	11	3.0	—	—	57	190
28104	Salsa, avocado	28.35 g	28	12	0	1	0	1	0.0	—	—	0	5
7204	Taco, chicken, soft	1 ea	128	238	17	15	0	12	4.0	—	—	74	120
49112	Tortilla, corn, 6"	1 ea	28	70	1	14	1	1	0.0	—	—	0	30
Hardees													
9280	Cheeseburger	1 ea	124	313	16	26	1	14	7.0	—	—	40	—
56412	Hamburger	1 ea	110	265	14	26	1	10	4.0	—	—	35	—
9286	Potatoes, french fries, Crispy Curls, reg svg	1 ea	96	340	5	41	0	18	4.0	—	—	0	—
6146	Potatoes, french fries, reg svg	1 ea	113	340	4	45	0	16	2.0	—	—	0	—
56418	Sandwich, roast beef, regular	1 ea	123	310	17	26	2	16	6.0	—	—	43	—

PAGE KEY: A-96 Granola Bars, Cereal Bars, Diet Bars, Scones, and Tarts   A-96 Meals and Dishes   A-100 Meats   A-106 Nuts, Seeds, and Products   A-108 Poultry   A-110 Salad Dressings, Dips, and Mayonnaise   A-110 Salads   A-110 Sandwiches   A-114 Sauces and Gravies   A-114 Snack Foods—Chips, Pretzels, Popcorn   A-116 Soups, Stews, and Chilis   A-118 Spices, Flavors, and Seasonings   A-120 Sports Bars and Drinks   A-120 Supplemental Foods and Formulas   A-122 Sweeteners and Sweet Substitutes   A-122 Vegetables and Legumes   A-136 Weight Loss Bars and Drinks   A-138 Miscellaneous

Thia (mg)	Ribo (mg)	Niac (mg NE)	Vit B6 (mg)	Vit B12 (µg)	Fol (µg)	Vit C (mg)	Vit D (IU)	Vit E (mg AT)	Cal (mg)	Iron (mg)	Magn (mg)	Phos (mg)	Pota (mg)	Sodi (mg)	Zinc (mg)	Wat (%)	Alco (g)	Caff (g)
—	—	—	—	—	—	1.2	—	—	10	1.08	—	—	—	880	—	—	0.00	0.00
—	—	—	—	—	—	2.4	—	—	16	1.29	—	—	—	462	—	—	0.00	0.00
—	—	—	—	—	—	6.6	—	—	440	2.88	—	—	—	5305	—	—	0.00	0.00
—	—	—	—	—	—	0.0	—	—	0	1.44	—	—	—	1335	—	—	0.00	0.00
—	—	—	—	—	—	0.0	—	—	180	6.48	—	—	—	675	—	—	0.00	0.00
—	—	—	—	—	—	10.8	—	—	130	4.50	—	—	—	1142	—	—	0.00	0.00
—	—	—	—	—	—	10.8	—	—	340	4.50	—	—	—	1595	—	—	0.00	0.00
—	—	—	—	—	—	6.6	—	—	290	3.05	—	—	—	1518	—	—	0.00	0.00
—	—	—	—	—	—	37.8	—	—	90	3.59	—	—	—	1360	—	—	0.00	0.00
—	—	—	—	—	—	4.8	—	—	40	1.25	—	—	—	2173	—	—	0.00	0.00
—	—	—	—	—	—	54.0	—	—	640	1.79	—	—	—	1982	—	—	0.00	0.00
—	—	—	—	—	—	13.2	—	—	120	4.32	—	—	—	1666	—	—	0.00	0.00
—	—	—	—	—	—	0.1	—	—	6	0.87	—	—	—	152	—	—	0.00	0.00
—	—	—	—	—	—	0.1	—	—	6	0.31	—	—	—	175	—	—	0.00	0.00
—	—	—	—	—	—	0.0	—	—	187	2.99	—	—	—	776	—	—	0.00	0.00
—	—	—	—	—	—	1.9	—	—	274	3.29	—	—	—	1102	—	51	0.00	0.00
—	—	—	—	—	—	0.1	—	—	279	3.40	—	—	—	1349	—	44	0.00	0.00
—	—	—	—	—	—	1.3	—	—	279	3.44	—	—	—	987	—	53	0.00	0.00
—	—	—	—	—	—	3.6	—	—	150	2.70	—	—	—	1050	—	—	0.00	0.00
—	—	—	—	—	—	2.4	—	—	0	0.72	—	—	—	260	—	—	0.00	0.00
—	—	—	—	—	—	3.6	—	—	0	1.44	—	—	—	270	—	—	0.00	—
—	—	—	—	—	—	1.2	—	—	0	1.08	—	—	—	350	—	—	0.00	0.00
—	—	—	—	—	—	1.2	—	—	0	0.36	—	—	—	200	—	—	0.00	0.00
—	—	—	—	—	—	0.0	—	—	0	1.44	—	—	—	320	—	—	0.00	0.00
—	—	—	—	—	—	24.0	—	—	250	2.70	—	—	—	1840	—	—	0.00	0.00
—	—	—	—	—	—	18.0	—	—	250	0.36	—	—	—	1050	—	83	0.00	0.00
—	—	—	—	—	—	2.4	—	—	0	0.72	—	—	—	340	—	—	0.00	0.00
—	—	—	—	—	—	0.0	—	—	100	2.70	—	—	—	1876	—	—	0.00	0.00
—	—	—	—	—	—	22.2	—	—	270	1.98	—	—	—	310	—	—	0.00	0.00
—	—	—	—	—	—	4.2	—	—	40	0.73	—	—	—	282	—	—	0.00	0.00
—	—	—	—	—	—	6.6	—	—	110	0.36	—	—	—	99	—	—	0.00	0.00
—	—	—	—	—	—	22.8	—	—	180	3.24	—	—	—	1175	—	—	0.00	0.00
—	—	—	—	—	—	7.2	—	—	0	0.18	—	—	—	204	—	92	0.00	0.00
—	—	—	—	—	—	10.2	—	—	181	1.62	—	—	—	631	—	—	0.00	0.00
—	—	—	—	—	—	0.0	—	—	10	0.36	—	—	—	35	—	42	0.00	0.00
—	—	—	—	—	—	—	—	—	—	—	—	—	—	895	—	—	0.00	0.00
—	—	—	—	—	—	—	—	—	—	—	—	—	—	663	—	—	0.00	0.00
—	—	—	—	—	—	—	—	—	—	—	—	—	—	950	—	—	0.00	0.00
—	—	—	—	—	—	—	—	—	—	—	—	—	—	390	—	41	0.00	0.00
—	—	—	—	—	—	—	—	—	—	—	—	—	—	804	—	—	0.00	0.00

PAGE KEY: A-46 Beverage and Beverage Mixes   A-48 Other Beverages   A-48 Beverages, Alcoholic   A-50 Candies and Confections, Gum   A-54 Cereals, Breakfast Type
A-58 Cheese and Cheese Substitutes   A-60 Dairy Products and Substitutes   A-62 Desserts   A-68 Dessert Toppings   A-68 Eggs, Substitutes, and Egg Dishes   A-70 Ethnic Foods
A-74 Fast Foods/Restaurants   A-88 Fats, Oils, Margarines, Shortenings, and Substitutes   A-88 Fish, Seafood, and Shellfish   A-90 Food Additives
A-90 Fruit, Vegetable, or Blended Juices   A-92 Grains, Flours, and Fractions   A-92 Grain Products, Prepared and Baked Goods

Code	Food Name	Unit/ Amt	Wt (g)	Energy (kcal)	Prot (g)	Carb (g)	Fiber (g)	Fat (g)	Sat (g)	Mono (g)	Poly (g)	Chol (mg)	Vit A (RE)
56404	Sandwich, sausage egg, w/biscuit	1 ea	156	617	19	44	—	41	12.9	—	—	224	—
56403	Sandwich, sausage, w/biscuit	1 ea	114	553	13	44	—	36	11.0	—	—	30	—
In-N-Out Burgers													
81119	Potatoes, french fries	1 ea	125	400	7	54	2	18	5.0	—	—	0	0
Jack in the Box													
56434	Cheeseburger	1 ea	116	300	14	31	2	13	6.0	—	—	40	40
15162	Chicken, strips, 5 pce svg	1 ea	150	360	27	24	1	17	3.0	—	—	80	40
62548	Dish, fish & chips	1 ea	281	780	19	86	6	39	9.0	—	—	45	20
56433	Hamburger	1 ea	104	250	12	30	2	9	3.5	—	—	30	0
2163	Milk Shake, chocolate, med, Jack in the Box	1 ea	332	630	11	85	1	27	16.0	—	—	85	150
2165	Milk Shake, vanilla, med, Jack in the Box	1 ea	332	610	12	73	0	31	18.0	—	—	95	150
56446	Onion Rings, svg	1 ea	120	450	7	50	3	25	5.0	—	—	0	40
56448	Salad, side	1 ea	86	50	2	3	1	3	1.5	—	—	10	75
69035	Sandwich, chicken	1 ea	164	400	15	38	3	21	3.0	—	—	40	40
56377	Taco	1 ea	90	170	7	12	2	10	3.5	—	—	15	60
Jamba Juice													
81280	Breadsticks, pizza, w/add prot, svg	1 ea	76	230	9	33	2	6	1.5	—	—	5	60
81227	Smoothie, Banana Berry, Jamba Juice	16 fl-oz	475	270	2	66	3	2	0.0	—	—	0	20
81245	Smoothie, Coldbuster, Jamba Juice	16 fl-oz	476	280	3	65	3	2	0.0	—	—	5	700
81266	Smoothie, Orange Dream Machine, Jamba Juice	16 fl-oz	504	410	15	84	1	2	1.0	—	—	5	80
81253	Smoothie, PowerBoost	16 fl-oz	519	280	4	67	6	1	0.0	—	—	0	600
81283	Smoothie, Razzmatazz, Jamba Juice	16 fl-oz	490	300	2	72	3	1	0.0	—	—	0	20
81362	Smoothie, strawberry banana	8 fl-oz	240	124	1	29	1	0	0.0	0.0	0.0	0	0
Kentucky Fried Chicken													
42331	Biscuit, buttermilk	1 ea	57	190	2	23	0	10	2.0	—	—	0	0
15163	Chicken, breast, original rec	1 ea	161	380	40	11	0	19	6.0	—	—	145	0
56451	Cole Slaw, svg	1 ea	130	190	1	22	3	11	2.0	—	—	5	250
6152	Corn, cob, large	1 ea	162	150	5	26	7	3	1.0	—	—	0	0
56453	Potatoes, mashed, w/gravy, svg	1 ea	136	130	2	18	1	4	1.0	—	—	0	20
6188	Potatoes, wedges, svg	1 ea	102	240	5	30	3	12	3.0	—	—	0	0
Long John Silvers													
91388	Cheese, cheesesticks, brd, fried, 0.5 oz ea	3 ea	45	140	4	12	1	8	2.0	—	—	10	40
56477	Cornbread, hush puppies, svg	1 ea	23	60	1	9	1	2	0.5	—	—	0	0
56461	Fish, batter dipped, reg, 3.3 oz	1 pce	92	230	11	16	0	13	4.0	—	—	30	0
69030	Sandwich, fish, batter dipped	1 ea	177	440	17	47	3	21	5.0	—	—	40	60
19108	Shrimp, battered	1 ea	14	45	2	3	0	3	1.0	—	—	15	0
McDonalds													
69009	Cheeseburger	1 ea	119	326	15	33	2	15	6.2	5.2	1.5	42	—
69010	Cheeseburger, Big Mac	1 ea	219	572	26	47	3	31	10.9	11.3	8.5	79	—
69012	Cheeseburger, Quarter Pounder	1 ea	199	535	30	39	2	29	13.8	12.1	2.6	96	—
15174	Chicken, nuggets, McNuggets, 4 pce svg	4 pce	72	190	10	13	1	11	2.5	—	—	35	0
47147	Cookie, McDonaldland, pkg	1 ea	57	230	3	38	1	8	2.0	—	—	0	0
19579	Eggs, scrambled, svg	1 ea	102	160	13	1	0	11	3.5	—	—	425	150
2171	Frozen Dessert, sundae, hot fudge, low fat	1 ea	179	340	8	52	1	12	9.0	—	—	30	100
69008	Hamburger	1 ea	105	270	13	32	2	10	3.6	4.1	1.3	27	—
69011	Hamburger, Quarter Pounder	1 ea	171	438	27	38	2	20	8.3	9.4	2.1	68	—
2169	Milk Shake, vanilla, sml, McDonalds	1 ea	293	360	11	59	0	9	6.0	—	—	40	60

PAGE KEY: A-96 Granola Bars, Cereal Bars, Diet Bars, Scones, and Tarts   A-96 Meals and Dishes   A-100 Meats   A-106 Nuts, Seeds, and Products   A-108 Poultry   A-110 Salad Dressings, Dips, and Mayonnaise   A-110 Salads   A-110 Sandwiches   A-114 Sauces and Gravies   A-114 Snack Foods—Chips, Pretzels, Popcorn   A-116 Soups, Stews, and Chilis   A-118 Spices, Flavors, and Seasonings   A-120 Sports Bars and Drinks   A-120 Supplemental Foods and Formulas   A-122 Sweeteners and Sweet Substitutes   A-122 Vegetables and Legumes   A-136 Weight Loss Bars and Drinks   A-138 Miscellaneous

Thia (mg)	Ribo (mg)	Niac (mg NE)	Vit B6 (mg)	Vit B12 (µg)	Fol (µg)	Vit C (mg)	Vit D (IU)	Vit E (mg AT)	Cal (mg)	Iron (mg)	Magn (mg)	Phos (mg)	Pota (mg)	Sodi (mg)	Zinc (mg)	Wat (%)	Alco (g)	Caff (g)
—	—	—	—	—	—	—	—	—	—	—	—	—	—	1359	—	—	0.00	0.00
—	—	—	—	—	—	—	—	—	—	—	—	—	—	1305	—	—	0.00	0.00
—	—	—	—	—	—	0.0	—	—	20	1.79	—	—	—	245	—	—	0.00	0.00
—	—	—	—	—	—	0.0	—	—	150	3.59	—	—	180	840	—	—	0.00	0.00
—	—	—	—	—	—	1.2	—	—	0	1.79	—	—	430	970	—	—	0.00	0.00
—	—	—	—	—	—	15.0	—	—	20	2.70	—	—	1060	1740	—	—	0.00	0.00
—	—	—	—	—	—	0.0	—	—	100	3.59	—	—	155	610	—	—	0.00	0.00
—	—	—	—	—	—	0.0	—	—	350	0.36	—	—	720	330	—	—	0.00	—
—	—	—	—	—	—	0.0	—	—	400	0.00	—	—	730	320	—	64	0.00	0.00
—	—	—	—	—	—	18.0	—	—	40	2.70	—	—	150	780	—	30	0.00	0.00
—	—	—	—	—	—	0.0	—	—	80	0.72	—	—	160	75	—	—	0.00	0.00
—	—	—	—	—	—	4.8	—	—	100	2.70	—	—	200	770	—	—	0.00	0.00
—	—	—	—	—	—	0.2	—	—	100	1.08	40.4	168	235	390	1.4	66	0.00	0.00
0.37	0.25	3.00	0.03	0.00	80.0	4.8	0.0	0.8	80	2.70	8.0	20	130	450	0.3	—	0.00	0.00
0.05	0.10	0.80	0.60	0.11	16.0	9.0	0.0	0.4	80	0.72	24.0	40	540	35	0.3	—	0.00	0.00
0.23	0.14	2.00	0.30	0.00	100.0	684.0	0.0	10.1	60	0.72	40.0	60	800	15	7.5	—	0.00	0.00
0.23	0.25	0.80	0.11	0.47	60.0	78.0	100.0	0.0	400	0.72	32.0	300	540	230	0.6	—	0.00	0.00
2.70	2.89	34.00	3.59	4.80	360.0	198.0	240.0	12.1	600	1.44	240.0	80	810	30	7.5	—	0.00	0.00
0.05	0.17	4.00	0.69	0.11	100.0	36.0	0.0	0.0	80	1.08	24.0	60	570	45	0.3	—	0.00	0.00
—	—	—	—	—	—	60.0	—	—	0	0.89	—	—	475	10	—	—	0.00	0.00
—	—	—	—	—	—	0.0	—	—	0	0.72	—	—	—	580	—	36	0.00	0.00
—	—	—	—	—	—	0.0	—	—	0	1.79	—	—	—	1150	—	55	0.00	0.00
—	—	—	—	—	—	24.0	—	—	40	0.00	—	—	—	300	—	—	0.00	0.00
—	—	—	—	—	—	6.0	—	—	60	1.08	—	—	—	10	—	—	0.00	0.00
—	—	—	—	—	—	2.4	—	—	0	0.36	—	—	—	380	—	—	0.00	0.00
—	—	—	—	—	—	3.6	—	—	20	1.79	—	—	—	830	—	—	0.00	0.00
—	—	—	—	—	—	0.0	—	—	100	0.72	—	—	—	320	—	—	0.00	0.00
—	—	—	—	—	—	0.0	—	—	20	0.36	—	—	—	200	—	43	0.00	0.00
—	—	—	—	—	—	4.8	—	—	20	1.79	—	—	—	700	—	54	0.00	0.00
—	—	—	—	—	—	9.0	—	—	60	3.59	—	—	—	1120	—	—	0.00	0.00
—	—	—	—	—	—	1.2	—	—	0	0.00	—	—	—	125	—	43	0.00	0.00
0.34	0.18	4.82	0.09	1.57	30.9	0.4	—	0.1	219	1.75	29.8	179	234	739	2.4	45	0.00	0.00
0.40	0.43	7.94	0.37	2.77	59.1	0.7	—	0.1	278	3.06	54.8	298	399	1062	4.7	51	0.00	0.00
0.23	0.51	8.06	0.18	3.48	31.8	0.6	—	0.4	356	2.02	51.7	364	444	1176	5.6	48	0.00	0.00
—	—	4.92	—	0.20	—	0.0	—	0.9	9	0.70	16.4	191	202	360	0.7	51	0.00	0.00
—	—	2.03	—	—	—	0.0	—	1.0	20	1.79	11.3	71	63	250	0.4	13	0.00	0.00
0.07	0.50	0.05	0.11	1.11	44.0	0.0	—	0.9	40	1.08	10.0	172	126	170	1.1	—	0.00	0.00
—	—	—	—	—	—	1.2	—	—	250	0.72	—	—	—	170	—	59	0.00	—
0.31	0.07	4.55	0.10	1.17	29.4	0.3	—	0.1	130	1.77	25.2	112	204	502	2.0	45	0.00	0.00
0.27	0.34	7.94	0.25	2.83	37.6	0.5	—	0.1	149	2.96	41.0	207	385	640	5.2	49	0.00	0.00
—	—	—	—	—	—	1.2	—	—	350	0.36	—	327	534	250	—	—	0.00	0.00

Code	Food Name	Unit/ Amt	Wt (g)	Energy (kcal)	Prot (g)	Carb (g)	Fiber (g)	Fat (g)	Sat (g)	Mono (g)	Poly (g)	Chol (mg)	Vit A (RE)
48136	Pie, apple	1 ea	77	260	3	34	1	13	3.5	—	—	0	—
6156	Potatoes, french fries, sml svg	1 ea	68	210	3	26	2	10	1.5	—	—	0	0
57764	Salad, chef, shaker	1 ea	206	150	17	5	2	8	3.5	—	—	95	300
56479	Salad, garden, shaker	1 ea	149	100	7	4	2	6	3.0	—	—	75	150
81097	Sandwich, chicken, crisp deluxe	1 ea	219	537	27	49	3	26	4.6	8.2	12.0	64	—
81098	Sandwich, chicken, grilled, McGrill	1 ea	213	422	31	39	3	16	3.1	4.5	8.2	70	—
69013	Sandwich, Filet O Fish	1 ea	141	415	16	40	2	21	4.7	6.4	10.1	45	—
49141	Sandwich, ham egg cheese, w/bagel	1 ea	218	550	26	58	2	23	8.0	—	—	255	150
69006	Sandwich, sausage cheese, w/muffin	1 ea	112	360	13	26	1	23	8.0	—	—	45	40
69007	Sandwich, sausage egg cheese, w/muffin	1 ea	162	440	19	27	1	28	10.0	—	—	255	100
69004	Sandwich, sausage egg, w/biscuit	1 ea	162	490	16	31	1	33	10.0	—	—	245	60
42747	Sweet Roll, cinnamon	1 ea	95	390	6	50	2	18	5.0	—	—	65	80
Olive Garden													
4836	Breadsticks	1 ea	50	140	5	26	—	2	0.0	—	—	0	—
4832	Dinner, chicken giardino	1 ea	611	460	36	59	—	8	3.0	—	—	60	—
4834	Dinner, shrimp primavera	1 ea	535	603	44	84	—	13	2.0	—	—	275	—
Pizza Hut													
92495	Chicken, wings, mild, 2 pce svg	2 pce	53	110	11	1	0	7	2.0	—	—	70	60
57787	Pizza, cheese, 6"	1 pce	63	160	7	18	1	7	3.0	—	—	15	40
56489	Pizza, cheese, med, 12"	1 pce	99	240	12	30	2	8	4.5	—	—	25	60
57372	Pizza, ham, med, 12"	1 pce	98	220	12	29	2	6	3.0	—	—	20	60
57383	Pizza, Meat Lover's, pan, med, 12"	1 pce	123	340	15	29	2	19	7.0	—	—	35	60
56482	Pizza, pepperoni, pan, med, 12"	1 pce	102	290	11	29	2	15	5.0	—	—	25	60
57376	Pizza, pork, med, 12"	1 pce	111	270	13	30	3	11	5.0	—	—	25	60
57377	Pizza, sausage, Italian, med, 12"	1 pce	111	290	13	30	2	12	6.0	—	—	30	60
57382	Pizza, Veggie Lovers, pan, med, 12"	1 pce	119	260	10	30	2	12	4.0	—	—	15	80
Subway													
91790	Chili, con carne	1 cup	240	310	17	28	9	14	5.0	—	—	35	150
91784	Chowder, clam, New England	1 cup	240	140	5	19	7	4	1.0	—	—	15	150
91786	Chowder, potato cheese	1 cup	240	210	7	22	2	10	7.0	—	—	25	300
52119	Salad, chicken, breast, rstd	1 ea	303	140	16	12	3	3	1.0	—	—	45	150
52115	Salad, club	1 ea	322	150	17	12	3	4	1.5	—	—	35	150
69119	Sandwich, beef steak cheese, w/white, 6"	1 ea	256	390	24	48	5	14	5.0	—	—	35	100
69125	Sandwich, chicken breast, rstd, w/white, 6"	1 ea	236	320	23	47	5	5	2.0	—	—	45	60
69115	Sandwich, ham, w/white, 6"	1 ea	232	290	18	46	4	5	1.5	—	—	25	60
69129	Sandwich, meatball, w/white, 6"	1 ea	287	530	24	53	6	26	10.0	—	—	55	150
69121	Sandwich, roast beef, w/white, 6"	1 ea	222	290	19	45	4	5	2.0	—	—	20	60
69137	Sandwich, turkey breast, w/ ham, w/white, 6"	1 ea	232	290	20	46	4	5	1.5	—	—	25	60
69111	Sandwich, turkey, w/white, 6"	1 ea	222	280	18	46	4	4	1.5	—	—	20	60
69109	Sandwich, veggie delite, w/white, 6"	1 ea	166	230	9	44	4	3	1.0	—	—	0	60
Taco Bell													
56519	Burrito, bean	1 ea	198	370	14	55	8	10	3.5	—	—	10	100
57678	Burrito, chicken, grilled, Stuft	1 ea	325	680	35	76	7	26	7.0	—	—	70	100
57677	Burrito, chili cheese	1 ea	156	390	16	40	3	18	9.0	—	—	40	150
45585	Dessert, cinnamon twists, svg	1 ea	35	160	1	28	0	5	1.0	—	—	0	0
57665	Gordita, beef, supreme	1 ea	153	310	14	30	3	16	7.0	—	—	35	100
56533	Nachos, svg	1 ea	99	320	5	33	2	19	4.5	—	—	5	0

PAGE KEY: A-96 Granola Bars, Cereal Bars, Diet Bars, Scones, and Tarts   A-96 Meals and Dishes   A-100 Meats   A-106 Nuts, Seeds, and Products   A-108 Poultry   A-110 Salad Dressings, Dips, and Mayonnaise   A-110 Salads   A-110 Sandwiches   A-114 Sauces and Gravies   A-114 Snack Foods—Chips, Pretzels, Popcorn   A-116 Soups, Stews, and Chilis   A-118 Spices, Flavors, and Seasonings   A-120 Sports Bars and Drinks   A-120 Supplemental Foods and Formulas   A-122 Sweeteners and Sweet Substitutes   A-122 Vegetables and Legumes   A-136 Weight Loss Bars and Drinks   A-138 Miscellaneous

Thia (mg)	Ribo (mg)	Niac (mg NE)	Vit B6 (mg)	Vit B12 (µg)	Fol (µg)	Vit C (mg)	Vit D (IU)	Vit E (mg AT)	Cal (mg)	Iron (mg)	Magn (mg)	Phos (mg)	Pota (mg)	Sodi (mg)	Zinc (mg)	Wat (%)	Alco (g)	Caff (g)
0.18	0.10	1.41	0.02	0.00	8.3	24.0	—	1.4	20	1.08	6.5	35	63	200	0.2	—	0.00	0.00
—	—	—	—	—	—	9.0	—	0.8	9	0.36	26.5	88	468	135	0.3	41	0.00	0.00
—	—	—	—	—	—	15.0	—	—	150	1.44	—	—	—	740	—	—	0.00	0.00
—	—	—	—	—	—	15.0	—	—	150	1.08	—	—	—	120	—	—	0.00	0.00
0.34	0.40	11.18	0.28	0.72	63.5	0.7	—	1.5	171	2.69	61.3	353	449	1424	2.2	51	0.00	0.00
0.37	0.36	11.31	0.28	0.69	57.5	0.6	—	0.9	175	2.39	59.6	343	505	1240	1.2	58	0.00	0.00
0.30	0.18	3.13	0.05	1.51	29.6	0.4	—	1.6	154	0.92	38.1	185	276	663	0.8	43	0.00	0.00
—	—	—	—	—	—	0.0	—		200	4.50	—	—	—	1490	—	—	0.00	0.00
—	—	—	—	—	15.7	0.0	—	0.7	200	1.79	21.7	156	191	740	1.5	—	0.00	0.00
—	—	—	—	—	30.0	0.0	—	1.1	250	2.70	26.0	273	250	890	2.1	52	0.00	0.00
—	—	3.76	—	—	25.7	0.0	—	1.5	80	2.70	19.4	475	258	1010	1.5	49	0.00	0.00
—	—	—	—	—	—	—	—	—	60	1.44	—	—	—	310	—	20	0.00	0.00
—	—	—	—	—	—	—	—	—	—	—	—	—	—	270	—	—	0.00	0.00
—	—	—	—	—	—	—	—	—	—	—	—	—	—	1180	—	—	0.00	0.00
—	—	—	—	—	—	—	—	—	—	—	—	—	—	1220	—	—	0.00	0.00
—	—	—	—	—	—	0.0	—	—	0	0.72	—	—	—	320	—	—	0.00	0.00
—	—	—	—	—	—	0.0	—	—	100	1.44	—	—	—	310	—	—	0.00	0.00
—	—	—	—	—	—	1.2	—	—	200	1.44	—	—	—	520	—	47	0.00	0.00
—	—	—	—	—	—	6.0	—	—	150	1.79	—	—	—	550	—	—	0.00	0.00
—	—	—	—	—	—	6.0	—	—	150	2.70	—	—	—	750	—	—	0.00	0.00
—	—	—	—	—	—	2.4	—	—	150	2.70	—	—	—	560	—	—	0.00	0.00
—	—	—	—	—	—	3.6	—	—	150	1.79	—	—	—	640	—	—	0.00	0.00
—	—	—	—	—	—	3.6	—	—	150	1.79	—	—	—	660	—	—	0.00	0.00
—	—	—	—	—	—	9.0	—	—	150	2.70	—	—	—	470	—	—	0.00	0.00
—	—	—	—	—	—	12.0	—	—	60	—	—	—	—	900	—	—	0.00	0.00
—	—	—	—	—	—	0.0	—	—	60	1.79	—	—	—	900	—	86	0.00	0.00
—	—	—	—	—	—	0.0	—	—	200	0.00	—	—	—	1010	—	—	0.00	0.00
—	—	—	—	—	—	30.0	—	—	40	1.08	—	—	—	800	—	—	0.00	0.00
—	—	—	—	—	—	30.0	—	—	40	18.00	—	—	—	1110	—	—	0.00	0.00
—	—	—	—	—	—	24.0	—	—	150	8.10	—	—	—	1210	—	—	0.00	0.00
—	—	—	—	—	—	21.0	—	—	60	5.40	—	—	—	1000	—	—	0.00	0.00
—	—	—	—	—	—	21.0	—	—	60	3.59	—	—	—	1270	—	—	0.00	0.00
—	—	—	—	—	—	27.0	—	—	150	5.40	—	—	—	1360	—	—	0.00	0.00
—	—	—	—	—	—	21.0	—	—	60	6.30	—	—	—	910	—	—	0.00	0.00
—	—	—	—	—	—	21.0	—	—	60	3.59	—	—	—	1220	—	—	0.00	0.00
—	—	—	—	—	—	21.0	—	—	60	3.59	—	—	—	1010	—	—	0.00	0.00
—	—	—	—	—	—	21.0	—	—	60	3.59	—	—	—	510	—	—	0.00	0.00
—	—	—	—	—	—	4.8	—	—	200	2.70	—	—	—	1200	—	—	0.00	0.00
—	—	—	—	—	—	6.0	—	—	300	3.59	—	—	—	1950	—	—	0.00	0.00
—	—	—	—	—	—	0.0	—	—	300	1.79	—	—	—	1080	—	—	0.00	0.00
—	—	—	—	—	—	0.0	—	—	0	0.36	—	—	—	150	—	—	0.00	0.00
—	—	—	—	—	—	4.8	—	—	150	2.70	—	—	—	590	—	—	0.00	0.00
—	—	—	—	—	—	0.0	—	—	80	0.72	—	—	—	530	—	40	0.00	0.00

PAGE KEY: A-46 Beverage and Beverage Mixes A-48 Other Beverages A-48 Beverages, Alcoholic A-50 Candies and Confections, Gum A-54 Cereals, Breakfast Type A-58 Cheese and Cheese Substitutes A-60 Dairy Products and Substitutes A-62 Desserts A-68 Dessert Toppings A-68 Eggs, Substitutes, and Egg Dishes A-70 Ethnic Foods A-74 Fast Foods/Restaurants A-88 Fats, Oils, Margarines, Shortenings, and Substitutes A-88 Fish, Seafood, and Shellfish A-90 Food Additives A-90 Fruit, Vegetable, or Blended Juices A-92 Grains, Flours, and Fractions A-92 Grain Products, Prepared and Baked Goods

Code	Food Name	Unit/ Amt	Wt (g)	Energy (kcal)	Prot (g)	Carb (g)	Fiber (g)	Fat (g)	Sat (g)	Mono (g)	Poly (g)	Chol (mg)	Vit A (RE)
56531	Pizza, Mexican	1 ea	216	550	21	46	7	31	11.0	—	—	45	150
57685	Quesadilla, cheese	1 ea	142	490	19	39	3	28	13.0	—	—	55	100
57689	Quesadilla, chicken	1 ea	184	540	28	40	3	30	13.0	—	—	80	150
56537	Salad, taco, w/salsa & shell	1 ea	533	790	31	73	13	42	15.0	—	—	65	300
53604	Sauce, border, mild, 1 oz svg	1 ea	28	5	0	1	0	0	0.0	0.0	0.0	0	60
56524	Taco	1 ea	78	170	8	13	3	10	4.0	—	—	25	60
56525	Taco, soft, beef	1 ea	90	191	9	19	2	9	4.1	—	—	23	55
56689	Taco, soft, chicken	1 ea	99	190	14	19	1	6	2.5	—	—	30	20
56528	Tostada	1 ea	170	250	11	29	7	10	4.0	—	—	15	100
Taco Johns													
57576	Burrito, bean, w/cheese	1 ea	187	380	15	53	10	12	5.0	—	—	15	—
57577	Burrito, beefy	1 ea	187	430	22	41	8	20	9.0	—	—	55	—
49127	Dessert, churros	1 ea	55	230	2	31	1	11	2.0	—	—	10	—
57585	Dish, chimi platter, beef & bean	1 ea	422	760	27	88	9	34	11.0	—	—	50	—
57586	Enchilada, double	1 ea	422	720	37	54	11	40	18.0	—	—	105	—
57589	Mexi Rolls	1 ea	213	480	20	33	3	30	10.0	—	—	50	—
57593	Nachos, svg	1 ea	142	380	6	38	1	23	6.0	—	—	10	—
57596	Taco Burger, w/cheese	1 ea	142	280	14	28	3	12	5.0	—	—	35	—
57600	Taco, crispy	1 ea	94	180	9	13	3	10	4.0	—	—	25	—
57601	Taco, soft shell	1 ea	113	220	11	21	4	10	5.0	—	—	25	—
Taco Time													
7141	Beans, refritos, svg	1 ea	201	326	18	44	13	10	5.0	—	—	22	44
56542	Burrito, bean, soft	1 ea	193	380	16	58	13	10	4.0	—	—	15	—
56621	Burrito, chicken, crisp	1 ea	150	422	17	32	2	25	8.0	—	—	54	—
56541	Burrito, meat, crispy	1 ea	163	552	34	39	7	30	10.0	—	—	58	—
56543	Burrito, meat, soft	1 ea	193	491	31	48	12	21	8.0	—	—	56	—
56620	Burrito, veggie	1 ea	321	491	21	70	10	16	6.0	—	—	24	—
56550	Cheeseburger, taco	1 ea	215	633	31	48	7	36	10.0	—	—	66	—
56551	Chimichanga, meat	1 ea	349	768	37	62	12	43	18.0	—	—	89	—
45586	Empanada, berry	1 ea	113	387	5	66	3	12	1.0	5.0	6.0	2	16
2488	Frozen Dessert, Choco Taco	1 ea	113	310	3	37	1	17	10.0	—	—	20	40
1696	Gordita, taco meat	1 ea	227	470	18	44	4	24	7.0	—	—	35	150
56554	Nachos, svg	1 ea	301	680	26	61	11	38	19.0	—	—	78	—
50979	Quesadilla, cheese	1 ea	93	205	11	17	1	11	6.0	—	—	30	—
56556	Salad, taco, w/o dressing, reg	1 ea	215	479	30	30	7	28	11.0	—	—	63	—
56545	Taco, crisp	1 ea	115	295	22	16	5	17	7.0	—	—	48	—
56674	Taco, fish	1 ea	231	470	19	32	2	29	8.0	—	—	60	—
56655	Taco, soft, value	1 ea	150	316	24	23	5	15	7.0	—	—	48	—
56856	Tostada, w/bean	1 ea	138	211	10	26	7	8	4.0	—	—	15	—
56548	Tostada, w/meat	1 ea	219	447	35	33	12	21	9.0	—	—	61	—
1705	Wrap, chicken, classic	1 ea	494	813	29	101	6	33	11.0	—	—	67	—
Wendy's													
56570	Cheeseburger, jr	1 ea	129	310	17	34	2	12	6.0	—	—	45	60
56571	Cheeseburger, w/bacon, jr	1 ea	165	380	20	34	2	19	7.0	—	—	55	80
15176	Chicken, nuggets, 5 pce svg	1 ea	75	220	11	13	0	14	3.0	—	—	35	0
50311	Chili, sml svg	1 ea	227	200	17	21	5	6	2.5	—	—	35	150
56579	Dish, baked potato bacon cheese	1 ea	380	580	18	79	7	22	6.0	—	—	40	100

PAGE KEY: A-96 Granola Bars, Cereal Bars, Diet Bars, Scones, and Tarts   A-96 Meals and Dishes   A-100 Meats   A-106 Nuts, Seeds, and Products   A-108 Poultry
A-110 Salad Dressings, Dips, and Mayonnaise   A-110 Salads   A-110 Sandwiches   A-114 Sauces and Gravies   A-114 Snack Foods—Chips, Pretzels, Popcorn
A-116 Soups, Stews, and Chilis   A-118 Spices, Flavors, and Seasonings   A-120 Sports Bars and Drinks   A-120 Supplemental Foods and Formulas
A-122 Sweeteners and Sweet Substitutes   A-122 Vegetables and Legumes   A-136 Weight Loss Bars and Drinks   A-138 Miscellaneous

Thia (mg)	Ribo (mg)	Niac (mg NE)	Vit B6 (mg)	Vit B12 (µg)	Fol (µg)	Vit C (mg)	Vit D (IU)	Vit E (mg AT)	Cal (mg)	Iron (mg)	Magn (mg)	Phos (mg)	Pota (mg)	Sodi (mg)	Zinc (mg)	Wat (%)	Alco (g)	Caff (g)
—	—	—	—	—	—	6.0	—	—	350	3.59	—	—	—	1030	—	—	0.00	0.00
—	—	—	—	—	—	0.0	—	—	500	1.44	—	—	—	1150	—	—	0.00	0.00
—	—	—	—	—	—	2.4	—	—	500	1.79	—	—	—	1380	—	—	0.00	0.00
—	—	—	—	—	—	21.0	—	—	400	6.30	—	—	—	1670	—	—	0.00	0.00
—	—	—	—	—	—	0.0	—	—	0	0.00	—	—	—	210	—	—	0.00	0.00
—	—	—	—	—	—	2.4	—	—	60	1.08	—	—	—	350	—	—	0.00	0.00
—	—	—	—	—	—	2.2	—	—	91	1.63	—	—	—	564	—	—	0.00	0.00
—	—	—	—	—	—	1.2	—	—	100	1.08	—	—	—	550	—	—	0.00	0.00
—	—	—	—	—	—	4.8	—	—	150	1.44	—	—	—	710	—	—	0.00	0.00
													—	830	—	—	0.00	0.00
—	—	—	—	—	—	—	—	—	—	—	—	—	—	870	—	—	0.00	0.00
—	—	—	—	—	—	—	—	—	—	—	—	—	—	120	—	—	0.00	0.00
—	—	—	—	—	—	—	—	—	—	—	—	—	—	1930	—	—	0.00	0.00
—	—	—	—	—	—	—	—	—	—	—	—	—	—	2090	—	—	0.00	0.00
—	—	—	—	—	—	—	—	—	—	—	—	—	—	1270	—	—	0.00	0.00
—	—	—	—	—	—	—	—	—	—	—	—	—	—	970	—	—	0.00	0.00
—	—	—	—	—	—	—	—	—	—	—	—	—	—	600	—	—	0.00	0.00
—	—	—	—	—	—	—	—	—	—	—	—	—	—	270	—	—	0.00	0.00
—	—	—	—	—	—	—	—	—	—	—	—	—	—	470	—	—	0.00	0.00
0.23	0.15	1.00	0.37	0.00	13.2	3.0	—	—	218	3.03	—	256	340	525	2.0	—	0.00	0.00
—	—	—	—	—	—	—	—	—	—	—	—	—	—	—	—	—	0.00	0.00
—	—	—	—	—	—	—	—	—	—	—	—	—	—	795	—	—	0.00	0.00
—	—	—	—	—	—	—	—	—	—	—	—	—	—	—	—	—	0.00	0.00
—	—	—	—	—	—	—	—	—	—	—	—	—	—	—	—	—	0.00	0.00
—	—	—	—	—	—	—	—	—	—	—	—	—	—	643	—	—	0.00	0.00
—	—	—	—	—	—	—	—	—	—	—	—	—	—	—	—	—	0.00	0.00
0.15	0.20	2.00	0.05	—	20.0	10.0	—	—	84	3.00	—	56	170	1	0.0	—	0.00	0.00
—	—	—	—	—	—	0.0	—	—	60	0.72	—	—	—	100	—	—	0.00	—
—	—	—	—	—	—	12.0	—	—	150	3.59	—	—	—	940	—	—	0.00	0.00
—	—	—	—	—	—	—	—	—	—	—	—	—	—	—	—	—	0.00	0.00
—	—	—	—	—	—	—	—	—	—	—	—	—	—	255	—	—	0.00	0.00
—	—	—	—	—	—	—	—	—	—	—	—	—	—	—	—	—	0.00	0.00
—	—	—	—	—	—	—	—	—	—	—	—	—	—	—	—	—	0.00	0.00
—	—	—	—	—	—	—	—	—	—	—	—	—	—	660	—	—	0.00	0.00
—	—	—	—	—	—	—	—	—	—	—	—	—	—	599	—	—	0.00	0.00
—	—	—	—	—	—	—	—	—	—	—	—	—	—	215	—	—	0.00	0.00
—	—	—	—	—	—	—	—	—	—	—	—	—	—	—	—	—	0.00	0.00
—	—	—	—	—	—	—	—	—	—	—	—	—	—	1688	—	—	0.00	0.00
—	—	—	—	—	—	3.6	—	—	150	3.59	—	—	230	820	—	49	0.00	0.00
—	—	—	—	—	—	9.0	—	—	150	3.59	—	—	320	890	—	—	0.00	0.00
—	—	—	—	—	—	1.2	—	—	20	0.72	—	—	190	480	—	48	0.00	0.00
—	—	—	—	—	—	2.4	—	—	80	1.79	—	—	470	870	—	—	0.00	0.00
—	—	—	—	—	—	42.0	—	—	200	3.59	—	—	1410	950	—	—	0.00	0.00

Code	Food Name	Unit/ Amt	Wt (g)	Energy (kcal)	Prot (g)	Carb (g)	Fiber (g)	Fat (g)	Sat (g)	Mono (g)	Poly (g)	Chol (mg)	Vit A (RE)
56580	Dish, baked potato broccoli cheese	1 ea	411	480	9	81	9	14	3.0	—	—	5	350
71834	Frozen Dessert, Frosty, dairy, jr	1 ea	113	170	4	28	0	4	2.5	—	—	20	80
2177	Frozen Dessert, Frosty, dairy, med	1 ea	298	440	11	73	0	11	7.0	—	—	50	200
56574	Hamburger, Big Bacon Classic	1 ea	282	570	34	46	3	29	12.0	—	—	100	150
71831	Potatoes, french fries, med, svg	1 ea	142	390	4	56	6	17	3.0	—	—	0	0
52080	Salad, caesar, w/o dressing, side	1 ea	99	70	7	2	1	4	2.0	—	—	15	450
56588	Salad, taco, supremo, w/o chips	1 ea	495	360	27	29	8	17	9.0	—	—	65	500
69059	Sandwich, chicken, grilled	1 ea	188	300	24	36	2	7	1.5	—	—	55	40

FATS, OILS, MARGARINES, SHORTENINGS, AND SUBSTITUTES

Fat Substitutes

Fats and Oils, Animal

Code	Food Name	Unit/ Amt	Wt (g)	Energy (kcal)	Prot (g)	Carb (g)	Fiber (g)	Fat (g)	Sat (g)	Mono (g)	Poly (g)	Chol (mg)	Vit A (RE)
8000	Butter, salted	1 Tbs	14	100	0	0	0	11	7.2	2.9	0.4	30	98
8003	Fat, bacon grease	1 tsp	4	39	0	0	0	4	1.7	1.9	0.5	4	0
8107	Fat, lard	1 Tbs	13	115	0	0	0	13	5.0	5.8	1.4	12	0

Fats and Oils, Vegetable

Code	Food Name	Unit/ Amt	Wt (g)	Energy (kcal)	Prot (g)	Carb (g)	Fiber (g)	Fat (g)	Sat (g)	Mono (g)	Poly (g)	Chol (mg)	Vit A (RE)
8084	Oil, canola	1 Tbs	14	124	0	0	0	14	1.0	8.2	4.1	0	0
8009	Oil, corn, salad or cooking	1 Tbs	14	120	0	0	0	14	1.8	3.8	7.4	0	0
8008	Oil, olive, salad or cooking	1 Tbs	14	119	0	0	0	14	1.8	10.0	1.4	0	0
90965	Oil, veg, pure	1 Tbs	14	120	0	0	0	14	1.5	6.0	6.0	0	0

Margarines and Spreads

Code	Food Name	Unit/ Amt	Wt (g)	Energy (kcal)	Prot (g)	Carb (g)	Fiber (g)	Fat (g)	Sat (g)	Mono (g)	Poly (g)	Chol (mg)	Vit A (RE)
8490	Margarine, soft, safflower oil	1 Tbs	14	100	0	0	0	11	1.0	8.0	2.0	0	100

Shortenings

Code	Food Name	Unit/ Amt	Wt (g)	Energy (kcal)	Prot (g)	Carb (g)	Fiber (g)	Fat (g)	Sat (g)	Mono (g)	Poly (g)	Chol (mg)	Vit A (RE)
8007	Shortening, household, hydrog soybean & cttnsd oil	1 Tbs	13	113	0	0	0	13	3.2	5.7	3.3	0	0

FISH, SEAFOOD, AND SHELLFISH

Code	Food Name	Unit/ Amt	Wt (g)	Energy (kcal)	Prot (g)	Carb (g)	Fiber (g)	Fat (g)	Sat (g)	Mono (g)	Poly (g)	Chol (mg)	Vit A (RE)
19049	Clams, bkd/brld, sml	15 ea	150	210	23	5	0	11	1.9	4.4	2.9	60	223
19151	Crab, imit	3 oz	85	99	11	11	0	1	0.1	0.1	0.3	42	6
17002	Fish Sticks, heated f/fzn, 4" x 1" x 1/2"	1 ea	28	76	4	7	0	3	0.9	1.4	0.9	31	9
17179	Fish, catfish, channel, fillet, bkd/brld, farmed	3 oz	85	129	16	0	0	7	1.5	3.5	1.2	54	13
17090	Fish, haddock, fillet, bkd/brld	3 oz	85	95	21	0	0	1	0.1	0.1	0.3	63	16
70260	Fish, halibut, battered, fzn	3 ea	113	330	13	22	0	21	3.0	8.0	1.5	20	—
17049	Fish, mackerel, Atlantic, fillet, bkd/brld	3 oz	85	223	20	0	0	15	3.6	6.0	3.7	64	46
17121	Fish, orange roughy, fillet, bkd/brld	3 oz	85	76	16	0	0	1	0.0	0.5	0.0	22	20
17093	Fish, perch, ocean, Atlantic, fillet, bkd/brld	3 oz	85	103	20	0	0	2	0.3	0.7	0.5	46	12
17171	Fish, salmon, pink, fillet, bkd/brld	3 oz	85	127	22	0	0	4	0.6	1.0	1.5	57	35
17068	Fish, sole, fillet, bkd/brld	3 oz	85	100	21	0	0	1	0.3	0.2	0.5	58	11
71139	Fish, sturgeon, filled, bkd/brld mixed species 4.5" x 2" 1/8" x 7/8"	3 oz	85	115	18	0	0	4	1.0	2.1	0.8	65	224
17101	Fish, tuna, bluefin, fillet, bkd/brld	3 oz	85	156	25	0	0	5	1.4	1.7	1.6	42	644
19056	Lobster, bkd/brld	1 ea	125	146	25	2	0	4	2.0	1.1	0.2	96	60
19061	Scallops, bkd/brld	4 ea	100	134	20	3	0	4	0.7	1.5	1.2	40	46
19065	Shrimp, bkd/brld, w/margarine & salt, med	2 ea	10	16	2	0	0	1	0.1	0.2	0.2	18	9
19401	Shrimp, cocktail	1 cup	230	218	28	21	5	3	0.5	0.4	1.0	196	72
70702	Shrimp, popcorn, breaded, fzn	20 ea	112	270	11	28	1	13	2.0	5.0	2.0	35	0

PAGE KEY: A-96 Granola Bars, Cereal Bars, Diet Bars, Scones, and Tarts   A-96 Meals and Dishes   A-100 Meats   A-106 Nuts, Seeds, and Products   A-108 Poultry   A-110 Salad Dressings, Dips, and Mayonnaise   A-110 Salads   A-110 Sandwiches   A-114 Sauces and Gravies   A-114 Snack Foods—Chips, Pretzels, Popcorn   A-116 Soups, Stews, and Chilis   A-118 Spices, Flavors, and Seasonings   A-120 Sports Bars and Drinks   A-120 Supplemental Foods and Formulas   A-122 Sweeteners and Sweet Substitutes   A-122 Vegetables and Legumes   A-136 Weight Loss Bars and Drinks   A-138 Miscellaneous

Thia (mg)	Ribo (mg)	Niac (mg NE)	Vit B6 (mg)	Vit B12 (µg)	Fol (µg)	Vit C (mg)	Vit D (IU)	Vit E (mg AT)	Cal (mg)	Iron (mg)	Magn (mg)	Phos (mg)	Pota (mg)	Sodi (mg)	Zinc (mg)	Wat (%)	Alco (g)	Caff (g)
—	—	—	—	—	—	72.0	—	—	200	4.50	—	—	1400	510	—	—	0.00	0.00
—	—	—	—	—	—	0.0	—	—	150	0.72	—	—	290	100	—	—	0.00	—
—	—	—	—	—	—	0.0	—	—	400	1.44	—	—	770	260	—	—	0.00	—
—	—	—	—	—	—	15.0	—	—	200	5.40	—	—	580	1460	—	—	0.00	0.00
—	—	—	—	—	—	3.6	—	—	20	1.44	—	—	770	340	—	—	0.00	0.00
—	—	—	—	—	—	21.0	—	—	150	1.08	—	—	280	250	—	—	0.00	0.00
—	—	—	—	—	—	27.0	—	—	350	3.59	—	—	950	1090	—	—	0.00	0.00
—	—	—	—	—	—	9.0	—	—	80	2.70	—	—	430	740	—	—	0.00	0.00
0.00	0.00	0.00	0.00	0.01	0.4	0.0	7.8	0.3	3	0.00	0.3	3	3	81	0.0	16	0.00	0.00
0.00	0.00	0.00	0.00	0.00	0.0	0.0	—	0.0	0	0.00	0.0	0	0	6	0.0	0	0.00	0.00
0.00	0.00	0.00	0.00	0.00	0.0	0.0	—	0.1	0	0.00	0.0	0	0	0	0.0	0	0.00	0.00
0.00	0.00	0.00	0.00	0.00	0.0	0.0	—	2.4	0	0.00	0.0	0	0	0	0.0	0	0.00	0.00
0.00	0.00	0.00	0.00	0.00	0.0	0.0	—	1.9	0	0.00	0.0	0	0	0	0.0	0	0.00	0.00
0.00	0.00	0.00	0.00	0.00	0.0	0.0	—	1.9	0	0.09	0.0	0	0	0	0.0	0	0.00	0.00
—	—	—	—	—	—	0.0	—	3.0	0	0.00	—	—	—	0	—	0	0.00	0.00
—	—	—	—	—	—	0.0	—	—	0	0.00	—	—	—	90	—	19	0.00	0.00
0.00	0.00	0.00	0.00	0.00	0.0	0.0	—	0.1	0	0.00	0.0	0	0	0	0.0	0	0.00	0.00
0.12	0.30	2.96	0.10	82.93	26.9	21.8	6.0	3.1	84	24.69	16.2	301	559	202	2.4	72	0.00	0.00
0.02	0.10	1.91	0.15	1.77	1.7	0.0	—	0.1	36	0.33	39.8	131	209	52	0.3	72	0.00	0.00
0.03	0.05	0.60	0.01	0.50	12.0	0.0	1.9	0.1	6	0.20	7.0	51	73	163	0.2	46	0.00	0.00
0.36	0.05	2.14	0.14	2.38	6.0	0.7	—	1.1	8	0.69	22.1	208	273	68	0.9	72	0.00	0.00
0.02	0.03	3.94	0.28	1.17	11.1	0.0	—	0.4	36	1.14	42.5	205	339	74	0.4	74	0.00	0.00
																48	0.00	0.00
0.14	0.34	5.82	0.38	16.15	1.7	0.3	—	1.6	13	1.34	82.5	236	341	71	0.8	53	0.00	0.00
0.10	0.15	3.10	0.28	1.96	6.8	0.0	—	0.5	32	0.20	32.3	218	327	69	0.8	69	0.00	0.00
0.10	0.10	2.06	0.23	0.98	8.5	0.7	—	1.4	117	1.00	33.2	236	298	82	0.5	73	0.00	0.00
0.17	0.05	7.25	0.20	2.94	4.3	0.0	—	1.1	14	0.83	28.1	251	352	73	0.6	70	0.00	0.00
0.07	0.10	1.85	0.20	2.13	7.7	0.0	—	0.6	15	0.28	49.3	246	293	89	0.5	73	0.00	0.00
0.07	0.07	8.59	0.20	2.13	14.5	0.0	—	0.5	14	0.76	38.3	230	310	59	0.5	70	0.00	0.00
0.23	0.25	8.96	0.44	9.25	1.7	0.0	—	1.1	9	1.11	54.4	277	275	43	0.7	59	0.00	0.00
0.00	0.07	1.29	0.09	3.77	13.6	0.0	7.0	1.3	75	0.47	42.5	225	428	492	3.5	74	0.00	0.00
0.00	0.05	1.33	0.17	1.75	18.5	3.5	4.0	1.7	30	0.34	68.0	266	392	231	1.2	71	0.00	0.00
0.00	0.00	0.28	0.00	0.12	0.3	0.2	14.0	0.1	6	0.28	4.5	25	23	21	0.1	68	0.00	0.00
0.10	0.10	4.30	0.25	1.26	47.7	25.7	147.2	3.5	91	3.76	59.4	307	576	1129	1.6	75	0.00	0.00
—	—	—	—	—	—	0.0	—	—	40	1.44	—	—	—	610	—	—	0.00	0.00

Code	Food Name	Unit/ Amt	Wt (g)	Energy (kcal)	Prot (g)	Carb (g)	Fiber (g)	Fat (g)	Sat (g)	Mono (g)	Poly (g)	Chol (mg)	Vit A (RE)
FOOD ADDITIVES													
ALGINATES													
Bases and Preps													
54032	Prep, consomme, chicken style, w/o msg, vgtrn, dry mix	1 cup	246	522	21	76	—	15	2.0	—	—	1	—
Chemicals													
Colors, Flavors, and Aromas													
26624	Flavor, vanilla extract	1 tsp	4	12	0	1	0	0	0.0	0.0	0.0	0	0
Gums, Fibers, Starches, Pectins, Emulsifiers													
30000	Cornstarch	1 Tbs	8	30	0	7	0	0	0.0	0.0	0.0	0	0
Ingredient Sweeteners													
Nutraceuticals													
Nutritional Additives													
JUICE—100% FRUIT, VEGETABLE, OR BLENDED													
3008	Juice, apple, unswtnd, cnd/btld	1 cup	248	117	0	29	0	0	0.0	0.0	0.1	0	0
3455	Juice, grapefruit, pink, fresh	1 cup	247	96	1	23	0	0	0.0	0.0	0.1	0	109
3090	Juice, orange, fresh	1 cup	248	112	2	26	0	0	0.1	0.1	0.1	0	50
3561	Juice, orange, fzn, conc	2.2 oz	63	110	1	27	0	0	0.0	0.0	0.0	0	0
Fruits													
3001	Apples, fresh, lrg, 3 1/4"	1 ea	212	110	1	29	5	0	0.1	0.0	0.1	0	13
3147	Applesauce, swtnd, unsalted, cnd	1 cup	255	194	0	51	3	0	0.1	0.0	0.1	0	5
3157	Apricots, fresh, whole	1 ea	35	17	0	4	1	0	0.0	0.1	0.0	0	67
3016	Avocado, avg, fresh	1 ea	201	322	4	17	13	29	4.3	19.7	3.7	0	28
3020	Banana, fresh, med, 7" to 7 7/8" long	1 ea	118	105	1	27	3	0	0.1	0.0	0.1	0	7
3029	Blueberries, fresh	0.5 cup	68	39	1	10	2	0	0.0	0.0	0.1	0	4
3026	Boysenberries, fresh	0.5 cup	72	31	1	7	4	0	0.0	0.0	0.2	0	16
3036	Cherries, sweet, fresh	1 ea	7	4	0	1	0	0	0.0	0.0	0.0	0	0
3191	Currants, red, fresh	1 cup	112	63	2	15	5	0	0.0	0.0	0.1	0	4
3676	Figs, fresh, lrg, 2 1/2"	1 ea	64	47	0	12	2	0	0.0	0.0	0.1	0	9
3203	Gooseberries, fresh	0.5 cup	75	33	1	8	3	0	0.0	0.0	0.2	0	22
3818	Grapefruit, pink, fresh, 3 3/4"	0.5 ea	123	52	1	13	2	0	0.0	0.0	0.0	0	143
3820	Grapefruit, red, fresh, 3 3/4"	0.5 ea	123	52	1	13	2	0	0.0	0.0	0.0	0	143
3638	Kiwi, fresh	1 cup	177	108	2	26	5	1	0.1	0.1	0.5	0	14
3067	Lemon Peel, fresh	1 Tbs	6	3	0	1	1	0	0.0	0.0	0.0	0	0
3071	Limes, peeled, fresh, 2"	1 ea	67	20	0	7	2	0	0.0	0.0	0.0	0	3
71769	Mandarin Oranges, fresh, med, 2 3/8"	1 ea	84	45	1	11	2	0	0.0	0.1	0.1	0	57
71774	Mandarin Oranges, w/light syrup, cnd	1 cup	252	154	1	41	2	0	0.0	0.0	0.1	0	212
3221	Mango, fresh, whole	0.5 ea	104	67	1	18	2	0	0.1	0.1	0.1	0	79
3076	Melon, cantaloupe, fresh, med, 5"	1 ea	552	188	5	45	5	1	0.3	0.0	0.4	0	1866
71102	Melon, honeydew, fresh, 5 1/4"	1 ea	1000	360	5	91	8	1	0.4	0.0	0.6	0	60
3309	Mulberries, fresh	10 ea	15	6	0	1	0	0	0.0	0.0	0.0	0	0
3215	Nectarines, fresh, 2 1/2"	1 ea	136	60	1	14	2	0	0.0	0.1	0.2	0	46
3082	Oranges, fresh, med, 2 5/8"	1 ea	131	62	1	15	3	0	0.0	0.0	0.0	0	29
3720	Papaya, fresh, lrg, 5 3/4" x 3 1/"4	1 ea	380	148	2	37	7	1	0.2	0.1	0.1	0	418
3096	Peaches, fresh, med, w/o skin, 2 1/2"	1 ea	98	38	1	9	1	0	0.0	0.1	0.1	0	31
3103	Pears, fresh, bartlett, med	1 ea	166	96	1	26	5	0	0.0	0.0	0.0	0	3
71114	Pineapple, chunks, w/juice, cnd, not drained	0.5 cup	124	75	1	20	1	0	0.0	0.0	0.0	0	5

PAGE KEY: A-96 Granola Bars, Cereal Bars, Diet Bars, Scones, and Tarts   A-96 Meals and Dishes   A-100 Meats   A-106 Nuts, Seeds, and Products   A-108 Poultry   A-110 Salad Dressings, Dips, and Mayonnaise   A-110 Salads   A-110 Sandwiches   A-114 Sauces and Gravies   A-114 Snack Foods—Chips, Pretzels, Popcorn   A-116 Soups, Stews, and Chilis   A-118 Spices, Flavors, and Seasonings   A-120 Sports Bars and Drinks   A-120 Supplemental Foods and Formulas   A-122 Sweeteners and Sweet Substitutes   A-122 Vegetables and Legumes   A-136 Weight Loss Bars and Drinks   A-138 Miscellaneous

Thia (mg)	Ribo (mg)	Niac (mg NE)	Vit B6 (mg)	Vit B12 (µg)	Fol (µg)	Vit C (mg)	Vit D (IU)	Vit E (mg AT)	Cal (mg)	Iron (mg)	Magn (mg)	Phos (mg)	Pota (mg)	Sodi (mg)	Zinc (mg)	Wat (%)	Alco (g)	Caff (g)
—	—	—	—	—	—	—	—	—	—	—	—	—	492	46494	—	—	0.00	0.00
0.00	0.00	0.01	0.00	0.00	0.0	0.0	—	0.0	0	0.00	0.5	0	6	0	0.0	53	1.49	0.00
0.00	0.00	0.00	0.00	0.00	0.0	0.0	—	0.0	0	0.03	0.2	1	0	1	0.0	8	0.00	0.00
0.05	0.03	0.25	0.07	0.00	0.0	2.2	—	0.0	17	0.92	7.4	17	295	7	0.1	88	0.00	0.00
0.10	0.05	0.49	0.10	0.00	24.7	93.9	0.0	0.1	22	0.49	29.6	37	400	2	0.1	90	0.00	0.00
0.21	0.07	0.99	0.10	0.00	74.4	124.0	—	0.1	27	0.50	27.3	42	496	2	0.1	88	0.00	0.00
0.00	—	0.00	0.00	—	10.0	78.0	—	0.0	20	0.00	—		430	5	—	53	0.00	0.00
0.03	0.05	0.18	0.09	0.00	6.4	9.8	—	0.4	13	0.25	10.6	23	227	2	0.1	86	0.00	0.00
0.02	0.07	0.47	0.07	0.00	2.5	4.3	—	0.5	10	0.88	7.6	18	156	8	0.1	80	0.00	0.00
0.00	0.00	0.20	0.01	0.00	3.1	3.5	—	0.3	5	0.14	3.5	8	91	0	0.1	86	0.00	0.00
0.12	0.25	3.49	0.51	0.00	162.8	20.1	—	4.2	24	1.11	58.3	105	975	14	1.3	73	0.00	0.00
0.03	0.09	0.77	0.43	0.00	23.6	10.3	—	0.1	6	0.31	31.9	26	422	1	0.2	75	0.00	0.00
0.02	0.02	0.28	0.03	0.00	4.1	6.6	—	0.4	4	0.18	4.1	8	52	1	0.1	84	0.00	0.00
0.00	0.01	0.46	0.01	0.00	18.0	15.1	—	0.8	21	0.44	14.4	16	117	1	0.4	88	0.00	0.00
0.00	0.00	0.00	0.00	0.00	0.3	0.5	—	0.0	1	0.01	0.7	1	15	0	0.0	82	0.00	0.00
0.03	0.05	0.10	0.07	0.00	9.0	45.9	—	0.1	37	1.12	14.6	49	308	1	0.3	84	0.00	0.00
0.03	0.02	0.25	0.07	0.00	3.8	1.3	—	0.1	22	0.23	10.9	9	148	1	0.1	79	0.00	0.00
0.02	0.01	0.23	0.05	0.00	4.5	20.8	—	0.3	19	0.23	7.5	20	148	1	0.1	88	0.00	0.00
0.05	0.03	0.25	0.07	0.00	16.0	38.4	—	0.2	27	0.10	11.1	22	166	0	0.1	88	0.00	0.00
0.05	0.03	0.25	0.07	0.00	16.0	38.4	—	0.2	27	0.10	11.1	22	166	0	0.1	88	0.00	0.00
0.05	0.03	0.60	0.10	0.00	44.2	164.1	—	2.6	60	0.55	30.1	60	552	5	0.2	83	0.00	0.00
0.00	0.00	0.01	0.00	0.00	0.8	7.7	—	0.0	8	0.05	0.9	1	10	0	0.0	82	0.00	0.00
0.01	0.00	0.12	0.02	0.00	5.4	19.5	—	0.1	22	0.40	4.0	12	68	1	0.1	88	0.00	0.00
0.05	0.02	0.31	0.07	0.00	13.4	22.4	—	0.2	31	0.12	10.1	17	139	2	0.1	85	0.00	0.00
0.12	0.10	1.12	0.10	0.00	12.6	49.9	—	0.3	18	0.93	20.2	25	197	15	0.6	83	0.00	0.00
0.05	0.05	0.60	0.14	0.00	14.5	28.7	—	1.2	10	0.12	9.3	11	161	2	0.0	82	0.00	0.00
0.23	0.10	4.05	0.40	0.00	115.9	202.6	—	0.3	50	1.15	66.2	83	1474	88	1.0	90	0.00	0.00
0.37	0.11	4.17	0.87	0.00	190.0	180.0	—	0.2	60	1.70	100.0	110	2280	180	0.9	90	0.00	0.00
0.00	0.01	0.09	0.00	0.00	0.9	5.5	0.0	0.1	6	0.28	2.7	6	29	2	0.0	88	0.00	0.00
0.05	0.03	1.52	0.02	0.00	6.8	7.3	—	1.0	8	0.37	12.2	35	273	0	0.2	88	0.00	0.00
0.10	0.05	0.37	0.07	0.00	39.3	69.7	—	0.2	52	0.12	13.1	18	237	0	0.1	87	0.00	0.00
0.10	0.11	1.27	0.07	0.00	144.4	234.8	—	2.8	91	0.37	38.0	19	977	11	0.3	89	0.00	0.00
0.01	0.02	0.79	0.01	0.00	3.9	6.5	—	0.7	6	0.25	8.8	20	186	0	0.2	89	0.00	0.00
0.01	0.03	0.25	0.05	0.00	11.6	7.0	—	0.2	15	0.28	11.6	18	198	2	0.2	84	0.00	0.00
0.11	0.01	0.34	0.09	0.00	6.2	11.8	—	0.0	17	0.34	17.4	7	152	1	0.1	84	0.00	0.00

PAGE KEY: A-46 Beverage and Beverage Mixes   A-48 Other Beverages   A-48 Beverages, Alcoholic   A-50 Candies and Confections, Gum   A-54 Cereals, Breakfast Type
A-58 Cheese and Cheese Substitutes   A-60 Dairy Products and Substitutes   A-62 Desserts   A-68 Dessert Toppings   A-68 Eggs, Substitutes, and Egg Dishes   A-70 Ethnic Foods
A-74 Fast Foods/Restaurants   A-88 Fats, Oils, Margarines, Shortenings, and Substitutes   A-88 Fish, Seafood, and Shellfish   A-90 Food Additives
A-90 Fruit, Vegetable, or Blended Juices   A-92 Grains, Flours, and Fractions   A-92 Grain Products, Prepared and Baked Goods

Code	Food Name	Unit/ Amt	Wt (g)	Energy (kcal)	Prot (g)	Carb (g)	Fiber (g)	Fat (g)	Sat (g)	Mono (g)	Poly (g)	Chol (mg)	Vit A (RE)
3112	Pineapple, fresh	1 ea	472	227	3	60	7	1	0.0	0.1	0.2	0	28
3121	Plums, fresh, 2 1/8"	1 ea	66	30	0	8	1	0	0.0	0.1	0.0	0	22
3197	Pomegranate, fresh, 3 3/8"	1 ea	154	105	1	26	1	0	0.1	0.1	0.1	0	15
3202	Raisins, golden, seedless, packed cup	0.25 cup	41	125	1	33	2	0	0.1	0.0	0.1	0	0
3209	Rhubarb, fresh, diced	0.5 cup	61	13	1	3	1	0	0.0	0.0	0.1	0	6
3134	Strawberries, fresh, whole	1 cup	144	46	1	11	3	0	0.0	0.1	0.2	0	3
3087	Tangelo, fresh, 2 3/8"	1 ea	96	45	1	11	2	0	0.0	0.0	0.0	0	21
3717	Tangerines, fresh, lrg, 2 1/2"	1 ea	98	52	1	13	2	0	0.0	0.1	0.1	0	67
3143	Watermelon, fresh, slice, 1/16 melon	1 pce	286	86	2	22	1	0	0.0	0.1	0.1	0	160

GRAINS, FLOURS, AND FRACTIONS

Code	Food Name	Unit/ Amt	Wt (g)	Energy (kcal)	Prot (g)	Carb (g)	Fiber (g)	Fat (g)	Sat (g)	Mono (g)	Poly (g)	Chol (mg)	Vit A (RE)
38650	Dish, wheat pilaf, dry mix	2 oz	57	184	6	42	5	1	0.2	0.1	0.4	0	7
28018	Flour, all purpose, self-rising, bleached, enrich	0.25 cup	30	100	3	22	0	0	0.0	0.0	0.0	0	0
38030	Flour, all purpose, white, bleached, enrich	0.25 cup	31	114	3	24	1	0	0.0	0.0	0.1	0	0
46086	Flour, cake, white, enrich, unsifted	0.25 cup	34	124	3	27	1	0	0.0	0.0	0.1	0	0
38032	Flour, whole wheat	0.25 cup	30	102	4	22	4	1	0.1	0.1	0.2	0	0
38017	Oats, old fash, dry	0.5 cup	40	148	5	27	4	3	0.4	0.8	0.9	0	0
38575	Oats, steel cut, Irish style, dry	0.25 cup	40	148	5	27	4	3	0.4	0.8	0.9	0	0
2730	Tapioca, dry	1.5 tsp	6	20	0	5	0	0	0.0	0.0	0.0	0	0
38027	Wheat, bulgur, dry	0.25 cup	35	120	4	27	6	0	0.1	0.1	0.2	0	0
38026	Wheat, germ, tstd	1 cup	113	432	33	56	17	12	2.1	1.7	7.5	0	11
38068	Wheat, sprouted	1 cup	108	214	8	46	1	1	0.2	0.2	0.6	0	0

GRAIN PRODUCTS, PREPARED AND BAKED GOODS

Bagels

Code	Food Name	Unit/ Amt	Wt (g)	Energy (kcal)	Prot (g)	Carb (g)	Fiber (g)	Fat (g)	Sat (g)	Mono (g)	Poly (g)	Chol (mg)	Vit A (RE)
71165	Bagel, egg, 3"	1 ea	57	158	6	30	1	1	0.2	0.2	0.4	14	19
8846	Bagel, plain, classic, 4 oz svg	1 ea	112	296	11	60	3	2	—	—	—	0	0

Biscuits

Code	Food Name	Unit/ Amt	Wt (g)	Energy (kcal)	Prot (g)	Carb (g)	Fiber (g)	Fat (g)	Sat (g)	Mono (g)	Poly (g)	Chol (mg)	Vit A (RE)
42001	Biscuit, buttermilk, prep f/recipe, 2 1/2"	1 ea	60	212	4	27	1	10	2.6	4.2	2.5	2	14
71195	Biscuit, plain, prep f/recipe, 2 1/2"	1 ea	60	212	4	27	1	10	2.6	4.2	2.5	2	14
42205	Biscuit, whole wheat	1 ea	63	199	6	30	5	7	1.7	3.0	2.2	2	14

Breads and Rolls

Code	Food Name	Unit/ Amt	Wt (g)	Energy (kcal)	Prot (g)	Carb (g)	Fiber (g)	Fat (g)	Sat (g)	Mono (g)	Poly (g)	Chol (mg)	Vit A (RE)
71024	Bread Crumbs, white, soft, enrich	1 cup	45	120	3	23	1	1	0.3	0.3	0.6	0	0
71021	Bread, 7 grain, slice	1 pce	26	65	3	12	2	1	0.2	0.4	0.2	0	0
42052	Bread, Boston brown, cnd, slice	1 pce	45	88	2	19	2	1	0.1	0.1	0.3	0	11
42042	Bread, cracked wheat, slice, reg	1 pce	25	65	2	12	1	1	0.2	0.5	0.2	0	0
71207	Bread, French, slice, lrg	1 pce	96	263	8	50	3	3	0.6	1.2	0.7	0	0
42049	Bread, oatmeal, slice	1 pce	27	73	2	13	1	1	0.2	0.4	0.5	0	1
42007	Bread, pita, white, enrich, lrg, 6 1/2"	1 ea	60	165	5	33	1	1	0.1	0.1	0.3	0	0
42051	Bread, raisin, enrich, slice	1 pce	26	71	2	14	1	1	0.3	0.6	0.2	0	0
57235	Bread, rye, mild	1 pce	32	70	3	13	4	0	0.0	—	—	0	0
42003	Bread, sourdough starter	1 cup	250	359	17	70	5	2	0.2	—	—	1	38
42012	Bread, wheat, slice	1 pce	25	65	2	12	1	1	0.2	0.4	0.2	0	0
42138	Bread, white, prep w/2% milk f/recipe, slice	1 pce	42	120	3	21	1	2	0.5	0.5	1.2	1	10
71020	Bread, whole grain, slice	1 pce	26	65	3	12	2	1	0.2	0.4	0.2	0	0
71939	Bread, wraps, thin thin	1 ea	35	110	4	21	0	1	0.0	—	—	0	0
42036	Breadsticks, plain, 7 5/8" x 5/8"	1 ea	10	41	1	7	0	1	0.1	0.4	0.4	0	0

PAGE KEY: A-96 Granola Bars, Cereal Bars, Diet Bars, Scones, and Tarts A-96 Meals and Dishes A-100 Meats A-106 Nuts, Seeds, and Products A-108 Poultry
A-110 Salad Dressings, Dips, and Mayonnaise A-110 Salads A-110 Sandwiches A-114 Sauces and Gravies A-114 Snack Foods—Chips, Pretzels, Popcorn
A-116 Soups, Stews, and Chilis A-118 Spices, Flavors, and Seasonings A-120 Sports Bars and Drinks A-120 Supplemental Foods and Formulas
A-122 Sweeteners and Sweet Substitutes A-122 Vegetables and Legumes A-136 Weight Loss Bars and Drinks A-138 Miscellaneous

Thia (mg)	Ribo (mg)	Niac (mg NE)	Vit B6 (mg)	Vit B12 (µg)	Fol (µg)	Vit C (mg)	Vit D (IU)	Vit E (mg AT)	Cal (mg)	Iron (mg)	Magn (mg)	Phos (mg)	Pota (mg)	Sodi (mg)	Zinc (mg)	Wat (%)	Alco (g)	Caff (g)
0.37	0.15	2.30	0.51	0.00	70.8	170.9	—	0.1	61	1.32	56.6	38	543	5	0.5	86	0.00	0.00
0.01	0.01	0.28	0.01	0.00	3.3	6.3	—	0.2	4	0.10	4.6	11	104	0	0.1	87	0.00	0.00
0.05	0.05	0.46	0.15	0.00	9.2	9.4	—	0.9	5	0.46	4.6	12	399	5	0.2	81	0.00	0.00
0.00	0.07	0.46	0.12	0.00	1.2	1.3	—	0.0	22	0.74	14.4	47	308	5	0.1	15	0.00	0.00
0.00	0.01	0.18	0.00	0.00	4.3	4.9	—	0.2	52	0.12	7.3	9	176	2	0.1	94	0.00	0.00
0.02	0.02	0.56	0.07	0.00	34.6	84.7	—	0.4	23	0.60	18.7	35	220	1	0.2	91	0.00	0.00
0.07	0.03	0.27	0.05	0.00	28.8	51.1	—	0.2	38	0.10	9.6	13	174	0	0.1	87	0.00	0.00
0.05	0.03	0.37	0.07	0.00	15.7	26.2	—	0.2	36	0.15	11.8	20	163	2	0.1	85	0.00	0.00
0.09	0.05	0.50	0.12	0.00	8.6	23.2	—	0.1	20	0.68	28.6	31	320	3	0.3	91	0.00	0.00
0.17	0.10	2.47	0.11	0.00	12.1	1.2	0.0	0.3	23	1.10	10.8	49	213	645	0.6	9	0.00	0.00
0.15	0.10	1.60	—	—	40.0	0.0	—	—	60	1.44	—	—	35	400	—	16	0.00	0.00
0.25	0.15	1.84	0.00	0.00	57.2	0.0	—	0.0	5	1.45	6.9	34	33	1	0.2	12	0.00	0.00
0.31	0.15	2.32	0.00	0.00	63.7	0.0	—	0.0	5	2.50	5.5	29	36	1	0.2	13	0.00	0.00
0.12	0.05	1.90	0.10	0.00	13.2	0.0	—	0.2	10	1.15	41.4	104	122	2	0.9	10	0.00	0.00
0.21	0.05	0.33	0.03	0.00	19.5	0.0	0.0	0.3	19	1.86	107.9	183	143	1	1.3	9	0.00	0.00
0.21	0.05	0.33	0.03	0.00	19.5	0.0	0.0	0.3	19	1.86	107.9	183	143	1	1.3	9	0.00	0.00
—	—	—	—	—	—	0.0	—	—	0	0.00	—	0	0	0	—	—	0.00	0.00
0.07	0.03	1.78	0.11	0.00	9.4	0.0	—	0.0	12	0.86	57.4	105	144	6	0.7	9	0.00	0.00
1.88	0.93	6.32	1.11	0.00	397.8	6.8	0.0	18.1	51	10.27	361.6	1295	1070	5	18.8	6	0.00	0.00
0.23	0.17	3.32	0.28	0.00	41.0	2.8	—	0.1	30	2.30	88.6	216	183	17	1.8	48	0.00	0.00
0.31	0.12	1.96	0.05	0.09	50.2	0.3	—	0.1	7	2.26	14.2	48	39	288	0.4	33	0.00	0.00
0.47	0.31	3.96	0.00	0.00	0.1	0.1	0.0	0.0	14	3.32	0.4	71	80	510	0.0	34	0.00	0.00
0.20	0.18	1.76	0.01	0.05	36.6	0.1	—	0.8	141	1.74	10.8	98	73	348	0.3	29	0.00	0.00
0.20	0.18	1.76	0.01	0.05	36.6	0.1	—	0.8	141	1.74	10.8	98	73	348	0.3	29	0.00	0.00
0.15	0.11	2.20	0.12	0.07	13.0	0.2	10.1	1.3	155	1.69	56.9	199	200	210	1.2	28	0.00	0.00
0.20	0.15	1.97	0.03	0.00	49.9	0.0	—	0.1	68	1.67	10.3	45	45	306	0.3	36	0.00	0.00
0.10	0.09	1.12	0.09	0.01	30.7	0.1	—	0.1	24	0.89	13.8	46	53	127	0.3	38	0.00	0.00
0.00	0.05	0.50	0.03	0.00	4.9	0.0	—	0.1	32	0.93	28.3	50	143	284	0.2	47	0.00	0.00
0.09	0.05	0.92	0.07	0.00	15.2	0.0	—	0.1	11	0.69	13.0	38	44	134	0.3	36	0.00	0.00
0.50	0.31	4.55	0.03	0.00	142.1	0.0	—	0.3	72	2.43	25.9	101	108	585	0.8	34	0.00	0.00
0.10	0.05	0.85	0.01	0.00	16.7	0.0	—	0.1	18	0.73	10.0	34	38	162	0.3	37	0.00	0.00
0.36	0.20	2.77	0.01	0.00	64.2	0.0	—	0.2	52	1.57	15.6	58	72	322	0.5	32	0.00	0.00
0.09	0.10	0.89	0.01	0.00	27.6	0.0	—	0.1	17	0.75	6.8	28	59	101	0.2	34	0.00	0.00
0.15	0.14	3.00	0.30	0.89	80.0	0.0	—	—	100	1.79	60.0	—	—	70	2.2	47	0.00	0.00
1.00	1.35	10.68	0.30	0.31	508.7	0.5	35.2	0.1	123	6.17	42.9	358	522	57	1.9	64	0.00	0.00
0.10	0.07	1.02	0.01	0.00	22.8	0.0	—	0.1	26	0.82	11.5	38	50	132	0.3	37	0.00	0.00
0.17	0.15	1.50	0.01	0.02	38.2	0.1	—	0.4	24	1.25	8.0	48	61	151	0.3	35	0.00	0.00
0.10	0.09	1.12	0.09	0.01	30.7	0.1	—	0.1	24	0.89	13.8	46	53	127	0.3	38	0.00	0.00
—	—	—	—	—	—	0.0	—	—	40	1.44	—	—	—	190	—	—	0.00	0.00
0.05	0.05	0.52	0.00	0.00	16.2	0.0	—	0.1	2	0.43	3.2	12	12	66	0.1	6	0.00	0.00

PAGE KEY: A-46 Beverage and Beverage Mixes   A-48 Other Beverages   A-48 Beverages, Alcoholic   A-50 Candies and Confections, Gum   A-54 Cereals, Breakfast Type   A-58 Cheese and Cheese Substitutes   A-60 Dairy Products and Substitutes   A-62 Desserts   A-68 Dessert Toppings   A-68 Eggs, Substitutes, and Egg Dishes   A-70 Ethnic Foods   A-74 Fast Foods/Restaurants   A-88 Fats, Oils, Margarines, Shortenings, and Substitutes   A-88 Fish, Seafood, and Shellfish   A-90 Food Additives   A-90 Fruit, Vegetable, or Blended Juices   A-92 Grains, Flours, and Fractions   A-92 Grain Products, Prepared and Baked Goods

Code	Food Name	Unit/Amt	Wt (g)	Energy (kcal)	Prot (g)	Carb (g)	Fiber (g)	Fat (g)	Sat (g)	Mono (g)	Poly (g)	Chol (mg)	Vit A (RE)
42020	Buns, hamburger	1 ea	43	120	4	21	1	2	0.5	0.5	0.8	0	0
42021	Buns, hot dog/frankfurter	1 ea	43	120	4	21	1	2	0.5	0.5	0.8	0	0
42649	Cornbread, homestyle, prep f/dry mix, 2" x 3" pce	1 pce	52	150	3	26	1	4	1.0	1.5	1.0	5	0
42015	Croissant, butter, med	1 ea	57	231	5	26	1	12	6.6	3.1	0.6	38	120
45520	Dumpling, plain	1 ea	32	40	1	7	0	1	0.3	0.4	0.3	1	4
43512	Matzoh Balls	3 ea	42	58	2	7	0	2	0.5	0.8	0.5	44	20
71886	Pretzels, soft, garlic	1 ea	120	320	9	66	2	1	0.0	—	—	0	0
42018	Rolls, dinner, brown & serve, browned	1 ea	28	84	2	14	1	2	0.5	1.0	0.3	0	0
42158	Rolls, dinner, prep f/recipe w/2% milk, 2 1/2"	1 ea	35	111	3	19	1	3	0.6	1.0	0.7	12	32
42022	Rolls, hard, 3 1/2"	1 ea	57	167	6	30	1	2	0.3	0.6	1.0	0	0
71358	Rolls, hoagie, whole wheat, med	1 ea	94	250	8	48	7	4	0.8	1.1	2.0	0	0
71359	Rolls, submarine, whole wheat, med	1 ea	94	250	8	48	7	4	0.8	1.1	2.0	0	0
Bread Crumbs, Croutons, Breading Mixes & Batters													
42004	Bread Crumbs, plain, grated, dry	1 Tbs	7	27	1	5	0	0	0.1	0.1	0.1	0	0
42016	Croutons, plain, dry	0.25 cup	8	31	1	6	0	0	0.1	0.2	0.1	0	0
Crackers													
43503	Cracker Crumbs, graham, plain	1 cup	84	355	6	65	2	8	1.3	3.4	3.2	0	0
71273	Crackers, cheese, 1" square	30 ea	30	151	3	17	1	8	2.8	3.6	0.7	4	9
11712	Crackers, club style	1 ea	7	32	1	5	0	1	0.3	—	—	0	0
11745	Crackers, ea, Town House	5 ea	16	83	1	9	0	5	0.9	—	—	0	1
47253	Crackers, graham, honey	3 ea	21	92	2	16	1	3	0.7	—	—	0	0
43535	Crackers, matzoh, egg, svg	1 oz	28	111	3	22	1	1	0.2	0.2	0.1	24	4
43509	Crackers, melba toast, plain, pce, 3 3/4" x 1 3/4" x 1/8"	1 pce	5	20	1	4	0	0	0.0	0.0	0.1	0	0
70963	Crackers, original, svg	5 ea	16	79	1	10	0	4	0.6	2.8	0.3	0	0
43506	Crackers, saltines	4 ea	12	51	1	9	0	1	0.2	0.8	0.1	0	0
43581	Crackers, wheat, original	16 ea	29	136	2	20	1	6	0.9	2.0	0.4	0	0
Muffins													
44585	English Muffin, traditional	1 ea	57	130	5	26	2	0	0.0	—	—	0	0
44515	Muffin, plain, prep f/recipe w/2% milk	1 ea	57	169	4	24	2	6	1.2	1.6	3.3	22	23
42295	Popover, unenrich, dry mix, 6 oz pkg	1 ea	170	631	18	121	—	7	1.7	3.4	1.4	0	0
Pancakes, French Toast, and Waffles													
45033	Crepe, suzette	1 ea	66	159	4	16	0	9	3.8	3.2	1.3	83	81
42156	French Toast, prep f/recipe w/2% milk	1 pce	65	149	5	16	1	7	1.8	2.9	1.7	75	84
45192	Pancakes, buttermilk	1 ea	43	99	3	16	0	3	0.6	1.3	0.9	5	73
45152	Waffles, buttermilk egg, 7" prep f/dry mix	1 ea	81	230	6	37	2	7	1.0	3.5	2.5	10	0
Pasta													
57411	Dish, ravioli, beef, square, preckd	9 pce	146	300	14	40	1	8	3.8	—	—	77	—
92216	Dish, tortellini, cheese filled	1 cup	108	332	15	51	2	8	3.9	2.2	0.5	45	42
91205	Pasta, acini di pepe, enrich, dry, all brands	3.6 oz	100	364	14	74	3	1	0.4	—	—	0	0
38365	Pasta, egg noodles	0.75 cup	68	200	8	33	1	4	1.0	—	—	40	0
38580	Pasta, elbow twist, semolina, dry	0.75 cup	56	201	7	41	2	1	0.3	0.2	0.8	0	0
91211	Pasta, lasagna noodles, enrich, dry, all brands	3.6 oz	100	364	14	74	3	1	0.4	—	—	0	0
38102	Pasta, macaroni noodles, enrich, ckd	1 cup	140	197	7	40	2	1	0.1	0.1	0.4	0	0
38551	Pasta, rice noodle, ckd	0.5 cup	88	96	1	22	1	0	0.0	0.0	0.0	0	0
38105	Pasta, shells, sml, enrich, ckd	0.5 cup	58	81	3	16	1	0	0.1	0.0	0.2	0	0
38118	Pasta, spaghetti noodles, enrich, ckd	0.5 cup	70	99	3	20	1	0	0.1	0.1	0.2	0	0

Thia (mg)	Ribo (mg)	Niac (mg NE)	Vit B6 (mg)	Vit B12 (μg)	Fol (μg)	Vit C (mg)	Vit D (IU)	Vit E (mg AT)	Cal (mg)	Iron (mg)	Magn (mg)	Phos (mg)	Pota (mg)	Sodi (mg)	Zinc (mg)	Wat (%)	Alco (g)	Caff (g)
0.17	0.14	1.78	0.02	0.09	47.7	0.0	—	0.0	59	1.42	9.0	27	40	206	0.3	35	0.00	0.00
0.17	0.14	1.78	0.02	0.09	47.7	0.0	—	0.0	59	1.42	9.0	27	40	206	0.3	35	0.00	0.00
—	—	—	—	—	—	0.0	—	—	9	0.49	—	90	40	280	—	35	0.00	0.00
0.21	0.14	1.25	0.02	0.09	50.2	0.1	—	0.5	21	1.15	9.1	60	67	424	0.4	23	0.00	0.00
0.05	0.05	0.41	0.00	0.01	1.8	0.1	—	0.1	45	0.43	3.0	28	20	66	0.1	72	0.00	0.00
0.02	0.07	0.31	0.01	0.09	4.5	0.0	—	0.3	6	0.43	3.3	26	22	13	0.2	72	0.00	0.00
—	—	—	—	—	—	0.0	—	—	20	2.16	—	—	—	830	—	—	0.00	0.00
0.14	0.09	1.12	0.01	0.01	27.4	0.0	—	0.1	33	0.87	6.4	32	37	146	0.2	32	0.00	0.00
0.14	0.14	1.21	0.01	0.05	31.5	0.1	—	0.3	21	1.03	6.7	44	53	145	0.2	29	0.00	0.00
0.27	0.18	2.42	0.01	0.00	54.1	0.0	—	0.2	54	1.87	15.4	57	62	310	0.5	31	0.00	0.00
0.23	0.14	3.46	0.18	0.00	28.2	0.0	—	0.8	100	2.26	79.9	211	256	449	1.9	33	0.00	0.00
0.23	0.14	3.46	0.18	0.00	28.2	0.0	—	0.8	100	2.26	79.9	211	256	449	1.9	33	0.00	0.00
0.07	0.02	0.44	0.00	0.01	7.2	0.0	—	0.0	12	0.33	2.9	11	13	49	0.1	7	0.00	0.00
0.05	0.01	0.40	0.00	0.00	9.9	0.0	—	0.0	6	0.31	2.3	9	9	52	0.1	6	0.00	0.00
0.18	0.25	3.46	0.05	0.00	38.6	0.0	—	0.3	20	3.13	25.2	87	113	508	0.7	4	0.00	0.00
0.17	0.12	1.39	0.17	0.14	45.6	0.0	—	0.0	45	1.42	10.8	65	44	298	0.3	3	0.00	0.00
—	—	—	—	—	—	0.0	—	—	2	0.15	—	—	—	70	—	7	0.00	0.00
—	—	—	—	—	—	0.2	—	—	4	0.47	—	—	—	155	—	—	0.00	0.00
—	—	—	—	—	—	0.0	—	—	17	0.73	—	—	—	114	—	3	0.00	0.00
0.21	0.18	1.44	0.01	0.05	6.8	0.0	—	0.3	11	0.76	6.8	42	43	6	0.2	6	0.00	0.00
0.01	0.00	0.20	0.00	0.00	6.2	0.0	—	0.0	5	0.18	3.0	10	10	41	0.1	5	0.00	0.00
0.03	0.05	0.61	0.00	0.00	9.6	0.0	—	—	24	0.64	3.2	48	15	124	0.2	3	0.00	0.00
0.00	0.05	0.62	0.00	0.00	16.7	0.0	—	0.1	8	0.68	2.6	12	18	129	0.1	5	0.00	0.00
0.09	0.09	1.15	0.02	—	12.2	0.0	—	—	23	1.07	15.1	60	56	168	—	2	0.00	0.00
—	—	—	—	—	—	0.0	—	—	80	1.08	—	—	—	250	—	43	0.00	0.00
0.15	0.17	1.32	0.01	0.09	29.1	0.2	—	1.0	114	1.36	9.7	87	69	266	0.3	38	0.00	0.00
0.17	0.03	1.76	0.07	0.14	42.5	0.2	—	1.8	54	1.38	42.5	170	170	1541	1.5	12	0.00	0.00
0.07	0.17	0.60	0.03	0.23	10.7	3.0	21.1	0.6	45	0.75	8.3	69	86	74	0.4	56	0.00	0.00
0.12	0.20	1.05	0.05	0.20	27.9	0.2	—	0.7	65	1.09	11.0	76	87	311	0.4	55	0.00	0.00
0.10	0.11	1.47	0.15	0.43	22.1	0.6	—	0.0	15	1.32	7.7	145	44	225	0.3	47	0.00	0.00
—	—	—	—	—	—	0.0	—	—	43	1.50	—	450	130	900	—	—	0.00	0.00
—	—	—	—	—	—	0.0	—	—	119	2.10	—	—	—	400	—	—	0.00	0.00
0.34	0.33	2.91	0.05	0.17	79.9	0.0	—	0.2	164	1.62	22.7	229	90	372	1.1	30	0.00	0.00
0.80	0.44	5.36	—	—	214.0	0.0	—	—	18	3.21	53.7	141	144	5	1.2	10	0.00	0.00
—	—	—	—	—	—	0.0	—	—	0	1.79	—	—	—	140	—	—	0.00	0.00
0.49	0.20	3.33	0.07	0.00	10.3	0.0	—	0.1	12	1.61	—	105	—	3	0.7	11	0.00	0.00
0.80	0.44	5.36	—	—	214.0	0.0	—	—	18	3.21	53.7	141	144	5	1.2	10	0.00	0.00
0.28	0.14	2.33	0.05	0.00	107.8	0.0	—	0.1	10	1.96	25.2	76	43	1	0.7	66	0.00	0.00
0.01	0.00	0.05	0.00	0.00	2.6	0.0	—	—	4	0.11	2.6	18	4	17	0.2	74	0.00	0.00
0.11	0.05	0.95	0.01	0.00	44.3	0.0	—	0.0	4	0.80	10.3	31	18	1	0.3	66	0.00	0.00
0.14	0.07	1.16	0.01	0.00	53.9	0.0	—	0.0	5	0.98	12.6	38	22	1	0.4	66	0.00	0.00

PAGE KEY: A-46 Beverage and Beverage Mixes A-48 Other Beverages A-48 Beverages, Alcoholic A-50 Candies and Confections, Gum A-54 Cereals, Breakfast Type A-58 Cheese and Cheese Substitutes A-60 Dairy Products and Substitutes A-62 Desserts A-68 Dessert Toppings A-68 Eggs, Substitutes, and Egg Dishes A-70 Ethnic Foods A-74 Fast Foods/Restaurants A-88 Fats, Oils, Margarines, Shortenings, and Substitutes A-88 Fish, Seafood, and Shellfish A-90 Food Additives A-90 Fruit, Vegetable, or Blended Juices A-92 Grains, Flours, and Fractions A-92 Grain Products, Prepared and Baked Goods

Code	Food Name	Unit/ Amt	Wt (g)	Energy (kcal)	Prot (g)	Carb (g)	Fiber (g)	Fat (g)	Sat (g)	Mono (g)	Poly (g)	Chol (mg)	Vit A (RE)
Rice													
38013	Rice, white, long grain, ckd	1 cup	158	205	4	45	1	0	0.1	0.1	0.1	0	0
Stuffing and Mixes													
38491	Baking Mix, dry, Bisquick	0.33 cup	40	162	3	24	1	6	1.6	2.5	0.5	0	0
42037	Stuffing, bread, prep f/dry mix	0.5 cup	100	178	3	22	3	9	1.7	3.8	2.6	0	125
Tortillas and Taco/Tostada Shells													
42359	Taco Shells	2 ea	27	130	2	18	2	6	1.0	3.8	1.2	0	0
Granola Bars, Cereal Bars, Diet Bars, Scones, and Tarts													
53227	Bar, cereal, mixed berry	1 ea	37	137	2	27	1	3	0.6	1.9	0.4	0	150
23100	Bar, granola, almond, hard	1 ea	24	117	2	15	1	6	3.0	1.8	0.9	0	1
47591	Bar, granola, cinnamon	2 ea	42	180	4	29	2	6	0.5	—	—	0	0
63342	Bar, granola, fruit & nut	3.6 oz	100	397	8	77	5	6	0.7	0.2	4.8	0	28
47592	Bar, granola, oats 'n honey	2 ea	42	180	4	29	2	6	0.5	—	—	0	0
23059	Bar, granola, plain, hard	1 ea	24	115	2	16	1	5	0.6	1.1	3.0	0	4
42071	Scones	1 ea	42	150	4	19	1	6	2.0	2.6	1.3	49	69
MEALS AND DISHES													
Canned Meals and Dishes													
92620	Dish, ravioli, beef, w/meat sauce, cnd	1 cup	212	260	11	39	5	7	3.0	—	—	10	100
FROZEN OR REFRIGERATED MEALS AND DISHES													
Frozen/Refrigerated Breakfasts													
70830	Eggs, scrambled, low fat	1 ea	170	240	12	18	2	13	3.0	—	—	40	225
70826	Sandwich, breakfast, sausage egg cheese, w/biscuit	1 ea	156	460	16	37	3	28	11.0	—	—	115	0
Frozen/Refrigerated Children's Meals													
Frozen/Refrigerated Dinners													
70023	Dinner, beef noodles, w/veg, fzn	1 ea	298	407	14	59	3	14	4.8	5.6	2.4	31	312
11118	Dinner, beef, pot roast, fzn, Healthy Choice	1 ea	312	300	20	41	8	6	2.0	—	—	40	250
15957	Dinner, chicken & noodles, homestyle, ckd f/fzn	1 cup	340	390	12	44	7	19	7.0	—	—	50	700

PAGE KEY: A-96 Granola Bars, Cereal Bars, Diet Bars, Scones, and Tarts   A-96 Meals and Dishes   A-100 Meats   A-106 Nuts, Seeds, and Products   A-108 Poultry
A-110 Salad Dressings, Dips, and Mayonnaise   A-110 Salads   A-110 Sandwiches   A-114 Sauces and Gravies   A-114 Snack Foods—Chips, Pretzels, Popcorn
A-116 Soups, Stews, and Chilis   A-118 Spices, Flavors, and Seasonings   A-120 Sports Bars and Drinks   A-120 Supplemental Foods and Formulas
A-122 Sweeteners and Sweet Substitutes   A-122 Vegetables and Legumes   A-136 Weight Loss Bars and Drinks   A-138 Miscellaneous

Thia (mg)	Ribo (mg)	Niac (mg NE)	Vit B6 (mg)	Vit B12 (µg)	Fol (µg)	Vit C (mg)	Vit D (IU)	Vit E (mg AT)	Cal (mg)	Iron (mg)	Magn (mg)	Phos (mg)	Pota (mg)	Sodi (mg)	Zinc (mg)	Wat (%)	Alco (g)	Caff (g)
0.25	0.01	2.32	0.15	0.00	91.6	0.0	—	0.1	16	1.89	19.0	68	55	2	0.8	68	0.00	0.00
0.20	0.15	1.67	—	—	—	0.0	—	—	60	1.39	—	—	50	499	—	—	0.00	0.00
0.14	0.10	1.48	0.03	0.00	39.0	0.0	—	1.4	32	1.09	12.0	42	74	543	0.3	65	0.00	0.00
—	—	—	—	—	—	0.0	—	—	40	0.72	—	—	63	190	—	2	0.00	0.00
0.37	0.40	4.98	0.51	0.00	40.0	0.0	—	0.0	14	1.80	9.6	36	70	110	1.5	14	0.00	0.00
0.07	0.01	0.14	0.00	0.00	2.8	0.0	—	0.4	8	0.58	19.1	54	64	60	0.4	3	0.00	0.00
—	—	—	—	—	—	0.0	—	—	0	1.08	—	—	—	160	—	—	0.00	0.00
0.49	0.43	5.11	0.80	0.00	160.0	0.0	—	1.1	36	5.30	85.0	243	238	251	1.9	7	0.00	0.00
—	—	—	—	—	—	0.0	—	—	0	1.08	—	—	—	160	—	—	0.00	0.00
0.05	0.02	0.38	0.01	0.00	5.6	0.2	—	0.3	15	0.72	23.8	68	82	72	0.5	4	0.00	0.00
0.15	0.15	1.21	0.02	0.10	7.9	0.1	6.7	0.7	80	1.32	7.1	74	49	171	0.3	27	0.00	0.00
0.15	0.17	4.00	—	—	60.0	0.0	—	—	40	1.79	—	—	—	1070	—	—	0.00	0.00
—	—	—	—	—	—	4.8	—	—	40	0.72	—	—	—	620	—	73	0.00	0.00
—	—	—	—	—	—	0.0	—	—	150	1.79	—	—	—	1060	—	46	0.00	0.00
0.25	0.25	3.44	0.20	0.87	38.0	16.5	—	1.3	116	2.02	43.5	210	466	2756	2.3	68	0.00	0.00
—	—	—	—	—	—	18.0	—	—	20	1.79	—	—	—	600	—	—	0.00	0.00
0.27	0.28	5.69	—	—	—	0.0	—	—	60	1.79	—	—	374	1080	—	—	0.00	0.00

PAGE KEY: A-46 Beverage and Beverage Mixes   A-48 Other Beverages   A-48 Beverages, Alcoholic   A-50 Candies and Confections, Gum   A-54 Cereals, Breakfast Type   A-58 Cheese and Cheese Substitutes   A-60 Dairy Products and Substitutes   A-62 Desserts   A-68 Dessert Toppings   A-68 Eggs, Substitutes, and Egg Dishes   A-70 Ethnic Foods   A-74 Fast Foods/Restaurants   A-88 Fats, Oils, Margarines, Shortenings, and Substitutes   A-88 Fish, Seafood, and Shellfish   A-90 Food Additives   A-90 Fruit, Vegetable, or Blended Juices   A-92 Grains, Flours, and Fractions   A-92 Grain Products, Prepared and Baked Goods

Code	Food Name	Unit/ Amt	Wt (g)	Energy (kcal)	Prot (g)	Carb (g)	Fiber (g)	Fat (g)	Sat (g)	Mono (g)	Poly (g)	Chol (mg)	Vit A (RE)
446	Dinner, egg roll, w/fried rice & chicken, ckd f/fzn	1 ea	241	330	12	51	5	9	3.0	—	—	60	200
70151	Dinner, enchilada, cheese, w/beans & rice, fzn	1 ea	340	515	19	71	14	18	7.8	6.7	2.3	32	121
1756	Dinner, fish, sticks, ckd f/fzn	1 ea	187	290	11	33	4	13	4.5	—	—	30	100
70766	Dinner, meatloaf, Swanson	1 ea	468	640	24	65	6	31	14.0	—	—	45	60
11071	Dinner, steak, salisbury, Swanson	1 ea	461	610	34	46	10	33	17.0	—	—	80	150
57293	Dinner, stir fry, teriyaki veg, fzn	1 cup	108	92	4	17	1	1	0.3	—	—	1	175
16912	Dinner, turkey, breast, traditional, fzn, Healthy Choice	1 ea	298	290	22	40	5	4	2.0	—	—	45	80

Frozen/Refrigerated Dishes

Code	Food Name	Unit/ Amt	Wt (g)	Energy (kcal)	Prot (g)	Carb (g)	Fiber (g)	Fat (g)	Sat (g)	Mono (g)	Poly (g)	Chol (mg)	Vit A (RE)
56668	Corn Dog	1 ea	175	460	17	56	—	19	5.2	9.1	3.5	79	61
16167	Dish, chicken & noodles, casserole, Swanson	1 ea	284	300	18	36	2	9	3.0	—	—	50	20
70749	Dish, fish & chips, Swanson	1 ea	156	350	16	38	4	15	4.5	—	—	30	40
16163	Dish, pot pie, chicken, Swanson	1 ea	198	410	10	43	2	22	9.0	—	—	25	200
16915	Dish, pot pie, turkey, Swanson	1 ea	198	400	10	42	3	21	8.0	—	—	25	100
57845	Dish, rice bowl, chicken & veg	1 ea	340	360	21	56	3	5	1.5	—	—	25	—
52165	Dish, rice bowl, chicken, sweet & sour	1 ea	340	360	17	65	2	3	0.5	—	—	30	—
83063	Dish, rice bowl, fried	1 ea	340	450	18	77	6	8	0.5	—	—	0	700
57140	Dish, tortellini, three cheese, fzn	2.9 oz	81	250	11	37	2	7	3.5	—	—	35	0

Frozen/Refrigerated Dinners/Dishes—Vegetarian

Code	Food Name	Unit/ Amt	Wt (g)	Energy (kcal)	Prot (g)	Carb (g)	Fiber (g)	Fat (g)	Sat (g)	Mono (g)	Poly (g)	Chol (mg)	Vit A (RE)
8869	Corn Dog, vegetarian	1 ea	71	159	8	22	1	4	0.5	1.2	2.5	0	0

Prepared Generic or Homemade Meals and Dishes

Code	Food Name	Unit/ Amt	Wt (g)	Energy (kcal)	Prot (g)	Carb (g)	Fiber (g)	Fat (g)	Sat (g)	Mono (g)	Poly (g)	Chol (mg)	Vit A (RE)
7037	Beans, baked, prep f/recipe	1 cup	253	382	14	54	14	13	4.9	5.4	1.9	13	0
56258	Chicken, liver, chopped, w/egg & oinon	1 cup	208	472	27	6	1	37	11.2	15.2	7.2	753	4581
11013	Dish, beef curry	1 cup	236	436	27	13	3	31	7.0	14.5	7.4	69	367
56195	Dish, chicken & noodles, w/cream sauce	1 cup	224	320	22	32	1	11	3.2	4.3	2.5	81	100
56200	Dish, chicken & noodles, w/tomato sauce	1 cup	224	291	20	31	2	9	2.1	3.8	2.5	74	143
15904	Dish, chicken cacciatore	1 cup	244	459	42	13	2	26	6.3	9.7	7.2	128	132
56213	Dish, chicken dumplings	1 cup	244	372	26	22	1	19	5.1	7.8	4.6	89	52
56287	Dish, egg foo young, chicken	1 ea	86	121	8	4	1	8	1.9	2.8	2.3	167	87
56110	Dish, egg roll, w/o meat	1 ea	64	101	3	10	1	6	1.2	2.9	1.3	30	16
11000	Dish, goulash, beef	1 cup	249	270	33	7	1	12	3.2	4.3	2.5	84	31
56239	Dish, jambalaya, shrimp	1 cup	243	310	27	28	1	9	1.8	3.8	2.8	181	133
56140	Dish, meatballs, Swedish, w/cream sauce	1 cup	246	406	31	17	1	23	9.5	9.0	1.3	163	94
56180	Dish, pork & potatoes, w/gravy	1 cup	252	255	21	21	2	10	3.2	4.3	1.1	57	1
56100	Dish, spaghetti w/meatballs, prep f/recipe	1 cup	248	362	18	28	3	18	4.8	—	—	65	164
57523	Dish, spring roll, fresh	1 ea	64	113	5	9	1	6	1.4	3.0	1.3	37	16
11008	Dish, stroganoff, beef	1 cup	256	408	26	16	1	27	10.6	7.9	6.3	85	99
56130	Dish, tortellini, meat	1 cup	190	373	25	33	1	15	5.4	5.7	2.1	240	134
56215	Dish, turkey & stuffing	1 cup	200	273	35	19	1	5	1.4	1.7	1.3	105	19
56242	Gumbo, w/rice, New Orleans style	1 cup	244	193	14	17	2	8	1.6	2.6	2.7	40	63
56150	Hash, beef	1 cup	190	312	21	21	2	16	4.9	5.7	3.3	57	0
56231	Pie, sheperds, w/beef	1 cup	243	278	17	32	3	9	2.6	4.0	1.7	37	78

Pizza

Code	Food Name	Unit/ Amt	Wt (g)	Energy (kcal)	Prot (g)	Carb (g)	Fiber (g)	Fat (g)	Sat (g)	Mono (g)	Poly (g)	Chol (mg)	Vit A (RE)
56995	Pizza, bagel, cheese & pepperoni, fzn	2 pce	22	52	3	6	1	2	0.8	—	—	4	20
56993	Pizza, bagel, cheese, extra, fzn	4 pce	88	190	11	24	3	6	2.0	—	—	10	80
81030	Pizza, Canadian bacon, fzn	1 ea	195	440	17	50	2	19	3.5	—	—	15	0

PAGE KEY: A-96 Granola Bars, Cereal Bars, Diet Bars, Scones, and Tarts   A-96 Meals and Dishes   A-100 Meats   A-106 Nuts, Seeds, and Products   A-108 Poultry
A-110 Salad Dressings, Dips, and Mayonnaise   A-110 Salads   A-110 Sandwiches   A-114 Sauces and Gravies   A-114 Snack Foods—Chips, Pretzels, Popcorn
A-116 Soups, Stews, and Chilis   A-118 Spices, Flavors, and Seasonings   A-120 Sports Bars and Drinks   A-120 Supplemental Foods and Formulas
A-122 Sweeteners and Sweet Substitutes   A-122 Vegetables and Legumes   A-136 Weight Loss Bars and Drinks   A-138 Miscellaneous

Thia (mg)	Ribo (mg)	Niac (mg NE)	Vit B6 (mg)	Vit B12 (µg)	Fol (µg)	Vit C (mg)	Vit D (IU)	Vit E (mg AT)	Cal (mg)	Iron (mg)	Magn (mg)	Phos (mg)	Pota (mg)	Sodi (mg)	Zinc (mg)	Wat (%)	Alco (g)	Caff (g)
—	—	—	—	—	—	0.0	—	—	40	1.08	—	—	—	1270	—	—	0.00	0.00
0.31	0.27	2.21	0.33	0.18	112.4	6.0	—	1.8	289	4.36	99.1	414	645	1967	2.7	66	0.00	0.00
—	—	—	—	—	—	3.6	—	—	60	1.79	—	—	—	820	—	—	0.00	0.00
—	—	—	—	—	—	18.0	—	—	150	5.40	—	—	—	1870	—	73	0.00	0.00
—	—	—	—	—	—	4.8	—	—	200	5.40	—	—	—	1620	—	74	0.00	0.00
—	—	—	—	—	—	10.2	—	—	73	0.58	—	—	—	717	—	—	0.00	0.00
0.44	0.25	6.00	—	—	—	36.0	—	—	20	1.44	—	270	540	460	—	—	0.00	0.00
0.28	0.69	4.15	0.09	0.43	103.2	0.0	—	0.7	102	6.17	17.5	166	262	973	1.3	47	0.00	0.00
—	—	—	—	—	—	0.0	—	—	200	3.59	—	—	—	940	—	76	0.00	0.00
—	—	—	—	—	—	1.2	—	—	150	1.44	—	—	—	930	—	54	0.00	0.00
—	—	—	—	—	—	1.2	—	—	20	1.79	—	—	—	780	—	—	0.00	0.00
—	—	—	—	—	—	2.4	—	—	20	1.79	—	—	—	700	—	62	0.00	0.00
—	—	—	—	—	—	—	—	—	—	—	—	—	—	1020	—	—	0.00	0.00
—	—	—	—	—	—	—	—	—	—	—	—	—	—	620	—	—	0.00	0.00
—	—	—	—	—	—	3.6	—	—	150	6.30	—	—	—	1090	—	—	0.00	0.00
—	—	—	—	—	—	0.0	—	—	0	0.00	—	—	—	300	—	30	0.00	0.00
0.10	0.05	0.00	—	—	—	0.0	—	—	12	0.64	—	113	66	527	0.2	49	0.00	0.00
0.34	0.11	1.02	0.23	0.00	121.4	2.8	—	1.3	154	5.03	108.8	276	906	1068	1.8	65	0.00	0.00
0.18	1.79	4.19	0.63	18.23	734.3	17.9	—	2.5	41	8.32	28.1	365	256	92	4.5	66	0.00	0.00
0.18	0.34	5.42	0.47	3.04	20.3	24.6	—	5.9	44	4.23	59.0	292	978	802	6.1	68	0.00	0.00
0.25	0.34	4.94	0.20	0.37	14.6	0.8	—	0.9	132	2.36	42.0	237	276	139	2.0	71	0.00	0.00
0.27	0.23	5.73	0.31	0.20	16.5	11.8	—	2.1	34	2.90	47.2	177	478	658	1.9	72	0.00	0.00
0.18	0.31	13.98	0.72	0.43	16.5	14.8	29.3	3.0	61	3.02	56.1	305	690	247	3.1	66	0.44	0.00
0.23	0.31	9.32	0.30	0.31	11.0	1.9	—	0.9	128	2.50	34.5	261	297	244	1.9	72	0.00	0.00
0.05	0.23	0.88	0.11	0.34	22.3	3.1	—	1.1	27	0.81	11.4	96	136	132	0.8	76	0.00	0.00
0.07	0.10	0.80	0.05	0.05	13.4	2.9	—	0.9	14	0.81	9.1	38	97	274	0.3	70	0.00	0.00
0.15	0.31	5.73	0.46	3.25	21.3	8.7	14.9	1.8	18	3.57	45.6	336	698	225	5.3	78	0.00	0.00
0.28	0.10	4.76	0.21	1.17	12.2	16.9	—	2.3	104	4.38	63.6	300	439	370	1.7	72	0.00	0.00
0.30	0.52	6.57	0.31	2.41	20.2	2.7	—	0.3	124	3.19	43.4	326	573	407	5.5	70	0.00	0.00
0.56	0.25	5.90	0.50	0.52	16.4	14.9	—	0.3	22	1.73	40.6	262	821	651	2.4	78	0.00	0.00
0.25	0.30	4.38	0.28	0.94	67.7	16.3	16.9	2.5	92	3.32	43.7	173	479	1133	3.4	71	0.00	0.00
0.15	0.12	1.27	0.09	0.11	9.9	2.1	—	0.8	15	0.82	10.0	57	124	274	0.5	66	0.00	0.00
0.18	0.38	4.51	0.28	2.60	20.2	1.8	—	2.4	92	3.64	40.4	308	556	677	4.9	72	0.00	0.00
0.46	0.56	4.48	0.21	0.89	29.1	0.0	—	1.1	178	3.11	28.1	290	231	437	2.2	61	0.00	0.00
0.23	0.31	13.10	0.44	0.36	28.7	2.9	—	0.6	43	2.27	47.5	293	403	511	2.5	70	0.00	0.00
0.20	0.15	4.51	0.20	2.41	45.6	13.5	—	1.4	71	2.60	40.1	152	446	542	15.2	83	0.00	0.00
0.15	0.20	3.74	0.49	1.79	16.5	7.1	—	1.2	19	2.46	36.4	204	587	470	5.0	69	0.00	0.00
0.20	0.18	3.90	0.58	1.25	21.1	16.4	—	1.3	40	2.18	46.9	193	764	312	3.9	75	0.00	0.00
—	—	—	—	—	—	2.2	—	—	25	0.36	—	—	38	162	—	—	0.00	0.00
—	—	—	—	—	—	9.0	—	—	150	0.72	—	—	150	490	—	—	0.00	0.00
—	—	—	—	—	—	0.0	—	—	150	3.59	—	—	—	1160	—	—	0.00	0.00

PAGE KEY: A-46 Beverage and Beverage Mixes   A-48 Other Beverages   A-48 Beverages, Alcoholic   A-50 Candies and Confections, Gum   A-54 Cereals, Breakfast Type
A-58 Cheese and Cheese Substitutes   A-60 Dairy Products and Substitutes   A-62 Desserts   A-68 Dessert Toppings   A-68 Eggs, Substitutes, and Egg Dishes   A-70 Ethnic Foods
A-74 Fast Foods/Restaurants   A-88 Fats, Oils, Margarines, Shortenings, and Substitutes   A-88 Fish, Seafood, and Shellfish   A-90 Food Additives
A-90 Fruit, Vegetable, or Blended Juices   A-92 Grains, Flours, and Fractions   A-92 Grain Products, Prepared and Baked Goods

Code	Food Name	Unit/ Amt	Wt (g)	Energy (kcal)	Prot (g)	Carb (g)	Fiber (g)	Fat (g)	Sat (g)	Mono (g)	Poly (g)	Chol (mg)	Vit A (RE)
56782	Pizza, cheese, for one, fzn	1 ea	184	497	21	48	4	24	—	—	—	40	—
56781	Pizza, deluxe, for one, fzn	1 ea	234	582	23	51	4	32	10.0	9.0	3.0	20	245
56779	Pizza, pepperoni, for one, fzn	1 ea	191	546	20	50	4	30	9.0	7.0	2.0	20	263
70898	Pizza, pepperoni, fzn, svg	1 ea	146	432	16	42	3	22	7.0	10.0	3.4	22	61
56778	Pizza, sausage, for one, fzn	1 ea	213	571	23	49	4	32	10.0	7.0	3.0	20	272
57178	Pizza, supreme, fzn, 1/5 of 12"	1 pce	130	300	14	30	3	14	6.0	—	—	30	60

MEATS
Beef

Code	Food Name	Unit/ Amt	Wt (g)	Energy (kcal)	Prot (g)	Carb (g)	Fiber (g)	Fat (g)	Sat (g)	Mono (g)	Poly (g)	Chol (mg)	Vit A (RE)
10820	Beef, average of all cuts, ckd, 1/8" trim	3 oz	85	247	22	0	0	17	6.6	7.2	0.6	74	0
10095	Beef, average of all cuts, ckd, choice, 1/4" trim	3 oz	85	274	22	0	0	20	8.0	8.6	0.7	75	0
10099	Beef, average of all cuts, ckd, prime, 1/4" trim	3 oz	85	274	22	0	0	20	8.1	8.6	0.7	71	0
10097	Beef, average of all cuts, ckd, select, 1/4" trim	3 oz	85	247	22	0	0	17	6.7	7.2	0.6	73	0
10705	Beef, average of all cuts, lean, ckd, 1/4" trim	3 oz	85	184	25	0	0	8	3.2	3.5	0.3	73	0
47441	Beef, chuck, ground, extra lean, raw	4 oz	113	130	22	0	0	5	2.0	2.0	0.5	60	0
10740	Beef, cubed patty	1 ea	91	251	15	2	0	20	8.1	—	—	64	11
58115	Beef, ground, hamburger, bkd, 10% fat	3 oz	85	182	23	0	0	9	3.7	4.0	0.3	73	0
58120	Beef, ground, hamburger, bkd, 15% fat	3 oz	85	204	22	0	0	12	4.6	5.3	0.4	77	0
58125	Beef, ground, hamburger, bkd, 20% fat	3 oz	85	216	21	0	0	14	5.9	6.1	0.4	77	0
58110	Beef, ground, hamburger, bkd, 5% fat	3 oz	85	148	23	0	0	5	2.5	2.4	0.3	62	0
10051	Beef, jerky, lrg pce	1 ea	20	81	7	2	0	5	2.1	2.2	0.2	10	0
53688	Beef, meat stick, spicy	0.63 oz	18	100	4	1	1	8	3.0	—	—	25	0
11019	Beef, meatballs	4 ea	112	240	19	7	0	14	5.1	6.3	0.7	93	21
11020	Beef, patty, brd, 3.6 oz	1 ea	101	216	17	6	0	13	4.6	5.7	0.7	84	19
11487	Beef, porterhouse steak, brld, 1/8" trim	3 oz	85	253	20	0	0	19	7.2	8.2	0.7	60	0
11407	Beef, prime rib, brld, 1/8" trim	3 oz	85	301	21	0	0	24	9.8	10.3	0.8	71	0
11386	Beef, rib pot roast, brld, 1/8" trim	3 oz	85	287	18	0	0	23	9.4	9.8	0.9	68	0
11015	Beef, ribs, w/bbq sauce	3 oz	85	148	18	2	0	7	2.6	2.9	0.3	52	16
11815	Beef, roast, Italian style, deli meat	2 oz	57	60	11	1	0	1	0.5	—	—	20	0
11681	Beef, roast, lean, rstd	3 oz	85	169	24	0	0	7	2.8	3.0	0.2	66	0
11680	Beef, roast, rstd	3 oz	85	227	22	0	0	15	5.8	6.3	0.5	68	0
10737	Beef, salisbury steak, patty, ckd, 3 oz	1 ea	85	280	12	5	0	23	10.7	—	—	59	7
11678	Beef, steak, brld/bkd	3.6 oz	100	255	28	0	0	15	5.9	6.3	0.5	83	0
11679	Beef, steak, lean, brld/bkd	3.6 oz	100	199	30	0	0	8	3.1	3.3	0.3	81	0
10049	Beef, stew meat, ckd	0.75 cup	105	322	29	0	0	22	8.5	9.4	0.8	106	0
10050	Beef, stew meat, lean, ckd	0.75 cup	105	248	33	0	0	12	4.5	5.2	0.4	107	0
10806	Beef, T-bone steak, brld, 0" trim	3 oz	85	210	21	0	0	14	5.2	6.1	0.5	51	0
10805	Beef, T-bone steak, brld, 1/4" trim	3 oz	85	260	20	0	0	19	7.6	8.6	0.7	55	0
11491	Beef, T-bone steak, brld, 1/8" trim	3 oz	85	238	21	0	0	17	6.4	7.3	0.6	53	0
10933	Beef, tenderloin, filet mignon, rstd, 1/8" trim	3 oz	85	276	20	0	0	21	8.3	8.7	0.9	72	0
10908	Beef, top round steak, brsd, 1/8" trim	3 oz	85	202	29	0	0	9	3.2	3.5	0.4	77	0
10943	Beef, top sirloin steak, raw, 1/8" trim	4 oz	113	228	23	0	0	14	5.8	6.2	0.5	53	0
11014	Beef, w/bbq sauce	1 cup	263	457	56	8	1	21	7.9	9.0	1.1	160	49
11016	Beef, w/sweet & sour	1 cup	252	336	16	28	2	18	6.1	7.2	2.6	54	33
10846	Beef, whole rib, brld, 1/8" trim	3 oz	85	287	19	0	0	23	9.2	9.7	0.8	70	0

PAGE KEY: A-96 Granola Bars, Cereal Bars, Diet Bars, Scones, and Tarts   A-96 Meals and Dishes   A-100 Meats   A-106 Nuts, Seeds, and Products   A-108 Poultry   A-110 Salad Dressings, Dips, and Mayonnaise   A-110 Salads   A-110 Sandwiches   A-114 Sauces and Gravies   A-114 Snack Foods—Chips, Pretzels, Popcorn   A-116 Soups, Stews, and Chilis   A-118 Spices, Flavors, and Seasonings   A-120 Sports Bars and Drinks   A-120 Supplemental Foods and Formulas   A-122 Sweeteners and Sweet Substitutes   A-122 Vegetables and Legumes   A-136 Weight Loss Bars and Drinks   A-138 Miscellaneous

Thia (mg)	Ribo (mg)	Niac (mg NE)	Vit B6 (mg)	Vit B12 (µg)	Fol (µg)	Vit C (mg)	Vit D (IU)	Vit E (mg AT)	Cal (mg)	Iron (mg)	Magn (mg)	Phos (mg)	Pota (mg)	Sodi (mg)	Zinc (mg)	Wat (%)	Alco (g)	Caff (g)
—	—	—	—	—	—	—	—	2.0	—	—	48.0	386	342	—	4.0	46	0.00	0.00
0.30	0.81	3.52	0.25	2.00	80.0	0.0	—	2.0	332	2.56	61.0	480	498	1367	5.0	53	0.00	0.00
0.25	0.70	2.57	0.20	2.00	97.0	0.0	—	4.0	336	2.03	53.0	443	416	1353	4.0	45	0.00	0.00
0.33	0.34	3.60	0.14	0.82	68.6	2.8	—	1.6	220	3.51	35.0	302	289	902	2.2	42	0.00	0.00
0.30	0.76	2.84	0.23	2.00	109.0	0.0	—	4.0	371	2.27	60.0	505	456	1363	0.0	48	0.00	0.00
—	—	—	—	—	—	0.0	—	—	150	1.44	—	—	—	690	—	—	0.00	0.00
0.07	0.18	3.16	0.28	2.09	6.0	0.0	—	0.2	8	2.27	19.6	177	271	54	5.1	53	0.00	0.00
0.07	0.18	3.03	0.27	2.04	6.0	0.0	10.2	0.1	9	2.19	18.7	169	260	52	4.9	50	0.00	0.00
0.07	0.18	3.64	0.31	2.07	6.8	0.0	—	0.2	8	2.07	20.4	168	295	53	4.6	51	0.00	0.00
0.07	0.18	3.11	0.28	2.07	6.0	0.0	—	0.1	9	2.25	19.6	174	269	53	5.1	52	0.00	0.00
0.09	0.20	3.50	0.31	2.25	6.8	0.0	—	0.1	8	2.53	22.1	198	306	57	5.9	59	0.00	0.00
—	—	5.00	—	2.40	—	0.0	—	—	0	1.79	—	—	—	65	4.5	—	0.00	0.00
0.10	—	—	—	—	—	8.0	—	—	17	1.89	—	—	—	53	—	58	0.00	0.00
0.02	0.15	4.44	0.30	2.13	5.1	0.0	—	0.3	11	2.46	17.9	164	255	52	5.7	61	0.00	0.00
0.02	0.15	4.19	0.28	2.11	5.1	0.0	—	0.4	15	2.32	17.0	158	243	54	5.5	59	0.00	0.00
0.03	0.14	3.94	0.28	2.10	6.0	0.0	—	0.4	20	2.19	16.2	152	230	57	5.3	58		0.00
0.02	0.15	4.69	0.30	2.13	5.1	0.0	—	0.3	7	2.58	18.7	169	268	49	5.8	65	0.00	0.00
0.02	0.02	0.34	0.03	0.20	26.5	0.0	—	0.1	4	1.07	10.1	81	118	438	1.6	23	0.00	0.00
—	—	—	—	—	—	0.0	—	—	0	0.72	—	—	—	350	—	23	0.00	0.00
0.07	0.28	4.17	0.15	1.72	12.4	0.6	—	0.1	45	2.10	23.3	167	306	138	3.8	62	0.00	0.00
0.07	0.25	3.75	0.12	1.54	11.2	0.6	—	0.1	40	1.89	21.0	151	276	124	3.4	62	0.00	0.00
0.09	0.18	3.46	0.30	1.83	6.0	0.0	—	0.2	7	2.32	19.6	159	273	54	3.9	53	0.00	0.00
0.07	0.15	3.46	0.28	2.50	6.0	0.0	—	0.2	11	1.89	18.7	151	282	54	4.9	47	0.00	0.00
0.05	0.14	2.35	0.20	2.46	5.1	0.0	—	0.2	9	1.86	16.2	155	263	54	4.3	49	0.00	0.00
0.05	0.12	2.61	0.20	2.19	5.8	1.3	—	0.3	12	2.08	19.9	150	295	204	4.1	66	0.00	0.00
—	—	—	—	—	—	0.0	—	—	0	1.08	—	—	—	360	—	73	0.00	0.00
0.07	0.18	3.42	0.28	2.17	6.9	0.0	10.2	0.1	5	2.19	22.3	191	321	57	5.5	62	0.00	0.00
0.07	0.17	3.06	0.27	2.03	6.1	0.0	10.2	0.2	6	1.98	19.6	173	290	53	4.8	56	0.00	0.00
0.07	—	—	—	—	—	4.0	—	—	51	1.20	—	—	—	621	—	—	0.00	0.00
0.09	0.21	4.57	0.38	2.45	8.3	0.0	12.0	0.1	9	2.61	25.4	209	365	61	5.2	55	0.00	0.00
0.10	0.23	5.26	0.46	2.53	9.3	0.0	12.0	0.1	9	2.75	28.8	228	411	66	5.9	60	0.00	0.00
0.07	0.25	3.10	0.30	2.58	7.3	0.0	12.6	0.2	11	3.27	21.6	231	265	66	7.9	50	0.00	0.00
0.07	0.28	3.35	0.31	2.76	8.2	0.0	12.6	0.1	11	3.73	24.6	259	291	70	9.3	56	0.00	0.00
0.09	0.20	3.63	0.31	1.86	6.0	0.0	—	0.2	4	2.84	20.4	169	257	57	4.0	58	0.00	0.00
0.07	0.18	3.36	0.28	1.80	6.0	0.0	—	0.2	6	2.63	18.7	157	240	57	3.7	52	0.00	0.00
0.09	0.18	3.51	0.30	1.85	6.0	0.0	—	0.2	7	2.41	20.4	164	286	56	4.0	55	0.00	0.00
0.07	0.21	2.54	0.20	2.08	6.8	0.0	—	0.2	8	2.65	18.7	173	282	48	3.4	48	0.00	0.00
0.05	0.20	3.09	0.23	2.23	7.7	0.0	—	0.1	4	2.69	20.4	183	271	38	3.7	55	0.00	0.00
0.07	0.10	6.78	0.62	1.19	12.5	0.0	—	0.4	27	1.67	23.8	212	357	59	4.0	66	0.00	0.00
0.15	0.40	8.10	0.61	6.76	17.9	4.0	—	0.9	36	6.44	61.6	463	913	632	12.7	66	0.00	0.00
0.11	0.18	2.61	0.31	1.59	12.7	21.6	—	1.2	27	2.69	33.7	151	336	930	3.9	74	0.00	0.00
0.07	0.14	2.77	0.23	2.46	5.1	0.0	—	0.2	9	1.86	17.0	152	268	54	4.5	48	0.00	0.00

PAGE KEY: A-46 Beverage and Beverage Mixes A-48 Other Beverages A-48 Beverages, Alcoholic A-50 Candies and Confections, Gum A-54 Cereals, Breakfast Type A-58 Cheese and Cheese Substitutes A-60 Dairy Products and Substitutes A-62 Desserts A-68 Dessert Toppings A-68 Eggs, Substitutes, and Egg Dishes A-70 Ethnic Foods A-74 Fast Foods/Restaurants A-88 Fats, Oils, Margarines, Shortenings, and Substitutes A-88 Fish, Seafood, and Shellfish A-90 Food Additives A-90 Fruit, Vegetable, or Blended Juices A-92 Grains, Flours, and Fractions A-92 Grain Products, Prepared and Baked Goods

Code	Food Name	Unit/ Amt	Wt (g)	Energy (kcal)	Prot (g)	Carb (g)	Fiber (g)	Fat (g)	Sat (g)	Mono (g)	Poly (g)	Chol (mg)	Vit A (RE)
Game Meats													
40559	Bison, ground, raw	4 oz	113	253	21	0	0	18	7.7	7.1	0.8	79	0
14009	Bison, rstd	3 oz	85	122	24	0	0	2	0.8	0.8	0.2	70	0
40565	Deer, ground, raw	4 oz	113	178	25	0	0	8	3.8	1.5	0.4	91	0
40551	Deer, rstd	3 oz	85	134	26	0	0	3	1.1	0.7	0.5	95	0
40560	Elk, ground, raw	4 oz	113	195	25	0	0	10	3.9	2.8	0.5	75	0
14014	Elk, rstd	3 oz	85	124	26	0	0	2	0.6	0.4	0.3	62	0
14068	Rabbit, brd, ckd	3.6 oz	100	245	28	6	0	11	2.9	4.0	2.8	86	0
14013	Venison, rstd	3 oz	85	134	26	0	0	3	1.1	0.7	0.5	95	0
Goat													
Lamb													
40354	Lamb, Austl, average of all cuts, ckd, 1/8" trim	3 oz	85	218	21	0	0	14	6.8	5.7	0.6	74	—
13628	Lamb, average of all cuts, ckd, choice, 1/8" trim	3 oz	85	230	22	0	0	15	6.3	6.5	1.1	82	0
13669	Lamb, ground, ckd	3.6 oz	100	283	25	0	0	20	8.1	8.3	1.4	97	0
Lunchmeats and Sausages													
13250	Frank, beef, fat free	1 ea	50	39	7	3	0	0	0.1	0.1	0.0	15	0
57967	Frank, beef, rducd fat	1 ea	49	120	6	0	0	10	4.5	—	—	25	0
13283	Frankfurter, beef	3.6 oz	100	326	13	2	0	29	12.3	14.0	1.4	64	0
13284	Frankfurter, beef & pork	3.6 oz	100	331	12	3	0	30	10.9	14.1	2.9	52	0
58290	Frankfurter, beef, low fat	1 cup	151	352	18	2	0	29	12.2	14.8	0.9	60	0
13318	Frankfurter, beef, low fat	1 ea	50	80	6	7	0	2	1.0	—	—	15	0
13260	Frankfurter, chicken	1 ea	45	116	6	3	0	9	2.5	3.8	1.8	45	18
13274	Frankfurter, low sod	1 ea	57	180	7	1	0	16	6.9	7.8	0.8	35	0
13012	Frankfurter, turkey	1 ea	45	102	6	1	0	8	2.7	2.5	2.2	48	0
13325	Hot Dog, fat free	1 ea	50	36	6	2	0	0	0.1	0.1	0.1	14	0
13000	Lunchmeat, beef, thin slice	1 oz	28	42	5	0	0	2	0.8	0.9	0.1	20	0
13177	Lunchmeat, bologna, beef	1 oz	28	90	3	1	0	8	3.6	4.3	0.3	18	0
58284	Lunchmeat, bologna, beef, low fat	1 cup	138	282	16	7	0	20	7.5	8.9	0.7	61	0
10439	Lunchmeat, bologna, beef, slice	1 pce	38	100	5	1	0	8	3.5	—	—	20	0
11829	Lunchmeat, bologna, chicken, slice	1 pce	38	100	4	1	0	9	2.5	—	—	45	20
13251	Lunchmeat, bologna, fat free, 1 oz svg	1 pce	28	22	4	2	0	0	0.1	0.1	0.0	7	0
13245	Lunchmeat, chicken breast, honey glazed, slice	1 oz	28	31	6	1	0	0	0.1	0.2	0.1	15	0
13257	Lunchmeat, chicken breast, oven rstd, fat free, slice	1 oz	28	24	5	0	0	0	0.0	0.0	0.0	12	0
58149	Lunchmeat, chicken breast, oven rstd, 1 oz slice	1 pce	28	20	5	0	0	0	0.0	0.0	0.0	10	—
58167	Lunchmeat, ham, brown sugar, deli, 0.8 oz slice	2 pce	45	60	8	4	0	1	0.0	—	—	10	0
13262	Lunchmeat, ham, extra lean, 5% fat, sliced	1 cup	135	148	23	4	0	4	1.2	1.7	0.5	65	0
11819	Lunchmeat, ham, smkd, deli meat	2 oz	57	60	9	2	0	2	0.5	—	—	30	0
58199	Lunchmeat, roast beef, choice, deli, 0.8 oz slice	2 pce	45	50	9	0	0	2	0.5	—	—	25	0
13114	Lunchmeat, turkey breast, oven rstd, fat free, slice	1 oz	28	24	4	1	0	0	0.1	0.1	0.0	9	0
13255	Lunchmeat, turkey breast, smkd, fat free, slice	1 oz	28	23	4	1	0	0	0.1	0.0	0.0	9	0
13020	Pastrami, turkey, slices	1 oz	28	35	5	1	0	1	0.3	0.4	0.3	19	1
13201	Salami, hard, slice	1 oz	28	104	7	0	0	8	3.1	4.2	0.8	27	2
58014	Salami, Italian, pork	3 oz	85	361	18	1	0	31	11.1	15.5	3.1	68	0
13025	Salami, turkey, ckd, 1 oz slice	2 pce	57	86	9	0	0	5	1.6	1.8	1.4	43	1
13182	Sausage, beef, smokies	1 ea	43	127	5	1	0	11	4.8	5.5	0.4	27	0

PAGE KEY: A-96 Granola Bars, Cereal Bars, Diet Bars, Scones, and Tarts   A-96 Meals and Dishes   A-100 Meats   A-106 Nuts, Seeds, and Products   A-108 Poultry
A-110 Salad Dressings, Dips, and Mayonnaise   A-110 Salads   A-110 Sandwiches   A-114 Sauces and Gravies   A-114 Snack Foods—Chips, Pretzels, Popcorn
A-116 Soups, Stews, and Chilis   A-118 Spices, Flavors, and Seasonings   A-120 Sports Bars and Drinks   A-120 Supplemental Foods and Formulas
A-122 Sweeteners and Sweet Substitutes   A-122 Vegetables and Legumes   A-136 Weight Loss Bars and Drinks   A-138 Miscellaneous

Thia (mg)	Ribo (mg)	Niac (mg NE)	Vit B6 (mg)	Vit B12 (μg)	Fol (μg)	Vit C (mg)	Vit D (IU)	Vit E (mg AT)	Cal (mg)	Iron (mg)	Magn (mg)	Phos (mg)	Pota (mg)	Sodi (mg)	Zinc (mg)	Wat (%)	Alco (g)	Caff (g)
0.15	0.25	5.57	0.40	2.02	12.5	0.0	—	0.3	12	2.95	21.5	205	348	75	4.9	64	0.00	0.00
0.09	0.23	3.16	0.34	2.43	6.8	0.0	—	0.3	7	2.91	22.1	178	307	48	3.1	67	0.00	0.00
0.62	0.33	6.46	0.52	2.11	4.5	0.0	—	0.5	12	3.30	23.8	228	374	85	4.8	71	0.00	0.00
0.15	0.50	5.71	0.31	2.70	4.0	0.0	—	0.2	6	3.79	20.4	192	285	46	2.3	65	0.00	0.00
0.14	0.28	5.55	0.37	2.42	7.9	0.0	—	0.3	14	3.11	24.9	221	365	90	6.1	69	0.00	0.00
—	—	—	—	5.53	7.7	0.0	—	0.0	4	3.08	20.4	153	279	52	2.7	66	0.00	0.00
0.10	0.15	6.55	0.30	5.65	9.5	0.0	12.0	1.4	35	3.26	24.3	212	291	103	2.2	52	0.00	0.00
0.15	0.50	5.71	0.31	2.70	4.0	0.0	—	0.2	6	3.79	20.4	192	285	46	2.3	65	0.00	0.00
0.10	0.28	4.63	0.31	2.44	—	—	—	—	14	1.63	18.7	166	256	65	4.0	59	0.00	0.00
0.09	0.21	5.57	0.11	2.19	16.2	0.0	—	0.1	14	1.63	20.4	164	270	61	4.0	56	0.00	0.00
0.10	0.25	6.69	0.14	2.60	19.0	0.0	—	0.2	22	1.78	24.0	201	339	81	4.7	55	0.00	0.00
—	—	—	—	—	—	0.0	—	—	10	0.98	9.5	64	234	464	1.2	78	0.00	0.00
—	—	—	—	—	—	0.0	—	—	0	0.72	—	—	—	360	—	64	0.00	0.00
0.05	0.10	2.30	0.10	1.38	3.6	0.0	—	0.2	21	1.51	3.0	88	168	1037	2.3	53	0.00	0.00
0.18	0.11	2.51	0.10	1.17	3.6	0.0	—	0.2	12	1.22	10.1	87	169	1132	2.0	52	0.00	0.00
0.07	0.15	3.47	0.15	2.10	6.0	1.5	—	0.3	12	1.74	16.6	288	195	1572	3.0	64	0.00	0.00
—	—	—	—	—	—	2.4	—	—	0	0.36	—	—	—	400	—	66	0.00	0.00
0.02	0.05	1.38	0.14	0.10	1.8	0.0	0.0	0.1	43	0.89	4.5	48	38	616	0.5	58	0.00	0.00
0.02	0.05	1.37	0.07	0.87	2.3	0.0	—	0.1	11	0.81	1.7	50	95	177	1.2	57	0.00	0.00
0.01	0.07	1.86	0.10	0.12	3.6	0.0	—	0.3	48	0.82	6.3	60	81	642	1.4	63	0.00	0.00
—	—	—	—	—	—	0.0	—	—	8	0.46	10.5	81	236	487	0.6	79	0.00	0.00
0.01	0.05	1.21	0.10	0.73	3.1	0.0	—	0.1	3	0.58	5.4	48	122	401	1.1	69	0.00	0.00
0.00	0.02	0.68	0.05	0.40	3.7	0.0	9.1	—	3	0.38	4.0	31	48	334	0.6	54	0.00	0.00
0.07	0.14	3.45	0.20	1.92	6.9	1.4	—	0.3	12	1.37	16.6	246	203	1628	2.5	65	0.00	0.00
—	—	—	—	—	—	0.0	—	—	0	0.36	—	—	—	340	—	60	0.00	0.00
—	—	—	—	—	—	1.2	—	—	40	0.72	—	—	—	350	—	60	0.00	0.00
—	—	—	—	—	—	0.0	—	—	4	0.25	6.2	43	44	274	0.3	78	0.00	0.00
—	—	—	—	—	1.1	0.0	—	—	3	0.31	10.2	82	93	408	0.2	70	0.00	0.00
—	—	—	—	—	—	0.0	—	—	3	0.37	10.2	73	90	352	0.2	76	0.00	0.00
—	—	—	—	—	—	—	—	—	—	—	—	—	—	240	—	77	0.00	0.00
—	—	—	—	—	—	0.0	—	—	0	0.36	—	—	—	490	—	—	0.00	0.00
1.25	0.30	6.75	0.02	1.00	5.4	0.0	—	0.4	12	1.08	23.0	294	472	1493	2.6	74	0.00	0.00
—	—	—	—	—	—	0.0	—	—	0	0.36	—	—	—	430	—	74	0.00	0.00
—	—	—	—	—	—	0.0	—	—	0	1.08	—	—	—	250	—	—	0.00	0.00
—	—	—	—	—	—	0.0	—	—	3	0.31	7.7	66	58	338	0.2	76	0.00	0.00
—	—	—	—	—	—	0.0	—	—	3	0.21	8.5	69	62	310	0.2	78	0.00	0.00
0.01	0.07	1.00	0.07	0.07	1.4	4.6	—	0.1	3	1.19	4.0	57	98	278	0.6	72	0.00	0.00
0.15	0.07	1.42	0.11	0.52	0.9	0.0	17.6	—	3	0.51	6.0	51	101	560	0.9	38	0.00	0.00
0.79	0.28	4.76	0.46	2.38	1.7	0.0	—	0.2	9	1.28	18.7	195	289	1607	3.6	35	0.00	0.00
0.23	0.17	2.25	0.23	0.56	5.7	0.0	13.3	0.1	23	0.70	12.5	151	122	569	1.3	72	0.00	0.00
—	—	—	—	—	4.7	0.0	—	—	5	0.75	6.5	99	74	416	1.3	56	0.00	0.00

PAGE KEY: A-46 Beverage and Beverage Mixes   A-48 Other Beverages   A-48 Beverages, Alcoholic   A-50 Candies and Confections, Gum   A-54 Cereals, Breakfast Type   A-58 Cheese and Cheese Substitutes   A-60 Dairy Products and Substitutes   A-62 Desserts   A-68 Dessert Toppings   A-68 Eggs, Substitutes, and Egg Dishes   A-70 Ethnic Foods   A-74 Fast Foods/Restaurants   A-88 Fats, Oils, Margarines, Shortenings, and Substitutes   A-88 Fish, Seafood, and Shellfish   A-90 Food Additives   A-90 Fruit, Vegetable, or Blended Juices   A-92 Grains, Flours, and Fractions   A-92 Grain Products, Prepared and Baked Goods

Code	Food Name	Unit/ Amt	Wt (g)	Energy (kcal)	Prot (g)	Carb (g)	Fiber (g)	Fat (g)	Sat (g)	Mono (g)	Poly (g)	Chol (mg)	Vit A (RE)
58242	Sausage, chicken & beef, smkd, pieces	1 cup	138	408	26	0	0	33	9.9	14.1	6.5	97	43
13021	Sausage, pepperoni, beef & pork, slice, 1 3/8" x 1/8"	1 pce	6	26	1	0	0	2	0.9	1.0	0.1	6	0
58353	Sausage, pork, link, USDA, ckd f/fzn	3.6 oz	100	267	20	0	0	20	5.5	8.7	2.3	98	15
13184	Sausage, smokies, links	1 ea	43	130	5	1	0	12	4.0	5.7	1.2	27	0
58232	Sausage, turkey, ckd	3.6 oz	100	196	24	0	0	10	2.3	3.0	2.7	92	15
Pork and Ham													
27096	Bacon Bits	1 Tbs	7	24	3	0	0	1	0.5	0.7	0.2	5	0
92207	Bacon, cured, microwv	1 pce	8	38	3	0	0	3	0.9	1.2	0.3	9	1
92208	Bacon, cured, pan fried	1 pce	8	42	3	0	0	3	1.0	1.4	0.4	9	1
28143	Canadian Bacon, 2 oz svg	1 ea	56	68	9	1	—	3	1.0	1.4	0.3	27	0
12118	Pork, avg of retail cuts, leg shoulder & loin, lean, ckd	3 oz	85	180	25	0	0	8	2.9	3.7	0.6	73	2
12309	Pork, avg of retail cuts, leg shoulder loin & sparerib, ckd	3 oz	85	232	23	0	0	15	5.3	6.5	1.2	77	2
12240	Pork, avg of retail cuts, loin & shoulder blade, ckd	3 oz	85	214	24	0	0	13	4.5	5.6	1.0	73	2
12311	Pork, avg of retail cuts, loin & shoulder blade, lean, ckd	3 oz	85	179	25	0	0	8	2.8	3.6	0.6	72	2
12184	Pork, chop, blade loin, brld	3 oz	85	272	19	0	0	21	7.9	9.1	1.9	73	2
12081	Pork, chop, breaded, brld/bkd, 3.6 oz svg	1 ea	100	259	25	6	0	14	5.1	6.2	1.5	72	2
12192	Pork, chop, center loin, brld	3 oz	85	204	24	0	0	11	4.1	5.0	0.8	70	3
12126	Pork, chop, w/bbq sauce	1 ea	116	209	23	3	0	11	3.7	4.9	1.2	65	23
12243	Pork, cured ham, dinner 3 oz slice, add wtr	1 ea	84	83	14	0	0	3	1.0	1.5	0.3	41	0
12307	Pork, cured ham, lean, 8% fat, rstd	1 cup	140	231	31	1	0	11	3.7	5.2	1.5	80	0
12099	Pork, ground, ckd	3 oz	85	253	22	0	0	18	6.6	7.9	1.6	80	2
12010	Pork, ribs, spareribs, brsd	3 oz	85	338	25	0	0	26	9.5	11.5	2.3	103	3
12060	Pork, roast, top loin, rstd	3 oz	85	192	25	0	0	10	3.5	4.5	0.7	66	2
92798	Pork, shred, w/original bbq sauce, ckd	0.25 cup	56	90	6	11	0	2	0.5	—	—	15	40
12900	Pork, sweet & sour	3 oz	85	87	6	9	1	3	0.8	1.2	0.9	14	12
12237	Pork, tenderloin, chop, brld	3 oz	85	171	25	0	0	7	2.5	2.8	0.6	80	2
Veal													
11531	Veal, avg of all cuts, ckd	3 oz	85	196	26	0	0	10	3.6	3.7	0.7	97	0
Variety Meats and By-Products													
10472	Beef, liver, brsd	3 oz	85	162	25	4	0	4	1.4	0.6	0.5	337	8042
Meat Substitutes, Soy Tofu and Vegetable													
27044	Bacon Bits, meatless	1 Tbs	7	33	2	2	1	2	0.3	0.4	0.9	0	0
7509	Bacon Substitute, vegetarian, strips	3 ea	15	46	2	1	0	4	0.7	1.1	2.3	0	1
7732	Beef Substitute, vegetarian, burger	0.25 cup	55	60	9	2	1	2	0.3	0.5	1.1	0	0
7558	Beef Substitute, vegetarian, fillet	1 ea	85	246	20	8	5	15	2.4	3.7	7.9	0	0
7561	Beef Substitute, vegetarian, patty	1 ea	56	110	12	4	3	5	0.8	1.2	2.6	0	0
7547	Chicken Substitute, vegetarian	1 cup	168	376	40	6	6	21	3.1	4.6	12.2	0	0
7549	Fish Sticks Substitute, vegetarian	1 ea	28	81	6	3	2	5	0.8	1.2	2.6	0	0
92148	Hot Dog Substitute	1 ea	70	163	14	5	3	10	1.4	2.7	5.5	0	0
7550	Hot Dog Substitute, vegetarian	1 ea	51	102	10	4	2	5	0.8	1.2	2.6	0	0
7551	Lunchmeat Substitute, vegetarian, 0.5 oz slice	1 pce	14	26	2	1	0	2	0.2	0.3	0.6	0	0
90626	Sausage Substitute, vegetarian, breakfast slices, 1 oz	1 ea	28	72	5	3	1	5	0.8	1.3	2.6	0	0
7564	Tempeh	0.5 cup	83	160	15	8	—	9	1.8	2.5	3.2	0	0
7519	Tofu, dried, fzn, 0.6 oz svg	1 pce	17	82	8	2	1	5	0.7	1.1	2.9	0	9
7522	Tofu, fermented & salted, block	3 oz	85	99	7	4	0	7	1.0	1.5	3.8	0	14
90040	Tofu, fermented & salted, w/calc sulfate, block, 0.4 oz	1 ea	11	13	1	1	0	1	0.1	0.2	0.5	0	2

PAGE KEY: A-96 Granola Bars, Cereal Bars, Diet Bars, Scones, and Tarts   A-96 Meals and Dishes   A-100 Meats   A-106 Nuts, Seeds, and Products   A-108 Poultry   A-110 Salad Dressings, Dips, and Mayonnaise   A-110 Salads   A-110 Sandwiches   A-114 Sauces and Gravies   A-114 Snack Foods—Chips, Pretzels, Popcorn   A-116 Soups, Stews, and Chilis   A-118 Spices, Flavors, and Seasonings   A-120 Sports Bars and Drinks   A-120 Supplemental Foods and Formulas   A-122 Sweeteners and Sweet Substitutes   A-122 Vegetables and Legumes   A-136 Weight Loss Bars and Drinks   A-138 Miscellaneous

Thia (mg)	Ribo (mg)	Niac (mg NE)	Vit B6 (mg)	Vit B12 (μg)	Fol (μg)	Vit C (mg)	Vit D (IU)	Vit E (mg AT)	Cal (mg)	Iron (mg)	Magn (mg)	Phos (mg)	Pota (mg)	Sodi (mg)	Zinc (mg)	Wat (%)	Alco (g)	Caff (g)
0.05	0.17	5.59	0.23	0.51	5.5	0.0	—	0.7	15	1.49	19.3	153	192	1408	2.4	56	0.00	0.00
0.02	0.00	0.30	0.01	0.09	0.3	0.0	0.5	0.0	1	0.07	1.0	10	17	98	0.2	31	0.00	0.00
0.73	0.23	2.79	0.28	0.88	1.0	0.0	—	0.7	9	1.14	19.0	190	239	540	2.8	59	0.00	0.00
—	—	—	—	—	—	0.0	—	—	4	0.50	7.3	103	77	433	0.9	56	0.00	0.00
0.07	0.25	5.71	0.31	1.23	6.0	0.7	—	0.2	22	1.49	21.0	202	298	665	3.9	65	0.00	0.00
—	—	—	—	—	—	0.0	—	—	2	0.20	4.6	43	39	224	0.3	35	0.00	0.00
0.03	0.01	0.75	0.02	0.11	0.2	0.0	—	0.0	1	0.10	2.3	36	37	155	0.3	16	0.00	0.00
0.03	0.01	0.91	0.02	0.10	0.2	0.0	—	0.0	1	0.10	2.8	44	47	192	0.3	12	0.00	0.00
—	—	—	—	—	—	0.8	—	—	3	0.50	10.6	—	156	569	1.0	73	0.00	0.00
0.72	0.28	4.40	0.37	0.63	0.9	0.3	—	0.2	18	0.93	22.1	202	319	50	2.5	60	0.00	0.00
0.64	0.28	4.19	0.34	0.64	5.1	0.3	—	0.2	21	0.93	20.4	197	301	53	2.5	55	0.00	0.00
0.72	0.28	4.21	0.34	0.62	5.1	0.3	10.2	0.2	20	0.83	20.4	193	308	48	2.2	57	0.00	0.00
0.74	0.28	4.46	0.37	0.63	5.1	0.3	—	0.4	19	0.91	22.1	199	321	48	2.4	60	0.00	0.00
0.55	0.25	3.49	0.31	0.70	3.4	0.6	—	0.3	25	0.79	18.7	180	293	60	2.9	52	0.00	0.00
0.81	0.30	4.75	0.41	0.62	5.8	0.5	12.0	0.4	24	1.00	26.8	240	400	415	2.2	52	0.00	0.00
0.91	0.23	4.46	0.36	0.62	5.1	0.3	—	0.3	28	0.68	21.3	197	304	49	1.9	58	0.00	0.00
0.73	0.28	4.90	0.36	0.64	5.0	1.9	—	0.5	19	1.30	24.1	221	373	860	2.4	65	0.00	0.00
0.60	0.18	3.93	0.31	0.40	—	0.0	—	—	4	1.01	16.9	203	221	1018	1.7	75	0.00	0.00
1.02	0.38	7.44	0.49	0.94	4.2	0.0	—	0.4	11	1.96	26.6	347	507	1939	3.7	66	0.00	0.00
0.60	0.18	3.57	0.33	0.46	5.1	0.6	10.2	0.2	19	1.10	20.4	192	308	62	2.7	53	0.00	0.00
0.34	0.31	4.65	0.30	0.92	3.4	0.0	—	0.3	40	1.57	20.4	222	272	79	3.9	40	0.00	0.00
0.51	0.25	4.36	0.31	0.46	6.8	0.3	—	0.3	4	0.68	19.6	183	291	37	1.9	59	0.00	0.00
—	—	—	—	—	—	0.0	—	—	0	0.72	—	—	—	380	—	—	0.00	0.00
0.20	0.07	1.37	0.15	0.12	3.9	7.4	10.2	0.4	11	0.54	12.9	56	145	316	0.6	77	0.00	0.00
0.81	0.31	4.30	0.43	0.82	5.1	0.9	—	0.3	4	1.17	29.8	247	378	54	2.5	61	0.00	0.00
0.05	0.27	6.78	0.25	1.34	12.8	0.0	—	0.3	19	0.98	22.1	203	276	74	4.0	57	0.00	0.00
0.15	2.91	14.90	0.86	60.02	215.2	1.6	—	0.4	5	5.55	17.9	423	299	67	4.5	59	0.00	0.00
0.03	0.00	0.10	0.00	0.07	8.9	0.1	—	0.5	7	0.05	6.7	15	10	124	0.1	8	0.00	0.00
0.66	0.07	1.12	0.07	0.00	6.3	0.0	—	1.0	3	0.36	2.9	10	26	220	0.1	49	0.00	0.00
0.12	0.10	1.96	0.23	1.13	—	0.0	—	—	4	1.73	—	56	25	269	0.4	71	0.00	0.00
0.93	0.75	10.19	1.27	3.56	86.7	0.0	—	2.9	81	1.70	19.6	382	510	416	1.2	45	0.00	0.00
0.50	0.34	5.59	0.67	1.34	43.7	0.0	—	1.0	16	1.17	10.1	193	101	308	1.0	58	0.00	0.00
1.14	0.40	2.44	1.17	3.66	127.7	0.0	—	4.5	59	5.48	28.6	563	91	1191	1.2	59	0.00	0.00
0.31	0.25	3.35	0.41	1.17	28.6	0.0	—	1.1	27	0.56	6.4	126	168	137	0.4	45	0.00	0.00
0.31	0.57	2.20	0.05	1.63	54.6	0.0	—	1.3	23	0.99	12.6	241	69	330	0.8	58	0.00	0.00
0.56	0.61	8.15	0.50	1.22	39.8	0.0	—	1.0	17	0.92	9.2	175	76	219	0.6	58	0.00	0.00
0.56	0.03	1.55	0.11	0.56	14.0	0.0	—	0.4	6	0.25	3.2	62	28	100	0.2	65	0.00	0.00
0.66	0.10	3.13	0.23	0.00	7.3	0.0	—	0.6	18	1.03	10.1	63	65	249	0.4	50	0.00	0.00
0.05	0.30	2.19	0.18	0.07	19.9	0.0	—	0.0	92	2.24	67.2	221	342	7	0.9	60	0.00	0.00
0.07	0.05	0.20	0.05	0.00	15.6	0.1	—	0.0	62	1.64	10.0	82	3	1	0.8	6	0.00	0.00
0.12	0.09	0.31	0.07	0.00	24.7	0.2	—	0.0	39	1.67	44.2	62	64	2443	1.3	70	0.00	0.00
0.01	0.00	0.03	0.00	0.00	3.2	0.0	—	0.0	135	0.21	6.4	8	8	316	0.2	70	0.00	0.00

Code	Food Name	Unit/ Amt	Wt (g)	Energy (kcal)	Prot (g)	Carb (g)	Fiber (g)	Fat (g)	Sat (g)	Mono (g)	Poly (g)	Chol (mg)	Vit A (RE)
NUTS, SEEDS, AND PRODUCTS													
4572	Almond Butter	1 cup	250	1582	38	53	9	148	14.0	95.9	31.0	0	0
4507	Coconut, fresh, shredded	1 cup	80	283	3	12	7	27	23.8	1.1	0.3	0	0
4559	Coconut, milk, cnd	2 Tbs	28	56	1	1	0	6	5.3	0.3	0.1	0	0
4575	Coconut, tstd f/dried	2 Tbs	9	55	0	4	1	4	3.9	0.2	0.0	0	0
4571	Nuts, almonds, dry rstd, salted, whole	22 ea	28	169	6	5	3	15	1.1	9.5	3.6	0	0
4549	Nuts, almonds, dry rstd, unsalted, whole	1 cup	138	824	30	27	16	73	5.6	46.4	17.5	0	0
4620	Nuts, almonds, oil rstd, salted	22 ea	28	172	6	5	3	16	1.2	9.9	3.8	0	0
4505	Nuts, almonds, oil rstd, unsalted	22 ea	28	172	6	5	3	16	1.2	9.9	3.8	0	0
4642	Nuts, beechnuts, dried	2 oz	57	327	4	19	2	28	3.2	12.4	11.4	0	0
4536	Nuts, Brazil, dried, lrg	6 ea	28	186	4	3	2	19	4.3	7.0	5.8	0	0
4750	Nuts, Brazil, dried, unblanched, shelled	1 cup	140	918	20	17	10	93	21.2	34.4	28.8	0	0
4519	Nuts, cashews, dry rstd, salted	0.25 cup	34	197	5	11	1	16	3.1	9.4	2.7	0	0
4621	Nuts, cashews, dry rstd, unsalted	0.25 cup	34	197	5	11	1	16	3.1	9.4	2.7	0	0
4596	Nuts, cashews, oil rstd, salted	0.25 cup	32	189	5	10	1	16	2.8	8.4	2.8	0	0
4622	Nuts, cashews, oil rstd, unsalted	0.25 cup	32	188	5	10	1	16	2.8	8.4	2.8	0	0
63431	Nuts, filberts, whole	1 cup	135	848	20	23	13	82	6.0	61.6	10.7	0	3
4513	Nuts, hazelnuts, whole	1 cup	135	848	20	23	13	82	6.0	61.6	10.7	0	3
4516	Nuts, macadamia, dried	11 ea	28	204	2	4	2	21	3.4	16.7	0.4	0	0
4595	Nuts, mixed, w/o peanuts, oil rstd, salted	0.25 cup	36	221	6	8	2	20	3.3	11.9	4.1	0	0
4594	Nuts, mixed, w/o peanuts, oil rstd, unsalted	0.25 cup	36	221	6	8	2	20	3.3	11.9	4.1	0	1
4592	Nuts, mixed, w/peanuts, dry rstd, salted	0.25 cup	34	203	6	9	3	18	2.4	10.8	3.7	0	0
4591	Nuts, mixed, w/peanuts, dry rstd, unsalted	0.25 cup	34	203	6	9	3	18	2.4	10.8	3.7	0	1
4593	Nuts, mixed, w/peanuts, oil rstd, salted	0.25 cup	36	219	6	8	3	20	3.1	11.3	4.7	0	0
4533	Nuts, mixed, w/peanuts, oil rstd, unsalted	0.25 cup	36	219	6	8	4	20	3.1	11.3	4.7	0	1
4541	Nuts, peanuts, dry rstd, salted	30 ea	30	176	7	6	2	15	2.1	7.4	4.7	0	0
4756	Nuts, peanuts, dry rstd, unsalted	30 ea	30	176	7	6	2	15	2.1	7.4	4.7	0	0
4763	Nuts, peanuts, oil rstd, salted	30 ea	27	162	8	4	3	14	2.3	7.0	4.1	0	0
4755	Nuts, peanuts, oil rstd, unsalted	32 ea	28	163	7	5	2	14	1.9	6.8	4.4	0	0
4542	Nuts, peanuts, oil rstd, unsalted, chpd	1 cup	133	773	35	25	9	66	9.1	32.5	20.7	0	0
4699	Nuts, peanuts, Spanish, oil rstd, salted	0.5 cup	74	426	21	13	7	36	5.6	16.2	12.5	0	0
4665	Nuts, peanuts, Spanish, oil rstd, unsalted	1 cup	147	851	41	26	13	72	11.1	32.4	25.0	0	0
4517	Nuts, peanuts, Spanish, raw	0.25 cup	36	208	10	6	3	18	2.8	8.1	6.3	0	0
4578	Nuts, pecans, halves	1 cup	108	746	10	15	10	78	6.7	44.1	23.3	0	6
4624	Nuts, pine	10 ea	1	7	0	0	0	1	0.1	0.2	0.3	0	0
4525	Nuts, walnuts, black, dried, chpd	1 cup	125	772	30	12	8	74	4.2	18.8	43.8	0	5
4626	Peanut Butter, chunky	2 Tbs	32	188	8	7	3	16	2.6	7.9	4.7	0	0
4576	Peanut Butter, chunky, unsalted	2 Tbs	32	188	8	7	3	16	2.6	7.9	4.7	0	0
4627	Peanut Butter, creamy	2 Tbs	32	188	8	6	2	16	3.3	7.6	4.4	0	0
63338	Peanut Butter, creamy, rducd fat	3.6 oz	100	520	26	36	5	34	7.4	16.2	10.3	0	0
4636	Peanut Butter, creamy, unsalted	2 Tbs	32	188	8	6	2	16	3.3	7.6	4.4	0	0
62939	Peanut Butter, crunchy, rducd fat	2 Tbs	36	190	8	15	2	12	2.5	—	—	0	0
4747	Peanut Butter, rducd fat	1 Tbs	16	81	4	5	1	5	1.0	2.8	1.6	0	—
62949	Peanut Butter, w/grape jelly, Goober	3 Tbs	53	230	7	24	2	13	2.0	—	—	0	—
4777	Seeds, flax/linseed	1 cup	155	763	30	53	43	53	5.0	10.6	34.8	0	0
4545	Seeds, sunflower, kernels, dried	1 cup	144	821	33	27	15	71	7.5	13.6	47.1	0	9

Thia (mg)	Ribo (mg)	Niac (mg NE)	Vit B6 (mg)	Vit B12 (µg)	Fol (µg)	Vit C (mg)	Vit D (IU)	Vit E (mg AT)	Cal (mg)	Iron (mg)	Magn (mg)	Phos (mg)	Pota (mg)	Sodi (mg)	Zinc (mg)	Wat (%)	Alco (g)	Caff (g)
0.33	1.52	7.19	0.18	0.00	162.5	1.8	—	65.0	675	9.25	757.5	1308	1895	1125	7.6	1	0.00	0.00
0.05	0.01	0.43	0.03	0.00	20.8	2.6	—	0.2	11	1.94	25.6	90	285	16	0.9	47	0.00	0.00
0.00	0.00	0.18	0.00	0.00	4.0	0.3	—	0.2	5	0.93	13.0	27	62	4	0.2	73	0.00	0.00
0.00	0.00	0.05	0.02	0.00	0.8	0.1	—	0.1	2	0.31	8.5	20	51	3	0.2	1	0.00	0.00
0.01	0.23	1.09	0.03	0.00	9.4	0.0	—	7.4	75	1.27	81.1	139	211	96	1.0	3	0.00	0.00
0.10	1.19	5.30	0.17	0.00	45.5	0.0	—	35.9	367	6.21	394.7	675	1029	1	4.9	3	0.00	0.00
0.02	0.21	1.03	0.02	0.00	7.7	2.6	—	7.4	82	1.03	77.7	132	198	96	0.9	3	0.00	0.00
0.02	0.21	1.03	0.02	0.00	7.7	0.0	—	7.4	82	1.03	77.7	132	198	0	0.9	3	0.00	0.00
0.17	0.20	0.50	0.38	0.00	64.1	8.8	—	—	1	1.38	0.0	0	577	22	0.2	7	0.00	0.00
0.17	0.00	0.07	0.02	0.00	6.2	0.2	—	1.6	45	0.68	106.6	206	187	1	1.2	3	0.00	0.00
0.86	0.05	0.40	0.14	0.00	30.8	1.0	—	8.0	224	3.40	526.4	1015	923	4	5.7	3	0.00	0.00
0.07	0.07	0.47	0.09	0.00	23.6	0.0	—	0.3	15	2.05	89.1	168	194	219	1.9	2	0.00	0.00
0.07	0.07	0.47	0.09	0.00	23.6	0.0	—	0.3	15	2.05	89.1	168	194	5	1.9	2	0.00	0.00
0.11	0.07	0.56	0.10	0.00	8.1	0.1	—	0.3	14	1.97	88.7	173	205	100	1.7	2	0.00	0.00
0.11	0.07	0.56	0.10	0.00	8.1	0.1	—	0.3	14	1.97	88.7	173	205	4	1.7	3	0.00	0.00
0.87	0.15	2.43	0.75	0.00	152.6	8.5	—	20.3	154	6.34	220.1	392	918	0	3.3	5	0.00	0.00
0.87	0.15	2.43	0.75	0.00	152.6	8.5	—	20.3	154	6.34	220.1	392	918	0	3.3	5	0.00	0.00
0.34	0.05	0.69	0.07	0.00	3.1	0.3	—	0.2	24	1.04	36.9	53	104	1	0.4	1	0.00	0.00
0.18	0.17	0.70	0.05	0.00	20.2	0.2	—	3.0	38	0.93	90.4	162	196	110	1.7	3	0.00	0.00
0.18	0.17	0.70	0.05	0.00	20.2	0.2	—	2.2	38	0.93	90.4	162	196	4	1.7	3	0.00	0.00
0.07	0.07	1.61	0.10	0.00	17.1	0.1	—	3.7	24	1.26	77.1	149	204	229	1.3	2	0.00	0.00
0.07	0.07	1.61	0.10	0.00	17.1	0.1	—	2.1	24	1.26	77.1	149	204	4	1.3	2	0.00	0.00
0.18	0.07	1.79	0.09	0.00	29.5	0.2	—	2.6	38	1.13	83.4	165	206	149	1.8	2	0.00	0.00
0.18	0.07	1.79	0.09	0.00	29.5	0.2	—	2.1	38	1.13	83.4	165	206	4	1.8	2	0.00	0.00
0.12	0.02	4.05	0.07	0.00	43.5	0.0	—	2.3	16	0.68	52.8	107	197	244	1.0	2	0.00	0.00
0.12	0.02	4.05	0.07	0.00	43.5	0.0	—	2.1	16	0.68	52.8	107	197	2	1.0	2	0.00	0.00
0.01	0.01	3.73	0.11	0.00	32.4	0.2	—	1.9	16	0.40	47.5	107	196	86	0.9	1	0.00	0.00
0.07	0.02	4.00	0.07	0.00	35.3	0.0	—	1.9	25	0.50	51.8	145	191	2	1.9	2	0.00	0.00
0.34	0.14	18.98	0.34	0.00	167.6	0.0	—	9.2	117	2.43	246.1	688	907	8	8.8	2	0.00	0.00
0.23	0.05	10.97	0.18	0.00	92.6	0.0	0.0	5.4	74	1.67	123.5	284	570	318	1.5	2	0.00	0.00
0.46	0.11	21.95	0.37	0.00	185.2	0.0	—	10.9	147	3.34	247.0	569	1141	9	2.9	2	0.00	0.00
0.25	0.05	5.80	0.12	0.00	87.6	0.0	—	2.7	39	1.42	68.6	142	272	8	0.8	6	0.00	0.00
0.70	0.14	1.25	0.23	0.00	23.8	1.2	—	1.5	76	2.73	130.7	299	443	0	4.9	4	0.00	0.00
—	—	—	—	0.00	—	0.0	—	—	0	0.05	—	—	—	0	—	2	0.00	0.00
0.07	0.15	0.58	0.73	0.00	38.8	2.1	—	2.2	76	3.90	251.2	641	654	2	4.2	5	0.00	0.00
0.02	0.03	4.38	0.12	0.00	29.4	0.0	0.0	2.0	14	0.61	51.2	102	238	156	0.9	1	0.00	0.00
0.02	0.03	4.38	0.12	0.00	29.4	0.0	—	2.0	14	0.61	51.2	102	230	5	0.9	1	0.00	0.00
0.01	0.02	4.28	0.17	0.00	23.7	0.0	—	2.9	14	0.60	49.3	115	208	147	0.9	2	0.00	0.00
0.27	0.05	14.60	0.31	0.00	60.0	0.0	—	6.7	35	1.89	170.0	369	669	540	2.8	1	0.00	0.00
0.01	0.02	4.28	0.17	0.00	23.7	0.0	—	2.9	14	0.60	49.3	115	208	5	0.9	2	0.00	0.00
—	—	5.00	0.11	0.00	24.0	0.0	—	—	0	0.72	60.0	—	—	220	0.9	—	0.00	0.00
—	—	2.07	—	0.00	—	—	—	—	6	0.31	—	59	115	89	—	3	0.00	0.00
—	—	—	—	0.00	—	0.0	—	—	0	0.36	—	—	—	160	—	—	0.00	0.00
0.25	0.25	2.17	1.44	0.00	430.9	2.0	—	0.5	308	9.64	561.1	772	1056	53	6.5	9	0.00	0.00
3.29	0.36	6.48	1.11	0.00	326.9	2.0	—	49.7	167	9.75	509.8	1015	992	4	7.3	5	0.00	0.00

PAGE KEY: A-46 Beverage and Beverage Mixes   A-48 Other Beverages   A-48 Beverages, Alcoholic   A-50 Candies and Confections, Gum   A-54 Cereals, Breakfast Type   A-58 Cheese and Cheese Substitutes   A-60 Dairy Products and Substitutes   A-62 Desserts   A-68 Dessert Toppings   A-68 Eggs, Substitutes, and Egg Dishes   A-70 Ethnic Foods   A-74 Fast Foods/Restaurants   A-88 Fats, Oils, Margarines, Shortenings, and Substitutes   A-88 Fish, Seafood, and Shellfish   A-90 Food Additives   A-90 Fruit, Vegetable, or Blended Juices   A-92 Grains, Flours, and Fractions   A-92 Grain Products, Prepared and Baked Goods

Code	Food Name	Unit/ Amt	Wt (g)	Energy (kcal)	Prot (g)	Carb (g)	Fiber (g)	Fat (g)	Sat (g)	Mono (g)	Poly (g)	Chol (mg)	Vit A (RE)
4597	Seeds, sunflower, kernels, dry rstd, salted	0.25 cup	32	186	6	8	3	16	1.7	3.0	10.5	0	0
4551	Seeds, sunflower, kernels, dry rstd, unsalted	0.25 cup	32	186	6	8	4	16	1.7	3.0	10.5	0	0
4546	Seeds, sunflower, kernels, oil rstd, unsalted	1 cup	135	799	27	31	14	69	9.5	10.9	46.3	0	1
4552	Seeds, sunflower, oil rstd, salted	0.25 cup	34	200	7	8	4	17	2.4	2.7	11.6	0	0
63261	Soy Nuts, wheat free	1.8 oz	50	241	20	14	6	11	1.7	—	—	1	4

POULTRY

Chicken—BBQ, Breaded, Fried, Glazed, Grilled, Raw

Code	Food Name	Unit/ Amt	Wt (g)	Energy (kcal)	Prot (g)	Carb (g)	Fiber (g)	Fat (g)	Sat (g)	Mono (g)	Poly (g)	Chol (mg)	Vit A (RE)
15064	Chicken, breast & wing, white meat, brd, fried	3 oz	85	258	19	10	1	15	4.1	6.4	3.5	77	30
81202	Chicken, breast, fillet, grilled	1 ea	85	100	20	1	0	2	—	—	—	45	0
81186	Chicken, breast, oven rstd, fat free, 0.75 oz slice	2 pce	42	33	7	1	0	0	0.1	0.1	0.0	15	0
15921	Chicken, breast, sweet & sour	1 ea	131	118	8	15	1	3	0.5	0.9	1.4	23	22
15915	Chicken, breast, teriyaki	3 oz	85	118	18	4	0	2	0.6	0.7	0.6	55	11
15057	Chicken, broiler/fryer, breast, w/o skin, fried	3 oz	85	159	28	0	0	4	1.1	1.5	0.9	77	6
15004	Chicken, broiler/fryer, breast, w/o skin, rstd	3 oz	85	140	26	0	0	3	0.9	1.1	0.7	72	5
15039	Chicken, broiler/fryer, breast, w/o skin, stwd	3 oz	85	128	25	0	0	3	0.7	0.9	0.6	65	5
15013	Chicken, broiler/fryer, breast, w/skin, batter fried	3 oz	85	221	21	8	0	11	3.0	4.6	2.6	72	17
15003	Chicken, broiler/fryer, breast, w/skin, flour fried	3 oz	85	189	27	1	0	8	2.1	3.0	1.7	76	13
15001	Chicken, broiler/fryer, breast, w/skin, rstd	3 oz	85	168	25	0	0	7	1.9	2.6	1.4	71	23
15113	Chicken, broiler/fryer, dark meat, w/skin, batter fried	3 oz	85	253	19	8	0	16	4.2	6.4	3.8	76	26
15079	Chicken, broiler/fryer, dark meat, w/skin, flour fried	3 oz	85	242	23	3	0	14	3.9	5.7	3.3	78	26
15080	Chicken, broiler/fryer, dark meat, w/skin, rstd	3 oz	85	215	22	0	0	13	3.7	5.3	3.0	77	51
15903	Chicken, buffalo wings, w/bone, spicy	1 pce	16	49	4	0	0	3	0.9	1.3	0.9	13	9
15063	Chicken, drumstick & thigh, dark meat, brd, fried	3 oz	85	247	17	9	1	15	4.1	6.3	3.6	95	38
81198	Chicken, ground, raw	4 oz	113	150	18	0	0	9	2.5	—	—	75	0
15243	Chicken, nuggets	4 pce	73	207	12	11	0	13	4.0	6.2	1.6	44	22
15902	Chicken, patty, brd, ckd	1 ea	75	213	12	11	0	13	4.1	6.4	1.7	45	22
15136	Chicken, roasting, dark meat, w/o skin, raw	4 oz	113	128	21	0	0	4	1.1	1.3	1.0	82	20
15134	Chicken, roasting, light meat, w/o skin, raw	4 oz	113	124	25	0	0	2	0.4	0.5	0.5	65	9
49158	Chicken, tenders, breast meat, fat free, bkd	3 ea	85	120	13	16	2	0	0.0	0.0	0.0	30	0
49171	Chicken, tenders, breast, ckd f/fzn	3 ea	85	240	11	16	1	14	4.0	—	—	25	0

Turkey

Code	Food Name	Unit/ Amt	Wt (g)	Energy (kcal)	Prot (g)	Carb (g)	Fiber (g)	Fat (g)	Sat (g)	Mono (g)	Poly (g)	Chol (mg)	Vit A (RE)
16086	Turkey, avg, breast, w/skin, rstd	3 oz	85	161	24	0	0	6	1.8	2.1	1.5	63	0
51101	Turkey, avg, dark meat, w/o skin, rstd	3 oz	85	159	24	0	0	6	2.1	1.4	1.8	72	0
16028	Turkey, avg, dark meat, w/skin, rstd	3 oz	85	188	23	0	0	10	3.0	3.1	2.6	76	0
16158	Turkey, avg, light meat, w/o skin, rstd	3 oz	85	134	25	0	0	3	0.9	0.5	0.7	59	0
16027	Turkey, avg, light meat, w/skin, rstd	3 oz	85	168	24	0	0	7	2.0	2.4	1.7	65	0
16071	Turkey, avg, skin, rstd	1 ea	496	2192	98	0	0	197	51.3	83.8	45.0	560	0
16000	Turkey, avg, w/o skin, rstd	3 oz	85	145	25	0	0	4	1.4	0.9	1.2	65	0
16204	Turkey, ground, 10% fat, raw	3 oz	85	137	16	0	0	8	2.6	3.1	2.5	73	0
51133	Turkey, ground, 99% fat free, raw	4 oz	113	120	28	0	0	2	—	—	—	45	0
16351	Turkey, jerky, original, Original California	1 oz	28	80	14	3	0	1	0.0	—	—	30	60

Duck, Emu, Ostrich and Other

Code	Food Name	Unit/ Amt	Wt (g)	Energy (kcal)	Prot (g)	Carb (g)	Fiber (g)	Fat (g)	Sat (g)	Mono (g)	Poly (g)	Chol (mg)	Vit A (RE)
15069	Cornish Game Hen, rstd	3 oz	85	221	19	0	0	15	4.3	6.8	3.1	111	27
16294	Duck, domesticated, whole, rstd, chpd	1 cup	140	472	27	0	0	40	13.5	18.1	5.1	118	88
16065	Goose, whole, w/o skin, raw	4 oz	113	183	26	0	0	8	3.2	2.1	1.0	95	14

PAGE KEY: A-96 Granola Bars, Cereal Bars, Diet Bars, Scones, and Tarts   A-96 Meals and Dishes   A-100 Meats   A-106 Nuts, Seeds, and Products   A-108 Poultry
A-110 Salad Dressings, Dips, and Mayonnaise   A-110 Salads   A-110 Sandwiches   A-114 Sauces and Gravies   A-114 Snack Foods—Chips, Pretzels, Popcorn
A-116 Soups, Stews, and Chilis   A-118 Spices, Flavors, and Seasonings   A-120 Sports Bars and Drinks   A-120 Supplemental Foods and Formulas
A-122 Sweeteners and Sweet Substitutes   A-122 Vegetables and Legumes   A-136 Weight Loss Bars and Drinks   A-138 Miscellaneous

Thia (mg)	Ribo (mg)	Niac (mg NE)	Vit B6 (mg)	Vit B12 (µg)	Fol (µg)	Vit C (mg)	Vit D (IU)	Vit E (mg AT)	Cal (mg)	Iron (mg)	Magn (mg)	Phos (mg)	Pota (mg)	Sodi (mg)	Zinc (mg)	Wat (%)	Alco (g)	Caff (g)
0.02	0.07	2.25	0.25	0.00	75.8	0.4	—	8.4	22	1.22	41.3	370	272	131	1.7	1	0.00	0.00
0.02	0.07	2.25	0.25	0.00	75.8	0.4	—	8.4	22	1.22	41.3	370	272	1	1.7	1	0.00	0.00
0.43	0.37	5.57	1.07	0.00	315.9	1.5	—	49.0	117	5.78	171.4	1538	652	4	7.0	2	0.00	0.00
0.10	0.09	1.38	0.27	0.00	79.0	0.4	—	12.3	29	1.44	42.9	384	163	138	1.8	2	0.00	0.00
—	—	—	—	0.00	—	0.0	—	—	105	3.20	—	—	—	—	—	2	0.00	0.00
0.07	0.15	6.25	0.30	0.34	15.3	0.0	—	0.8	31	0.76	19.6	160	295	509	0.8	46	0.00	0.00
—	—	—	—	—	—	0.0	—	—	0	1.08	—	—	—	410	—	—	0.00	0.00
0.00	0.00	1.44	0.05	0.03	0.4	0.0	—	0.0	3	0.12	3.8	25	28	457	0.1	77	0.00	0.00
0.05	0.07	3.08	0.18	0.07	5.8	12.1	—	0.7	15	0.83	20.8	75	185	506	0.7	79	0.00	0.00
0.05	0.12	5.82	0.31	0.18	8.1	2.1	—	0.2	18	1.13	23.4	132	205	1118	1.3	67	0.56	0.00
0.07	0.10	12.56	0.54	0.31	3.4	0.0	—	0.4	14	0.97	26.4	209	235	67	0.9	60	0.00	0.00
0.05	0.10	11.65	0.50	0.28	3.4	0.0	—	0.2	13	0.87	24.7	194	218	63	0.9	65	0.00	0.00
0.03	0.10	7.19	0.28	0.20	2.6	0.0	—	0.2	11	0.75	20.4	140	159	54	0.8	68	0.00	0.00
0.10	0.11	8.94	0.37	0.25	12.8	0.0	—	0.9	17	1.05	20.4	157	171	234	0.8	52	0.00	0.00
0.07	0.10	11.68	0.49	0.28	5.1	0.0	—	0.5	14	1.00	25.5	198	220	65	0.9	57	0.00	0.00
0.05	0.10	10.81	0.47	0.27	3.4	0.0	—	0.2	12	0.91	23.0	182	208	60	0.9	62	0.00	0.00
0.10	0.18	4.76	0.20	0.23	15.3	0.0	—	1.0	18	1.22	17.0	123	157	251	1.8	49	0.00	0.00
0.07	0.20	5.82	0.27	0.25	9.4	0.0	—	0.7	14	1.27	20.4	150	196	76	2.2	51	0.00	0.00
0.05	0.18	5.40	0.25	0.25	6.0	0.0	—	0.5	13	1.15	18.7	143	187	74	2.1	59	0.00	0.00
0.00	0.01	1.02	0.07	0.03	0.5	0.0	1.9	0.1	2	0.20	3.0	24	29	13	0.3	53	0.00	0.00
0.07	0.25	4.13	0.18	0.47	14.5	0.0	—	0.8	20	0.92	21.3	138	256	434	1.9	49	0.00	0.00
—	—	—	—	—	—	0.0	—	—	0	0.00	—	—	—	65	—	—	0.00	0.00
0.07	0.10	4.90	0.23	0.21	8.0	0.3	8.8	1.4	12	0.91	14.6	146	180	388	0.8	49	0.00	0.00
0.07	0.10	5.03	0.23	0.23	8.2	0.3	9.0	1.5	12	0.93	15.0	150	184	399	0.8	49	0.00	0.00
0.07	0.20	6.67	0.36	0.38	10.2	0.0	—	0.2	10	1.29	23.8	202	257	108	1.9	75	0.00	0.00
0.07	0.10	11.59	0.62	0.43	4.5	0.0	—	0.2	12	1.00	28.4	253	286	58	0.7	74	0.00	0.00
—	—	—	—	—	—	0.0	—	—	0	0.72	—	—	—	480	—	—	0.00	0.00
—	—	—	—	—	—	0.0	—	—	20	0.72	—	—	—	450	—	—	0.00	0.00
0.05	0.10	5.40	0.40	0.31	5.1	0.0	—	0.2	18	1.19	23.0	179	245	54	1.7	63	0.00	0.00
0.05	0.20	3.09	0.31	0.31	7.7	0.0	—	0.5	27	1.98	20.4	174	247	67	3.8	63	0.00	0.00
0.05	0.20	3.00	0.27	0.31	7.7	0.0	—	0.5	28	1.92	19.6	167	233	65	3.5	60	0.00	0.00
0.05	0.10	5.82	0.46	0.31	5.1	0.0	—	0.1	16	1.14	23.8	186	259	54	1.7	66	0.00	0.00
0.05	0.10	5.34	0.40	0.30	5.1	0.0	—	0.1	18	1.20	22.1	177	242	54	1.7	63	0.00	0.00
0.10	0.72	13.17	0.40	1.19	19.8	0.0	—	2.6	174	8.88	79.4	680	794	263	10.3	40	0.00	0.00
0.05	0.15	4.63	0.38	0.31	6.0	0.0	—	0.3	21	1.50	22.1	181	253	60	2.6	65	0.00	0.00
—	—	—	—	—	—	0.0	—	—	22	1.28	22.9	140	207	109	2.5	71	0.00	0.00
—	—	—	—	—	—	0.0	—	—	0	1.44	—	—	—	65	—	—	0.00	0.00
—	—	—	—	—	—	0.0	—	—	20	1.08	—	—	—	550	—	31	0.00	0.00
0.05	0.17	5.01	0.25	0.23	1.7	0.4	10.2	0.2	11	0.76	15.3	124	208	54	1.3	59	0.00	0.00
0.23	0.37	6.75	0.25	0.41	8.4	0.0	—	1.0	15	3.77	22.4	218	286	83	2.6	52	0.00	0.00
0.15	0.43	4.84	0.73	0.56	35.2	8.2	—	1.3	15	2.91	27.2	354	476	99	2.7	68	0.00	0.00

Code	Food Name	Unit/ Amt	Wt (g)	Energy (kcal)	Prot (g)	Carb (g)	Fiber (g)	Fat (g)	Sat (g)	Mono (g)	Poly (g)	Chol (mg)	Vit A (RE)
16064	Goose, whole, w/skin, raw	4 oz	113	421	18	0	0	38	11.1	20.2	4.3	91	19
81168	Ostrich, ground, brld	3 oz	85	149	22	0	0	6	1.5	1.8	0.6	71	0
51148	Pheasant, whole, ckd	3 oz	85	210	28	0	0	10	3.0	4.8	1.3	76	48
SALAD DRESSINGS, DIPS, MAYONNAISE, OR SPREADS													
Dips													
53685	Dip, bean	2 Tbs	35	40	2	6	0	1	0.5	—	—	5	0
27138	Dip, creamy ranch	2 Tbs	31	60	1	3	0	4	3.0	—	—	0	0
53554	Dip, French onion	2 Tbs	33	60	1	4	0	5	3.0	—	—	15	20
27136	Dip, green onion	2 Tbs	31	60	1	4	0	4	3.0	—	—	0	0
27132	Dip, guacamole	2 Tbs	32	60	1	4	0	4	3.0	—	—	0	0
90861	Dip, salsa con queso, medium	2 Tbs	32	42	1	5	1	2	0.5	—	—	5	19
44415	Dip, salsa, grande	2 Tbs	28	50	1	1	0	5	3.0	—	—	15	40
27143	Dip, spinach	2 Tbs	28	140	0	3	0	14	2.0	—	—	10	80
44414	Dip, Veggie	2 Tbs	28	50	1	2	0	5	3.0	—	—	15	60
44425	Guacamole, med	2 Tbs	28	57	1	3	2	5	1.0	—	—	0	10
Mayonnaise													
8069	Mayonnaise, fat free	1 Tbs	16	11	0	2	0	0	0.1	—	—	2	3
4070	Mayonnaise, light	1 Tbs	15	50	0	2		5	0.0	2.5	1.5	5	0
44719	Mayonnaise, rducd cal, cholest free	1 Tbs	15	49	0	1	0	5	0.7	1.1	2.8	0	0
8503	Mayonnaise, real	1 Tbs	14	100	0	0	0	11	1.5	—	—	5	0
Salad Dressings—Lower Calorie/Fat/Sodium/Cholest													
44731	Dip, hummus, low fat, dry mix	2 Tbs	15	75	3	8	2	3	0.0	—	—	0	0
44727	Salad Dressing, blue cheese, fat free	1 Tbs	17	20	0	4	1	0	0.0	0.0	0.1	1	1
44722	Salad Dressing, blue cheese, rducd cal	1 Tbs	16	14	0	2	0	0	0.1	0.2	0.1	2	11
44465	Salad Dressing, buttermilk, light	3.6 oz	100	225	1	16	1	17	1.3	5.4	4.3	21	19
8138	Salad Dressing, caesar, low cal	1 Tbs	15	16	0	3	0	1	0.1	0.2	0.4	0	0
44729	Salad Dressing, French, rducd cal	1 Tbs	16	32	0	4	0	2	0.3	0.5	1.2	0	3
44699	Salad Dressing, Italian	2 Tbs	31	70	0	0	0	8	1.0	—	—	0	0
44498	Salad Dressing, Italian, fat free	1 Tbs	14	7	0	1	0	0	0.0	0.0	0.0	0	1
44720	Salad Dressing, Italian, rducd cal	1 Tbs	14	28	0	1	0	3	0.4	0.7	1.6	0	0
44497	Salad Dressing, thousand island, fat free	1 Tbs	16	21	0	5	1	0	0.0	0.1	0.1	1	0
8545	Salad Dressing, vinaigrette, Italian, fat free	2 Tbs	35	35	0	8	0	0	0.0	0.0	0.0	0	0
8546	Salad Dressing, vinaigrette, raspberry, fat free	2 Tbs	35	35	0	8	0	0	0.0	0.0	0.0	0	0
Salad Dressings—Regular													
44705	Salad Dressing, caesar	2 Tbs	29	155	0	1	0	17	2.6	4.0	9.7	1	1
8015	Salad Dressing, French, cmrcl	2 Tbs	31	143	0	5	0	14	1.8	2.6	6.6	0	14
8569	Salad Dressing, French, creamy	2 Tbs	32	160	0	5	0	15	2.5	—	—	0	250
8579	Salad Dressing, honey dijon	2 Tbs	31	110	0	6	0	10	1.5	—	—	0	0
8612	Salad Dressing, Italian, zesty	2 Tbs	31	109	0	2	0	11	1.2	—	—	0	2
8479	Salad Dressing, Miracle Whip	1 Tbs	15	70	0	2	0	7	1.0	—	—	5	0
44590	Salad Dressing, ranch, cmrcl	1 oz	28	137	0	2	0	15	2.3	3.2	8.0	9	3
8024	Salad Dressing, thousand island, cmrcl	1 Tbs	16	58	0	2	0	5	0.8	1.2	2.8	4	4
SPREADS—CRACKER OR SANDWICH													
Salads													
57482	Cole Slaw, prep f/recipe	0.5 cup	60	41	1	7	1	2	0.2	0.4	0.8	5	39
56118	Salad, bean, three	0.5 cup	75	70	2	7	3	4	0.6	0.9	2.2	0	10

PAGE KEY: A-96 Granola Bars, Cereal Bars, Diet Bars, Scones, and Tarts   A-96 Meals and Dishes   A-100 Meats   A-106 Nuts, Seeds, and Products   A-108 Poultry   A-110 Salad Dressings, Dips, and Mayonnaise   A-110 Salads   A-110 Sandwiches   A-114 Sauces and Gravies   A-114 Snack Foods—Chips, Pretzels, Popcorn   A-116 Soups, Stews, and Chilis   A-118 Spices, Flavors, and Seasonings   A-120 Sports Bars and Drinks   A-120 Supplemental Foods and Formulas   A-122 Sweeteners and Sweet Substitutes   A-122 Vegetables and Legumes   A-136 Weight Loss Bars and Drinks   A-138 Miscellaneous

Thia (mg)	Ribo (mg)	Niac (mg NE)	Vit B6 (mg)	Vit B12 (µg)	Fol (µg)	Vit C (mg)	Vit D (IU)	Vit E (mg AT)	Cal (mg)	Iron (mg)	Magn (mg)	Phos (mg)	Pota (mg)	Sodi (mg)	Zinc (mg)	Wat (%)	Alco (g)	Caff (g)
0.10	0.28	4.09	0.43	0.38	4.5	4.8	—	2.0	14	2.83	20.4	265	349	83	2.0	50	0.00	0.00
0.18	0.23	5.57	0.43	4.88	11.9	0.0	—	0.2	7	2.92	19.6	191	275	68	3.7	67	0.00	0.00
0.05	0.15	6.40	0.63	0.61	4.3	2.0	—	0.2	14	1.22	18.7	206	230	37	1.2	54	0.00	0.00
—	—	—	—	—	—	0.0	—	—	0	0.36	—	—	—	140	—	70	0.00	0.00
—	—	—	—	—	—	0.0	—	—	0	0.00	—	—	20	210	—	—	0.00	0.00
—	—	—	—	—	—	0.0	—	—	0	0.00	—	—	—	230	—	—	0.00	0.00
—	—	—	—	—	—	0.0	—	—	0	0.00	—	0	20	190	—	—	0.00	0.00
—	—	—	—	—	—	0.0	—	—	0	0.00	—	0	25	240	—	—	0.00	0.00
—	—	—	—	—	—	0.0	—	—	19	0.00	—	—	—	254	—	—	0.00	0.00
—	—	—	—	—	—	1.2	—	—	20	0.00	—	—	—	130	—	—	0.00	0.00
—	—	—	—	—	—	0.0	—	—	0	0.36	—	—	—	200	—	—	0.00	0.00
—	—	—	—	—	—	0.0	—	—	20	0.00	—	—	—	125	—	—	0.00	0.00
—	—	—	—	—	—	1.8	—	—	10	0.18	—	—	—	147	—	66	0.00	0.00
—	—	—	—	—	—	0.0	—	0.5	1	0.01	—	4	8	120	—	82	0.00	0.00
—	—	—	—	—	—	—	—	0.6	—	—	—	—	—	125	—	51	0.00	0.00
0.00	0.00	0.00	0.00	0.00	0.0	0.0	—	0.9	0	0.00	0.0	0	10	107	0.0	56	0.00	0.00
—	—	—	—	—	—	0.0	—	0.4	0	0.00	—	0	0	75	—	20	0.00	0.00
—	—	—	—	—	—	0.0	—	—	0	0.54	—	—	—	240	—	—	0.00	0.00
0.00	0.01	0.00	0.00	0.03	1.0	0.0	—	0.0	12	0.00	1.5	18	33	136	0.0	68	0.00	0.00
0.00	0.00	0.00	0.00	0.01	4.5	0.0	—	0.1	11	0.01	0.6	8	8	258	0.0	78	0.00	0.00
0.01	0.02	0.00	0.02	0.00	4.0	0.7	4.9	1.6	125	0.87	6.0	193	132	932	0.6	62	0.00	0.00
0.00	0.00	0.00	0.00	0.00	0.3	0.0	—	0.1	4	0.02	0.3	3	4	162	0.0	73	0.00	0.00
0.00	0.00	0.00	0.00	0.00	0.3	0.0	—	0.5	2	0.05	0.0	2	13	160	0.0	59	0.00	0.00
—	—	—	—	—	—	0.0	—	—	0	0.00	—	—	—	350	—	71	0.00	0.00
0.00	0.00	0.01	0.00	0.03	1.7	0.1	—	0.1	4	0.05	0.7	15	14	158	0.1	86	0.00	0.00
0.00	0.00	0.00	0.00	0.00	0.4	0.1	—	0.1	1	0.01	0.3	1	5	199	0.0	70	0.00	0.00
0.03	0.00	0.03	0.00	0.00	1.9	0.0	—	0.1	2	0.03	0.6	0	20	117	0.0	66	0.00	0.00
—	—	—	—	—	—	0.0	—	—	0	—	—	—	—	280	—	—	0.00	0.00
—	—	—	—	—	—	0.0	—	—	0	—	—	—	—	35	—	—	0.00	0.00
0.00	0.00	0.00	0.00	0.00	0.9	0.0	—	1.5	7	0.05	0.6	6	9	317	0.0	34	0.00	0.00
0.00	0.01	0.05	0.60	0.03	0.0	0.0	—	1.6	7	0.25	1.6	6	21	261	0.1	37	0.00	0.00
—	—	—	—	—	—	0.0	—	—	0	0.00	—	0	20	270	—	35	0.00	0.00
—	—	—	—	—	—	0.0	—	—	0	0.00	—	0	35	210	—	—	0.00	0.00
—	—	—	—	—	—	0.2	—	—	1	0.05	—	4	9	505	—	53	0.00	0.00
—	—	—	—	—	—	0.0	—	0.0	0	0.00	—	0	0	95	—	—	0.00	0.00
0.02	0.01	0.00	0.00	0.09	1.1	1.0	0.8	1.3	9	0.18	1.4	46	18	231	0.1	38	0.00	0.00
0.23	0.00	0.07	0.00	0.00	0.0	0.0	—	0.6	3	0.18	1.2	4	17	135	0.0	47	0.00	0.00
0.03	0.03	0.15	0.07	0.00	16.2	19.6	—	0.1	27	0.34	6.0	19	109	14	0.1	82	0.00	0.00
0.03	0.05	0.21	0.01	0.00	28.0	2.0	—	0.9	18	0.74	13.7	38	123	260	0.3	81	0.00	0.00

PAGE KEY: A-46 Beverage and Beverage Mixes   A-48 Other Beverages   A-48 Beverages, Alcoholic   A-50 Candies and Confections, Gum   A-54 Cereals, Breakfast Type
A-58 Cheese and Cheese Substitutes   A-60 Dairy Products and Substitutes   A-62 Desserts   A-68 Dessert Toppings   A-68 Eggs, Substitutes, and Egg Dishes   A-70 Ethnic Foods
A-74 Fast Foods/Restaurants   A-88 Fats, Oils, Margarines, Shortenings, and Substitutes   A-88 Fish, Seafood, and Shellfish   A-90 Food Additives
A-90 Fruit, Vegetable, or Blended Juices   A-92 Grains, Flours, and Fractions   A-92 Grain Products, Prepared and Baked Goods

Code	Food Name	Unit/ Amt	Wt (g)	Energy (kcal)	Prot (g)	Carb (g)	Fiber (g)	Fat (g)	Sat (g)	Mono (g)	Poly (g)	Chol (mg)	Vit A (RE)
52061	Salad, chicken	0.5 cup	100	250	10	9	2	20	4.0	—	—	55	20
56253	Salad, crab	1 cup	208	282	27	11	1	14	2.0	3.5	7.1	142	37
56003	Salad, egg	1 cup	183	584	17	3	0	56	10.5	17.4	23.9	581	263
3312	Salad, fruit, w/citrus, fresh	1 cup	175	99	1	25	3	1	0.1	0.0	0.1	0	14
3311	Salad, fruit, w/o citrus, fresh	1 cup	175	101	1	26	4	1	0.1	0.1	0.2	0	34
69160	Salad, gelatin, fruity, prep f/recipe	1 ea	192	376	5	41	2	22	9.5	—	—	35	94
52029	Salad, macaroni, elbow, classic	0.5 cup	106	197	3	25	2	9	1.5	—	—	8	—
69196	Salad, Mediterranean Blend	2 cup	100	90	1	5	1	8	1.0	—	—	0	225
5637	Salad, mixed greens, raw	1 cup	55	9	1	2	1	0	0.0	0.0	0.1	0	150
4839	Salad, pasta, Greek, w/feta cheese	0.66 cup	140	200	6	27	3	8	2.0	—	—	5	—
56005	Salad, potato, prep f/recipe	0.5 cup	125	179	3	14	2	10	1.8	3.1	4.7	85	44
56257	Salad, seafood	0.5 cup	104	164	13	2	0	11	1.6	8.0	1.2	66	25
56256	Salad, shrimp	1 cup	182	282	27	6	1	17	2.6	4.5	8.4	206	42
5537	Salad, spinach, w/o dressing	1 cup	74	108	5	11	2	5	1.4	2.2	0.7	77	176
56643	Salad, taco	1.5 cup	198	279	13	24	—	15	6.8	5.2	1.7	44	93
52060	Salad, tuna	0.5 cup	100	260	12	9	2	19	3.0	—	—	30	20
SANDWICHES													
56647	Cheeseburger, reg, w/condiments	1 ea	113	295	16	27	—	14	6.3	5.3	1.1	37	97
66004	Hot Dog, plain, w/bun	1 ea	98	242	10	18	—	15	5.1	6.9	1.7	44	0
56667	Hot Dog, w/chili & bun	1 ea	114	296	14	31	—	13	4.9	6.6	1.2	51	7
56009	Sandwich, BLT, w/white	1 ea	124	318	10	29	2	18	4.1	—	—	20	49
56010	Sandwich, BLT, w/whole wheat	1 ea	137	339	12	29	5	20	4.9	—	—	23	56
56281	Sandwich, bologna	1 ea	83	256	7	26	1	13	4.1	6.3	2.1	16	37
56000	Sandwich, chicken, fillet, plain	1 ea	182	515	24	39	—	29	8.5	10.4	8.4	60	31
70755	Sandwich, egg cheese, medium	1 ea	119	350	12	30	1	20	8.0	—	—	110	0
56657	Sandwich, egg cheese, large	1 ea	146	340	16	26	—	19	6.6	8.3	2.6	291	201
66010	Sandwich, fish, w/tartar sauce	1 ea	158	431	17	41	0	23	5.2	7.7	8.2	55	33
56013	Sandwich, grilled cheese, w/white	1 ea	119	399	17	30	1	23	11.9	—	—	53	167
56014	Sandwich, grilled cheese, w/whole wheat	1 ea	132	431	20	30	4	27	13.8	—	—	60	192
56272	Sandwich, gyro	1 ea	105	170	12	21	1	4	1.5	1.4	0.4	34	11
56664	Sandwich, ham cheese	1 ea	146	352	21	33	—	15	6.4	6.7	1.4	58	96
56274	Sandwich, ham cheese, grilled	1 ea	141	381	21	30	1	20	7.9	7.9	2.4	54	106
56029	Sandwich, ham, w/white	1 ea	157	365	24	30	2	16	3.3	—	—	54	6
56030	Sandwich, ham, w/whole wheat	1 ea	169	379	27	29	4	18	3.9	—	—	59	7
56267	Sandwich, pastrami	1 ea	134	331	14	27	2	18	6.2	8.7	1.0	51	3
56040	Sandwich, peanut butter & jam, w/white	1 ea	101	348	11	47	3	14	2.7	—	—	1	0
56041	Sandwich, peanut butter & jam, w/whole wheat	1 ea	114	398	13	51	5	17	3.6	—	—	0	1
56277	Sandwich, pork	1 ea	136	324	26	32	1	9	2.9	4.1	1.0	62	1
56266	Sandwich, reuben	1 ea	181	464	21	30	3	29	9.9	9.7	6.7	82	94
66003	Sandwich, roast beef, plain	1 ea	139	346	22	33	—	14	3.6	6.8	1.7	51	22
56669	Sandwich, roast beef, w/cheese	1 ea	176	473	32	45	—	18	9.0	3.7	3.5	77	58
56286	Sandwich, salami	1 ea	82	234	8	25	1	11	3.4	5.2	1.9	19	35
56261	Sandwich, sloppy joe, w/bun	1 ea	186	358	18	36	2	15	5.0	6.6	1.4	46	73
56670	Sandwich, steak	1 ea	204	459	30	52	—	14	3.8	5.3	3.3	73	39
56048	Sandwich, tuna salad, w/white	1 ea	122	326	13	35	1	14	1.9	—	—	13	15
56052	Sandwich, turkey, w/white	1 ea	156	346	24	29	1	14	1.9	—	—	43	8
56053	Sandwich, turkey, w/whole wheat	1 ea	169	360	27	29	4	16	2.3	—	—	47	8

Thia (mg)	Ribo (mg)	Niac (mg NE)	Vit B6 (mg)	Vit B12 (µg)	Fol (µg)	Vit C (mg)	Vit D (IU)	Vit E (mg AT)	Cal (mg)	Iron (mg)	Magn (mg)	Phos (mg)	Pota (mg)	Sodi (mg)	Zinc (mg)	Wat (%)	Alco (g)	Caff (g)
—	—	—	—	—	—	1.2	—	—	40	0.36	—	—	—	600	—	—	0.00	0.00—
0.15	0.09	4.50	0.28	9.76	79.4	6.9	—	2.8	157	1.45	48.6	292	536	700	5.7	74	0.00	0.00
0.09	0.66	0.09	0.46	1.57	61.1	0.0	—	7.7	74	1.80	13.5	238	181	464	1.4	57	0.00	0.00
0.07	0.05	0.41	0.23	0.00	14.1	29.2	0.0	0.6	16	0.31	17.4	18	309	1	0.1	84	0.00	0.00
0.07	0.07	0.88	0.20	0.00	13.7	14.5	0.0	0.7	13	0.41	19.7	21	328	1	0.2	84	0.00	0.00
0.09	0.07	0.18	0.03	0.14	7.1	8.0	2.3	0.8	36	0.99	17.8	70	91	149	0.8	64	0.00	0.00
—	—	—	—	—	—	—	—	—	—	—	—	—	—	560	—	—	0.00	0.00
—	—	—	—	—	—	18.0	—	—	40	0.72	—	—	—	180	—	—	0.00	0.00
0.03	0.05	0.23	0.03	0.00	63.6	8.9	0.0	0.4	30	0.72	13.2	18	174	14	0.2	94	0.00	0.00
—	—	—	—	—	—	—	—	—	—	—	—	—	—	780	—	—	0.00	0.00
0.10	0.07	1.11	0.18	0.00	8.8	12.5	—	2.3	24	0.81	18.8	65	318	661	0.4	76	0.00	0.00
0.03	0.05	1.17	0.09	0.92	15.7	6.2	—	2.0	46	0.99	27.1	141	251	176	1.7	73	0.00	0.00
0.05	0.05	3.25	0.27	1.30	15.5	5.7	—	3.4	87	3.39	51.6	280	367	392	1.5	72	0.00	0.00
0.12	0.28	1.66	0.10	0.20	59.9	6.7	0.0	0.9	46	1.46	27.1	83	242	227	0.6	70	0.00	0.00
0.10	0.36	2.46	0.21	0.62	83.2	3.6	—	—	192	2.27	51.5	143	416	762	2.7	72	0.00	0.00
—	—	—	—	—	—	0.0	—	—	20	0.36	—	—	—	580	—	—	0.00	0.00
0.25	0.23	3.72	0.10	0.93	54.2	1.9	—	0.5	111	2.43	20.3	176	223	616	2.1	48	0.00	0.00
0.23	0.27	3.65	0.05	0.50	48.0	0.1	—	0.3	24	2.30	12.7	97	143	670	2.0	54	0.00	0.00
0.21	0.40	3.74	0.05	0.30	73.0	2.7	—	—	19	3.27	10.3	192	166	480	0.8	48	0.00	0.00
0.40	0.25	3.69	0.15	0.34	66.3	6.0	6.8	2.3	68	2.20	22.0	123	239	631	1.0	52	0.00	0.00
0.37	0.20	3.97	0.25	0.37	45.0	6.8	7.5	2.9	51	2.53	60.7	216	346	690	1.9	52	0.00	0.00
0.28	0.20	2.73	0.07	0.37	18.7	0.0	—	0.8	60	1.96	15.4	74	112	598	0.9	41	0.00	0.00
0.33	0.23	6.80	0.20	0.37	100.1	8.9	—	—	60	4.67	34.6	233	353	957	1.9	47	0.00	0.00
—	—	—	—	—	—	1.2	—	—	150	1.79	—	—	—	890	—	45	0.00	0.00
0.25	0.56	2.06	0.12	1.13	97.8	1.5	—	—	225	2.98	21.9	302	188	804	1.6	56	0.00	0.00
0.33	0.21	3.40	0.10	1.07	85.3	2.8	—	0.9	84	2.60	33.2	212	340	615	1.0	47	0.00	0.00
0.28	0.40	2.36	0.07	0.40	60.4	0.0	9.7	1.0	407	2.00	26.5	470	162	1155	2.0	37	0.00	0.00
0.23	0.36	2.46	0.15	0.46	36.6	0.0	10.8	1.4	439	2.31	68.2	619	264	1291	3.1	38	0.00	0.00
0.23	0.20	3.14	0.12	0.89	17.8	3.8	—	0.3	46	1.85	20.9	116	209	272	2.3	64	0.00	0.00
0.31	0.47	2.69	0.20	0.54	75.9	2.8	—	0.3	130	3.24	16.1	152	291	771	1.4	51	0.00	0.00
0.70	0.43	5.01	0.27	0.81	16.4	0.0	—	1.1	233	2.41	32.4	343	337	1465	2.5	47	0.00	0.00
0.89	0.43	6.82	0.38	0.61	59.8	0.1	25.1	2.5	76	3.09	32.1	270	384	1237	2.6	52	0.00	0.00
0.89	0.38	7.30	0.50	0.66	34.6	0.2	27.5	3.1	58	3.47	72.4	378	502	1339	3.7	53	0.00	0.00
0.28	0.27	4.76	0.12	0.97	21.2	2.0	—	0.3	68	2.64	23.1	135	243	1335	2.7	53	0.00	0.00
0.28	0.23	5.44	0.15	0.01	79.0	1.7	4.9	2.6	76	2.28	51.8	143	240	429	1.1	27	0.00	0.00
0.28	0.20	6.42	0.20	0.00	76.3	2.1	0.0	3.2	80	2.66	75.2	201	336	465	1.5	27	0.00	0.00
0.91	0.46	6.25	0.34	0.55	26.4	0.2	—	0.4	85	2.75	34.1	229	343	392	2.5	49	0.00	0.00
0.23	0.34	3.45	0.21	1.34	37.2	4.1	—	0.8	299	2.92	38.7	291	261	1348	4.0	53	0.00	0.00
0.37	0.31	5.86	0.25	1.22	57.0	2.1	—	0.2	54	4.23	30.6	239	316	792	3.4	49	0.00	0.00
0.38	0.46	5.90	0.33	2.05	63.4	0.0	—	—	183	5.05	40.5	401	345	1633	5.4	44	0.00	0.00
0.30	0.28	2.96	0.09	1.07	17.2	0.0	—	0.7	58	2.25	16.1	80	117	612	0.9	44	0.00	0.00
0.28	0.27	5.73	0.23	1.51	21.8	5.8	—	1.3	92	3.63	35.5	149	368	1008	3.2	61	0.00	0.00
0.40	0.37	7.30	0.37	1.57	89.8	5.5	—	—	92	5.15	49.0	298	524	798	4.5	51	0.00	0.00
0.30	0.23	5.88	0.12	0.66	62.5	1.1	72.0	2.8	76	2.40	24.5	152	168	588	0.7	46	0.00	0.00
0.31	0.28	9.27	0.41	1.74	60.3	0.0	15.0	3.3	72	2.18	30.9	250	306	1586	1.3	54	0.00	0.00
0.25	0.21	10.06	0.52	1.91	35.4	0.0	16.4	3.9	53	2.46	71.2	356	417	1734	2.2	54	0.00	0.00

PAGE KEY: A-46 Beverage and Beverage Mixes   A-48 Other Beverages   A-48 Beverages, Alcoholic   A-50 Candies and Confections, Gum   A-54 Cereals, Breakfast Type
A-58 Cheese and Cheese Substitutes   A-60 Dairy Products and Substitutes   A-62 Desserts   A-68 Dessert Toppings   A-68 Eggs, Substitutes, and Egg Dishes   A-70 Ethnic Foods
A-74 Fast Foods/Restaurants   A-88 Fats, Oils, Margarines, Shortenings, and Substitutes   A-88 Fish, Seafood, and Shellfish   A-90 Food Additives
A-90 Fruit, Vegetable, or Blended Juices   A-92 Grains, Flours, and Fractions   A-92 Grain Products, Prepared and Baked Goods

Code	Food Name	Unit/Amt	Wt (g)	Energy (kcal)	Prot (g)	Carb (g)	Fiber (g)	Fat (g)	Sat (g)	Mono (g)	Poly (g)	Chol (mg)	Vit A (RE)
SAUCES AND GRAVIES													
Gravies													
53564	Gravy, beef, fat free	0.25 cup	60	20	0	5	0	0	0.0	0.0	0.0	5	0
53006	Gravy, beef, prep f/recipe	0.5 cup	135	107	3	7	1	8	1.9	3.4	2.0	3	150
53022	Gravy, chicken, can	0.25 cup	60	47	1	3	0	3	0.8	1.5	0.9	1	1
53565	Gravy, chicken, fat free	0.25 cup	60	15	1	3	0	0	0.0	0.0	0.0	5	20
53401	Gravy, country, dry mix	1 Tbs	6	22	1	4	0	1	0.1	0.4	0.0	0	0
53038	Gravy, mushroom, dry mix, svg	1 ea	21	70	2	14	1	1	0.5	0.3	0.0	1	0
53403	Gravy, onion, dry mix	1 Tbs	5	18	1	3	1	0	0.1	0.2	0.0	0	0
53044	Gravy, turkey, dry mix, svg	1 ea	7	26	1	5	—	1	0.1	0.2	0.2	1	1
Sauces													
53591	Marinade, cooking sauce, mesquite	1 Tbs	17	10	0	3	0	0	0.0	0.0	0.0	0	0
53587	Marinade, cooking sauce, teriyaki	1 Tbs	18	25	1	5	0	0	0.0	0.0	0.0	0	0
9559	Sauce, alfredo	0.25 cup	61	110	1	2	0	10	3.5	—	—	30	40
53000	Sauce, barbecue	1 cup	250	188	4	32	3	4	0.7	1.9	1.7	0	5
53320	Sauce, barbecue, sweet & sour	2 Tbs	34	45	0	10	0	0	0.0	0.0	0.0	0	0
53420	Sauce, barbecue, teriyaki	2 Tbs	36	60	0	12	0	0	0.0	0.0	0.0	0	0
9558	Sauce, cheese, cheddar, rts	0.25 cup	61	90	2	2	0	8	2.5	—	—	25	20
53523	Sauce, cheese, rts	0.25 cup	63	110	4	4	0	8	3.8	2.4	1.6	18	52
53474	Sauce, fish, rts	2 Tbs	36	13	2	1	0	0	0.0	0.0	0.0	0	1
53356	Sauce, Italian, rts	1 ea	1956	1917	33	362	27	37	5.1	23.3	5.3	0	1545
9425	Sauce, pasta, alfredo, classic	0.25 cup	61	110	1	3	0	10	3.5	—	—	25	100
53627	Sauce, pasta, garlic & herb, cnd	0.5 cup	126	50	2	10	2	0	0.0	0.0	0.0	0	40
53623	Sauce, pasta, garlic & onion, cnd	0.5 cup	125	40	2	9	2	0	0.0	0.0	0.0	0	30
53629	Sauce, pasta, traditional, cnd	0.5 cup	126	50	2	11	2	0	0.0	0.0	0.0	0	30
53540	Sauce, peanut	1 cup	240	749	31	29	8	63	12.8	30.0	17.1	0	1
7479	Sauce, picante, mild	2 Tbs	32	10	0	2	1	0	0.0	0.0	0.0	0	20
53284	Sauce, picante, med	2 Tbs	30	10	0	2	0	0	0.0	0.0	0.0	0	20
53221	Sauce, picante, hot	2 Tbs	30	10	0	2	0	0	0.0	0.0	0.0	0	0
53363	Sauce, pizza, deluxe, rts	0.25 cup	63	34	1	5	1	1	0.3	0.3	0.1	2	42
53425	Sauce, sloppy joe, cnd	0.25 cup	73	50	2	11	2	0	0.0	0.0	0.0	0	150
1709	Sauce, spaghetti, meatless, USDA, cnd	3.6 oz	100	48	1	9	—	1	0.2	0.2	0.5	0	34
51016	Sauce, spaghetti, traditional, cnd	0.5 cup	125	60	2	15	3	1	0.0	—	—	0	75
53011	Sauce, spaghetti, w/meat, cnd	1 cup	250	178	7	19	4	8	1.8	3.3	1.8	15	176
53524	Sauce, spaghetti/marinara, rts	0.5 cup	125	92	2	14	0	3	0.4	1.0	1.2	0	68
92310	Sauce, steak	1 Tbs	16	5	0	1	0	0	0.0	0.0	0.0	0	0
53352	Sauce, stir fry, all purpose, rts	1 Tbs	15	16	0	2	0	1	0.1	0.2	0.3	0	1
8983	Sauce, tartar	2 Tbs	28	139	0	1	0	15	2.7	0.7	2.3	11	6
90268	Sauce, white, dehyd, svg	1 ea	20	92	2	10	1	5	1.3	2.4	1.4	0	0
5181	Tomato Paste, unsalted, 6 oz can	1 ea	170	139	7	32	8	1	0.2	0.1	0.3	0	259
5180	Tomato Sauce, cnd	0.5 cup	122	39	2	9	2	0	0.0	0.0	0.1	0	42
SNACK FOODS—CHIPS, PRETZELS, POPCORN													
44061	Chips, bagel	5 pce	70	298	6	52	4	7	1.3	2.1	3.4	0	0
44256	Chips, corn, original	11 pce	28	140	2	19	2	6	0.5	—	—	0	0
44278	Chips, corn, original	32 pce	28	158	2	15	1	10	1.0	2.5	6.4	0	0
61236	Chips, potato, bkd	1 oz	28	133	1	20	1	5	0.7	2.8	1.2	0	0
43703	Chips, potato, classic	20 pce	28	150	2	15	1	10	3.0	—	—	0	0

PAGE KEY: A-96 Granola Bars, Cereal Bars, Diet Bars, Scones, and Tarts   A-96 Meals and Dishes   A-100 Meats   A-106 Nuts, Seeds, and Products   A-108 Poultry
A-110 Salad Dressings, Dips, and Mayonnaise   A-110 Salads   A-110 Sandwiches   A-114 Sauces and Gravies   A-114 Snack Foods—Chips, Pretzels, Popcorn
A-116 Soups, Stews, and Chilis   A-118 Spices, Flavors, and Seasonings   A-120 Sports Bars and Drinks   A-120 Supplemental Foods and Formulas
A-122 Sweeteners and Sweet Substitutes   A-122 Vegetables and Legumes   A-136 Weight Loss Bars and Drinks   A-138 Miscellaneous

Thia (mg)	Ribo (mg)	Niac (mg NE)	Vit B6 (mg)	Vit B12 (µg)	Fol (µg)	Vit C (mg)	Vit D (IU)	Vit E (mg AT)	Cal (mg)	Iron (mg)	Magn (mg)	Phos (mg)	Pota (mg)	Sodi (mg)	Zinc (mg)	Wat (%)	Alco (g)	Caff (g)
—	—	—	—	—	—	0.0	—	—	0	0.00	—	—	—	308	—	90	0.00	0.00
0.01	0.05	0.60	0.00	0.14	2.7	0.0	1.0	0.2	27	0.62	2.7	39	147	779	1.1	85	0.00	0.00
0.00	0.02	0.25	0.00	0.05	1.2	0.0	—	0.1	12	0.28	1.2	17	65	343	0.5	85	0.00	0.00
—	—	—	—	—	—	0.0	—	—	0	0.00	—	—	—	318	—	92	0.00	0.00
0.00	0.00	0.00	0.00	0.00	—	0.0	—	—	1	0.02	—	7	7	249	0.0	7	0.00	0.00
0.03	0.09	0.79	0.01	0.15	6.6	1.5	—	0.0	49	0.20	7.2	43	56	1402	0.3	3	0.00	0.00
0.02	0.01	0.00	0.01	0.00	—	0.0	—	—	1	0.10	—	10	25	229	0.0	8	0.00	0.00
0.00	0.02	0.18	0.00	0.03	5.7	0.0	—	0.0	10	0.23	3.1	18	30	307	0.1	5	0.00	0.00
—	—	—	—	—	—	1.8	—	—	0	0.00	—	—	25	400	—	—	0.00	0.00
—	—	—	—	—	—	3.0	—	—	0	0.00	—	—	40	480	—	64	0.00	0.00
—	—	—	—	—	—	0.0	—	—	40	0.00	—	—	—	390	—	76	0.00	0.00
0.07	0.05	2.25	0.18	0.00	10.0	17.5	—	0.0	48	2.25	45.0	50	435	2038	0.5	81	0.00	0.00
—	—	—	—	—	—	0.0	—	—	0	0.00	—	—	—	420	—	—	0.00	0.00
—	—	—	—	—	—	0.0	—	—	0	0.36	—	—	—	440	—	63	0.00	0.00
—	—	—	—	—	—	0.0	—	—	60	0.00	—	—	—	480	—	78	0.00	0.00
0.00	0.07	0.01	0.00	0.09	2.5	0.3	—	0.2	116	0.12	5.7	99	19	522	0.6	70	0.00	0.00
0.00	0.01	0.82	0.14	0.17	18.4	0.2	—	0.0	15	0.28	63.0	3	104	2779	0.1	71	0.00	0.00
2.41	1.42	35.63	5.40	0.00	508.6	131.1	—	37.8	1076	12.13	625.9	1350	11892	9584	8.2	76	0.00	0.00
—	—	—	—	—	—	0.0	—	—	40	—	—	—	—	340	—	75	0.00	0.00
—	—	—	—	—	—	6.0	—	—	40	1.08	—	—	—	390	—	88	0.00	0.00
—	—	—	—	—	—	6.0	—	—	40	1.08	—	—	—	390	—	89	0.00	0.00
—	—	—	—	—	—	6.0	—	—	40	1.08	—	—	—	390	—	87	0.00	0.00
0.11	0.14	16.63	0.58	0.00	99.2	27.1	—	12.4	52	2.29	200.9	460	901	580	3.7	47	0.00	0.00
—	—	—	—	—	—	0.0	—	—	0	0.00	—	—	—	230	—	92	0.00	0.00
—	—	—	—	—	—	0.0	—	—	0	0.00	—	—	—	230	—	91	0.00	0.00
—	—	—	—	—	—	19.8	—	—	0	0.00	—	—	—	260	—	91	0.00	0.00
0.03	0.02	0.89	0.09	0.00	6.3	7.1	—	1.6	34	0.56	13.2	32	223	117	0.2	87	0.00	0.00
—	—	—	—	—	—	0.0	—	—	0	0.72	—	—	—	420	—	—	0.00	0.00
0.02	0.11	0.73	0.05	0.00	—	3.9	—	—	20	0.89	13.0	25	292	590	0.2	87	0.00	0.00
—	—	—	—	—	—	9.0	—	—	40	1.44	—	—	—	590	—	84	0.00	0.00
0.12	0.11	3.47	0.31	0.49	25.0	18.8	1.2	3.0	54	2.09	43.2	104	742	982	1.3	85	0.00	0.00
0.02	0.07	4.90	0.21	0.00	13.8	3.9	—	2.5	34	1.05	26.2	45	470	601	0.7	82	0.00	0.00
—	—	—	—	—	—	0.0	—	—	0	0.00	—	—	—	200	—	90	0.00	0.00
0.00	0.00	0.14	0.00	0.00	0.6	0.7	—	0.0	2	0.10	1.5	4	8	233	0.0	74	0.00	0.00
—	—	—	—	—	—	0.7	—	—	6	0.14	—	—	38	153	—	39	0.00	0.00
0.03	0.07	0.14	0.01	0.15	6.7	0.6	—	0.1	133	0.10	7.7	49	73	675	0.2	2	0.00	0.00
0.10	0.25	5.23	0.37	0.00	20.4	37.3	—	7.3	61	5.07	71.4	141	1725	167	1.1	74	0.00	0.00
0.02	0.07	1.19	0.11	0.00	11.0	8.6	—	2.5	16	1.25	19.6	32	405	642	0.2	89	0.00	0.00
0.12	0.11	1.62	0.15	0.00	46.0	0.0	—	1.7	9	1.38	39.2	145	167	419	0.9	3	0.00	0.00
0.05	0.15	0.50	—	—	—	0.0	—	—	0	0.36	—	70	75	115	0.0	2	0.00	0.00
0.00	0.03	0.33	—	—	—	0.0	—	—	44	0.37	—	54	54	104	0.0	3	0.00	0.00
0.10	0.01	1.15	0.14	0.00	0.0	0.0	—	0.6	35	0.23	12.2	78	204	260	0.1	1	0.00	0.00
—	—	—	—	—	—	6.0	—	—	0	0.00	—	—	—	180	—	1	0.00	0.00

PAGE KEY: A-46 Beverage and Beverage Mixes   A-48 Other Beverages   A-48 Beverages, Alcoholic   A-50 Candies and Confections, Gum   A-54 Cereals, Breakfast Type
A-58 Cheese and Cheese Substitutes   A-60 Dairy Products and Substitutes   A-62 Desserts   A-68 Dessert Toppings   A-68 Eggs, Substitutes, and Egg Dishes   A-70 Ethnic Foods
A-74 Fast Foods/Restaurants   A-88 Fats, Oils, Margarines, Shortenings, and Substitutes   A-88 Fish, Seafood, and Shellfish   A-90 Food Additives
A-90 Fruit, Vegetable, or Blended Juices   A-92 Grains, Flours, and Fractions   A-92 Grain Products, Prepared and Baked Goods

Code	Food Name	Unit/ Amt	Wt (g)	Energy (kcal)	Prot (g)	Carb (g)	Fiber (g)	Fat (g)	Sat (g)	Mono (g)	Poly (g)	Chol (mg)	Vit A (RE)
61253	Chips, potato, fat free	100 g	100	379	10	84	8	1	0.2	0.0	0.3	0	2
44230	Chips, potato, original	18 pce	28	148	2	15	1	10	3.0	1.9	5.0	0	0
44241	Chips, potato, rducd fat	16 pce	28	128	2	18	1	7	1.0	1.6	4.1	0	0
44238	Chips, potato, unsalted	19 pce	28	158	2	16	1	10	3.0	—	—	0	0
44301	Chips, tortilla, blue corn	18 pce	28	110	3	22	2	2	0.0	—	—	0	0
44224	Chips, tortilla, cooler ranch	15 pce	28	138	2	18	1	7	1.5	1.9	2.2	0	0
61156	Chips, tortilla, light, bkd	10 ea	16	74	1	12	1	2	0.5	1.0	0.8	0	1
44225	Chips, tortilla, nacho cheesier	15 pce	28	138	2	17	1	7	1.5	1.9	2.2	0	0
4039	Chips, tortilla, salsa verde	12 pce	28	150	2	19	1	7	1.5	3.0	2.5	0	0
44223	Chips, tortilla, tstd corn	13 pce	28	138	2	18	1	7	1.5	—	—	0	0
44298	Chips, tortilla, yellow corn	18 pce	28	110	3	22	2	2	0.0	—	—	0	0
44087	Corn Cake, butter flvr	1 ea	9	34	1	7	0	0	0.1	0.1	0.1	0	4
44308	Corn Cake, caramel flvrd	1 ea	13	50	1	12	0	0	0.0	0.1	0.1	0	4
44031	Corn Nuts, plain	1 oz	28	126	2	20	2	4	0.7	2.7	0.9	0	0
44212	Fruit Leather, bar	1 ea	23	81	0	18	1	1	0.9	0.1	0.0	0	3
23404	Fruit Leather, roll, lrg	1 ea	21	78	0	18	1	1	0.1	0.3	0.1	0	3
44022	Popcorn Cake	1 ea	10	38	1	8	0	0	0.0	0.1	0.1	0	1
44014	Popcorn, caramel coated, w/o peanuts	1 oz	28	122	1	22	1	4	1.0	0.8	1.3	1	1
44038	Popcorn, cheese flvrd	1 cup	11	58	1	6	1	4	0.7	1.1	1.7	1	5
43701	Popcorn, Cracker Jacks, original	0.5 cup	28	120	2	23	1	2	0.0	—	—	0	0
44065	Popcorn, microwv	1 ea	87	435	8	50	9	24	4.3	7.1	11.7	0	13
44013	Popcorn, oil popped	1 cup	11	55	1	6	1	3	0.5	0.9	1.5	0	2
44072	Popcorn, white, air popped	1 cup	8	31	1	6	1	0	0.0	0.1	0.2	0	0
44015	Pretzels, hard	5 pce	30	114	3	24	1	1	0.2	0.4	0.4	0	0
44215	Pretzels, hard, chocolate coated	1 ea	11	50	1	8	0	2	0.8	0.6	0.2	0	0
61182	Pretzels, soft, med	1 ea	115	389	9	80	2	4	0.8	1.2	1.1	3	0
60899	Rice Cake, brown	1 ea	20	74	1	16	0	0	0.1	0.2	0.2	—	0
44017	Rice Cake, caramel corn, mini	1 ea	3	13	0	3	0	0	0.1	0.0	0.0	0	1
44016	Rice Cake, plain	1 ea	9	35	1	7	0	0	0.1	0.1	0.1	0	0
44032	Snack Mix, Chex	1 cup	42	181	5	28	2	7	2.4	3.9	1.1	0	6
57096	Snack, cheese n' crackers, pkg	1 ea	27	100	2	10	0	6	2.0	—	—	10	20
44248	Snack, cheese puffs, Cheetos	29 pce	28	158	2	15	1	10	2.5	2.7	3.1	0	0
44058	Trail Mix, regular	0.25 cup	38	173	5	17	2	11	2.1	4.7	3.6	0	1
44060	Trail Mix, tropical	1 cup	140	570	9	92	9	24	11.9	3.5	7.2	0	6
44059	Trail Mix, w/chocolate chips, salted nuts & seeds	0.25 cup	36	175	5	16	2	12	2.2	4.9	4.1	1	1

SOUPS, STEWS AND CHILIS

Canned/Frozen/Prepared Soups, Stews and Chilis

Code	Food Name	Unit/ Amt	Wt (g)	Energy (kcal)	Prot (g)	Carb (g)	Fiber (g)	Fat (g)	Sat (g)	Mono (g)	Poly (g)	Chol (mg)	Vit A (RE)
50595	Bouillon/Broth, beef, clear, cnd	1 cup	198	15	2	0	0	0	0.0	—	—	0	0
50596	Broth, chicken, clear, rts, cnd	1 cup	198	15	1	1	0	0	0.0	—	—	5	0
50312	Chili, con carne	1 cup	253	256	25	22	—	8	3.4	3.4	0.5	134	167
7760	Chili, vegetarian, cnd	1 cup	230	176	16	26	13	1	0.2	0.2	0.5	1	47
56001	Chili, w/beans, cnd	1 cup	256	287	15	30	11	14	6.0	6.0	0.9	44	87
50901	Chili, w/beef, rts, cnd	1 cup	245	190	16	34	8	2	0.5	—	—	5	100
28167	Chili, w/o beans, cnd	100 g	100	118	8	6	—	7	2.3	2.5	0.5	21	—
50406	Chowder, clam, New England, rts, cnd	1 cup	244	117	5	20	1	2	0.5	0.7	0.4	5	49

Thia (mg)	Ribo (mg)	Niac (mg NE)	Vit B6 (mg)	Vit B12 (µg)	Fol (µg)	Vit C (mg)	Vit D (IU)	Vit E (mg AT)	Cal (mg)	Iron (mg)	Magn (mg)	Phos (mg)	Pota (mg)	Sodi (mg)	Zinc (mg)	Wat (%)	Alco (g)	Caff (g)
1.08	0.11	6.44	0.80	0.00	45.0	9.3	—	0.0	35	3.56	70.0	167	1628	643	0.7	2	0.00	0.00
0.05	0.03	1.09	—	0.00	—	5.9	—	—	6	0.44	—	44	489	178	0.4	2	0.00	0.00
0.03	0.05	1.09	—	0.00	—	5.9	—	—	0	0.36	—	45	356	158	0.3	2	0.00	0.00
—	—	—	—	0.00	—	5.9	—	—	0	0.00	—	—	—	15	—	—	0.00	0.00
—	—	—	—	—	—	0.0	—	—	60	0.36	—	—	—	140	—	4	0.00	—
0.02	0.02	0.49	—	—	—	0.0	—	—	40	0.41	—	64	69	168	0.0	2	0.00	0.00
0.03	0.03	0.07	0.02	0.00	2.6	0.0	—	0.6	25	0.25	15.5	51	44	160	0.2	1	0.00	0.00
0.02	0.02	0.40	—	—	—	0.0	—	—	43	0.41	—	59	64	188	0.0	6	0.00	0.00
0.02	0.00	0.43	—	—	—	0.0	—	—	20	0.00	—	18	38	210	0.2	—	0.00	0.00
—	—	—	—	—	—	0.0	—	—	40	0.00	—	—	—	119	—	2	0.00	0.00
—	—	—	—	—	—	0.0	—	—	60	0.36	—	—	—	160	—	3	0.00	—
0.01	0.00	0.34	0.02	0.00	3.0	0.0	0.0	0.0	1	0.07	8.9	20	17	45	0.1	6	0.00	0.00
0.02	0.00	0.31	0.03	0.00	3.0	0.0	—	0.0	1	0.07	8.9	20	15	28	0.1	3	0.00	0.00
0.00	0.03	0.47	0.05	0.00	0.0	0.0	—	0.6	3	0.46	32.0	78	79	156	0.5	1	0.00	0.00
0.00	0.00	0.01	0.07	0.00	0.9	16.1	—	0.1	7	0.18	5.1	13	32	18	0.0	14	0.00	0.00
0.01	0.00	0.01	0.05	0.00	0.8	25.2	—	0.1	7	0.20	4.2	7	62	67	0.0	10	0.00	0.00
0.00	0.01	0.60	0.01	0.00	1.8	0.0	—	0.0	1	0.18	15.9	28	33	29	0.4	5	0.00	0.00
0.01	0.01	0.62	0.00	0.00	1.4	0.0	—	0.3	12	0.49	9.9	24	31	58	0.2	3	0.00	0.00
0.00	0.02	0.15	0.02	0.05	1.2	0.1	—	0.0	12	0.25	10.0	40	29	98	0.2	2	0.00	0.00
—	—	—	—	—	—	0.0	—	—	0	0.00	—	—	—	70	—	—	0.00	0.00
0.11	0.11	1.35	0.18	0.00	14.8	0.3	—	0.1	9	2.42	94.0	218	196	769	2.3	3	0.00	0.00
0.00	0.00	0.17	0.01	0.00	1.9	0.0	—	0.6	1	0.31	11.9	28	25	97	0.3	3	0.00	0.00
0.01	0.01	0.15	0.01	0.00	1.8	0.0	—	0.0	1	0.20	10.5	24	24	0	0.3	4	0.00	0.00
0.14	0.18	1.58	0.02	0.00	51.3	0.0	—	0.1	11	1.29	10.5	34	44	514	0.3	3	0.00	0.00
0.00	0.01	0.09	0.01	0.00	1.0	0.1	—	0.0	8	0.21	4.5	16	25	63	0.1	2	0.00	—
0.46	0.33	4.90	0.01	0.00	27.6	0.0	—	0.6	26	4.51	24.1	91	101	1615	1.1	15	0.00	0.00
—	—	—	—	—	—	0.0	—	—	5	0.15	—	—	67	57	—	5	0.00	0.00
0.00	0.00	0.10	0.00	0.00	0.6	0.0	0.0	0.0	1	0.02	2.6	6	6	14	0.0	2	0.00	0.00
0.03	0.00	0.58	0.05	0.00	1.8	0.0	0.0	0.0	1	0.12	14.2	33	25	14	2.0	3	0.00	0.00
0.66	0.20	7.15	0.66	5.26	21.2	20.2	—	0.1	15	10.50	26.8	79	114	432	0.9	4	0.00	0.00
—	—	—	—	—	—	0.0	—	—	60	0.36	—	—	—	331	—	—	0.00	0.00
0.10	0.05	0.72	—	—	—	0.0	—	—	22	0.58	—	15	20	365	0.0	2	0.00	0.00
0.17	0.07	1.76	0.10	0.00	26.6	0.5	—	1.3	29	1.13	59.2	129	257	86	1.2	9	0.00	0.00
0.62	0.15	2.06	0.46	0.00	58.8	10.6	—	3.1	80	3.70	134.4	260	993	14	1.6	9	0.00	0.00
0.15	0.07	1.60	0.09	0.00	23.6	0.5	—	3.9	40	1.23	58.4	140	235	44	1.1	7	0.00	2.18
—	—	—	—	—	—	0.0	—	—	0	0.00	—	—	—	890	—	98	0.00	0.00
—	—	—	—	—	—	0.0	—	—	0	0.00	—	—	—	960	—	—	0.00	0.00
0.12	1.13	2.48	0.33	1.13	45.5	1.5	—	1.6	68	5.19	45.5	197	691	1007	3.6	77	0.00	0.00
0.00	0.15	0.00	—	0.00	—	0.0	—	—	40	3.68	—	237	645	1144	0.6	79	0.00	0.00
0.11	0.27	0.92	0.34	0.00	58.9	4.4	—	1.5	120	8.77	115.2	394	934	1336	5.1	76	0.00	0.00
—	—	—	—	—	—	2.4	—	—	100	4.50	—	—	—	480	—	—	0.00	0.00
0.02	0.10	1.25	0.12	1.01	—	1.8	—	—	30	2.00	20.0	77	185	389	1.1	78	0.00	0.00
0.05	0.09	0.86	0.09	6.17	29.3	5.1	—	0.6	17	0.89	12.2	59	283	529	0.4	89	0.00	0.00

PAGE KEY: A-46 Beverage and Beverage Mixes A-48 Other Beverages A-48 Beverages, Alcoholic A-50 Candies and Confections, Gum A-54 Cereals, Breakfast Type A-58 Cheese and Cheese Substitutes A-60 Dairy Products and Substitutes A-62 Desserts A-68 Dessert Toppings A-68 Eggs, Substitutes, and Egg Dishes A-70 Ethnic Foods A-74 Fast Foods/Restaurants A-88 Fats, Oils, Margarines, Shortenings, and Substitutes A-88 Fish, Seafood, and Shellfish A-90 Food Additives A-90 Fruit, Vegetable, or Blended Juices A-92 Grains, Flours, and Fractions A-92 Grain Products, Prepared and Baked Goods

Code	Food Name	Unit/ Amt	Wt (g)	Energy (kcal)	Prot (g)	Carb (g)	Fiber (g)	Fat (g)	Sat (g)	Mono (g)	Poly (g)	Chol (mg)	Vit A (RE)
50907	Chowder, clam, New England, rts, cnd	1 cup	251	120	5	24	4	2	1.0	—	—	10	0
50647	Soup, bean & pork, cond, cnd, cmrcl	1 cup	269	347	16	46	16	12	3.1	4.4	3.7	5	180
50003	Soup, beef noodle, prep f/cnd w/water, cmrcl	1 cup	244	83	5	9	1	3	1.1	1.2	0.5	5	12
50399	Soup, beef vegetable, rts, cnd	1 cup	241	154	10	25	6	2	0.6	0.6	0.2	14	415
50686	Soup, chicken mushroom, cond, cnd, cmrcl	1 cup	251	274	9	19	1	18	4.8	8.1	4.6	20	25
50080	Soup, chicken mushroom, prep f/cnd w/water, cmrcl	1 cup	244	132	4	9	0	9	2.4	4.0	2.3	10	112
50982	Soup, chicken noodle, chunky, rts, cnd, svg	1 ea	243	114	8	14	—	3	0.8	1.2	0.6	24	262
50400	Soup, chicken noodle, rts, cnd	1 cup	237	76	6	9	1	2	0.4	0.6	0.4	19	182
50020	Soup, chicken rice, prep f/cnd w/water, cmrcl	1 cup	241	60	4	7	1	2	0.5	0.9	0.4	7	43
50091	Soup, chicken vegetable, prep f/cnd w/water, cmrcl	1 cup	241	75	4	9	1	3	0.8	1.3	0.6	10	193
50402	Soup, cream of broccoli, rts, cnd	1 cup	244	88	2	13	2	3	0.7	0.9	0.6	5	59
50654	Soup, cream of chicken, cond, cnd, cmrcl	1 cup	251	223	6	18	0	14	4.0	5.1	2.6	20	113
50666	Soup, cream of mushroom, cond, cnd, cmrcl	1 cup	251	213	4	17	0	15	3.4	2.8	3.6	0	20
50049	Soup, cream of mushroom, prep f/cnd w/water, cmrcl	1 cup	244	129	2	9	0	9	2.4	1.7	4.2	2	17
50197	Soup, cream of potato, prep f/cnd w/water, cmrcl	1 cup	244	73	2	11	0	2	1.2	0.6	0.4	5	76
50999	Soup, gumbo, zesty, rts, cnd	1 cup	244	100	6	15	3	2	1.0	—	—	10	40
50404	Soup, lentil, rts, cnd	1 cup	242	126	8	20	6	2	0.3	0.8	0.2	0	191
50405	Soup, minestrone, rts, cnd	1 cup	241	123	5	20	1	3	0.4	0.9	1.0	0	272
50486	Soup, onion, French, cond, cnd	0.5 cup	119	45	2	6	1	2	0.5	—	—	5	0
50403	Soup, pasta & garlic, rts, cnd	1 cup	243	100	4	20	3	1	0.3	0.4	0.5	5	311
50050	Soup, pea, green, prep f/cnd w/water, cmrcl	1 cup	250	165	9	26	3	3	1.4	1.0	0.4	0	20
50407	Soup, split pea, rts, cnd	1 cup	253	180	10	30	5	2	0.8	0.9	0.4	5	142
50504	Soup, tomato, cond, cnd	0.5 cup	122	90	2	20	1	0	0.0	0.0	0.0	0	100
50409	Soup, vegetable, rts, cnd	1 cup	238	81	4	13	1	1	0.3	0.4	0.3	5	640
57659	Stew, beef, cnd, svg	1 ea	232	218	11	16	3	12	5.2	5.5	0.5	37	385
7559	Stew, vegetarian	1 cup	247	304	42	17	3	7	1.2	1.8	3.8	0	232
Dry and Prepared Soups and Chilis													
90243	Broth, beef, dry cube, svg	1.33 ea	5	8	1	1	0	0	0.1	0.1	0.0	0	0
90247	Broth, chicken, cube, dry svg	1 ea	6	13	1	2	0	0	0.1	0.1	0.1	1	0
50037	Soup, chicken noodle, prep f/dehyd w/water	1 cup	252	58	2	9	0	1	0.3	0.5	0.4	10	5
50036	Soup, cream of chicken, prep f/dehyd w/water	1 cup	261	107	2	13	0	5	3.4	1.2	0.4	3	42
90346	Soup, minestrone, prep f/pkt w/water	1 ea	1142	354	20	54	—	8	3.7	3.3	0.5	11	137
50039	Soup, mushroom, prep f/dehyd w/water, pkt	1 ea	194	74	2	9	1	4	0.6	1.7	1.2	0	14
50040	Soup, onion, prep f/dehyd w/water, pkt	1 ea	184	20	1	4	1	0	0.1	0.2	0.1	0	0
92163	Soup, ramen noodle, any flvr, dry	3.6 oz	100	453	9	66	2	17	7.6	6.4	2.6	0	2
50042	Soup, tomato, prep f/dry w/water, pkt	1 ea	199	78	2	15	0	2	0.8	0.7	0.2	0	66
50044	Soup, vegetable beef, prep f/dry w/water	1 cup	253	53	3	8	1	1	0.6	0.5	0.1	0	25
Homemade/Generic Soups and Chilis													
50709	Broth, vegetable	1 cup	235	16	2	2	0	0	—	—	—	0	1
92757	Chili, con carne, w/beans & chicken	1 cup	254	217	17	27	7	5	1.2	1.9	1.5	33	124
50211	Chowder, fish	1 cup	244	194	24	12	1	5	2.4	1.9	0.6	56	63
50077	Soup, chicken gumbo, prep f/cnd w/water, cmrcl	1 cup	244	56	3	8	2	1	0.3	0.7	0.3	5	15
SPICES, FLAVORS, AND SEASONINGS													
90622	Salt Substitute, Mrs. Dash, original blend	0.25 tsp	1	0	0	0	0	0	0.0	0.0	0.0	0	0
26632	Salt Substitute, Nu-Salt, no sod, pkt	1 g	1	0	0	0	0	0	0.0	0.0	0.0	0	0
26014	Salt, table	0.25 tsp	2	0	0	0	0	0	0.0	0.0	0.0	0	0

Thia (mg)	Ribo (mg)	Niac (mg NE)	Vit B6 (mg)	Vit B12 (µg)	Fol (µg)	Vit C (mg)	Vit D (IU)	Vit E (mg AT)	Cal (mg)	Iron (mg)	Magn (mg)	Phos (mg)	Pota (mg)	Sodi (mg)	Zinc (mg)	Wat (%)	Alco (g)	Caff (g)
—	—	—	—	—	—	4.8	—	—	20	0.72	—	—	—	480	—	86	0.00	0.00
0.17	0.07	1.12	0.07	0.07	64.6	3.2	—	2.3	161	4.11	88.8	264	807	1907	2.1	70	0.00	0.00
0.07	0.05	1.07	0.03	0.20	19.5	0.2	—	0.7	15	1.10	4.9	46	100	952	1.5	92	0.00	0.00
0.10	0.11	2.80	0.25	0.31	24.1	4.6	—	0.5	14	1.77	31.3	99	605	405	1.3	85	0.00	0.00
0.05	0.23	3.25	0.10	0.12	5.0	0.0	—	1.6	58	1.75	17.6	55	316	1940	2.0	80	0.00	0.00
0.01	0.10	1.62	0.05	0.05	0.0	0.0	—	1.2	29	0.87	9.8	27	154	942	1.0	90	0.00	0.00
—	—	—	—	—	—	—	—	—	—	1.19	—	—	—	875	—	89	0.00	0.00
0.10	0.10	3.44	0.05	0.20	33.2	0.7	—	0.1	19	1.11	9.5	85	209	460	0.4	92	0.00	0.00
0.01	0.01	1.12	0.01	0.14	0.0	0.2	—	0.1	17	0.75	0.0	22	101	815	0.3	94	0.00	0.00
0.03	0.05	1.23	0.05	0.11	4.8	1.0	—	0.4	17	0.87	7.2	41	154	945	0.4	93	0.00	0.00
0.02	0.05	0.31	0.07	0.00	29.3	5.9	—	0.4	41	1.22	14.6	39	161	578	0.3	92	0.00	0.00
0.02	0.11	0.98	0.00	0.00	5.0	0.3	—	1.4	35	2.66	10.0	78	123	1644	0.7	83	0.00	0.00
0.10	0.10	1.05	0.00	0.00	5.0	0.0	—	2.0	30	2.78	10.0	65	156	1619	0.5	84	0.00	0.00
0.05	0.09	0.72	0.00	0.05	4.9	1.0	—	1.0	46	0.50	4.9	49	100	881	0.6	90	0.00	0.00
0.02	0.03	0.54	0.03	0.05	2.4	0.0	—	0.0	20	0.49	2.4	46	137	1000	0.6	92	0.00	0.00
—	—	—	—	—	—	3.6	—	—	40	0.72	—	—	—	480	—	88	0.00	0.00
0.10	0.09	0.69	0.15	0.00	101.6	1.0	—	0.6	41	2.66	41.1	128	336	443	1.0	88	0.00	0.00
0.15	0.07	1.02	0.14	0.00	60.3	0.7	—	0.7	39	1.69	31.3	87	306	470	0.7	87	0.00	0.00
—	—	—	—	—	—	0.0	—	—	20	0.00	—	—	—	900	—	90	0.00	0.00
0.23	0.12	2.03	0.10	0.00	63.2	0.0	—	0.5	51	0.87	34.0	87	299	450	0.6	88	0.00	0.00
0.10	0.07	1.24	0.05	0.00	2.5	1.8	—	0.4	28	1.95	40.0	125	190	918	1.7	83	0.00	0.00
0.18	0.07	1.15	0.18	0.02	50.6	0.0	—	0.5	43	1.95	35.4	137	463	420	1.0	82	0.00	0.00
—	—	—	—	—	—	6.0	—	—	0	0.72	—	—	—	710	—	80	0.00	0.00
0.07	0.07	1.83	0.07	0.07	28.6	1.4	—	0.1	31	1.51	21.4	74	290	466	0.4	91	0.00	0.00
0.17	0.14	2.85	0.30	0.86	25.5	10.2	—	0.2	28	1.64	32.5	128	404	947	1.9	82	0.00	0.00
1.73	1.48	29.63	2.72	5.42	254.4	0.0	—	1.2	77	3.21	313.7	543	296	988	2.7	70	0.00	0.00
0.00	0.00	0.15	0.00	0.05	1.5	0.0	—	0.0	3	0.10	2.4	11	19	1152	0.0	3	0.00	0.00
0.00	0.01	0.25	0.00	0.01	2.0	0.1	0.0	0.0	12	0.11	3.6	12	24	1536	0.0	2	0.00	0.00
0.20	0.07	1.09	0.02	0.05	17.7	0.0	—	0.1	5	0.50	7.6	30	33	578	0.2	94	0.00	0.00
0.10	0.20	2.60	0.05	0.25	5.2	0.5	—	0.6	76	0.25	5.2	97	214	1185	1.6	91	0.00	0.00
0.34	0.23	4.57	0.46	0.00	159.9	4.6	—	0.2	171	4.57	34.3	274	1531	4616	3.4	92	0.00	0.00
0.21	0.09	0.37	0.01	0.18	3.9	0.8	—	0.4	50	0.38	3.9	58	153	782	0.1	92	0.00	0.00
0.01	0.03	0.36	0.00	0.00	1.8	0.2	—	0.0	9	0.10	3.7	22	48	635	0.0	96	0.00	0.00
0.66	0.43	5.40	0.05	0.00	147.0	0.0	—	2.0	16	4.26	24.0	108	120	1160	0.6	5	0.00	0.00
0.05	0.03	0.58	0.07	0.05	6.0	3.4	—	0.4	40	0.31	9.9	50	221	708	0.2	90	0.00	0.00
0.02	0.03	0.46	0.05	0.25	7.6	1.3	—	0.2	13	0.86	22.8	35	76	1002	0.3	94	0.00	0.00
0.00	0.01	0.54	0.01	0.11	3.8	0.0	—	0.0	7	0.11	7.0	38	54	3114	0.0	95	0.00	0.00
0.21	0.23	5.17	0.36	0.11	58.0	21.4	—	1.7	58	2.68	53.1	195	682	874	1.5	79	0.00	0.00
0.17	0.25	2.88	0.36	1.25	16.3	7.3	—	0.4	148	0.70	49.1	298	711	180	1.1	83	0.00	0.00
0.01	0.05	0.66	0.05	0.01	4.9	4.9	—	0.4	24	0.89	4.9	24	76	954	0.4	94	0.00	0.00
—	—	—	—	0.00	—	0.0	—	—	0	0.00	—	—	—	0	—	—	0.00	0.00
—	—	—	—	—	—	0.0	—	0.0	0	—	0.0	—	530	0	—	—	0.00	0.00
0.00	0.00	0.00	0.00	0.00	0.0	0.0	—	0.0	0	0.00	0.0	0	0	581	0.0	0	0.00	0.00

Code	Food Name	Unit/ Amt	Wt (g)	Energy (kcal)	Prot (g)	Carb (g)	Fiber (g)	Fat (g)	Sat (g)	Mono (g)	Poly (g)	Chol (mg)	Vit A (RE)
53439	Sea Salt	100 g	100	0	0	0	0	0	0.0	0.0	0.0	0	0
669	Seasoning, garlic salt	0.25 tsp	1	0	0	0	0	0	0.0	0.0	0.0	—	—
26604	Seasoning, lemon pepper	1 tsp	2	2	0	0	0	0	0.0	0.0	0.0	0	0
26028	Seasoning, poultry	1 tsp	2	5	0	1	0	0	0.0	0.0	0.0	0	4
26004	Spice Blend, curry, pwd	1 tsp	2	6	0	1	1	0	0.0	0.1	0.1	0	2
26001	Spice, basil, ground	1 tsp	1	4	0	1	1	0	0.0	0.0	0.0	0	13
26524	Spice, chili pepper, ground, domestic	1 tsp	2	6	0	1	1	0	—	—	—	—	42
26002	Spice, chili pepper, pwd	1 tsp	3	8	0	1	1	0	0.1	0.1	0.2	0	77
7395	Spice, cilantro, dehyd	100 g	100	265	31	34	11	8	0.2	3.7	0.5	0	3670
26003	Spice, cinnamon, ground	1 tsp	2	6	0	2	1	0	0.0	0.0	0.0	0	1
26019	Spice, clove, ground	1 tsp	2	7	0	1	1	0	0.1	0.0	0.1	0	1
26109	Spice, dill seed	1 tsp	2	6	0	1	0	0	0.0	0.2	0.0	0	0
26065	Spice, garlic powder	1 tsp	3	8	0	2	1	0	—	—	—	0	0
26008	Spice, onion, powder	1 tsp	2	7	0	2	0	0	0.0	0.0	0.0	0	0
26009	Spice, oregano, ground	1 tsp	2	5	0	1	1	0	0.0	0.0	0.1	0	10
26010	Spice, paprika	1 tsp	2	6	0	1	1	0	0.0	0.0	0.2	0	111
26522	Spice, pepper, black, ground	1 tsp	2	7	0	1	1	0	—	—	—	—	2
26628	Spice, peppermint, fresh	2 Tbs	3	2	0	0	0	0	0.0	0.0	0.0	0	14
26015	Spice, poppy seed	1 tsp	3	15	1	1	0	1	0.1	0.2	0.9	0	0
26631	Spice, spearmint, dried	1 Tbs	2	5	0	1	0	0	0.0	0.0	0.1	0	17
26033	Spice, thyme, ground	1 tsp	1	4	0	1	1	0	0.0	0.0	0.0	0	5
SPORTS BARS AND DRINKS													
62275	Bar, energy, apple cinnamon	1 ea	65	230	10	45	3	2	0.5	1.5	0.5	0	0
62714	Bar, energy, carrot cake	1 ea	68	234	10	41	5	4	1.8	—	—	0	884
62278	Bar, energy, chocolate	1 ea	65	230	10	45	3	2	0.5	0.5	1.0	0	0
62715	Bar, energy, chocolate almond fudge	1 ea	68	231	10	38	5	5	0.9	—	—	0	276
62709	Bar, energy, chocolate chip	1 ea	68	238	10	42	5	4	0.9	—	—	0	278
62831	Bar, energy, chocolate fudge brownie	1 ea	78	290	24	38	4	5	4.0	—	—	5	0
62561	Bar, energy, chocolate peanut butter	1 ea	65	230	10	45	3	3	0.5	1.5	1.0	0	0
62716	Bar, energy, cookies & cream	1 ea	68	225	10	39	5	4	1.5	—	—	0	277
62725	Bar, energy, honey peanut	1 ea	50	200	14	22	1	6	3.5	—	—	3	500
62710	Bar, energy, peanut butter	1 ea	68	240	12	38	5	5	0.8	—	—	0	277
62205	Bar, energy, peanut butter, Tiger's Milk	1 ea	35	140	6	18	1	5	1.0	—	—	0	150
62821	Bar, energy, vanilla crisp	1 ea	65	230	9	45	3	2	0.5	1.5	0.5	0	0
62833	Carbohydrate Gel, chocolate, pkt	1 ea	41	120	0	28	0	2	1.0	—	—	0	0
63031	Drink, protein, Max Whey, all flvrs, pwd, scoop	1 ea	27	88	20	3	0	1	—	—	—	25	0
62995	Formula, Myoplex Pro, vanilla, rtd	0.33 ea	250	110	15	8	2	2	0.5	—	—	13	168
20142	Sports Drink, btld	1 cup	241	60	0	15	0	0	0.0	0.0	0.0	0	0
20558	Sports Drink, grape, can/btl	1 cup	247	73	0	19	0	0	0.0	0.0	0.0	0	0
20559	Sports Drink, lemon lime, can/btl	1 cup	247	72	0	19	0	0	0.0	0.0	0.0	0	0
SUPPLEMENTAL FOODS AND FORMULAS—CHILD/ADULT													
Medical Nutritionals													
63162	Instant Breakfast, supplement, chocolate, rtu	1 ea	260	390	12	44	0	12	2.0	—	—	5	250
62761	Instant Breakfast, supplement, straw, liquid, rts	8 fl-oz	250	250	12	33	0	8	—	—	—	18	250
62760	Instant Breakfast, supplement, van, liquid, rts	8 fl-oz	250	250	12	33	0	8	—	—	—	18	250

PAGE KEY: A-96 Granola Bars, Cereal Bars, Diet Bars, Scones, and Tarts   A-96 Meals and Dishes   A-100 Meats   A-106 Nuts, Seeds, and Products   A-108 Poultry
A-110 Salad Dressings, Dips, and Mayonnaise   A-110 Salads   A-110 Sandwiches   A-114 Sauces and Gravies   A-114 Snack Foods—Chips, Pretzels, Popcorn
A-116 Soups, Stews, and Chilis   A-118 Spices, Flavors, and Seasonings   A-120 Sports Bars and Drinks   A-120 Supplemental Foods and Formulas
A-122 Sweeteners and Sweet Substitutes   A-122 Vegetables and Legumes   A-136 Weight Loss Bars and Drinks   A-138 Miscellaneous

Thia (mg)	Ribo (mg)	Niac (mg NE)	Vit B6 (mg)	Vit B12 (μg)	Fol (μg)	Vit C (mg)	Vit D (IU)	Vit E (mg AT)	Cal (mg)	Iron (mg)	Magn (mg)	Phos (mg)	Pota (mg)	Sodi (mg)	Zinc (mg)	Wat (%)	Alco (g)	Caff (g)
0.00	0.00	0.00	0.00	0.00	0.0	0.0	0.0	0.0	12	380.00	500.0	0	260	32000	870.0	7	0.00	0.00
—	—	—	—	0.00	—	—	—	—	—	—	—	—	—	240	—	11	0.00	0.00
0.00	0.00	0.00	0.00	0.00	0.0	0.0	0.0	0.0	3	0.10	0.8	1	6	461	0.0	2	0.00	0.00
0.00	0.00	0.03	0.01	0.00	2.1	0.2	0.0	0.0	15	0.52	3.4	3	10	0	0.0	9	0.00	0.00
0.00	0.00	0.07	0.01	0.00	3.1	0.2	0.0	0.4	10	0.58	5.1	7	31	1	0.1	10	0.00	0.00
0.00	0.00	0.10	0.02	0.00	3.8	0.9	0.0	0.1	30	0.58	5.9	7	48	0	0.1	6	0.00	0.00
—	—	—	—	0.00	—	0.7	—	—	4	0.23	—	—	—	3	—	14	0.00	0.00
0.00	0.01	0.20	0.10	0.00	2.6	1.7	0.0	0.8	7	0.37	4.4	8	50	26	0.1	8	0.00	0.00
0.93	1.59	9.68	1.46	0.00	137.0	139.0	—	—	1300	25.89	345.0	478	7189	371	6.0	4	0.00	0.00
0.00	0.00	0.02	0.00	0.00	0.7	0.7	0.0	0.0	28	0.87	1.3	1	12	1	0.0	10	0.00	0.00
0.00	0.00	0.02	0.00	0.00	2.0	1.7	0.0	0.2	14	0.18	5.5	2	23	5	0.0	7	0.00	0.00
0.00	0.00	0.05	0.00	0.00	0.2	0.4	0.0	0.0	32	0.34	5.4	6	25	0	0.1	8	0.00	0.00
0.00	0.00	0.01	—	0.00	—	0.1	—	—	3	0.01	—	—	38	1	—	6	0.00	0.00
0.00	0.00	0.00	0.02	0.00	3.5	0.3	0.0	0.0	8	0.05	2.6	7	20	1	0.0	5	0.00	0.00
0.00	0.00	0.09	0.01	0.00	4.1	0.8	0.0	0.3	24	0.66	4.0	3	25	0	0.1	7	0.00	0.00
0.00	0.03	0.31	0.07	0.00	2.2	1.5	0.0	0.6	4	0.50	3.9	7	49	1	0.1	10	0.00	0.00
—	—	—	—	0.00	—	0.0	—	—	8	0.15	—	—	—	0	—	12	0.00	0.00
0.00	0.00	0.05	0.00	0.00	3.6	1.0	—	0.0	8	0.15	2.6	2	18	1	0.0	79	0.00	0.00
0.01	0.00	0.02	0.00	0.00	1.6	0.1	0.0	0.0	41	0.25	9.3	24	20	1	0.3	7	0.00	0.00
0.00	0.01	0.10	0.03	0.00	8.5	0.0	—	0.0	24	1.39	9.6	4	31	6	0.0	11	0.00	0.00
0.00	0.00	0.07	0.00	0.00	3.8	0.7	0.0	0.1	26	1.73	3.1	3	11	1	0.1	8	0.00	0.00
1.50	1.70	20.00	2.00	6.00	400.0	60.0	—	18.4	300	6.30	140.0	350	110	90	5.2	—	0.00	0.00
0.37	0.28	3.54	0.41	0.98	87.0	67.1	—	20.2	275	5.32	103.2	298	246	170	3.2	17	0.00	0.00
1.50	1.70	20.00	2.00	6.00	400.0	60.0	—	18.4	300	6.30	140.0	350	145	90	5.2	—	0.00	15.00
0.38	0.31	3.63	0.43	0.98	84.6	65.7	—	20.8	278	5.73	128.3	304	232	139	3.7	19	0.00	0.00
0.34	0.28	3.49	0.38	0.98	85.6	66.1	—	20.3	265	5.21	95.5	286	206	76	3.5	15	0.00	—
1.50	1.70	20.00	2.00	6.00	400.0	60.0	—	18.3	300	6.30	140.0	350	—	150	5.2	—	0.00	—
1.50	1.70	20.00	2.00	6.00	400.0	60.0	—	18.3	300	6.30	140.0	350	140	95	5.2	—	0.00	—
0.34	0.27	3.45	0.43	0.98	85.1	66.2	—	20.3	279	5.23	102.6	266	212	179	3.2	20	0.00	0.00
0.60	0.50	9.00	0.60	1.20	80.0	60.0	80.0	13.6	100	3.59	40.0	100	115	220	3.0	—	0.00	—
0.40	0.30	6.25	0.41	0.98	96.2	65.8	—	20.4	268	5.30	113.7	305	301	289	3.6	15	0.00	0.00
1.26	0.60	3.00	0.60	1.50	—	6.0	60.0	—	300	2.70	100.0	100	—	75	—	—	0.00	0.00
1.50	1.70	20.00	2.00	6.00	400.0	60.0	—	18.3	300	6.30	140.0	350	110	90	5.2	—	0.00	0.00
—	—	—	—	—	—	9.0	—	2.8	0	0.00	—	—	40	50	—	—	0.00	25.00
—	—	—	—	—	—	0.0	—	—	0	0.00	—	—	35	—	10	0.00	—
0.25	0.33	3.32	0.33	1.33	120.0	15.0	66.7	4.5	110	—	59.3	141	167	177	2.5	—	0.00	0.00
0.00	0.00	0.00	0.00	0.00	0.0	0.0	0.0	0.0	0	0.11	2.4	22	26	96	0.0	94	0.00	0.00
—	—	—	—	—	—	0.0	—	—	0	0.00	—	—	32	28	—	—	0.00	0.00
—	—	—	—	—	—	0.0	—	—	0	0.00	—	—	32	28	—	—	0.00	0.00
0.37	0.43	5.00	0.50	1.50	100.0	15.0	—	—	250	4.50	100.0	250	430	120	3.8	—	0.00	—
0.37	0.43	5.00	0.50	1.50	1000.0	15.0	100.0	3.4	300	4.50	60.0	300	480	190	3.8	—	0.00	0.00
0.37	0.43	5.00	0.50	1.50	1000.0	15.0	100.0	3.4	300	4.50	60.0	300	480	190	3.8	—	0.00	0.00

PAGE KEY: A-46 Beverage and Beverage Mixes   A-48 Other Beverages   A-48 Beverages, Alcoholic   A-50 Candies and Confections, Gum   A-54 Cereals, Breakfast Type
A-58 Cheese and Cheese Substitutes   A-60 Dairy Products and Substitutes   A-62 Desserts   A-68 Dessert Toppings   A-68 Eggs, Substitutes, and Egg Dishes   A-70 Ethnic Foods
A-74 Fast Foods/Restaurants   A-88 Fats, Oils, Margarines, Shortenings, and Substitutes   A-88 Fish, Seafood, and Shellfish   A-90 Food Additives
A-90 Fruit, Vegetable, or Blended Juices   A-92 Grains, Flours, and Fractions   A-92 Grain Products, Prepared and Baked Goods

Code	Food Name	Unit/ Amt	Wt (g)	Energy (kcal)	Prot (g)	Carb (g)	Fiber (g)	Fat (g)	Sat (g)	Mono (g)	Poly (g)	Chol (mg)	Vit A (RE)
62136	Pudding, supplement, rtu, 5 oz can	1 ea	142	240	7	32	0	9	1.5	—	—	5	150
62795	Supplement Drink, Hi Protein, vanilla, rtu	1 cup	256	240	15	33	0	6	0.5	—	—	10	250
62796	Supplement Drink, Plus, vanilla, rtu	8 fl-oz	260	360	14	45	1	14	1.5	—	—	10	250
62162	Supplement Drink, vanilla, rtu	1 cup	256	240	10	41	0	4	0.5	—	—	5	250

Soy Nutritionals

SWEETENERS AND SWEET SUBSTITUTES

Jams and Jellies

Code	Food Name	Unit/ Amt	Wt (g)	Energy (kcal)	Prot (g)	Carb (g)	Fiber (g)	Fat (g)	Sat (g)	Mono (g)	Poly (g)	Chol (mg)	Vit A (RE)
90974	Fruit Spread, apricot, 100% fruit	1 Tbs	19	40	0	10	0	0	0.0	0.0	0.0	0	0
90976	Fruit Spread, blueberry, 100% fruit	1 Tbs	19	40	0	10	0	0	0.0	0.0	0.0	0	0
90984	Fruit Spread, concord grape, 100% fruit	1 Tbs	19	40	0	10	0	0	0.0	0.0	0.0	0	0
90978	Fruit Spread, red raspberry, 100% fruit	1 Tbs	19	40	0	10	0	0	0.0	0.0	0.0	0	0
90979	Fruit Spread, strawberry, 100% fruit	1 Tbs	19	40	0	10	0	0	0.0	0.0	0.0	0	0
23054	Jam	1 Tbs	20	56	0	14	0	0	0.0	0.0	0.0	0	0
23205	Jam, apricot	1 Tbs	20	48	0	13	0	0	0.0	0.0	0.0	0	6
23288	Jam, concord grape	1 Tbs	20	50	0	13	0	0	0.0	0.0	0.0	0	0
92262	Jam, red raspberry	1 Tbs	20	50	0	13	0	0	0.0	0.0	0.0	0	0
23286	Jam, strawberry	1 Tbs	20	50	0	13	0	0	0.0	0.0	0.0	0	0
23003	Jelly	1 Tbs	19	51	0	13	0	0	0.0	0.0	0.0	0	0
23285	Jelly, apple	1 Tbs	20	50	0	13	0	0	0.0	0.0	0.0	0	0
23293	Jelly, concord grape	1 Tbs	20	50	0	13	0	0	0.0	0.0	0.0	0	0
90881	Jelly, mixed fruit	1 Tbs	20	50	0	13	0	0	0.0	0.0	0.0	0	0
23294	Jelly, strawberry	1 Tbs	20	50	0	13	0	0	0.0	0.0	0.0	0	0
23005	Marmalade, orange	1 Tbs	20	49	0	13	0	0	0.0	0.0	0.0	0	1
92229	Preserves	1 Tbs	20	56	0	14	0	0	0.0	0.0	0.0	0	0
92232	Preserves, apricot	1 Tbs	20	48	0	13	0	0	0.0	0.0	0.0	0	6
90891	Preserves, blueberry	1 Tbs	20	50	0	13	0	0	0.0	0.0	0.0	0	0
23297	Preserves, red raspberry	1 Tbs	20	50	0	13	0	0	0.0	0.0	0.0	0	0
23301	Preserves, strawberry	1 Tbs	20	50	0	13	0	0	0.0	0.0	0.0	0	0

Sugars, Sugar Substitutes, and Syrups

Code	Food Name	Unit/ Amt	Wt (g)	Energy (kcal)	Prot (g)	Carb (g)	Fiber (g)	Fat (g)	Sat (g)	Mono (g)	Poly (g)	Chol (mg)	Vit A (RE)
25309	Honey, light	1 Tbs	21	64	0	17	0	0	0.0	0.0	0.0	0	0
25003	Molasses	1 Tbs	20	59	0	15	0	0	0.0	0.0	0.0	0	0
25201	Sugar, brown, unpacked	1 cup	145	547	0	141	0	0	0.0	0.0	0.0	0	0
63415	Sugar, powdered	0.25 cup	37	140	0	37	0	0	0.0	0.0	0.0	0	
25006	Sugar, white, granulated	1 tsp	4	16	0	4	0	0	0.0	0.0	0.0	0	0
25007	Sugar, white, granulated, pkt	1 ea	6	23	0	6	0	0	0.0	0.0	0.0	0	0
25010	Syrup, corn, dark	2 Tbs	41	117	0	32	0	0	0.0	0.0	0.0	0	0
25000	Syrup, corn, light	1 cup	328	961	0	261	0	0	0.0	0.0	0.0	0	0
63334	Syrup, dietetic	1 Tbs	15	6	0	7	0	0	0.0	0.0	0.0	0	0
23042	Syrup, pancake	1 Tbs	20	47	0	12	0	0	0.0	0.0	0.0	0	0
23090	Syrup, pancake, w/butter	1 cup	315	932	0	233	0	5	3.2	1.5	0.2	13	47

VEGETABLES AND LEGUMES

VEGETABLES

Fresh Vegetables

Code	Food Name	Unit/ Amt	Wt (g)	Energy (kcal)	Prot (g)	Carb (g)	Fiber (g)	Fat (g)	Sat (g)	Mono (g)	Poly (g)	Chol (mg)	Vit A (RE)
5010	Alfalfa Sprouts, fresh	0.5 cup	16	5	1	1	0	0	0.0	0.0	0.1	0	3
7440	Artichokes, Calif, fresh	1 ea	340	85	7	20	10	0	0.0	0.0	0.0	0	0
5001	Asparagus, fresh	0.5 cup	67	13	1	3	1	0	0.0	0.0	0.1	0	51

PAGE KEY: A-96 Granola Bars, Cereal Bars, Diet Bars, Scones, and Tarts   A-96 Meals and Dishes   A-100 Meats   A-106 Nuts, Seeds, and Products   A-108 Poultry   A-110 Salad Dressings, Dips, and Mayonnaise   A-110 Salads   A-110 Sandwiches   A-114 Sauces and Gravies   A-114 Snack Foods—Chips, Pretzels, Popcorn   A-116 Soups, Stews, and Chilis   A-118 Spices, Flavors, and Seasonings   A-120 Sports Bars and Drinks   A-120 Supplemental Foods and Formulas   A-122 Sweeteners and Sweet Substitutes   A-122 Vegetables and Legumes   A-136 Weight Loss Bars and Drinks   A-138 Miscellaneous

Thia (mg)	Ribo (mg)	Niac (mg NE)	Vit B6 (mg)	Vit B12 (µg)	Fol (µg)	Vit C (mg)	Vit D (IU)	Vit E (mg AT)	Cal (mg)	Iron (mg)	Magn (mg)	Phos (mg)	Pota (mg)	Sodi (mg)	Zinc (mg)	Wat (%)	Alco (g)	Caff (g)
0.23	0.25	3.00	0.30	0.89	60.0	9.0	60.0	2.0	230	2.70	60.0	230	320	120	2.3	65	0.00	0.00
0.37	0.43	5.00	0.69	2.09	140.0	60.0	150.0	13.6	330	4.50	105.0	310	380	170	4.5	78	0.00	0.00
0.37	0.43	5.00	0.69	2.09	140.0	60.0	150.0	13.6	330	4.50	105.0	310	380	170	4.5	72	0.00	0.00
0.37	0.43	5.00	0.69	2.09	140.0	60.0	100.0	13.6	300	3.59	100.0	250	400	130	4.5	78	0.00	0.00
—	—	—	—	—	—	0.0	—	—	0	0.00	—	—	—	0	—	47	0.00	0.00
—	—	—	—	—	—	0.0	—	—	0	0.00	—	—	—	0	—	47	0.00	0.00
—	—	—	—	—	—	0.0	—	—	0	0.00	—	—	—	0	—	47	0.00	0.00
—	—	—	—	—	—	0.0	—	—	0	0.00	—	—	—	0	—	47	0.00	0.00
—	—	—	—	—	—	0.0	—	—	0	0.00	—	—	—	0	—	47	0.00	0.00
0.00	0.01	0.00	0.00	0.00	2.2	1.8	—	0.0	4	0.10	0.8	4	15	6	0.0	30	0.00	0.00
0.00	0.00	0.00	0.00	0.00	6.6	1.8	—	0.0	4	0.10	0.8	2	15	8	0.0	34	0.00	0.00
—	—	—	—	—	—	0.0	—	—	0	0.00	—	—	—	0	—	35	0.00	0.00
—	—	—	—	—	—	0.0	—	—	0	0.00	—	—	—	0	—	35	0.00	0.00
—	—	—	—	—	—	0.0	—	—	0	0.00	—	—	—	0	—	35	0.00	0.00
0.00	0.00	0.00	0.00	0.00	0.4	0.2	—	0.0	1	0.03	1.1	1	10	6	0.0	30	0.00	0.00
—	—	—	—	—	—	0.0	—	—	0	0.00	—	—	—	0	—	35	0.00	0.00
—	—	—	—	—	—	0.0	—	—	0	0.00	—	—	—	0	—	35	0.00	0.00
—	—	—	—	—	—	0.0	—	—	0	0.00	—	—	—	0	—	35	0.00	0.00
—	—	—	—	—	—	0.0	—	—	0	0.00	—	—	—	0	—	35	0.00	0.00
0.00	0.00	0.00	0.00	0.00	1.8	1.0	—	0.0	8	0.02	0.4	1	7	11	0.0	33	0.00	0.00
0.00	0.01	0.00	0.00	0.00	2.2	1.8	—	0.0	4	0.10	0.8	4	15	6	0.0	30	0.00	0.00
0.00	0.00	0.00	0.00	0.00	6.6	1.8	—	0.0	4	0.10	0.8	2	15	8	0.0	34	0.00	0.00
—	—	—	—	—	—	0.0	—	—	0	0.00	—	—	—	0	—	35	0.00	0.00
—	—	—	—	—	—	0.0	—	—	0	0.00	—	—	—	0	—	35	0.00	0.00
—	—	—	—	—	—	0.0	—	—	0	0.00	—	—	—	0	—	35	0.00	0.00
0.00	0.05	0.05	0.00	0.00	2.1	0.1	0.0	0.0	1	0.05	0.4	1	10	1		17	0.00	0.00
0.00	0.00	0.18	0.14	0.00	0.0	0.0	—	0.0	42	0.97	49.6	6	300	8	0.1	22	0.00	0.00
0.00	0.00	0.11	0.03	0.00	1.5	0.0	—	0.0	123	2.76	42.1	32	502	57	0.3	2	0.00	0.00
—	—	—	—	—	—	—	—	—	—	—	—	—	—	0	—	0	0.00	0.00
0.00	0.00	0.00	0.00	0.00	0.0	0.0	—	0.0	0	0.00	0.0	0	0	0	0.0	0	0.00	0.00
0.00	0.00	0.00	0.00	0.00	0.0	0.0	—	0.0	0	0.00	0.0	0	0	0	0.0	0	0.00	0.00
0.00	0.00	0.00	0.00	0.00	0.0	0.0	0.0	0.0	7	0.15	3.3	5	18	64	0.0	22	0.00	0.00
0.03	0.02	0.07	0.02	0.00	0.0	0.0	0.0	0.0	10	0.15	6.6	7	13	397	0.1	20	0.00	0.00
0.00	0.00	0.00	0.00	0.00	0.0	0.0	—	0.0	0	0.00	0.0	0	0	3	0.0	50	0.00	0.00
0.00	0.00	0.00	0.00	0.00	0.0	0.0	—	0.0	1	0.00	0.4	2	3	16	0.0	38	0.00	0.00
0.02	0.02	0.05	0.00	0.00	0.0	0.0	—	0.1	6	0.28	6.3	32	9	309	0.1	24	0.00	0.00
0.00	0.01	0.07	0.00	0.00	5.9	1.4	—	0.0	5	0.15	4.5	12	13	1	0.2	91	0.00	0.00
0.10	0.11	2.72	0.14	—	136.0	20.4	—	1.4	68	2.45	136.0	204	578	255	—	91	0.00	0.00
0.10	0.09	0.66	0.05	0.00	34.8	3.8	—	0.8	16	1.42	9.4	35	135	1	0.4	93	0.00	0.00

PAGE KEY: A-46 Beverage and Beverage Mixes   A-48 Other Beverages   A-48 Beverages, Alcoholic   A-50 Candies and Confections, Gum   A-54 Cereals, Breakfast Type   A-58 Cheese and Cheese Substitutes   A-60 Dairy Products and Substitutes   A-62 Desserts   A-68 Dessert Toppings   A-68 Eggs, Substitutes, and Egg Dishes   A-70 Ethnic Foods   A-74 Fast Foods/Restaurants   A-88 Fats, Oils, Margarines, Shortenings, and Substitutes   A-88 Fish, Seafood, and Shellfish   A-90 Food Additives   A-90 Fruit, Vegetable, or Blended Juices   A-92 Grains, Flours, and Fractions   A-92 Grain Products, Prepared and Baked Goods

Code	Food Name	Unit/ Amt	Wt (g)	Energy (kcal)	Prot (g)	Carb (g)	Fiber (g)	Fat (g)	Sat (g)	Mono (g)	Poly (g)	Chol (mg)	Vit A (RE)
5572	Beets, fresh, whole, 2"	1 ea	82	35	1	8	2	0	0.0	0.0	0.1	0	3
5678	Broccoflower, fresh	1 cup	100	32	3	6	3	0	0.0	0.0	0.1	0	7
6757	Broccoli, fresh	1 cup	71	24	2	5	2	0	0.0	0.0	0.0	0	47
5036	Cabbage, fresh, shredded	1 cup	70	17	1	4	2	0	0.0	0.0	0.0	0	13
5042	Cabbage, red, fresh, shredded	0.5 cup	35	11	1	3	1	0	0.0	0.0	0.0	0	39
9329	Carrots, baby, fresh	0.75 cup	85	40	1	9	2	0	0.0	0.0	0.0	0	1250
90429	Carrots, fresh, slices	1 pce	3	1	0	0	0	0	0.0	0.0	0.0	0	36
5049	Cauliflower, fresh	0.5 cup	50	12	1	3	1	0	0.0	0.0	0.0	0	1
90436	Celery, stalk, sml, 5" long, fresh	1 ea	17	2	0	1	0	0	0.0	0.0	0.0	0	7
7927	Chili Peppers, banana, fresh	1 cup	124	33	2	7	4	1	0.1	0.0	0.3	0	42
5359	Chives, fresh	1 Tbs	3	1	0	0	0	0	0.0	0.0	0.0	0	13
5560	Corn, white, sweet, kernels f/one ear, ckd, drained	1 ea	77	83	3	19	2	1	0.2	0.3	0.5	0	0
6015	Corn, white, sweet, kernels, fresh	1 cup	154	132	5	29	4	2	0.3	0.5	0.9	0	0
5379	Corn, yellow, sweet, kernels, ckd, drained	0.5 cup	82	89	3	21	2	1	0.2	0.3	0.5	0	21
5378	Corn, yellow, sweet, kernels, fresh	0.5 cup	77	66	2	15	2	1	0.1	0.3	0.4	0	15
7921	Cucumber, w/o skin, fresh, sliced	1 pce	7	1	0	0	0	0	0.0	0.0	0.0	0	1
5071	Cucumber, w/skin, fresh, slices	0.5 cup	52	8	0	2	0	0	0.0	0.0	0.0	0	5
5371	Eggplant, fresh, cubes	1 cup	82	20	1	5	3	0	0.0	0.0	0.1	0	2
26005	Garlic, cloves, fresh	4 ea	12	18	1	4	0	0	0.0	0.0	0.0	0	0
7081	Hummus, prep f/recipe	1 cup	246	435	12	49	10	21	2.8	12.1	5.1	0	1
5208	Kale, fresh, chpd	1 cup	67	34	2	7	1	0	0.1	0.0	0.2	0	1030
4851	Lettuce, crisphead, fresh, chpd	1 cup	55	8	0	2	1	0	0.0	0.0	0.0	0	28
5083	Lettuce, iceberg, fresh, chpd	1 cup	55	8	0	2	1	0	0.0	0.0	0.0	0	28
9316	Lettuce, iceberg, shredded	1.5 cup	100	15	1	3	1	0	0.0	0.0	0.0	0	20
5088	Lettuce, romaine, fresh, chpd	1 cup	56	10	1	2	1	0	0.0	0.0	0.1	0	325
5090	Mushrooms, fresh, pces/slices	0.5 cup	35	8	1	1	0	0	0.0	0.0	0.0	0	0
6494	Mushrooms, fresh, whole	1 cup	96	21	3	3	1	0	0.0	0.0	0.1	0	0
5099	Okra, ckd, drained, slices	0.5 cup	80	18	1	4	2	0	0.0	0.0	0.0	0	22
5775	Okra, fresh	0.5 cup	50	16	1	4	2	0	0.0	0.0	0.0	0	19
7498	Onion, red, fresh, chpd	1 cup	160	67	2	16	2	0	0.0	0.0	0.1	0	0
9548	Onion, sweet, fresh	100 g	100	32	1	8	1	0	—	—	—	0	0
5101	Onion, white, fresh, chpd	0.5 cup	80	34	1	8	1	0	0.0	0.0	0.0	0	0
7499	Onion, yellow, fresh, chpd	0.5 cup	80	34	1	8	1	0	0.0	0.0	0.0	0	0
26012	Parsley, fresh, chpd	0.5 cup	30	11	1	2	1	0	0.0	0.1	0.0	0	253
5124	Peppers, bell, green, sweet, fresh, chpd	0.5 cup	74	15	1	3	1	0	0.0	0.0	0.0	0	27
5128	Peppers, bell, red, sweet, fresh, chpd	0.5 cup	74	19	1	4	1	0	0.0	0.0	0.1	0	234
9242	Peppers, bell, yellow, sweet, fresh, chpd	0.5 cup	74	20	1	5	1	0	0.0	0.0	0.1	0	15
5143	Radishes, fresh, med, 3/4" to 1"	10 ea	45	7	0	2	1	0	0.0	0.0	0.0	0	0
7214	Rutabaga, fresh, cubes	0.5 cup	70	25	1	6	2	0	0.0	0.0	0.1	0	0
6861	Soybean Sprouts, mature, fresh	10 ea	10	12	1	1	0	1	0.1	0.2	0.4	0	0
5146	Spinach, fresh, chpd	1 cup	30	7	1	1	1	0	0.0	0.0	0.0	0	281
6863	Spinach, fresh, leaf	1 ea	10	2	0	0	0	0	0.0	0.0	0.0	0	94
7369	Squash, banana, fresh	0.75 cup	85	30	1	7	1	0	0.0	0.0	0.0	0	350
5801	Squash, butternut, fresh, cubes	0.5 cup	120	54	1	14	2	0	0.0	0.0	0.1	0	1277
90537	Squash, summer, all types, fresh, med	1 ea	196	31	2	7	2	0	0.1	0.0	0.2	0	39

PAGE KEY: A-96 Granola Bars, Cereal Bars, Diet Bars, Scones, and Tarts   A-96 Meals and Dishes   A-100 Meats   A-106 Nuts, Seeds, and Products   A-108 Poultry
A-110 Salad Dressings, Dips, and Mayonnaise   A-110 Salads   A-110 Sandwiches   A-114 Sauces and Gravies   A-114 Snack Foods—Chips, Pretzels, Popcorn
A-116 Soups, Stews, and Chilis   A-118 Spices, Flavors, and Seasonings   A-120 Sports Bars and Drinks   A-120 Supplemental Foods and Formulas
A-122 Sweeteners and Sweet Substitutes   A-122 Vegetables and Legumes   A-136 Weight Loss Bars and Drinks   A-138 Miscellaneous

Thia (mg)	Ribo (mg)	Niac (mg NE)	Vit B6 (mg)	Vit B12 (µg)	Fol (µg)	Vit C (mg)	Vit D (IU)	Vit E (mg AT)	Cal (mg)	Iron (mg)	Magn (mg)	Phos (mg)	Pota (mg)	Sodi (mg)	Zinc (mg)	Wat (%)	Alco (g)	Caff (g)
0.02	0.02	0.27	0.05	0.00	89.4	4.0	—	0.0	13	0.66	18.9	33	266	64	0.3	88	0.00	0.00
0.07	0.10	0.80	0.20	0.00	57.0	74.0	0.0	0.3	32	0.07	20.0	64	322	23	0.5	90	0.00	0.00
0.05	0.07	0.44	0.11	0.00	44.7	63.3	—	0.6	33	0.51	14.9	47	224	23	0.3	89	0.00	0.00
0.03	0.02	0.20	0.07	0.00	30.1	22.5	—	0.1	33	0.40	10.5	16	172	13	0.1	92	0.00	0.00
0.01	0.01	0.15	0.07	0.00	6.3	19.9	—	0.0	16	0.28	5.6	10	85	9	0.1	90	0.00	0.00
—	—	—	—	—	—	6.0	—	—	20	0.00	—	—	—	45	—	88	0.00	0.00
0.00	0.00	0.02	0.00	0.00	0.6	0.2	—	0.0	1	0.00	0.4	1	10	2	0.0	88	0.00	0.00
0.02	0.02	0.25	0.10	0.00	28.5	23.2	—	0.0	11	0.21	7.5	22	152	15	0.1	92	0.00	0.00
0.00	0.00	0.05	0.00	0.00	6.1	0.5	—	0.0	7	0.02	1.9	4	44	14	0.0	95	0.00	0.00
0.10	0.07	1.53	0.43	0.00	36.0	102.5	—	0.9	17	0.56	21.1	40	317	16	0.3	92	0.00	0.00
0.00	0.00	0.01	0.00	0.00	3.1	1.7	—	0.0	3	0.05	1.3	2	9	0	0.0	91	0.00	0.00
0.17	0.05	1.24	0.05	0.00	35.4	4.8	0.0	0.1	2	0.46	24.6	79	192	13	0.4	70	0.00	0.00
0.31	0.09	2.61	0.07	0.00	70.8	10.5	—	0.1	3	0.80	57.0	137	416	23	0.7	76	0.00	0.00
0.18	0.05	1.32	0.05	0.00	37.7	5.1	—	0.1	2	0.50	26.2	84	204	14	0.4	70	0.00	0.00
0.15	0.05	1.30	0.03	0.00	35.4	5.2	—	0.1	2	0.40	28.5	69	208	12	0.3	76	0.00	0.00
0.00	0.00	0.00	0.00	0.00	1.0	0.2	—	0.0	1	0.01	0.8	1	10	0	0.0	97	0.00	0.00
0.00	0.01	0.05	0.01	0.00	3.6	1.5	—	0.0	8	0.15	6.8	12	76	1	0.1	95	0.00	0.00
0.02	0.02	0.52	0.07	0.00	18.0	1.8	—	0.2	7	0.20	11.5	20	189	2	0.1	92	0.00	0.00
0.01	0.00	0.07	0.15	0.00	0.4	3.7	—	0.0	22	0.20	3.0	18	48	2	0.1	59	0.00	0.00
0.21	0.12	0.98	0.98	0.00	145.1	19.4	—	1.8	121	3.85	71.3	271	426	595	2.7	65	0.00	0.00
0.07	0.09	0.67	0.18	0.00	19.4	80.4	—	0.5	90	1.13	22.8	38	299	29	0.3	84	0.00	0.00
0.01	0.00	0.07	0.01	0.00	16.0	1.5	—	0.1	10	0.23	3.9	11	78	6	0.1	96	0.00	0.00
0.01	0.00	0.07	0.01	0.00	16.0	1.5	—	0.1	10	0.23	3.9	11	78	6	0.1	96	0.00	0.00
—	—	—	—	—	—	3.6	—	—	0	0.00	—	—	—	10	—	96	0.00	0.00
0.03	0.03	0.18	0.03	0.00	76.2	13.4	—	0.1	18	0.54	7.8	17	138	4	0.1	95	0.00	0.00
0.02	0.15	1.35	0.03	0.00	5.6	0.8	26.6	0.0	1	0.18	3.1	30	110	1	0.2	92	0.00	0.00
0.09	0.40	3.70	0.10	0.03	15.4	2.3	73.0	0.0	3	0.50	8.6	82	301	4	0.5	92	0.00	0.00
0.10	0.03	0.69	0.15	0.00	36.8	13.0	—	0.2	62	0.21	28.8	26	108	5	0.3	93	0.00	0.00
0.10	0.02	0.50	0.10	0.00	44.0	10.6	—	0.2	40	0.40	28.5	32	152	4	0.3	90	0.00	0.00
0.07	0.03	0.12	0.23	0.00	30.4	10.2	—	0.0	35	0.30	16.0	43	230	5	0.3	89	0.00	0.00
0.03	0.01	0.12	0.12	—	23.0	4.8	—	0.0	20	0.25	9.0	27	119	8	0.1	91	0.00	0.00
0.03	0.01	0.07	0.11	0.00	15.2	5.1	—	0.0	18	0.15	8.0	22	115	2	0.1	89	0.00	0.00
0.03	0.01	0.07	0.11	0.00	15.2	5.1	—	0.0	18	0.15	8.0	22	115	2	0.1	89	0.00	0.00
0.02	0.02	0.38	0.02	0.00	45.6	39.9	—	0.2	41	1.86	15.0	17	166	17	0.3	88	0.00	0.00
0.03	0.01	0.36	0.17	0.00	8.2	59.9	—	0.3	7	0.25	7.4	15	130	2	0.1	94	0.00	0.00
0.03	0.05	0.73	0.21	0.00	13.4	141.6	—	1.2	5	0.31	8.9	19	157	1	0.2	92	0.00	0.00
0.01	0.01	0.66	0.12	0.00	19.4	136.7	0.0	0.5	8	0.34	8.9	18	158	1	0.1	92	0.00	0.00
0.00	0.01	0.10	0.11	0.00	11.2	6.7	—	0.0	11	0.15	4.5	9	105	18	0.1	95	0.00	0.00
0.05	0.02	0.49	0.07	0.00	14.7	17.5	—	0.2	33	0.36	16.1	41	236	14	0.2	90	0.00	0.00
0.02	0.00	0.10	0.01	0.00	17.2	1.5	—	0.0	7	0.20	7.2	16	48	1	0.1	69	0.00	0.00
0.01	0.05	0.21	0.05	0.00	58.2	8.4	—	0.6	30	0.81	23.7	15	167	24	0.2	91	0.00	0.00
0.00	0.01	0.07	0.01	0.00	19.4	2.8	—	0.2	10	0.27	7.9	5	56	8	0.1	91	0.00	0.00
—	—	—	—	0.00	—	9.0	—	—	20	0.36	—	—	—	0	—	90	0.00	0.00
0.11	0.01	1.44	0.18	0.00	32.4	25.2	—	1.7	58	0.83	40.8	40	422	5	0.2	86	0.00	0.00
0.09	0.28	0.94	0.43	0.00	56.8	33.3	—	0.2	29	0.68	33.3	74	514	4	0.6	95	0.00	0.00

PAGE KEY: A-46 Beverage and Beverage Mixes A-48 Other Beverages A-48 Beverages, Alcoholic A-50 Candies and Confections, Gum A-54 Cereals, Breakfast Type
A-58 Cheese and Cheese Substitutes A-60 Dairy Products and Substitutes A-62 Desserts A-68 Dessert Toppings A-68 Eggs, Substitutes, and Egg Dishes A-70 Ethnic Foods
A-74 Fast Foods/Restaurants A-88 Fats, Oils, Margarines, Shortenings, and Substitutes A-88 Fish, Seafood, and Shellfish A-90 Food Additives
A-90 Fruit, Vegetable, or Blended Juices A-92 Grains, Flours, and Fractions A-92 Grain Products, Prepared and Baked Goods

Code	Food Name	Unit/ Amt	Wt (g)	Energy (kcal)	Prot (g)	Carb (g)	Fiber (g)	Fat (g)	Sat (g)	Mono (g)	Poly (g)	Chol (mg)	Vit A (RE)
90538	Squash, summer, all types, fresh, sml	1 ea	118	19	1	4	1	0	0.1	0.0	0.1	0	24
5833	Squash, winter, all types, fresh, cubes	0.5 cup	58	20	1	5	1	0	0.0	0.0	0.0	0	79
90604	Squash, zucchini, baby, med, fresh	1 ea	11	2	0	0	0	0	0.0	0.0	0.0	0	0
5519	Tomatoes, green, fresh, chpd	0.5 cup	90	21	1	5	1	0	0.0	0.0	0.1	0	58
3973	Tomatoes, orange, fresh	1 ea	111	18	1	4	1	0	0.0	0.0	0.1	0	166
90530	Tomatoes, red, cherry, fresh, year round avg	1 ea	17	3	0	1	0	0	0.0	0.0	0.0	0	14
5178	Tomatoes, red, ckd f/fresh w/o salt	0.5 cup	120	22	1	5	1	0	0.0	0.0	0.1	0	58
5177	Tomatoes, red, ckd f/fresh w/o salt, med	1 ea	123	22	1	5	1	0	0.0	0.0	0.1	0	59
5170	Tomatoes, red, fresh, year round avg, chpd/sliced	0.5 cup	90	16	1	4	1	0	0.0	0.0	0.1	0	76
6492	Tomatoes, roma, fresh, year round avg, fresh	1 ea	62	11	1	2	1	0	0.0	0.0	0.1	0	52
5547	Turnip Greens, chpd, fresh	1 cup	55	18	1	4	2	0	0.0	0.0	0.1	0	0
5183	Turnips, ckd, drained, cubes	0.5 cup	78	17	1	4	2	0	0.0	0.0	0.0	0	0
5306	Yams, fresh, cubes	0.5 cup	75	88	1	21	3	0	0.0	0.0	0.1	0	10
Cooked Vegetables													
4437	Artichokes, French, hearts, ckd, drained	0.5 cup	84	42	3	9	5	0	0.0	0.0	0.1	0	15
5000	Artichokes, globe, ckd, drained, med	1 ea	120	60	4	13	6	0	0.0	0.0	0.1	0	22
5003	Asparagus, ckd, drained	0.5 cup	90	20	2	4	2	0	0.1	0.0	0.1	0	90
5249	Bamboo Shoots, slices, ckd, drained	1 cup	120	14	2	2	1	0	0.1	0.0	0.1	0	0
5025	Beet Greens, ckd, drained	1 cup	144	39	4	8	4	0	0.0	0.1	0.1	0	1103
5022	Beets, ckd, drained, sliced	0.5 cup	85	37	1	8	2	0	0.0	0.0	0.1	0	3
5407	Borage, ckd, drained	100 g	100	25	2	4	1	1	0.2	0.2	0.1	0	438
5028	Broccoli, chpd, ckd, drained	0.5 cup	78	27	2	6	3	0	0.1	0.0	0.1	0	153
6092	Broccoli, spears, ckd f/fzn w/salt, drained	0.5 cup	92	26	3	5	3	0	0.0	0.0	0.1	0	103
5234	Broccoli, spears, ckd f/fzn, drained	0.5 cup	92	26	3	5	3	0	0.0	0.0	0.1	0	103
5653	Broccoli, stmd	1 cup	156	44	5	8	5	1	0.1	0.0	0.3	0	228
5033	Brussels Sprouts, ckd, drained, cup	0.5 cup	78	28	2	6	2	0	0.1	0.0	0.2	0	61
5038	Cabbage, ckd, drained, shredded	1 cup	150	33	2	7	3	1	0.1	0.0	0.3	0	21
5238	Cabbage, red, ckd, drained, shredded	0.5 cup	75	22	1	5	2	0	0.0	0.0	0.0	0	3
5358	Carrots, ckd f/fzn w/o salt, drained, slices	0.5 cup	73	27	0	6	2	0	0.1	0.0	0.2	0	1213
5889	Carrots, ckd f/fzn w/salt, drained, slices	0.5 cup	73	27	0	6	2	0	0.1	0.0	0.2	0	1213
5656	Carrots, stir fried	1 cup	156	67	2	16	5	0	0.0	0.0	0.1	0	3955
5655	Carrots, stmd	1 cup	156	67	2	16	5	0	0.0	0.0	0.1	0	3955
5052	Cauliflower, florets, ckd, drained	3 ea	54	12	1	2	1	0	0.0	0.0	0.1	0	1
7266	Cauliflower, green, ckd, head	0.2 ea	90	29	3	6	3	0	0.0	0.0	0.1	0	13
5894	Celery, ckd w/salt, drained, diced	0.5 cup	75	14	1	3	1	0	0.0	0.0	0.1	0	44
5056	Celery, ckd, drained, diced	1 cup	150	27	1	6	2	0	0.1	0.0	0.1	0	87
6093	Collards, chpd, ckd w/salt, drained	1 cup	190	49	4	9	5	1	0.1	0.0	0.3	0	1543
5061	Collards, chpd, ckd, drained	0.5 cup	80	21	2	4	2	0	0.0	0.0	0.1	0	650
6917	Corn, white, sweet, cob, ckd f/fzn w/salt, drained	1 ea	63	59	2	14	2	0	0.1	0.1	0.2	0	0
5567	Corn, white, sweet, cob, ckd f/fzn, drained	1 ea	63	59	2	14	1	0	0.1	0.1	0.2	0	0
6019	Corn, white, sweet, kernels, ckd f/fzn w/salt, drained	0.5 cup	82	66	2	16	2	0	0.1	0.1	0.2	0	0
5393	Corn, white, sweet, kernels, ckd f/fzn, drained	0.5 cup	82	66	2	16	2	0	0.1	0.1	0.2	0	0
6964	Corn, yellow, sweet, kernels, ckd f/fzn cob w/salt, drnd	0.5 cup	82	76	3	18	2	1	0.1	0.2	0.3	0	20
5365	Corn, yellow, sweet, kernels, ckd f/fzn cob, drained	0.5 cup	82	76	3	18	2	1	0.1	0.2	0.3	0	20
5639	Cucumber, ckd	1 cup	180	29	2	6	2	0	0.1	0.0	0.1	0	42
5456	Dish, broccoli, w/cheese sauce, ckd	0.5 cup	114	115	7	6	2	8	3.6	2.5	1.1	16	152

PAGE KEY: A-96 Granola Bars, Cereal Bars, Diet Bars, Scones, and Tarts   A-96 Meals and Dishes   A-100 Meats   A-106 Nuts, Seeds, and Products   A-108 Poultry   A-110 Salad Dressings, Dips, and Mayonnaise   A-110 Salads   A-110 Sandwiches   A-114 Sauces and Gravies   A-114 Snack Foods—Chips, Pretzels, Popcorn   A-116 Soups, Stews, and Chilis   A-118 Spices, Flavors, and Seasonings   A-120 Sports Bars and Drinks   A-120 Supplemental Foods and Formulas   A-122 Sweeteners and Sweet Substitutes   A-122 Vegetables and Legumes   A-136 Weight Loss Bars and Drinks   A-138 Miscellaneous

Thia (mg)	Ribo (mg)	Niac (mg NE)	Vit B6 (mg)	Vit B12 (µg)	Fol (µg)	Vit C (mg)	Vit D (IU)	Vit E (mg AT)	Cal (mg)	Iron (mg)	Magn (mg)	Phos (mg)	Pota (mg)	Sodi (mg)	Zinc (mg)	Wat (%)	Alco (g)	Caff (g)
0.05	0.17	0.56	0.25	0.00	34.2	20.1	—	0.1	18	0.40	20.1	45	309	2	0.3	95	0.00	0.00
0.01	0.03	0.28	0.09	0.00	13.9	7.1	—	0.1	16	0.34	8.1	13	203	2	0.1	90	0.00	0.00
0.00	0.00	0.07	0.01	0.00	2.2	3.8	0.0	0.0	2	0.09	3.6	10	50	0	0.1	93	0.00	0.00
0.05	0.03	0.44	0.07	0.00	8.1	21.1	—	0.3	12	0.46	9.0	25	184	12	0.1	93	0.00	0.00
0.05	0.03	0.66	0.07	0.00	32.2	17.8	—	—	6	0.51	8.9	32	235	47	0.2	95	0.00	0.00
0.00	0.00	0.10	0.00	0.00	2.5	2.2	—	0.1	2	0.05	1.9	4	40	1	0.0	94	0.00	0.00
0.03	0.02	0.63	0.09	0.00	15.6	27.4	—	0.7	13	0.81	10.8	34	262	13	0.2	94	0.00	0.00
0.03	0.02	0.64	0.10	0.00	16.0	28.0	—	0.7	14	0.83	11.1	34	268	14	0.2	94	0.00	0.00
0.02	0.01	0.52	0.07	0.00	13.5	11.4	—	0.5	9	0.23	9.9	22	213	4	0.2	94	0.00	0.00
0.01	0.01	0.37	0.05	0.00	9.3	7.9	—	0.3	6	0.17	6.8	15	147	3	0.1	94	0.00	0.00
0.03	0.05	0.33	0.14	0.00	106.7	33.0	—	1.6	104	0.61	17.1	23	163	22	0.1	90	0.00	0.00
0.01	0.01	0.23	0.05	0.00	7.0	9.0	—	0.0	26	0.14	7.0	20	138	12	0.1	94	0.00	0.00
0.07	0.01	0.40	0.21	0.00	17.2	12.8	—	0.3	13	0.40	15.8	41	612	7	0.2	70	0.00	0.00
0.05	0.05	0.83	0.09	0.00	42.8	8.4	—	0.2	38	1.08	50.4	72	297	80	0.4	84	0.00	0.00
0.07	0.07	1.20	0.12	0.00	61.2	12.0	—	0.2	54	1.54	72.0	103	425	114	0.6	84	0.00	0.00
0.15	0.12	0.98	0.07	0.00	134.1	6.9	—	1.3	21	0.81	12.6	49	202	13	0.5	93	0.00	0.00
0.01	0.05	0.36	0.11	0.00	2.4	0.0	—	0.8	14	0.28	3.6	24	640	5	0.6	96	0.00	0.00
0.17	0.41	0.72	0.18	0.00	20.2	35.9	—	2.6	164	2.74	97.9	59	1309	347	0.7	89	0.00	0.00
0.01	0.02	0.28	0.05	0.00	68.0	3.1	—	0.0	14	0.67	19.6	32	259	65	0.3	87	0.00	0.00
0.05	0.17	0.93	0.09	0.00	10.0	32.5	—	—	102	3.64	57.0	55	491	88	0.2	92	0.00	0.00
0.05	0.10	0.43	0.15	0.00	84.2	50.6	—	1.1	31	0.51	16.4	52	229	32	0.4	89	0.00	0.00
0.05	0.07	0.41	0.11	0.00	27.6	36.9	—	1.2	47	0.56	18.4	51	166	239	0.3	91	0.00	0.00
0.05	0.07	0.41	0.11	0.00	27.6	36.9	—	1.2	47	0.56	18.4	51	166	22	0.3	91	0.00	0.00
0.09	0.18	0.93	0.21	0.00	93.9	123.4	0.0	0.7	75	1.37	39.0	103	505	42	0.6	91	0.00	0.00
0.07	0.05	0.46	0.14	0.00	46.8	48.4	—	0.3	28	0.93	15.6	44	247	16	0.3	89	0.00	0.00
0.09	0.07	0.41	0.17	0.00	30.0	30.2	—	0.2	46	0.25	12.0	22	146	12	0.1	94	0.00	0.00
0.05	0.03	0.28	0.17	0.00	18.0	8.1	—	0.1	32	0.50	12.8	25	196	6	0.2	91	0.00	0.00
0.01	0.02	0.30	0.05	0.00	8.0	1.7	—	0.7	26	0.38	8.0	23	140	43	0.3	90	0.00	0.00
0.01	0.02	0.30	0.05	0.00	8.0	1.7	0.0	0.3	26	0.38	8.0	23	140	215	0.3	90	0.00	0.00
0.14	0.09	1.37	0.21	0.00	20.7	11.6	0.0	0.7	42	0.77	23.4	69	504	55	0.3	88	0.00	0.00
0.14	0.09	1.37	0.21	0.00	20.7	10.9	0.0	0.7	42	0.77	23.4	69	504	55	0.3	88	Alco	0.00
0.01	0.02	0.21	0.09	0.00	23.8	23.9	—	0.0	9	0.18	4.9	17	77	8	0.1	93	0.00	0.00
0.05	0.09	0.61	0.18	0.00	36.9	65.3	—	0.0	29	0.64	17.1	51	250	21	0.6	89	0.00	0.00
0.02	0.03	0.23	0.05	0.00	16.5	4.6	0.0	0.3	32	0.31	9.0	19	213	245	0.1	94	0.00	0.00
0.05	0.07	0.47	0.12	0.00	33.0	9.1	—	0.5	63	0.62	18.0	38	426	136	0.2	94	0.00	0.00
0.07	0.20	1.09	0.23	0.00	176.7	34.6	0.0	1.7	266	2.20	38.0	57	220	479	0.4	92	0.00	0.00
0.02	0.07	0.46	0.10	0.00	74.4	14.6	—	0.7	112	0.93	16.0	24	93	13	0.2	92	0.00	0.00
0.10	0.03	0.95	0.14	0.00	19.5	3.0	—	0.0	2	0.37	18.3	47	158	151	0.4	73	0.00	0.00
0.10	0.03	0.95	0.14	0.00	19.5	3.0	—	0.0	2	0.37	18.3	47	158	3	0.4	73	0.00	0.00
0.07	0.05	1.07	0.10	0.00	25.4	2.5	—	0.1	3	0.28	15.6	47	121	201	0.3	77	0.00	0.00
0.07	0.05	1.07	0.10	0.00	25.4	2.5	—	0.1	3	0.28	15.6	47	121	4	0.3	77	0.00	0.00
0.14	0.05	1.24	0.18	0.00	25.4	3.9	—	0.1	2	0.50	23.8	62	206	197	0.5	73	0.00	0.00
0.14	0.05	1.24	0.18	0.00	25.4	3.9	—	0.1	2	0.50	23.8	62	206	3	0.5	73	0.00	0.00
0.03	0.05	0.43	0.07	0.00	20.2	9.4	0.0	0.2	30	0.55	23.2	40	288	4	0.4	95	0.00	0.00
0.05	0.18	0.54	0.11	0.14	39.4	54.0	—	1.7	161	0.79	25.0	138	268	202	0.8	81	0.00	0.00

PAGE KEY: A-46 Beverage and Beverage Mixes A-48 Other Beverages A-48 Beverages, Alcoholic A-50 Candies and Confections, Gum A-54 Cereals, Breakfast Type A-58 Cheese and Cheese Substitutes A-60 Dairy Products and Substitutes A-62 Desserts A-68 Dessert Toppings A-68 Eggs, Substitutes, and Egg Dishes A-70 Ethnic Foods A-74 Fast Foods/Restaurants A-88 Fats, Oils, Margarines, Shortenings, and Substitutes A-88 Fish, Seafood, and Shellfish A-90 Food Additives A-90 Fruit, Vegetable, or Blended Juices A-92 Grains, Flours, and Fractions A-92 Grain Products, Prepared and Baked Goods

Code	Food Name	Unit/ Amt	Wt (g)	Energy (kcal)	Prot (g)	Carb (g)	Fiber (g)	Fat (g)	Sat (g)	Mono (g)	Poly (g)	Chol (mg)	Vit A (RE)
5457	Dish, broccoli, w/cream sauce, ckd	0.5 cup	114	87	4	8	2	5	1.3	2.0	1.4	3	154
5989	Dish, succotash, ckd w/salt, drained	0.5 cup	96	110	5	23	5	1	0.1	0.1	0.4	0	29
5642	Eggplant, batter dipped, fried	1 pce	50	75	1	6	1	5	1.1	2.3	1.7	8	4
5072	Eggplant, ckd, drained, 1" cubes	0.5 cup	50	17	0	4	1	0	0.0	0.0	0.0	0	2
5673	Eggplant, stmd	1 cup	96	25	1	6	2	0	0.0	0.0	0.1	0	8
5640	Hominy, ckd	1 cup	165	119	2	24	4	1	0.2	0.4	0.7	0	0
7957	Hummus, cmrcl	1 cup	250	415	20	36	15	24	3.6	10.1	9.0	0	10
5075	Kale, ckd, drained	0.5 cup	65	18	1	4	1	0	0.0	0.0	0.1	0	885
5514	Mushrooms, batter dipped, fried	5 ea	70	156	2	11	1	12	1.5	3.6	6.0	2	6
5924	Mushrooms, ckd w/salt, drained, pieces	0.5 cup	78	22	2	4	2	0	0.0	0.0	0.1	0	0
5092	Mushrooms, ckd, drained	0.5 cup	78	22	2	4	2	0	0.0	0.0	0.1	0	0
5384	Mushrooms, shiitake, ckd, whole	4 ea	72	40	1	10	2	0	0.0	0.0	0.0	0	0
5657	Mushrooms, stmd	1 cup	156	39	3	7	2	1	0.1	0.0	0.3	0	0
5643	Mushrooms, stuffed	2 ea	48	138	5	13	1	7	2.2	3.1	1.6	6	50
5096	Mustard Greens, ckd, drained	1 cup	140	21	3	3	3	0	0.0	0.2	0.1	0	885
5644	Okra, batter dipped, fried	1 cup	92	175	2	14	2	13	1.7	3.1	7.1	2	39
5932	Okra, ckd f/fzn w/salt, drained, slices	0.5 cup	92	26	2	5	3	0	0.1	0.0	0.1	0	31
70623	Onion Rings	6 ea	88	222	3	27	—	12	1.9	4.1	5.1	0	9
6074	Onion, ckd w/salt, drained	0.5 cup	105	46	1	11	1	0	0.0	0.0	0.1	0	0
5529	Onion, pearl, ckd, whole	3 ea	45	20	1	5	1	0	0.0	0.0	0.0	0	0
7811	Onion, red, ckd, drained, chpd	0.5 cup	105	46	1	11	1	0	0.0	0.0	0.1	0	0
5650	Onion, stir fried	1 cup	210	80	2	18	4	0	0.1	0.0	0.1	0	0
5649	Onion, stmd	1 cup	210	80	2	18	4	0	0.1	0.0	0.1	0	0
5108	Onion, white, ckd, drained, chpd	0.5 cup	105	46	1	11	1	0	0.0	0.0	0.1	0	0
7812	Onion, yellow, ckd, drained, chpd	0.5 cup	105	46	1	11	1	0	0.0	0.0	0.1	0	0
5212	Parsnips, ckd, drained	1 cup	156	111	2	27	6	0	0.1	0.2	0.1	0	0
5662	Peppers, bell, green, sweet, chpd, stir fried	0.5 cup	68	18	1	4	1	0	0.0	0.0	0.1	0	39
5661	Peppers, bell, green, sweet, chpd, stmd	0.5 cup	68	18	1	4	1	0	0.0	0.0	0.1	0	41
9549	Peppers, bell, green, sweet, sauteed	100 g	100	127	1	4	2	12	1.6	2.3	5.9	0	28
5663	Peppers, bell, red, sweet, chpd, stmd	0.5 cup	68	18	1	4	1	0	0.0	0.0	0.1	0	368
5229	Poi	0.5 cup	120	134	0	33	0	0	0.0	0.0	0.1	0	7
9366	Potatoes, white, baby, ckd	0.5 cup	85	70	2	15	1	0	0.0	0.0	0.0	0	0
9368	Potatoes, yukon gold, ckd	0.5 cup	85	70	2	15	1	0	0.0	0.0	0.0	0	0
5426	Purslane, ckd, drained	0.5 cup	58	10	1	2	—	0	0.0	0.0	0.0	0	107
7226	Rutabaga, ckd, drained, mashed	0.5 cup	120	47	2	10	2	0	0.0	0.0	0.1	0	0
5459	Soybean Sprouts, mature, stmd	0.5 cup	47	38	4	3	0	2	0.3	0.5	1.2	0	2
6227	Spinach, chpd, fzn	0.33 cup	85	20	3	3	2	0	0.1	—	—	0	681
5972	Spinach, ckd w/salt, drained	0.5 cup	90	21	3	3	2	0	0.0	0.0	0.1	0	943
5147	Spinach, ckd, drained	0.5 cup	90	21	3	3	2	0	0.0	0.0	0.1	0	943
5670	Spinach, stmd	0.5 cup	95	21	3	3	3	0	0.1	0.0	0.1	0	607
5316	Squash, acorn, ckd, mashed	0.5 cup	122	42	1	11	3	0	0.0	0.0	0.0	0	100
5317	Squash, butternut, bkd, cubes	0.5 cup	102	41	1	11	3	0	0.0	0.0	0.0	0	1144
5455	Squash, spaghetti, bkd/ckd, drained	0.5 cup	78	21	1	5	1	0	0.0	0.0	0.1	0	9
6922	Squash, spaghetti, ckd w/salt, drained	0.5 cup	78	21	1	5	1	0	0.0	0.0	0.1	0	9
5975	Squash, summer, all types, ckd w/salt, drained	0.5 cup	90	18	1	4	1	0	0.1	0.0	0.1	0	20

PAGE KEY: A-96 Granola Bars, Cereal Bars, Diet Bars, Scones, and Tarts   A-96 Meals and Dishes   A-100 Meats   A-106 Nuts, Seeds, and Products   A-108 Poultry   A-110 Salad Dressings, Dips, and Mayonnaise   A-110 Salads   A-110 Sandwiches   A-114 Sauces and Gravies   A-114 Snack Foods—Chips, Pretzels, Popcorn   A-116 Soups, Stews, and Chilis   A-118 Spices, Flavors, and Seasonings   A-120 Sports Bars and Drinks   A-120 Supplemental Foods and Formulas   A-122 Sweeteners and Sweet Substitutes   A-122 Vegetables and Legumes   A-136 Weight Loss Bars and Drinks   A-138 Miscellaneous

Thia (mg)	Ribo (mg)	Niac (mg NE)	Vit B6 (mg)	Vit B12 (µg)	Fol (µg)	Vit C (mg)	Vit D (IU)	Vit E (mg AT)	Cal (mg)	Iron (mg)	Magn (mg)	Phos (mg)	Pota (mg)	Sodi (mg)	Zinc (mg)	Wat (%)	Alco (g)	Caff (g)
0.07	0.14	0.50	0.10	0.12	22.7	27.6	—	1.3	89	0.56	20.0	83	194	180	0.4	84	0.00	0.00
0.15	0.09	1.26	0.10	0.00	31.7	7.9	—	0.3	16	1.46	50.9	112	394	243	0.6	68	0.00	0.00
0.05	0.03	0.46	0.03	0.02	7.4	0.6	—	0.8	14	0.34	7.6	23	106	15	0.1	74	0.00	0.00
0.03	0.00	0.30	0.03	0.00	6.9	0.6	—	0.2	3	0.11	5.4	7	61	0	0.1	90	0.00	0.00
0.05	0.02	0.55	0.07	0.00	15.5	1.4	0.0	0.0	7	0.25	13.4	21	208	3	0.1	92	0.00	0.00
0.00	0.00	0.05	0.00	0.00	1.6	0.0	0.0	0.1	16	1.01	26.4	58	15	346	1.7	83	0.00	0.00
0.44	0.15	1.46	0.50	0.00	207.5	0.0	—	—	95	6.09	177.5	440	570	948	4.6	67	0.00	0.00
0.02	0.05	0.31	0.09	0.00	8.4	26.6	0.0	0.6	47	0.57	11.7	18	148	15	0.2	91	0.00	0.00
0.10	0.25	2.25	0.03	0.02	8.3	1.2	—	2.3	15	1.22	6.8	119	154	112	0.4	63	0.00	0.00
0.05	0.23	3.48	0.07	0.00	14.0	3.1	59.3	0.0	5	1.36	9.4	68	278	186	0.7	91	0.00	0.00
0.05	0.23	3.48	0.07	0.00	14.0	3.1	—	0.0	5	1.36	9.4	68	278	2	0.7	91	0.00	0.00
0.02	0.11	1.08	0.10	0.00	15.1	0.2	—	0.0	2	0.31	10.1	21	84	3	1.0	83	0.00	0.00
0.14	0.67	6.13	0.14	0.00	28.1	4.7	0.0	0.2	8	1.92	15.6	162	577	6	1.1	92	0.00	0.00
0.15	0.25	2.64	0.07	0.10	11.0	2.8	25.0	0.8	100	1.49	14.3	107	209	298	0.7	43	0.07	0.00
0.05	0.09	0.61	0.14	0.00	102.2	35.4	—	1.7	104	0.98	21.0	57	283	22	0.2	94	0.00	0.00
0.18	0.14	1.44	0.11	0.03	38.1	10.3	11.0	3.0	61	1.25	35.8	122	190	122	0.5	67	0.00	0.00
0.09	0.10	0.72	0.03	0.00	134.3	11.2	—	0.3	88	0.62	46.9	42	215	220	0.6	91	0.00	0.00
0.07	0.03	1.05	—	0.00	—	4.2	—	—	18	0.82	—	—	161	200	—	52	0.00	0.00
0.03	0.01	0.17	0.14	0.00	15.7	5.5	—	0.0	23	0.25	11.5	37	174	251	0.2	88	0.00	0.00
0.01	0.00	0.07	0.05	0.00	6.8	2.3	0.0	0.1	10	0.10	4.9	16	75	1	0.1	88	0.00	0.00
0.03	0.01	0.17	0.14	0.00	15.7	5.5	—	0.0	23	0.25	11.5	37	174	3	0.2	88	0.00	0.00
0.07	0.03	0.30	0.23	0.00	32.3	10.9	0.0	0.7	42	0.46	21.0	69	330	6	0.4	90	0.00	0.00
0.07	0.03	0.30	0.23	0.00	32.3	10.2	0.0	0.7	42	0.46	21.0	69	330	6	0.4	90	0.00	0.00
0.03	0.01	0.17	0.14	0.00	15.7	5.5	—	0.0	23	0.25	11.5	37	174	3	0.2	88	0.00	0.00
0.03	0.01	0.17	0.14	0.00	15.7	5.5	—	0.0	23	0.25	11.5	37	174	3	0.2	88	0.00	0.00
0.12	0.07	1.12	0.15	0.00	90.5	20.3	—	1.6	58	0.89	45.2	108	573	16	0.4	80	0.00	0.00
0.03	0.01	0.33	0.15	0.00	12.0	51.7	0.0	0.5	6	0.31	6.8	13	120	1	0.1	92	0.00	0.00
0.03	0.01	0.33	0.15	0.00	12.7	51.7	0.0	0.5	6	0.31	6.8	13	120	1	0.1	92	0.00	0.00
0.03	0.05	0.57	0.20	0.00	2.0	177.0	—	1.4	8	0.30	8.0	15	134	17	0.1	83	0.00	0.00
0.03	0.01	0.33	0.15	0.00	12.7	110.2	0.0	0.5	6	0.31	6.8	13	120	1	0.1	92	0.00	0.00
0.15	0.05	1.32	0.33	0.00	25.2	4.8	—	2.8	19	1.05	28.8	47	220	14	0.3	72	0.00	0.00
—	—	—	—	—	—	18.0	—	—	0	0.72	—	—	—	5	—	79	0.00	0.00
—	—	—	—	—	—	18.0	—	—	0	0.72	—	—	—	5	—	79	0.00	0.00
0.01	0.05	0.25	0.03	0.00	5.2	6.0	—	—	45	0.43	38.5	21	281	25	0.1	94	0.00	0.00
0.10	0.05	0.86	0.11	0.00	18.0	22.6	—	0.4	58	0.63	27.6	67	391	24	0.4	89	0.00	0.00
0.10	0.01	0.50	0.05	0.00	37.6	3.9	—	0.1	28	0.62	28.2	63	167	5	0.5	79	0.00	0.00
0.07	0.12	0.34	0.09	0.00	26.1	18.5	—	—	90	1.75	40.0	33	260	79	—	91	0.00	0.00
0.09	0.20	0.43	0.21	0.00	131.4	8.8	0.0	1.9	122	3.21	78.3	50	419	275	0.7	91	0.00	0.00
0.09	0.20	0.43	0.21	0.00	131.4	8.8	—	1.9	122	3.21	78.3	50	419	63	0.7	91	0.00	0.00
0.05	0.17	0.62	0.17	0.00	120.7	16.1	0.0	1.8	89	2.44	75.0	40	494	75	0.5	92	0.00	0.00
0.11	0.00	0.64	0.14	0.00	13.5	8.0	—	0.1	32	0.68	31.9	33	322	4	0.1	90	0.00	0.00
0.07	0.01	0.99	0.12	0.00	19.5	15.5	—	1.3	42	0.62	29.7	28	291	4	0.1	88	0.00	0.00
0.02	0.01	0.62	0.07	0.00	6.2	2.7	—	0.1	16	0.25	8.5	11	91	14	0.2	92	0.00	0.00
0.02	0.01	0.62	0.07	0.00	6.2	2.7	—	0.1	16	0.25	8.5	11	91	197	0.2	92	0.00	0.00
0.03	0.03	0.46	0.05	0.00	18.0	4.9	—	0.1	24	0.31	21.6	35	173	213	0.4	94	0.00	0.00

PAGE KEY: A-46 Beverage and Beverage Mixes   A-48 Other Beverages   A-48 Beverages, Alcoholic   A-50 Candies and Confections, Gum   A-54 Cereals, Breakfast Type   A-58 Cheese and Cheese Substitutes   A-60 Dairy Products and Substitutes   A-62 Desserts   A-68 Dessert Toppings   A-68 Eggs, Substitutes, and Egg Dishes   A-70 Ethnic Foods   A-74 Fast Foods/Restaurants   A-88 Fats, Oils, Margarines, Shortenings, and Substitutes   A-88 Fish, Seafood, and Shellfish   A-90 Food Additives   A-90 Fruit, Vegetable, or Blended Juices   A-92 Grains, Flours, and Fractions   A-92 Grain Products, Prepared and Baked Goods

Code	Food Name	Unit/ Amt	Wt (g)	Energy (kcal)	Prot (g)	Carb (g)	Fiber (g)	Fat (g)	Sat (g)	Mono (g)	Poly (g)	Chol (mg)	Vit A (RE)
5152	Squash, summer, all types, ckd, drained, slices	0.5 cup	90	18	1	4	1	0	0.1	0.0	0.1	0	20
5153	Squash, winter, ckd w/salt	1 cup	240	94	2	21	7	2	0.3	0.1	0.6	0	854
5667	Squash, zucchini, slices, stmd	0.5 cup	90	13	1	3	1	0	0.0	0.0	0.1	0	29
5327	Squash, zucchini, w/skin, ckd, drained, slices	0.5 cup	90	14	1	4	1	0	0.0	0.0	0.0	0	101
5059	Swiss Chard, ckd, drained, chpd	0.5 cup	88	18	2	4	2	0	0.0	0.0	0.0	0	536
5544	Taro, ckd, slices, Tahitian, Colocassia	0.5 cup	68	30	3	5	1	0	0.1	0.0	0.2	0	121
7277	Tempeh, ckd	3.6 oz	100	197	18	9	—	11	3.4	3.7	2.6	—	—
5536	Tomatoes, green, ckd/frd	1 ea	144	284	5	19	1	22	4.6	9.4	6.4	41	82
5628	Tomatoes, red, fried	1 ea	101	168	3	12	1	13	2.7	5.5	3.8	24	57
5185	Turnip Greens, chpd, ckd, drained	0.5 cup	72	14	1	3	3	0	0.0	0.0	0.1	0	549
6004	Turnip Greens, ckd w/salt, drained, chpd	0.5 cup	72	14	1	3	3	0	0.0	0.0	0.1	0	549
6233	Vegetables, mixed, broccoli cauliflower carrots, fzn	0.5 cup	92	25	2	5	2	0	0.0	—	—	0	500
6644	Vegetables, mixed, broccoli cauliflower, fzn	0.5 cup	91	22	2	4	—	0	0.1	—	—	0	41
5187	Vegetables, mixed, ckd f/fzn w/o salt, drnd, 10 oz pkg	1 cup	182	118	5	24	8	0	0.1	0.0	0.1	0	779
6007	Vegetables, mixed, ckd f/fzn w/salt, drained	0.5 cup	91	54	3	12	4	0	0.0	0.0	0.1	0	389
6224	Vegetables, mixed, fzn	0.33 cup	85	52	2	12	3	0	0.1	—	—	0	582
6010	Yams, ckd/bkd w/salt, cubes	0.5 cup	68	79	1	19	3	0	0.0	0.0	0.0	0	8
5168	Yams, ckd/bkd, cubes	0.5 cup	68	79	1	19	3	0	0.0	0.0	0.0	0	8
Frozen, Dehydrated, and Dried Vegetables													
5361	Asparagus, spears, fzn	4 pce	58	14	2	2	1	0	0.0	0.0	0.1	0	55
6388	Broccoli, cuts, fzn	0.66 cup	90	25	2	4	2	0	0.0	0.0	0.0	0	40
6551	Broccoli, florets, select, fzn	1.33 cup	83	25	2	4	2	0	0.0	0.0	0.0	0	50
5740	Carrots, fzn, slices	0.5 cup	64	23	0	5	2	0	0.0	0.0	0.2	0	719
70617	Corn, cob, fzn	1 ea	174	212	6	45	—	6	1.1	0.2	0.3	0	59
6706	Corn, cob, Nibblers, fzn	1 ea	61	70	2	14	1	0	0.0	—	—	0	0
56958	Corn, cream style, fzn	0.5 cup	118	110	2	23	2	1	0.0	—	—	0	0
6392	Corn, niblets, fzn	0.66 cup	96	80	3	17	3	0	0.0	—	—	0	0
6018	Corn, white, sweet, kernels, fzn	0.5 cup	82	72	2	17	2	1	0.1	0.2	0.3	0	0
338	Dish, mixed vegetables, skillet, fzn	0.66 cup	82	25	2	4	2	0	0.0	0.0	0.0	0	200
6558	Mushrooms, dehyd	100 g	100	285	24	53	9	5	0.7	0.1	2.0	0	0
90491	Onion Rings, breaded, par fried, heated f/fzn	1 cup	48	195	3	18	1	13	4.1	5.2	2.5	0	11
5492	Onion, green, dehyd	100 g	100	295	20	66	10	2	0.3	0.3	0.6	0	5900
1830	Spinach, 80% ckd, fzn	3 oz	85	20	2	3	2	0	0.0	0.0	0.0	0	600
5446	Tomatoes, sun dried	0.5 cup	27	70	4	15	3	1	0.1	0.1	0.3	0	24
5821	Turnip Greens, fzn, chpd/dices, 10 oz pkg	0.5 cup	82	18	2	3	2	0	0.1	0.0	0.1	0	507
6395	Vegetables, stew style, fzn	0.5 cup	65	38	1	8	0	0	0.0	0.0	0.0	0	49
Canned Vegetables													
7867	Artichokes, hearts, cnd, pieces	3 pce	80	30	2	5	0	0	0.0	0.0	0.0	0	10
6261	Asparagus, spears, cnd	128 g	128	20	2	3	1	0	0.0	0.0	0.0	0	40
6607	Beets, slices, cnd	0.5 cup	121	35	1	8	2	0	0.0	0.0	0.0	0	0
5199	Carrots, cnd, drained, slices	1 ea	3	1	0	0	0	0	0.0	0.0	0.0	0	31
7933	Chili Peppers, green, cnd	0.5 cup	70	15	1	3	1	0	0.0	0.0	0.1	0	8
6268	Corn, cnd	0.33 cup	77	70	2	15	2	0	0.0	0.0	0.0	0	0
6265	Corn, cream style, cnd	0.5 cup	127	100	2	22	1	0	0.0	—	—	0	20
51031	Corn, golden, cream style, cnd	0.5 cup	125	90	2	20	2	1	0.0	—	—	0	0

PAGE KEY: A-96 Granola Bars, Cereal Bars, Diet Bars, Scones, and Tarts   A-96 Meals and Dishes   A-100 Meats   A-106 Nuts, Seeds, and Products   A-108 Poultry   A-110 Salad Dressings, Dips, and Mayonnaise   A-110 Salads   A-110 Sandwiches   A-114 Sauces and Gravies   A-114 Snack Foods—Chips, Pretzels, Popcorn   A-116 Soups, Stews, and Chilis   A-118 Spices, Flavors, and Seasonings   A-120 Sports Bars and Drinks   A-120 Supplemental Foods and Formulas   A-122 Sweeteners and Sweet Substitutes   A-122 Vegetables and Legumes   A-136 Weight Loss Bars and Drinks   A-138 Miscellaneous

Thia (mg)	Ribo (mg)	Niac (mg NE)	Vit B6 (mg)	Vit B12 (µg)	Fol (µg)	Vit C (mg)	Vit D (IU)	Vit E (mg AT)	Cal (mg)	Iron (mg)	Magn (mg)	Phos (mg)	Pota (mg)	Sodi (mg)	Zinc (mg)	Wat (%)	Alco (g)	Caff (g)
0.03	0.03	0.46	0.05	0.00	18.0	4.9	—	0.1	24	0.31	21.6	35	173	1	0.4	94	0.00	0.00
0.20	0.05	1.67	0.17	0.00	67.2	23.0	—	0.3	34	0.79	19.2	48	1049	2	0.6	89	0.00	0.00
0.05	0.02	0.34	0.07	0.00	16.9	6.9	0.0	0.1	14	0.37	19.8	29	223	3	0.2	95	0.00	0.00
0.03	0.03	0.38	0.07	0.00	15.3	4.1	—	0.1	12	0.31	19.8	36	228	3	0.2	95	0.00	0.00
0.02	0.07	0.31	0.07	0.00	7.9	15.8	—	1.7	51	1.98	75.2	29	480	157	0.3	93	0.00	0.00
0.02	0.14	0.33	0.07	0.00	4.8	26.0	—	1.8	102	1.07	34.9	46	427	37	0.1	86	0.00	0.00
0.05	0.36	2.13	0.20	0.14	21.0	—	—	—	96	2.13	77.0	253	401	14	1.6	60	0.00	0.00
0.15	0.18	1.36	0.10	0.14	12.7	20.9	9.2	3.0	101	1.50	17.1	102	254	134	0.4	68	0.00	0.00
0.10	0.11	0.97	0.07	0.07	11.8	13.4	6.5	1.8	55	0.93	12.6	62	200	78	0.2	72	0.00	0.00
0.02	0.05	0.30	0.12	0.00	85.0	19.7	—	1.4	99	0.57	15.8	21	146	21	0.1	93	0.00	0.00
0.02	0.05	0.30	0.12	0.00	85.0	19.7	0.0	1.4	99	0.57	15.8	21	146	191	0.1	93	0.00	0.00
0.05	0.07	0.46	0.15	0.00	50.0	43.7	—	—	31	0.51	12.9	39	192	28	—	—	0.00	0.00
—	—	—	—	0.00	—	—	54.7	—	29	0.44	—	—	—	22	—	—	0.00	0.00
0.12	0.21	1.54	0.12	0.00	34.6	5.8	—	0.8	46	1.49	40.0	93	308	64	0.9	83	0.00	0.00
0.05	0.10	0.76	0.07	0.00	17.3	2.9	0.0	0.3	23	0.75	20.0	46	154	247	0.4	83	0.00	0.00
0.09	0.05	1.01	0.11	0.00	23.8	7.6	—	—	20	0.72	16.1	47	167	37	—	83	0.00	0.00
0.05	0.01	0.37	0.15	0.00	10.9	8.2	—	0.3	10	0.34	12.2	33	456	166	0.1	70	0.00	0.00
0.05	0.01	0.37	0.15	0.00	10.9	8.2	—	0.3	10	0.34	12.2	33	456	5	0.1	70	0.00	0.00
0.07	0.07	0.69	0.05	0.00	110.8	18.4	—	1.2	14	0.41	8.1	37	147	5	0.3	92	0.00	0.00
—	—	—	—	0.00	—	42.0	—	—	20	0.72	—	—	—	150	—	93	0.00	0.00
—	—	—	—	—	—	36.0	—	—	0	0.00	—	—	—	20	—	92	0.00	0.00
0.02	0.01	0.30	0.05	0.00	6.4	1.6	—	0.5	23	0.28	7.7	21	150	44	0.2	90	0.00	0.00
0.14	0.14	4.30	—	0.00	—	14.9	—	—	—	1.66	—	—	532	26	—	67	0.00	0.00
—	—	—	—	0.00	—	2.4	—	—	0	0.00	—	—	—	5	—	72	0.00	0.00
—	—	—	—	—	—	40.0	—	—	0	0.00	—	—	—	330	—	—	0.00	0.00
—	—	—	—	0.00	—	1.2	—	—	0	0.36	—	—	—	60	—	78	0.00	0.00
0.07	0.05	1.41	0.15	0.00	29.5	5.2	0.0	0.0	3	0.34	14.8	57	172	2	0.3	75	0.00	0.00
—	—	—	—	—	—	18.0	—	—	0	0.00	—	—	—	30	—	—	0.00	0.00
1.13	5.13	47.00	1.13	0.00	241.0	40.0	—	—	57	14.19	114.0	1187	4224	46	8.3	6	0.00	0.00
0.12	0.07	1.73	0.03	0.00	31.7	0.7	—	0.3	15	0.81	9.1	39	62	180	0.2	28	0.00	0.00
0.82	1.64	2.35	0.00	0.00	162.0	531.0	—	—	708	22.29	236.0	390	3034	47	5.2	4	0.00	0.00
—	—	—	—	—	—	6.0	—	—	60	0.36	—	—	—	115	—	93	0.00	0.00
0.14	0.12	2.44	0.09	0.00	18.4	10.6	—	0.0	30	2.45	52.4	96	925	566	0.5	15	0.00	0.00
0.03	0.07	0.31	0.07	0.00	60.7	22.0	—	1.9	97	1.24	22.1	22	151	10	0.1	93	0.00	0.00
0.05	0.01	1.05	—	0.00	—	2.3	—	—	0	0.00	—	—	152	38	—	85	0.00	0.00
—	—	—	—	0.00	—	3.6	—	—	0	1.08	—	—	0	200	—	91	0.00	0.00
—	—	—	—	—	—	12.0	—	—	0	0.36	—	—	—	450	—	95	0.00	0.00
—	—	—	—	—	—	0.0	—	—	0	1.08	—	—	—	260	—	92	0.00	0.00
0.00	0.00	0.01	0.00	0.00	0.3	0.1	—	0.0	1	0.01	0.2	1	5	7	0.0	93	0.00	0.00
0.00	0.01	0.43	0.07	0.00	37.5	23.8	—	—	25	0.92	2.8	8	79	276	0.1	93	0.00	0.00
—	—	—	—	—	—	2.4	—	—	0	0.00	—	—	—	230	—	77	0.00	0.00
—	—	—	—	—	—	2.4	—	—	0	0.00	—	—	—	430	—	80	0.00	0.00
—	—	—	—	—	—	2.4	—	—	0	0.36	—	—	—	360	—	81	0.00	0.00

PAGE KEY: A-46 Beverage and Beverage Mixes   A-48 Other Beverages   A-48 Beverages, Alcoholic   A-50 Candies and Confections, Gum   A-54 Cereals, Breakfast Type   A-58 Cheese and Cheese Substitutes   A-60 Dairy Products and Substitutes   A-62 Desserts   A-68 Dessert Toppings   A-68 Eggs, Substitutes, and Egg Dishes   A-70 Ethnic Foods   A-74 Fast Foods/Restaurants   A-88 Fats, Oils, Margarines, Shortenings, and Substitutes   A-88 Fish, Seafood, and Shellfish   A-90 Food Additives   A-90 Fruit, Vegetable, or Blended Juices   A-92 Grains, Flours, and Fractions   A-92 Grain Products, Prepared and Baked Goods

Code	Food Name	Unit/ Amt	Wt (g)	Energy (kcal)	Prot (g)	Carb (g)	Fiber (g)	Fat (g)	Sat (g)	Mono (g)	Poly (g)	Chol (mg)	Vit A (RE)
51059	Corn, golden, whole kernel, cnd	0.5 cup	125	90	2	18	3	1	0.0	—	—	0	0
7855	Corn, whole kernel, cnd	0.5 cup	125	90	2	14	2	1	0.0	—	—	0	0
38077	Hominy, white, cnd	0.5 cup	82	59	1	12	2	1	0.1	0.2	0.3	0	0
5094	Mushrooms, cnd, drained, pces/slices	0.5 cup	78	20	1	4	2	0	0.0	0.0	0.1	0	0
5095	Mushrooms, cnd, drained, whole, med	1 ea	12	3	0	1	0	0	0.0	0.0	0.0	0	0
27169	Olives, black, jumbo, cnd	1 ea	8	7	0	0	0	1	0.1	0.4	0.0	0	3
9539	Olives, green, pickled, cnd	100 g	100	145	1	4	3	15	2.0	11.3	1.3	0	40
92209	Pickles, bread & butter	1 ea	8	6	0	1	0	0	0.0	0.0	0.0	0	1
90583	Pickles, dill, chpd/diced	1 cup	143	26	1	6	2	0	0.1	0.0	0.1	0	26
27028	Pickles, dill, low sod, med	1 ea	65	12	0	3	1	0	0.0	0.0	0.1	0	21
27039	Pickles, dill, rducd salt	1 ea	65	7	0	1	1	0	0.0	0.0	0.1	0	10
27013	Pickles, dill, slices	5 pce	35	6	0	1	1	0	0.0	0.0	0.0	0	6
27025	Pickles, sour	1 cup	155	17	1	4	2	0	0.1	0.0	0.1	0	22
90585	Pickles, sweet, slices	1 ea	7	8	0	2	0	0	0.0	0.0	0.0	0	1
5227	Pimentos, cnd	1 Tbs	12	3	0	1	0	0	0.0	0.0	0.0	0	32
5142	Pumpkin, cnd, unsalted	0.5 cup	122	42	1	10	4	0	0.2	0.0	0.0	0	1906
5964	Pumpkin, cnd, w/salt	0.5 cup	122	42	1	10	4	0	0.2	0.0	0.0	0	2702
27063	Relish, pickle, hotdog	1 Tbs	15	18	0	4	0	0	0.0	0.0	0.1	0	1
27052	Relish, pickle, sweet	1 cup	245	318	1	86	3	1	0.1	0.5	0.3	0	44
6393	Sauerkraut, crisp	30 g	30	5	0	1	1	0	0.0	0.0	0.0	0	0
5595	Spinach, cnd, not drained	0.5 cup	117	22	2	3	2	0	0.1	0.0	0.2	0	753
5599	Squash, zucchini, Italian style, cnd	0.5 cup	114	33	1	8	2	0	0.0	0.0	0.1	0	61
51000	Tomatoes, chunky, chili style, cnd	0.5 cup	128	30	1	8	2	0	0.0	0.0	0.0	0	50
51001	Tomatoes, chunky, pasta style, cnd	0.5 cup	128	45	1	11	2	0	0.0	0.0	0.0	0	50
6927	Tomatoes, crushed, cnd	0.5 cup	50	16	1	4	1	0	0.0	0.0	0.1	0	35
51005	Tomatoes, dices, cnd	0.5 cup	126	25	1	6	2	0	0.0	0.0	0.0	0	50
5630	Tomatoes, green, pickled	0.5 cup	71	26	1	6	1	0	0.0	0.1	0.1	0	59
6394	Tomatoes, pickled, halves	1 oz	28	5	0	1	1	0	0.0	0.0	0.0	0	0
6293	Tomatoes, puree, cnd	0.25 cup	63	20	1	4	0	0	0.0	0.0	0.0	0	50
9169	Tomatoes, stwd, cnd	0.5 cup	121	35	1	8	1	0	0.0	0.0	0.0	0	30
51020	Tomatoes, stwd, Italian recipe, cnd	0.5 cup	126	30	1	8	2	0	0.0	0.0	0.0	0	50
51022	Tomatoes, stwd, original recipe, cnd	0.5 cup	126	35	1	9	2	0	0.0	0.0	0.0	0	50
7885	Tomatoes, stwd, unsalted, cnd	0.5 cup	123	35	1	7	2	0	0.0	0.0	0.0	0	50
7896	Tomatoes, whole, peeled, cnd	0.5 cup	121	25	1	4	1	0	0.0	0.0	0.0	0	50
9520	Turnip Greens, cnd, unsalted	1 cup	144	27	2	4	2	0	0.1	0.0	0.2	0	858
51044	Vegetables, mixed, cnd	0.5 cup	124	40	2	8	2	0	0.0	0.0	0.0	0	225
5305	Vegetables, mixed, cnd, drained	0.5 cup	82	40	2	8	2	0	0.0	0.0	0.1	0	949
9522	Vegetables, mixed, cnd, unsalted	1 cup	182	67	3	13	6	0	0.1	0.0	0.2	0	2118
7873	Vegetables, peas & carrots, cnd	0.5 cup	123	50	4	10	3	0	0.0	0.0	0.0	0	500
Legumes													
7165	Beans, bbq	0.5 cup	100	160	6	32	6	2	0.5	—	—	—	—
7042	Beans, black turtle soup, mature, cnd	0.5 cup	120	109	7	20	8	0	0.1	0.0	0.2	0	0
7012	Beans, black, mature, ckd	1 cup	172	227	15	41	15	1	0.2	0.1	0.4	0	1
5213	Beans, blackeyed, immature, ckd, drained	0.5 cup	82	80	3	17	4	0	0.1	0.0	0.1	0	66
4450	Beans, blackeyed, mature, ckd	1 cup	172	200	13	36	11	1	0.2	0.1	0.4	0	3

PAGE KEY: A-96 Granola Bars, Cereal Bars, Diet Bars, Scones, and Tarts   A-96 Meals and Dishes   A-100 Meats   A-106 Nuts, Seeds, and Products   A-108 Poultry   A-110 Salad Dressings, Dips, and Mayonnaise   A-110 Salads   A-110 Sandwiches   A-114 Sauces and Gravies   A-114 Snack Foods—Chips, Pretzels, Popcorn   A-116 Soups, Stews, and Chilis   A-118 Spices, Flavors, and Seasonings   A-120 Sports Bars and Drinks   A-120 Supplemental Foods and Formulas   A-122 Sweeteners and Sweet Substitutes   A-122 Vegetables and Legumes   A-136 Weight Loss Bars and Drinks   A-138 Miscellaneous

Thia (mg)	Ribo (mg)	Niac (mg NE)	Vit B6 (mg)	Vit B12 (µg)	Fol (µg)	Vit C (mg)	Vit D (IU)	Vit E (mg AT)	Cal (mg)	Iron (mg)	Magn (mg)	Phos (mg)	Pota (mg)	Sodi (mg)	Zinc (mg)	Wat (%)	Alco (g)	Caff (g)
—	—	—	—	—	—	3.6	—	—	0	0.36	—	—	—	360	—	82	0.00	0.00
—	—	—	—	0.00	—	2.4	—	—	0	0.36	—	—	0	340	—	85	0.00	0.00
0.00	0.00	0.02	0.00	0.00	0.8	0.0	—	0.0	8	0.50	13.2	29	7	173	0.9	83	0.00	0.00
0.07	0.01	1.24	0.05	0.00	9.4	0.0	—	0.0	9	0.62	11.7	51	101	332	0.6	91	0.00	0.00
0.00	0.00	0.18	0.00	0.00	1.4	0.0	—	0.0	1	0.09	1.8	8	15	51	0.1	91	0.00	0.00
0.00	0.00	0.00	0.00	0.00	0.0	0.1	0.0	0.1	8	0.28	0.3	0	1	75	0.0	84	0.00	0.00
0.01		0.23	0.02	0.00	3.0	0.0	—	3.8	52	0.49	11.0	4	42	1556	0.0	75	0.00	0.00
0.00	0.00	0.00	0.00	0.00	0.3	0.7	—	0.0	3	0.02	0.2	2	16	54	0.0	79	0.00	0.00
0.01	0.03	0.09	0.01	0.00	1.4	2.7	—	0.1	13	0.75	15.7	30	166	1833	0.2	92	0.00	0.00
0.00	0.01	0.03	0.00	0.00	0.6	1.2	—	0.1	6	0.34	7.1	14	75	12	0.1	92	0.00	0.00
0.00	0.00	0.00	0.00	0.00	0.5	0.6	—	0.0	0	0.25	2.6	9	15	12	0.0	94	0.00	0.00
0.00	0.00	0.01	0.00	0.00	0.3	0.7	—	0.0	3	0.18	3.8	7	41	449	0.0	92	0.00	0.00
0.00	0.01	0.00	0.00	0.00	1.5	1.5	—	0.1	0	0.62	6.2	22	36	1872	0.0	94	0.00	0.00
0.00	0.00	0.00	0.00	0.00	0.1	0.1	—	0.0	0	0.03	0.3	1	2	66	0.0	65	0.00	0.00
0.00	0.00	0.07	0.02	0.00	0.7	10.2	—	0.1	1	0.20	0.7	2	19	2	0.0	93	0.00	0.00
0.02	0.07	0.44	0.07	0.00	14.7	5.1	—	1.3	32	1.70	28.2	43	252	6	0.2	90	0.00	0.00
0.02	0.07	0.44	0.07	0.00	14.7	5.1	—	1.2	32	1.70	28.2	43	252	295	0.2	90	0.00	0.00
0.00	0.00	0.00	0.00	0.00	0.8	0.9	0.0	0.0	4	0.20	3.2	3	31	81	0.0	69	0.00	0.00
0.00	0.07	0.56	0.03	0.00	2.5	2.5	—	0.2	7	2.13	12.2	34	61	1987	0.3	62	0.00	0.00
—	—	—	—	—	—	3.6	—	—	0	0.00	—	—	—	220	—	94	0.00	0.00
0.01	0.11	0.31	0.09	0.00	67.9	15.8	—	1.3	97	1.85	65.5	37	269	373	0.5	93	0.00	0.00
0.05	0.05	0.60	0.17	0.00	34.0	2.6	0.0	0.1	19	0.76	15.9	33	311	424	0.3	91	0.00	0.00
—	—	—	—	—	—	9.0	—	—	20	0.36	—	—	—	670	—	92	0.00	0.00
—	—	—	—	—	—	9.0	—	—	20	0.36	—	—	—	560	—	—	0.00	0.00
0.03	0.02	0.62	0.07	0.00	6.6	4.6	—	0.3	17	0.66	10.1	16	148	67	0.1	89	0.00	0.00
—	—	—	—	—	—	9.0	—	—	20	0.36	—	—	—	160	—	—	0.00	0.00
0.03	0.01	0.28	0.05	0.00	5.3	20.0	0.0	0.2	11	0.36	7.5	19	128	89	0.1	90	0.00	0.00
—	—	—	—	—	—	0.0	—	—	0	0.00	—	—	—	324	—	—	0.00	0.00
—	—	—	—	—	—	9.0	—	—	0	0.36	—	—	—	15	—	91	0.00	0.00
—	—	—	—	—	—	15.0	—	—	60	1.08	—	—	—	390	—	—	0.00	0.00
—	—	—	—	—	—	9.0	—	—	20	0.36	—	—	—	420	—	—	0.00	0.00
—	—	—	—	—	—	9.0	—	—	20	0.36	—	—	—	360	—	—	0.00	0.00
—	—	—	—	0.00	—	12.0	—	—	40	1.44	—	—	150	15	—	93	0.00	0.00
—	—	—	—	0.00	—	12.0	—	—	20	0.72	—	—	200	220	—	95	0.00	0.00
0.00	0.09	0.51	0.05	0.00	132.5	22.3	—	2.1	170	2.17	28.8	30	203	42	0.3	95	0.00	0.00
—	—	—	—	—	—	2.4	—	—	20	0.72	—	—	—	360	—	91	0.00	0.00
0.03	0.03	0.46	0.05	0.00	19.6	4.1	—	0.3	22	0.86	13.0	34	237	121	0.3	87	0.00	0.00
0.05	0.07	0.87	0.15	0.00	32.8	6.9	—	0.6	38	1.17	27.3	67	251	47	0.9	90	0.00	0.00
—	—	—	—	0.00	—	9.0	—	—	20	1.08	—	—	0	330	—	88	0.00	0.00
—	—	—	—	—	—	—	—	—	—	—	—	—	—	640	—	—	0.00	0.00
0.17	0.14	0.74	0.07	0.00	73.2	3.2	—	0.3	42	2.27	42.0	130	370	461	0.6	76	0.00	0.00
0.41	0.10	0.87	0.11	0.00	256.3	0.0	—	0.1	46	3.60	120.4	241	611	2	1.9	66	0.00	0.00
0.07	0.11	1.15	0.05	0.00	104.8	1.8	—	0.2	106	0.92	42.9	42	345	3	0.8	75	0.00	0.00
0.34	0.09	0.85	0.17	0.00	357.8	0.7	—	0.5	41	4.32	91.2	268	478	7	2.2	70	0.00	0.00

PAGE KEY: A-46 Beverage and Beverage Mixes A-48 Other Beverages A-48 Beverages, Alcoholic A-50 Candies and Confections, Gum A-54 Cereals, Breakfast Type A-58 Cheese and Cheese Substitutes A-60 Dairy Products and Substitutes A-62 Desserts A-68 Dessert Toppings A-68 Eggs, Substitutes, and Egg Dishes A-70 Ethnic Foods A-74 Fast Foods/Restaurants A-88 Fats, Oils, Margarines, Shortenings, and Substitutes A-88 Fish, Seafood, and Shellfish A-90 Food Additives A-90 Fruit, Vegetable, or Blended Juices A-92 Grains, Flours, and Fractions A-92 Grain Products, Prepared and Baked Goods

Code	Food Name	Unit/ Amt	Wt (g)	Energy (kcal)	Prot (g)	Carb (g)	Fiber (g)	Fat (g)	Sat (g)	Mono (g)	Poly (g)	Chol (mg)	Vit A (RE)
7027	Beans, broad, mature, ckd	1 cup	170	187	13	33	9	1	0.1	0.1	0.3	0	3
7056	Beans, catjang cowpeas, ckd	1 cup	171	200	14	35	6	1	0.3	0.1	0.5	0	3
4441	Beans, chickpea, mature, ckd	0.5 cup	82	134	7	22	6	2	0.2	0.5	0.9	0	2
4465	Beans, cowpeas, immature, ckd, drained	1 cup	165	160	5	34	8	1	0.2	0.1	0.3	0	132
7018	Beans, cowpeas, mature, ckd	0.5 cup	86	100	7	18	6	0	0.1	0.0	0.2	0	2
4444	Beans, fava, mature, ckd	1 cup	170	187	13	33	9	1	0.1	0.1	0.3	0	3
7045	Beans, French, mature, ckd	1 cup	177	228	12	43	17	1	0.1	0.1	0.8	0	1
7175	Beans, garbanzo, cnd	0.5 cup	130	100	6	16	4	2	0.0	—	—	0	0
7001	Beans, garbanzo, mature, ckd	1 cup	164	269	15	45	12	4	0.4	1.0	1.9	0	3
7031	Beans, goa, mature, ckd	1 cup	172	253	18	26	4	10	1.4	3.7	2.7	0	0
7219	Beans, golden gram, mature, ckd	0.5 cup	101	106	7	19	8	0	0.1	0.1	0.1	0	2
7021	Beans, great northern, mature, ckd	1 cup	177	209	15	37	12	1	0.2	0.0	0.3	0	0
6219	Beans, green, cut, fzn	0.5 cup	83	25	1	6	2	0	0.0	—	—	0	44
6220	Beans, green, French cut, fzn	0.5 cup	83	25	1	6	2	0	0.0	—	—	0	38
5013	Beans, green, snap, ckd f/fzn, drained	1 cup	135	38	2	9	4	0	0.1	0.0	0.1	0	76
5856	Beans, green, snap, ckd w/salt, drained	1 cup	125	44	2	10	4	0	0.1	0.0	0.2	0	88
5009	Beans, green, snap, fresh	0.5 cup	55	17	1	4	2	0	0.0	0.0	0.0	0	38
6198	Beans, green, whole, deluxe, fzn	10 ea	40	11	1	2	1	0	0.0	—	—	0	27
6241	Beans, green, whole, fzn	21 ea	84	22	1	5	2	0	0.0	—	—	0	58
7008	Beans, kidney, all types, mature, ckd	1 cup	177	225	15	40	11	1	0.1	0.1	0.5	0	0
7047	Beans, kidney, red, mature, ckd	1 cup	177	225	15	40	13	1	0.1	0.1	0.5	0	0
7006	Beans, lentils, ckd f/dry w/o salt	0.5 cup	99	115	9	20	8	0	0.1	0.1	0.2	0	1
90019	Beans, lentils, mature, ckd w/salt	1 cup	198	230	18	40	16	1	0.1	0.1	0.3	0	2
6222	Beans, lima, baby, fzn	0.5 cup	94	126	7	24	6	0	0.1	—	—	0	22
7058	Beans, lima, baby, mature, ckd	0.5 cup	91	115	7	21	7	0	0.1	0.0	0.2	0	0
7010	Beans, lima, lrg, mature, ckd	1 cup	188	216	15	39	13	1	0.2	0.1	0.3	0	0
7059	Beans, mung, mature, ckd	0.5 cup	101	106	7	19	8	0	0.1	0.1	0.1	0	2
7022	Beans, navy, mature, ckd	1 cup	182	255	15	47	19	1	0.1	0.2	0.6	0	0
7050	Beans, pink, mature, ckd	1 cup	169	252	15	47	9	1	0.2	0.1	0.4	0	0
7013	Beans, pinto, mature, ckd	1 cup	171	245	15	45	15	1	0.2	0.2	0.3	0	0
7053	Beans, white, mature, ckd	1 cup	179	249	17	45	11	1	0.2	0.1	0.3	0	0
57290	Dish, green beans, French cut, w/toasted almonds, fzn	0.66 cup	81	51	2	6	2	3	0.3	—	—	0	33
5939	Peas, green, ckd f/fzn w/salt, drained	0.5 cup	80	62	4	11	4	0	0.0	0.0	0.1	0	53
5938	Peas, green, ckd w/salt, drained	0.5 cup	80	67	4	13	4	0	0.0	0.0	0.1	0	64
5116	Peas, green, fresh	1 cup	145	117	8	21	7	1	0.1	0.1	0.3	0	110
6226	Peas, green, fzn	0.5 cup	89	71	5	13	5	0	0.1	—	—	0	62
7020	Peas, split, ckd	1 cup	196	231	16	41	16	1	0.1	0.2	0.3	0	1
6364	Peas, sweet, fzn	0.66 cup	94	60	4	12	4	0	0.0	0.0	0.0	0	30
5971	Soybeans, green, ckd w/salt, drained	0.5 cup	90	127	11	10	4	6	0.7	1.1	2.7	0	14
7015	Soybeans, mature, ckd	1.25 cup	215	372	36	21	13	19	2.8	4.3	10.9	0	2
90028	Soybeans, mature, ckd w/salt	1.25 cup	215	372	36	21	13	19	2.8	4.3	10.9	0	2
5123	Vegetables, peas & carrots, ckd f/fzn, drnd	0.5 cup	80	38	2	8	2	0	0.1	0.0	0.2	0	749
Potatoes													
6179	Dish, baked potato & broccoli, w/cheese sauce	1 ea	339	403	14	47	—	21	8.5	7.7	4.2	20	315
5464	Dish, mashed potatoes, flakes, prep f/dry w/milk & butter	0.5 cup	105	102	2	11	1	5	2.9	1.2	0.1	15	46
5138	Dish, mashed potatoes, flakes, prep f/dry w/milk & margarine	0.5 cup	105	119	2	16	2	6	1.5	2.4	1.6	4	52

PAGE KEY: A-96 Granola Bars, Cereal Bars, Diet Bars, Scones, and Tarts   A-96 Meals and Dishes   A-100 Meats   A-106 Nuts, Seeds, and Products   A-108 Poultry   A-110 Salad Dressings, Dips, and Mayonnaise   A-110 Salads   A-110 Sandwiches   A-114 Sauces and Gravies   A-114 Snack Foods—Chips, Pretzels, Popcorn   A-116 Soups, Stews, and Chilis   A-118 Spices, Flavors, and Seasonings   A-120 Sports Bars and Drinks   A-120 Supplemental Foods and Formulas   A-122 Sweeteners and Sweet Substitutes   A-122 Vegetables and Legumes   A-136 Weight Loss Bars and Drinks   A-138 Miscellaneous

Thia (mg)	Ribo (mg)	Niac (mg NE)	Vit B6 (mg)	Vit B12 (µg)	Fol (µg)	Vit C (mg)	Vit D (IU)	Vit E (mg AT)	Cal (mg)	Iron (mg)	Magn (mg)	Phos (mg)	Pota (mg)	Sodi (mg)	Zinc (mg)	Wat (%)	Alco (g)	Caff (g)
0.15	0.15	1.21	0.11	0.00	176.8	0.5	—	0.0	61	2.54	73.1	212	456	8	1.7	72	0.00	0.00
0.28	0.07	1.22	0.15	0.00	242.8	0.7	—	0.6	44	5.21	164.2	243	641	32	3.2	70	0.00	0.00
0.10	0.05	0.43	0.10	0.00	141.0	1.1	—	0.3	40	2.36	39.4	138	239	6	1.3	60	0.00	0.00
0.17	0.23	2.30	0.10	0.00	209.6	3.6	—	0.4	211	1.85	85.8	84	690	7	1.7	75	0.00	0.00
0.17	0.05	0.43	0.09	0.00	178.9	0.3	—	0.2	21	2.16	45.6	134	239	3	1.1	70	0.00	0.00
0.15	0.15	1.21	0.11	0.00	176.8	0.5	—	0.0	61	2.54	73.1	212	456	8	1.7	72	0.00	0.00
0.23	0.10	0.97	0.18	0.00	132.8	2.1	—	0.2	112	1.90	99.1	181	655	11	1.1	67	0.00	0.00
—	—	—	—	0.00	—	0.0	—	—	40	1.44	—	—	—	340	—	—	0.00	0.00
0.18	0.10	0.86	0.23	0.00	282.1	2.1	—	0.6	80	4.73	78.7	276	477	11	2.5	60	0.00	0.00
0.50	0.21	1.42	0.07	0.00	17.2	0.0	—	0.2	244	7.44	92.9	263	482	22	2.5	67	0.00	0.00
0.17	0.05	0.57	0.07	0.00	160.6	1.0	—	0.2	27	1.40	48.5	100	269	2	0.8	73	0.00	0.00
0.28	0.10	1.21	0.20	0.00	180.5	2.3	—	0.5	120	3.76	88.5	292	692	4	1.6	69	0.00	0.00
0.03	0.07	0.02	0.03	0.00	10.8	8.9	—	—	35	0.70	16.6	22	128	3	—	—	0.00	0.00
0.05	0.07	0.25	0.03	0.00	11.1	7.6	—	—	38	0.79	18.3	21	141	3	—	—	0.00	0.00
0.05	0.11	0.51	0.07	0.00	31.1	5.5	—	0.5	66	1.19	32.4	42	170	12	0.6	91	0.00	0.00
0.09	0.11	0.76	0.07	0.00	41.2	12.1	—	0.6	58	1.60	31.2	49	374	299	0.5	89	0.00	0.00
0.05	0.05	0.40	0.03	0.00	20.4	9.0	—	0.2	20	0.56	13.8	21	115	3	0.1	90	0.00	0.00
0.01	0.03	0.11	0.01	0.00	4.7	4.3	—	—	15	0.31	8.0	10	71	1	—	—	0.00	0.00
0.05	0.07	0.25	0.03	0.00	9.8	9.1	—	—	32	0.64	16.8	21	149	2	—	—	0.00	0.00
0.28	0.10	1.01	0.20	0.00	230.1	2.1	—	0.1	62	3.93	74.3	244	717	2	1.8	67	0.00	0.00
0.28	0.10	1.01	0.20	0.00	230.1	2.1	—	1.5	50	5.19	79.7	251	713	4	1.9	67	0.00	0.00
0.17	0.07	1.04	0.18	0.00	179.2	1.5	—	0.1	19	3.29	35.6	178	365	2	1.3	70	0.00	0.00
0.33	0.14	2.09	0.34	0.00	358.4	3.0	—	0.2	38	6.59	71.3	356	731	471	2.5	70	0.00	0.00
0.09	0.07	1.12	0.15	0.00	83.2	18.0	—	—	32	1.85	45.1	96	471	114	0.9	65	0.00	0.00
0.15	0.05	0.60	0.07	0.00	136.5	0.0	—	0.2	26	2.18	48.2	116	365	3	0.9	67	0.00	0.00
0.30	0.10	0.79	0.30	0.00	156.0	0.0	—	0.3	32	4.48	80.8	209	955	4	1.8	70	0.00	0.00
0.17	0.05	0.57	0.07	0.00	160.6	1.0	—	0.2	27	1.40	48.5	100	269	2	0.8	73	0.00	0.00
0.43	0.11	1.17	0.25	0.00	254.8	1.6	—	0.0	126	4.30	96.5	262	708	0	1.9	64	0.00	0.00
0.43	0.10	0.95	0.30	0.00	283.9	0.0	—	1.7	88	3.89	109.9	279	859	3	1.6	61	0.00	0.00
0.33	0.10	0.54	0.38	0.00	294.1	1.4	—	1.6	79	3.56	85.5	251	746	2	1.7	63	0.00	0.00
0.20	0.07	0.25	0.17	0.00	145.0	0.0	—	1.7	161	6.61	112.8	202	1004	11	2.5	63	0.00	0.00
—	—	—	—	0.00	—	6.6	—	—	42	1.08	—	—	—	347	—	—	0.00	0.00
0.23	0.07	1.17	0.09	0.00	47.2	7.9	—	0.1	19	1.25	23.2	72	134	258	0.8	80	0.00	0.00
0.20	0.11	1.62	0.17	0.00	50.4	11.4	—	0.1	22	1.23	31.2	94	217	191	1.0	78	0.00	0.00
0.38	0.18	3.02	0.25	0.00	94.2	58.0	—	0.2	36	2.13	47.9	157	354	7	1.8	79	0.00	0.00
0.28	0.09	1.96	0.11	0.00	49.2	17.8	—	—	21	1.41	22.2	79	152	125	0.9	79	0.00	0.00
0.37	0.10	1.74	0.09	0.00	127.4	0.8	—	0.1	27	2.52	70.6	194	710	4	2.0	69	0.00	0.00
—	—	—	—	0.00	—	6.0	—	—	0	1.08	—	—	—	200	—	—	0.00	0.00
0.23	0.14	1.12	0.05	0.00	99.9	15.3	—	0.0	130	2.25	54.0	142	485	225	0.8	69	0.00	0.00
0.33	0.61	0.86	0.50	0.00	116.1	3.7	—	0.8	219	11.05	184.9	527	1107	2	2.5	63	0.00	0.00
0.33	0.61	0.86	0.50	0.00	116.1	3.7	—	0.8	219	11.05	184.9	527	1107	510	2.5	63	0.00	0.00
0.18	0.05	0.92	0.07	0.00	20.8	6.5	—	0.4	18	0.75	12.8	39	126	54	0.4	86	0.00	0.00
0.27	0.27	3.58	0.77	0.34	61.0	48.5	—	—	336	3.31	78.0	346	1441	485	2.0	70	0.00	0.00
0.14	0.05	0.80	0.10	0.11	6.3	10.6	12.9	0.1	30	0.17	11.5	41	170	172	0.2	81	0.00	0.00
0.11	0.05	0.69	0.00	0.00	7.3	10.2	—	0.7	51	0.23	18.9	59	245	349	0.2	76	0.00	0.00

PAGE KEY: A-46 Beverage and Beverage Mixes A-48 Other Beverages A-48 Beverages, Alcoholic A-50 Candies and Confections, Gum A-54 Cereals, Breakfast Type A-58 Cheese and Cheese Substitutes A-60 Dairy Products and Substitutes A-62 Desserts A-68 Dessert Toppings A-68 Eggs, Substitutes, and Egg Dishes A-70 Ethnic Foods A-74 Fast Foods/Restaurants A-88 Fats, Oils, Margarines, Shortenings, and Substitutes A-88 Fish, Seafood, and Shellfish A-90 Food Additives A-90 Fruit, Vegetable, or Blended Juices A-92 Grains, Flours, and Fractions A-92 Grain Products, Prepared and Baked Goods

Code	Food Name	Unit/ Amt	Wt (g)	Energy (kcal)	Prot (g)	Carb (g)	Fiber (g)	Fat (g)	Sat (g)	Mono (g)	Poly (g)	Chol (mg)	Vit A (RE)
66107	Dish, mashed potatoes, real, premium, prep	0.5 cup	108	63	2	13	1	1	0.1	0.4	0.1	0	0
5137	Dish, mashed potatoes, w/whole milk	0.5 cup	105	87	2	18	2	1	0.3	0.1	0.1	2	4
5569	Dish, mashed potatoes, w/whole milk & butter	0.5 cup	105	119	2	18	2	4	1.8	1.3	0.2	12	38
5272	Dish, mashed potatoes, w/whole milk & margarine	0.5 cup	105	119	2	18	2	4	1.0	1.8	1.3	1	45
5786	Dish, potatoes au gratin, prep f/recipe w/butter	1 cup	245	323	12	28	4	19	11.6	5.3	0.7	56	164
5275	Dish, potatoes au gratin, prep f/recipe w/margarine	1 cup	245	323	12	28	4	19	8.6	6.3	2.6	37	167
70605	Dish, potatoes o'brien	0.5 cup	78	56	1	12	2	0	0.0	0.0	0.0	0	0
5787	Dish, potatoes o'brien, fzn	0.5 cup	97	74	2	17	2	0	0.0	0.0	0.1	—	14
5268	Dish, potatoes o'brien, prep f/recipe	1 cup	97	79	2	15	1	1	0.8	0.3	0.1	4	93
57362	Dish, potatoes, au gratin, prep f/dry	3 oz	85	90	3	14	—	2	—	—	—	—	—
70612	Dish, twice baked potatoes, w/butter	1 ea	143	204	4	27	4	9	3.1	3.1	0.5	0	86
5948	Potatoes, baked, peeled, salted	0.5 cup	61	57	1	13	1	0	0.0	0.0	0.0	0	0
5130	Potatoes, baked, peeled, unsalted	0.5 cup	61	57	1	13	1	0	0.0	0.0	0.0	0	0
6996	Potatoes, baked, salted	0.5 cup	61	57	2	13	1	0	0.0	0.0	0.0	0	1
5334	Potatoes, baked, unsalted, med, 2 1/4" to 3 1/4"	1 ea	173	161	4	37	4	0	0.1	0.0	0.1	0	3
7259	Potatoes, dehyd	100 g	100	367	8	81	3	1	—	—	—	—	0
5691	Potatoes, french fries, battered, shoestring, 80% ckd, fzn	3 oz	85	170	4	17	1	10	2.5	—	—	0	0
8900	Potatoes, french fries, crinkle, 1/2" x 1/2", 80% ckd, fzn	3 oz	85	170	3	24	2	7	2.0	—	—	0	0
5790	Potatoes, french fries, fzn	10 ea	65	101	2	16	2	4	0.6	2.4	0.4	0	0
5592	Potatoes, french fries, heated f/fzn w/o salt	10 ea	50	100	2	16	2	4	0.6	2.4	0.4	0	0
6413	Potatoes, french fries, waffle style	15 pce	84	140	2	22	2	5	1.5	2.0	0.0	0	0
6851	Potatoes, fresh, w/skin, med, 2 1/4" to 3 1/4"	1 ea	213	164	4	37	5	0	0.1	0.0	0.1	0	0
70611	Potatoes, hash browns, box, microwv	3.6 oz	100	193	2	23	1	10	2.6	3.5	0.0	0	0
70603	Potatoes, hash browns, shredded	0.5 cup	78	62	2	14	1	5	1.9	2.1	0.6	0	0
6402	Potatoes, patty, golden	1 ea	71	140	1	16	1	7	1.5	3.5	0.5	0	0
9250	Potatoes, red, w/skin, baked, med, 2 1/4" to 3 1/4"	1 ea	173	154	4	34	3	0	0.0	0.0	0.1	0	3
5512	Potatoes, rstd	1 ea	93	132	3	30	3	0	0.0	0.0	0.1	0	0
57368	Potatoes, scalloped, prep	3 oz	85	90	2	16	—	2	—	—	—	—	—
5339	Potatoes, skin, bkd	1 ea	58	115	2	27	5	0	0.0	0.0	0.0	0	1
70598	Potatoes, tater tots	0.5 cup	62	107	1	16	1	6	1.1	1.8	0.0	0	0
9247	Potatoes, w/skin, baked, med, 2 1/4"–3 1/4"	1 ea	173	163	4	36	4	0	0.0	0.0	0.1	0	3
7906	Potatoes, wedges, USDA, fzn	3 oz	85	105	2	22	2	2	0.5	1.2	0.1	0	0
5162	Sweetpotatoes, mashed f/cnd	1 cup	256	259	5	59	4	1	0.1	0.0	0.2	0	0
WEIGHT LOSS BARS & DRINKS													
Weight Loss Bars													
63408	Bar, diet, chocolate chip	1 ea	50	200	16	17	0	8	4.0	—	—	3	350
63370	Bar, diet, cranberry apple, granola	1 ea	56	220	8	35	1	5	3.5	—	—	5	150
8975	Bar, diet, hi prot & low carbohydrate, peanut butter	1 ea	50	190	22	2	0	5	2.5	—	—	0	0
62875	Bar, diet, hi prot, peanut butter	1 ea	70	250	30	11	2	6	3.5	—	—	0	0
62855	Bar, diet, oatmeal raisin	1 ea	56	220	8	36	2	5	3.5	—	—	3	350
62639	Bar, diet, peanut butter, breakfast & lunch	1 ea	34	150	5	19	2	6	2.5	—	—	5	250
63372	Bar, diet, peanut butter, granola	1 ea	56	220	8	35	1	6	3.5	—	—	5	150
Weight Loss Drinks													
62854	Drink, diet, cappuccino, milk base, rtd can	1 ea	345	220	10	42	5	1	0.5	0.5	0.0	5	350
62648	Drink, diet, choc fudge, milk base, rtd can	1 ea	345	220	10	42	5	3	1.0	1.5	0.5	5	350
63359	Drink, diet, chocolate, soy prot, rtd can	1 ea	345	230	12	39	5	3	1.0	1.5	0.5	0	350

PAGE KEY: A-96 Granola Bars, Cereal Bars, Diet Bars, Scones, and Tarts   A-96 Meals and Dishes   A-100 Meats   A-106 Nuts, Seeds, and Products   A-108 Poultry
A-110 Salad Dressings, Dips, and Mayonnaise   A-110 Salads   A-110 Sandwiches   A-114 Sauces and Gravies   A-114 Snack Foods—Chips, Pretzels, Popcorn
A-116 Soups, Stews, and Chilis   A-118 Spices, Flavors, and Seasonings   A-120 Sports Bars and Drinks   A-120 Supplemental Foods and Formulas
A-122 Sweeteners and Sweet Substitutes   A-122 Vegetables and Legumes   A-136 Weight Loss Bars and Drinks   A-138 Miscellaneous

Thia (mg)	Ribo (mg)	Niac (mg NE)	Vit B6 (mg)	Vit B12 (µg)	Fol (µg)	Vit C (mg)	Vit D (IU)	Vit E (mg AT)	Cal (mg)	Iron (mg)	Magn (mg)	Phos (mg)	Pota (mg)	Sodi (mg)	Zinc (mg)	Wat (%)	Alco (g)	Caff (g)
0.05	0.00	1.19	—	—	—	2.6	—	—	17	0.27	7.8	23	189	245	—	84	0.00	0.00
0.09	0.05	1.17	0.23	0.07	8.4	6.5	6.4	0.0	23	0.28	18.9	48	311	317	0.3	79	0.00	0.00
0.09	0.05	1.12	0.23	0.07	8.4	6.3	8.7	0.1	23	0.27	18.9	47	298	333	0.3	76	0.00	0.00
0.10	0.05	1.23	0.25	0.07	9.4	11.0	6.0	0.4	21	0.27	19.9	50	342	350	0.3	75	0.00	0.00
0.15	0.28	2.43	0.43	0.00	27.0	24.3	—	0.5	292	1.57	49.0	277	970	1061	1.7	74	0.00	0.00
0.15	0.28	2.43	0.43	0.00	27.0	24.3	—	1.3	292	1.57	49.0	277	970	1061	1.7	74	0.00	0.00
0.07	0.01	1.19	—	—	—	3.7	—	—	0	0.00	—	—	148	14	—	82	0.00	0.00
0.05	0.03	1.10	0.20	0.00	7.8	11.0	—	0.2	13	1.00	17.5	48	242	32	0.3	80	0.00	0.00
0.07	0.05	0.98	0.20	0.00	7.8	16.2	—	0.1	35	0.46	17.5	48	258	210	0.3	80	0.00	0.00
0.02	0.07	0.80	—	0.00	—	2.4	—	—	40	0.36	16.0	60	265	340	—	75	0.00	0.00
0.09	0.10	3.03	—	0.00	—	21.4	—	—	57	1.02	—	—	601	357	—	—	0.00	0.00
0.05	0.00	0.85	0.18	0.00	5.5	7.8	—	0.0	3	0.20	15.2	30	239	147	0.2	75	0.00	0.00
0.05	0.00	0.85	0.18	0.00	5.5	7.8	—	0.0	3	0.20	15.2	30	239	3	0.2	75	0.00	0.00
0.03	0.02	0.86	0.18	0.00	17.1	5.9	—	0.0	9	0.66	17.1	43	326	149	0.2	75	0.00	0.00
0.10	0.07	2.44	0.54	0.00	48.4	16.6	—	0.1	26	1.87	48.4	121	926	17	0.6	75	0.00	0.00
0.23	0.15	3.70	—	0.00	—	11.0	—	—	27	2.79	—	200	922	8	—	6	0.00	0.00
—	—	—	—	—	—	3.6	—	—	0	0.36	—	—	—	190	—	63	0.00	0.00
—	—	—	—	—	—	9.0	—	—	0	1.08	—	—	—	25	—	59	0.00	0.00
0.07	0.00	1.11	0.15	0.00	7.8	6.4	—	0.1	4	0.62	11.0	42	212	15	0.2	67	0.00	0.00
0.05	0.00	1.03	0.15	0.00	6.0	5.1	0.0	0.1	4	0.62	11.0	41	209	15	0.2	57	0.00	0.00
—	—	—	—	0.00	—	2.4	—	—	0	1.44	—	—	290	35	—	—	0.00	0.00
0.17	0.07	2.25	0.62	0.00	34.1	42.0	0.0	0.0	26	1.65	49.0	121	897	13	0.6	79	0.00	0.00
0.07	—	1.57	—	0.00	—	0.0	—	—	0	0.00	—	—	246	263	—	64	0.00	0.00
—	—	—	—	—	—	7.1	—	—	6	0.58	—	—	355	25	—	73	0.00	0.00
—	—	—	—	0.00	—	0.0	—	—	0	0.00	—	—	120	280	—	—	0.00	0.00
0.11	0.09	2.75	0.37	0.00	46.7	21.8	—	0.1	16	1.21	48.4	125	943	14	0.7	77	0.00	0.00
0.11	0.05	2.34	0.40	0.00	19.2	26.3	0.0	0.1	12	1.26	35.0	77	905	10	0.7	62	0.00	0.00
0.02	0.07	0.80	—	0.00	—	2.4	—	—	40	0.36	16.0	60	245	300	—	75	0.00	0.00
0.07	0.05	1.77	0.36	0.00	12.8	7.8	—	0.0	20	4.07	24.9	59	332	12	0.3	47	0.00	0.00
—	—	—	—	—	—	0.7	—	—	0	0.00	—	—	162	251	—	61	0.00	0.00
0.07	0.07	2.64	0.37	0.00	65.7	21.8	—	0.1	17	1.11	46.7	130	941	12	0.6	75	0.00	0.00
0.09	0.02	1.30	0.30	0.00	—	9.5	—	—	13	0.60	16.2	74	335	42	0.3	68	0.00	0.00
0.07	0.23	2.44	0.60	0.00	28.2	13.3	—	0.7	77	3.40	61.4	133	538	192	0.5	74	0.00	0.00
0.21	0.60	7.00	0.69	2.09	60.0	21.0	140.0	4.8	300	2.70	140.0	400	400	200	2.2	—	0.00	—
0.21	0.60	7.00	0.69	2.09	60.0	21.0	140.0	4.8	300	2.70	140.0	400	400	230	2.2	—	0.00	0.00
—	—	—	—	—	—	0.0	—	—	160	1.00	—	—	—	120	—	—	0.00	—
—	—	—	—	—	—	0.0	—	—	200	1.10	—	—	—	120	—	—	0.00	—
0.21	0.60	7.00	0.69	2.09	60.0	21.0	140.0	4.8	300	2.70	140.0	250	170	100	2.2	—	0.00	0.00
0.37	0.43	5.00	0.40	1.50	40.0	15.0	80.0	3.4	100	4.50	16.0	100	115	65	3.8	—	0.00	—
0.21	0.60	7.00	0.69	2.09	60.0	21.0	140.0	4.8	3000	2.70	140.0	400	400	320	2.2	—	0.00	—
0.51	0.60	7.00	0.69	2.09	120.0	60.0	140.0	13.6	400	2.70	140.0	400	600	220	2.2	—	0.00	—
0.51	0.60	7.00	0.69	2.09	120.0	60.0	140.0	13.6	400	2.70	140.0	400	600	220	2.2	—	0.00	—
0.44	0.50	6.00	0.60	2.09	160.0	30.0	120.0	3.4	400	4.50	100.0	300	700	420	3.8	—	0.00	—

PAGE KEY: A-46 Beverage and Beverage Mixes A-48 Other Beverages A-48 Beverages, Alcoholic A-50 Candies and Confections, Gum A-54 Cereals, Breakfast Type A-58 Cheese and Cheese Substitutes A-60 Dairy Products and Substitutes A-62 Desserts A-68 Dessert Toppings A-68 Eggs, Substitutes, and Egg Dishes A-70 Ethnic Foods A-74 Fast Foods/Restaurants A-88 Fats, Oils, Margarines, Shortenings, and Substitutes A-88 Fish, Seafood, and Shellfish A-90 Food Additives A-90 Fruit, Vegetable, or Blended Juices A-92 Grains, Flours, and Fractions A-92 Grain Products, Prepared and Baked Goods

Code	Food Name	Unit/ Amt	Wt (g)	Energy (kcal)	Prot (g)	Carb (g)	Fiber (g)	Fat (g)	Sat (g)	Mono (g)	Poly (g)	Chol (mg)	Vit A (RE)
62650	Drink, diet, milk choc, milk base, rtd can	1 ea	345	220	10	40	5	3	1.0	1.5	0.5	5	350
62646	Drink, diet, orange pineapple, rtd can	1 ea	360	220	7	46	5	1	0.0	0.0	0.0	5	500
62649	Drink, diet, straw cream, milk base, rtd can	1 ea	345	220	10	40	5	2	0.5	1.5	0.5	5	350
63374	Drink, diet, vanilla cream, low carb, rtd can	1 ea	350	190	20	7	5	9	1.5	6.0	1.5	15	350
63024	Shake, weight management, chocolate fudge, rtd	1 ea	250	100	15	5	—	2	0.0	—	—	15	150
63025	Shake, weight management, vanilla, rtd	1 ea	250	90	15	3	1	2	0.0	—	—	15	150

MISCELLANEOUS

Baking Chips, Chocolates, Coatings, and Cocoas

Code	Food Name	Unit/ Amt	Wt (g)	Energy (kcal)	Prot (g)	Carb (g)	Fiber (g)	Fat (g)	Sat (g)	Mono (g)	Poly (g)	Chol (mg)	Vit A (RE)
23519	Baking Chips, chocolate	31 pce	15	72	1	9	1	4	3.0	—	—	0	1
23012	Baking Chips, chocolate, semi sweet	10 pce	5	23	0	3	0	1	0.8	0.5	0.0	0	0
23200	Baking Chips, chocolate, semi sweet, w/butter	60 pce	28	135	1	18	2	8	5.0	2.8	0.3	5	2
23423	Baking Chips, M & M's, milk chocolate, mini bits	1 Tbs	14	71	1	10	0	3	2.1	1.1	0.1	2	6
23444	Baking Chips, milk chocolate, mini kisses	11 ea	15	80	1	9	0	4	3.0	—	—	5	0
4153	Baking Chips, Nestle Crunch, pieces	1.5 Tbs	15	80	1	10	0	4	2.0	—	—	0	0
23446	Baking Chips, Reese's peanut butter	1 Tbs	15	80	3	7	—	4	4.0	—	—	0	0
28299	Baking Chips, white chocolate, chunks	15 g	15	80	1	9	0	5	3.0	—	—	5	0
23401	Baking Chocolate, bar, semi sweet	0.5 oz	14	70	1	8	1	4	2.5	—	—	0	0
28063	Baking Chocolate, bar, unswtnd	0.5 oz	14	70	2	4	2	7	4.5	—	—	0	0
4355	Baking Chocolate, bar, white, premium	0.5 oz	14	80	1	8	0	4	3.0	—	—	5	0
28208	Baking Chocolate, unswntd, liquid	1 Tbs	15	71	2	5	3	7	3.8	1.4	1.6	0	0
28200	Cocoa Powder, unswntd	1 cup	86	197	17	47	29	12	6.9	3.9	0.4	0	0

Baking Ingredients

Code	Food Name	Unit/ Amt	Wt (g)	Energy (kcal)	Prot (g)	Carb (g)	Fiber (g)	Fat (g)	Sat (g)	Mono (g)	Poly (g)	Chol (mg)	Vit A (RE)
28006	Baking Powder, low sod	1 tsp	5	5	0	2	0	0	0.0	0.0	0.0	0	0
28003	Baking Soda	1 tsp	5	0	0	0	0	0	0.0	0.0	0.0	0	0
51150	Candied Fruit	3.6 oz	100	321	0	83	2	0	0.0	0.0	0.0	0	2
26017	Cream of Tartar	1 tsp	3	8	0	2	0	0	0.0	0.0	0.0	0	0
3977	Pineapple, slices, natural glace	1 pce	63	180	0	46	0	0	0.0	0.0	0.0	0	0
28149	Yeast, active, dry	3.6 oz	100	333	39	43	24	5	1.2	2.6	0.8	0	0
28000	Yeast, baker's, dry active	1 tsp	4	12	2	2	1	0	0.0	0.1	0.0	0	0

Condiments

Code	Food Name	Unit/ Amt	Wt (g)	Energy (kcal)	Prot (g)	Carb (g)	Fiber (g)	Fat (g)	Sat (g)	Mono (g)	Poly (g)	Chol (mg)	Vit A (RE)
9149	Catsup	1 Tbs	15	15	0	4	0	0	0.0	0.0	0.0	0	14
27032	Catsup, low sod	1 Tbs	15	16	0	4	0	0	0.0	0.0	0.0	0	16
90602	Catsup, low sod, pkt	1 ea	6	6	0	2	0	0	0.0	0.0	0.0	0	6
27004	Horseradish, prep	1 tsp	5	2	0	1	0	0	0.0	0.0	0.0	0	0
27000	Ketchup	1 Tbs	15	15	0	4	0	0	0.0	0.0	0.0	0	14
9151	Ketchup, low sod	1 Tbs	15	16	0	4	0	0	0.0	0.0	0.0	0	16
9152	Ketchup, low sod, pkt	1 ea	6	6	0	2	0	0	0.0	0.0	0.0	0	6
90931	Mustard, deli	100 g	100	113	5	10	6	7	0.3	—	—	0	4
27058	Mustard, dijon, Grey Poupon	0.5 cup	125	151	8	13	1	11	0.5	3.9	3.0	0	12
53254	Mustard, honey	1 ea	14	50	0	3	0	4	0.5	—	—	10	2
91801	Mustard, honey, fat free	1.5 Tbs	21	30	0	7	0	0	0.0	0.0	0.0	0	0
27070	Mustard, hot, pkt	1 ea	28	60	1	7	1	4	0.0	—	—	5	4
435	Mustard, yellow, prep	1 tsp	5	3	0	0	0	0	0.0	0.1	0.0	0	1
90211	Mustard, yellow, prep, pkt	1 ea	5	3	0	0	0	0	0.0	0.1	0.0	0	1
7523	Sauce, soy, dark	0.5 tsp	3	0	0	0	0	0	0.0	0.0	0.0	0	0

PAGE KEY: A-96 Granola Bars, Cereal Bars, Diet Bars, Scones, and Tarts   A-96 Meals and Dishes   A-100 Meats   A-106 Nuts, Seeds, and Products   A-108 Poultry
A-110 Salad Dressings, Dips, and Mayonnaise   A-110 Salads   A-110 Sandwiches   A-114 Sauces and Gravies   A-114 Snack Foods—Chips, Pretzels, Popcorn
A-116 Soups, Stews, and Chilis   A-118 Spices, Flavors, and Seasonings   A-120 Sports Bars and Drinks   A-120 Supplemental Foods and Formulas
A-122 Sweeteners and Sweet Substitutes   A-122 Vegetables and Legumes   A-136 Weight Loss Bars and Drinks   A-138 Miscellaneous

Thia (mg)	Ribo (mg)	Niac (mg NE)	Vit B6 (mg)	Vit B12 (µg)	Fol (µg)	Vit C (mg)	Vit D (IU)	Vit E (mg AT)	Cal (mg)	Iron (mg)	Magn (mg)	Phos (mg)	Pota (mg)	Sodi (mg)	Zinc (mg)	Wat (%)	Alco (g)	Caff (g)
0.51	0.60	7.00	0.69	2.09	120.0	60.0	140.0	13.6	400	2.70	140.0	400	600	220	2.2	—	0.00	—
0.51	0.60	7.00	0.69	2.09	120.0	60.0	140.0	13.6	350	2.70	140.0	400	500	180	2.2	—	0.00	0.00
0.51	0.60	7.00	0.69	2.09	120.0	60.0	140.0	13.6	400	2.70	140.0	400	600	220	2.2	—	0.00	0.00
0.51	0.60	2.00	0.20	0.60	120.0	60.0	140.0	13.6	400	2.70	140.0	400	400	200	2.2	—	0.00	0.00
0.30	0.34	0.40	—	1.50	120.0	15.0	—	4.1	100	0.00	80.0	150	280	170	3.0	—	0.00	—
0.30	0.34	—	0.40	1.50	120.0	—	—	4.1	100	0.00	80.0	150	170	170	3.0	—	0.00	0.00
—	—	—	—	—	—	0.0	—	—	5	2.00	—	—	—	31	—	4	0.00	—
0.00	0.00	0.01	0.00	0.00	0.1	0.0	—	0.0	2	0.15	5.4	6	17	1	0.1	1	0.00	2.93
0.01	0.02	0.11	0.00	0.00	0.9	0.0	—	0.3	9	0.88	32.6	37	103	3	0.5	1	0.00	17.57
0.00	0.02	0.02	0.00	0.03	0.7	0.1	—	0.1	16	0.17	6.5	24	42	10	0.2	2	0.00	2.50
—	—	—	—	—	—	0.0	—	—	20	0.00	—	—	—	15	—	2	0.00	—
—	—	—	—	—	—	0.0	—	—	0	0.00	—	—	—	25	—	2	0.00	—
—	—	—	—	—	—	0.0	—	—	0	0.00	—	—	—	35	—	—	0.00	0.00
—	—	—	—	—	—	0.0	—	—	20	0.00	—	—	—	15	—	0	0.00	—
—	—	—	—	—	—	0.0	—	—	0	0.72	—	—	—	0	—	3	0.00	—
—	—	—	—	—	—	0.0	—	—	0	1.44	—	—	—	0	—	4	0.00	—
—	—	—	—	—	—	0.0	—	—	20	0.00	—	—	—	15	—	3	0.00	—
0.00	0.03	0.31	0.00	0.00	2.9	0.0	—	0.9	8	0.62	39.8	51	175	2	0.6	1	0.00	7.05
0.07	0.20	1.87	0.10	0.00	27.5	0.0	—	0.1	110	11.92	429.1	631	1311	18	5.9	3	0.00	197.80
0.00	0.00	0.00	0.00	0.00	0.0	0.0	—	0.0	217	0.40	1.5	343	505	4	0.0	6	0.00	0.00
0.00	0.00	0.00	0.00	0.00	0.0	0.0	—	0.0	0	0.00	0.0	0	0	1259	0.0	0	0.00	0.00
0.00	0.00	0.00	0.00	0.00	0.0	0.0	—	0.0	18	0.17	4.0	5	57	98	0.1	17	0.00	0.00
0.00	0.00	0.00	0.00	0.00	0.0	0.0	—	0.0	0	0.10	0.1	0	495	2	0.0	2	0.00	0.00
—	—	—	—	0.00	—	0.0	—	—	0	0.00	—	—	5	40	—	27	0.00	0.00
10.00	5.00	41.00	—	—	—	6.0	—	—	73	6.00	—	898	1361	259	—	8	0.00	0.00
0.09	0.21	1.59	0.05	0.00	93.6	0.0	—	0.0	3	0.66	3.9	52	80	2	0.3	8	0.00	0.00
0.00	0.07	0.23	0.01	0.00	1.5	2.3	—	0.2	3	0.07	2.9	5	57	166	0.0	68	0.00	0.00
0.00	0.00	0.20	0.02	0.00	2.2	2.3	—	0.2	3	0.10	3.3	6	72	3	0.0	67	0.00	0.00
0.00	0.00	0.07	0.00	0.00	0.9	0.9	—	0.1	1	0.03	1.3	2	29	1	0.0	67	0.00	0.00
0.00	0.00	0.01	0.00	0.00	2.9	1.2	—	0.0	3	0.01	1.4	2	12	16	0.0	85	0.00	0.00
0.00	0.07	0.23	0.01	0.00	1.5	2.3	—	0.2	3	0.07	2.9	5	57	166	0.0	68	0.00	0.00
0.00	0.00	0.20	0.02	0.00	2.2	2.3	—	0.2	3	0.10	3.3	6	72	3	0.0	67	0.00	0.00
0.00	0.00	0.07	0.00	0.00	0.9	0.9	—	0.1	1	0.03	1.3	2	29	1	0.0	67	0.00	0.00
—	—	—	—	—	—	0.0	—	—	113	2.09	—	—	—	1553	—	74	0.00	0.00
0.17	0.11	2.55	0.10	0.00	0.0	1.0	—	—	170	3.25	—	273	222	3030	1.9	70	0.00	0.00
0.00	0.00	0.00	0.00	0.02	0.9	0.1	0.0	0.7	3	0.03	0.2	4	6	85	0.0	—	0.00	0.00
—	—	—	—	—	—	0.0	—	—	0	0.00	—	—	—	140	—	—	0.00	0.00
0.00	0.00	0.14	—	—	—	0.0	—	—	7	0.72	—	17	27	240	—	—	0.00	0.00
0.00	0.00	0.01	0.00	0.00	0.4	0.1	—	0.0	4	0.09	1.9	4	8	56	0.0	82	0.00	0.00
0.00	0.00	0.01	0.00	0.00	0.4	0.1	—	0.0	4	0.09	1.9	4	8	56	0.0	82	0.00	0.00
—	—	—	—	—	—	0.0	—	—	0	0.00	—	—	—	150	—	—	0.00	0.00

Code	Food Name	Unit/ Amt	Wt (g)	Energy (kcal)	Prot (g)	Carb (g)	Fiber (g)	Fat (g)	Sat (g)	Mono (g)	Poly (g)	Chol (mg)	Vit A (RE)
53614	Sauce, soy, light	1 Tbs	18	10	1	1	0	0	0.0	0.0	0.0	0	0
53530	Sauce, soy, low sod	1 Tbs	16	8	1	1	0	0	0.0	0.0	0.0	0	0
53471	Sauce, tabasco, rts	1 tsp	5	1	0	0	0	0	0.0	0.0	0.0	0	8
53099	Sauce, worcestershire	1 Tbs	17	11	0	3	0	0	0.0	0.0	0.0	0	2
53457	Vinegar, balsamic	1 Tbs	15	10	0	2	—	0	0.0	0.0	0.0	0	—
27007	Vinegar, cider	1 Tbs	15	2	0	1	0	0	0.0	0.0	0.0	0	0
92153	Vinegar, distilled	1 Tbs	17	2	0	1	0	0	0.0	0.0	0.0	0	0
27204	Vinegar, red wine	1 Tbs	16	0	0	0	0	0	0.0	0.0	0.0	0	0
Salsas													
92617	Salsa, lime & garlic	2 Tbs	32	15	0	3	1	0	0.0	0.0	0.0	0	40
92618	Salsa, rstd peppers & garlic	2 Tbs	32	10	0	2	1	0	0.0	0.0	0.0	0	40
53466	Salsa, rts	2 Tbs	32	9	0	2	1	0	0.0	0.0	0.0	0	10

PAGE KEY: A-96 Granola Bars, Cereal Bars, Diet Bars, Scones, and Tarts   A-96 Meals and Dishes   A-100 Meats   A-106 Nuts, Seeds, and Products   A-108 Poultry   A-110 Salad Dressings, Dips, and Mayonnaise   A-110 Salads   A-110 Sandwiches   A-114 Sauces and Gravies   A-114 Snack Foods—Chips, Pretzels, Popcorn   A-116 Soups, Stews, and Chilis   A-118 Spices, Flavors, and Seasonings   A-120 Sports Bars and Drinks   A-120 Supplemental Foods and Formulas   A-122 Sweeteners and Sweet Substitutes   A-122 Vegetables and Legumes   A-136 Weight Loss Bars and Drinks   A-138 Miscellaneous

Thia (mg)	Ribo (mg)	Niac (mg NE)	Vit B6 (mg)	Vit B12 (µg)	Fol (µg)	Vit C (mg)	Vit D (IU)	Vit E (mg AT)	Cal (mg)	Iron (mg)	Magn (mg)	Phos (mg)	Pota (mg)	Sodi (mg)	Zinc (mg)	Wat (%)	Alco (g)	Caff (g)
—	—	—	—	—	—	0.0	—	—	0	0.00	—	—	—	605	—	—	0.00	0.00
0.00	0.01	0.54	0.02	0.00	2.5	0.0	—	0.0	3	0.31	5.4	18	29	533	0.1	71	0.00	0.00
0.00	0.00	0.00	0.00	0.00	0.0	0.2	—	—	1	0.05	0.6	1	6	30	0.0	95	0.00	0.00
0.00	0.01	0.11	0.00	0.00	1.4	2.2	—	0.0	18	0.89	2.2	10	136	167	0.0	79	0.00	0.00
—	—	—	—	—	—	—	—	—	—	—	—	—	—	5	—	—	—	0.00
0.00	0.00	0.00	0.00	0.00	0.0	0.0	—	0.0	1	0.09	3.3	1	15	0	0.0	94	0.00	0.00
0.00	0.00	0.00	0.00	0.00	0.0	0.0	—	0.0	0	0.00	3.7	0	3	0	0.0	95	0.00	0.00
—	—	—	—	—	—	0.0	—	—	0	0.00	—	—	0	0	—	100	0.00	0.00
—	—	—	—	—	—	1.8	—	—	0	0.00	—	—	—	210	—	89	0.00	0.00
—	—	—	—	—	—	0.0	—	—	0	0.00	—	—	—	230	—	92	0.00	0.00
0.00	0.00	0.01	0.05	0.00	1.3	0.6	—	0.4	9	0.15	4.9	10	96	194	0.1	90	0.00	0.00

absorption The process by which substances are taken up from the GI tract and enter the bloodstream or the lymph. p. 88

absorptive cells A class of cells, that line the villi; these cells participate in nutrient absorption. p. 93

acesulfame-K (ay-SUL-fame) An alternative sweetener that yields no energy to the body; it is 200 times sweeter than sucrose. p. 119

$$\text{acid group} \; -\overset{\overset{\textstyle O}{\|}}{C}-OH \quad \text{p. 148}$$

acquired immunodeficiency syndrome (AIDS) A disorder in which a virus (human immunodeficiency virus [HIV]) infects specific types of immune system cells. This leaves the person with reduced immune function and, in turn, defenseless against numerous infectious agents; typically contributes to the person's death. p. 575

active absorption Absorption using a carrier and expending energy. In this way, the absorptive cell absorbs nutrients, such as glucose, when a high concentration of the nutrient is already present in the absorptive cells. p. 94

acute alcohol intoxication A temporary deterioration in mental function, accompanied by lack of coordination and partial paralysis, arising from drinking large amounts of alcoholic beverages rapidly. p. 229

additives Substances added to foods, such as preservatives. p. 540

adenosine diphosphate (ADP) (ah-DEN-o-scene di-FOS-fate) A breakdown product of ATP. ADP is synthesized into ATP using energy from foodstuffs and a phosphate group (abbreviated Pi). p. 379

adenosine triphosphate (ATP) (ah-DEN-o-scene tri-FOS-fate) The main energy currency for cells. ATP energy is used to promote ion pumping, enzyme activity, and muscular contraction. p. 379

Adequate Intake (AI) Recommendations for nutrient intake when not enough information is available to establish an RDA. AIs are based on observed or experimentally determined estimates of the average nutrient intake that appears to maintain a defined nutritional state (e.g., bone health) in a specific population. Used when no RDA can be set. p. 59

adipose tissue (ad-i-POSE) A group of fat-storing cells. p. 19

aerobic (air-ROW-bic) Requiring oxygen. p. 76

air displacement A method for estimating body composition that makes use of the volume of space taken up by a body inside a small chamber. p. 345

alcohol Ethyl alcohol or ethanol (CH_3CH_2OH). p. 13

alcohol abuse Excessive alcohol consumption that leads to severe alcohol-related health and other problems, such as recurrent sickness, an inability to fulfill major obligations, use in hazardous situations (e.g., when driving), related legal problems, or use despite social and interpersonal difficulties. p. 219

alcohol dehydrogenase (dee-high-DRO-jen-ase) An enzyme used in alcohol (ethanol) metabolism. p. 221

alcohol dependence The person experiences repeated alcohol-related difficulties, such as an inability to control use, spending a great deal of time associated with alcohol use, continued use of alcohol despite physical or psychological consequences, persistent desire or unsuccessful efforts to cut down or control alcohol use, and withdrawal symptoms. Tolerance is also seen. p. 230

aldosterone (al-DOS-ter-own) A hormone produced by the adrenal glands that acts on the kidneys to cause conservation of sodium (and, therefore, water). p. 290

allergen A foreign protein, or antigen, that induces excess production of certain immune system antibodies; subsequent exposure to the same protein leads to allergic symptoms. Whereas all allergens are antigens, not all antigens are allergens. p. 483

allergy A hypersensitive immune response that occurs when antibodies produced by the body react with a protein foreign to the body (an antigen). p. 474, 483

alpha-linolenic acid (AL-fah-lin-oh-LE-nik) An essential omega-3 fatty acid with 18 carbons and 3 double bonds. p. 151

alpha-tocopherol (to-ca-FUR-all) The most potent form of vitamin E in terms of antioxidant function in humans. p. 251

amino acid (ah-MEE-noh) The building block for proteins containing a central carbon atom with nitrogen and other atoms attached. p. 9

amniotic fluid (am-nee-OTT-ik) Fluid contained in a sac within the uterus. This fluid surrounds and protects the fetus during development. p. 288

amphetamine (am-FET-ah-mean) A group of medications that induce stimulation of the central nervous system, among other effects. Abuse is linked to physical and psychological dependence. p. 363

amylase (AM-uh-lace) Starch-digesting enzyme from the salivary glands or pancreas. p. 91, 121

amylopectin (AM-uh-low-pek-tin) A digestible branched-chain type of starch composed of multiple glucose units. p. 114

amylose (AM-uh-los) A digestible straight-chain type of starch made of multiple glucose units. p. 114

anaerobic (AN-ah-ROW-bic) Not requiring oxygen. p. 75

analog (AN-a-log) A chemical compound that differs slightly from another, usually natural, compound. Analogs generally contain extra or altered chemical groups and may have similar or opposite metabolic effects compared with the native compound. Also spelled *analogue*. p. 245

anal sphincters A group of two sphincters (inner and outer) that help control expulsion of feces from the body. p. 97

anaphylactic shock (an-ah-fih-LAK-tic) A severe allergic response that results in lowered blood pressure and respiratory and gastrointestinal distress. This can be fatal. p. 483

anemia (ah-NEM-ee-a) Generally refers to a decreased oxygen-carrying capacity of the blood. This can be caused by many factors, such as iron deficiency or blood loss. p. 310

animal model Study of disease in animals that duplicates human disease. This can be used to understand more about human disease. p. 25

anorexia nervosa (an-oh-REX-ee-uh ner-VOH-sah) An eating disorder involving a psychological loss or denial of appetite, followed by self-starvation, related in part to a distorted body image and to various social pressures commonly associated with puberty. p. 412

anthropometric assessment (an-throw-PO-meh-trik) Pertaining to the measurement of body weight and the lengths, circumferences, and thicknesses of parts of the body. p. 42

antibody (AN-tih-bod-ee) Blood protein (immunoglobulin) that binds foreign proteins found in the body. This helps prevent and control infections. p. 87

antidiuretic hormone (an-tie-dye-u-RET-ik) A hormone secreted by the pituitary gland that acts on the kidney to cause a decrease in water excretion. p. 290

antigen (AN-ti-jen) Any substance that induces a state of sensitivity and/or resistance to microorganisms or toxic substances after a lag period; substance that stimulates a specific aspect of the immune system. p. 87, 483

antioxidant (an-tie-OX-ih-dant) Generally a compound that stops the damaging effects of reactive substances seeking an electron (i.e., oxidizing agent). This prevents the breakdown of substances in food or the body, particularly lipids. Some antioxidants are able to donate electrons to electron-seeking compounds. This in turn reduces breakdown of unsaturated fatty acids and other cell components by oxidizing agents. p. 164

anus (A-nus) Last portion of the GI tract; serves as an outlet for that organ. p. 97

appetite The primarily psychological (external) influences that encourage us to find and eat food, often in the absence of obvious hunger. p. 18

arachidonic acid (ar-a-kih-DON-ik) An omega-6 fatty acid with 20 carbon atoms and 4 carbon-carbon double bonds. p. 167

artery A blood vessel that carries blood away from the heart. p. 82

aseptic processing (ah-SEP-tik) A method by which food and containers are simultaneously sterilized; it allows manufacturers to produce boxes of milk that can be stored at room temperature. Variations of this process are also known as *ultrahigh temperature (UHT)* packaging. p. 533

aspartame (AH-spar-tame) An alternative sweetener made of two amino acids and methanol; it is about 180 times sweeter than sucrose. p. 119

atherosclerosis (ath-e-roh-scle-ROH-sis) A buildup of fatty material (plaque) in the arteries, including those surrounding the heart. p. 161

atom Smallest combining unit of an element. p. 6

axon (ax-ON) The part of a nerve cell that conducts impulses away from the main body of the cell. p. 84

bacteria Single-cell microorganisms, some of which produce poisonous substances that cause illness in humans. They contain only one chromosome and lack many of the organelles found in human cells. Some can live without oxygen and survive harsh conditions by means of spore formation. p. 84, 529

basal metabolism The minimal amount of calories the body requires to support itself in a fasting state when resting (e.g., 12 hours for both) and awake in a warm, quiet environment. It amounts to roughly 1 kcal per kilogram per hour for men and 0.9 kcal per kilogram per hour for women; these estimates are often referred to as basal metabolic rate (BMR). p. 338

benign Noncancerous; tumors that do not spread. p. 509

beriberi (BEAR-ee-BEAR-ee) The thiamin deficiency disorder characterized by muscle weakness, loss of appetite, nerve degeneration, and sometimes edema. p. 257

BHA Butylated hydroxyanisol, a synthetic antioxidant added to food. p. 173

BHT Butylated hydroxytoluene, a synthetic antioxidant added to food. p. 173

bile A liver secretion that is stored in the gallbladder and released through the common bile duct into the first segment of the small intestine. It is essential for the absorption of fat. p. 97

bile acids Emulsifiers synthesized by the liver and released by the gallbladder during digestion; they have a cholesterol-like structure. p. 91

binge-eating disorder An eating disorder characterized by recurrent binge eating and feelings of loss of control over eating that has lasted at least 6 months. Binge episodes can be triggered by frustration, anger, depression, anxiety, self-permission to eat forbidden foods, and excessive hunger. p. 412

bioavailability The degree to which an ingested nutrient is absorbed and available to the body. p. 255, 291

biochemical assessment Assessment focusing on reduced biochemical function (e.g., low concentrations of nutrient by-products or enzyme activities in the blood or urine) resulting from a nutritional deficiency. p. 42

bioelectrical impedance A method to estimate total body fat that uses a low-energy electrical current. The more fat storage a person has, the more impedance (resistance) to electrical flow will be exhibited. p. 345

biotechnology A collection of processes that involve the use of advanced scientific techniques to alter and, ideally, improve characteristics of animals, plants, and other forms of life. p. 579

bisphosphonates (bis-FOS-foh-nates) Compounds primarily composed of carbon and phosphorus that bind to bone mineral and in turn reduce bone breakdown. Examples are alendronate (Fosamax) and risedronate (Actonel). p. 328

blood doping A technique by which an athlete's red blood cell count is increased. Blood is taken from the athlete, and the red blood cells are concentrated and then later reinjected into the athlete. Alternately, a hormone may be injected to increase red blood cell synthesis (erythropoietin [Epogen]). p. 403

body mass index (BMI) Weight (in kilograms) divided by height (in meters) squared. A normal value is 18.5 to 24.9. A value of 25 and above indicates overweight and a value of 30 and above indicates obesity. A BMI of 25 and above increases the risk for weightrelated health disorders, such as type 2 diabetes and cardiovascular disease. 1 BMI unit equals 6 to 7 pounds. p. 16, 175, 342

bolus A moistened mass of food that is swallowed from the oral cavity into the pharynx. p. 91

bomb calorimeter (kal-oh-RIM-eh-ter) An instrument used to measure the calorie content of a food. p. 337

bond A linkage formed by the sharing of electrons, charges, or attractions between two atoms. p. 7

bone mass Total mineral substance (such as calcium or phosphorus) in a cross section of bone, generally expressed as grams per centimeter of length. p. 326

bone mineral density Total mineral content of bone at a specific bone site divided by the width of the bone at that site, generally expressed as grams per cubic centimeter. p. 326

branched-chain amino acids Amino acids with a branching carbon backbone; these are leucine, isoleucine, and valine. All are essential amino acids. p. 188

brown adipose tissue (ADD-ih-pose) A specialized form of adipose tissue that produces large amounts of heat by metabolizing energy-yielding nutrients without synthesizing much useful energy for the body. The unused energy is released as heat. p. 340

buffers Compounds that cause a solution to resist changes in acid-base conditions. p. 202

bulimia nervosa (boo-LEEM-ee-uh) An eating disorder in which large quantities of food are eaten at one time (binge eating) and then purged from the body by vomiting, or misuse of laxatives, diuretics, or enemas. Alternate means to counteract the caloric excess are fasting and excessive exercise. p. 412

cancer A condition characterized by uncontrolled growth of abnormal body cells. p. 4

capillary bed (KAP-ill-air-ee) Network of vessels one cell thick that create a junction between arterial and venous circulation. It is here that gas and nutrient exchange occurs between body cells and the blood. p. 82, 200

carbohydrate (kar-bow-HIGH-drate) A compound containing carbon, hydrogen, and oxygen atoms; most are known as *sugars*, *starches*, and *fibers*. p. 5

carbohydrate loading A process in which a very high carbohydrate intake is consumed for 6 days before an athletic event while tapering exercise duration in an attempt to increase muscle glycogen stores. p. 389

carbon skeleton Amino acid after the amino group ($-NH_2$) has been removed. p. 201

carcinogenic Describes a compound with the potential to cause cancer. p. 511

cardiac muscle Muscle that makes up the walls of the heart. Produces rhythmical involuntary contractions. p. 77

cardiovascular disease A general term that refers to any disease of the heart and circulatory system. The disease is generally characterized by the deposition of fatty material in the blood vessels (hardening of the arteries), which in turn can lead to heart damage and death. Also termed *coronary heart disease (CHD)*, as the vessels of the heart are the primary site of disease. p. 4

cardiovascular system The body system consisting of the heart, blood vessels, and blood. This system transports nutrients, waste products, gases, and hormones throughout the body and plays an important role in immune responses and regulation of body temperature. p. 81

carnitine (CAR-nih-teen) A compound used to shuttle fatty acids from the cytoplasm of the cell into mitochondria. p. 279, 403

carotenoids (kah-ROT-en-oyds) Pigment materials in fruits and vegetables that range in color from yellow to orange to red; 3 yield vitamin A activity in humans and thus are called provitamin A. Many have antioxidant properties as well. One example is beta-carotene. p. 243

cartilage Connective tissue, usually part of the skeleton, that is composed of cells in a flexible network. p. 77

case-control study Individuals who have the condition in question, such as lung cancer, are compared with individuals who do not have the condition. p. 25

celiac disease (SEE-lee-ak) An allergic reaction to the protein gluten in certain cereals, such as wheat and rye. The effect is to destroy the intestinal absorptive cells, resulting in a much reduced surface area due to flattening of the villi. Elimination of wheat, rye, and certain other grains from the diet typically restores the intestinal surface. p. 105

cell A minute structure; the living basis of plant and animal organization. In animals it is bounded by a cell membrane. Cells contain both genetic material and systems for synthesizing energy-yielding compounds. Cells have the ability to take up compounds from and excrete compounds into their surroundings. p. 7

cell body Main structure of a nerve cell that contains the organelles. p. 84

cell-mediated immunity A process in which white blood cells come in actual contact with the invading cells in order to destroy them. p. 88

cell nucleus An organelle bound by its own double membrane and containing chromosomes, the genetic information for cell protein synthesis and cell replication. p. 76

cellulose (SELL-you-los) An insoluble straight-chain polysaccharide made of glucose molecules that is undigestible. p. 114

Celsius A centigrade measure of temperature. For conversion: (degrees in Fahrenheit − 32) × 5/9 = °C; (degrees in Celsius × 9/5) + 32 = °F. p. 14

cerebrovascular accident (CVA) (se-REE-bro-VAS-cue-lar) Death of part of the brain tissue due typically to a blood clot; also termed a *stroke.* p. 162

chain-breaking Breaking the link between two or more actions that encourage overeating such as snacking while watching television. p. 357

chemical reaction An interaction between two chemicals that changes both chemicals. p. 10

cholecystokinin (CCK) (ko-la-sis-toe-KY-nin) A hormone that participates in enzyme release from the pancreas, bile release from the gallbladder, and hunger regulation. p. 19, 91

cholesterol (ko-LES-te-rol) A waxy lipid found in all body cells. It has a structure containing multiple chemical rings that is found only in foods that contain animal products. p. 7, 91, 147

chromosome A single large DNA molecule and its associated proteins; contains many genes to store and transmit genetic information. p. 76

chronic (KRON-ik) Long-standing, developing over time. When referring to disease, this term indicates that the disease progress, once developed, is slow and lasting. A good example is cardiovascular disease. p. 4

chylomicron (kye-lo-MY-kron) Lipoprotein made of dietary fats that are surrounded by a shell of cholesterol, phospholipids, and protein. Chylomicrons are formed in the absorptive cells in the small intestine after fat absorption and travel through the lymphatic system to the bloodstream. p. 159

chyme (KIME) A mixture of stomach secretions and partially digested food. p. 92

cirrhosis (see-ROH-sis) A loss of functioning liver cells, which are replaced by nonfunctioning connective tissue. Any substance that poisons liver cells can lead to cirrhosis. The most common cause is chronic, excessive alcohol intake. Exposure to certain industrial chemicals also can lead to cirrhosis. p. 221

cis **fatty acid** A form of unsaturated fatty acid that has the hydrogens lying on the same side of the carbon-carbon double bond. p. 151

clinical assessment An assessment that focuses on one's general appearance of skin, eyes, and tongue; evidence of rapid hair loss; sense of touch; and ability to cough and walk. p. 42

Clostridium botulinum **(klo-STRID-ee-um BOT-you-LY-num)** A bacterium that can cause a fatal type of foodborne illness. p. 534

coagulation Blood clotting; essentially a transition from a liquid into a solid, gel-like form. p. 253

coenzyme An organic compound that combines with an inactive enzyme to form a catalytically active form. In this manner, coenzymes aid in enzyme function. p. 239

cofactor A mineral or other substance that binds to a specific region on a protein, such as an enzyme, and is necessary for the protein's function. p. 290

cognitive behavior therapy Psychological therapy in which the person's assumptions about dieting, body weight, and related issues are challenged. New ways of thinking are explored and then practiced by the person. In this way, the person can learn new ways to control disordered eating behaviors and related life stress. p. 421

cognitive restructuring Changing one's frame of mind regarding eating—for example, instead of using a difficult day as an excuse to overeat, substituting other pleasures for rewards, such as a relaxing walk with a friend. p. 357

colostrum (ko-LAHS-trum) The first fluid secreted by the breast during late pregnancy and the first few days after birth. This thick fluid is rich in immune factors and protein. p. 458

complementary proteins Two food protein sources that make up for each other's inadequate supply of specific essential amino acids; together they yield a sufficient amount of all nine and so provide high-quality (complete) protein for the diet. p. 190

complete proteins Proteins that contain ample amounts of all nine essential amino acids. p. 189

complex carbohydrate A term that describes carbohydrates with multiple sugar units, such as starch. p. 7

compound A group of different types of atoms bonded together in definite proportion (see also molecule). p. 13

conjugated linoleic acid Isomers of an essential fatty acid that may affect fat and protein synthesis and reduce cancer risk. Animal fats are a source as it is synthesized by bacteria in an animal's digestive tract. p. 403

connective tissue Protein tissue that holds different structures in the body together. Some structures are made up of connective tissue—notably, tendons and cartilage. Connective tissue also forms part of bone and the nonmuscular structures of arteries and veins. p. 77

constipation A condition characterized by infrequent bowel movements. p. 100

contingency management Forming a plan of action to respond to a situation in which overeating is likely, such as when snacks are within arm's reach at a party. p. 359

control group Participants in an experiment who are not given the treatment being tested. p. 25

cortical bone (KORT-ih-kal) Tightly packed bone; also called compact or dense bone. p. 325

creatine (CREE-a-tin) An organic molecule in muscle cells that serves as a part of a high-energy compound (termed creatine phosphate or phosphocreatine) capable of synthesizing ATP from ADP. p. 383

cretinism (KREET-in-ism) The stunting of body growth and poor mental development in the offspring that results from inadequate maternal intake of iodide during pregnancy. p. 317

cystic fibrosis (SIS-tik figh-BRO-sis) A disease that often leads to overproduction of mucus. Mucus can invade the pancreas, decreasing enzyme output. The lack of lipase enzyme output from the pancreas then contributes to severe fat malabsorption. p. 95

cytoplasm (SITE-o-plas-um) The fluid and organelles (except the nucleus) in a cell. p. 75

Daily Values (DV) A set of standard nutrient-intake values developed by FDA and used as a reference for expressing nutrient content on nutrition labels. p. 62

Delaney Clause A clause to the 1958 Food Additives Amendment of the Pure Food and Drug Act in the United States that prevents the intentional (direct) addition to foods of a compound that has been shown to cause cancer in laboratory animals or humans. p. 544

dementia (de-MEN-sha) General loss or decrease in mental function. p. 259

denaturation (dee-NAY-ture-a-shun) Alteration of a protein's three-dimensional structure, usually because of treatment by heat, enzymes, acid or alkaline solutions, or agitation. p. 193

dendrite (DEN-dright) A relatively short, highly branched nerve cell process that carries electrical activity to the main body of the nerve cell. p. 84

dental caries (KARE-ees) Erosions in the surface of a tooth caused by acids made by bacteria as they metabolize sugars. p. 136

deoxyribonucleic acid (DNA) The site of hereditary information in cells; DNA directs the synthesis of cell proteins. p. 76

DEXA scan DEXA stands for dual energy x-ray absorptiometry. Method to measure bone mass and density and other aspects of body composition using a small amount of x-ray radiation. p. 327

diabetes (DYE-uh-BEET-eez) A group of diseases characterized by high blood glucose. Type 1 diabetes involves a lack of release of the hormone insulin by the pancreas and requires daily insulin therapy. Type 2 diabetes results from either insufficient release of insulin or general inability of insulin to act on certain body cells, such as muscle cells. People with type 2 diabetes may or may not require insulin therapy. p. 4, 126

diastolic blood pressure (dye-ah-STOL-ik) The pressure in the arterial blood vessels when the heart is between beats. p. 165

dietary assessment An assessment that focuses on the typical food choices of the person, relying mostly on a recounting of one's usual intake or a record of one's previous days' meals. p. 42

dietary fiber Fiber naturally found in food. p. 115

Dietary Guidelines for Americans General goals for nutrient intake and diet composition set by USDA and the U.S. Department of Health and Human Services. p. 52

Dietary Reference Intakes (DRIs) The overarching frameworks for nutrient recommendations made by the Food and Nutrition Board, a part of the National Academy of Sciences. p. 59

dietitian See *registered dietitian (R.D.).* p. 29

digestion The process by which large ingested molecules are mechanically and chemically broken down to produce basic nutrients that can be absorbed across the wall of the GI tract. p. 88

digestive system The body system consisting of the gastrointestinal tract and accessory structures such as the liver, gallbladder, and pancreas. This system performs the mechanical and chemical processes of digestion, absorption of nutrients, and elimination of wastes. p. 88

diglyceride A breakdown product of a triglyceride consisting of two fatty acids bonded to a glycerol backbone. p. 151

direct calorimetry (kal-oh-RIM-eh-tree) A method of measuring a body's energy use based on the heat that is released from the body, usually using an insulated chamber. p. 340

disaccharides (dye-SACK-uh-rides) Class of sugars formed by the chemical bonding of two monosaccharides. p. 7, 113

discretionary calories The calories allowed in a diet after the person has met overall nutrition needs. p. 45

disordered eating Mild and short-term changes in eating patterns that occur in relation to a stressful event, an illness, or desire to modify one's diet for a variety of health and personal appearance reasons. p. 412

distillation (dis-te-LAY-shun) A physical method used to separate liquids based on their boiling points. p. 220

diuretic (dye-u-RET-ik) A substance that, when ingested, increases the flow of urine. p. 296

diverticula (DYE-ver-TIK-you-luh) Pouches that protrude through the exterior wall of the large intestine. p. 130

diverticulitis (DYE-ver-tik-you-LITE-us) An inflammation of the diverticula caused by acids produced by bacterial metabolism inside the diverticula. p. 130

diverticulosis (DYE-ver-tik-you-LOW-sus) The condition of having many diverticula in the large intestine. p. 130

docosahexaenoic acid (DHA) (DOE-co-sa-hex-ee-no-ik) An omega-3 fatty acid with 22 carbons and 6 carbon-carbon double bonds. It is present in large amounts in fatty fish and is slowly synthesized in the body from alpha-linolenic acid. DHA is especially present in the retina and brain. p. 166

dopamine (DOE-pah-mean) A type of neurotransmitter in the central nervous system that leads to feelings of euphoria, among other functions. p. 230

double-blind study An experiment in which neither the participants nor the researchers are aware of the participant's assignment (test or placebo) or the outcome of the study until it is completed. An independent third party holds the code and the data until the study is completed. p. 25

dual energy X-ray absorptiometry (DEXA) A highly accurate method of measuring body composition and bone mass and density using multiple low-energy X rays. p. 327, 346

early childhood caries Tooth decay that results from formula or juice (and even human milk) bathing the teeth as the child sleeps with a bottle in his or her mouth. The upper teeth are mostly affected, as the lower teeth are protected by the tongue; formerly called *nursing bottle syndrome* and *baby bottle tooth decay*. p. 480

eating disorder Severe alterations in eating patterns linked to physiological changes. The alterations are associated with food restricting, binge eating, purging, and fluctuations in weight. They also involve a number of emotional and cognitive changes that affect the way a person perceives and experiences his or her body. p. 412

eclampsia See *pregnancy-induced hypertension*. p. 454

economic assessment An assessment that focuses on the ability of the person to purchase, transport, and cook food. The person's weekly budget for food purchases is a key factor. p. 42

edema (uh-DEE-muh) The buildup of excess fluid in extracellular spaces. p. 201

eicosapentaenoic acid (EPA) (eye-KOH-sah-pen-tah-ee-NO-ik) An omega-3 fatty acid with 20 carbons and 5 carbon-carbon double bonds. It is present in large amounts in fatty fish and is slowly synthesized in the body from alpha-linolenic acid. p. 166

electrolytes (ih-LEK-tro-lites) Substances that separate into ions in water and, in turn, are able to conduct an electrical current. These include sodium, chloride, and potassium. p. 10, 285

element A substance that cannot be separated into simpler substances by chemical processes. Common elements in nutrition include carbon, oxygen, hydrogen, nitrogen, calcium, phosphorus, and iron. p. 6

elimination diet A restrictive diet that systematically tests foods that may cause an allergic response by first eliminating them for 1 to 2 weeks and then adding them back, one at a time. p. 484

embryo (EM-bree-oh) In humans, the developing offspring from about the beginning of the third to the end of the eighth week after conception. p. 438

emulsifier (ee-MULL-sih-fire) A compound that can suspend fat in water by isolating individual fat droplets, using a shell of water molecules or other substances to prevent the fat from coalescing. p. 169

endocrine gland (EN-doh-krin) A hormone-producing gland. p. 85

endocrine system (EN-doh-krin) The body system consisting of the various glands and the hormones these glands secrete. This system has major regulatory functions in the body, such as in reproduction and cell metabolism. p. 85

endometrium (en-doh-ME-tree-um) The membrane that lines the inside of the uterus. It increases in thickness during the menstrual cycle until ovulation occurs. The surface layers are shed during menstruation if conception does not take place. p. 510

endoplasmic reticulum (ER) (en-doh-PLAZ-mik re-TIK-u-lum) An organelle in the cytoplasm composed of a network of canals running through the cystoplasm. Part of the endoplasmic reticulum contains ribosomes. p. 76

endorphins (en-DOR-fins) Natural body tranquilizers that may be involved in the feeding response and function in pain reduction. p. 19, 411

energy balance A state in which energy intake, in the form of food, beverages, and alcohol (if used), matches the energy expended, primarily through basal metabolism and physical activity. p. 335

energy density A comparison of the calorie content of a food with the weight of the food. An energy-dense food is high in calories but weighs very little (e.g., many fried foods), whereas a food low in energy density has few calories but weighs a lot, such as an orange. p. 38

enriched A term generally meaning that the vitamins thiamin, niacin, riboflavin, and folic acid and the mineral iron have been added to a grain product to improve nutritional quality. p. 63

enterohepatic circulation (EN-ter-oh-heh-PAT-ik) The recycling of compounds between the small intestine and the liver over and over again, as happens with certain bile constituents. p. 97

enzyme (EN-zime) A compound that speeds the rate of a chemical process but is not altered by that process. Almost all enzymes are proteins. p. 8, 74

epidemiology (ep-uh-dee-me-OLL-uh-gee) The study of how disease patterns vary among different population groups. p. 24

epiglottis (ep-ih-GLOT-iss) Flap that folds down over the trachea during swallowing. p. 91

epinephrine (ep-ih-NEF-rin) A hormone also known as *adrenaline*; it is released by the adrenal glands (located on each kidney) at times of stress. It acts to increase glycogen breakdown in the liver, among other functions. p. 85, 125

epithelial cells (ep-ih-THEE-lee-ul) The cells that line the outside of the body and the inside of all external passages within it, such as the GI tract. p. 244

epithelial tissue (ep-ih-THEE-lee-ul) The surface tissue that lines the outside of the body and all external passages within it. p. 77

ergogenic (ur-go-JEN-ic) Work-producing. An ergogenic aid is a mechanical, nutritional, psychological, pharmacological, or physiological substance or treatment that is intended to directly improve exercise performance. p. 401

erythrocyte (eh-RITH-row-site) Mature red blood cell. These have no nucleus and a life span of about 120 days; they contain hemoglobin, which transports oxygen and carbon dioxide. p. 263

erythropoietin (eh-REE-throw-POY-eh-tin) A hormone secreted mostly by the kidneys that enhances red blood cell synthesis and stimulates red blood cell release from bone marrow. p. 103

esophagus (eh-SOF-ah-gus) A tube in the GI tract that connects the pharynx with the stomach. p. 91

essential amino acids Amino acids that cannot be synthesized by humans in sufficient amounts or at all and therefore must be included in the diet; there are nine essential amino acids. These are also called indispensable amino acids. p. 189

essential fatty acids Fatty acids that must be supplied by the diet to maintain health. Currently only linoleic acid and alpha-linolenic acid are classified as essential. p. 151

essential nutrient In nutritional terms, a substance that, when left out of a diet, leads to signs of poor health. The body either cannot produce this nutrient or cannot produce it fast enough to meet its needs. Then, if added back to a diet before permanent damage occurs, the affected aspects of health are restored. p. 3

Estimated Energy Requirement (EER) Estimate of average calorie needs for various ages and genders; these are set by the Food and Nutrition Board of the National Academy of Sciences. p. 59

ethanol Chemical term for the form of alcohol found in alcoholic beverages. p. 219

exchange The serving size of a food on a specific exchange list. p. A-10

Exchange System A system for classifying foods into numerous lists based on their macronutrient composition and establishing serving sizes, so that one serving of each food on a list contains the same amount of carbohydrate, protein, fat, and calorie content. p. A-10

experiment A test made to examine the validity of a hypothesis. p. 23

extracellular fluid Fluid present outside the cells; represents one-third of all body fluid. p. 285

extracellular space The space outside cells. p. 200

facilitated diffusion The carrier-mediated transport of molecules through the cell membrane along the direction of their concentration gradients. It does not require the expenditure of energy. p. 94

famine An extreme shortage of food that leads to massive starvation in a population; often associated with crop failures, war, and political unrest. p. 562

fasting hypoglycemia (HIGH-po-gligh-SEE-me-ah) Low blood glucose that follows after about a day of fasting. p. 129

fat-soluble vitamins Vitamins that dissolve in such substances as ether and benzene, but not readily in water. These vitamins are A, D, E, and K. p. 10, 239

fatty acid Major part of most lipids; composed of a chain of carbons flanked by hydrogen. These have an

$$\overset{O}{\overset{\|}{}}$$

acid group (—C—OH) at one end and a methyl group (–CH₃) at the other. p. 7

feces (FEE-seas) Substances discharged from the bowel during defecation, consisting of the undigested residue of food, dead GI tract cells, mucus, bacteria, and other waste material. Another term for feces is *stool*. p. 96

female athlete triad A condition characterized by disordered eating, lack of menstrual periods (amenorrhea), and osteoporosis. p. 427

fermentation The conversion, without the use of oxygen, of carbohydrates to alcohols, acids, and carbon dioxide. p. 113

fetal alcohol effect (FAE) Hyperactivity, attention deficit disorder, poor judgment, sleep disorders, and delayed learning as a result of being prenatally exposed to alcohol. p. 450

fetal alcohol syndrome (FAS) A group of irreversible physical and mental abnormalities in the infant that result from the mother's consuming alcohol during pregnancy. p. 449

fetus (FEET-us) The developing life form from about the beginning of the ninth week after conception until birth. p. 247, 438

fiber Substances in plant foods that are not digested by the processes that take place in the human stomach or small intestine. These add bulk to feces. Fiber naturally found in foods is also called *dietary fiber*. p. 7, 111

foodborne illness Sickness caused by the ingestion of food containing toxic substances produced by microorganisms. p. 529

food insecurity A condition of anxiety regarding running out of either food or money to buy more food. p. 350, 559

food intolerance An adverse reaction to food that does not involve an allergic reaction. p. 483

food sensitivity A mild reaction to a substance in a food that might be expressed as slight itching or redness of the skin. p. 483

fortified A term generally meaning that vitamins, minerals, or both have been added to a food product in excess of what was originally found in the product. p. 63

free radicals Short-lived form of compounds that exist with an unpaired electron, causing it to seek an electron from another compound. Free radicals can be very destructive to electron-dense components, such as DNA and cell membranes. p. 227

fructose (FROOK-tose) A six-carbon monosaccharide that usually exists in a ring form; found in fruits and honey; also known as fruit sugar. p. 112

fruitarian (froot-AIR-ee-un) A person who consumes primarily fruits, nuts, honey, and vegetable oils. p. 207

functional fiber Fiber added to foods that has shown to provide health benefits. p. 115

functional foods Foods that provide health benefits beyond those supplied by the traditional nutrients they contain. For example, a tomato contains the phytochemical lycopene, so it can be called a functional food. p. 36

fungi Simple parasitic life forms, including molds, mildews, yeasts, and mushrooms. They live on dead or decaying organic matter. Fungi can grow as single cells, like yeast, or as multicellular colonies, as seen with molds. p. 529

galactose (gah-LAK-tos) A six-carbon monosaccharide that usually exists in a ring form; closely related to glucose. p. 112

gallbladder An organ attached to the underside of the liver; site of bile storage, concentration, and eventual excretion. p. 97

gastrin (GAS-trin) A hormone that stimulates enzyme and acid secretion in the stomach. p. 91

gastroesophageal reflux disease (GERD) (gas-troh-eh-SOF-ah-jee-al) A disease that results from stomach acid backing up into the esophagus. The acid irritates the lining of the esophagus, causing pain. p. 99

gastrointestinal (GI) tract The main sites in the body used for digestion and absorption of nutrients. It consists of the mouth, esophagus, stomach, small intestine, large intestine, rectum, and anus. Also called the digestive tract. p. 18, 19, 88

gastroplasty (GAS-troh-plas-tee) Gastric bypass surgery performed on the stomach to limit its volume to approximately 30 milliliters. Also referred to as stomach stapling. p. 365

gene expression Use of DNA information on a gene to produce a protein. Thought to be a major determinant of cell development. p. 76, 245

generally recognized as safe (GRAS) A list of food additives that in 1958 were considered safe for consumption. Manufacturers were allowed to continue to use these additives, without special clearance, when needed for food products. FDA bears responsibility for proving they are not safe, but can remove unsafe products from the list. p. 541

genes (JEANs) A specific segment on a chromosome. Genes provide the blueprint for the production of cell proteins. p. 13, 76

genetic engineering Manipulation of the genetic makeup of any organism with recombinant DNA technology. p. 579

genetically modified organism (GMO) Any organism created by genetic engineering. p. 580

gestation (jes-TAY-shun) The period of intrauterine development of offspring, from conception to birth; in humans, gestation lasts for about 40 weeks after the woman's last menstrual period. p. 441

gestational diabetes (jes-TAY-shun-al) Elevated blood glucose that develops during pregnancy and returns to normal after birth; one cause is placental production of hormones that interfere with the regulation of blood glucose by insulin. p. 454

ghrelin A hormone produced in the stomach that increases the desire to eat. p. 19

glucagon (GLOO-kuh-gon) A hormone made by the pancreas that stimulates the breakdown of glycogen in the liver into glucose; this increases blood glucose. Glucagon also performs other functions. p. 91, 125

glucose (GLOO-kos) A six-carbon monosaccharide that usually exists in a ring form; found as such in blood, and in table sugar bound to fructose; also known as *dextrose*, it is one of the simple sugars. p. 4, 112

glycemic index (GI) (gli-SEA-mik) The blood glucose response of a given food, compared to a standard (typically, glucose or white bread). Glycemic index of a food is influenced by starch structure, fiber content, food processing, physical structure, and macronutrients in the meal, such as fat. p. 137

glycemic load (GL) The amount of carbohydrate in a food multiplied by the glycemic index of that carbohydrate. The result is then divided by 100. p. 139

glycerol (GLIS-er-ol) A three-carbon alcohol used to form triglycerides. p. 147

glycogen (GLI-ko-jen) A carbohydrate made of multiple units of glucose with a highly branched structure; sometimes known as *animal starch*. It is the storage form of glucose in humans and is synthesized (and stored) in the liver and muscles. p. 111

goiter (GOY-ter) An enlargement of the thyroid gland that can be caused by insufficient iodide in the diet. p. 316

Golgi complex (GOAL-jee) The cell organelle near the nucleus that processes newly synthesized protein for secretion or distribution to other organelles. p. 76

gout Joint inflammation caused by accumulation of a body compound called uric acid. Obesity is a risk factor for developing gout. p. 224

green revolution Increases in crop yields accompanying the introduction of new agricultural technologies in less developed countries, beginning in the 1960s. The key technologies were high-yielding, disease-resistant strains of rice, wheat, and corn; greater use of fertilizer and water; and improved cultivation practices. p. 573

growth hormone A pituitary hormone that stimulates body growth and release of fat from storage; it also has other effects. p. 403

gruels A thin mixture of grains or legumes in milk or water. p. 211

gums A soluble fiber containing chains of galactose, glucuronic acid, and other monosaccharides; characteristically found in exudates from plant stems. p. 115

H₂ blockers Medications, such as cimetidine (Tagamet), that block the stimulation of stomach acid production caused by histamine. p. 99

heart attack Rapid fall in heart function caused by reduced blood flow through the heart's blood vessels. Often part of the heart dies in the process. Technically called a *myocardial infarction*. p. 44

heartburn A pain emanating from the esophagus, caused by stomach acid backing up into the esophagus and irritating the esophageal tissue. p. 99

heart disease See *cardiovascular disease*.

heat cramps A frequent complication of heat exhaustion. They usually occur in individuals exercising for several hours in a hot climate who have experienced large sweat losses and have consumed a large volume of plain water. The cramps occur in skeletal muscles and consist of contractions for 1 to 3 minutes at a time. p. 395

heat exhaustion The first stage of heat-related illness that occurs because of depletion of blood volume from fluid loss by the body. This increases body temperature and can lead to headache, dizziness, muscle weakness, and visual disturbances, among other effects. p. 394

heatstroke Heatstroke can occur when internal body temperature reaches 104°F. Sweating generally ceases if left untreated, and blood circulation is greatly reduced. Nervous system damage may ensue and death is likely.

Often in individuals who suffer heatstroke the skin is hot and dry. p. 395

hematocrit (hee-MAT-oh-krit) The percentage of total blood volume made up of red blood cells. p. 310

heme iron (HEEM) Iron provided from animal tissues as hemoglobin and myoglobin. Approximately 40% of the iron in meat is heme iron; it is readily absorbed. p. 309

hemicellulose (hem-ih-SELL-you-los) A soluble fiber containing xylose, galactose, glucose, and other monosaccharides bonded together. p. 115

hemochromatosis (heem-oh-krom-ah-TOE-sis) A disorder of iron metabolism characterized by increased iron absorption and deposition in the liver and heart tissue. This eventually poisons the cells in those organs. p. 312

hemoglobin (HEEM-oh-glow-bin) The iron-containing part of the red blood cell that carries oxygen to the cells and some carbon dioxide away from the cells. The heme iron portion is also responsible for the red color of blood. p. 309

hemolysis (hee-MOL-ih-sis) Destruction of red blood cells caused by the breakdown of the red blood cell membranes. This causes the cell contents to leak into the fluid portion (plasma) of the blood. p. 251

hemorrhage (hem-OR-ij) An escape of blood from blood vessels. p. 252

hemorrhagic stroke (hem-oh-RAJ-ik) Damage to part of the brain resulting from rupture of a blood vessel and subsequent bleeding within or over the internal surface of the brain. p. 167

hemorrhoid (HEM-or-oid) A pronounced swelling in a large vein, particularly veins found in the anal region. p. 101, 130

high-density lipoprotein (HDL) The lipoprotein in the blood that picks up cholesterol from dying cells and other sources and transfers it to the other lipoproteins in the bloodstream, as well as directly to the liver; low HDL increases the risk for cardiovascular disease. p. 161

high-fructose corn syrup A corn syrup that has been manufactured to contain between 40% and 90% fructose. p. 112

high-quality (complete) proteins Dietary proteins that contain ample amounts of all nine essential amino acids. p. 189

histamine A breakdown product of the amino acid histidine that stimulates acid secretion by the stomach and has other effects on the body, such as contraction of smooth muscles, increased nasal secretions, relaxation of blood vessels, and changes in relaxation of airways. p. 99

homocysteine (homo-CYS-ti-ene) An amino acid not used in protein synthesis, but instead arises during metabolism of the amino acid methionine. Homocysteine is likely toxic to many cells, such as those that line blood vessels. p. 163

hormone A compound secreted into the bloodstream by one type of cell that acts to control the function of another type of cell. For example, certain cells in the pancreas produce insulin, which in turn acts on muscle and other types of cells to promote the uptake of nutrients from the blood. p. 19

hospice units (HAHS-pis) A facility offering care that emphasizes comfort and dignity in death. p. 521

human immunodeficiency virus (HIV) The virus that leads to acquired immune deficiency syndrome (AIDS). p. 571

hunger The primarily physiological (internal) drive to find and eat food, mostly regulated by innate cues to eating. p. 18, 559

hydrogen peroxide Chemically, H_2O_2. p. 76

hydrogenation (high-dro-jen-AY-shun) Addition of hydrogen to a carbon-carbon double bond, producing a single carbon-carbon bond with two hydrogens attached. Because hydrogenation of unsaturated fatty acids in a vegetable oil increases its hardness, this process is used to convert liquid oils into more solid fats, which are used in making margarine and shortening. *Trans* fatty acids are a by-product of hydrogenation of vegetable oils. p. 171

hyperglycemia (HIGH-per-gligh-SEE-me-uh) High blood glucose, above 125 milligrams per 100 milliliters of blood. p. 125

hypertension (high-per-TEN-shun) A condition in which blood pressure remains persistently elevated. Obesity, inactivity, excess alcohol intake, excess salt intake, and genetics may each contribute to the problem. p. 4

hypoglycemia (HIGH-po-gligh-SEE-me-uh) Low blood glucose, below 40 to 50 milligrams per 100 milliliters of blood. p. 125

hypothalamus (high-po-THALL-uh-mus) A region at the base of the brain that contains cells that play a role in the regulation of hunger, respiration, body temperature, and other body functions. p. 19

hypothesis (high-POTH-eh-sis) An tentative explanation by a scientist to explain a phenomenon. p. 23

identical twins Two offspring that develop from a single ovum and sperm and, consequently, have the same genetic makeup. p. 349

ileocecal sphincter (ill-ee-oh-SEE-kal SFINK-ter) The ring of smooth muscle between the end of the small intestine and the large intestine. p. 95

immune system The body system consisting of white blood cells, lymph glands and vessels, and various other body tissues. The immune system provides defense against foreign invaders, primarily due to the production of various types of white blood cells. p. 87

immunoglobulins (em-you-no-GLOB-you-lins) Proteins found in the blood that bind to specific antigens, also called *antibodies*. The five major classes of immunoglobins play different roles in antibody-related immunity. p. 87

incidence The number of new cases of a disease in a defined population over a specific period of time, such as 1 year. p. 25

incidental food additives Additives that appear in food products indirectly, from environmental contamination of food ingredients or during the manufacturing process. p. 541

incomplete (lower-quality) protein Food protein that lacks ample amount of one or more of the essential amino acids needed to support human protein needs. p. 189

indirect calorimetry (kal-oh-RIM-eh-tree) A method to estimate the energy use by the body by measuring oxygen uptake. Formulas are then used to convert this gas exchange value into energy use. p. 340

infancy Earliest stage of childhood—from birth to 1 year of age. p. 469

infectious disease (in-FEK-shus) Any disease caused by an invasion of the body by microorganisms, such as bacteria, fungi, or viruses. p. 25

infrastructure (IN-fra-struck-sure) The basic framework of a system or organization. For society, this includes roads, bridges, telephones, and other basic technologies. p. 570

inorganic (in-or-GAN-ik) Any substance lacking carbon atoms linked to hydrogen atoms in the chemical structure. p. 10

insoluble fibers Fibers that mostly do not dissolve in water and are not metabolized by bacteria in the large intestine. These include cellulose, some hemicelluloses, and lignins. Also called poorly fermented fibers. p. 115

insulin (IN-su-lynn) A hormone produced by the pancreas. Among other processes, insulin increases the synthesis of glycogen in the liver and the movement of glucose from the bloodstream into body cells. p. 86, 91, 125

intentional food additive Additives knowingly (directly) incorporated into food products by manufacturers. p. 541

international unit (IU) A crude measure of vitamin activity, often based on the growth rate of animals in response to the vitamin. Today IUs have largely been replaced by more precise milligram or microgram measures. p. 246

intracellular fluid Fluid contained within a cell; represents about two-thirds of all body fluid. p. 285

intrinsic factor (in-TRIN-zik) A protein-like compound produced by the stomach that enhances vitamin B-12 absorption. p. 93, 266

ion (EYE-on) An atom with an unequal number of electrons and protons. Negative ions have more electrons than protons; positive ions have more protons than electrons. p. 13

irradiation (ir-RAY-dee-AY-shun) A process in which radiation energy is applied to foods, creating compounds (free radicals) within the food that destroy cell membranes, break down DNA, link proteins together, limit enzyme activity, and alter a variety of other proteins and cell functions of microorganisms that would otherwise lead to food spoilage. This process does not make the food radioactive. p. 533

ischemic stroke (ih-SKI-mik) A stroke caused by the absence of blood flow to a part of the brain. p. 223

isomers (EYE-so-mers) Different chemical structures for compounds that share the same chemical formula. p. 251

ketone bodies (KEE-tone) Incomplete breakdown products of fat containing three or four carbons. p. 124

ketosis (kee-TOE-sis) The condition of having a high concentration of ketone bodies and related breakdown products in the bloodstream and tissues. p. 124

kidney nephrons (NEF-rons) The units of kidney cells that filter wastes from the bloodstream and deposit them in the urine. p. 507

kilocalorie (kill-oh-KAL-oh-ree) (kcal) Unit that describes the energy content of food, specifically, the heat energy needed to raise the temperature of 1000 grams (1 liter) of water 1 degree Celsius. Also written as Calories, with a capital *C*. p. 4

kwashiorkor (kwash-ee-OR-core) A disease occurring primarily in young children who have an existing disease and who consume a marginal amount of calories and insufficient protein in relation to needs, especially in response to concurrent infections. The child exhibits edema, poor growth, weakness, and an increased susceptibility to further illness. p. 210

lactase An enzyme made by absorptive cells of the small intestine; this enzyme digests lactose into glucose and galactose. p. 123

lactation The period of milk secretion by the breast. p. 441

lacteal (LACK-tee-al) A small lymphatic duct associated with a villus of the small intestine. p. 84

lactic acid (LAK-tik) A three-carbon acid formed during anaerobic cell metabolism; a partial breakdown product of glucose; also called *lactate.* p. 383

Lactobacillus bifidus factor **(lak-toe-bah-SIL-us BIFF-id-us)** A protective factor secreted in the colostrum that encourages growth of beneficial bacteria in the newborn's intestines. p. 458

lactoovovegetarian (lak-toe-o-vo-vej-eh-TEAR-ree-an) A person who consumes plant products, dairy products, and eggs. p. 207

lactose (LAK-tose) Glucose bonded to another sugar galactose; also known as *milk sugar.* p. 112

lactose intolerance A condition where significant symptoms such as abdominal gas and bloating appear as a result of severe lactose maldigestion. p. 140

lactose maldigestion (primary and secondary) Primary lactose maldigestion occurs when production of the enzyme lactase declines for no apparent reason. Secondary lactose maldigestion occurs when a specific cause, such as long-standing diarrhea, results in a decline in lactase production. When significant symptoms develop after lactose intake, it is then called *lactose intolerance.* p. 140

lactovegetarian (lak-toe-vej-eh-TEAR-ree-an) A person who consumes plant products and dairy products. p. 207

lanugo (lah-NEW-go) Downlike hair that appears after a person has lost much body fat through semi-starvation. The hair stands erect and traps air, acting as insulation for the body to compensate for the relative lack of body fat, which usually functions as insulation. p. 418

laxative A medication or other substance that stimulates evacuation of the intestinal tract. p. 101

lean body mass Body weight minus fat storage weight equals lean body mass. This includes organs such as the brain, muscles, and liver, as well as blood and other body fluids. p. 338

lecithin (LESS-uh-thin) A group of compounds that are major components of cell membranes. p. 71, 152, 271

leptin (LEP-tin) A hormone made by adipose tissue in proportion to total fat mass in the body that influences long-term regulation of fat mass. Leptin also influences reproductive functions, as well as other body processes, such as release of the hormone insulin. p. 19

let-down reflex A reflex stimulated by infant suckling that causes the release (ejection) of milk from milk ducts in the mother's breasts, also called *milk ejection reflex.* p. 457

life expectancy The average length of life for a given group of people born in a certain year, such as this year. p. 505

life span The potential oldest age to which a person can reach. p. 505

lignins (LIG-nins) An insoluble fiber made up of a multiringed alcohol (noncarbohydrate) structure. p. 115

limiting amino acid The essential amino acid in the lowest concentration in a food or diet relative to body needs. p. 190

linoleic acid (lin-oh-LEE-ik) An essential omega-6 fatty acid with 18 carbons and 2 double bonds. p. 151

lipase (LYE-pase) Fat-digesting enzyme; lipase is produced by the stomach, salivary glands, and the pancreas. p. 91, 157

lipid (LIP-id) A compound composed of much carbon and hydrogen, little oxygen, and sometimes other elements. Lipids dissolve in ether or benzene, but not water, and include fats, oils, and cholesterol. p. 5

lipoprotein (ly-poh-PRO-teen) A compound found in the bloodstream containing a core of lipids with a shell composed of protein, phospholipid, and cholesterol. p. 158

lipoprotein lipase An enzyme attached to the cells that form the inner lining of blood vessels; it breaks down triglycerides into free fatty acids and glycerol. p. 159

liter (LEE-ter) (L) A measure of volume in the metric system. One liter equals 0.96 quarts. p. 12

liver Largest organ in the body, located in the abdominal cavity below the diaphragm; performs many vital functions that maintain balance in blood composition. p. 95

lobules (LOB-you-els) Saclike structures in the breast that store milk. p. 456

long-chain fatty acid Fatty acid that contains 12 or more carbons. p. 150

low birth weight (LBW) Referring to any infant weighing less than 5.5 pounds (2.5 kilograms) at birth; most commonly results from preterm birth. p. 441

low-density lipoprotein (LDL) The lipoprotein in the blood containing primarily cholesterol; elevated LDL is strongly linked to cardiovascular disease risk. p. 160

lower-body (gynecoid, gynoid) obesity The type of obesity, in which fat storage is primarily located in the buttocks and thigh area. p. 348

lower esophageal sphincter (eh-sof-ah-GEE-al SFINK-ter) A circular muscle that constricts the opening of the esophagus to the stomach. Also called gastroesophageal sphincter. p. 92

lower-quality (incomplete) proteins Dietary proteins that are low in or lack one or more essential amino acids. p. 189

lumen (LOO-men) The inside cavity of a tube, such as the GI tract. p. 92

lymph (limf) A clear fluid that flows through lymph vessels; carries most forms of fat after their absorption by the small intestine. p. 82

lymphatic system (lim-FAT-ick) System of vessels and lymph that accepts fluid surrounding cells and large particles, such as products of fat absorption. Lymph fluid eventually passes into the bloodstream from the lymphatic system. p. 81, 82

lysosome (LYE-so-som) A cellular organelle that contains digestive enzymes for use inside the cell for turnover of cell parts. p. 76

lysozyme (LYE-so-zime) An enzyme produced by a variety of cells; it can destroy bacteria by rupturing cell membranes. p. 87

macrocytic anemia (mack-ro-SIT-ik ah-NEM-ee-a) Anemia characterized by the presence of abnormally large red blood cells. p. 263

macronutrient A nutrient need in gram quantities in the diet. p. 6

macular degeneration A painless condition leading to disruption of the central part of the retina (in the eye) and, in turn, blurred vision. p. 244

major mineral A mineral vital to health that is required in the diet in amounts greater than 100 milligrams per day. p. 10, 291

malignant (ma-LIG-nant) Malicious; in reference to a tumor, the property of spreading locally and to distant sites. p. 509

malnutrition Failing health that results from long-standing dietary practices that do not coincide with nutritional needs. p. 40, 560

maltase (MALL-tase) An enzyme made by the absorptive cells of the small intestine; this enzyme digests maltose to two glucoses. p. 123

maltose (MALL-tos) Glucose bonded to glucose. p. 113

marasmus (ma-RAZ-mus) A disease that results from consuming a minimal amount of protein and calories; one of the diseases classed as protein-calorie malnutrition. Victims have little or no fat stores, little muscle mass, and poor strength. Death from infections is common. p. 210

medium-chain fatty acid A fatty acid that contains 6 to 10 carbons. p. 403

megadose Intake of a nutrient beyond estimates of needs or what would be found in a balanced diet; 2 to 10 times human needs is a starting point for such a dosage. p. 28, 239

megaloblast (MEG-ah-low-blast) A large, immature red blood cell that results from the inability of a cell to divide normally. p. 263

menarche (men-AR-kee) The onset of menstruation. Menarche usually occurs around age 13, 2 or 3 years after the first signs of puberty start to appear. p. 448

menopause (MEN-oh-paws) The cessation of menses in women, usually beginning at about 50 years of age. p. 161

metabolic syndrome A condition in which the person has poor blood glucose regulation, hypertension, increased blood triglycerides, and other health problems. This condition is usually accompanied by obesity, lack of physical activity, and a diet high in refined carbohydrates. Also called *Syndrome X.* p. 139, 165

metabolism (meh-TAB-oh-lizm) Chemical processes in the body by which food energy is converted into useful forms, and vital activities are sustained. p. 10

metastasis (ma-TAS-tah-sis) The spreading of disease from one part of the body to another, even to parts of the body that are remote from the site of original tumor. Cancer cells can spread via blood vessels, the lymphatic system, or direct growth of the tumor. p. 509

meter A measure of length in the metric system. One meter equals 39.4 inches. p. 11

methyl group —CH_3 p. 148

micronutrient A nutrient needed in milligram or microgram quantities in a diet. p. 6

microorganism Bacteria, virus, or other organism that is invisible to the naked eye, some of which can cause disease. Also called *microbes*. p. 23

mineral Element used in the body to promote chemical reactions and to form body structures. p. 5

mitochondria (my-toe-KON-dree-ah) The main sites for synthesizing a form of energy cells can use. They also contain the pathway for using fat for fuel, among other metabolic pathways. p. 75

monoglyceride (mon-oh-GLIS-er-ide) A breakdown product of a triglyceride consisting of one fatty acid bonded to a glycerol backbone. p. 151

monosaccharide (mon-oh-SACK-uh-ride) A simple sugar, such as glucose, that is not broken down further during digestion. p. 7, 112

monounsaturated fatty acid (mon-oh-un-SAT-ur-ated) A fatty acid containing one carbon-carbon double bond. p. 150

motility Generally, the ability to move spontaneously. It also refers to movement of food through the GI tract. p. 89

mottling (MOT-ling) The discoloration or marking of the surface of teeth from fluorosis. p. 318

mucilages (MYOU-sih-laj) A soluble fiber consisting of chains of galactose, mannose, and other monosaccharides; characteristically found in seaweed. p. 115

mucosal membranes (MYOO-co-sul) Consisting of mucus-forming cells and supporting connective tissue. This lines cavities that open to the outside of the body, such as the stomach and intestine. p. 87

mucus (MYOO-cuss) A thick fluid secreted by many cells throughout the body. It contains a compound that has both carbohydrate and protein parts. It acts as a lubricant and means of protection for cells. p. 91, 244

muscle tissue A type of tissue adapted to contract in order to cause movement. p. 77

mutation (myoo-TAY-shun) A change in the chemistry of a gene that remains in subsequent divisions of the cell in which it occurred; a change in the sequence of the DNA. p. 509

myelin sheath (MY-eh-lyn) A lipid and protein combination that covers nerve fibers. p. 85

myocardial infarction (MY-oh-CARD-ee-ahl in-FARK-shun) Death of part of the heart muscle. Also termed *heart attack*. p. 44, 162

myoglobin (my-oh-GLOW-bin) Iron-containing protein that binds oxygen in muscle tissue. p. 309

narcotic An agent that reduces sensations or consciousness. p. 226

near infrared reactance A method of estimating body fat content based on differential reactions of fat and lean tissue to a beam of light. p. 346

negative energy balance The state in which calorie intake is less than energy expended, resulting in weight loss. p. 335

negative protein balance The state in which protein losses from the body exceed intake, as in cases of starvation. p. 203

neotame A general purpose nonnutritive sweetener that is approximately 7000 to 13,000 times sweeter than table sugar. It has a chemical structure similar to aspartame. Neotame is heat stable and can be used as a tabletop sweetener as well as in cooking applications. It is

not broken down to its amino acid components in the body after consumption. p. 119

nervous system The body system consisting of the brain, spinal cord, nerves, and sensory receptors. This system detects sensations, directs movement, and controls physiological and intellectual functions. p. 84

nervous tissue Tissue composed of highly branched, elongated cells, which transport nerve impulses from one part of the body to another. p. 77

neural tube defect A defect in the formation of the neural tube occurring during early fetal development. This type of defect results in various nervous system disorders, such as spina bifida. Folate deficiency in the pregnant woman increases the risk of the fetus developing this disorder. p. 263

neuron (NYOUR-on) The structural and functional unit of the nervous system. Consists of cell body, dendrites, and axon. p. 84

neuropeptide Y (nyoo-row-PEP-tide) A chemical substance made in the hypothalamus that stimulates food intake. The hormone leptin inhibits neuropeptide Y production. p. 19

neurotransmitter (nyoo-row-TRANS-mit-er) A compound made by a nerve cell that allows for communication between it and other cells. p. 85

night blindness A vitamin A deficiency condition in which the retina (in the eye) cannot adjust to low amounts of light. p. 244

nitrate (NI-trait) A nitrogen-containing compound used to cure meats. Its use contributes a pink color to meats and confers some resistance to bacterial growth. p. 511

nitrosamine (ni-TROH-sa-mean) A carcinogen formed from nitrates and breakdown products of amino acids; can lead to stomach cancer. p. 512

nonessential amino acids Amino acids that can be synthesized by a healthy body in sufficient amounts; there are 11 nonessential amino acids. These are also termed *dispensable amino acids*. p. 188

nonheme iron (non-HEEM) Iron provided from plant sources and animal tissues other than hemoglobin and myoglobin. Nonheme iron is less efficiently absorbed than heme iron; absorption is closely dependent on body needs. p. 309

nonspecific immunity Defenses that stop the invasion of pathogens, and requires no previous encounter with a pathogen. p. 87

norepinephrine (nor-ep-ih-NEF-rin) A neurotransmitter from nerve endings and a hormone from the adrenal gland. It is released in times of stress and is involved in hunger regulation, blood glucose regulation, and other body processes. p. 85

NSAIDS Nonsteroidal anti-inflamatory drugs; includes aspirin, ibuprofen, and naproxen. p. 99

nucleolus (NEW-klee-o-lus) Center for production of ribosomes within the cell nucleus. p. 75

nutrient density The ratio derived by dividing a food's contribution to nutrient needs by its contribution to calorie needs. When its contribution to nutrient needs exceeds its calorie contribution, the food is considered to have a favorable nutrient density. p. 38

nutrients Chemical substances in food that contribute to health, many of which are essential parts of a diet. Nutrients nourish us by providing calories to fulfill

energy needs; materials for building body parts, and factors to regulate necessary chemical processes in the body. p. 3

nutrition The science of food; the nutrients and the substances therein; their action, interaction, and balance in relation to health and disease; and the process by which the organism (i.e., body) ingests, digests, absorbs, transports, utilizes, and excretes food substances." p. 3

nutritional state The nutritional health of a person as determined by anthropometric measures (height, weight, circumferences, and so on), biochemical measures of nutrients or their by-products in blood and urine, a clinical (physical) examination, a dietary analysis, and a review of economic status; also called *nutritional status*. p. 40

obesity (oh-BEES-ih-tee) A condition characterized by excess body fat. p. 4

oleic acid (oh-LAY-ik) An omega-9 fatty acid with 18 carbons and one carbon-carbon double bond. p. 151

omega-3 (ω-3) fatty acid Unsaturated fatty acid with the first carbon-carbon double bond on the third carbon atom from the methyl end ($-CH_3$). p. 150

omega-6 (ω-6) fatty acid Unsaturated fatty acid with the first carbon-carbon double bond on the sixth carbon atom from the methyl end ($-CH_3$). p. 150

organ A group of tissues designed to perform a specific function—for example, the heart. It contains muscle tissue, nerve tissue, and so on. p. 73

organelles (OAR-gan-ells) A compartment, particle, or filament that performs specialized functions within a cell. p. 74

organic Any substance that contains carbon atoms linked to hydrogen atoms in the chemical structure. p. 10

organ system A collection of organs that work together to perform an overall function. p. 73

osmosis (oz-MO-sis) The passage of a solvent such as water through a semipermeable membrane from a less concentrated solution to a more concentrated compartment. p. 285

osteomalacia (OS-tee-oh-mal-AY-shuh) Adult form of rickets. The weakening of the bones that is seen in this disease is caused by low calcium content. A reduction in the amount of the vitamin D hormone in the body is one cause. p. 248

osteoporosis (os-tee-oh-po-ROH-sis) Decreased bone mass related to the effects of aging, genetic background, and poor diet in both genders, and hormonal effects of menopause in women. p. 4, 298

overnutrition A state in which nutritional intake greatly exceeds the body's needs. p. 40

ovum (OH-vum) The egg cell from which a fetus eventually develops if the egg is fertilized by a sperm cell. p. 438

oxalic acid (oxalate) An organic acid found in spinach, rhubarb, and other leafy green vegetables that can depress the absorption of certain minerals present in the food, such as calcium. p. 29

oxidation (ox-ih-DAY-shun) Loss of an electron by an atom or a molecule; in metabolism, often associated with a gain of oxygen or loss of hydrogen. Oxidation (loss of an electron) and reduction (gain of an electron) take place simultaneously in metabolism, because an electron that is lost by one atom is accepted by another. p. 164

oxidative stress The damage to lipids, proteins, and DNA in the body produced by the excessive production of free radicals. p. 393

oxidize (OX-ih-dize) In the most basic sense, the loss of an electron or gain of an oxygen. This change typically alters the shape and/or function of the substance. p. 164

oxytocin (ok-si-TO-sin) A hormone secreted by the pituitary gland. It causes contraction of the musclelike cells surrounding the ducts of the breasts and the smooth muscle of the uterus. p. 457

pancreas (pan-KREE-us) Endocrine organ, located near the stomach, that secretes digestive enzymes into the small intestine and produces hormones, notably insulin. p. 97

parasite An organism that lives in or on another organism and derives nourishment from it. p. 529

parathyroid hormone (PTH) A hormone made by the parathyroid glands that increases synthesis of the vitamin D hormone and aids calcium release from bone and calcium conservation by the kidneys, among other functions. p. 248

passive diffusion (transport) Absorption that uses no energy. It requires permeability for the substance through the wall of the small intestine and a concentration gradient higher in the lumen of the intestine than in the absorptive cell. The higher concentration of the substance in the lumen of the intestine in comparison with that in the absorptive cells promotes the absorption of the nutrient. p. 94

pasteurizing (PAS-tur-i-zing) Heating food products rapidly to kill pathogenic microorganisms and to reduce the total number of bacteria. p. 529

pectin (PEK-tin) A soluble fiber containing chains of galacturonic acid and other monosaccharides; characteristically found between plant cell walls. p. 115

peer-reviewed journal A journal that publishes research only after two or three scientists who were not part of the study agree it was well conducted and the results are fairly represented. Thus, the research has been approved by peers of the research team. p. 26

pellagra (peh-LAHG-rah) A deficiency disease characterized by inflammation of the skin, diarrhea, and eventual mental incapacity; results from an insufficient amount of the vitamin niacin in the diet. p. 23

pepsin (PEP-sin) A protein-digesting enzyme produced by the stomach. p. 198

peptide bond A chemical bond formed between amino acids in a protein. p. 191

percentile Classification of a measurement of a unit into divisions of 100 units. p. 471

peristalsis (per-ih-STALL-sis) A coordinated muscular contraction that is used to propel food down the gastrointestinal tract. p. 91

pernicious anemia The anemia that results from a lack of vitamin B-12 absorption; it is pernicious because of associated degeneration that can result in eventual paralysis and death. p. 267

peroxisome (per-OK-si-som) A cell organelle that destroys toxic products within the cell. p. 76

pesticide A general term for an agent that can destroy bacteria, fungi, insects, rodents, or other pests. p. 550

pH A measure of relative acidity or alkalinity of a solution. The pH scale is 0–14. A ph below 7 is acidic; a pH above 7 is alkaline. p. 103

phagocytes (fag-oh-SITE) Cells that engulf substances; these cells include neutrophils and macrophages. p. 88

phagocytosis (FAG-oh-sigh-TOW-sis) A process in which a cell forms an indentation, and particles or fluids entering the indentation are then engulfed by the cell. p. 88, 95

pharynx (FAIR-ingks) The organ of the digestive tract and respiratory tract located at the back of the oral and nasal cavities, commonly known as the *throat*. p. 91

phenylalanine (fen-ihl-AL-ah-neen) An essential (indispensable) amino acid. p. 120

phenylketonuria (PKU) (fen-ihl-kee-toh-NEW-ree-ah) A disease caused by a defect in the ability of the liver to metabolize the amino acid phenylalanine into the amino acid tyrosine. Toxic by-products of phenylalanine can then build up in the body and lead to mental retardation. p. 120

phosphocreatine (PCr) (fos-fo-CREE-a-tin) A high-energy compound that can be used to reform ATP. It is used primarily during bursts of activity, such as lifting weights and jumping. p. 379

phospholipid Any of a class of fat-related substances that contain phosphorus, fatty acids, and a nitrogen-containing component. Phospholipids are an essential part of every cell. p. 74, 147

photosynthesis (foto-SIN-tha-sis) The process by which plants use energy from the sun to produce energy-yielding compounds, such as glucose. p. 112

physiological anemia The normal increase in blood volume in pregnancy that dilutes the concentration of red blood cells, resulting in anemia; also called *hemodilution*. p. 454

phytic acid (phytate) (FY-tick, FY-tate) A constituent of plant fibers that has multiple phosphate groups. p. 292

phytochemical A chemical found in plants. Some phytochemicals may contribute to a reduced risk of cancer or cardiovascular disease in people who consume them regularly. p. 36

pica (PIE-kah) The practice of eating nonfood items, such as dirt, laundry starch, or clay. p. 446

pinocytosis (pee-no-sigh-TOE-sis) Formation of a vesicle that brings molecules into a cell; also called *cell drinking*. p. 95

placebo (plah-SEE-bo) A fake medicine used to disguise the treatments given to the participants in an experiment. p. 26

placenta (plah-SEN-tah) An organ that forms in the uterus of pregnant women. Through this organ, oxygen and nutrients from the mother's blood are transferred to the fetus and fetal wastes are removed. The placenta also releases hormones that maintain the state of pregnancy. p. 438

plaque (PLACK) A cholesterol-rich substance deposited in the blood vessels; it contains various white blood cells, smooth muscle cells, various proteins, cholesterol and other lipids, and eventually calcium. p. 162

plasma The fluid, extracellular portion of the blood that results when blood is centrifuged but is not allowed to clot beforehand. This includes the blood serum plus all blood-clotting factors. In contrast, serum is the fluid that remains after clotting factors have been removed from plasma. p. 82

polypeptide (POL-ee-PEP-tide) A group of amino acids bonded together; from 50 to 2000 or more. p. 191

polysaccharide (POL-ee-SACK-uh-ride) Large carbohydrates containing many glucose units, from 10 to 1000 or more. p. 7, 113

polyunsaturated fatty acid A fatty acid containing two or more carbon-carbon double bonds. p. 150

pool The amount of a nutrient stored within the body that can be easily mobilized when needed. p. 201

portal circulation The portion of the circulatory system that utilizes a large vein to carry nutrient-rich blood from capillaries in the intestines and portions of the stomach to the liver. p. 82

portal vein A large vein that distributes blood from the intestine to the liver through capillaries. p. 82

positive energy balance State in which calorie intake is greater than energy expended, generally resulting in weight gain. p. 335

positive protein balance A state in which protein intake exceeds related losses. This causes a net gain of protein in the body, such as when tissue protein is gained during growth. p. 203

prebiotic A substance that stimulates bacterial growth in the large intestines. p. 95

preeclampsia (pre-ee-KLAMP-see-ah) Part of the disease pregnancy-induced hypertension. This serious disorder can include high blood pressure, kidney failure, convulsions, and even death of the mother and fetus. Mild cases are known as *preeclampsia;* more severe cases are called *eclampsia,* formerly called *toxemia.* p. 454

pregnancy-induced hypertension A serious disorder that can include high blood pressure, kidney failure, convulsions, and even death of the mother and fetus. Although its exact cause is not known, an adequate diet (especially adequate calcium intake) and obtaining prenatal care may prevent or limit its severity. Mild cases are known as *preeclampsia;* more severe cases are called *eclampsia* (formerly called *toxemia*). p. 454

premenstrual syndrome (PMS) A disorder found in some women a few days before menstrual periods begin. It is characterized by depression, anxiety, headache, bloating, and mood swings. Severe cases are currently termed *premenstrual dysphoric disorder (PDD)*. p. 262

preservatives Compounds that extend the shelf life of foods by inhibiting microbial growth or minimizing the destructive effect of oxygen and metals. p. 544

preterm An infant born before 37 weeks of gestation; also referred to as *premature.* p. 212, 441

primary disease A disease process that is not simply caused by another disease process. p. 140

probiotic (PRO-bye-ah-tic) A product that contains specific types of bacteria. Use is intended to colonize the large intestine with the specific bacteria in the product. An example is yogurt. p. 95

prolactin (pro-LACK-tin) A hormone secreted by the mother that stimulates the synthesis of milk. p. 456

prostate cancer A form of cancer found in the prostate gland. p. 79

prostate gland (PROS-tait) A solid, chestnut-shaped organ surrounding the first part of the urinary tract in the male. The prostate gland secretes substances into the semen. p. 245

protease (PRO-tea-ace) Protein-digesting enzyme, such as pepsin (stomach) and trypsin (secreted by pancreas and acts in the small intestine). p. 91

protein Food and body components made of amino acids; proteins contain carbon, hydrogen, oxygen, nitrogen, and sometimes other atoms, in a specific configuration. Proteins contain the form of nitrogen most easily used by the human body. p. 5

protein-calorie malnutrition (PCM) A condition resulting from regularly consuming insufficient amounts of calories and protein. The deficiency eventually results in body wasting of primarily lean tissue and an increased susceptibility to infections. p. 210

protein equilibrium A state in which protein intake and all evidence of protein loss are equal. The person is said to be in protein balance. p. 203

protein turnover The process of breaking down proteins and then resynthesizing new proteins by cells. In this way the cell will have the proteins it needs to function at that time. p. 200

proton pump inhibitor A medication that inhibits the ability of gastric cells to secrete hydrogen ions. p. 99

provitamin A A substance that can be made into a vitamin. p. 243

pyloric sphincter (pi-LOR-ik SFINK-ter) Ring of smooth muscle between the stomach and the small intestine. p. 93

pyruvic acid A three-carbon compound formed during glucose metabolism; also called *pyruvate*. p. 383

radiation Literally, energy that is emitted from a center in all directions. Various forms of radiation energy include X rays and ultraviolet rays from the sun. p. 533

rancid (RAN-sid) Containing products of decomposed fatty acids that have an unpleasant flavor and odor. p. 167

reactive hypoglycemia (HIGH-po-gligh-SEE-mee-uh) Low blood glucose that may follow a meal high in simple sugars, with corresponding symptoms of irritability, headache, nervousness, sweating, and confusion; also called *postprandial hypoglycemia.* p. 129

receptor (ri-SEP-ter) A site in a cell at which compounds (such as hormones) bind. Cells that contain receptors for a specific compound are partially controlled by that compound. p. 86

recombinant DNA technology (re-KOM-bih-nant) A test tube technology that rearranges DNA sequences in an organism by cutting the DNA, adding or deleting a DNA sequence, and then rejoining DNA molecules with a series of enzymes. p. 580

Recommended Dietary Allowances (RDAs) Recommended intakes of nutrients that meet the needs of nearly all (97% to 98%) healthy individuals of similar age and gender. These are established by the Food and Nutrition Board of the National Academy of Sciences. p. 59, A-1

rectum Terminal portion of the large intestine. p. 97

registered dietitian (R.D.) (dye-eh-TISH-shun) A person who has completed a baccalaureate degree program approved by the American Dietetic Association, performed at least 900 hours of supervised professional practice, and passed a registration examination. p. 29

relapse prevention A series of strategies used to help prevent and cope with weight-control lapses, such as recognizing high-risk situations and deciding beforehand on appropriate responses. p. 359

reserve capacity The extent to which an organ can preserve essentially normal function despite decreasing cell number or cell activity. p. 506

resting metabolism The amount of calories the body uses when the person has not eaten in 4 hours and is resting (e.g., 15 to 30 minutes) and awake in a warm, quiet environment. It is roughly 6% higher than basal metabolism due to the less strict criteria for the test; the rate of calorie use per minute is referred to as *resting metabolic rate.* p. 338

retinoids (RET-ih-noyds) Chemical forms of preformed vitamin A; one source is animal foods; biologically active forms of vitamin A, including retinol, retinal, and retinoic acid. p. 243

ribonucleic acid (RNA) (RI-bow-new-CLAY-ik) The single-stranded nucleic acid involved in the transcription of genetic information and translation of that information into protein structure. p. 76

ribose (RIGH-bos) A five-carbon sugar found in genetic material—specifically, RNA. p. 402

ribosomes (RI-bow-soms) Cytoplasmic particles that participate in the linking together of amino acids to form proteins; may exist freely in the cytoplasm or attach to endoplasmic reticulum. p. 76

rickets (RIK-its) A disease characterized by poor mineralization of bones because of low calcium content. This deficiency disease arises in infants and children with a poor vitamin D status. p. 248

risk factor A term used frequently when discussing factors contributing to the development of a disease. A risk factor is an aspect of our lives—such as heredity, lifestyle choices (e.g., smoking), or nutritional habits—that make us more likely to develop a disease. p. 4

saccharin (SACK-ah-rin) An alternate sweetener that yields no energy to the body; it is 300 times sweeter than sucrose. p. 119

saliva (sah-LIGH-vah) A watery fluid, produced by the salivary glands in the mouth, that contains lubricants, enzymes, and other substances. p. 90

salivary amylase (SAL-ih-var-ee AM-ih-lace) Starch-digesting enzyme produced by salivary glands. p. 90, 91

salt Generally refers to a compound of sodium and chloride in a 40:60 ratio. p. 16

satiety (suh-TIE-uh-tee) State in which there is no longer a desire to eat; a feeling of satisfaction. p. 18

saturated fatty acid A fatty acid containing no carbon-carbon double bonds. p. 7, 148

scavenger cells Specific form of white blood cells that can bury themselves in the artery wall and accumulate LDL. As these cells take up LDL, they contribute to the development of atherosclerosis. p. 161

scurvy (SKER-vee) The deficiency disease that results after a few weeks to months of consuming a diet that lacks vitamin C; pinpoint sites of bleeding on the skin are an early sign. p. 24

secretin (SEE-kreh-tin) A hormone that causes bicarbonate ion release from the pancreas. p. 91

secretory vesicles (see-KRE-tor-ee VES-ih-kels) Membrane-bound vesicles produced by the Golgi apparatus; contains protein and other compounds to be secreted by the cell. p. 76

segmentation Contractions of the circular muscles in the intestines that lead to a dividing and mixing of the intestinal contents. This action aids digestion and absorption of nutrients. p. 92

self-monitoring Tracking foods eaten and conditions affecting eating; actions are usually recorded in a diary, along with location, time, and state of mind. This can be a tool to help people understand more about their eating habits. p. 359

semiessential amino acids Amino acids that, when consumed, spare the need to use an essential amino acid for their synthesis. Tyrosine in the diet, for example, spares the need to use phenylalanine for tyrosine synthesis. p. 188

sequestrants (see-KWES-ter-ants) Compounds that bind free metal ions. By so doing, they reduce the ability of ions to cause rancidity in foods containing fat. p. 547

serotonin (ser-oh-TONE-in) A neurotransmitter synthesized from the amino acid tryptophan that affects mood (sense of calmness), behavior, appetite, and induces sleep. p. 19, 230

serum (SEER-um) The portion of the blood fluid remaining after (1) the blood is allowed to clot and (2) the red and white blood cells and other solid matter are removed by centrifugation. p. 82

set point Often refers to the close regulation of body weight. It is not known what cells control this set point or how it actually functions in weight regulation. There is evidence, however, that mechanisms exist that help regulate weight. p. 350

sickle cell disease (sickle cell anemia) An illness that results from a malformation of the red blood cell because of an incorrect structure in part of its hemoglobin protein chains. The disease can lead to episodes of severe bone and joint pain, abdominal pain, headache, convulsions, paralysis, and even death. p. 192

simple sugar Term used to describe the group of typical sugars in our diets: glucose, fructose, and sucrose. p. 6, 113

skeletal muscle Muscle responsible for voluntary body movements. p. 77

slough (SLUF) To shed or cast off. p. 200

small for gestational age (SGA) (jes-TAY-shun-al) Referring to infants who weigh less than the expected weight for their length of gestation. This corresponds to less than 5.5 pounds (2.5 kilograms) in a full-term newborn. A preterm infant who is also SGA will most likely develop some medical complications. p. 441

smooth muscle Muscle under involuntary control; found in GI tract, artery walls, respiratory passages, urinary tract, and reproductive tract. p. 77

sodium bicarbonate (SO-dee-um bi-KAR-bow-nait) An alkaline substance made basically of sodium and carbon dioxide (NaHCO₃). p. 402

soluble fibers (SOL-you-bull) Fibers that either dissolve or swell in water and are metabolized (fermented) by bacteria in the large intestine. These include pectins, gums, and mucilages. Also called *viscous fibers.* p. 115

solvent A liquid substance in which other substances dissolve. p. 10, 285

sorbitol (SOR-bih-tol) An alcohol derivative of glucose. p. 119

specific immunity Function of white blood cells directed at specific antigens. p. 87

spontaneous abortion Any cessation of pregnancy and expulsion of the embryo or nonviable fetus as the result of natural causes, such as a genetic defect or developmental problem; also called *miscarriage.* p. 440

spores Dormant reproductive cells capable of turning into adult organisms without the help of another cell. Various fungi and bacteria form spores. p. 529

sports anemia (ah-NEE-me-ah) A decrease in the blood's ability to carry oxygen, found in athletes, which may be caused by iron loss through perspiration and feces or increased blood volume. p. 393

starch A carbohydrate made of multiple units of glucose linked together in a form the body can digest; also known as *complex carbohydrate*. p. 7, 111

sterol (STARE-ol) A compound containing a multi-ring (steroid) structure and a hydroxyl group (–OH). p. 147

stimulus control Altering the environment to minimize the stimuli for eating—for example, removing foods from sight and storing them in kitchen cabinets. p. 357

stress fracture A fracture that occurs from repeated jarring of a bone. Common sites include bones of the foot. p. 394

stroke A decrease or loss in blood flow to the brain that results from a blood clot or other change in the brain. This in turn causes the death of brain tissue. Also called a *cerebrovascular accident*. p. 5

subclinical Stage of a disease or disorder that is not severe enough to produce symptoms that can be detected or diagnosed. p. 41

sucralose (SOO-kra-los) An alternative sweetener that has chlorines in place of three hydroxyl (–OH) groups on sucrose. It is 600 times sweeter than sucrose. p. 119

sucrase An enzyme made by the absorptive cells of the small intestine; this enzyme digests sucrose to glucose and fructose. p. 123

sucrose (SOO-kros) Fructose bonded to glucose; table sugar. p. 112

sugar Simple carbohydrate form with a chemical composition $(CH_2O)_n$. Most sugars form ringed structures when in solution. The primary sugar in the diet is sucrose, which is made up of glucose and fructose. p. 111

symptom A change in health status noted by the person with the problem, such as a stomach pain. p. 41

synapse (SIN-aps) The space between one neuron and another neuron (or cell). p. 85

Syndrome X See *metabolic syndrome*.

systolic blood pressure (sis-TOL-lik) The pressure in the arterial blood vessels associated with the pumping of blood from the heart. p. 165

tagatose A slightly altered form of fructose that is poorly absorbed and so only yields 1.5 kcal/g to the body. It is 90% as sweet as sucrose. p. 120

tendon (TEN-don) Dense connective tissue that attaches a muscle to a bone. p. 77

tetany (TET-ah-nee) A state marked by sharp contraction of muscles with failure to relax afterward; usually caused by abnormal calcium metabolism. p. 298

theory An explanation for a phenomenon that has numerous lines of evidence to support it. p. 23

thermic effect of food (TEF) The increase in metabolism that occurs during the digestion, absorption, and metabolism of energy-yielding nutrients. This represents 5% to 10% of calories consumed. p. 339

thermogenesis This term encompasses the ability of humans to regulate body temperature within narrow limits (thermoregulation). Two visible examples of thermogenesis are fidgeting and shivering when cold. Other terms used to describe thermogenesis include *adaptive thermogenesis* and *nonexercise activity thermogenesis (NEAT)*. p. 339

thrifty metabolism A metabolism that characteristically conserves more energy than normal, such that it increases risk of weight gain and obesity. p. 347

thyroid hormones Hormones produced by the thyroid gland that among their functions increase the rate of overall metabolism in the body. p. 86

tissue (TISH-you) Collection of cells adapted to perform a specific function. p. 73

tocopherols (tuh-KOFF-er-alls) The chemical name for some forms of vitamin E. The alpha form is the most potent form. p. 251

Tolerable Upper Intake Level (UL) Maximum chronic daily intake of a nutrient that is unlikely to cause adverse health effects in almost all people in a population. This number applies to a chronic daily use. p. 60

total fiber Combination of dietary fiber and functional fiber in a food. Also just called *fiber*. p. 115

total parenteral nutrition The intravenous provision of all necessary nutrients, including the most basic forms of protein, carbohydrates, lipids, vitamins, minerals, and electrolytes. p. 167

toxemia See *pregnancy-induced hypertension*.

toxic Poisonous; caused by a poison. p. 541

toxicity The capacity of a substance to produce injury or illness at some dosage. p. 541

toxin Poisonous compounds produced by an organism that can cause disease in a different organism. p. 530

trabecular bone (trah-BEK-you-lar) Bone tissue with a latticelike structure; also called *spongy* or *cancellous* bone. p. 325

trace mineral A mineral vital to health that is required in the diet in amounts less than 100 milligrams per day. p. 10, 291

trans **fatty acids** A form of an unsaturated fatty acid, usually a monounsaturated one when found in food, in which the hydrogens on both carbons forming that double bond lie on opposite sides of that bond, rather than on the same side (the latter is typical of fatty acids). Stick margarine, shortenings, and deep-fat fried foods in general are rich sources. p. 7, 151

transgenic (trans-JEN-ick) Organism that contains genes originally present in another organism. p. 580

triglyceride (try-GLISS-uh-ride) The major form of lipid in the body and in food. It is composed of three fatty acids bonded to glycerol, an alcohol. p. 7, 147

trimesters Three 13- to 14-week periods into which the normal pregnancy of about 37 to 41 weeks is divided somewhat arbitrarily for purposes of discussion and analysis. Development of the embryo and fetus, however, is continuous throughout pregnancy, with no specific physiological markers demarcating the transition from one trimester to the next. p. 439

trypsin (TRIP-sin) A protein-digesting enzyme secreted by the pancreas to act in the small intestine. p. 198

tumor Mass of cells; may be cancerous (malignant) or noncancerous (benign). p. 509

type 1 diabetes A form of diabetes that is prone to ketosis and requires insulin therapy. p. 126

type 2 diabetes A form of diabetes in which ketosis is not commonly seen. Insulin therapy can be used but often is not required. This form of the disease is often associated with obesity. p. 126

ulcer (UL-sir) Erosion of the tissue lining, usually in the stomach or the upper small intestine. As a group, these are generally referred to as *peptic ulcers*. p. 23, 98

umami (you-MA-mee) A brothy, meaty, savory flavor in some foods. Monosodium glutamate enhances this flavor when added to foods. p. 90

undernutrition Failing health that results from a long-standing dietary intake that is not enough to meet nutritional needs. p. 40, 470, 560

underwater weighing A method of estimating total body fat by weighing the individual on a standard scale and then weighing him or her again submerged in water. The difference between the two weights is used to estimate total body fat. p. 345

underweight A body mass index below 18.5. The cutoff is less precise than for obesity because this condition has been studied less. p. 366

unsaturated fatty acid A fatty acid with one or more carbon-carbon double bonds. p. 7

upper-body obesity The type of obesity, also called *android*, in which fat is stored primarily in the abdominal area; defined as a waist circumference greater than 40 inches (102 centimeters) in men and greater than 35 inches (89 centimeters) in women; closely associated with a high risk of cardiovascular disease, hypertension, and type 2 diabetes. p. 346

Upper Level (UL) See *Tolerable Upper Intake Level (UL)*.

urea (yoo-REE-ah) Nitrogen-containing waste product of protein metabolism; major source of nitrogen in the urine, chemically $NH_2{-}\overset{\displaystyle O}{\overset{\|}{C}}{-}NH_2$. p. 81, 201, 287

ureter (YOUR-ih-ter) Tube that transports urine from the kidney to the urinary bladder. p. 103

urethra (yoo-REE-thra) Tube that transports urine from the urinary bladder to the outside of the body. p. 103

urinary system The body system consisting of the kidneys, urinary bladder, and the ducts that carry urine. This system removes waste products from the circulatory system and regulates blood acid-base balance, overall chemical balance, and water balance in the body. p. 103

vegan (VEE-gun) A person who consumes only plant foods. p. 176, 207

vegetarian A person who avoids eating animal products to a varying degree, ranging from consuming no animal products to simply not consuming four-footed animal products. p. 205

vein A blood vessel that carries blood to the heart. p. 82

very-low-calorie diet (VLCD) Known also as *protein-sparing modified fast (PSMF)*, this diet allows a person 400 to 800 kcal per day, often in liquid form. Of this, 120 to 480 kcals are carbohydrate, and the rest is mostly high-quality protein. p. 364

very-low-density lipoprotein (VLDL) The lipoprotein created in the liver that carries both the cholesterol and lipids taken up from the bloodstream by the liver, as well as that newly synthesized by the liver. p. 160

villi (VIL-eye) (singular, *villus*) The fingerlike protrusions into the small intestine that participate in digestion and absorption of food. p. 93

virus (VI-rus) The smallest known type of infectious agent, many of which cause disease in humans. Viruses do not metabolize, grow, or move by themselves. They reproduce only with the aid of a living cellular host. A virus is essentially a piece of genetic material surrounded by a coat of protein. p. 529

vitamin Compound needed in very small amounts in the diet to help regulate and support chemical reactions in the body. p. 5, 239

water The universal solvent of life; chemically, H_2O. The body is composed of about 60% water. Water (fluid) needs are about 9 cups (women) to 11 cups (men) per day; needs are greater if one exercises heavily. p. 5

water-soluble vitamins Vitamins that dissolve in water. These vitamins are the B vitamins and vitamin C. p. 10, 239

white blood cells One of the formed elements of the circulating blood system; also called *leukocytes*. Five types of leukocytes are lymphocytes, monocytes, neutrophils, basophils, and eosinophils. White blood cells are able to squeeze through intracellular spaces and migrate. Leukocytes phagocytize bacteria, fungi, and viruses, as well as detoxify proteins that may result from allergic reactions, cellular injury, and other immune system cells. p. 88

whole grains Grains containing the entire seed of the plant, including the bran, germ, and endosperm (starchy interior). Examples are whole wheat and brown rice. p. 115

xerophthalmia (zer-op-THAL-mee-uh) Literally, "dry eye." This is a cause of blindness that results from a vitamin A deficiency. The specific cause is a lack of mucus production by the eye, which then leaves it more vulnerable to surface dirt and bacteria. p. 244

xylitol (ZIGH-lih-tol) An alcohol derivative of a five-carbon monosaccharide, called xylose. p. 119

zygote (ZIGH-goat) The fertilized ovum; the cell resulting from union of an egg cell (ovum) and sperm until it divides. p. 438

Photo Credits

Chapter 1

Opener 1: © PhotoDisc Website; p. 4: © PhotoDisc Website; p. 5: MHHE Image Library; 1-1 (left): © CORBIS/Vol. 609; 1-1 (middle): © PhotoDisc/Vol. 20; 1-1 (right): © CORBIS/Vol. 192; Table 1-4 (bread): © CORBIS/Vol. 83; (potatoes): © CORBIS/Vol. 83; (apples): © CORBIS/Vol. 83; (oil): © PhotoDisc/EO006; (steak): © CORBIS/Vol. 83; (eggs): © CORBIS/Vol. 83; (beans): © CORBIS/Vol. 83; (water): © PhotoDisc/Vol. 30; (broccoli): © CORBIS/Vol. 83; (strawberries): © CORBIS/Vol. 83; (lettuce): © CORBIS/RF website; (milk): © CORBIS/Vol. 83; (cereal): © CORBIS/RF website; (bananas): © CORBIS/Vol. 83; (tofu): © PhotoDisc/OS49; (salmon): © CORBIS/Vol. 83; (nuts): © PhotoDisc/OS49; (Wheat&Flour): © CORBIS/RF website; p. 13: Ken Halfmann/Photographics; 1.2 (both): © PhotoDisc website; p. 13: © CORBIS/RF website; p. 16: © CORBIS/Vol. 130; p. 17: © Ohio State University Communications Photo Service; p. 19: © CORBIS/Vol. 115; 20&21: © CORBIS/Vol. 4; p. 22: © CORBIS/Vol. 27; p. 26: © CORBIS/Vol. 154; p. 29: © CORBIS/Vol. 275; p. 30: © PhotoDisc Website

Chapter 2

Opener: © CORBIS/Vol. 589; p. 36: Reproduction with permission. © Culinary Hearts Kitchen, 1982; p. 37: Courtesy of U.S. Rice Federation; p. 38: © Quaker Oats; p. 39: © PhotoDisc/Vol. 67; 2.3a: © CORBIS/Vol. 76; 2.3b: © PhotoDisc/Vol. 29; 2.3c: © PhotoDisc Website; 2.3d: © CORBIS/Vol. 102; 2.3e: © CORBIS/ Vol. 130; p. 44: © CORBIS/Vol. 154; p. 48: © CORBIS/Vol. 192; 2.6 (golf): © CORBIS/Vol. 127; (tennis): © PhotoDisc/OS25; (yo-yo): © CORBIS/RF website; (mouse): © CORBIS/Vol. 127; (baseball): © PhotoDisc/OS25; (fist): © PhotoDisc/OS02; p. 50: © CORBIS/RF website; p. 51: © PhotoDisc/OS49; p. 57: © PhotoDisc/Vol 67; p. 58 (top): © CORBIS/Vol. 589; p. 60: © Vol. 130/CORBIS; p. 61: © PhotoDisc/Vol. 110; p. 64: © PhotoDisc/Vol. 25; p. 65: © PhotoDisc/Vol. 192

Chapter 3

Opener: © PhotoDisc Website; 3-1: © PhotoDisc/Vol. 36; p. 75: © CORBIS/CDRPHOTO; p. 79: © CORBIS/Vol. 40; p. 82: © PhotoDisc; p. 93: © CORBIS/Vol. 40; p. 97: Courtesy of National Cattlemen's Beef Association; p. 100 (left): © Gordon Wardlaw; p. 100 (right): © PhotoDisc Website; p. 104: © PhotoDisc/Vol. 83

Chapter 4

Opener: © Getty Images/Eyewire; p. 111: © PhotoDisc/OS49; p. 114: © Greg Kidd and Joanne Scott; p. 117: Courtesy of The Sugar Association, Inc., Washington, D.C.; p. 118: © CORBIS/Vol. 83; p. 121: USDA Rice Federation; p. 123: Beano® is a registered trademark of AkPharma Inc.; p. 128: © CORBIS/ Vol. 108; p. 129: © PhotoDisc/Vol. 70; p. 132: Quaker® Oats; p. 133: Courtesy of Wheat Foods Council; p. 137: © The Ohio State University Communications Photo Service; p. 138: © CORBIS/Vol. 83; p. 140: © PhotoDisc/Vol. 49; p. 141: © Getty Images/Eyewire

Chapter 5

Opener: © PhotoDisc/Vol. 66; p. 151: © Greg Kidd and Joanne Scott; p. 152: © PhotoDisc/OS49; p. 154: © PhotoDisc/Vol. 12; p. 155: © PhotoDisc/Vol. 4; p. 164: © PhotoDisc/SS42; p. 167: Courtesy National Fisheries Institute; p. 168: © CORBIS/Vol. 19; p. 170: © PhotoDisc/Vol. 02; p. 172: © Saffola Quality Foods, Inc.; p. 173: © CORBIS/Vol. 4; p. 174: National Cancer Institute; p. 177: © Mark Kempf; p. 178: © William Wardlaw; p. 179: © PhotoDisc/Vol. 66

Chapter 6

Opener: © PhotoDisc/Vol. 38; p. 187: Courtesy of Florida Tomato Committee; p. 190: © PhotoDisc/Vol. 20; p. 191: © PhotoDisc; 6-3 (both): © Bill Longcore/SPL/Photo Researchers; 6-6: © CORBIS/Vol. 83; p. 196: © CORBIS/Vol. 130; p. 197: Courtesy of Walnut Marketing Board; 6-11a: © CORBIS/Vol. 116; 6-11b: © CORBIS/Vol. 589; 6-11c: © CORBIS/Vol. 52; p. 206: © Gordon Wardlaw; p. 207: © Getty Images/ Vol. 49/Steve Mason; p. 208: © Greg Kidd and Joanne Scott; p. 209 (top): © PhotoDisc/Vol. 38; p. 209 (bottom): © The Ohio State University Communications Photo Service; 6-12 (left): © Kevin Fleming/Corbis; (right): © Peter Turnley/Corbis

Chapter 7

Opener: © PhotoDisc/Vol. 66; p. 219: © CORBIS/RF website; p. 220: © CORBIS/Vol. 192; p. 221: © CORBIS/RF website; p. 223 (top): © PhotoDisc/Vol. 20; p. 223 (bottom): © CORBIS/Vol. 554; p. 225 (top): © CORBIS/Vol. 94; p. 225 (bottom): © PhotoDisc Website; 7-3 (both): Arthur Glauberman/Photo Researchers, Inc.; p. 229: © PhotoDisc/Vol. 94; p. 231 © PhotoDisc Website; p. 233 (top): © PhotoDisc website; p. 233 (bottom): © PhotoDisc/Vol. 66

Chapter 8

Opener: © PhotoDisc/Vol. 94; 8-2a,b: © A Color Atlas and Text of Nutritional Disorders by Dr. Donald D. McLaren/Mosby-Woolfe Europe, Ltd.; 8-2c: © BioPhoto Associates/ SPL/Photo Researchers; 8-2d-f: © A Color Atlas and Text of Nutritional Disorders by Dr. Donald D. McLaren/Mosby-Woolfe Europe, Ltd.; p. 242: © PhotoDisc/OS49; p. 243: Reproduced with permission. © Culinary Hearts Kitchen, 1982 © America Heart Association; p. 247: © PhotoDisc/OS49; p. 248: © CORBIS/Vol 262; p. 250: © Greg Kidd and Joanne Scott; p. 255: © CORBIS/Vol. 83; p. 258: Courtesy of National Park Producers Council; p. 259: © CORBIS/ Vol. 43; p. 262: © CORBIS/Vol. 130; p. 265: © CORBIS/Vol. 202; p. 268: © CORBIS/Vol. 30; p. 270 (top): © The Ohio State University Communications Photo Service, Jodi Miller; (bottom): © PhotoDisc/Vol. 12; 8-12: © RBHT Human Type/Getty; p. 272 (top): © CORBIS/RF website; (bottom): © PhotoDisc/ Vol. 94; p. 275: © The Ohio State University Communications Photo Service, Jodi Miller; p. 276: © PhotoDisc/Vol. 67; 8-14 (bottom): © PhotoDisc/OS49; 8-14 (middle): © CORBIS/Vol. 83; 8-14 (top): © PhotoDisc/EO006

Chapter 9

Opener: © Getty Images/Digital Vision; p. 288: © PhotoDisc; p. 291 & 292: MHHE Image Library; p. 294: © CORBIS/Vol. 43; p. 295: © CORBIS/Vol. 552; p. 297: © PhotoDisc; p. 298: MHHE Image Library; p. 300: © CORBIS/Vol. 130; p. 302 (top): © Getty Images/Digital Vision; p. 302 (bottom): © CORBIS/ Vol. 43; p. 304: © CORBIS/RF website; p. 306: © PhotoDisc/Vol. 40; p. 309: Courtesy of Florida Tomato Committee; p. 310 (bottom): Courtesy National Cattlemen's Beef Association; p. 313: © The Ohio State University Communications Photo Service; p. 316: © A Color Atlas and Text of Nutritional Disorders by Dr. Donald D. McLaren/Mosby-Woolfe Europe, Ltd.; p. 318 (top): Courtesy of Fishery Products International, Danver, MA; (bottom): © Paul Casamassimo, DDS, MS; p. 319 (top): © PhotoDisc/Vol. 02; (bottom): © CORBIS/RF website; p. 320: Photo courtesy of Almond Board of California; 9-10: © RBHT Human Type/Getty; p. 327: © Yoav Levy/Phototake; p. 328: © CORBIS/Vol. 61

Chapter 10

Opener: © CORBIS/RF website; p. 337: © CORBIS/Vol. 130; p. 339: © CORBIS/Vol. 529; 10-4: Medical Graphics, Inc.; 10-6: © Rick O'Quihn University of Georgia; 10-7: Courtesy of Life Measurement Instruments; 10-8: © Diana Linsley/Linsley Photographics; 10-9: © Gordon Wardlaw; 10-10: DEXA; p. 348: © CORBIS/RF website; p. 349: © The Ohio State University Communications Photo Service, Jodi Miller; p. 351: © PhotoDisc/Vol. 82; p. 352: © PhotoDisc/Getty Images/Vol. 190; p. 356 (top): © Royalty-free/Corbis/Vol. 306; (bottom): © PhotoDisc/Vol. 20; p. 358: © PhotoDisc/Vol. 20; p. 359 © Royalty-free/Corbis/Vol 306; p. 362: © PhotoDisc/Vol. 67; p. 363: © CORBIS/RF website

Chapter 11

Opener: © PhotoDisc/EP040; p. 377&378: PhotoDisc/EP040; p. 381: © Getty Images/
Vol. 67/Duncan Smith; p. 382: © CORBIS/Vol. 223; p. 379: © PhotoDisc/Sports
Metaphors; p. 387: © CORBIS/Vol. 20; p. 388: © James Mulligan; p. 389:
© CORBIS/RF website; p. 392 (top): © Gordon Wardlaw; (bottom): © PhotoDisc/
DV287; p. 394: © PhotoDisc/Vol. 51; p. 395: © CORBIS/Vol. 103; p. 398: © Getty
Images/Vol. 1/Photolink; p. 401: © CORBIS/Vol. 20; p. 403: © PhotoDisc/EP040

Chapter 12

Opener: © PhotoDisc/Vol. 67; p. 413 (top): © PhotoDisc Website; p. 413 (bottom):
© PhotoDisc Website; p. 414: © CORBIS/Vol. 75; p. 415: © Getty Images/Eyewire;
p. 416: © PhotoDisc website; p. 418: © PhotoDisc/Vol. 95; p. 421 (top): © Tom
Stewart Photography/CORBIS; (bottom): © PhotoDisc/Vol. 67; p. 423: © PhotoDisc
website; 12-2: © PhotoDisc/EP047; 12-3: © Paul Casamassimo, DDS, MS; p. 426:
© CORBIS/RF website; p. 428: © PhotoDisc website; p. 429: © CORBIS/Vol. 552;
p. 430: © Photodisc/Vol. 45

Chapter 13

Opener: PhotoDisc/Vol. 46; p. 440 (top): © CORBIS/Vol. 19; p. 440 (bottom): © Gordon
Wardlaw, photographer Greg Wolff; p. 442&443: USDA; p. 446&447: © CORBIS/RF
website; p. 449: USDA; p. 452 (top): USDA; (bottom): © PhotoDisc/Vol. 46; p. 453:
© CORBIS/Vol. 83; p. 455: USDA; p. 459: © PhotoDisc/Vol. 192; p. 461:
© PhotoDisc/EP039; p. 462: © CORBIS/Vol. 52

Chapter 14

Opener: © PhotoDisc/Vol. 61; p. 469: © PhotoDisc/EP077; p. 472: © PhotoDisc/Vol. 113;
p. 473: © CORBIS/Vol. 135; p. 476: © CORBIS/Vol. 9; p. 477 (top): © PhotoDisc/
Vol. 58; (bottom): © PhotoDisc/Vol. 113; p. 478: © CORBIS/Vol. 26; p. 480:
© PhotoDisc/Vol. 113; 14-3: © Paul Casamassimo, DDS, MS; p. 481 (top): © Gordon
Wardlaw; (bottom): © CORBIS/Vol. 552; p. 482: © PhotoDisc/Vol. 61; p. 484: © Greg
Kidd & Joanne Scott; p. 486: © Joanne Scott; p. 489: USDA Photo by: Ken Hammond;
p. 490: MH Digital Library; p. 491: © CORBIS/Vol. 124; p. 492: © CORBIS/Vol. 552;
p. 493: © CORBIS/Vol. 527; p. 494: © CORBIS/RF website; p. 495: © PhotoDisc/
Vol. 95; p. 496: © PhotoDisc Website

Chapter 15

Opener: © PhotoDisc Website; p. 503: © CORBIS/Vol. 141; p. 504: © David Craddock;
p. 504: © PhotoDisc/Vol. 83; p. 506: © CORBIS/RF website; p. 507: © CORBIS/
Vol. 36; p. 508: © CORBIS/RF website; p. 510: © PhotoDisc/OS49; p. 514: © CORBIS/
Vol. 81; p. 515: © Gordon Wardlaw; p. 517: © PhotoDisc/Vol. 48; p. 518: © CORBIS/
Vol. 81; p. 519: © PhotoDisc/EP038; p. 520: © Getty Images/Digital Vision; p. 522:
© PhotoDisc/Vol. 58; p. 522 © PhotoDisc Website; p. 526: © PhotoDisc/SS45

Chapter 16

Opener: © PhotoDisc Website; p. 532: © CORBIS/Vol. 12; p. 537: © Gregg Wolff; p. 538:
© PhotoDisc/Vol. 48; p. 535: © PhotoDisc Website; p. 542: © CORBIS/Vol. 43;
p. 544: © Greg Kidd and Joanne Scott; p. 545: © CORBIS/Vol. 83; p. 546: © CORBIS/
Vol. 192; 16-3a&b: © Gordon Wardlaw; p. 548: © The Ohio State University Com-
munications Photo Service; p. 550: © The Ohio State University Communications
Photo Service, Lloyd Lemmermann; p. 551: © PhotoDisc website; p. 552 (top):
© PhotoDisc/Vol. 49; (bottom): © CORBIS/Vol. 552

Chapter 17

Opener: © PhotoDisc Website; p. 559: © CORBIS/RF website; 17-1 (boy reading):
MHHE Image Library; 17-1 (all others): AP Wide World Photos; p. 563 (both):
© The Ohio State University Commnications Photo Service; p. 564: © CORBIS/RF
website; p. 565 (top): © PhotoDisc Website; (bottom): USDA photo by Peter
Manzelli; p. 568: © Royalty Free/CORBIS; p. 569: © PhotoDisc/Vol. 25;
p. 571&572: MHHE Image Library; p. 573: © Getty Images/Digital Vision; p. 574:
© CORBIS/RF website; p. 576: © CORBIS/Vol. 25; p. 578: MHHE Image Library;
p. 580: © CORBIS/Vol. 609; p. 581: © The Ohio State University Communications
Photo Service, Jodi Miller

Dietary Reference Intakes (DRIs): Recommended Intakes for Individuals, Electrolytes and Water

Food and Nutrition Board, Institute of Medicine, National Academies

Life Stage Group	Sodium (mg/d)	Potassium (mg/d)	Chloride (mg/d)	Water (L/d)
Infants				
0–6 mo	120*	400*	180ᴬ	0.7*
7–12 mo	370*	700*	570*	0.8*
Children				
1–3 y	1,000*	3,000*	1,500*	1.3*
4–8 y	1,200*	3,800*	1,900*	1.7*
Males				
9–13 y	1,500*	4,500*	2,300*	2.4*
14–18 y	1,500*	4,700*	2,300*	3.3*
19–30 y	1,500*	4,700*	2,300*	3.7*
31–50 y	1,500*	4,700*	2,300*	3.7*
51–70 y	1,300*	4,700*	2,000*	3.7*
> 70 y	1,200*	4,700*	1,800*	3.7*
Females				
9–13 y	1,500*	4,500*	2,300*	2.1*
14–18 y	1,500*	4,700*	2,300*	2.3*
19–30 y	1,500*	4,700*	2,300*	2.7*
31–50 y	1,500*	4,700*	2,300*	2.7*
51–70 y	1,300*	4,700*	2,000*	2.7*
> 70 y	1,200*	4,700*	1,800*	2.7*
Pregnancy				
14–18 y	1,500*	4,700*	2,300*	3.0*
19–50 y	1,500*	4,700*	2,300*	3.0*
Lactation				
14–18 y	1,500*	5,100*	2,300*	3.8*
19–50 y	1,500*	5,100*	2,300*	3.8*

NOTE: The table is adapted from the DRI reports. See www.nap.edu. Adequate Intakes (AIs) are followed by an asterisk(*). These may be used as a goal for individual intake. For healthy breastfed infants, the AI is the average intake. The AI for other life stage and gender groups is believed to cover the needs of all individuals in the group, but lack of data prevent being able to specify with confidence the percentage of individuals covered by this intake; therefore, no Recommended Dietary Allowance (RDA) was set.

SOURCE: *Dietary Reference Intakes for Water, Potassium, Sodium, Chloride, and Sulfate.* This report may be accessed via www.nap.edu.

Acceptable Macronutrient Distribution Ranges

| Macronutrient | Range (percent of energy) | | |
	Children, 1–3 y	Children, 4–18 y	Adults
Fat	30–40	25–35	20–35
omega-6 polyunsaturated fats (linoleic acid)	5–10	5–10	5–10
omega-3 polyunsaturated fatsᵃ (α-linolenic acid)	0.6–1.2	0.6–1.2	0.6–1.2
Carbohydrate	45–65	45–65	45–65
Protein	5–20	10–30	10–35

ᵃApproximately 10% of the total can come from longer-chain n-3 fatty acids.

SOURCE: *Dietary Reference Intakes for Energy, Carbohydrate, Fiber, Fat, Fatty Acids, Cholesterol, Protein, and Amino Acids* (2002). The report may be accessed via www.nap.edu.

Dietary Reference Intakes (DRIs): Tolerable Upper Intake Levels (UL[a]), Vitamins

Food and Nutrition Board, Institute of Medicine, National Academies

Life Stage Group	Vitamin A (μg/d)[b]	Vitamin C (mg/d)	Vitamin D (μg/d)	Vitamin E (mg/d)[c,d]	Vitamin K	Thiamin	Riboflavin	Niacin (mg/d)[d]	Vitamin B-6 (mg/d)	Folate (μg/d)[d]	Vitamin B-12	Pantothenic Acid	Biotin	Choline (g/d)	Carotenoids[e]
Infants															
0–6 mo	600	ND[f]	25	ND	ND	ND	ND	ND	ND	ND	ND	ND	ND	ND	ND
7–12 mo	600	ND	25	ND	ND	ND	ND	ND	ND	ND	ND	ND	ND	ND	ND
Children															
1–3 y	600	400	50	200	ND	ND	ND	10	30	300	ND	ND	ND	1.0	ND
4–8 y	900	650	50	300	ND	ND	ND	15	40	400	ND	ND	ND	1.0	ND
Males, Females															
9–13 y	1,700	1,200	50	600	ND	ND	ND	20	60	600	ND	ND	ND	2.0	ND
14–18 y	2,800	1,800	50	800	ND	ND	ND	30	80	800	ND	ND	ND	3.0	ND
19–70 y	3,000	2,000	50	1,000	ND	ND	ND	35	100	1,000	ND	ND	ND	3.5	ND
>70 y	3,000	2,000	50	1,000	ND	ND	ND	35	100	1,000	ND	ND	ND	3.5	ND
Pregnancy															
≤18 y	2,800	1,800	50	800	ND	ND	ND	30	80	800	ND	ND	ND	3.0	ND
19–50 y	3,000	2,000	50	1,000	ND	ND	ND	35	100	1,000	ND	ND	ND	3.5	ND
Lactation															
≤18 y	2,800	1,800	50	800	ND	ND	ND	30	80	800	ND	ND	ND	3.0	ND
19–50 y	3,000	2,000	50	1,000	ND	ND	ND	35	100	1,000	ND	ND	ND	3.5	ND

[a]UL = The maximum level of daily nutrient intake that is likely to pose no risk of adverse effects. Unless otherwise specified, the UL represents total intake from food, water, and supplements. Due to lack of suitable data, ULs could not be established for vitamin K, thiamin, riboflavin, vitamin B-12, pantothenic acid, biotin, or carotenoids. In the absence of ULs, extra caution may be warranted in consuming levels above recommended intakes.

[b]As preformed vitamin A only.

[c]As α-tocopherol; applies to any form of supplemental α-tocopherol.

[d]The ULs for vitamin E, niacin, and folate apply to synthetic forms obtained from supplements, fortified foods, or a combination of the two.

[e]β-Carotene supplements are advised only to serve as a provitamin A source for individuals at risk of vitamin A deficiency.

[f]ND = Not determinable due to lack of data of adverse effects in this age group and concern with regard to lack of ability to handle excess amounts. Source of intake should be from food only to prevent high levels of intake.

SOURCES: Dietary Reference Intakes for Calcium, Phosphorus, Magnesium, Vitamin D, and Fluoride (1997); Dietary Reference Intakes for Thiamin, Riboflavin, Niacin, Vitamin B-6, Folate, Vitamin B-12, Pantothenic Acid, Biotin, and Choline (1998); Dietary Reference Intakes for Vitamin C, Vitamin E, Selenium, and Carotenoids (2000); and Dietary Reference Intakes for Vitamin A, Vitamin K, Arsenic, Boron, Chromium, Copper, Iodine, Iron, Manganese, Molybdenum, Nickel, Silicon, Vanadium, and Zinc (2001). These reports may be accessed via www.nap.edu.